PRIMARY EYECARE IN SYSTEMIC DISEASE

NOTICE

PRIMARY EYECARE IN SYSTEMIC DISEASE

SECOND EDITION

Edited by

Kelly H. Thomann, OD, FAAO
Chief, Optometry Service
VA Hudson Valley Healthcare System
Montrose, New York
Adjunct Assistant Clinical Professor
State University of New York
State College of Optometry
New York, New York
Adjunct Clinical Professor
New England College of Optometry
Boston, Massachusetts
Adjunct Assistant Professor
Illinois College of Optometry
Chicago, Illinois

Esther S. Marks, OD, FAAO
Consultant and Lecturer
Lynbrook, New York

Diane T. Adamczyk, OD, FAAO
Director of Residencies & External Programs
Associate Professor
State University of New York
State College of Optometry
New York, New York

McGraw-Hill
Medical Publishing Division

New York Chicago San Francisco Lisbon London Madrid Mexico City
Milan New Delhi San Juan Seoul Singapore Sydney Toronto

McGraw-Hill
A Division of The McGraw-Hill Companies

PRIMARY EYECARE IN SYSTEMIC DISEASE
Second Edition

1234567890 KGPKGP 09876543210

ISBN 0-8385-8176-5

This book was set in Palatino by York Graphic Services, Inc.
The editors were Sally Barhydt and John M. Morriss.
The production supervisor was Catherine Saggese.
The cover was designed by Aimee Nordin.
The color insert was designed by Marsha Cohen.
Quebecor Printing/Kingsport was printer and binder.

This book is printed on recycled, acid-free paper.

Library of Congress Cataloging-in-Publication Data

Primary eyecare in systemic disease / [edited by] Kelly H. Thomann, Esther S. Marks, Diane T. Adamczyk. — 2nd ed.
p. ; cm.
Includes bibliographical references and index.
ISBN 0-8385-8176-5 (hd : alk. paper)
1. Ocular manifestations of general diseases. I. Thomann, Kelly H. II. Marks, Esther S. III. Adamczyk, Diane T.
[DNLM: 1. Eye Manifestations. WW 275 P952 2001]
RE65 .P75 2001
617.7—dc21

To our families, with thanks for their constant support, encouragement, and patience.

Contents

Section VII
SKELETAL AND CONNECTIVE TISSUE DISORDERS

Section VIII
PHAKOMATOSES

Section IX
DERMATOLOGIC DISORDERS

Color plates appear between pages 426 and 427.

Contributors*

DIANE T. ADAMCZYK, O.D., F.A.A.O. [13–15, 47, 48, 52]
Director of Residencies & External Programs
Associate Professor
State University of New York
State College of Optometry
New York, New York

ELIZABETH B. AKSIONOFF, O.D., F.A.A.O. [35–37]
Scarsdale, New York

DAVID S. ALTENDERFER, O.D. [45]
Staff Optometrist
The Eye Institute
Pennsylvania College of Optometry
Philadelphia, Pennsylvania

SHERRY J. BASS, O.D., F.A.A.O. [59]
Clinical Professor
State University of New York
State College of Optometry
New York, New York

DEBRA BEZAN, O.D., F.A.A.O. [40, 41]
Adjunct Professor
NSW College of Optometry
Tulsa, Oklahoma

BERNARD H. BLAUSTEIN, O.D. [5]
Associate Professor
The Eye Institute
Pennsylvania College of Optometry
Philadelphia, Pennsylvania

DAVID C. BRIGHT, O.D., F.A.A.O. [45]
Professor
Southern California College of Optometry
Fullerton California
Chief
Optometry Section
DVA Greater Los Angeles Healthcare System

HARRIETTE MOUTOPOULOS CANELLOS, O.D. [27]
Assistant Clinical Professor
State University of New York
State College of Optometry
New York, New York

TANYA L. CARTER, O.D. [64, 65]
Assistant Clinical Professor
State University of New York
State College of Optometry
New York, New York

ANTHONY CAVALLERANO, O.D. [16]
Staff Optometrist
Beetham Eye Institute
Joslin Diabetes Center
Boston, Massachusetts

JERRY CAVALLERANO, O.D., Ph.D. [16]
Staff Optometrist
Beetham Eye Institute
Joslin Diabetes Center
Boston, Massachusetts

MICHAEL CHAGLASIAN, O.D. [38, 39]
Associate Professor
Chief, Center for Advanced Opthalmic Care
Illinois Eye Institute
Illinois College of Optometry
Chicago, Illinois

CONNIE L. CHRONISTER, O.D., F.A.A.O. [45]
Associate Professor
Pennsylvania College of Optometry
Chief, Primary Care Module 2
The Eye Institute of Optometry
Staff Optometrist/Low Vision Specialist
Philadelphia Veterans Administration Medical Center
Fellow of American Academy of Optometry

JOHN E. CONTO, O.D. [11, 12, 23]
Associate Professor of Optometry
Illinois College of Optometry
Chief of Staff
Illinois Eye Institute
Chicago, Illinois

GINA DELL'ARCIPRETE [21]
Assistant Clinical Professor
State University of New York
State College of Optometry
New York, New York

BERNARD J. DOLAN, O.D., M.S. [17–19]
Staff Optometrist
Department of Veterans Affairs Medical Center
San Francisco, CA
Clinical Professor
School of Optometry
University of California, Berkeley
Berkeley, California

*The numbers in brackets following each contributor's name indicate the chapter(s) written or co-written by that contributor.

MITCHELL W. DUL, O.D., M.S. [2–4]
Associate Professor
Chairman/Department of Clinical Services
State University of New York
State College of Optometry
New York, New York

CHRISTINE DUMESTRE, O.D. [46]
Assistant Clinical Professor
State University of New York
State College of Optometry
New York, New York
East New York Diagnostic and Treatment Center
Brooklyn, New York

THU-HA DAO EASTER, O.D., M.S. [62]
Apple Hill Eye Center
York, Pennsylvania

SHARON L. FELDMAN, O.D. [65]
Assistant Clinical Professor
State College of Optometry
State University of New York
New York, New York

FELICIA A. FODERA, O.D., F.A.A.O. [54]
Staff Optometrist
Optometry Service
VA Hudson Valley Healthcare System
Castle Point, New York
Adjunct Assistant Clinical Professor
State University of New York
State College of Optometry
New York, New York
Adjunct Clinical Professor
New England College of Optometry
Boston, Massachusetts
Adjunct Assistant Professor
Illinois College of Optometry
Chicago, Illinois

CHARLES HASKES, O.D., M.S., F.A.A.O. [4]
Assistant Chief/Residency Program Supervisor
Optometry Section
Veterans Administration Connecticut Healthcare System
West Haven Campus
West Haven, Connecticut
Adjunct Clinical Professor
New England College of Optometry
Boston, Massachusetts
Adjunct Assistant Clinical Professor
Department of Clinical Services
State University of New York
State College of Optometry
New York, New York

JEAN Y. JUNG, O.D., M.S., F.A.A.O. [66]
Staff Optometrist
Optometry Service
VA Hudson Valley Healthcare System
Montrose, New York
Adjunct Assistant Clinical Professor
Department of Clinical Sciences
State University of New York
State College of Optometry
New York, New York
Adjunct Clinical Professor
New England College of Optometry
Boston, Massachusetts
Adjunct Clinical Professor
Illinois College of Optometry
Chicago, Illinois

DAVID M. KRUMHOLZ [1]
Associate Clinical Professor
State University of New York
State College of Optometry
New York, New York

TERESA A. LOWE [20]
Assistant Clinical Professor
State University of New York
State College of Optometry
New York, New York

RICHARD J. MADONNA, O.D., M.A., F.A.A.O. [26]
Associate Professor
Chief Ocular Disease and Special Testing Service
Acting Chief, Primary Care Service
State University of New York
State College of Optometry
New York, New York

ESTHER S. MARKS, O.D., F.A.A.O. [28, 42, 58, 61]
Consultant and Lecturer
Lynbrook, New York

TARYN MATTHEWS [49, 50]
Lubbock, Texas

JANICE M. McMAHON [11]
Assistant Professor of Optometry
Illinois College of Optometry
Attending Optometrist
Illinois Eye Institute
Chicago, Illinois

MARGARET McNELIS, O.D. [30–33]
Warrenville, Illinois

LEONARD V. MESSNER, O.D. [6]
Associate Professor of Optometry
Illinois College of Optometry
Vice President for Patient Care Services
Illinois Eye Institute
Chicago, Illinois

TRICIA L. NEWMAN [6]
Illinois College of Optometry
Illinois Eye Institute
Chicago, Illinois

SUSAN C. OLESZEWSKI, O.D., M.A., F.A.A.O. [8–10]
Associate Professor
Pennsylvania College of Optometry
Philadelphia, Pennsylvania

LEONARD J. OSHINSKIE, O.D., F.A.A.O. [56, 57]
Chief, Optometry Section
Veterans Administration Connecticut Health Care System
Newington, Connecticut
Adjunct Clinical Professor of Optometry
New England College of Optometry
Boston, Massachusetts

JOAN K. PORTELLO, O.D., F.A.A.O. [34]
Associate Clinical Professor
State University of New York
State College of Optometry
New York, New York

LORI R. REMINICK, O.D. [53, 55]
Associate Clinical Professor
New York Harbor Health Care System
Brooklyn Campus
Surgical Service/Optometry (112)
Brooklyn, New York

MIRIAM ROLF, O.D., M.S., F.A.A.O. [22]
Supervisor of Optometric Externs
Optometry Service
VA Hudson Valley Healthcare System
Montrose, New York
Adjunct Assistant Clinical Professor
State University of New York
State College of Optometry
New York, New York
Adjunct Clinical Professor
New England College of Optometry
Boston, Massachusetts
Adjunct Assistant Professor
Illinois College of Optometry
Chicago, Illinois

SUSAN P. SCHUETTENBERG, O.D., F.A.A.O. [29]
Assistant Clinical Professor
State University of New York
State College of Optometry
New York, New York

JEROME SHERMAN, O.D., F.A.A.O. [59]
Distinguished Teaching Professor
State University of New York
State College of Optometry
New York, New York

CHUNG YONG SONG, O.D. [24]
Staff Optometrist
Optometry Service
VA Hudson Valley Healthcare System
Montrose, New York
Adjunct Assistant Clinical Professor
State University of New York
State College of Optometry
New York, New York
Adjunct Clinical Professor
New England College of Optometry
Boston, Massachusetts
Adjunct Assistant Professor
Illinois College of Optometry
Chicago, Illinois

ELLIOT STERNTHAL, M.D., F.A.C.P., F.A.C.E. [16]
Instructor in Medicine
Harvard Medical School
Senior Physician
Joslin Clinic
Boston, Massachusetts

BRAD M. SUTTON, O.D., F.A.A.O. [51]
Associate Professor
Indiana University
Clinic Director
Indianapolis Eyecare Center
Indianapolis, Indiana

KELLY H. THOMANN, O.D., F.A.A.O. [7, 43, 44, 60]
Chief, Optometry Service
VA Hudson Valley Healthcare System
Montrose, New York
Adjunct Assistant Clinical Professor
State University of New York
State College of Optometry
New York, New York
Adjunct Clinical Professor
New England College of Optometry
Boston, Massachusetts
Adjunct Assistant Professor
Illinois College of Optometry
Chicago, Illinois

DAWN N. TOMASINI, O.D., F.A.A.O. [64]
Staff Optometrist
Optometry Service
VA Hudson Valley Healthcare System
Castle Point, New York
Adjunct Assistant Clinical Professor
State University of New York
State College of Optometry
New York, New York
Adjunct Clinical Professor
New England College of Optometry
Boston, Massachusetts
Adjunct Assistant Professor
Illinois College of Optometry
Chicago, Illinois

JULIE K. TORBIT, O.D., F.A.A.O. [51]
Indianapolis Eyecare Center
Indianapolis, Indiana

CATHERINE PACE WATSON [21]
Assistant Clinical Professor
State University of New York
State College of Optometry
New York, New York

LYNDON C. WONG, O.D., F.A.A.O., F.C.O.V.D. [63]
Assistant Clinical Professor
State University of New York
State College of Optometry
New York, New York

NANCY N. WONG, O.D., M.S., F.A.A.O. [25]
Supervisor of Optometric Residents
Optometry Service
VA Hudson Valley Healthcare System
Montrose, New York
Adjunct Assistant Clinical Professor
State University of New York
State College of Optometry
New York, New York
Adjunct Clinical Professor
New England College of Optometry
Boston, Massachusetts
Adjunct Assistant Professor
Illinois College of Optometry
Chicago, Illinois

Foreword

The real voyage of discovery consists not in seeking new landscapes but in having new eyes.

Marcel Proust

Doctors of Optometry are primary health care professionals; we are the eye and vision care experts. Our roots are long and deep in those areas of patient care for which our profession is uniquely qualified — refraction, contact lenses, binocular vision, functional vision, vision therapy, and sports vision, to name a few. The quality of life for countless numbers of patients has been immeasurably enhanced thanks to the care delivered by doctors of optometry in these vitally important areas.

As the scope of optometric practice has expanded over the past three decades, I do not believe that we have abandoned our professional "roots." Rather, we have come to view our patients through "new eyes." In doing so, we understand that in innumerable ways the delivery of primary eye and vision care services is inextricably linked to the patient's systemic health. It is to this premise that the second edition of *Primary Eyecare in Systemic Disease* is dedicated by the editors and authors.

In the clinical setting, we can all recall countless numbers of patients for whom this link has been a vitally important one: the 8-year-old boy who presents with strabismus caused by a midbrain tumor; the 72-year-old man with amaurosis fugax caused by cerebrovascular disease; the 62-year-old man with a blood pressure reading of 160/110 and hypertensive retinopathy; the 31-year-old woman with anterior uveitis related to inflammatory bowel disease. It is to these patients and their doctors of optometry that the editors and authors additionally dedicate their work.

Dr. Kelly Thomann, Dr. Esther Marks, and Dr. Diane Adamczyk are talented and dedicated clinicians, educators, and colleagues. Their work on a project of this magnitude and breadth is reflective of their commitment to the profession and the patients it serves. Their contributions to the profession of optometry, both individually and collectively, have been outstanding; this volume is an enduring tribute to those contributions. Similarly, Drs. Thomann, Marks, and Adamczyk have assembled a distinguished group of knowledgeable and accomplished contributing authors. All of their efforts are deserving of high praise from the profession.

When the first edition of *Primary Eyecare in Systemic Disease* was published in 1995, it was a landmark text within the optometric literature. It readily earned this stature, not only for the quality and nature of its content with its inherent positive impact on how we care for patients, but also for the quality of its presentation and format. Modifications found in the second edition are exciting in their scope and nature. Yet, the focus of the text remains on usability for the reader and an emphasis on "must-know" systemic conditions without comprising scope and depth of the material.

I encourage all who read this text — from the student just launching his or her "voyage of discovery" to the established practitioner committed to lifelong learning — to actively utilize its contents. Do so with the same enthusiasm, dedication, and knowledge demonstrated by its editors and contributing authors. From the most fundamental standpoint, your patients are counting on your ability and willingness to do so. On another level, your own lives will continue to be enriched beyond measure by the gratitude expressed by those patients and their families whom you have served in ways they likely did not imagine when they first crossed the threshold of your optometric practice.

Linda Casser, OD, FAAO
Associate Dean for Academic Programs
Pacific University College of Optometry
Forest Grove, Oregon

Preface

When we signed our original contract for the first edition of *Primary Eyecare in Systemic Disease,* we knew that we had taken on an extensive project. Our goal was to produce a clinically oriented textbook for eyecare providers that would be a concise, user-friendly guide and would bridge the gap in information between systemic diseases and their ocular manifestations. After the book was published, we felt confident that we had successfully accomplished this major goal.

As we began work on the second edition of *Primary Eyecare in Systemic Disease,* we kept our original goal in mind, added new goals, and incorporated helpful suggestions from our colleagues. We have updated every chapter, improved the format of the book, and streamlined the contents by the appropriate deletion, redesign, or addition of chapter topics. In this second edition, every chapter has been updated in order to keep the textbook current on new medical findings, diagnostic tests, or treatment strategies.

Ten chapters, including those on patient assessment, HIV and AIDS, Lyme disease, diabetes, hematologic disorders, systemic lupus erythematosus, and drug and alcohol abuse, have been completely rewritten and expanded. A new chapter on Down syndrome, sorely missing from the first edition, has been added. Also new to this edition is the full-color insert of over 70 images.

We have improved the book format through the addition of new tables. Therefore, along with the established tables in each chapter (systemic manifestations, ocular manifestations, and management protocols), we have added differential diagnoses and laboratory test tables. Useful **clinical pearls,** which highlight pertinent medical facts, have been added to almost every chapter. Again, in an effort to streamline the book, chapters on systemic conditions unlikely to be encountered in clinical practice were deleted. Chapters covering uncommon systemic conditions but conditions we felt were useful to include were redesigned into a bulleted outline format for easy reference. Lastly, Appendix I, which cross-references ocular manifestations to systemic diseases, was expanded and updated.

Each chapter in the textbook follows the format of the first edition, beginning with an introduction and disease epidemiology. The natural history section has been renamed "pathophysiology/disease process" because our intent is to help the reader understand how and why the disease occurs, as well as to provide clues for diagnosis. The treatment and management section and conclusion follow.

Once again, we set high goals for *Primary Eyecare in Systemic Disease,* and we feel confident that we have attained them. We hope that this book continues to be a valuable reference and resource for practitioners and for students intent on providing the highest quality eyecare possible.

Kelly H. Thomann, O.D., F.A.A.O.
Esther S. Marks, O.D., F.A.A.O.
Diane T. Adamczyk, O.D., F.A.A.O.

Section I

INTRODUCTION

Chapter 1

PATIENT ASSESSMENT

David M. Krumholz

Primary eyecare encompasses more than examining only the ocular structures. In order to fully evaluate the patient, it is often necessary to assess components of systemic health. In addition to formal laboratory testing and imaging studies, there are many simple, noninvasive diagnostic procedures that the eyecare practitioner can easily perform in the office. These may yield important information regarding the presence of systemic conditions so that their interrelationship with the visual system may be evaluated.

This chapter discusses physical diagnostic procedures that can be performed with a minimum of specialized equipment in an eyecare office. In addition, selected blood tests and imaging studies that may assist the eyecare practitioner are discussed.

CASE HISTORY

The patient history is probably the most powerful diagnostic tool possessed by clinicians. The history focuses the diagnostic workup and allows the clinician to assess the probability that the patient is suffering from a certain disease and develop a differential diagnostic list. It can also help to assess the effectiveness of therapy, monitor the progress of a disease, and allow other risk factors to be assessed. Although the history actually begins when the clinician first greets the patient, and lasts throughout the entire encounter, a good rule of thumb is that by the end of the formal case history the clinician should have *ample* information with which to begin a directed examination.

AMPLE is an acronym to help remember important aspects of the patient history. *A* stands for allergies, most importantly to medications. The goal is to prevent adverse drug reactions at all times.

M stands for medications. Knowledge of the patient's current medications helps point the clinician to certain ongoing systemic conditions. This information also makes it possible to rule out adverse drug effects as an etiology of the patient's complaint, and allows the clinician to be aware of any possible drug–drug interactions.

P stands for past history. This includes all previous illnesses and contact with other healthcare providers not directly related to the current illness or reason for visit.

L stands for last intervention, which is the last time the patient had contact with a healthcare provider, whether it was for hospitalization, surgery, other treatment, or just a checkup.

E is for the extenuating circumstances that brought the patient in for an ocular examination. This is the *chief complaint* (CC). There are three general categories of chief complaints. A problem-related CC is one given by a patient who notices a need to seek care, eg, a red eye. The administrative CC is one given by a patient who does not have a specific symptom but has returned for a clinician-requested visit, eg, a glaucoma follow-up. A preventive CC is one given by a patient who feels well and is not experiencing any acute symptoms but desires to rule out a given condition for one reason or another. These are patients who may be at risk for certain systemic diseases that affect the eye, or with a family history of heritable diseases requiring periodic monitoring.

The CC is generally followed by a section of the history called the *history of present illness* (HPI), which is a detailed chronological description of the course of the CC prior to the current visit. For patients with a problem-related CC with specific symptoms, the HPI attempts to begin the differential diagnostic process. Here, in addition to a chronological sequence of events, risk factors are assessed, and clues consisting of pertinent positive and pertinent negative findings are listed. For each symptom that patient complains of, the onset and course should be ascertained. Additional attributes to investigate include symptom location, quality or severity, timing, setting (environmental factors, personal activities, other circumstances), alleviating or exacerbating factors, and any other associated manifestations. The clinician should also inquire about any previous episodes and treatments (including medications), which would assist in uncovering iatrogenic illnesses, such as adverse drug reactions. This gives a "profile" of the complaint that the clinician can then match against known conditions to see which diagnosis, if any, fits best.

If the patient is already under care and has an administrative CC in which the disease is already known, then all that is required for the HPI is a brief, organized summary of the patient status since last seen. It may be useful to make a comment regarding the current status and any complications either of the disease or therapy, including compliance with the treatment plan.

If the patient presents without symptoms, for a preventive visit, very little is required in the way of the HPI. Risk factors that may have some bearing on the patient's concerns should be assessed. These are usually investigated in the personal and/or family medical histories.

Following the HPI, it is important to gather other information about the patient that, while not directly related to the CC, may still be important. Past medical history describes any previous illnesses or health problems unrelated to the presenting symptom. Similarly, the family medical history reveals similar illnesses or symptoms in blood relatives, as well as risk factors for common heritable conditions. A personal and social history may be indicated to gather information regarding diet and nutrition, smoking, alcohol or drug use, and environmental conditions.

A full, thorough, and comprehensive case history includes a review of systems. This includes all important, but not immediately applicable, data about all the organ systems in the body (Table 1–1).

Although the history does not end until the patient is dismissed, the clinician should have enough information at this point to perform a directed examination to work through a differential diagnostic list.

PHYSICAL EXAMINATION

Gross Observation

The examination really begins the moment the patient is first seen. Age, gender, and race provide an initial template for differential diagnoses. Further gross observations provide additional information. For example, complexion, dress, grooming, and personal hygiene may help determine whether a patient appears "well" or "sick." Any striking physical abnormality, such as missing limbs, the need for supportive devices (canes, wheelchairs), or abnormal stature, postures, or deformities should be noted. For example, patients with osteoporosis may have a characteristic stooped (kyphotic) posture; unusually tall or short stature may indicate certain endocrine disorders or poor nutritional status.

The patient's gait is observed for characteristic abnormalities, such as the slow shuffling gait and tremor of Parkinsonism, or the unsteady wide-based gait of an ataxic patient. Key signs of certain diseases, such as body type, hair distribution, skin pigmentations and rashes, nodules, xanthomas, edema, venous distentions, pallor, jaundice, cyanosis, and plethora, should be noted. Speech, affect, orientation, and intellectual function also should be noted. These observations, in addition to the patient history, will help direct the examination.

Certain disorders can often be diagnosed at a glance, but only if the clinician is aware of what to look for. For example, an elderly man with an oily, expressionless face and coarse tremor, who shuffles along with small steps, bent over, with arms and legs slightly flexed, should be suspected to have Parkinson's disease. The recognition of Graves' disease, Down syndrome, and Cushing's syndrome can occur in the same way. This is called *pattern recognition*, or recognition by *gestalt*. The more the disease processes are understood and the greater the clinician's knowledge base, the easier it becomes to recognize these patterns and make a diagnosis.

TABLE 1–1. REVIEW OF SYSTEMS

General
Usual state of health
Fever
Chills
Usual weight
Change in weight
Weakness
Fatigue
Sweats
Hot or cold intolerance
History of anemia
Bleeding tendencies
Blood transfusions and possible reactions
Exposure to radiation

Skin
Rashes
Itching
Hives
Easy bruisability
History of eczema
Dryness
Changes in skin color
Changes in hair texture
Changes in nail texture
Changes in nail appearance
History of previous skin disorders
Lumps
Use of hair dyes

Head
"Dizziness"
Headaches
Pain
Fainting
History of head injury
Stroke

Eyes
Use of eyeglasses
Current vision
Change in vision
Double vision
Excessive tearing
Pain
Recent eye examination
Pain when looking at light
Unusual sensations
Redness
Discharge
Infections
History of glaucoma
Cataracts
Injuries

Ears
Hearing impairment
Use of hearing aid
Discharge
"Dizziness"
Pain
Ringing in ears
Infections

Nose
Nosebleeds
Infections
Discharge
Frequency of colds
Nasal obstruction
History of injury
Sinus infections
Hay fever

Mouth and Throat
Condition of teeth
Last dental appointment
Condition of gums
Bleeding gums
Frequent sore throats
Burning of tongue
Hoarseness
Voice changes
Postnasal drip

Neck
Lumps
Goiter
Pain on movement
Tenderness
History of "swollen glands"
Thyroid trouble

Chest
Cough
Pain
Shortness of breath
Sputum production (quantity, appearance)
Tuberculosis
Asthma
Pleurisy
Bronchitis
Coughing up blood
Wheezing
Last x-ray
Last test for tuberculosis
History of BCG vaccination

Cardiac
Pain
High blood pressure
Palpitations
Shortness of breath with exertion
Shortness of breath when lying flat
Sudden shortness of breath while sleeping
History of heart attack
Rheumatic fever
Heart murmur
Last ECG
Other tests for heart function

Vascular
Pain in legs, calves, thighs, or hips while walking
Swelling of legs
Varicose veins
Thrombophlebitis
Coolness of extremity
Loss of hair on legs
Discoloration of extremity
Ulcers

Breasts
Lumps
Discharge
Pain
Tenderness
Self-examination

Gastrointestinal
Appetite
Excessive hunger
Excessive thirst
Nausea
Swallowing
Constipation
Diarrhea
Heartburn
Vomiting
Abdominal pain
Change in stool color
Change in stool caliber
Change in stool consistency
Frequency of bowel movements
Vomiting up blood
Rectal bleeding
Black, tarry stools
Laxative or antacid use
Excessive belching
Food intolerance
Change in abdominal size
Hemorrhoids
Infections
Jaundice
Rectal pain
Previous abdominal x-rays
Hepatitis
Liver disease
Gallbladder disease

Urinary
Frequency
Urgency
Difficulty in starting the stream
Incontinence
Excessive urination
Pain on urination
Burning
Blood in urine
Infections
Stones
Bed wetting
Flank pain
Awakening at night to urinate
History of retention
Urine color
Urine odor

Male Genitalia
Lesions on penis
Discharge
Impotence
Pain
Scrotal masses
Hernias
Frequency of intercourse
Ability to enjoy sexual relations
Fertility problems
Prostate problems
History of venereal disease and treatment

Female Genitalia
Lesions on external genitalia
Itching
Discharge
Last Pap smear and result
Pain on intercourse
Frequency of intercourse
Birth control methods
Ability to enjoy sexual relations
Fertility problems
Hernias
History of venereal disease and treatment
History of DES exposure
Age at menarche
Interval between periods
Duration of periods
Amount of flow
Date of last period
Bleeding between periods
Number of pregnancies
Abortions
Term deliveries
Complications of pregnancies
Description(s) of labor
Number of living children
Menstrual pain
Age at menopause
Menopausal symptoms
Postmenopausal bleeding

Musculoskeletal
Weakness
Paralysis
Muscle stiffness
Limitation of movement
Joint pain
Joint stiffness
Arthritis
Gout
Back problems
Muscle cramps
Deformities

Neurologic
Fainting
"Dizziness"
"Blackouts"
Paralysis
Strokes
"Numbness"
Tingling
Burning
Tremors
Loss of memory
Psychiatric disorders
Mood changes
Nervousness
Speech disorders
Unsteadiness of gait
General behavioral change
Loss of consciousness
Hallucinations
Disorientation

Reprinted with permission from Swartz MH. Textbook of Physical Diagnosis: History and Examination. *Philadelphia; Saunders, 1989.*

When recognizing diseases by their characteristic patterns, it is important to keep three points in mind:

1. "Common diseases occur commonly." Simply because common diseases are more prevalent, consider the simplest diagnoses first, and the esoteric ones last.
2. "Uncommon manifestations of common diseases are more common than common manifestations of uncommon diseases." If diagnostic reasoning is based upon what is common in the population, there exists a better chance of making a correct diagnosis.
3. "It isn't rare if it's in your chair." No disease is rare to the patient who has it. After ruling out the more common conditions, do not overlook the rarer possibilities. Think common, but remember rare.

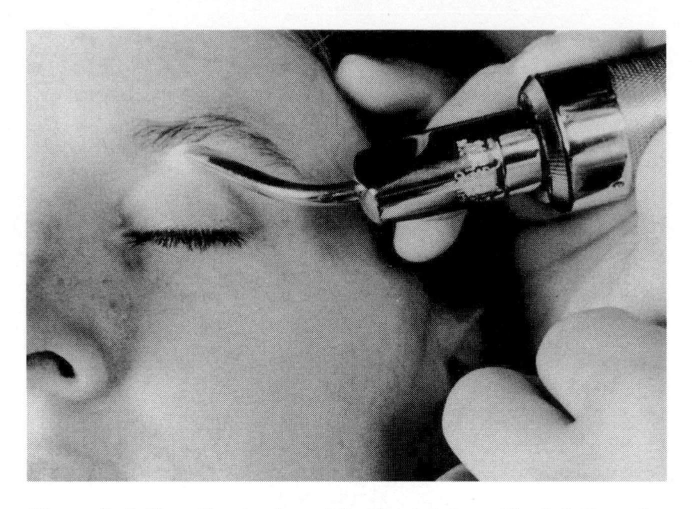

Figure 1–1. Transillumination of the frontal sinus. The light from the transilluminator is directed behind the bone of the superior orbital rim and the patient's forehead viewed in a completely dark room.

DIAGNOSTIC PROCEDURES

The following are some diagnostic procedures that may easily be performed in the office to assess various aspects of a patient's health status.

Sinus Evaluation

The maxillary and frontal sinuses may be grossly evaluated in patients with suspected sinus infection, congestion, or mass. The examination room must be as dark as possible. A bright transilluminator should be gently placed up under the superior orbital rim. The light should be directed up and slightly posterior, into the frontal sinus, not anteriorly into the skin of the forehead, and may be moved around gently for full transillumination. A red glow outlining the sinus may be observed on the forehead if the sinus is unobstructed. Repeat the procedure with the other orbit (Figure 1–1).

The maxillary sinuses may be transilluminated by tilting the patient's head back, and asking the patient to open the mouth. The transilluminator should be placed inside the center of the infraorbital rim and directed down into the sinus. Here also, the light may be moved around gently for full sinus transillumination. The clinician should look for a red glow in the roof of the patient's mouth. Repeat the procedure with the other orbit. Any asymmetry in transillumination should be noted.

The frontal and maxillary sinuses also may be evaluated by gently tapping over the sinus (forehead for frontal, cheekbone for maxillary). Tapping on an infected or congested sinus will cause discomfort or pain. Sinus transillumination and tapping are gross evaluations. Any suspected pathology warrants further evaluation (e.g., x-rays of the paranasal sinuses).

Thyroid Evaluation

Thyroid palpation should be performed on patients with suspected thyroid eye disease, or with notable thyroid gland enlargement. The best examiner position for palpating the thyroid is from behind the patient. The examiner should place the fingers of both hands just below the thyroid cartilage (cricoid) on the slightly extended neck of the patient (Figure 1–2). The patient should be asked to swallow to allow the examiner to feel the thyroid isthmus against the trachea as it rises and falls with the swallowing action. Next, the examiner's fingers should be rotated down and out to either side to palpate the lateral lobes as the patient swallows.

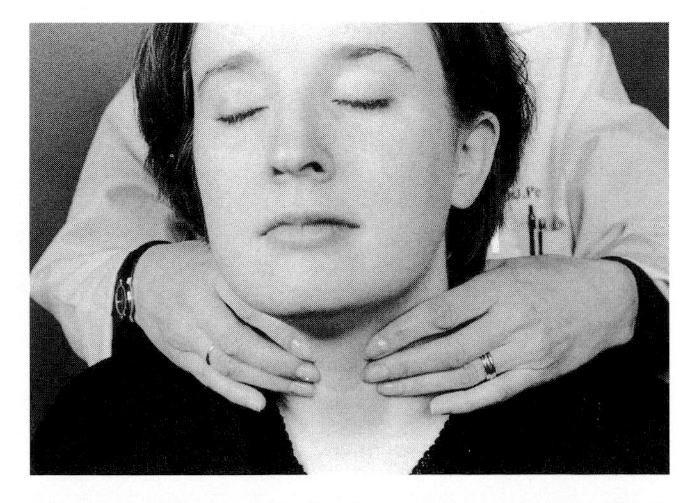

Figure 1–2. Palpation of the thyroid gland. Having the patient swallow may help in locating the isthmus.

The normal thyroid is either nonpalpable or feels rubbery or muscle-like, without palpable nodules. An enlarged thyroid gland (a goiter) is found in patients with thyroid disease. A firm nodule within the gland may indicate a neoplastic process, or scarring, and warrants further investigation.

Lymph Node Evaluation

Patients presenting with anterior segment ocular inflammation or infection may have involvement of the lymph nodes of the head and neck. Lymph node assessment is a relatively straightforward examination procedure requiring simultaneous palpation of both sides of the head and neck, but it is important to perform the examination in an organized fashion due to the large number of nodes present. Starting over the occipital area, the examiner should feel for palpable occipital and postauricular lymph nodes by rolling the pads of two or three fingers over the area (Figure 1–3). The clinician should then examine the posterior cervical chain located behind the sternocleidomastoid muscle, followed by the superficial and deep cervical chains over and under the sternocleidomastoid muscle, respectively. Next, the clinician should palpate the angle of the jaw for tonsillar nodes, under the jaw for submaxillary nodes, and under the tip of the chin in search of submental nodes. The fingers should next palpate up in front of the ears for preauricular nodes, which are the nodes most likely to become involved with ocular infections. Finally, the examiner should stand behind the patient and palpate for supraclavicular nodes (just behind the clavicles) as the patient inhales deeply, since these are most likely to be involved with metastatic disease from an apical lung tumor. Any palpable nodes should be noted for consistency, mobility, and tenderness. Inflammation or infection is usually indicated by tender, enlarged nodes. Fixed, hard nodes may indicate a malignancy and so warrant further evaluation.

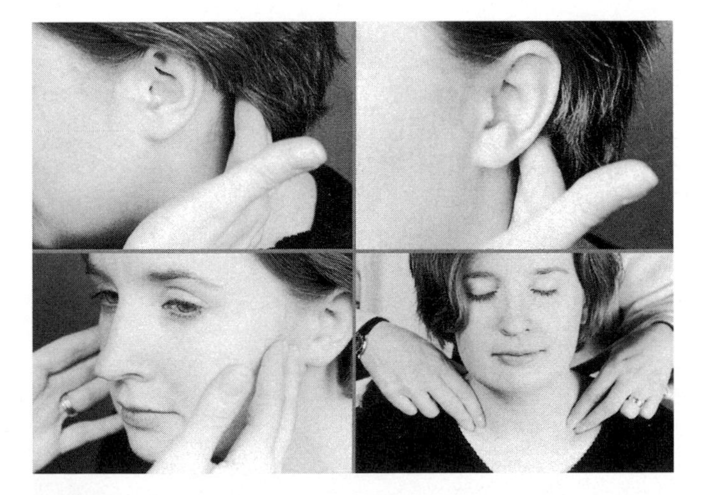

Figure 1–3. Lymph node palpation. All the lymph nodes in the head and neck, and the supraclavicular nodes, should be assessed in an orderly manner: back to front, and top to bottom. Start with the occipital nodes (upper left), move forward to the posterior auricular (top right), then to the preauricular (bottom left), the posterior, deep, and superficial cervical chains, tonsillar, submandibular, and submental (not shown), and finish with the supraclavicular (bottom right).

Vascular Evaluation

Certain facets of the vascular system can be easily assessed in the office with minimal additional equipment. These tests may include arterial pulse assessment, carotid artery auscultation, ophthalmodynamometry, and sphygmomanometry.

There are many indications for evaluating pulses in an eyecare setting. For example, a pulse may be taken before and after prescribing ophthalmic medications with systemic side effects (e.g., beta-blockers for glaucoma), in patients suspected of having carotid artery or cerebrovascular disease, or as part of taking a blood pressure measurement.

The arterial pulse is actually the shock wave traveling along the arterial tree produced by the heart ejecting blood into the aorta. It may be felt anywhere an artery is close to the surface of the skin, underneath which lies some firm structure. The most common pulses for the eyecare practitioner to assess are the radial and carotid arteries.

To assess the radial pulse, the examiner's second, third, and fourth fingers are placed into the groove between the radius and the flexor tendon on the lateral aspect of the patient's wrist just below the ball of the thumb, directly over the radial artery (Figure 1–4). The thumb should not be used because the thumb's pulse may be confused with the patient's radial pulse. With firm pressure, the artery can be felt pulsating and several factors can be simultaneously assessed. These include the *rate* (most accurately measured by counting the full 60 seconds), *rhythm* (regular versus irregular), *volume/strength* (normal/full versus weak/thready), and the *condition of the vessel wall* (palpable, tender, or rigid). The results are recorded as artery tested, rate, rhythm, and volume/strength; for example: *Right radial 55, irregular and thready.*

An average pulse rate for adults is between 60 and 100 beats/minute (although athletes and the elderly may have slower pulses), and for children between 90 and 140 beats/minute. If the pulse rate is elevated, the clinician should recheck it at the end of the examination, as it may be temporarily elevated for reasons other than disease (eg, nervousness).

To evaluate the carotid pulse, the examiner's first two fingers should be placed at the angle of the jaw,

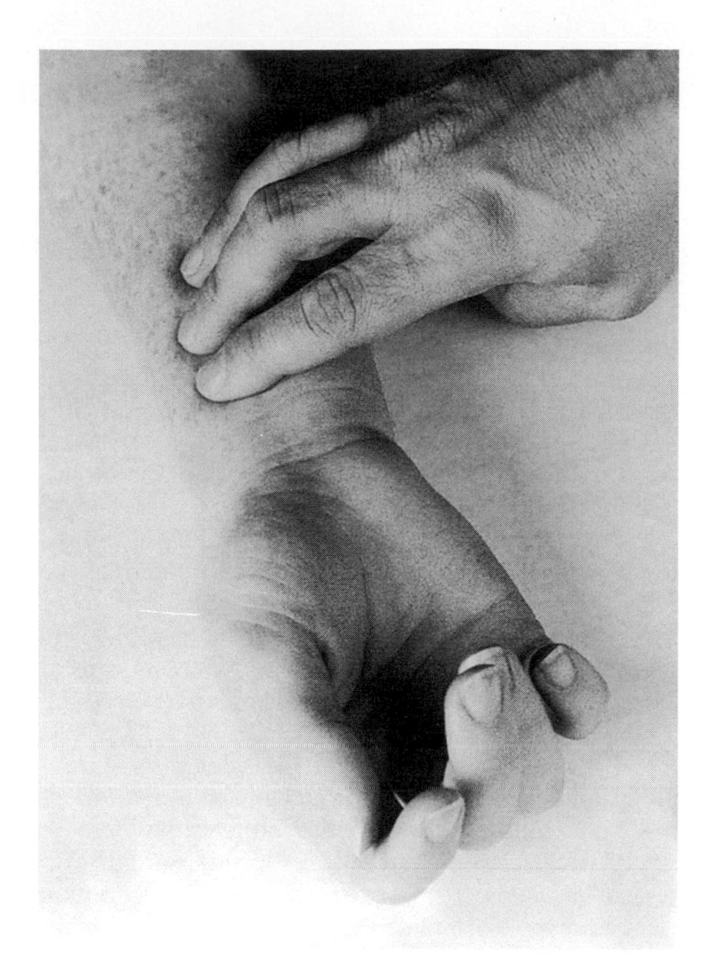

Figure 1–4. Assessing the radial pulse. The examiner's fingers are placed on the lateral aspect of the patient's wrist and gently pressed into the groove between the radius and the flexor tendon.

and then slid down into the sulcus formed between the sternocleidomastoid muscle and the trachea (Figure 1–5). Palpation should be gentle to avoid stimulating the carotid sinus, which may cause a drop in blood pressure and heart rate. In addition, both carotids should not be palpated simultaneously, since this may significantly obstruct blood flow to the brain.

The carotid pulse is evaluated in the same manner as the radial pulse; however, the carotid artery is often evaluated further because it is commonly affected by atherosclerosis. Palpation and auscultation are indicated in patients with symptoms of amaurosis fugax, transient ischemic attacks, retinal emboli, retinal occlusive disease, asymmetric diabetic retinopathy, ocular ischemic syndrome, or history of carotid artery or vertebrobasilar disease. Palpation of the carotid pulse may provide an indication of gross asymmetry in blood flow, in addition to providing a gross assessment of the condition of the carotid artery walls.

Auscultation is done to detect bruits, which are caused by blockages within the carotid arteries. As the blood squirts through a partially occluded vessel, it becomes turbulent and makes a sound called a *bruit*. This noise may be audible with a stethoscope, but only if there is enough constriction to generate sufficient turbulence yet still enough blood flow to produce adequate volume. This typically happens when the vessel is more than 50% but less than 90% occluded.

To auscultate the carotid arteries, the patient should elevate the chin slightly, turning their head *slightly* away from the side to be auscultated first. Too much chin elevation and/or head turn can actually constrict the carotid artery and artificially induce a bruit. The bell (or diaphragm) of the stethoscope is placed just below the angle of the jaw, where the common carotid bifurcates. Due to the nearness of the heart, the pulse beat can be heard, which indicates that the stethoscope head is in the proper position. The bruit, if present, is a very soft sound and may only be heard during periods of silence. Therefore, the procedure must be done in a very quiet environment, and the patient must hold his or her breath while the examiner listens for any rushing or whooshing sounds *in between* the pulse beats. The stethoscope should be moved up and down the neck since the bruit, if present, might only be heard if the stethoscope is placed directly over the area of occlusion, and might not be audible elsewhere along the artery (Figure 1–6).

The same procedure should be repeated on the other side. Although the presence of a bruit is highly suggestive of significant carotid artery occlusive disease, the absence of a bruit does not rule it out, since a bruit will not be loud enough to hear once the occlusion exceeds 90%, or if the occlusion is in a different portion of the artery. Therefore, any patient suspected of carotid artery occlusive arterial disease, with or without an audible bruit, requires a vascular workup.

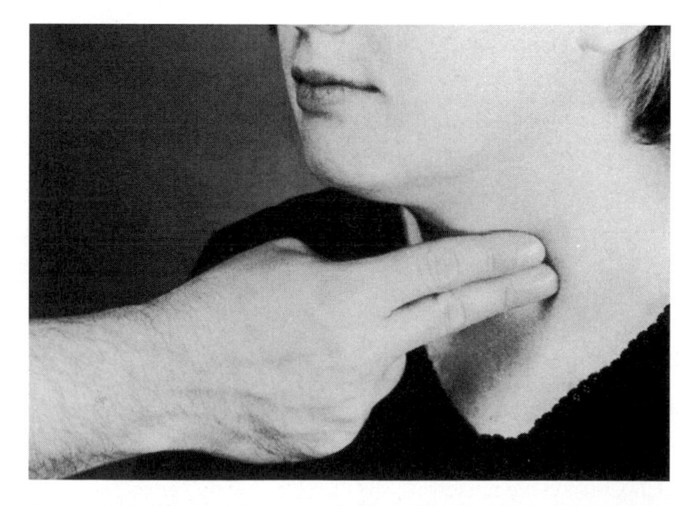

Figure 1–5. Assessing the carotid pulse. The examiner's fingers are gently pressed into the sulcus between the trachea and the sternocleidomastoid muscle.

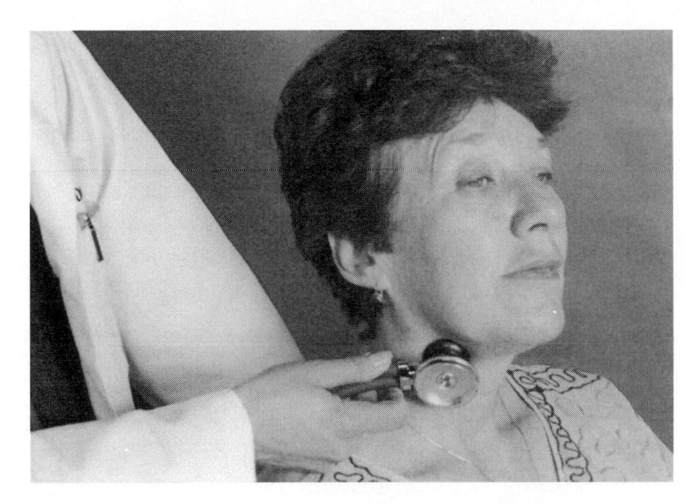

Figure 1–6. Assessing for a carotid bruit. The procedure must be performed in a quiet room, and the patient must hold his or her breath while the examiner listens for sounds between beats. The stethoscope head is held by the tubing to insulate it acoustically from the examiner's fingers.

Another in-office procedure that can help detect carotid artery disease is ophthalmodynamometry (ODM). This measures the relative central retinal artery pressure between the two eyes, which is dependent upon the ophthalmic artery pressure, which in turn is dependent upon the pressures in the carotid arteries. This procedure has the same indications as carotid artery auscultation, but is contraindicated in patients with a recent history of repair of retinal detachment or tears, recent intraocular surgery, recent penetration or blunt injury to the globe, ectopia lentis, or neovascularization. Both the systolic pressure (peak of the cardiac cycle) and the diastolic pressure (resting phase of the cardiac cycle) may be measured, but since this procedure is mainly used to rule out an asymmetry between the eyes, usually only the diastolic reading for each eye is taken.

The ophthalmodynamometer has a scale (usually a dial) at one end and a footplate at the other. The footplate is placed on the anesthetized sclera, and gentle pressure is applied directly in toward the exact center of the globe (Figure 1–7). At the same time the optic nerve head is visualized via either direct or indirect ophthalmoscopy. The amount of pressure (read off the dial) required to cause the central retinal artery to *begin* to pulsate corresponds to its diastolic pressure. The amount of pressure required to *collapse* the central retinal artery completely corresponds to its systolic pressure. The total pressure exerted on the central retinal artery is the sum of the pressure applied by the ODM and the eye's intraocular pressure. A difference in the readings of 15 to 20% or more between the two eyes is considered clinically significant, after the intraocular pressure has been taken into account. Although the absolute numerical values provide useful information, it is the asymmetry between the eyes that is particularly important, since it suggests carotid artery disease on the side with the lower pressure.

Blood pressure assessment should be routine for many eyecare practitioners. Clinically, the indirect technique of sphygmomanometry is used to screen for systemic hypertension and monitor known hypertensives, as well as to monitor the effects of some ophthalmic medications (e.g., topical sympathomimetics, beta-blockers) and aid in the diagnosis of certain ocular conditions (e.g., hypertensive retinopathy). A sphygmomanometer is a device consisting of a cloth cuff containing an inflatable rubber bladder, connected to a rubber bulb with a valve (to inflate or deflate the cuff), and a manometer (pressure gauge). The manometer may be an actual column of mercury, or it may be of the aneroid type, which is calibrated in millimeters of mercury (mm Hg) (Figure 1–8).

To perform sphygmomanometry (Figure 1–9), the patient should be seated or reclined in a quiet, relaxed environment. The arm to be tested should be bare, extended, and well supported at the level of the heart either by having the examiner hold the arm or by resting the arm on a firm support. The cuff is secured around the patient's biceps about 1 inch above the antecubital fossa, with the inflatable bladder over the brachial artery. It is important to choose an appropriate cuff size, since a cuff that is significantly too large or too small can give erroneous results. Next, the stethoscope head is placed over the brachial artery. At this point, no pulse beat should be audible due to the distance from the heart. The valve screw is turned

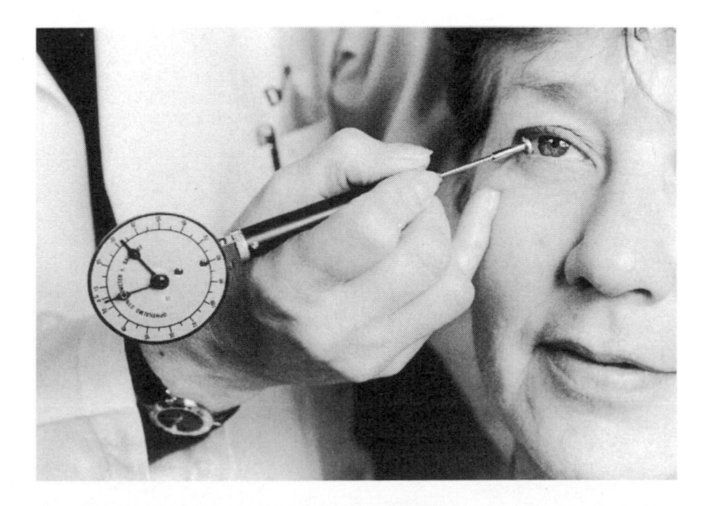

Figure 1–7. The ophthalmodynamometer is placed against the anesthetized sclera so that the force is directed directly in toward the center of the globe. The optic nerve head is observed for an induced arterial pulsation (not shown).

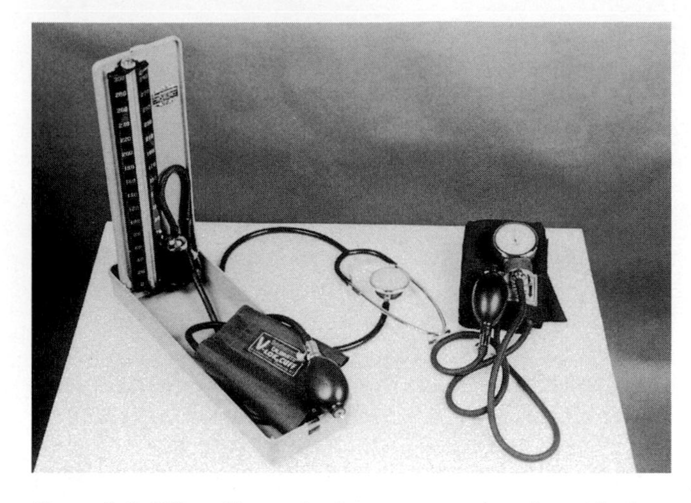

Figure 1–8. Different types of sphygmomanometers. Aneroid sphygmomanometers should be calibrated against a mercury sphygmomanometer periodically.

clockwise until snug to close the valve, and air is pumped into the bladder while palpating the radial artery. When the radial pulse is no longer palpable, several more pumps are administered to ensure that the artery is completely occluded. The clinician then holds the head of the stethoscope firmly against the brachial artery. The valve screw is turned slightly counterclockwise to allow air to escape the bladder very slowly. The pressure gauge is monitored carefully. The scale should indicate that the pressure is dropping no faster than 5 mmHg/second.

At this point, the pressure in the cuff has totally occluded the brachial artery, cutting off all blood flow. As the pressure in the cuff decreases, it reaches a point at which it is unable to stop the blood flow during the

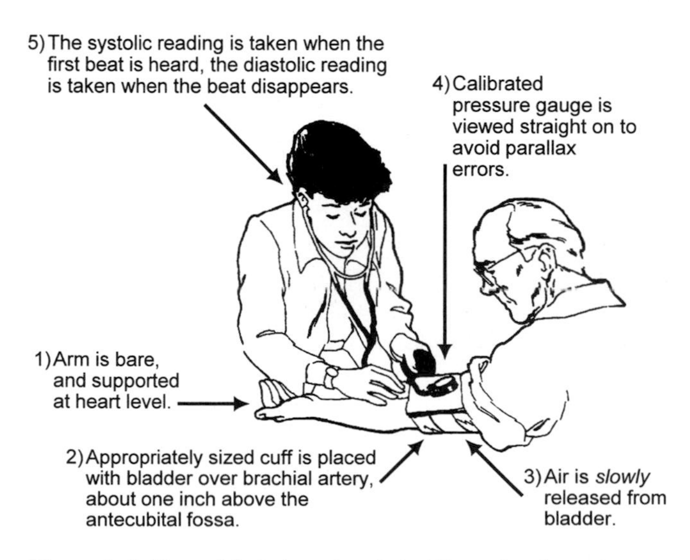

Figure 1–9. Key points to keep in mind while performing sphygmomanometry.

peak of the cardiac cycle, or systole. As the blood squirts through the partially occluded vessel, the turbulence produces noise that can be picked up by the stethoscope. It is at this point, where this first audible beat is heard, that the reading on the scale is noted. This represents the systolic blood pressure reading.

As the cuff deflation continues, there will be increased blood flow, and more turbulence, resulting in louder Korotkoff sounds, named after the Russian physician who first described them. When the pressure in the cuff falls low enough so the blood is able to flow through the vessel unimpeded and without turbulence, these sounds will fade. The scale reading at which the audible beat disappears is taken as the diastolic reading. This represents the pressure at which the artery remains open even during the trough of the cardiac cycle, or diastole. This is shown graphically in Figure 1–10.

After the sound has faded, the valve is opened even more to rapidly deflate the cuff. The finding is recorded as the systolic reading over the diastolic reading, with the limb tested, posture, and time noted; for example: *120/80 right arm sitting, 11AM.* Sources of errors are listed in Table 1–2. Normal values and interpretation are given in Table 1–3.

Nervous System Evaluation

The eyecare provider may be in a position to uncover neurological disease because so much of the brain is either involved with vision directly, or is located close to structures that are involved with the visual system. Careful observation of gait and posture, as well as interaction with the patient during the history, will often provide many clues regarding neurological status without explicit testing. Often, in-office screening tests can provide further information needed to direct the examination and determine the need for a formal neurological evaluation.

A complete neurological examination requires the evaluation of seven areas: mental status, cranial nerve function, motor function, sensory function, station and gait, cerebellar function, and reflexes. Although a full discussion of each of these areas is beyond the scope of this chapter, each is discussed briefly, and simple screening tests, which do not require much specialized equipment, are presented. Emphasis should be placed on detecting asymmetry, which may indicate neurological dysfunction. The clinician may then investigate whether the lesion is in the central or peripheral nervous system.

Mental Status

Mental status can be screened by use of the mnemonic FOGS. The patient's level of consciousness (alert and

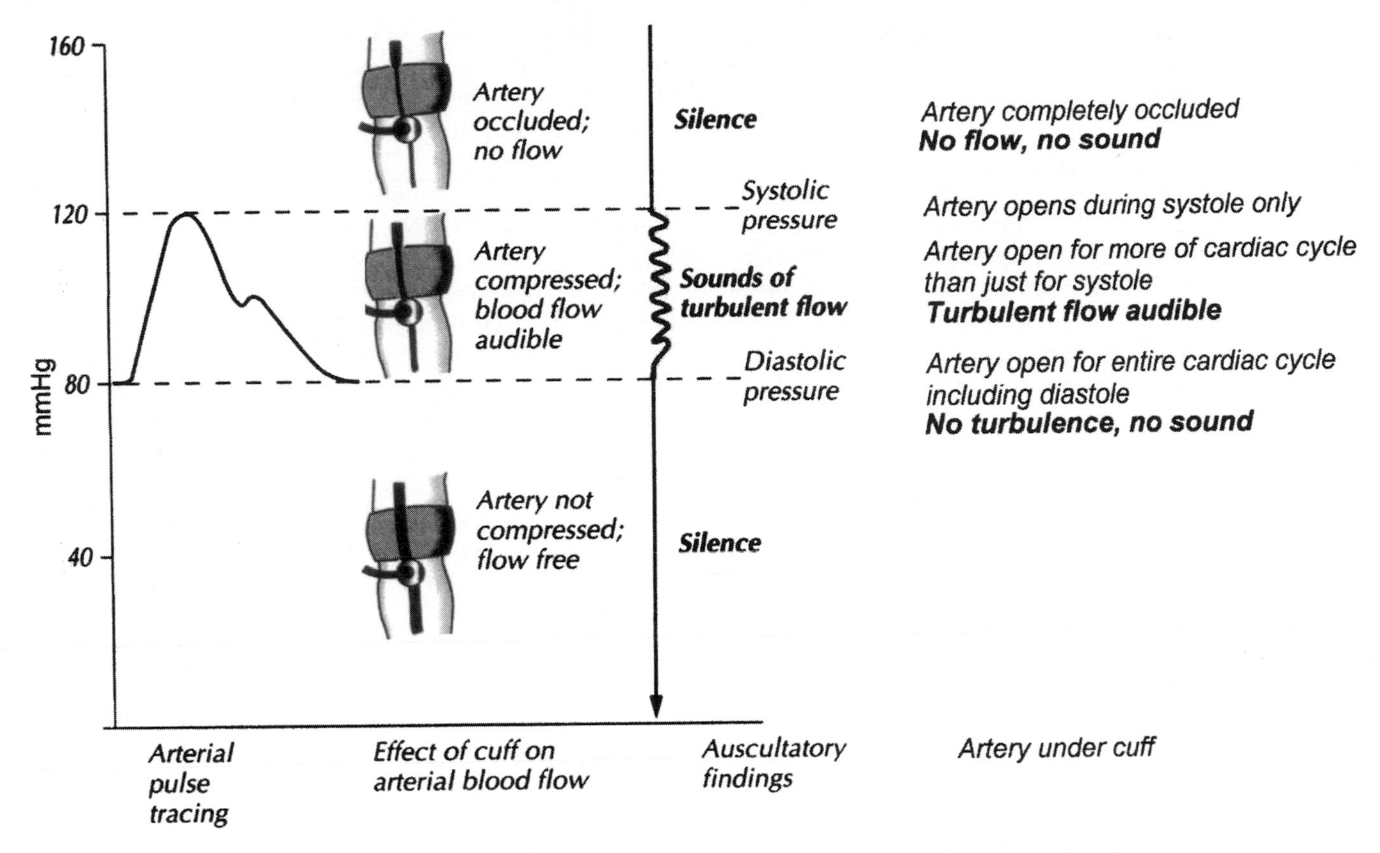

Figure 1–10. The sounds heard during sphygmomanometry and how they are produced.

TABLE 1–2. SOURCES OF ERROR IN SPHYGMOMANOMETRY

False high readings may result from the following:
Anxious patient
Cuff deflation too slow (causing venous congestion)
Cuff wrapped too loosely
Cuff too small
Physical activity just prior to reading
Tobacco use or caffeinated beverage just prior to reading

False low readings may result from the following:
Auscultatory gap
Constrictive clothing
Cuff deflation too rapid
Cuff too large
Patient's arm unsupported
Poor reaction time
Poor hearing acuity

Other sources of error:
Aneroid manometer not calibrated
Mercury manometer tilted
Parallax error while reading scale
Repeated BP measurements

TABLE 1–3. SPHYGMOMANOMETRY—EXPECTED VALUES

Blood Pressure Range (mmHg)	Category	Management
Diastolic		
< 85	Normal	Recheck within 2 years
85–89	High normal	Recheck within 1 year
90–104	Mild hypertension	Confirm within 2 months
105–114	Moderate hypertension	Confirm or refer within 2 weeks
> 115	Severe hypertension	Immediate referral
Systolic, when diastolic < 90		
< 140		Recheck within 2 years
140–199		Confirm within 2 months
> 200		Confirm or refer within 2 weeks

Reprinted with permission from Good GW, Aughburger AR. Role of optometrists in combatting high blood pressure. J Am Optom Assoc. *1989; 60:352–355.*

attentive versus "foggy" or lethargic) should be immediately apparent upon history taking. Other factors to evaluate include Family history, Orientation, General information/memory, and Speech/spelling. Often the patient's family can provide valuable information about changes in the patient's mental status, which include characteristics such as intellect, mood, affect, and attention. Disorientation is common with impaired memory and attention span; therefore, evaluation of the patient's orientation to person, place, and time is important. This can be accomplished informally during the case history, or more formally by asking patients directly *who* they are, *where* they are, and *when* they are (for example: "What is your name?, Where are we now?, What is today's date?").

To report on general information, the patient must have intact orientation, memory, and abstract thought. A good way to test this is to ask about current events, but the questions must be tailored to the individual's education and socioeconomic level. Recent memory can be tested by asking patients to recall a few common objects that they were specifically told to remember earlier in the exam. Remote memory is evaluated by asking about well-known events that happened in the past.

Speech is constantly evaluated during the course of the exam, noting any difficulties in producing certain sounds or misnaming of common objects. Also, a simple spelling test in which the patient is asked to spell the word WORLD forward and backward (a five-number sequence may be used instead with an illiterate patient) may provide information regarding mental status. For example, a patient with short-term memory loss might have difficulty spelling WORLD backwards.

Cranial Nerve Function

Four cranial nerves are directly and thoroughly evaluated during a routine eye examination (II, III, IV, and VI). Additionally, four others are indirectly evaluated (V, VII, VIII, and X). Patients must be able to hear the clinician's questions (CN VIII) and respond verbally (CN X). When eyedrops are instilled, stinging is felt (CN V), and the immediate protective reaction is to shut the eyes (CN VII).

For formal testing purposes it makes sense to group the cranial nerves together by function, instead of testing in numerical order. The *ocular group* (CN II, III, IV, and VI) is tested extensively by the eye examination. Therefore, only screening tests for the remaining eight cranial nerves will be briefly presented. As noted previously, symmetry is the most important aspect to assess.

The *motor group* consists of the motor root of CN V, and nerves VII, IX, X, XI, and XII. It is evaluated by testing jaw movement, facial movements, the gag reflex, head turning, shoulder elevation, and tongue strength, respectively. The *sensory group* (CN I, V, and VIII) is evaluated by testing smell, corneal and facial sensation, and hearing, respectively.

Motor Group. The trigeminal nerve (CN V) has a motor root that controls the muscles of mastication. By having patients clench their jaws and by palpating the masseter muscles, the clinician can feel for any muscle atrophy, which would occur if the muscle is not being innervated properly. As patients open their mouths, deviation of the jaw to one side or the other should be noted. Patients may also be asked to move their jaws to each side as the clinician presses a hand against the jawbone to assess strength (Figure 1–11).

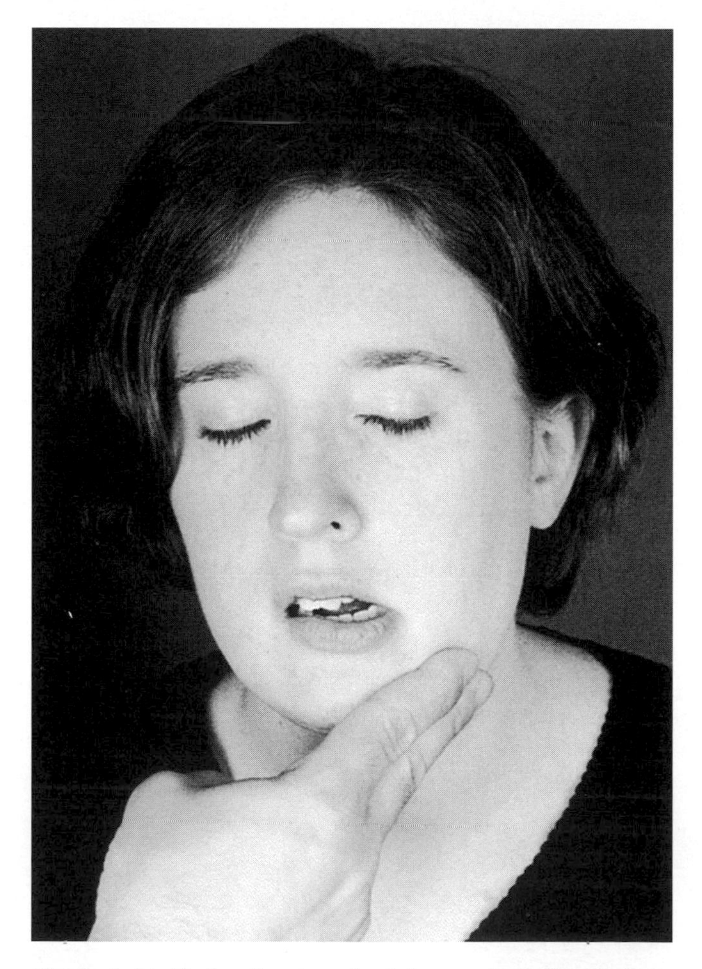

Figure 1–11. Testing the strength of the muscles of mastication, which are innervated by the motor root of the trigeminal nerve (CN V). Care must be taken to press only against the patient's jaw, the muscles of which are innervated by CN V, and not the patient's cheek, the muscles of which are innervated by CN XI.

The facial nerve (CN VII) has two subnuclei in its nucleus. One subnucleus controls the upper half of the face, and the other controls the lower half of the face. Each subnucleus gets input from cortical centers on the opposite side of the brain. However, the subnucleus that controls the upper half of the face also gets input from the ipsilateral side of the brain. Therefore, both sides of the brain have input to the upper half of the face, whereas only one side of the brain has input to the contralateral lower half of the face. In other words, if anything is wrong with either the upper motor neuron (UMN) or the lower motor neuron (LMN) of the facial nerve, it will show up in the lower half of the face, but only LMN dysfunction will also show up in the upper half of the face. Accordingly, to fully test the facial nerve, only the lower half of the face need be tested. This is most easily accomplished by having patients smile widely and bare their teeth. If the smile is normal and symmetric, the nerve and nucleus are intact. However, if one side of a patient's mouth is weak and droops, testing of the upper half of the face becomes necessary to determine the location of the lesion. Patients are asked to look up and raise their eyebrows. Wrinkles should appear across their foreheads. If the resulting wrinkles go all the way across, then the facial nerve itself is intact and the lesion must be supranuclear (UMN) on the side opposite the weakness. On the other hand, if the forehead wrinkles stop at the midline, the lesion has affected all fibers to that side of the face, upper and lower, and therefore, it must be in the nerve after it leaves the brainstem (LMN) on the same side as the weakness. This is a peripheral, or Bell's, palsy (Figure 1–12).

The glossopharyngeal and vagus nerves (CN IX and X) are usually tested together as a reflex arc. The soft palate is innervated by the glossopharyngeal nerve for sensation, and the vagus for movement. If each side of the soft palate is touched lightly with a cotton-tipped applicator, there should be prompt symmetric elevation of the palate. If there is a motor weakness, the palate will deviate to the stronger side no matter which side is touched. If there is a sensory deficit, there will be no response when the affected side is touched, but a bilateral response when the normal side is touched (Figure 1–13).

The spinal accessory nerve (CN XI) controls head position by innervating the trapezius and sternocleidomastoid muscles. The nerve may be tested by asking patients to elevate their shoulders against manual resistance. Patients can also turn their heads from side to side against manual resistance on the cheekbone. In both instances, the examiner assesses muscle strength and symmetry.

The hypoglossal nerve innervates the muscles of the tongue, which are pushing muscles. Patients should be asked to stick their tongues straight out while the clinician observes for any deviation or muscle wasting. The tongue will always deviate to the weaker side. If the tongue deviates to one side but that side is not atrophic, a UMN lesion is indicated, because muscle wasting, or atrophy, is a sign that the muscle is not innervated properly and typically occurs in LMN lesions.

Sensory Group. Before testing the olfactory nerve (CN I), the clinician must check the nasal passages to ensure they are patent. The patient covers each nostril in turn and attempts to breath freely through each side. The patient is then asked to close his or her eyes and occlude one nostril. A familiar, nonirritating substance is placed near the unoccluded nostril and the patient asked to identify the odor. The other side is then tested. It is important to use a familiar smell, such as coffee or chocolate, and one that is not irritating because irritating vapors can stimulate sensory branches of the trigeminal nerve (which also innervates the nasal mucosa), and may produce a false-positive response.

The trigeminal nerve (CN V) supplies sensation to the face through its three sensory divisions. The most useful test determines if patients can differentiate between a sharp and a dull stimulus. A cotton swab is broken in half. The broken end is used as the sharp stimulus and the cotton end as the dull stimulus. The procedure should first be demonstrated to patients so that they recognize what the stimuli feel like. The procedure is then repeated with the patients' eyes closed, and they are asked to correctly identify the stimulus for each division on each side.

The trigeminal nerve can also be tested together with the facial nerve (CN VII) in the corneal reflex arc. The end of a sterile cotton swab is teased out so that a thin wisp of cotton is formed. While patients look up and away from the swab, the cornea (not the eyelashes or conjunctiva) is gently touched. There should be a brisk blink response of both eyes. This is repeated on the other side. A sensory deficit produces no motor response on either side when the affected side is touched, and a bilateral motor response when the unaffected side is touched. A motor deficit results in no response on the affected side no matter which side is touched (Figure 1–14).

The vestibulocochlear nerve (CN VIII) senses both hearing and the vestibular sense, which is involved in balance. Of the two, hearing is easier to assess. The patient is asked to keep his or her eyes closed. The examiner then produces a soft sound by rubbing fingers

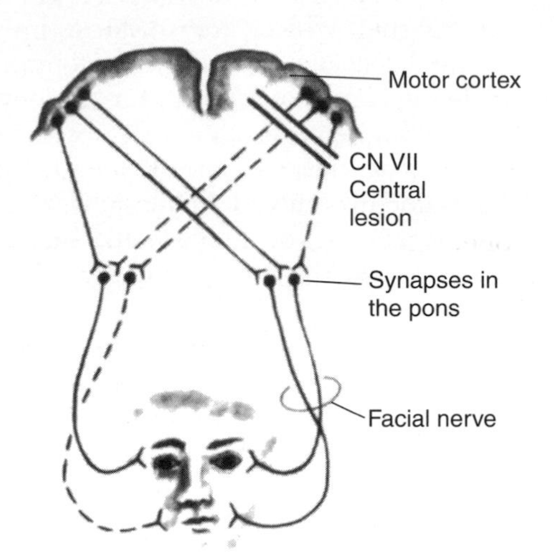

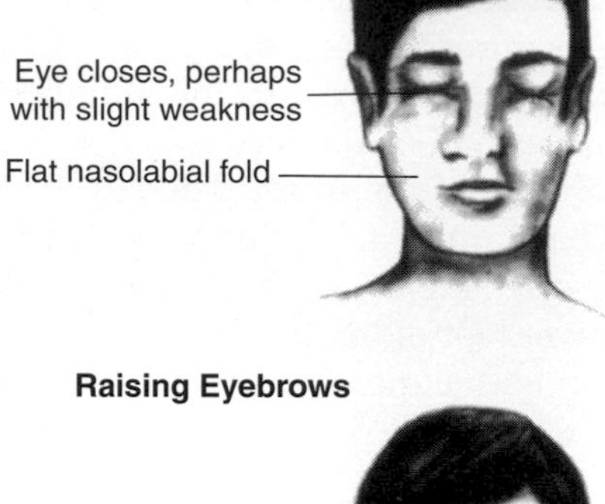

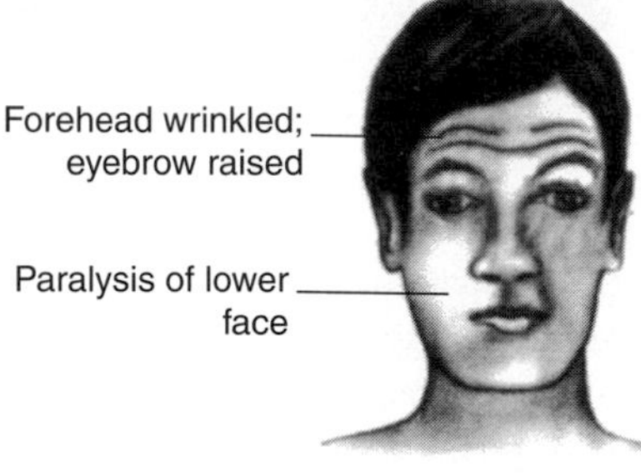

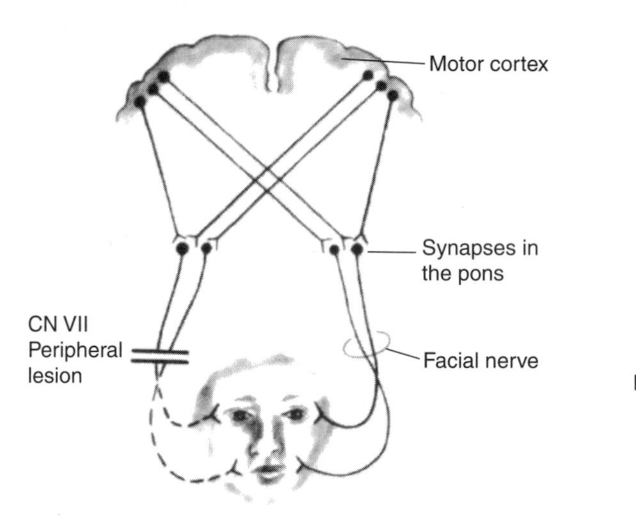

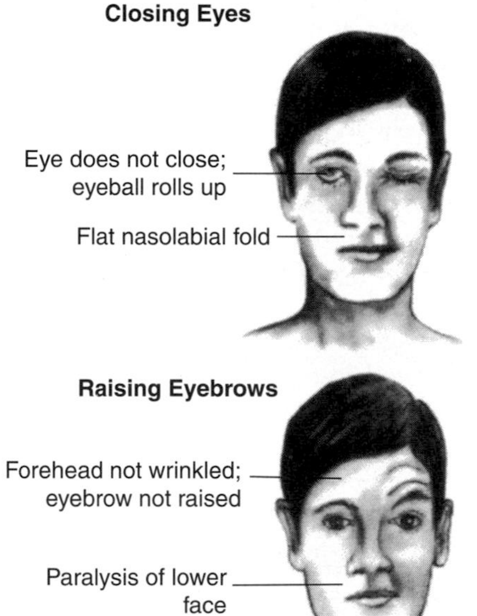

Figure 1–12. Differentiating upper (top) versus lower (bottom) motor neuron facial nerve palsies (CN VII). (*Reprinted with permission from Bickley LS, Hoekelman RA, Bates B.* Bates' Guide to Physical Examination and History Taking. *7th ed. Philadelphia: Lippincott; 1999.*)

together on the right side of the patient's head. The sound is slowly brought closer to the patient's right ear until heard. The distance between the examiner's fingers and the patient's ear is noted. The procedure is then repeated on the left side. If there is a gross asymmetry in the two distances, there may be hearing loss on the side with the shorter distance. Before assuming that the hearing loss is sensorineural, it is important to rule out a conductive deficit, such as wax buildup in the ear canal, or a problem with the ear itself. An ear problem should be referred to an otolaryngologist, but a sensorineural problem should go to a neurologist.

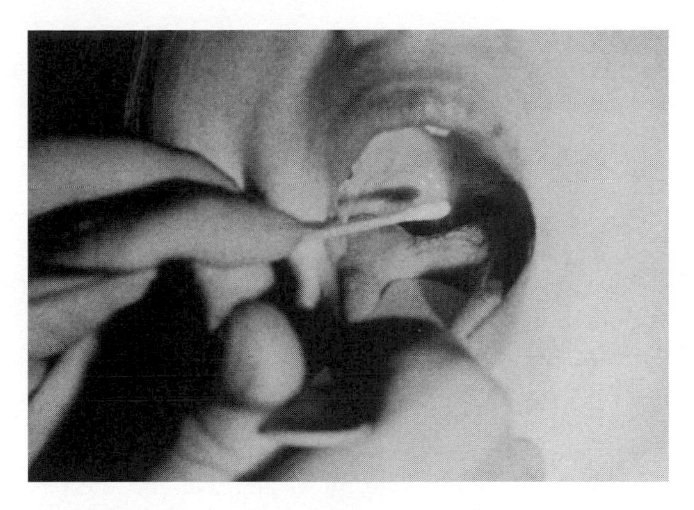

Figure 1–13. Lightly touching the soft palate tests the glossopharyngeal (CN IX) and the vagus (CN X) nerves together in a reflex arc.

There are two tests that can help differentiate between conductive and sensorineural hearing loss. The Rinne test compares air conduction to bone conduction. A 512-Hz tuning fork is struck and held with the handle placed firmly on the mastoid process. This transmits the sound directly to the inner ear via bone conduction, bypassing the middle and outer ears. The patient indicates when the sound fades, at which point the vibrating end of the tuning fork is held near to the outer ear on the same side. If the outer and middle ears are working normally, the patient will be able to hear the sound via air conduction because the outer and middle ears work as an amplifier for sound coming through the air. If the patient cannot hear the sound when the vibrating end of the tuning fork is placed near to the ear, then it points to a problem with the ear itself, a conduction deficit. If air conduction is better than bone conduction on both sides (which is considered normal), the patient most likely has a sensorineural deficit on the side with the hearing loss; if the nerve is damaged, the sound will be less on the affected side no matter how the sound gets in, via air or bone. If bone conduction is better on the affected side, there is most likely a problem with the ear itself because the patient responds to the sound only when it is transmitted via the bone, since the sound is blocked when coming in through the air (Figure 1–15).

In the Weber test, bone conduction between the two ears is compared. The handle of a vibrating 512-Hz tuning fork is placed on the patient's head midway between the two ears. The patient is asked to localize the sound. A normal response is when the patient is unable to localize the sound, or localizes it to the middle. If the patient has hearing loss from a conduction deficit, that ear will have room noise filtered out, and the only sound it will hear will be that of the tuning fork transmitted via bone. Therefore, the sound will appear to be louder on the side affected by a conduction deficit. On the other hand, if the patient has sensorineural hearing loss, the affected side will hear the sound more softly, no matter how the sound gets there, via air or bone. In this case, the sound will be louder on the normal side (Figure 1–16).

Motor Function

Motor function is assessed by evaluating muscle tone, strength, and bulk. A muscle that is not innervated properly will become atrophic and may show visible muscle wasting. Any abnormal movements, such as

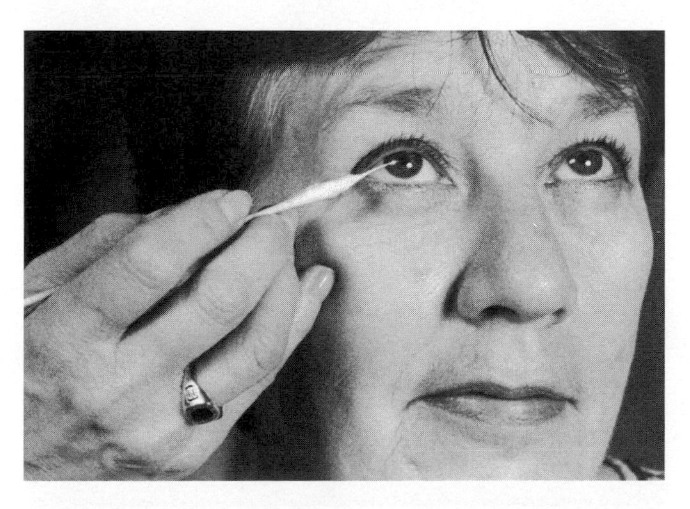

Figure 1–14. Touching the cornea with a fine cotton wisp tests the trigeminal (CN V) and facial (CN VII) nerves together in a reflex arc. Care must be taken to keep the cotton swab outside of the patient's view, and to touch only the cornea, not the conjunctiva or lashes.

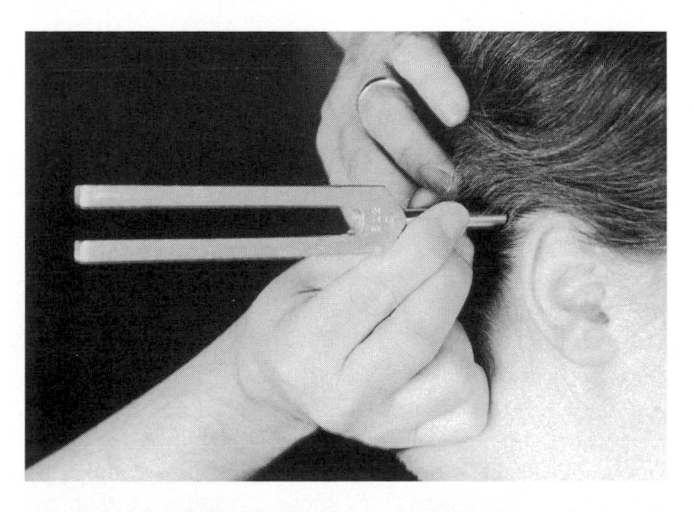

Figure 1–15. The Rinne test compares sound conduction through the air versus through bone on each side. The handle of the vibrating 512-Hz tuning fork should be placed directly on the mastoid process.

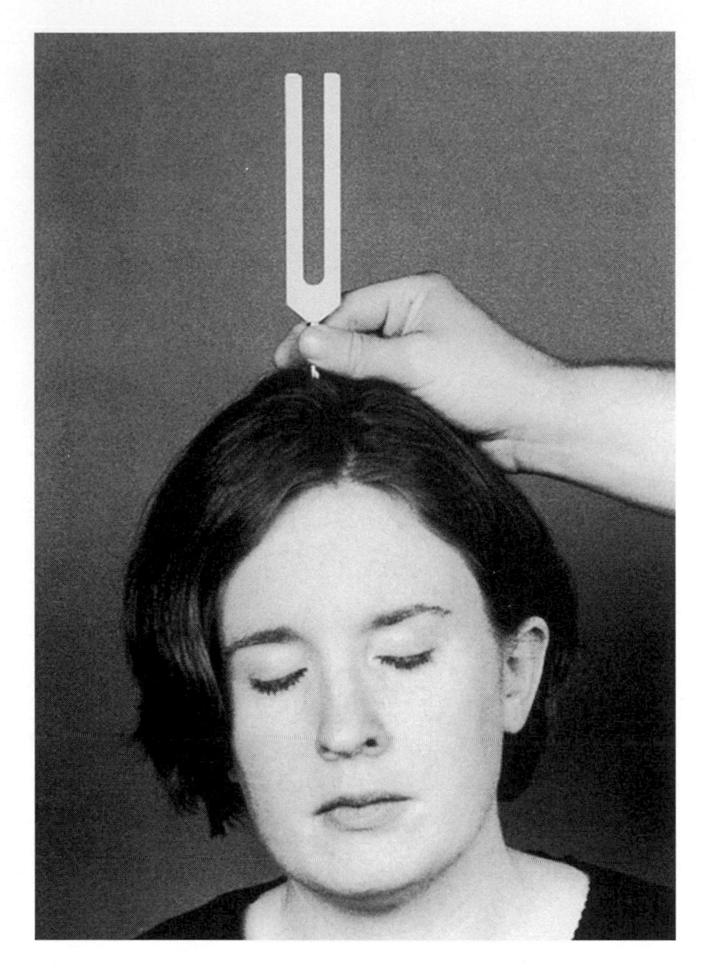

Figure 1–16. The Weber test compares bone conduction between the two ears. The tuning fork handle is pressed firmly against the patient's forehead or the middle of the patient's head.

tremors, tics, fasciculations, or other dyskinesias should be noted. To screen for these, the clinician can ask the patient to hold the arms straight out, directly in front of his or her body, with the palms facing up and eyes closed. The clinician looks for the ability to maintain arm position, any drifts or weakness (such as pronator drift), and symmetry of muscle bulk. The patient can also grasp the examiner's hands and squeeze to allow the examiner to directly assess relative strength between the two sides of the body. The patient's dominant side may normally be slightly stronger than his or her nondominant side.

Sensory Function

Sensory function can be broken down into primary and secondary sensory modalities. The primary sense modalities include light touch, pain, vibration, and position sense. The secondary sense modalities are stereognosis, graphesthesia, and two-point discrimination. These are integrative, providing information regarding primary sensory modalities and higher cortical (parietal lobe) function. The identification of common objects through touch (e.g., by placing a paper clip in the patient's hand) will assess stereognosis. Agraphesthesia is the inability to identify traced figures on the skin of a limb in the presence of normal primary sensory modalities.

Light touch and pain are assessed in the same manner utilized in the assessment of the trigeminal nerve; however, the backs of the hands and tops of the feet are tested instead. Vibration sense is examined by touching the handle of a vibrating low-frequency (128 Hz) tuning fork to a bony prominence of the terminal digits of the upper and lower limbs (Figure 1–17). To test position sense (proprioception), the clinician manipulates the patient's thumb or big toe, and the patient (with eyes closed) attempts to accurately determine if the digit has been moved up or down. Care must be taken to grasp the digit from the sides rather than the top and bottom in order to avoid any clues as to which way the clinician is pressing. The procedure should be visually demonstrated first (Figure 1–18).

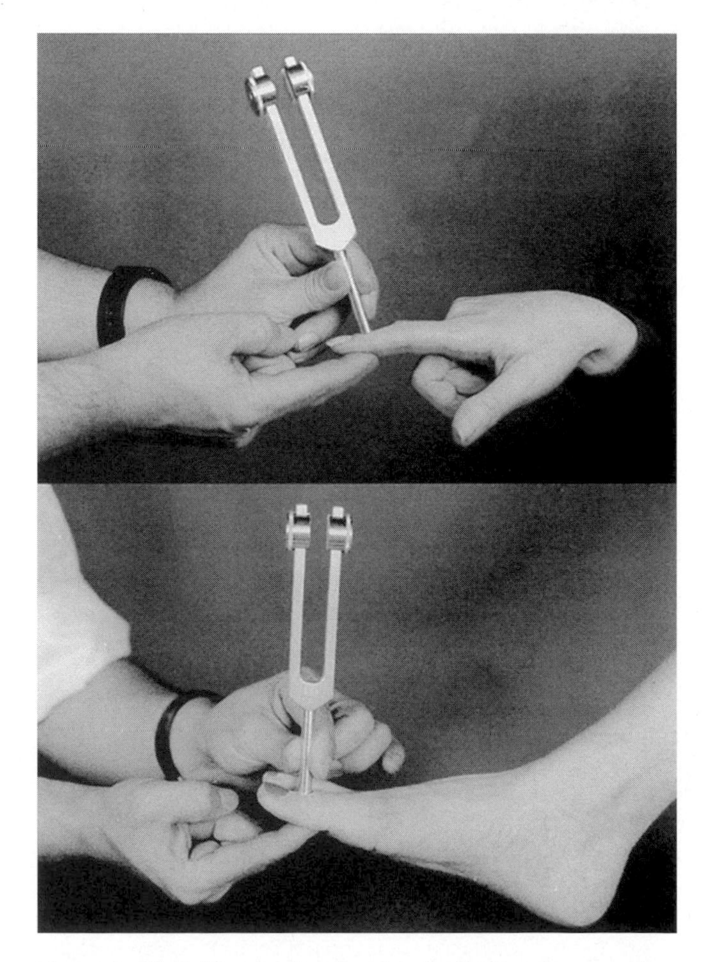

Figure 1–17. Holding the handle of a vibrating low-frequency tuning fork directly against the bone of a terminal digit tests vibration sense.

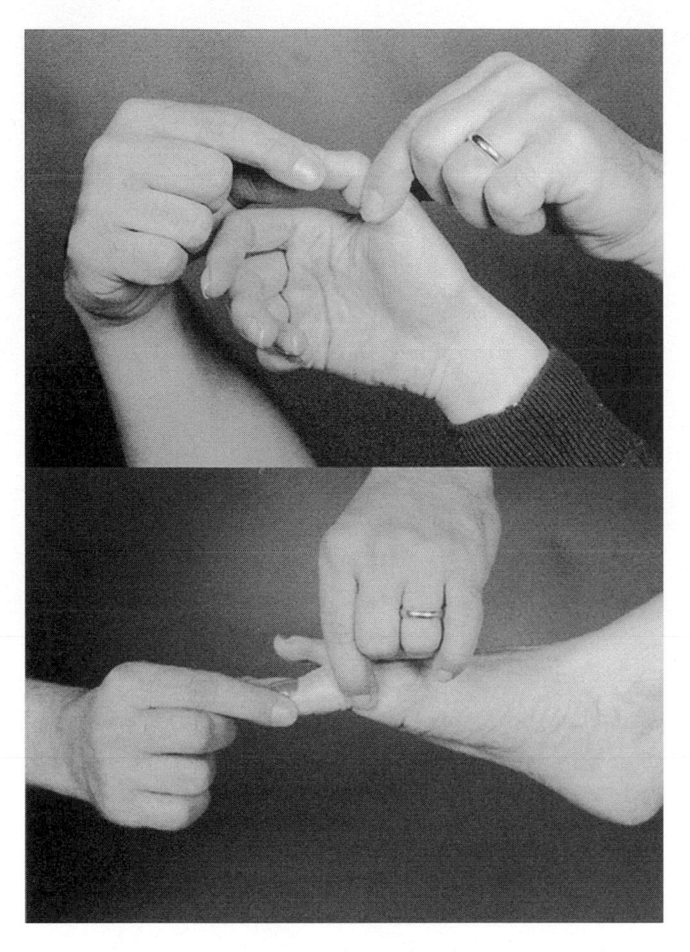

Figure 1–18. Gently grasping a patient's terminal digit from the side and bending it up or down allows the examiner to test the patient's proprioception, or position sense.

Station and Gait

Station (the position assumed in standing) and gait (the manner or style of walking) are easily assessed by scrutinizing the patient as he or she enters the examination room. The examiner should note any characteristic deficiencies of station (abnormal posture), balance (such as swaying to one side), or gait (ataxic gait, parkinsonian gait, etc.) (Figure 1–19).

The Romberg test is a useful tool to assess balance. Three senses are involved in maintaining balance: vision, proprioception, and vestibular sense. However, only two of the three are necessary to maintain balance. If there is a deficiency in one of the three, and one of the remaining two is removed, balance cannot be maintained. Since vision is the easiest sense to remove, the patient is instructed to stand straight with feet shoulder width apart and eyes closed. If both proprioception and the vestibular sense are intact, the patient should be able to maintain balance without difficulty. If either proprioception or the vestibular sense are deficient, the patient will start to sway with eyes closed. The swaying may be pronounced and the patient may even fall, so the clinician must be positioned to catch the patient in case of a fall. The Romberg test does not differentiate between a deficit in proprioception or vestibular sense, but indicates that there is a problem with one of them. Other testing (described earlier) would be necessary to determine which sense is affected.

Cerebellar Function

The function of the cerebellum is to integrate senses, primarily vision, vestibular sense, and proprioception. Cerebellar dysfunction is characterized by awkwardness of intentional movements. Cerebellar function can be assessed through specific tests of coordination.

Any rapid, alternating movement (diadochokinesia) may be used to uncover cerebellar dysfunction. Among the easiest test to perform is that in which patients rapidly and repeatedly alternate between touching the examiner's outstretched finger and their own noses (Figure 1–20). After several cycles this may be done with the patients' eyes closed. Patients with cerebellar disease may become inaccurate with their eyes closed (past pointing). Patients can also be asked to rapidly pat their knees while flipping their hands each time. The inability to perform rapid alternating movements is called dysdiadochokinesia.

Reflexes

The final portion of the neurological examination tests patient reflexes. The most important item to note when testing any reflex is the symmetry of the response between the two sides of the body. There are a number of different types of reflexes. A *visceral* reflex (e.g., the pupillary light reflex) has already been tested during the eye examination. A *superficial* reflex (eg, the corneal reflex) was described under sensory testing. *Deep tendon* reflexes can be elicited when certain muscle tendons are stretched. Although there are many deep tendon reflexes, only the biceps, patellar (knee), and Achilles (ankle) are described here. A *pathological* reflex is an abnormal response (one that should not be present) and is typified by the Babinski reflex, which has been called probably the most useful sign in clinical neurology.

The deep tendon reflexes use stimulation of stretch receptors in the muscle's tendon to send an afferent signal to the spinal cord where it synapses directly with the efferent neuron, causing that muscle to contract. It is a simple, two-neuron reflex loop, performed completely at the level of the spinal column. In order to produce this type of reflex, the muscle being tested must not be under voluntary contraction.

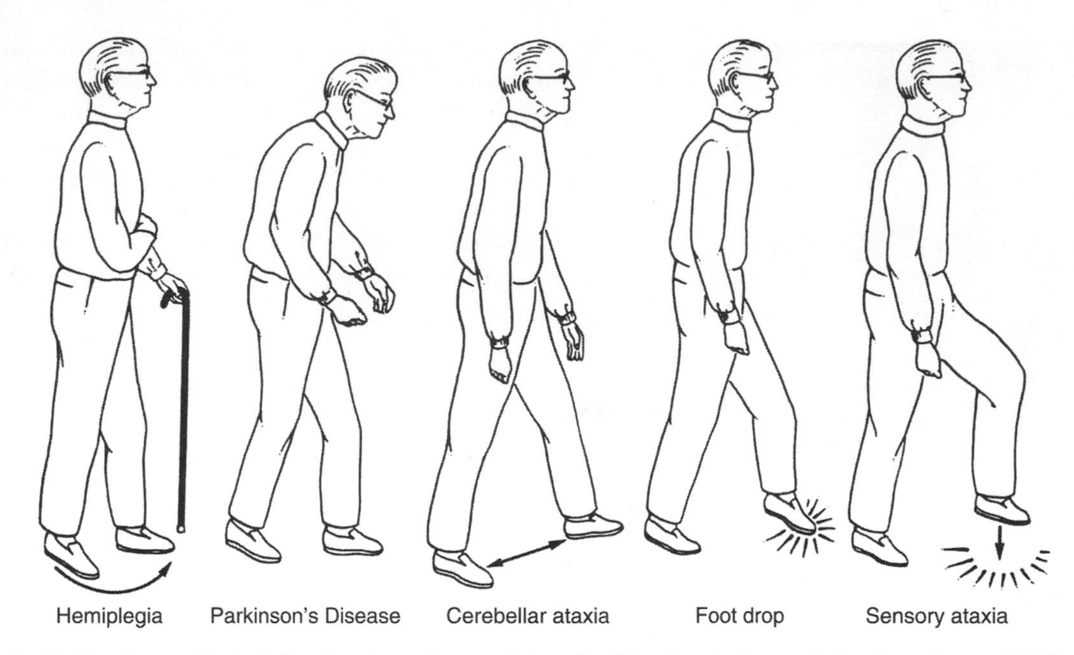

Figure 1–19. Certain neurological disorders have characteristic gaits. (*Reprinted with permission from Swartz MH.* Textbook of Physical Diagnosis: History and Examination, *2nd ed. Philadelphia: Saunders; 1994.*)

Therefore, it is very important to support the limb being tested so that the muscle is completely relaxed. The reflex hammer is held between the thumb and forefinger and swung by the wrist, not the elbow. It is important to tap the tendon, not strike it with undue force. When the tendon is struck with a reflex hammer, the tendon is stretched, inducing the reflex. It helps if the examiner palpates the muscle being tested, because often the positive response is not enough to produce an obvious movement of the limb, but the muscle contraction can be felt.

Reflex symmetry is critical. Although higher cortical centers play a role in inhibiting or enhancing reflexes, they generally should be equal. If not normal, reflexes can be described as hyporeflexive (a subnormal response) or hyperreflexive (a supranormal response). Hyperreflexia is commonly associated with a UMN lesion (between cortex and spinal cord). Hyporeflexia is often associated with an LMN lesion such as peripheral nerve disease (between spinal cord and muscle). Remember that LMN lesions are also associated with muscle wasting and atrophy (Table 1–4).

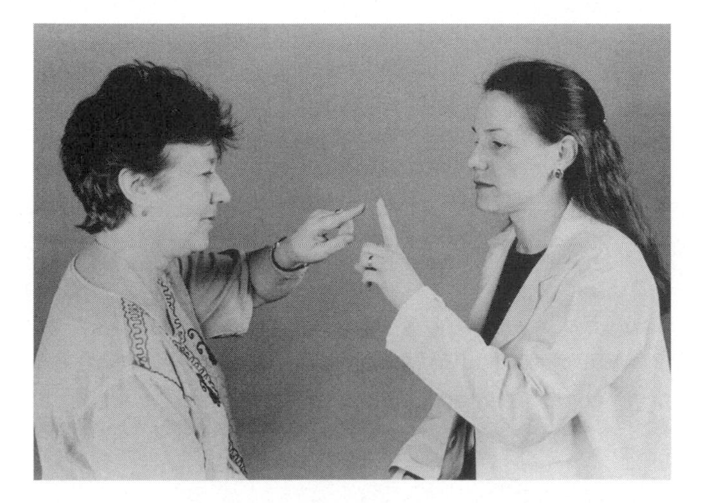

Figure 1–20. Having patients rapidly touch your finger and their noses repeatedly tests cerebellar function.

To test the biceps reflex, the patient's arm is held, flexed slightly, draped over the clinician's arm, and supported so that the biceps muscle is fully relaxed. Because the biceps tendon is buried deep in the tissues of the elbow joint, the clinician should locate it using the thumb, and then keep the thumb placed directly on the tendon. The thumb is then struck with the pointed end of the reflex hammer to transmit force to the tendon. The clinician should be able to feel the biceps muscle contract, even if there is no discernible limb movement. The other arm must be tested in order to compare responses (Figure 1–21).

TABLE 1–4. FEATURES OF MOTOR NEURON LESIONS

Upper	Lower
Muscle weakness	Muscle weakness
Increased deep tendon reflexes	Decreased deep tendon reflexes
Positive Babinski reflex	Normal plantar reflex
Spasticity	Flaccidity
Normal bulk	Muscle wasting

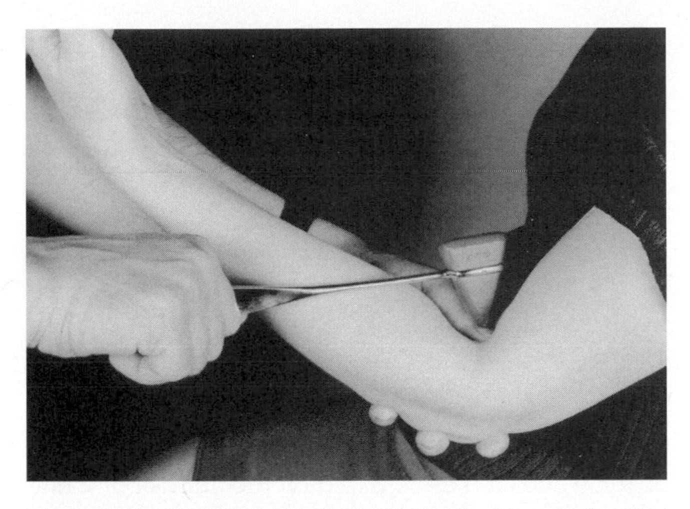

Figure 1–21. Proper positioning for testing the biceps reflex. The patient's arm is well supported, and the examiner's thumb is on the biceps tendon. The examiner strikes his or her own thumb with the pointed end of the reflex hammer.

When the patellar, or knee, reflex is tested, the patient should be seated with the thighs well supported but the calves allowed to swing free. With one hand on the patient's quadriceps muscle, the clinician strikes the patellar tendon (between the patella and tibia), where the tendon is unsupported. Since the tendon is not buried within tissue like the biceps tendon, the broad end of the reflex hammer is held at right angles to the tendon and used to strike the tendon directly. Again, because the clinician's hand is on the quadriceps muscle, any muscle contraction should be felt even if the leg itself does not move (Figure 1–22).

The Achilles, or ankle, reflex is tested with the patient in the same position as the patellar reflex test. Making sure that the patient's limb is relaxed, the clinician lifts the front of the patient's foot very slightly, just enough to take up the slack of the Achilles tendon. The tendon then is struck with the broad end of the reflex hammer at right angles to the tendon, and the foot is observed for a downward motion. Note that when the tendon is struck, the foot will move down slightly just due to mechanics; striking the tendon mechanically elevates the heel, which depresses the front of the foot. This is not the actual reflex. The reflex takes place a few hundred milliseconds later because the signal has to travel all the way up the leg to the spinal cord, synapse in the spinal cord, and then travel all the way back down the leg to stimulate the muscle to contract, all of which takes time. With a hand on the patient's foot, the clinician will notice this because it is only shortly after striking the tendon that the front of the patient's foot pushes down as the gastrocnemius muscle contracts (Figure 1–23).

The Babinski reflex is tested by stroking the lateral aspect of the sole of the patient's foot with a firm object, such as the handle of a reflex hammer. A normal response would be for the patient's toes to flex, or bend downward (the plantar reflex). A normal response is also for the patient to pull his or her foot away from this noxious stimulus. Therefore, the clinician should keep one hand on top of the patient's foot, both to prevent the patient from pulling away and to feel what the toes are doing. An abnormal response is when the toes fan out and the big toe extends up (a

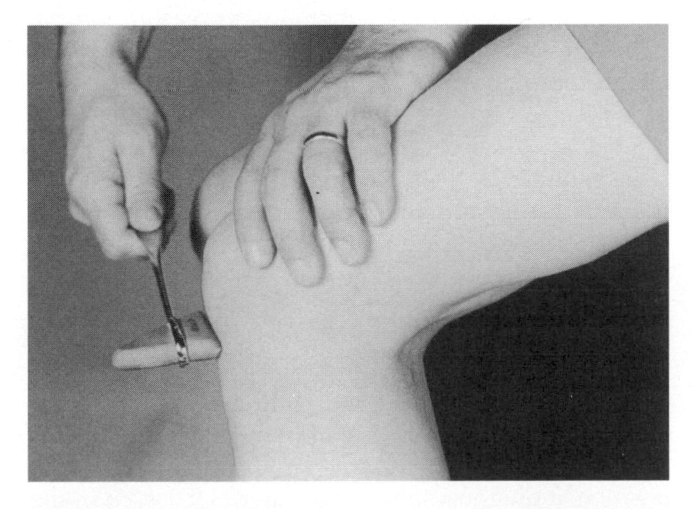

Figure 1–22. Proper positioning for testing the patellar reflex. The patellar tendon is struck with the broad end of the reflex hammer held at right angles to the tendon's direction. With the examiner's hand on the patient's quadriceps muscle, he or she can feel the muscle contract even if the leg does not visibly move.

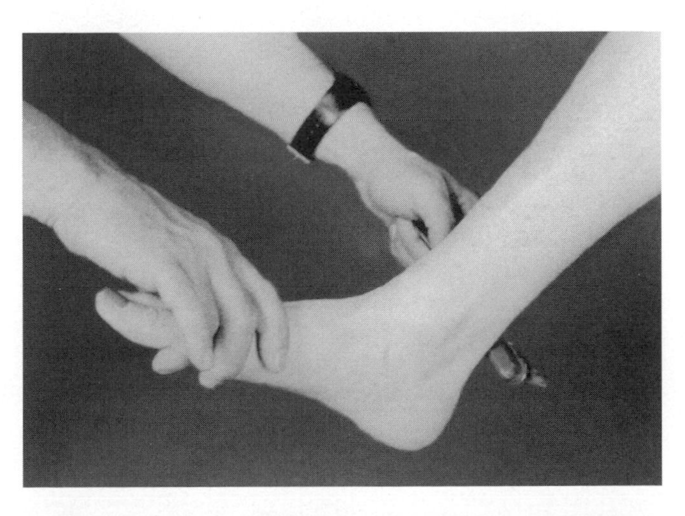

Figure 1–23. Proper positioning for testing the ankle reflex. With the front of the patient's foot supported just enough to take up the slack in the Achilles tendon, the tendon is struck with the broad end of the reflex hammer held at right angles to the tendon. The examiner can feel the reflex muscle contraction as it pushes the front of the foot down.

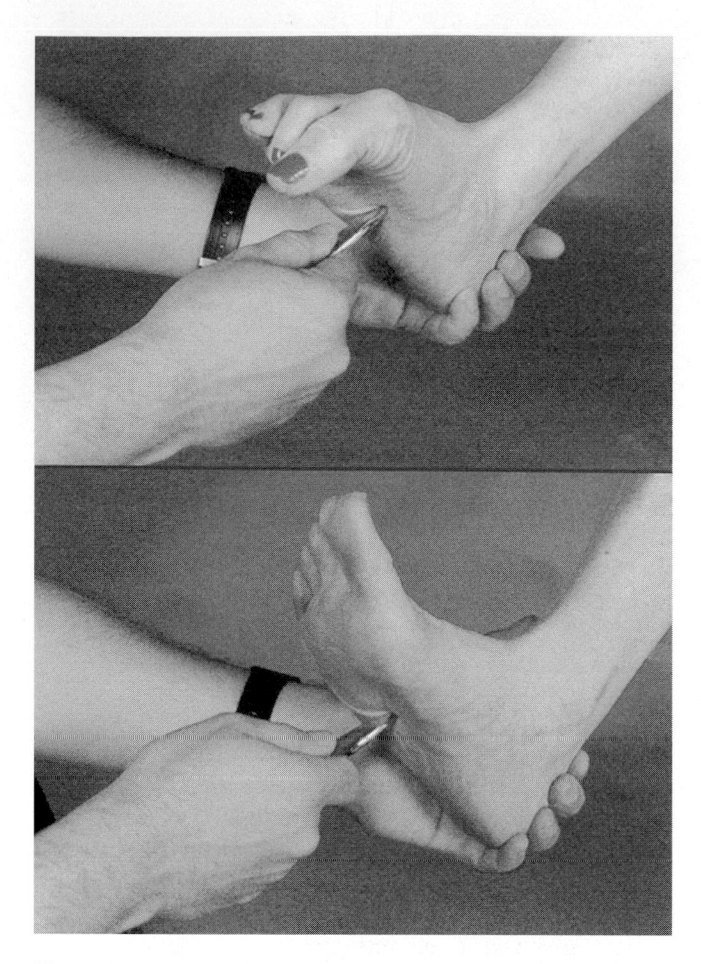

Figure 1–24. Normal (top) plantar flexion versus abnormal (bottom) Babinski sign. An upgoing toe suggests an upper motor neuron lesion.

positive Babinski) (Figure 1–24). This indicates a UMN lesion of the pyramidal system at any level from the motor cortex through the descending corticospinal pathways. However, a positive Babinski reflex is a normal response in a young infant. It is only when the myelinization of the spinal column is complete that toes will flex downward in response to stroking the sole of the foot.

LABORATORY TESTING

Laboratory testing refers to examining the patient's blood, cerebrospinal fluid, urine, or other bodily fluids to obtain information unavailable by other methods. Lab tests may be obtained to help confirm a clinical impression and support a given diagnosis, to rule out (r/o) a given disease or diagnosis, to follow the course of a disease or the effectiveness of its treatment, or to screen for occult disease. Some lab tests are quite specialized and are useful for only a single condition, whereas others may screen several body systems at once. Only rarely do lab tests establish a diagnosis in and of themselves; rather, they adjust the probability of a given diagnosis up or down depending on the result of the test. They provide one piece of information that must be integrated with the case history and physical examination to obtain a complete picture of the patient's condition.

Lab test results can be either qualitative or quantitative. Qualitative results are reported as being either positive or negative. An example would be results from a pregnancy test—a patient is either pregnant or not. Quantitative results are reported as a number that is compared to a reference range. An example would be the white cell count. Based on the number of white blood cells in the patient's sample, the count indicates either too many, too few, or the right amount. The reference range is calculated as the arithmetic mean of a disease-free population plus or minus (+/−) two standard deviation units. Although reference ranges are widely published, each laboratory will calculate its own reference range, so the actual numbers may vary slightly from lab to lab. As a result, each lab will report its reference range when reporting the patient's results.

A reference range that encompasses all results within two standard deviations of a mean value will include 95% of all "normal" values. However, that still leaves 5% of the values that fall outside of this reference range. Yet, because they are taken from a population that does not have the disease in question, they are still "normal" by definition; that is, they do not represent a diseased state. Since 1 in 20 patients may have a result outside the reference range on any given lab test yet still be "normal," it stands to reason that the more lab tests that are done the more likely it is to get one or more test results that fall outside the reference range, yet do not represent disease. This is why it is important to select tests wisely rather than order a large number of tests indiscriminately. Once an "abnormal" test result is reported, it must be addressed, even if only to decide that it is not clinically significant. Therefore, correlation with the patient's history and physical exam is critical to interpreting the lab results.

Lab test results can also be classified into either *decision-level* or *confirmatory* findings. Decision-level findings help diagnose a condition in and of themselves. An example would be an HIV antibody test. If positive, it diagnoses the patient with HIV even in the absence of other clinical signs or symptoms. Far more common are confirmatory findings. These help confirm a provisional diagnosis that was established by other means such as history, physical exam, or other lab tests. An example of this type of result would be measuring the amount of angiotensin-converting enzyme (ACE) in the blood. ACE is an enzyme that normally is present in the lungs, and plays a role in blood pressure control by converting angiotensin I into angiotensin II. Approximately 85% of patients with active sarcoidosis will have elevated ACE levels. Fifteen percent will have normal ACE levels. Other conditions can cause elevated ACE levels as well, so although an elevated ACE level is clearly not pathognomonic for sarcoidosis, it does serve as a good marker for the disease. If the ACE is performed as a screening test and comes back positive, it tells the clinician where to focus diagnostic efforts. If the test is positive in the presence of other clinical signs and symptoms, it helps confirm the diagnosis.

Blood Testing

The blood can be examined for materials that are normally present, such as metabolites, which should be present in certain concentrations. For example, creatinine is a byproduct of muscle metabolism and is normally cleared from the blood by the kidney. It can therefore be used as an indicator of kidney function. If creatinine levels are elevated, decreased kidney function can be suspected. Certain materials are not present in the blood normally, but may leak into the blood from damaged tissue. For example, in liver damage certain enzymes leak into the blood and are measurable. Therefore, elevated levels of certain liver enzymes imply liver damage. There may also be materials present in the blood that are normal, but are present in abnormal concentrations. As an illustration, consider thyroid-stimulating hormone (TSH). In cases of thyroid disease, this hormone may not have the desired effect on the thyroid gland. Depending on whether the defect lies in the thyroid gland itself or in another part of the feedback mechanism, this hormone may be present at abnormal levels. Again, it is important to correlate this finding with other lab results and the patient's clinical condition before a firm diagnosis is established.

Ideally, each test should correctly identify all patients who have the disease it is testing for, and exclude all patients who do not. Realistically, there is no such test. All lab tests are limited by their *sensitivity* and *specificity*. Sensitivity is the ability of a test to show a positive result in patients who actually do have the disease in question. A highly sensitive test is most likely to detect every patient with the disease and may even be positive in patients who do not, in fact, have that particular disease, but it is negative in patients who do *not* have the disease. The test is *positive in disease* (PID). This type of test is most useful for ruling out a diagnosis because if *negative,* the patient most likely does *not* have the disease in question. Specificity, on the other hand, is the ability of a test to show a negative result in a patient who does not have the disease in question. It is *negative in health* (NIH). A highly specific test is one that is most likely to be negative in patients without that particular disease, so it is most useful for confirming a diagnosis because if the test is *positive,* then the patient most likely *does* have the disease in question.

Many tests screen for disease indirectly, by detecting substances the body may produce in response to that disease, or other possibly related diseases. Although screening tests may result in false-positive results, they are usually cost-effective and easy to perform. As an example, the rapid plasma reagin (RPR) tests for the presence of the antibody reagin in the blood, which is produced in response to infection with a number of organisms, including *Treponema pallidum,* the spirochete that causes syphilis. If used to screen for syphilis, the test will give a number of false-positive results, because it will be positive in patients who produce reagin for reasons other than in response to infection with *T. pallidum.* This test has a high false-positive rate. This is an advantage for a screening test, as it will be positive in almost all patients with active syphilis even though it can also be positive in some of those without syphilis. Most positive results on screening tests require a follow-up confirmatory test to rule out the false-positives.

A confirmatory test is often more complex, with numerous steps to the procedure, and the opportunity for error at every step. Therefore, a confirmatory test can yield a negative result in a diseased patient due to test error. These are termed *false-negatives* because the negative result is due to some reason other than health. An example would be the fluorescent treponemal antibody absorption test (FTA-Abs), which is the confirmatory test for syphilis. The advantage to this test is that it tests only for the antibody specific to the *Treponema* organism. The disadvantage is that there are many complex steps involved. Therefore, a negative result could mean either that the patient does not have syphilis, or that something went wrong while performing the test. Running both the RPR and the FTA-Abs makes it is possible to use each as a check on the other to increase confidence in the findings.

Certain tests have a high positive predictive value; a positive result correlates highly with having the disease in question. A test with a high negative predictive value indicates that the patient most likely does not have the disease in question. The erythrocyte sedimentation rate (ESR) determines the rate at which red blood cells (RBCs) will settle to the bottom of a graduated cylinder over an hour's time. Any inflammatory, necrotic, or malignant condition in the body can alter the proteins in the red blood cell membrane, resulting in a loss of negative charge. This allows the RBCs to clump together and thus settle faster. Therefore, if the ESR is elevated, it indicates that there is indeed some inflammatory, necrotic, or malignant process going on somewhere in the body, but not which one it is or where it is. Thus, the ESR has limited positive predictive value. However, if the ESR is normal, it usually rules out any significant inflammatory, necrotic, or malignant process—it has a high negative predictive value.

There are an overwhelming number of tests that can be performed on blood. Presented here are only some of those that have direct relevance to the topics covered in this book, or that are so common that the clinician should have some familiarity with them. Blood testing can be organized into four main categories. The complete blood count (CBC) investigates the cellular component of the blood, whereas the serum chemistry examines the aqueous component. Serological testing checks immune system function, whereas the endocrine function tests look at the function of various endocrine organs and their feedback mechanisms. Information can be obtained regarding several important areas: blood production, metabolic function, hemostasis, infection, and immune status.

Hematological Testing

The CBC counts the number and types of blood cells, whereas the peripheral blood smear looks at their morphology. The RBC count and indices help classify different types of anemias. The count is reported as the number of cells per cubic millimeter of blood. The RBC indices measure the size of the cells and the amount of hemoglobin they contain. The hemoglobin concentration (Hgb) is the amount of hemoglobin present in each RBC and is reported as grams per deciliter of blood. The hematocrit (Hct) is the proportion of whole blood made up of RBCs, expressed as a percentage. Taken together these values can give an indication of the oxygen-carrying capabilities of the blood and also are used to classify the different types of anemias.

To further classify the anemias, the hemoglobin can be examined directly by hemoglobin electrophoresis. Here, the different types of hemoglobins are separated out according to molecular weight by electrophoresis. Abnormal hemoglobins or abnormal concentrations of hemoglobins may be accurately determined by this method. This same technique can be used to investigate other proteins in the blood as well.

The white blood cell (WBC) count and differential is often used to determine the presence of infection, allergic reaction, and malignancies. The count is reported as the number of WBCs per cubic millimeter of blood, and the differential is reported as the percentage of each type of WBC (neutrophils, lymphocytes, monocytes, eosinophils, and basophils) that contributes to the total.

The platelet count reports the number of platelets present per cubic millimeter of blood. This value is used to diagnose and treat certain clotting or bleeding disorders. Two other tests also measure the blood's ability to clot: the prothrombin time (PT) and the partial thromboplastin time (PTT). The PT tests the extrinsic and common coagulation pathways whereas the PTT tests the intrinsic and common coagulation pathways. Testing both makes it possible to localize a defect to either the extrinsic coagulation pathway (if only the PT is abnormal), the intrinsic coagulation pathway (if only the PTT is abnormal), or the common coagulation pathway (if both are abnormal). This is an example of how testing the same entity multiple ways can give more detailed information regarding a defect.

The ESR, mentioned earlier, is used as a nonspecific indicator of inflammation. It is important to note that this is one test where the results are age- and sex-dependent. It is normally higher in the elderly, and normally slightly higher for females than for males of the same age. Thus, it is important to calculate clinical norms for the individual patient. For males, the upper limit of the normal ESR is represented by the patient's age divided by 2. In females, the upper limit of the normal ESR is age plus 10, divided by 2.

In cases of acute infection or inflammation certain proteins are released in what is known as the *acute-phase response.* One of these proteins, C-reactive protein (CRP), has been shown to more accurately indicate immune system activity than the ESR. Therefore, it may be a better test to rule out a systemic inflammatory condition.

Serum Chemistry

There are many substances dissolved in the aqueous component of the blood that can be assayed. Serum chemistry is evaluated to monitor fluid and electrolyte balance, and to investigate the function of certain organs, such as the liver, kidney, parathyroid, and heart. These tests are usually ordered in a battery of about 6 to 20 tests that are all done by automated equipment, and are organized according to the aspect of the patient's status being investigated: electrolytes, kidney function, liver function, acute myocardial infarction enzymes, metabolic bone disease, lipid profile, and diabetes. Of these, the two areas that have the most immediate relevance to eye care are the lipid profile and the diabetes tests.

A lipid profile is used to diagnose, manage, and treat lipid disorders and their sequelae (eg, atherosclerosis). This profile usually includes total lipids, cholesterol, triglycerides, and lipoproteins (classified by density: HDL = high-density lipoprotein, LDL = low-density lipoprotein, and VLDL = very-low-density lipoprotein). The National Heart Blood and Lung Institute has developed guidelines for determining the risk of developing coronary heart disease in adults over 20 years of age. It is based upon three categories: measures of the total cholesterol level and LDL cholesterol level, and the calculated atherosclerosis risk ratios (LDL/HDL and total cholesterol/HDL).

The two diabetes tests of importance are the fasting blood glucose and the hemoglobin A_{1c}. The fasting blood glucose measures the amount of glucose present in the blood after an 8-hour fast. The value only indicates the glucose level at the time when the blood was drawn, and does not reflect what the blood glucose was at other times. To get an indication of what the average blood glucose levels run, the amount of protein glycosylation can be measured.

Glucose is normally present in the blood, and it will normally bind to proteins in a process known as glycosylation. This binding is irreversible and is dependent on both time and glucose concentration. The higher the glucose level, the more protein becomes glycosylated over a set period of time. One of the easier proteins to measure is hemoglobin, both because it is readily obtained, and because it remains in the body for a known period of time—the life of an RBC, about 3 months. Therefore, with time being relatively constant, the amount of glycosylated hemoglobin is indicative of the glucose concentration in the blood over the life of that RBC. This amount is expressed as a percentage of the total hemoglobin that is glycosylated, and is normally around 6%. There are different types (and subtypes) of hemoglobin. The amount of glycosylation of the subtype of hemoglobin A with the subscript designation 1C is the subtype that is most highly correlated with diabetic retinopathy. Therefore, measuring the amount of glycosylated HbA_{1c} is clinically the most useful measure because elevated HbA_{1c} levels have been correlated with a poorer prognosis and worsening diabetic retinopathy.

Serologic Tests

Serologic tests look for the presence of immunologically active proteins (antibodies, immunoglobulins, and antigens). The main types of tests are flocculation, agglutination, immunofluorescent antibody, and human leukocyte antigen typing. When an antibody is mixed directly with an immunoglobulin, an immune complex may form that is visible to the naked eye as lacy strands in the solution. This is called *flocculation* (Figure 1–25). Rheumatoid factor, a substance found in patients with rheumatoid arthritis and other autoimmune diseases, is tested by flocculation.

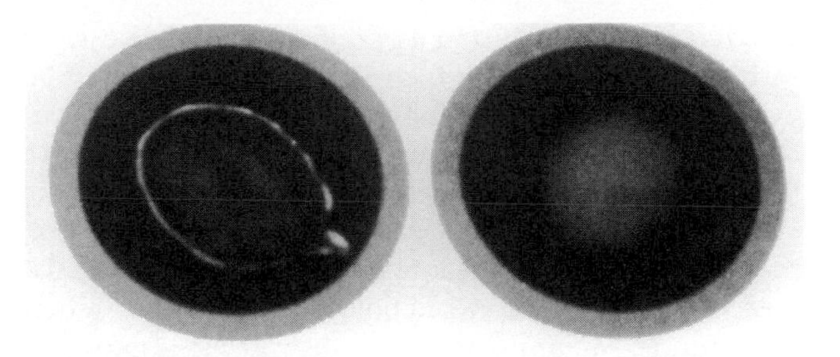

Figure 1–25. Flocculation appears as visible lacy white strands. (*Reprinted with permission from Sacher RA, McPherson RA.* Widman's Clinical Interpretation of Laboratory Tests. *10th ed. Philadelphia: FA Davis; 1991.*)

Agglutination is similar to flocculation. The patient's serum is mixed together with antigen-coated latex or charcoal particles. If the antibody is present in the patient's serum, it will react with the antigen, forming immune complexes that are visible as large clumps in the test solution. This result can be reported as a *titer,* which is a successive dilution of the sample until the antigen–antibody reaction no longer occurs (Figure 1–26). Active disease states have higher concentrations of antibodies in the blood, and thus can be diluted more and still produce a positive response (a higher titer). An example of a test that uses agglutination and is reported as a titer is the RPR.

Immunofluorescent antibody testing is a complex multistep process that looks for the presence of certain specific antibodies. A sample from the patient is incubated with a substrate containing antigens for the an-

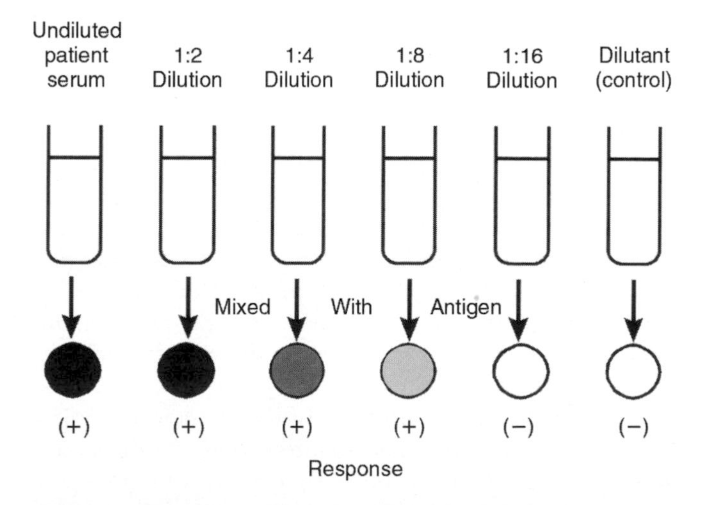

Figure 1–26. A titer is the successive dilution of a sample until a positive response is no longer noted.

tibodies in question. After a period of time the patient's serum is washed off and the substrate incubated again, this time with immunoglobulins that bind to the antibodies bound to the antigens in the substrate. These immunoglobulins are labeled with fluorescein, so the substrate is examined under ultraviolet light to look for fluorescence. Any fluorescence indicates that a labeled immunoglobulin has bound to an antibody that has bound to an antigen in the substrate. This may also be reported as a titer. The FTA-Abs is one example of an immunofluorescent antibody test. Others include the antinuclear antibody (ANA) test, which looks for antibodies produced against the patient's own WBC nuclei, and a Lyme titer, which tests for antibodies produced against *Borrelia burgdorferi,* the spirochete that causes Lyme disease.

Human leukocyte antigen (HLA) typing relates to histocompatibility and immune responsiveness—it does not test for a disease process directly. It was originally used for tissue typing in organ transplantation, and now is used for paternity testing and disease risk assessment as well. There are strong associations between certain diseases and certain HLA types; however, the HLA types do not cause disease in and of themselves.

Endocrine Function Tests

Testing for diabetes has already been covered under serum chemistry. Another prevalent endocrine disorder that can be diagnosed by blood testing is thyroid disease. Thyroxine (T_4), and several other hormones that are involved in the feedback mechanisms that control the production of T_4, can be measured. These include levels of thyroid-stimulating hormone (TSH) and thyrotropin-releasing factor (TRF), and the T_3 resin uptake (T_3RU), which indirectly estimates the number of binding sites available on thyroid-binding globulin that transports the thyroid hormones in the blood.

Skin Testing

Often it is necessary to determine if a patient has been exposed to tuberculosis. This may be done indirectly by a skin test in which a small amount of a purified protein derivative (PPD) of the tuberculosis organism is injected intradermally. The amount of antigen injected is not enough to cause antibody production, but if antibodies are already present in the blood (from previous exposure to TB), an antigen–antibody reaction will occur causing induration of the injected area. The amount of induration is measured 48 to 72 hours after injection and graded. A positive response suggests previous exposure to the TB organism and is followed up with more definitive testing to rule out active TB.

Cerebrospinal Fluid Testing

A lumbar puncture allows evaluation of the cerebrospinal fluid (CSF) (eg, for color, protein, glucose, cells, and immunoglobulins) as well as the measurement of intracranial pressure (ICP) in millimeters of water.

Urinalysis

Urinalysis is a specific measure of kidney function, as well as an indicator of liver, cardiovascular, and/or metabolic disorders. Abnormal test results may occur with certain diseases, diets, and medications. The standard urinalysis measures several parameters. Specific gravity is a measure of the kidneys' ability to concentrate urine. The appearance of urine should be clear to slightly hazy. The normal color of urine (indicating the concentration) is yellow to pale amber, and varies with its specific gravity. Medications can alter the color of urine (e.g., the sodium fluorescein used in fluorescein angiography will discolor urine to a vivid orange-yellow). The pH of urine is between 4.6 and 8, with the average being about 6. The presence of protein or albumin is an indication of a kidney disorder because the kidney filter spaces are normally too small to allow the passage of protein. If glucose is present in urine, it indicates that the renal glucose threshold was exceeded. Ketones or acetone are not normally found in the urine. In uncontrolled type 1 diabetes the body turns to stored fat to burn for fuel, and ketones (or acetone), formed as byproducts, are spilled into the urine. The presence of blood, leukocyte esterase, and nitrite may indicate infection of the urinary tract. The presence of bilirubin may indicate liver dysfunction. Sediment analysis (looking for trace cells, casts, and crystals in the urine sediment) may be done if urinary tract infections or kidney disorders are suspected.

IMAGING

Imaging studies may be necessary to aid in the diagnosis of certain ocular conditions. This discussion is limited to the more frequently used diagnostic imaging tests. Common radiographic studies include plain films, computerized tomography (CT), and radiography with contrast media (e.g., angiography). Other imaging studies include ultrasonography (eg, duplex scan), magnetic resonance imaging, and nuclear medicine studies.

Radiography

X-Rays

Radiographs use electromagnetic waves of very short wavelength (x-rays). As the x-rays pass through the body, their intensity is reduced by absorption. Denser tissue, such as bone, absorbs more and therefore appears whiter on the film, whereas soft tissue, which is less dense, absorbs less and therefore appears darker on the film. Contrast media may be used to enhance or highlight detail not normally seen on plain film. These may be radiopaque (which fully block x-ray transmission) or radiolucent (which partially block x-ray transmission), but are imaged directly and serve to increase contrast of structures they outline or fill. Potential contraindications to contrast media include allergic reaction, which may be mild (hives) to severe (anaphylaxis).

X-rays are transilluminations of body structures that yield information about shape and density only. A structure's edge will be distinct only if it differs significantly in density from the surrounding tissue. Four basic densities can be distinguished on an x-ray: air, fat, tissue/fluid, and bone. They are based on the tissue's ability to attenuate the x-ray beam. The shadow profile obtained will depend on the structure's position relative to the film and the angle of view (Figure 1–27).

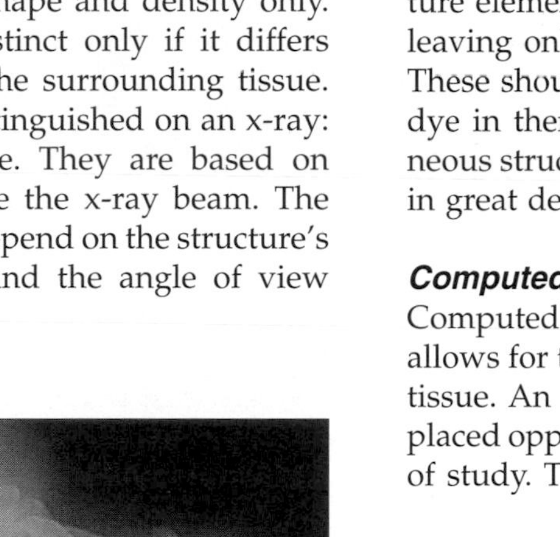

Figure 1–27. On an x-ray, air appears black, bone appears white, and soft tissue shows as various shades of gray. The large mass in the center of this chest film is the cardiac shadow. It appears white because of attenuation of the x-ray beam by the large mass of muscle. (*Courtesy Barbara Zeifer, MD, The New York Eye & Ear Infirmary.*)

Angiography

Angiography involves a rapid series of x-rays obtained after an injection of a radiopaque contrast dye in order to study major arteries and their branches, as well as tumors. Angiography may be used to study the cardiac, cerebral, carotid, and pulmonary arterial systems. Angiography is associated with a certain amount of morbidity and mortality, due both to the contrast media employed and the injection procedure itself.

Digital subtraction angiography (DSA) enhances an angiogram by eliminating the surrounding anatomy from the view. A preinjection "mask" image is stored digitally and compared with postinjection "live" images. A computer digitally removes all picture elements that were unchanged between the two, leaving only the picture elements that have changed. These should be only those picture elements that had dye in them for the live image. Removing the extraneous structures allows the blood vessels to be imaged in great detail (Figure 1–28).

Computed Tomography

Computed tomography (CT) is an x-ray procedure that allows for the examination of a single layer or plane of tissue. An x-ray source and an array of detectors are placed opposite each other and rotated around the area of study. This allows the detectors to obtain multiple

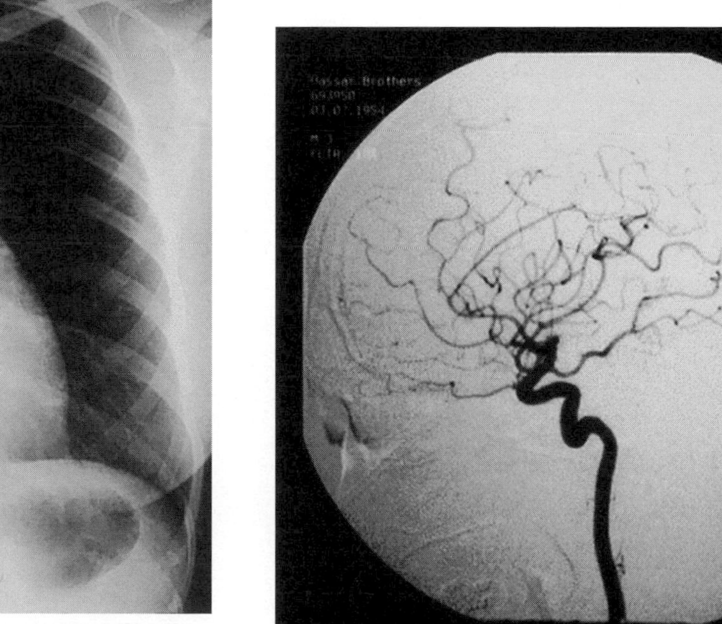

Figure 1–28. A digital subtraction angiogram (DSA) removes extraneous information digitally so that only the image of the blood vessel remains. (*Courtesy Richard Madonna, OD, SUNY State College of Optometry.*)

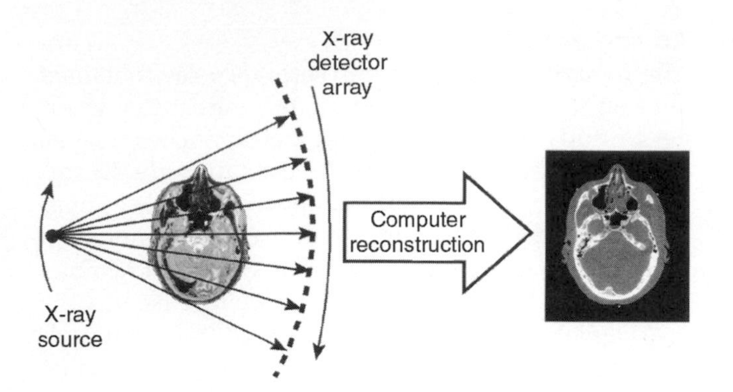

Figure 1–29. CT scanning examines a structure from many angles with x-rays to determine its internal structure.

readings of that slice from many different angles. These readings indicate the degree of x-ray beam attenuation at each angle; they are not images of the structures. The computer then calculates what the structure would have to look like in order to produce the patterns of x-ray beam attenuation at the angles measured, and displays this image on a screen (Figure 1–29).

The significant advantages of CT scanning over conventional x-ray films are the imaging of soft tissue, and localization (Figure 1–30). Since each CT image represents a slice through the body, it is possible to know exactly from where the image is taken. Bone, calcified lesions, and some soft tissue structures show up well on CT. Taking multiple slices close together makes it possible to build up a three-dimensional mental picture of the patient's anatomy. Since the images are created from data stored in a computer, it is also possible to reconstruct different image views after the fact. Contrast media can be used in CT scanning in much the same way as they are used in plain x-ray films. A CT image is still based on attenuation of an x-ray beam, so structures that either do not attenuate x-rays well or structures that are surrounded by bone do not image well on CT.

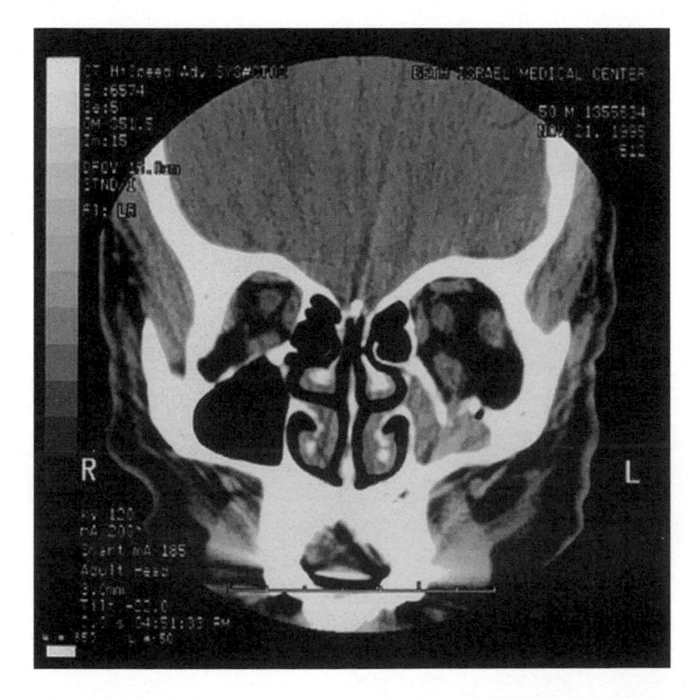

Figure 1–30. CT scan of a blowout fracture of the left orbital floor. This coronal section shows extraocular muscle and other soft tissue entrapment. (*Courtesy Barbara Zeifer, MD, The New York Eye & Ear Infirmary.*)

The main disadvantage of CT scanning is that it still uses ionizing radiation. This limits the number of slices that can be obtained during a study, and their resolution. Each slice of a CT scan can be anywhere from 1 to 5 mm in thickness, and spaced anywhere from 1 to 10 mm apart. The thinner the slice, the greater the resolution of the scan, but as more slices are required to cover the same area, radiation exposure increases. The slices can be made thicker with a corresponding decrease in resolution, or they can be kept thin and placed farther apart with the risk that a small lesion falling in between adjacent slices may be missed. Accordingly, a plain x-ray film of the area in question may be taken first in order to direct the scan, especially in some conditions such as a foreign body (Figure 1–31).

Nuclear Medicine Studies

Nuclear medicine studies or scans are used to visualize organs and regions within organs that cannot be seen with regular x-rays. Various radiopharmaceuticals may be injected or ingested depending upon the tissue or structure being imaged (e.g., thyroid, bone, brain). A scanning device is passed over the tissue or body part to be examined to pick up emitted radiation in order to determine the distribution of the substance. Tissues with abnormal metabolic activity (necrosis, tumors, granulomas) take up excessive amounts of the radioisotope and show up as hot spots on the scan. In contrast to the imaging procedures already mentioned, these scans give information regarding function, from which structural information can then be obtained. Contraindications to nuclear scans include certain prosthetic devices in the body, which can absorb radioisotopes and distort the scanning process, and a history of allergies to radioisotopes (Figure 1–32).

Radiation Hazard

There is a radiation hazard with radiographic studies, and, to a lesser degree, nuclear scans. Therefore, pregnant or nursing mothers should not undergo these procedures unless absolutely necessary. Genetic and somatic damage (tissue burn) may occur, depending on the type and length of exposure.

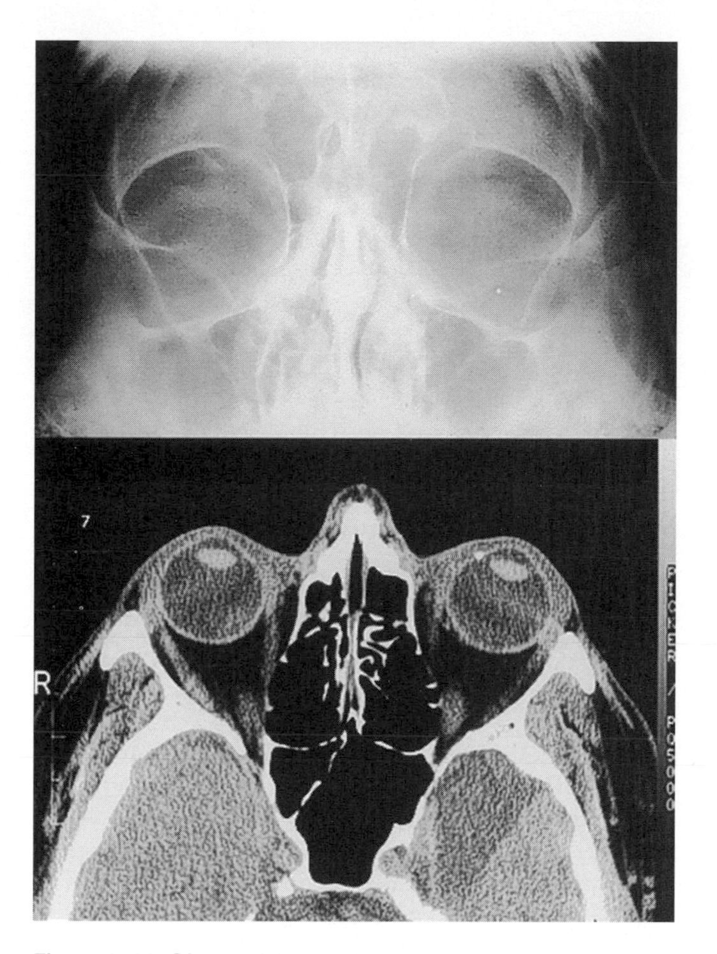

Figure 1–31. Often a plain x-ray is taken of an area to direct a CT scan. In the plain film (top) a small foreign body is barely visible in the left orbital region. It cannot be further localized without additional views. A CT scan (bottom) allows the foreign body to be localized to the left globe, approximately at the nasal limbus. (*Courtesy Barbara Zeifer, MD, The New York Eye & Ear Infirmary.*)

Magnetic Resonance Imaging

Magnetic resonance imaging (MRI) has fast become one of the most useful imaging tests available. However, due to cost and time factors, MRI scans are not routine. MRI uses the intrinsic magnetic properties of certain atoms that have an odd number of protons, and how they interact with an external magnetic field. Although a number of atoms have this property, clinically MRI uses hydrogen because it is the most ubiquitous atom in the body that will interact with an external magnetic field.

One property that an atomic nucleus has is *spin,* which is dependent on the atomic number and atomic weight of an atom. Each spinning atom will have its own tiny magnetic vector. Normally, these spinning atoms are not aligned; that is, they are all pointing in random directions. Therefore, there is no overall net magnetic vector. If these atoms are placed in a very strong external magnetic field, they will all line up oriented along the magnetic field. All the individual magnetic vectors from the individual atoms will now add together to form an overall net magnetic vector in the direction of the external magnetic field. If a radio pulse of a specific frequency is applied, it will knock these atoms out of their alignment with the external magnetic field; they will stabilize 90° away from it. Once the radio pulse is stopped, they will come back into alignment with the external magnetic field in a process known as *precession.*

This whole procedure takes place inside a large coil of wire that acts as an antenna. As the atoms, which can be thought of as tiny magnets, move within the coil of wire, they generate a small electrical current in the receiving antenna. Both the rate of precession and the exact frequency generated depend on the local environment. The signal the hydrogen ion radiates as it comes back into alignment with the external magnetic field can be localized in space by varying the exciting

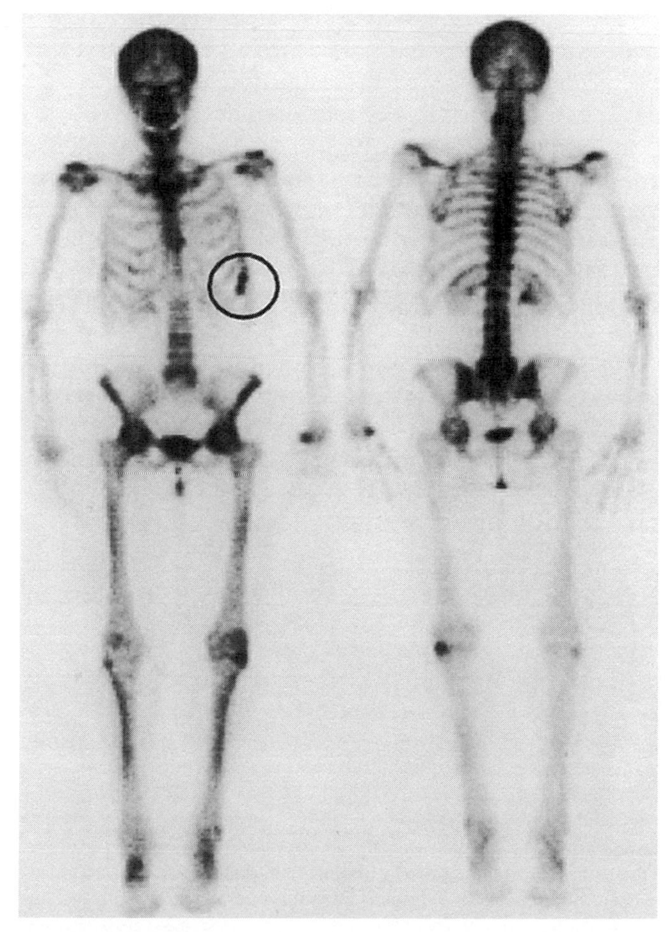

Figure 1–32. Whole body bone scan of patient with breast cancer that has metastasized to a rib (circle). (*Courtesy J. Anthony Parker, MD PhD, Harvard Medical School.*)

radio frequency (RF) pulse and by superimposing an additional gradient magnetic field over the main external magnetic field. The signal is processed by computer and displayed on a screen as a plot of hydrogen ion concentration (Figure 1–33).

There are two parameters of precession that contribute to the signal and can be measured. After the RF pulse has been applied, the hydrogen atoms will come back into alignment with the external magnetic field at a certain rate, dependent upon the tissue. The time it takes for 63% of them to decay and realign with the external magnetic field is called the *T_1 relaxation time.* Before they realign with the external magnetic field, they lose cohesion in the direction they were all pointing when the RF pulse was stopped. The time required for 63% of the atoms to lose this cohesion is called the *T_2 relaxation time.*

The T_1 and T_2 relaxation times are known quantities for each tissue—they are a property intrinsic to that tissue. The scan can selectively tune in the T_1 or the T_2 signal, a process called *image weighting.* Images can be weighted by varying the time between successive RF pulses (repetition time, or TR) and the time between the RF pulse and data acquisition (echo time, or TE). This enables MRI to image soft tissue in a way never before possible. Because the same tissue may appear hypointense on one type of scan and hyperintense on another, the TR and TE values are printed directly on the scan and need to be interpreted before the scan can be read properly (Figure 1–34).

MRI is particularly useful for delineating soft tissue (e.g., demyelinating plaques in the central nervous system, aneurysms, tumors). A contrast medium (gadolinium) may be used to enhance the image; however, rather than being directly imaged, the gadolinium works by changing local electrochemical properties to enhance the image. Contraindications to MRI include metallic foreign bodies (pacemakers, metallic vascular clips, metallic plates) and claustrophobia. Unlike other imaging techniques, MRI requires up to an hour to complete and is particularly loud as it generates the magnetic field. Therefore, patients should be educated prior to this test about the length of time, as well as the intensity of noise the instrument produces during the test. It is unknown whether pregnancy is a contraindication for MRI; therefore, it should be used on pregnant women only when absolutely necessary.

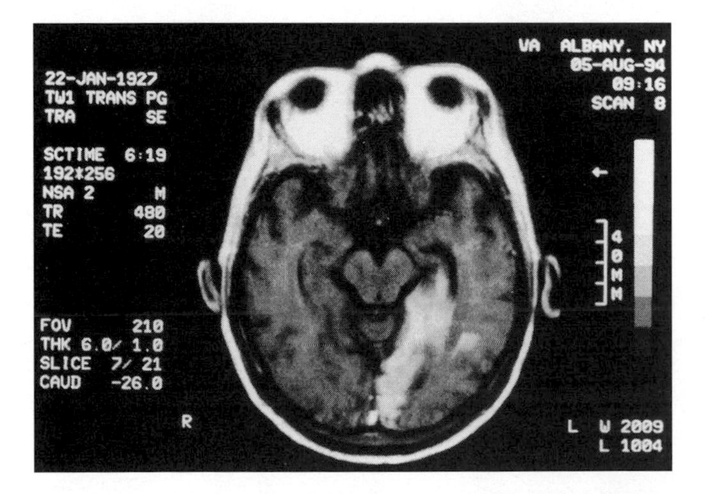

Figure 1–33. Fourier transformation allows signals from individual hydrogen nuclei to be extracted from the overall signal from the entire area under study. The resulting image is displayed on a screen. This patient has an intracerebral hemorrhage on the left side. (*Courtesy Richard Madonna, OD, SUNY State College of Optometry.*)

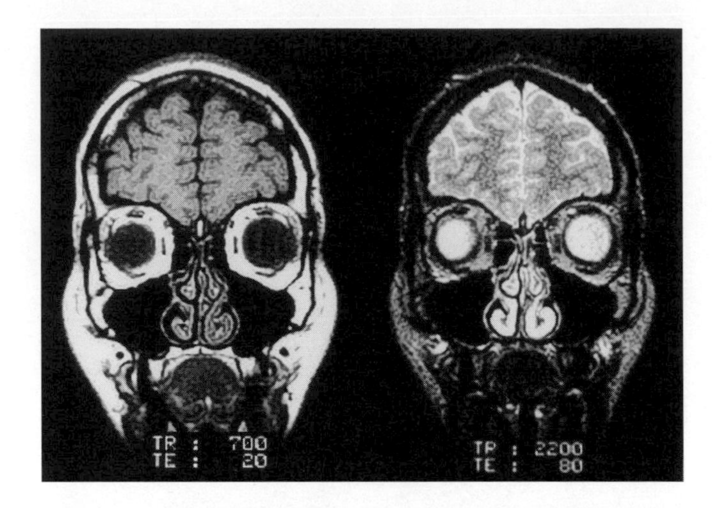

Figure 1–34. Short TR and TE times yield a T_1 weighted image (left), and long TR and TE times yield a T_2 weighted image (right). As the same structure can appear hypointense on one and hyperintense on the other, always look for the TR and TE values before reading an MRI scan. (*Courtesy Barbara Zeifer, MD, The New York Eye & Ear Infirmary.*)

Ultrasonography

Ultrasonography (echography) is a noninvasive procedure used to visualize soft tissue structures. An ultrasound beam is directed into the body part to be examined. Propagated by vibration, the sound waves are reflected differently depending upon tissue density. The reflected sound waves, or echoes, are electronically processed and imaged. The reflected ultrasound waves are interpreted by the instrument and displayed on a screen. Photography and videotaping are two common methods available to record the displayed image. There are several different procedures and display techniques depending on the structure to be imaged. A-mode ultrasonography (amplitude modulated) gives information regarding time and amplitude of the sound waves

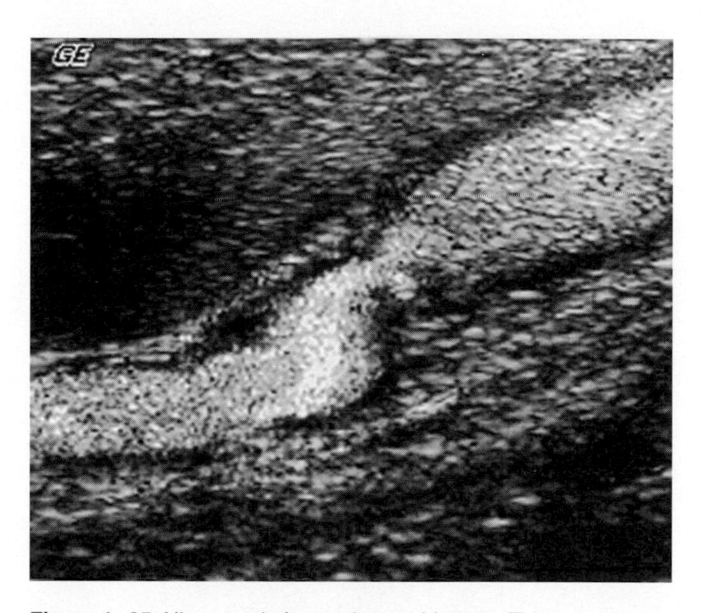

Figure 1–35. Ultrasound of stenotic carotid artery. This type of study gives anatomical information only, without any data regarding blood flow. (*Courtesy GE Medical Systems.*)

reflected from the structure studied (eg, distance between the cornea and retina for determination of the power of an intraocular lens). A-mode does not provide an image; however, it is from this that all other modes of ultrasound are derived. B-mode (brightness modulated) provides two-dimensional or cross-sectional information, thus forming an image of the structure studied as well as the movement of tissues (Figure 1–35). To study the movement of blood flow through vessels and cardiac valves, the Doppler principle is applied. This interprets the change in frequency in the movement of objects (red blood cells through the vessels or valves). Duplex scans are used to evaluate occlusive vessel disease (e.g., carotid arteries). This method combines Doppler ultrasound and B-mode sonography into one instrument. Echocardiograms utilize this method to assess the vessels and valves of the heart.

CONCLUSION

Primary eyecare in systemic disease mandates an overall evaluation of the patient. Incorporation of patient history, ocular and physical examinations, laboratory diagnostic tests, and imaging studies is vital for comprehensive evaluation of the patient. Referrals to or consultations with other specialties should be used in the management of a patient with ocular manifestations of a systemic disease.

REFERENCES

Berman EL, Jonathan D. Imaging. In: Stamper RL, ed. *Ophthalmology Clinics of North America.* Philadelphia: Saunders; 1994.

Bickley LS, Hoekelman RA, Bates B. *Bates' Guide to Physical Examination and History Taking.* 7th ed. Philadelphia: Lippincott; 1999.

Brown MA, Semelka RC. *MRI: Basic Principles and Applications.* New York: Wiley-Liss; 1999.

Classe JG. Clinicolegal aspects of practice record keeping and documentation in clinical practice. *South J Optom.* 1987; 5:11–25.

Cutler P. *Problem Solving in Clinical Medicine: From Data to Diagnosis.* Philadelphia: Williams & Wilkins; 1998.

Epstein O. *Clinical Examination.* Philadelphia: Mosby; 1997.

Fingeret M, Casser L, Woodcombe HI. *Atlas of Primary Eyecare Procedures.* Norwalk, CT: Appleton & Lange; 1990.

Fischbach F. *A Manual of Laboratory Diagnostic Tests.* 3rd ed. Philadelphia: Lippincott; 1988.

Judge RD, Wolliscroft JO, Zelenock GB, Zuidema GD. *The Michigan Manual of Clinical Diagnosis.* Philadelphia: Lippincott-Raven; 1998.

Kutty K, Sebastian JL. *Kochar's Concise Textbook of Medicine.* Baltimore: Williams & Wilkins; 1998.

Levin LA. Clinical signs and symptoms requiring computed tomography and magnetic resonance imaging evaluation. *Neuroimaging Clin N Am.* 1996;6(1):1–14.

Mackay RS. *Medical Images and Displays: Comparisons of Nuclear Magnetic Resonance, Ultrasound, X-rays, and Other Modalities.* New York: Wiley; 1984.

Ravel R. *Clinical Laboratory Medicine: Clinical Application of Laboratory Data.* 5th ed. Chicago: Yearbook; 1989.

Roberts SP. Optometric utilization of clinical laboratory tests. In: Abplanalp PL, ed. *Problems in Optometry: Modern Diagnostic Technology.* Philadelphia: Lippincott; 1991; 72–91.

Swartz MH. *Textbook of Physical Diagnosis: History and Examination.* Philadelphia: Saunders; 1994.

Thomann KH, Dul MW. The optometric assessment of neurologic function. *J Am Optom Assoc.* 1993;64:421–431.

Traub SL. *Basic Skills in Interpreting Laboratory Data: Illustrated with Case Studies.* Bethesda: American Society of Health-System Pharmacists; 1996.

Wirtschafter JD, Berman EL, McDonald CS. *Magnetic Resonance Imaging and Computed Tomography: Clinical Neuro-Orbital Anatomy.* San Francisco: American Academy of Ophthalmology; 1992.

Section II

CARDIOVASCULAR DISORDERS

Chapter 2

HYPERTENSION

Mitchell W. Dul

Hypertension accounts for the greatest number of office visits to healthcare providers in the United States. In a given individual, blood pressure can vary with the time of day, level of anxiety, and a host of other factors. A diagnosis of hypertension is therefore reserved for those individuals who, in a relaxed atmosphere, demonstrate diastolic pressure exceeding 90 mmHg or whose systolic pressure exceeds 140 mmHg on two or three separate occasions. Hypertension can be divided into two general categories: primary (essential) hypertension, accounting for approximately 95% of all cases, and secondary hypertension. Although a common ailment, the etiology of primary hypertension is not fully understood. Secondary hypertension is generally a sequela of kidney or endocrine disorders. Ocular complications may occur in the presence of long-standing systemic hypertension or may result from acute severe episodes. The vasculature of the retina, choroid, and optic nerves is affected differently by hypertension.

EPIDEMIOLOGY

Systemic

Hypertension affects over 60 million Americans, roughly 30% of the adult population over the age of 40 and more than 50% of the population over the age of 60. It is the leading indication for physician office visits, one of the leading causes of cardiovascular morbidity and mortality, and a major risk factor for renal disease. The risk of stroke is four times greater in persons with hypertension, and the risk of stroke increases with the elevation in systolic pressure.

Ocular

It is difficult to calculate the actual incidence of hypertensive retinopathy, but it is second only to diabetic retinopathy as the most common retinal vascular disease encountered in general practice. Its clinical presentation varies with the severity and duration of hypertension and the degree of blood pressure control. Hypertension is the most commonly associated systemic disease in the presence of a branch retinal vein occlusion.

PATHOPHYSIOLOGY/DISEASE PROCESS

Systemic

The etiology of essential hypertension is unknown, and probably no singular mechanism accounts for its development. It is likely to result from a combination of causes whose cumulative effect results in poor blood pressure control. Risk factors include male sex, increased age, family history, the affects of the renin–angiotensin system, and sympathetic nervous system overactivity. Alcohol abuse, obesity, sedentary life style, and cigarette smoking also may contribute to hypertension. Salt intake, while commonly associated with an increased risk, applies primarily to patients with established hypertension or those with a family history of the disease.

> Approximately 95% of all cases of hypertension are primary (essential) hypertension.

The renin–angiotensin system and sympathetic nervous system overactivity, although not primarily implicated in the pathogenesis of essential hypertension, are noteworthy in order to better understand both treatment options and the etiology of the more common types of secondary hypertension.

Renin–Angiotensin System

The renin–angiotensin system serves to maintain normal regulation of blood pressure via its influence on sympathetic activity, renal sodium and water balance, and peripheral resistance. Peripheral resistance is provided primarily by the arterioles, which are also known as resistance vessels. The interaction between peripheral resistance and cardiac output determines the arterial pressure (arterial pressure = cardiac output × total peripheral resistance). Therefore, any increase or decrease in either of these variables will produce a corresponding increase or decrease in arterial pressure.

The release of renin by the juxtaglomerular cells may be triggered by any number of conditions including decreased renal perfusion pressure, decreased intravascular volume, circulating catecholamines, and increased sympathetic nervous system activity. The release of renin precipitates a sequence of biochemical reactions that results in the formation of angiotensin II, a potent vasoconstrictor. Vasoconstriction increases peripheral resistance, which correspondingly increases arterial pressure, a short-lived effect. A prolonged effect from angiotensin II results from its direct action on the kidneys and the adrenal glands. Angiotensin II causes the kidneys to retain salt and water and the adrenal glands to release aldosterone, which results in retention of salt and water by the kidney. This increases extracellular fluid volume, which ultimately causes increased arterial pressure and increased blood flow from the heart to body tissues. The resulting local vasoconstriction in turn increases peripheral resistance, which further increases the arterial pressure. The increase in arterial pressure increases the renal glomerular filtration rate, thus promoting the release and subsequent excretion of salt and water. This is called *pressure diuresis* or *pressure natriuresis.* Pressure diuresis decreases extracellular fluid volume and, by means of the previously reported cascade of events, normalizes blood pressure.

In addition to being present in the renal renin–angiotensin system, angiotensin-converting enzyme (ACE), which converts angiotensin I to angiotensin II, is found in tissues, including the vasculature, heart, and brain, among others. Angiotensin II is a potent vasoconstrictor that can stimulate vascular smooth muscle cell growth, causing hypertrophy of the blood vessels. Over time, vascular hypertrophy reduces blood flow to tissues and increases pressure within the vessels or peripheral resistance. Arteriosclerosis, which decreases the size of the lumen through which blood must flow, is now thought to result from injury to the vessel endothelium that subsequently sets off a cascade of events and the release of growth factors and angiotensin II from the endothelium, as well as an influx of plasma growth factors and lipids to the site of injury. The increase in growth factors and lipids decreases the size of the lumen and increases peripheral resistance.

Sympathetic Nervous System Overactivity

Sympathetic nervous system overactivity increases the heart rate up to 250 beats per minute and increases the strength of ventricular contractions up to 100%. At the same time, it decreases the duration of systolic contractions to allow for greater filling time during diastole. Direct stimulation of blood vessels under sympathetic control leads to vasoconstriction and increased peripheral resistance, thereby increasing arterial pressure.

The systemic manifestations of hypertension (Table 2–1) vary with the severity of blood pressure elevation and the organs affected. Although most patients are asymptomatic and are diagnosed as an incidental finding, acute hypertension often is associated with headaches, nausea, vomiting, and loss of consciousness. Prolonged, poorly controlled hypertension compromises the ability of the cardiovascular system to transport oxygenated blood to vital organs (especially the heart, brain, and kidneys). Therefore, the clinical picture is variable.

Heart

Early in the course of hypertension, cardiac output is increased by approximately 15%. Resistance vessels attempt to compensate for the increase in cardiac output and intravascular volume by constricting in order to reduce tissue blood flow to normal, although resistance may remain normal at rest. In patients with longstanding hypertension, cardiac output usually is normal, and peripheral vascular resistance is increased. The increase in peripheral vascular resistance serves to

TABLE 2–1. SYSTEMIC MANIFESTATIONS OF PRIMARY HYPERTENSION

Chronic Hypertension
Asymptomatic
Acute Hypertension
Headaches
Nausea
Vomiting
Loss of consciousness
Long-term complications
Heart
• Coronary artery disease
• Atherosclerosis
• Left ventricular hypertrophy and heart failure
• Angina
• Myocardial infarction
• Sudden death
Brain
• Cerebrovascular accident
• Encephalopathy
Kidneys
• Renal artery stenosis
• Renal insufficiency

maintain the elevation in blood pressure. As an important cardiovascular risk factor, hypertension initiates and promotes the progression of a series of events in the cardiovascular disease continuum, from coronary artery disease and atherosclerosis to end-stage heart disease (Figure 2–1).

Left ventricular hypertrophy is a common sequela of prolonged hypertension and results in a significant increase in risk of mortality and morbidity at any level of blood pressure. The ventricles must contract with sufficient force to move blood out of the ventricle into the circulation. The ventricles must work against the pressure of the blood already in the arteries—the greater the pressure or peripheral resistance, the harder the ventricles must work. Like skeletal muscle, one way in which the myocardium responds to a prolonged increase in workload is to increase in size (hypertrophy). Muscle hypertrophy causes an increase in oxygen demand that may not be met, particularly in the presence of concurrent atherosclerosis or previous myocardial infarct with subsequent tissue necrosis. Inadequate oxygen supply manifests clinically as angina, myocardial infarct, or sudden death.

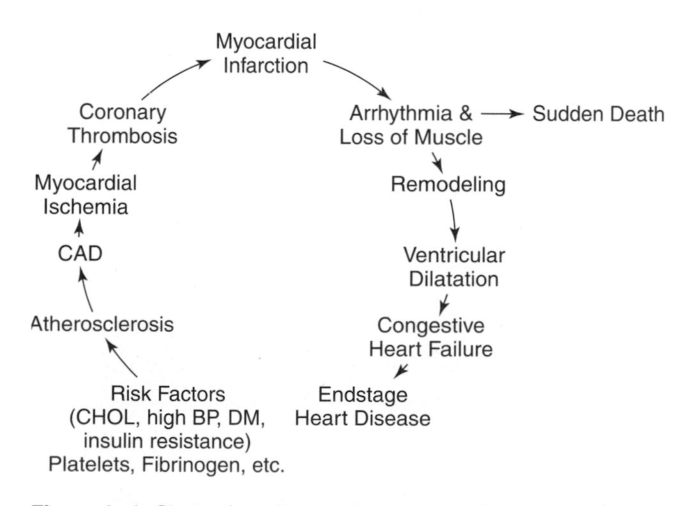

Figure 2–1. Chain of cardiovascular events initiated by risk factors. (*Adapted with permission from Dzauv, Braunwald E. Resolved and unresolved issues in the prevention and treatment of coronary artery disease: A workshop consensus statement.* Am Heart J. 1991;131: 1244–1263.)

Other limitations from ventricular hypertrophy include heart failure. If the arterial pressure is high enough, the hypertrophied ventricle may not pump out its full load of blood with each beat. Therefore, some blood remains in the heart (referred to as forward failure) at the expense of both the oxygen demand by the body's tissues and the capacity of the ventricle (which cannot adequately hold all of the new blood arriving from the atria). The latter causes a hematologic logjam (backward failure), which backs up into the pulmonary vein (on the left side) or the vena cava (on the right). Right ventricular failure results in peripheral edema, distended neck veins, abdominal distension, and hepatomegaly. Left ventricular failure is characterized by difficult or labored breathing (dyspnea) and low cardiac output, which may be exacerbated when the patient lies down due to further increases in pulmonary blood volume. Some patients may have difficulty breathing, except in the upright position (orthopnea).

Long-standing pulmonary venous hypertension can promote anastomoses between the pulmonary and bronchial veins. This is analogous to the collateral vessels that develop between the central retinal vein and choroidal circulation in the presence of a central retinal vein occlusion. These bronchial anastomoses or submucosal varices (enlarged and tortuous vessels) often rupture, causing the patient to expectorate blood or blood-stained sputum (hemoptysis). In the presence of left ventricular hypertrophy, rales (any abnormal respiratory sound) and gallop rhythms (an accentuated extra cardiac sound) may be audible with the stethoscope.

Brain

The effects of hypertension and associated atherosclerosis are responsible for the majority of cerebral vascular accidents (CVAs) by hemorrhagic, thrombotic, or embolic causes, and account for significant mortality and morbidity (see Chapter 5). Approximately 40% of all CVAs are attributable to systolic blood pressure greater than 140 mm Hg. Intracerebral hemorrhage almost always occurs secondary to a sustained elevation in systolic blood pressure.

Hypertensive encephalopathy is associated with a rapid rise in blood pressure and probably results from acute capillary congestion and exudation, which causes cerebral edema. These changes usually are reversible as blood pressure is brought under control. Patients with hypertensive encephalopathy present with symptoms of headache, nausea, vomiting, or loss of consciousness, as well as severe hypertensive retinopathy and renal insufficiency. In general, diastolic blood pressure exceeds 130 mmHg, although there are often exceptions to this.

Kidneys

Prolonged hypertension also is commonly implicated in the pathogenesis of renal artery stenosis and may lead to renal insufficiency. In general, controlling or normalizing elevated blood pressure minimizes the incidence of associated complications. Most treated patients occasionally will experience a mild to moderate increase in blood pressure that is either short-lived or responsive to modifications in therapy. Complications do not typically occur without a prolonged period of increased pressure that directly impacts the heart (left ventricular hypertrophy), the vessels, and their respective end organs (formation of aneurysms or hemorrhage). Indirect complications may occur as a result of atherosclerosis, which is often accompanied and exacerbated by unchecked hypertension. The degree of pressure increase leading to end-organ damage varies from patient to patient.

Malignant Hypertension

A small percentage (5%) of patients with essential hypertension will develop malignant hypertension, which is defined as a systolic pressure greater than or equal to 200 mmHg and a diastolic pressure greater than or equal to 120 mmHg with concurrent evidence of end-organ damage (systemic: renal failure, left ventricular failure; ocular: disc edema, hemorrhage, exudate, hypertensive encephalopathy). Typically these patients are males in their late 30s to early 40s with high levels of renin, angiotensin II, and aldosterone. An association may exist between malignant hypertension and human leukocyte antigen (HLA) B15. The etiology of malignant hypertension is unknown.

Secondary Hypertension

Hypertension may develop secondary to a number of disorders or diseases as well as to drug use (Table 2–2). The most common specific cause of secondary hypertension is the use of oral contraceptives (estrogen), which increase the activity of the renin–angiotensin system. Most women experience some rise in blood pressure, but only approximately 5% have an increase in blood pressure above 140/90 mmHg. Clinically significant increases in blood pressure are more common in obese women and in those over the age of 35. This phenomenon is not known to occur in postmenopausal women on estrogen therapy.

> A secondary form of hypertension should be suspected in a patient younger than age 30 years or older than age 50 at the time of onset.

Another common cause of secondary hypertension is stenosis of the renal artery either from atherosclerosis (generally in patients over the age of 50) or fibromuscular hyperplasia (generally in women under the age of 50). Fibromuscular hyperplasia accounts for approximately 30% of renal disease. Stenosis of the renal artery causes decreased renal blood flow and perfusion pressure, which triggers the release of renin and results in an increase in blood pressure. Less commonly, adrenal tumors may produce secondary hypertension. Primary hyperaldosteronism (usually a result of an adrenal adenoma with subsequent hypersecretion of aldosterone) is present in less than 0.5% of all cases of hypertension. Pheochromocytoma, a rare condition, usually results from an adrenal tumor with subsequent hypersecretion of catecholamine. The typical clinical picture includes intermittent or sustained hypertension with fluctuations, headache, palpitations, pallor, sweating, orthostatic hypotension, and hyperglycemia. Treatment is surgical removal of the pheochromocytoma.

> Most cases of secondary hypertension result from endocrine or kidney disorders.

> The retinal, choroidal, and optic nerve head vasculature are differently affected by high blood pressure.

Ocular

The retina, optic nerve, and choroidal vasculature are affected differentially by hypertension (summarized in Table 2–3).

TABLE 2–2. CAUSES OF SECONDARY HYPERTENSION

Renal Disorders
Volume overload secondary to renal failure
Chronic renal failure (parenchymal disease)
  Polycystic kidneys
  Chronic glomerulonephritis
Obstructive uropathy
Primary abnormality in salt excretion
  Gordon syndrome
  Liddle syndrome
Renovascular disease
  Atherosclerosis
  Fibromuscular dysplasia
  Other (aortic arch syndrome, polyarteritis nodosa)
Tumors
  Renin-secreting (pericytoma)
  Wilms'
  Adenocarcinoma

Endocrine Disorders
Adrenal disease
  Mineralocorticoid excess
  Primary hyperaldosteronism
  11,17-hydroxylase deficiency
  Cushing syndrome
  Pheochromocytoma
Pituitary disease
  Acromegaly
  Cushing syndrome
Thyroid disease
  Hypothyroidism
  Hyperthyroidism
  Hyperparathyroidism (hypercalcemia)

Drug Use
Hormonal
  Estrogen/progestogen contraceptive
  Exogenous ACTH
  Anabolic steroids
  Glucocorticoids
Nonhormonal
  Licorice
  Cocaine/crack
  Amphetamines

Other Causes
Excess ethanol intake
Ethanol or drug withdrawal
Pregnancy
Aortic coarctation
Neurologic disorders
  Increased intracranial pressure
  Familial dysautonomia
  Quadriplegia
  Guillain-Barré syndrome
Pain
Acute stress
Porphyria
Endothelin-producing tumor

Reprinted with permission from Nasir M, Eisner GM: Reversible hypertension in adults. Hospital Med *1992;28:23.*

Retinal Vasculature

The retinal vasculature (the central retinal artery and its tributaries) provides blood to the inner portion of the retina. Zonulae occludens between cells create a blood–tissue barrier similar to that of the circulatory system of the brain. Anterior to the lamina cribrosa, they are not under sympathetic nervous system control. These vessels respond to increases in blood pressure by autoregulation.

TABLE 2–3. OCULAR MANIFESTATIONS OF HYPERTENSION

Retinal Vasculature
- Vasoconstriction
- Sclerosis
- Exudation
- Complications of sclerosis

Optic Nerve Vasculature
- Bilateral disc edema
- Variable concurrent retinal vascular changes
- Exudation

Choroidal Vasculature
- Elschnig spots
- Siegrist spots
- Fluorescein leak in late phase
- Possible serous RD or macular star

Vasoconstrictive Phase of Hypertensive Retinopathy. The initial response to increased pressure inside a retinal artery is vasoconstriction. This is accomplished by myogenic and metabolic autoregulation and is not under autonomic nervous system control. The myogenic autoregulatory system is regulated by pacemaker cells in the walls of the vessels that are stimulated by changes in perfusion pressure (a function of transmural pressure and the intraocular pressure). For instance, vasodilation occurs in the presence of increased intraocular pressure or low retinal arterial transmural pressure, and is a compensatory response intended to maintain a steady flow of uninterrupted blood under manageable pressure. Metabolic autoregulation is a function of the balanced concentration of metabolites and nutrients (excess O_2 produces vasoconstriction, whereas excess CO_2 produces vasodilation). Retinal vascular autoregulation is negatively impacted by age, hypertension, hyperglycemia, and other systemic conditions—so much so that a patient may have difficulty adapting to even normal changes in retinal perfusion pressure. Retinal arterial vasoconstriction is best appreciated beyond the second branch of the central retinal artery. In fact, the primary site of vasoconstriction is the precapillary arterioles. The goal of retinal vasoconstriction is to stabilize the intraluminal pressure, thereby supplying the tissue that is fed by the retinal capillary beds with a constant source of oxygenated blood under pressure that will not damage the vessel walls.

Sclerotic Phase of Hypertensive Retinopathy. Prolonged elevated hypertension will result in retinal arterial damage, specifically, intimal hyalinization, medial hypertrophy, and endothelial hyperplasia. This translates to a thickening of the arterial wall and is clinically appreciated as attenuation of the arteries, widening of the arterial light reflex, and nicking/banking changes at arterial–venous crossings. This phase of hypertensive retinopathy is considered the sclerotic phase (Figure 2–2), and it is clinically and histopathologically indistinguishable from the arteriolosclerotic retinal arterial changes described in Chapter 3. Retinal arterial sclerosing is not thought of as a reversible pathologic change. Sclerosing may be segmental, which is evident as retinal arteries of irregular caliber. This may be particularly apparent during subsequent vasoconstriction of the retinal arteries (in response to a rise in blood pressure).

> Retinal vessel sclerosing (hyalinization), retinal aneurysm, and branch vein occlusion suggest chronic uncontrolled hypertension.

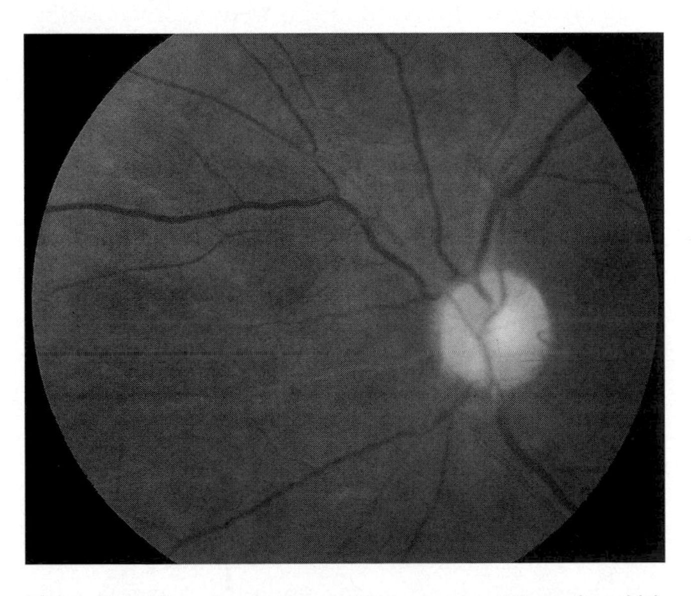

Figure 2–2. The sclerotic phase of hypertensive retinopathy, which is clinically and histopathologically indistinguishable from arteriolosclerotic retinal arterial changes (Chapter 3).

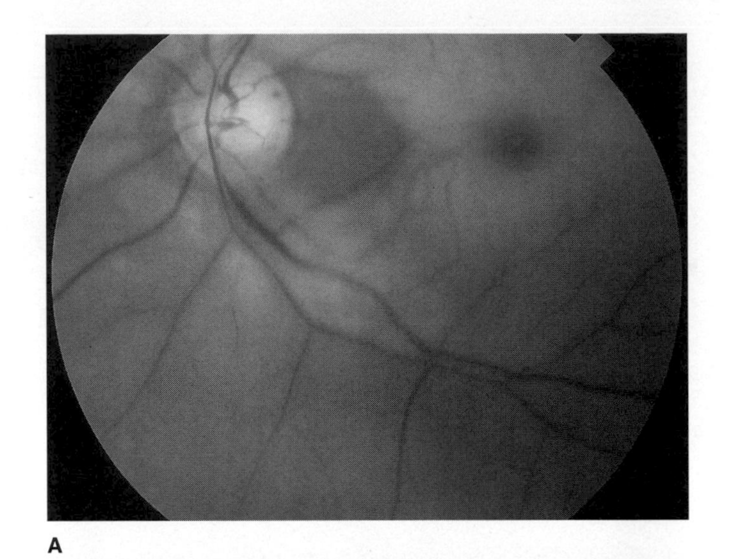

A

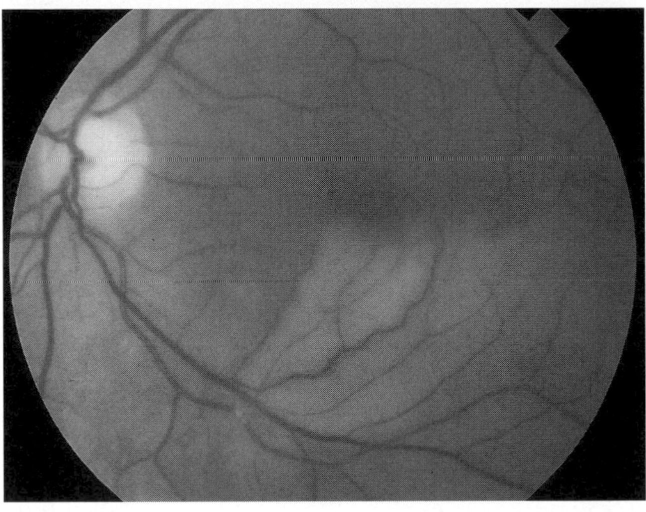

B

Figure 2–3. A. Central retinal artery occlusion. **B.** Branch retinal artery occlusion.

Complications of the Sclerotic Phase. Complications of the sclerotic phase include central and branch artery occlusion (Figure 2–3), retinal macroaneurysm (outpouching of the compromised vessel wall in the presence of high intraluminal pressure; Figure 2–4), and central and branch retinal vein occlusion (Figure 2–5). Branch retinal vein occlusion results from the compression of the venous branch at an arterial–venous crossing. Retinal ischemia resulting from either central or branch vein and arterial occlusions may produce retinal, optic nerve, and/or anterior segment neovascularization, as well as vitreal hemorrhage and rhegmatogenous retinal detachment. The probability of neovascularization, and in particular of rubeosis iridis secondary to central retinal artery occlusion, may be as high as 20% (approximating that of central retinal vein occlusion). When it does occur, its peak incidence

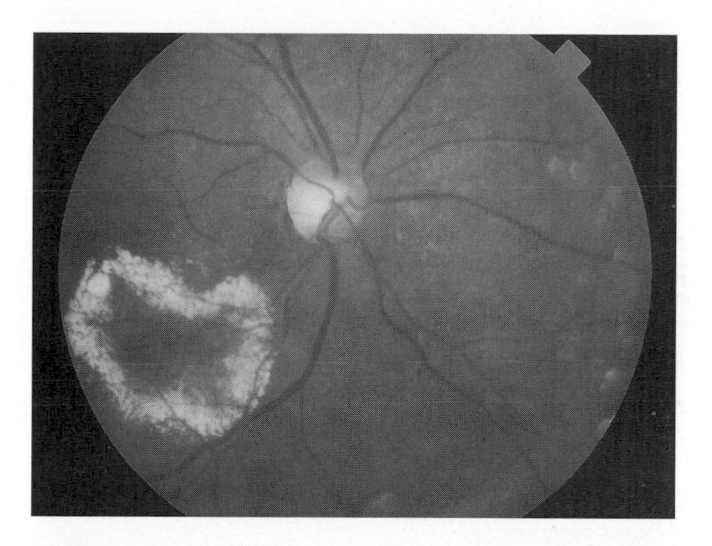

Figure 2–4. A complication of the sclerotic phase: retinal macroaneurysm.

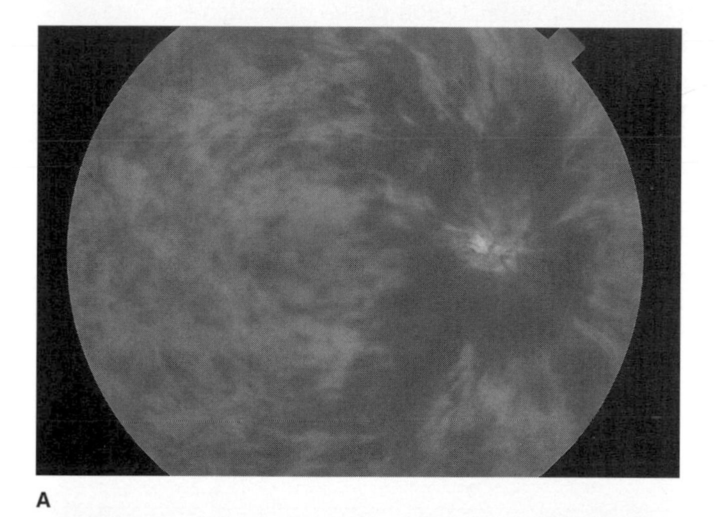

A

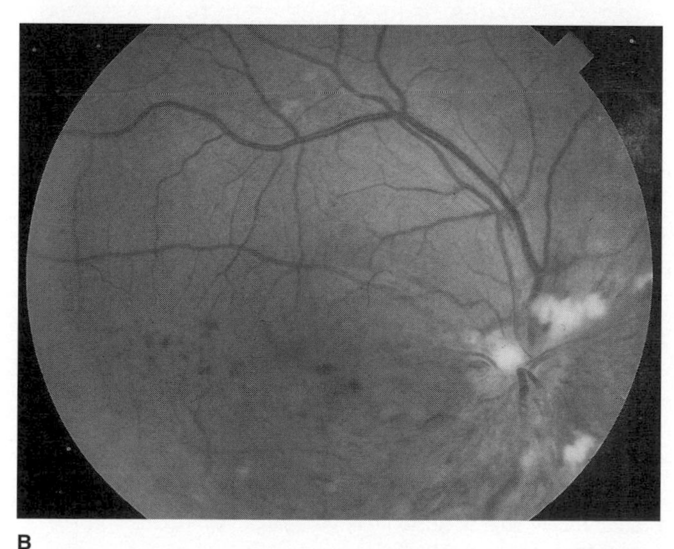

B

Figure 2–5. Complications of the sclerotic phase. **A.** Central retinal vein occlusion. **B.** Branch retinal vein occlusion.

is approximately 4 weeks following the occlusion versus an average of 5 months following a central retinal vein occlusion. Panretinal photocoagulation has proven to be beneficial in some of these patients, although those who go on to develop neovascularization generally require additional treatment modalities such as cyclocryotherapy or YAG laser cyclophotocoagulation.

Exudative Phase of Hypertensive Retinopathy. If the pressure of blood inside the retinal artery acutely rises or remains elevated over a prolonged period of time, it may exceed the limits for which vasoconstriction and sclerosis can compensate. This leads to a compromise in the integrity of the endothelial zonulae occludens, which results in the vessel leaking blood products. The leaking of red blood cells is seen clinically as flame-shaped (on the precapillary side) or dot/blot hemorrhages (on the postcapillary side). Plasma lipoprotein, phospholipid, cholesterol, and triglycerides may leak, and are clinically seen as hard exudates. In the case of acute or severe hypertension, the change is so rapid that the response of the vessel progresses from the vasoconstrictive phase directly to this exudative phase (Figure 2–6). If the hypertension is not brought under control, the vessel wall becomes necrotic. This results in loss of autoregulation and a resultant dilation of the vessel. Without the benefit of the protection afforded by vasoconstriction, the capillary beds are subject to the high pressure. The result is capillary damage and leakage, which impairs the flow of blood to the retina. This is seen clinically as retinal nerve fiber layer ischemia (cotton-wool spots). If the underlying hypertension is brought under control during the vasoconstrictive or exudative phase, the arterial supply returns

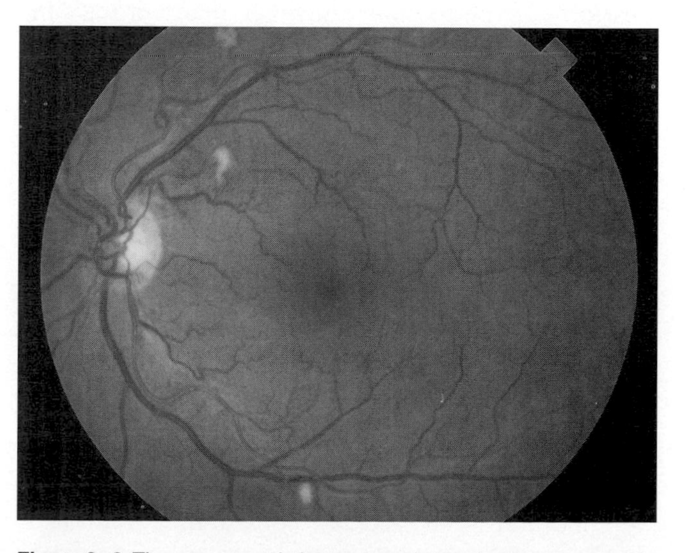

Figure 2–6. The vasoconstrictive and exudative phases concurrently present due to a prolonged episode of acute hypertension.

to its normal caliber and the retinal hemorrhages, exudates, and ischemia eventually resolve.

> Vasoconstriction of the retinal arteries, retinal exudates, and ischemia suggests acute high blood pressure.

Shortcomings of Hypertensive Retinopathy Grading Systems. Appreciation of constricted retinal arteries relies on accurate and dependable knowledge of the normal retinal arterial caliber. Using the caliber of the retinal veins and describing the two vessels as a ratio is a common practice that can be misleading, because the caliber of retinal veins is variable. Furthermore, this technique offers poor interobserver reliability. It is also not uncommon to see arterial attenuation and even arterial–venous crossing changes in elderly patients with no evidence of hypertension. It would better serve the practitioner to develop an appreciation for normal retinal vascular caliber and use this as a reference when assessing vasoconstrictive changes in the retina. Over the years, several grading systems were established in an effort to judge the efficacy of treatment and the progression of hypertension. However, many of the clinical signs are found in a nonhypertensive population and may represent normal age-related changes. For instance, debris accumulating in the perivascular sheath, a normal age-related phenomenon, may appear clinically as a widening of the arterial reflex. Also, most grading systems do not consider the dynamics of the retinal arterial response to increased intraluminal pressure. For example, focusing on the sclerotic component alone (as in previous classification systems) narrows the clinical utility of this examination. When the clinician is familiar with the dynamic response of the retinal vasculature to increased pressure, more useful information can be generated from a retinal examination. For instance, the presence of recurrent vasoconstriction in a patient with "stable" hypertension suggests that the condition is, in fact, not consistently controlled. This is useful information to a practitioner who is basing the success of treatment in large part on an in-office reading of blood pressure, which is often an inaccurate measure of long-term stability. Hypertensive retinopathy has also been classified by several clinical grading systems that, in many cases, supply the clinician with little if any useful information that might affect the treatment of the patient. It would be more useful to incorporate what is known about the physiologic response of the retinal vasculature to increased blood pressure into a classification system that would provide practitioners with some degree of evidence of improper control of hypertension. Such a classification system has been postulated by Tso and associates (1991) and is summarized in Table 2–4.

> Grading systems for hypertensive eye findings offer poor inter-observer reliability, lack specificity (because it includes normal age-related changes), and provide little or no prognostic value.

Optic Nerve Vasculature

The blood supply of the optic nerve head is composed of a complex network of vessels derived from the posterior ciliary, retinal, and pial circulations. The pial circulation is primarily composed of branches of the ophthalmic artery or recurrent branches from the posterior ciliary arteries. These three sources, in addition to their individual contributions, anastomose and in some individuals form an incomplete intrascleral circle that surrounds the optic nerve known as the *circle of Zinn–Haller.* Because the optic nerve receives a blood supply from sources regulated by sympathetic tone and autoregulation, it is subject to each of these forms of intraluminal pressure regulation. Like the blood–retina barrier in the retinal vasculature, the blood supply to the optic nerve is characterized as having tight endothelial junctions, muscular walls, and thick basement membranes that provide an effective blood–

TABLE 2–4. STAGES OF RESPONSE OF RETINAL ARTERIAL SUPPLY TO INCREASES IN BLOOD PRESSURE

Vasconstriction
Initial response to hypertension
Transient
Controlled by autoregulation
Beyond second branch of central retinal artery

Sclerosis
Results from prolonged hypertension
Irreversible
Damage and thickening of arterial wall
May mimic normal age-related changes

Exudation
Results from prolonged hypertension or abrupt acute hypertension
Integrity of tight junctions compromised
Blood produces leak into retina

Complications of Sclerosis
Branch retinal vein occlusion, central retinal vein occlusion (ischemic and nonischemic)
Central retinal artery occlusion, branch retinal artery occlusion
Retinal macroaneurysm

nerve barrier. Although it is unlikely that direct anastomoses exist between the choriocapillaris and the capillaries of the optic nerve, the border tissue of Elschnig, which separates these two systems, does not offer an effective blood–nerve barrier. It is capable of leaking choroidal fluid, which may contribute to disc edema. In secondary hypertension, the release of renin leads to the production of angiotensin II. It is theorized that this potent vasoconstictor is able to pass through the fenestrations of the choriocapillaris to produce vasoconstriction of the muscular arteriolar walls of the choroid. From the choriocapillaris, it may also be able to cross the border tissue of Elschnig to produce vasoconstriction in the vessels of the optic nerve.

The vasculature of the optic nerve head is most prominently affected in the presence of acute, severe hypertension. The ocular presentation of malignant hypertension is characterized by bilateral disc edema (Figure 2–7), with or without hypertensive retinal vascular changes, and venous engorgement. Visual acuities may be unaffected or dramatically reduced. Retinal exudation may appear in the macula in the form of a star pattern (consistent with the architecture of the Henle layer) (Figure 2–8), and hypertensive encephalopathy may be present. In animal models, the order of appearance of fundus lesions is (1) focal intraretinal periarteriolar transudates; (2) acute focal retinal pigment epithelial lesions, macular edema, and disc edema; and (3) focal nerve fiber layer ischemia (cotton-wool spots).

Disc edema may be secondary to the ingress of choroidal fluid or angiotensin II through the border tissue of Elschnig, direct damage of the vascular supply of the optic nerve with secondary ischemia, or in the presence of hypertensive encephalopathy, a corresponding elevation in cerebral spinal fluid pressure. It is important to note that, contrary to previously held assertions, disc edema can be present in the absence of encephalopathy, and the extent of disc edema is not an indication of the patient's visual or general prognosis. Generally, these patients are concurrently treated for the underlying increase in blood pressure. However, if the blood pressure is lowered too abruptly, the perfusion pressure to the nerve may become so low as to cause further irreparable damage. The same is true regarding the perfusion pressure to the brain.

Choroidal Circulation

The choroidal circulation is a fenestrated system that lacks a tight blood–tissue barrier. It is derived primarily from the short posterior ciliary arteries. There is also some lesser contribution from the peripapillary blood vessels. Its response to changes in intraluminal pressure is regulated by the sympathetic nervous system.

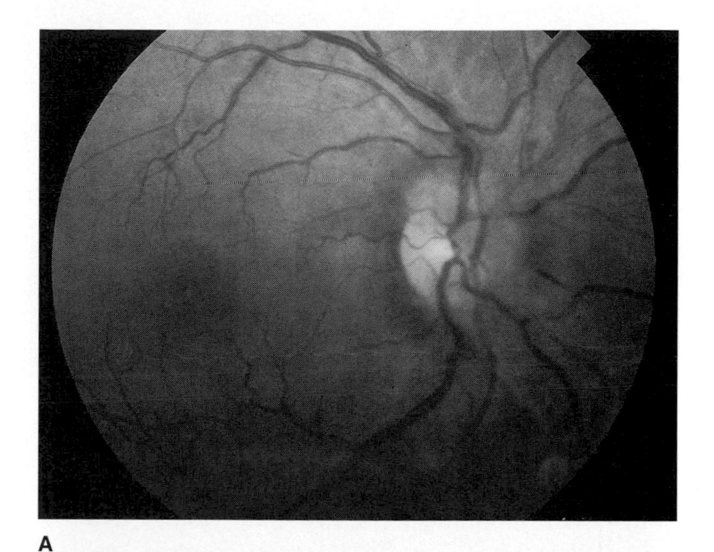

A

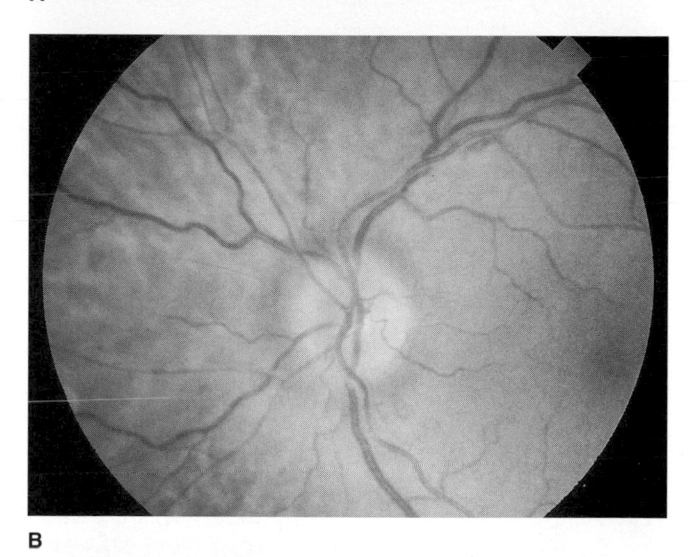

B

Figure 2–7. Bilateral disc edema secondary to malignant hypertension. **A.** Right eye. **B.** Left eye.

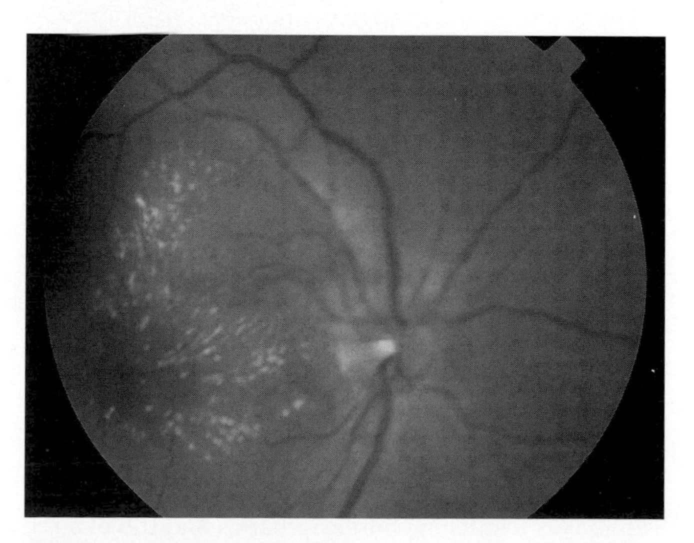

Figure 2–8. Hypertensive macular star.

Unlike the retinal vasculature, the choroid responds to sympathetic stimulation. In addition, the fenestrated choriocapillaris may allow angiotensin II and/or other substrates to pass into the choroidal stroma to stimulate choroidal arteriolar muscular walls. The choroidal circulation is also influenced by the intraocular pressure. Elevation of intraocular pressure increases choroidal vascular resistance possibly due to pressure translated to the vortex veins as they pass through the oblique scleral canal.

The majority of cases of hypertensive choroidopathy (HC) are found in young patients and result from acute hypertension (pregnancy induced, renal diseases, pheochromocytoma, malignant hypertension). Ocular signs include retinal pigmented epithelium (RPE) disruption and retinal vascular changes.

> Hypertensive choroidopathy is generally found in young patients and results from acute and secondary forms of hypertension.

The choriocapillaris is vulnerable to increased blood pressure because of the relatively short course and scant branching of the choroidal arteries. Vasoconstriction of these arteries protects the nearby choriocapillaris but may produce local ischemia to the RPE. The result is focal necrosis of the RPE in a pattern corresponding to the structural arrangement of the choriocapillaris. The ensuing window defect will typically leak fluorescein during the late phase. There also may be a corresponding serous retinal detachment and/or macular star formation.

The structural arrangement of the choriocapillaris varies with its location. In the posterior pole, an arteriole supplies oxygenated blood to the center of a lobular network of capillaries, which is drained circumferentially. The benefit of this lobular arrangement appears to be greater blood flow to this region. In the posterior pole, the RPE disruption is termed an *Elschnig spot,* and the pattern is lobular in shape. This suggests that each lobule is an independent functioning vascular unit. In time, these areas will develop a pigmented center surrounded by a depigmented halo, and there will no longer be fluorescein leakage in the late phase.

In the equator, the medium-sized choroidal arteries travel anteriorly and join the choroidal veins, which are traveling in the same direction toward the vortex veins. This results in choriocapillaries that travel a relatively straight course in a spindle-shaped arrangement. Here, the lesion is termed a *Siegrist spot* (Figure 2–9). It is typically larger in area. Multiple spots may follow the course of a choroidal vessel.

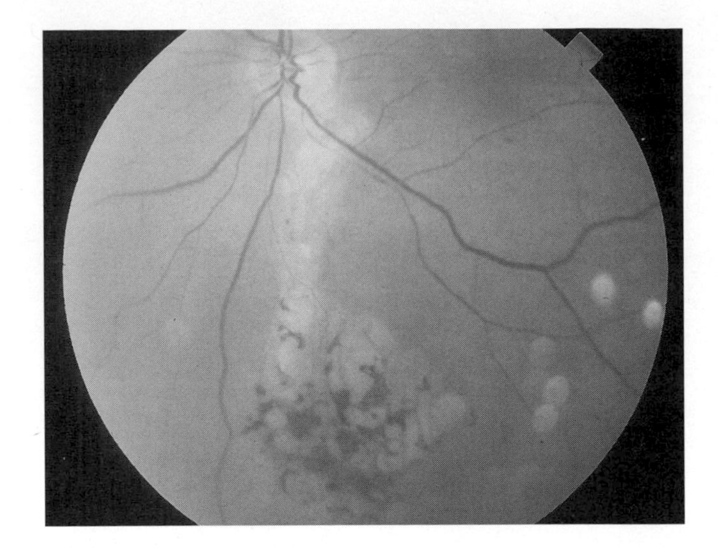

Figure 2–9. Siegrist spot.

In the periphery, the choroidal arteries and veins are relatively parallel and travel perpendicular to the ora serrata. They are connected by a network of capillaries that run between them at right angles. The result is a ladder-shaped configuration. These spots are generally triangular in shape with the base toward the ora serrata.

DIAGNOSIS

Systemic

An exhaustive workup is not required in the diagnosis of hypertension. The initial evaluation includes a determination of arterial blood pressure. A systolic pressure greater than 140 mmHg or diastolic greater than 90 mmHg on at least two (preferably three) occasions (taken in as stress-free an environment as possible) constitutes hypertension. Other components of the initial evaluation include a physical examination, an assessment of end-organ damage, screening for secondary causes of hypertension, identification of other cardiovascular risk factors, and characterization of the patient (age, sex, race, lifestyle, concomitant illnesses) to aid in selection of therapy.

Laboratory tests (Table 2–5) are generally recommended before starting antihypertensive therapy to determine the presence of end-organ damage and evidence of secondary causes. They also serve as baseline measurements for monitoring antihypertensive therapy. There is some controversy as to how in depth

TABLE 2–5. BASIC TESTS FOR INITIAL EVALUATION OF PATIENTS WITH HYPERTENSION

Should Include:
- Urinalysis
- Hematocrit
- Serum potassium
- Serum creatinine and/or blood urea nitrogen
- Electrocardiogram

May Include:
- Microscopic urine analysis
- White blood cell count
- Plasma/blood glucose, cholesterol, HDL cholesterol, and triglycerides
- Serum calcium, phosphate, and uric acid
- Chest x-ray; echocardiogram

From Williams, Gordon H., Fauci AS, et al, eds. Approach to the patient with hypertension. In: Harrison's Principles of Internal Medicine. New York: McGraw-Hill; *14th ed. 1998: 204.*

laboratory analysis should be for secondary forms of hypertension. In general, basic laboratory studies should be performed for all patients. Additional testing should be sought when basic tests suggest secondary causes or if blood pressure is not brought under control following medical management. Basic testing should include urine for protein, blood (suggestive of renal disease), and glucose (suggestive of diabetes); hematocrit (to detect anemia); serum potassium (hyperaldosteronism); serum creatinine and/or blood urea nitrogen (for renal function); and an electrocardiogram. Additional testing could include serum calcium (to detect hyperparathyroidism), sodium levels (for baseline), fasting glucose and glycosolated hemoglobin (to detect diabetes or evidence of pheochromocytoma and as a baseline because some antihypertensive medications such as diuretics can raise blood sugar levels), fasting triglycerides and low-density lipoprotein cholesterol (to assess the risk of atherosclerosis), microscopic examination of the urine (for renal status), serum uric acid levels (to detect hyperuricemia—found in some patients with renal disease and essential hypertension), and thyroid-stimulating hormone (TSH) (to assist in ruling out thyroid dysfunction). A limited echocardiography and chest x-ray to determine the presence of left ventricular hypertrophy can also be helpful.

The differential diagnosis of hypertension includes primary hypertension and secondary hypertension (Table 2–6). Diagnostic studies for secondary causes of hypertension generally are not warranted since it accounts for less than 5% of all cases of hypertension. However, these studies are warranted in the following patients: (1) those in whom routine history, physical examination, or laboratory test results suggest a specific secondary cause of hypertension; (2) those less than 30 years of age, since they are the group most likely to have correctable secondary hypertension; (3) those with poor or inadequate response to drug therapy; (4) those with sudden worsening of their hypertension; and (5) older patients who develop new onset of hypertension or patients with sudden onset of hypertension.

TABLE 2–6. CLINICAL FINDINGS SUGGESTIVE OF HYPERTENSION

Primary Hypertension

History
Age at onset 30–50 years
Presence of family history

Physical Examination
Diastolic pressure exceeding 90 mmHg or systolic exceeding 140 mmHg on two or three separate occasions

Secondary Hypertension

History
Age at onset < 20 or > 50 years
Absence of family history
Poor BP control on 3-drug regimen
Uncontrolled BP after period of good control
Palpitations, tremors, excessive sweating, weight loss, glucose intolerance
Peripheral vascular disease, cerebrovascular disease, or myocardial infarction
Ethanol intake > 3 drinks/day
Hormonal contraceptive use
Use of cocaine, amphetamines, or similar drugs
Genitourinary or renal disease
Possible malignancy
Deterioration in renal function induced by ACE inhibitors
Muscle pain or weakness, especially after diuretic use
Symptoms of Cushing syndrome

Physical Examination
Difference in BP in upper extremities
Difference in BP and pulse in upper and lower extremities
Abdominal bruit
Abdominal mass
Peripheral cyanosis or gangrene
Peripheral edema
Needle marks
Perforated nasal septum
Thyroid enlargement
Immature secondary sex characteristics

BP, Blood pressure.
Modified with permission from Nasir M, Eisner GM: Reversible hypertension in adults. Hospital Med. *1992;28:26.*

Most tests for renovascular hypertension are neither highly sensitive nor specific. Renal hypertension should be suspected if the age of onset is less than 20 years or greater than 50, in the presence of concurrent atherosclerotic disease elsewhere, or if renal function is dramatically compromised following angiotensin-converting enzyme (ACE) inhibitor therapy. Abdominal bruits,

TABLE 2-7. DIFFERENTIAL DIAGNOSIS OF HYPERTENSIVE RETINOPATHY

Retinal Vasculature
Branch artery occlusion
Diabetic retinopathy
Retinal telangiectasia
Central retinal vein occlusion
Branch retinal vein occlusion
Old branch retinal artery occlusion
Hypoperfusion retinopathy
Arteriolosclerotic retinopathy
Retinitis pigmentosa

Optic Nerve Head Vasculature
Macular star
- Retinal angioma
- Macular neuroretinitis
- Papillitis
- Papilledema

Swollen disc central retinal vein occlusion
- Hypoperfusion retinopathy
- Diabetic papillopathy
- Ischemic optic neuropathy
- Pseudotumor cerebri
- Optic nerve compression (e.g., nerve sheath memingioma)
- Optic nerve infection (e.g., meningitis)
- Optic nerve inflammation (e.g., optic neuritis, papillitis)
- Toxic optic nerve disease (e.g., acute methanol poisoning)

Choroidal Vasculature
Retinal dystrophy (e.g., hereditary macular degeneration)
Retinal degeneration (e.g., macular degeneration, focal choroiditis)
Retinal atrophy (pavingstone degeneration)
Previous retinal inflammation (e.g., toxoplasmosis)
Previous retinal trauma (e.g., retinal dialysis)

particularly those that lateralize to the renal areas or have a diastolic component, suggest renovascular disease.

Ocular

The diagnosis of the ocular manifestations of hypertension are based on the funduscopic and fluorescein angiographic appearance previously described (Table 2–3). The most common differential diagnoses are summarized in Table 2–7.

TREATMENT AND MANAGEMENT

Systemic

The goals of antihypertensive therapy are to reduce overall cardiovascular risk and morbidity and mortality. The decision to initiate antihypertensive therapy is governed by the extent of blood pressure elevation, presence or absence of other risk factors or target organ damage/clinical cardiovascular disease, or both (Table 2–8). Risk factors of importance are smoking, dyslipidemia, diabetes, age greater than 60 years, sex (men and postmenopausal women), and family history of cardiovascular disease (women less than age 65 or men less than age 55 years). Target organ damage includes stroke or transient ischemic attack, nephropathy, peripheral arterial disease, and retinopathy. Cardiovascular disease includes left ventricular hypertrophy, angina or prior myocardial infarction, prior coronary revascularization, and heart failure.

TABLE 2–8. CLASSIFICATION, RISK STRATIFICATION, AND TREATMENT OF HIGH BLOOD PRESSURE IN ADULTS AGED 18 YEARS AND ABOVE

Classification of Blood Pressure (mm Hg)	Risk Stratification[a] and Treatment		
	Risk Group A	*Risk Group B*	*Risk Group C*
Optimum (<120/<80)	—	—	—
Normal (<130/<85)	—	—	—
High normal (130–139/85–89)	Lifestyle modification	Lifestyle modification	Drug therapy[b,c]
Stage 1 hypertension (140–159/90–99)	Lifestyle modification (up to 12 months)	Lifestyle modification[d] (up to 6 months)	Drug therapy[b]
Stage 2 and 3 hypertension (160–179/100–109; >180/ >110)	Drug therapy[b]	Drug therapy[b]	Drug therapy[b]

[a]Definition of risk groups: A = no cardiovascular risk factors, no target organ damage or clinical cardiovascular disease; B = at least one other cardiovascular risk factor not including diabetes, no target organ damage or clinical cardiovascular disease; C = target organ damage/clinical cardiovascular disease and/or diabetes, with or without other cardiovascular risk factors.
[b]Lifestyle modification is adjunctive therapy in all patients for whom pharmacologic therapy is recommended.
[c]In patients with heart failure, renal insufficiency, or diabetes.
[d]For patients with multiple cardiovascular risk factors, drugs are considered as initial therapy as well as lifestyle modifications.
Modified with permission from The Sixth Report of the Joint National Committee on Prevention, Detection, Evaluation, and Treatment of High Blood Pressure. Arch Intern Med. *1997;157:2413–2446.*

The Sixth Report of the Joint National Committee (JNC VI) on Prevention, Detection, Evaluation, and Treatment of High Blood Pressure (1997) provides the currently accepted treatment recommendations (Figure 2–10). Initial treatment of mild hypertension consists of lifestyle modifications, including weight reduction, moderation of alcohol intake, cessation of cigarette smoking, regular physical activity, and dietary changes (moderation of sodium intake; adequate potassium, calcium, and magnesium intake; and reduction in saturated fat and cholesterol intake). Pharmacologic therapy is recommended for patients not achieving goal blood pressure levels with lifestyle modifications and for those with moderate to severe hypertension.

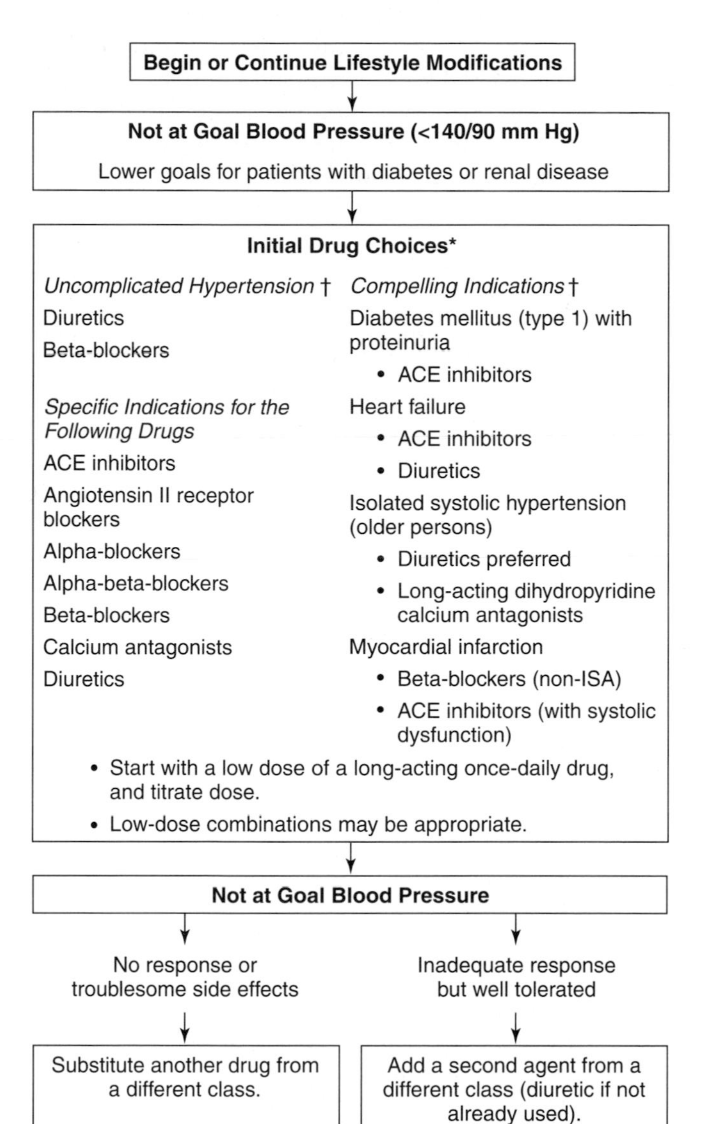

Figure 2–10. Algorithm for the treatment of hypertension. (*Modified with permission from The Sixth Report of the Joint National Committee on Prevention, Detection, Evaluation, and Treatment of High Blood Pressure.* Arch Intem Med. 1997;157:2413–2446.)

Ample evidence indicates that reducing blood pressure with drug therapy, regardless of the extent of elevation, will reduce cardiovascular morbidity and mortality, particularly stroke, coronary events, heart failure, progression of renal disease, and progression to more severe hypertension (Psaty et al., 1997). Optimum protection against the occurrence of major cardiovascular events and a better quality of life appear to be achieved when blood pressure is in the range of 80 to 85 mm Hg for diastolic and 130 to 140 mm Hg for systolic blood pressure (Hansson, 1999).

General principles of drug therapy include the following: (1) initiate therapy with a low dose and slowly titrate the dose upward based on age, response, and occurrence of adverse events; (2) select drug formulations that provide efficacy over a 24-hour period to improve compliance with therapy, to provide smooth blood pressure control, and to protect against the risk of sudden death, stroke, or heart attack from a sudden increase in blood pressure upon arising; (3) add a drug with a different mechanism of action if blood pressure is not controlled adequately after reasonable therapeutic trial; and (4) slowly attempt to decrease the dosage and number of antihypertensive agents after blood pressure has been controlled for at least 1 year.

The most commonly prescribed antihypertensive agents include diuretics, beta-blockers, ACE inhibitors, and calcium channel blockers. Newer classes of antihypertensive agents include combined alpha-beta blockers and angiotensin II receptor blockers (ARBs). Classes of antihypertensive agents no longer prescribed routinely (and not discussed in detail herein) include peripheral adrenergic drugs (e.g., guanethidine, reserpine), central alpha-agonists (e.g., clonidine, methyldopa), direct vasodilators (e.g., hydralazine, minoxidil), and alpha-blockers (e.g., doxazosin, prazosin, terazosin).

In general, at least 50% of patients respond to monotherapy with any class of antihypertensive agent, but over time, a substantial proportion of patients require multiple drugs to adequately control their blood pressure. Diuretic- and beta-blocker–based regimens seem to reduce blood pressure to lower levels than regimens based on newer classes of drugs. The JNC VI recommends diuretics or beta-blockers as the initial drug of choice for patients with uncomplicated hypertension (Figure 2–10) because these classes have been shown in long-term clinical trials to reduce morbidity and mortality. The specific indications for initiating therapy with other classes of antihypertensive agents are summarized in Table 2–9. Studies published since the JNC VI report generally provide confirmation of its recommendations. A study of 20,000 patients with hypertension found a 25% higher incidence of major cardiovascular disease events in patients treated with an alpha-blocker compared to a diuretic, prompting the discontinuation of the alpha-blocker treatment arm (The ALLHAT Officers and Coordinators, 2000).

Certain patient groups may have a greater response with some antihypertensive agents than with others (Table 2–10). In general, patients with increased plasma volume and/or low plasma renin activity (African-Americans, geriatric patients, and obese patients) tend to respond more favorably to diuretics and calcium channel blockers; combined alpha-beta blockers also effectively lower blood pressure in African-Americans. Combination therapy with a diuretic and a calcium channel blocker has less of an additive

TABLE 2–9. CONSIDERATIONS FOR INDIVIDUALIZING ANTIHYPERTENSIVE DRUG THERAPY

Consideration/Indication	Drug Therapy
Compelling Indications Unless Contraindicated	
Diabetes mellitus, type 1, with proteinuria	ACE inhibitor
Heart failure	ACE inhibitor, diuretic
Isolated systolic hypertension (older patients)	Diuretic (preferred), CCB (long-acting dihydropyridine)
Myocardial infarction	Beta-blocker (non-ISA), ACE inhibitor (with systolic dysfunction)
May Have Favorable Effects on Comorbid Conditions[a]	
Angina	Beta-blocker, CCB
Atrial tachycardia and fibrillation	Beta-blocker, CCB (nondihydropyridine)
Cyclosporine-induced hypertension	CCB
Diabetes mellitus, types 1 and 2, with proteinuria	ACE inhibitor (preferred), CCB
Diabetes mellitus, type 2	Diuretic, low dose
Dyslipidemia	Alpha-blocker
Essential tremor	Beta-blocker (non-CS)
Heart failure	ACE inhibitor, combined alpha-beta blocker, ARB
Hyperthyroidism	Beta-blocker
Migraine	Beta-blocker (non-CS), CCB (nondihydropyridine)
Myocardial infarction	CCB (nondihydropyridine)
Osteoporosis	Thiazide diuretic
Preoperative hypertension	Beta-blocker
Prostatism (BPH)	Alpha-blocker
Renal insufficiency (caution in renovascular hypertension, creatinine ≥ 3 mg/dL)	ACE inhibitor
May Have Unfavorable Effects on Comorbid Conditions[b]	
Bronchospastic disease	Beta-blocker[c]
Depression	Beta-blocker, central alpha-agonist, reserpine[c]
Diabetes mellitus, types 1 and 2	Beta-blocker, high-dose diuretic
Dyslipidemia	Beta-blocker (non-ISA), high-dose diuretic
Gout	Diuretic
Second- or third-degree heart block	Beta-blocker,[c] CCB (nondihydropyridine)[c]
Heart failure	Beta-blocker (except carvedilol), CCB (except amlodipine besylate, felodipine)
Liver disease	Labetalol, methyldopa[c]
Peripheral vascular disease	Beta-blocker
Pregnancy	ACE inhibitor[c], ARB[c]
Renal insufficiency	Potassium-sparing agents
Renovascular disease	ACE inhibitor, ARB

[a]Considerations/indications and drugs listed alphabetically.
[b]Drugs listed may be used with special monitoring unless contraindicated.
[c]Contraindicated.
Abbreviations: ACE = angiotensin-converting enzyme; ARB = angiotensin II receptor blocker; BPH = benign prostatic hyperplasia; CCB = calcium channel blocker; CS = cardioselective; ISA = intrinsic sympathomimetic activity.
Modified with permission from The Sixth Report of the Joint National Committee on Prevention, Detection, Evaluation, and Treatment of High Blood Pressure. Arch Intern Med. *1997;157:2413–2446.*

TABLE 2–10. OVERVIEW OF ANTIHYPERTENSIVE DRUG CLASSES

Parameter	Diuretics	Beta-Blockers	ACE Inhibitors	Calcium Channel Blockers	Alpha-Beta Blockers	Angiotensin II Receptor Blockers
Patient type best suited for	African-Americans Elderly Obese	Caucasians Younger ages	Caucasians Younger ages (Less effective in African-Americans, elderly)	All demographic groups	Caucasians	Caucasians (Less effective in African-Americans)
Pressure-lowering effects	Initially ⇓ plasma volume Subsequent ⇓ in peripheral vascular resistance by an unknown mechanism	⇓ Heart rate ⇓ Cardiac output ⇓ Renin release	Inhibit RAAS Inhibit bradycardia Stimulate vasodilating prostaglandin synthesis	Inhibit influx of Ca^{++} during membrane depolarization Cause peripheral vasodilation with less reflex tachycardia (⇑ myocardial contractility and fluid retention)	⇓ Cardiac output ⇓ Peripheral vascular resistance Cause vasodilation	Inhibit receptor binding of angiotensin II Block angiotensin II–induced vasoconstriction and aldosterone secretion
Other favorable effects	⇓ Morbidity and mortality Useful in heart failure	⇓ Morbidity and mortality Cardioprotective	Cardioprotective Useful in heart failure Anti-ischemic effects Potent combined with diuretic, calcium channel blocker	Combination with ACE inhibitor potent Antianginal effects	⇓ Tachycardia	
Side effects	⇓ K^+, Mg^{++} ⇑ Glucose ⇑ LDL ⇑ Uric acid	Bradycardia Fatigue Bronchospasm Sleep disturbance Impotence ⇑ Triglycerides ⇑ HDL	Few side effects (dry cough, skin rash, and taste alterations with captopril) Angioneurotic edema ($<1\%$)	Headache Peripheral edema Bradycardia Constipation (verapamil)	Fatigue Dizziness ⇑ Glucose Diarrhea Bradycardia Hypotension	Few side effects (no cough as with ACE inhibitors)
Contraindications	Reasonably safe Anuria (thiazide and loop) Hyperkalemia (K^+-sparing) Hypokalemia (carbonic anhydrase inhibitors)	Congestive heart failure Bronchospasm Peripheral vascular disease Relative contraindication: type 1 diabetes (⇓ gluconeogenesis; may ⇑ hypoglycemic episodes)	Reasonably safe	Concomitant paroxysmal supraventricular tachycardia Nondihydropyridines: heart block or sick sinus syndrome unless pacemaker; systolic hypotension (<90 mmHg)	Severe heart failure Bronchospastic conditions Heart block or sick sinus syndrome unless pacemaker Severe bradycardia Cardiogenic shock	Reasonably safe

Abbreviations: ACE = angiotensin-converting enzyme; Ca^{++} = calcium; HDL = high-density lipoprotein cholesterol; K^+ = potassium; LDL = low-density lipoprotein cholesterol; Mg^{++} = magnesium; RAAS = renin–angiotensin–aldosterone system.

effect than if either is combined with an ACE inhibitor or a beta-blocker. Patients who generally have elevated plasma renin activity (young, Caucasian) tend to benefit more from the use of an ACE inhibitor or a beta-blocker. ACE inhibitors generally are preferred in this population because of their relative lack of adverse effects. The ARBs also affect the renin–angiotensin system and may be beneficial in the same patient groups as ACE inhibitors. However, experience with this new class of agents is limited compared to that with ACE inhibitors.

Antihypertensive agents may have benefits in addition to blood pressure lowering in the presence of concurrent disease or they may worsen a concurrent condition. Because beta-blockers lower both cardiac output and heart rate, they are often prescribed for patients with previous myocardial infarction and angina, and they may prevent coronary artery disease. In addition, beta-blockers are useful for patients with migraine headaches and for somatic manifestations of anxiety. However, a patient with hypertension, angina, and chronic obstructive pulmonary disease (COPD) would not be a candidate for a beta-blocker (or a combined alpha-beta blocker) because its vasoconstrictive and bronchospasm effects are likely to exacerbate COPD. Calcium channel blockers may be beneficial in patients with concurrent angina, diabetes, or COPD, and nondihydropryidine calcium channel blockers (diltiazem, verapamil) may be useful in patients with atrial arrhythmias. The ACE inhibitors are beneficial in patients with diabetes, renal insufficiency, and heart failure or left ventricular hypertrophy because they help restore endothelial function.

Clearly, there is no one drug or cookbook approach to the treatment of hypertension. Each patient requires an individualized plan based on the extent of blood pressure elevation, presence or absence of other risk factors or target organ damage/clinical cardiovascular disease, or both, as well as the properties of specific antihypertensive drug(s).

Ocular

The management of the ocular complications of hypertension is summarized in Table 2–11 and, in general, centers around the treatment of the underlying systemic hypertension. Treatment specific to the eye is generally limited to the complications of the sclerotic phase of the retinal vasculature.

CONCLUSION

Undoubtedly, many patients live a long and "healthy" life with undiagnosed hypertension. It is clear, however,

TABLE 2–11. MANAGEMENT OF THE PATIENT WITH KNOWN OR SUSPECTED HYPERTENSION BASED ON OCULAR FINDINGS

Retinal Finding	Clinical Suggestion	Management
Vasoconstriction	**Known Hypertensive** Suggests noncompliance or failure of current treatment regimen	Take blood pressure Consult with internist
	Undiagnosed Hypertensive Suggests hypertension	Hypertension history: risk factors; family history; signs/symptoms (although generally none) Take blood pressure: if elevated, reschedule patient and repeat in a relaxed atmosphere or consult with internist; if "normal," schedule follow-up in 3–6 months for repeat blood pressure, funduscopy, and photos Photodocument
Exudative phase	Suggests rapid, prolonged, significant elevation of blood pressure (if concurrent vasoconstriction present, this suggests a relatively recent onset; if vasoconstriction absent, this suggests the onset was greater than 1–2 months)	Take blood pressure Hypertension history including recent headaches, vomiting, nausea Consult with internist Return in 3 months for follow-up
Sclerotic phase	Suggests prolonged, uncontrolled hypertension	Take blood pressure Consult with internist Photodocument
Complications of the sclerotic phase	Suggests prolonged, uncontrolled hypertension	Take blood pressure Consult with internist Photodocument Monitor as indicated for complications of ocular ischemia (e.g., neovascularization)

that high blood pressure poses a significant increased risk for developing atherosclerosis, stroke, heart disease, and a host of other conditions that can be easily reduced with proper intervention. Despite the multiple potentially deleterious effects from hypertension, in the United States most patients with hypertension die from complications of coronary artery disease (atherosclerosis).

Although the cause of hypertension is unknown in the overwhelming majority of cases (primary or essential hypertension), a small but significant percentage of patients with hypertension have a definable cause (secondary hypertension). Patients with hypertension generally are asymptomatic, which may delay diagnosis and complicate compliance with treatment regimens and follow-up. Compliance also is complicated by the cost of medications, the need for chronic or life-long treatment, side effects from medications, and disruption in daily routine and quality of life due to treatment.

Delay in diagnosis and inadequate treatment may result in the more serious sequelae of hypertension noted above. Measurement of blood pressure should, therefore, be as publicly accessible as possible and part of the routine assessment of all patients. The ocular effects of hypertension, which are a function of the amplitude and duration of increased blood pressure, are easily assessed by a trained eyecare practitioner and provide valuable clinical information regarding the status of these patients.

REFERENCES

Alexander L. *Primary Care of the Posterior Segment.* 2nd ed. Norwalk, CT: Appleton & Lange; 1994:171–276.

Casser-Locke L. Ocular manifestations of hypertension. *Optom Clin.* 1992;2:47–76.

Dzau V, Braunwald E. Resolved and unresolved issues in the prevention and treatment of coronary artery disease: A workshop consensus statement. *Am Heart J.* 1991;131:1244–1263.

Hansson L. The Hypertension Optimal Treatment study and the importance of lowering blood pressure. *J Hypertens.* 1999;17(suppl 1):S9–S13.

Joint National Committee on Prevention, Detection, Evaluation, and Treatment of High Blood Pressure. The Sixth Report of the Joint National Committee on Prevention, Detection, Evaluation, and Treatment of High Blood Pressure. *Arch Intern Med.* 1997;157:2413–2446.

Kaplan NM, Gifford RW Jr. Choice of initial therapy for hypertension. *JAMA.* 1996;275:1577–1580.

Psaty BM, Smith NL, Siscovick DS, et al. Health outcomes associated with antihypertensive therapies used as first-line agents: A systematic review and meta-analysis. *JAMA.* 1997;277:739–745.

Robbins SL, Cotron RS, Kumar V. *Pathologic Basis of Disease.* 3rd ed. Philadelphia: Saunders; 1984:1041–1048.

The ALLHAT Officers and Coordinators for the ALLHAT Collaborative Research Group. Major cardiovascular events in hypertensive patients randomized to doxazosin vs chlorthalidone: The Antihypertensive and Lipid-Lowering Treatment to Prevent Heart Attack Trial (ALLHAT). *JAMA.* 2000;283:1967–1975.

Tso M, Abrams G, Jampol L. Hypertensive retinopathy, choroidopathy, and optic neuropathy: A clinical and pathophysiological approach to classification. In: Singerman LJ, Jampol LM, eds. *Retinal and Choroidal Manifestations of Systemic Disease.* Baltimore: Williams & Wilkins; 1991:79–127.

Williams HW. The eye in malignant hypertension. *Clin Eye Vision Care.* 1990;2:172–185.

Chapter 3

ARTERIOSCLEROSIS

Mitchell W. Dul

Arteriosclerosis is a general term defined as the thickening or hardening of the artery wall and loss of elasticity of the artery wall. In general, there are two important variations of arteriosclerosis: atherosclerosis and arteriolosclerosis. Atherosclerosis is a slow, mostly silent, progressive inflammation of the intima of large- and medium-sized arteries. It results from an accumulation of lipids and hard, collagen-rich sclerotic tissue in the arterial wall; hence the name characterizes the component parts, atherosis and sclerosis. Arteriolosclerosis is characterized by hyalinization of the walls of small arteries and arterioles and is implicated in nephrosclerosis and the intraocular manifestations of arteriosclerosis. In the eye, arteriolosclerosis negatively affects retinal vessel autoregulation, exacerbates retinal ischemic disease, and contributes to occlusions of retinal veins.

Thickening of the arterial wall due to arteriosclerosis leads to a progressive narrowing of the lumen that may prevent an adequate supply of blood from reaching various tissues. Clinical manifestations of lumen narrowing are ischemia or ischemic atrophy. Atherosclerosis also may cause abrupt occlusion of a vessel lumen as a result of thrombus formation or an internal hemorrhage in an atheromatous plaque. The fibrin–platelet covering of an atherosclerotic plaque may become compromised and expose its cholesterol-rich contents to the arterial circulation. Emboli may then travel downstream, potentially occluding the arterial supply of a tissue. The loss of elasticity of arterial walls, another result of arteriosclerosis, increases peripheral resistance and arterial pressure. Damage to the vessel itself can lead to formation of an aneurysm or frank rupture. Arteriosclerosis commonly occurs in the arteries of the heart, brain, abdomen, and legs, with clinical manifestations varying by the artery or end organ affected.

EPIDEMIOLOGY

Systemic

Atherosclerosis is pervasive in the Western world. It is the leading cause of heart disease, accounting for 90% of all cases of coronary artery disease (CAD). Approximately 50% of all deaths in the United States are attributable to atherosclerosis-related disease, primarily myocardial infarction, which accounts for 20 to 25% of deaths. It is a slowly progressive disease beginning in adolescence, and the majority of the population has some evidence of atherosclerosis by the fifth decade of life.

Ocular

The prevalence of arteriolosclerosis in the ocular vasculature is difficult to assess because the clinical sign, widening of the arterial reflex, also occurs as a normal age-related change in the retinal vasculature. However, it appears to be more prevalent and more severe in patients with long-standing hypertension and/or diabetes irrespective of age.

PATHOPHYSIOLOGY/DISEASE PROCESS

The pathogenesis of atherosclerosis is not completely understood. Specific risk factors, including hypertension, hypercholesterolemia, diabetes, smoking, age, gender, and genetic predisposition, contribute to its development. The evidence for a link between serum lipid levels and atherosclerosis is compelling: most normal species fed cholesterol-rich diets will develop atherosclerosis. Chronic injury to the endothelium is also considered an early initiator of atherosclerosis. According to the response to injury hypothesis, an injury to the endothelium can result from prolonged exposure to subtle abuse such as turbulent blood flow created at a bifurcation; the insult to the endothelium is compounded by risk factors such as hypertension, dyslipidemia, diabetes, and smoking. It is not known how these risk factors influence the development and progression of atherosclerosis, only that they influence the extent of disease (percentage of artery surface containing mature plaques). It is also not known whether hypercholesterolemia or endothelial injury is the precipitating factor for initiating the atherosclerotic process.

Types of Atherosclerotic Lesions

Atherosclerosis, which begins with the accumulation of lipids, progresses slowly through characteristic stages (Figure 3–1). The stages correspond to six lesion types that are characterized according to their form and morphology or structure. Lesion types I to IV grow mainly by accumulation of lipids. Lesion type V has a high fibrous component, which helps to stabilize it, whereas lesion type VI does not, making it unstable and likely to rupture. The earliest lesions of atherosclerosis precede the more advanced lesions, but they do not necessarily progress to advanced lesions. Progression of a lesion tends to require a further stimulus, such as continued lipid accumulation.

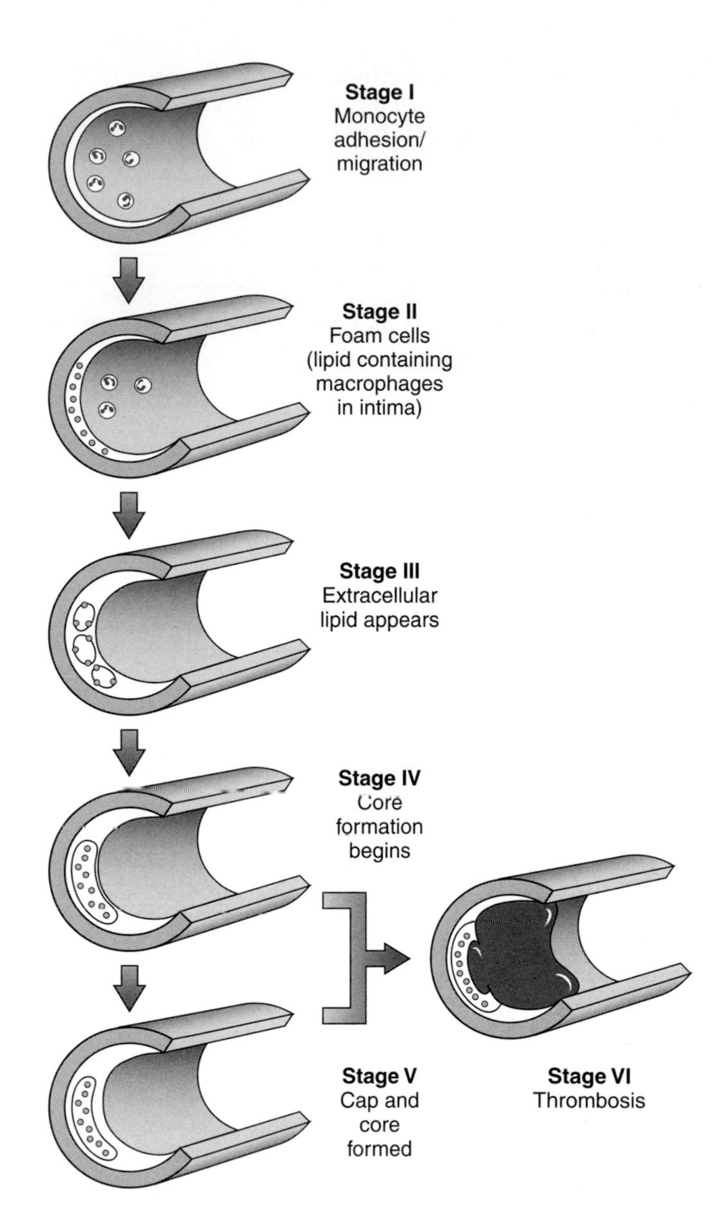

Figure 3–1. Schema of the American Heart Association Plaque Nomenclature that provides both the nomenclature and the proposed evolutionary progression of atherosclerotic plaques. (*Reprinted with permission from Davies MJ.* Atlas of Coronary Artery Disease. *Philadelphia: Lippincott-Raven; 1999:24–61.*)

> Early or initial atherosclerotic lesions frequently occur in children.

Early or initial atherosclerotic lesions (type I) frequently occur in children and may represent adaptive intimal thickening (normal physiologic adaptation to local changes in blood flow or arterial wall tension) at vessel bifurcations. There is microscopically detectable accumulation of lipids in the intima of the artery wall. These lesions may progress to precursor atherosclerotic lesions (type II) that often are visible fatty streaks with intracellular accumulation of lipids. Type II lesions have foam cells in stratified layers, and smooth muscle cells in the intima contain lipid deposits. Mechanical forces on the artery wall determine whether a type II lesion progresses to an intermediate lesion or preatheroma (type III). The type III lesion serves as a bridge between precursor lesions and more advanced ones and contains small pools of lipid that disrupt smooth muscle cells. The first of the advanced lesions, an atheroma (type IV), contains a lipid core and disrupts the organization of the intimal layer. Another advanced lesion is the fibrous plaque or fibroatheroma (type V) that is characterized by a fibrous tissue cover with smooth muscle cells and collagen over the lipid core. It may affect vessel wall layers other than the intima (e.g., adventitia, media), and it may be susceptible to developing fissures. The complicated lesion (type VI) is a fibrous plaque that has fissured and may have hemorrhaged or have thrombotic deposits in the surface. These lesions are responsible for the morbidity and mortality associated with atherosclerosis.

The Atherosclerotic Process

The endothelium is permeable to all plasma lipoproteins and selectively allows passage of nutrients into the arterial wall. Chronic endothelial injury makes the arterial wall more permeable to lipoproteins, primarily cholesterol-rich low-density lipoprotein (LDL), which enter and accumulate in the intima of the artery. Once accumulated in the intima, endothelial cells oxidize LDL particles, which is the start of an inflammatory process. In response, monocytes circulating in the blood are recruited to the site of inflammation (where there is oxidized LDL), attach to the endothelium, and enter the arterial wall. Once in the vessel wall, monocytes are converted into macrophages that enter the intima and take up the oxidized LDL particles. The lipid-laden macrophages grow in size to become foam cells, which accumulate to form a fatty streak, the beginning of the crescent-shaped lesion characteristic of atherosclerosis. A fatty streak, however, does not obstruct blood flow.

As the inflammatory atherosclerotic process continues, the once smooth endothelial surface becomes bumpy and irregular in shape. Circulating platelets are attracted to the lesion site where they aggregate, adhere to the surface, and become activated. The activated platelets, endothelial cells, and macrophages release growth factors that cause smooth muscle cells to migrate and proliferate, eventually forming an extracellular matrix. This proliferative response is the body's attempt to heal the atherosclerotic lesion. If the proliferative response is predominant, the lesion may not progress. If the accumulation of lipids and macrophages is more predominant than the proliferative response, the lesion progresses to the first of the advanced atherosclerotic lesions, an atheroma (derived from the Greek word for gruel, *athere*). The atheroma contains a soft lipid core resembling porridge or gruel (created when foam cells in the center of the lesion die) covered by a fibrous cap containing smooth muscle cells and collagen. If the cap is dense and fibrous with hard collagen-rich tissue, the plaque may be at low risk of rupturing and of causing an acute clinical event; this is a so-called *stable plaque.*

Atheromas that have only a thin fibrous cap separating them from the arterial lumen are considered vulnerable or unstable, as they are likely to fissure or rupture at the shoulders (ends of the crescent shape). When a plaque ruptures, its atheromatous material spills into the blood where it is exposed to coagulation substances (e.g., fibrin), which leads to the development of a blood clot or thrombus. Local risk factors for thrombus formation include degree of plaque disruption and stenosis, more lipid-rich plaque, recurrent thrombus, and vasoconstriction. Systemic risk factors for thrombus formation may include smoking, stress, the renin–angiotensin system, high cholesterol levels, diabetes, and impaired fibrinolysis. A complicated lesion (one that has ruptured) is responsible for symptoms and acute clinical events. The thrombus also can be incorporated into the lesion (healed lesion) and covered over with a layer of endothelial cells. The process of rupture, thrombus formation, and healing can be repeated causing growth of the complicated lesion into a stenotic or fibrotic lesion. Fibrotic lesions are not prone to rupture; therefore, they do not cause clinical symptoms until the vessel lumen is completely occluded. Myocardial infarction (MI) is a clinical manifestation of a complete occlusion in a coronary artery.

Systemic

Atherosclerosis generally affects large and medium-sized muscular arteries (coronary artery, carotid artery, and arteries of the lower extremities) and large elastic arteries (aorta and iliac arteries). Early in the disease process, atherosclerotic plaques are widely distributed in relatively predictable locations throughout the circulatory system. In descending order, atherosclerotic plaques are most likely to appear in the following arteries: abdominal aorta (especially near the ostia of its major branches), coronary arteries (especially within the first 6 cm), popliteal arteries (supply blood to the calf and foot), descending thoracic aorta, internal carotid arteries, and the vessels of the circle of Willis. Affected less often are the vessels of the upper extremities and the mesenteric and renal arteries (except at their ostia). As atherosclerosis progresses, the plaques encroach on the lumen of the vessel and weaken it, setting the stage for the subsequent formation of an aneurysm, a complication of atherosclerosis. Other complications of atherosclerosis noted previously include calcification, thrombus formation, hemorrhage, and ulceration (fissuring).

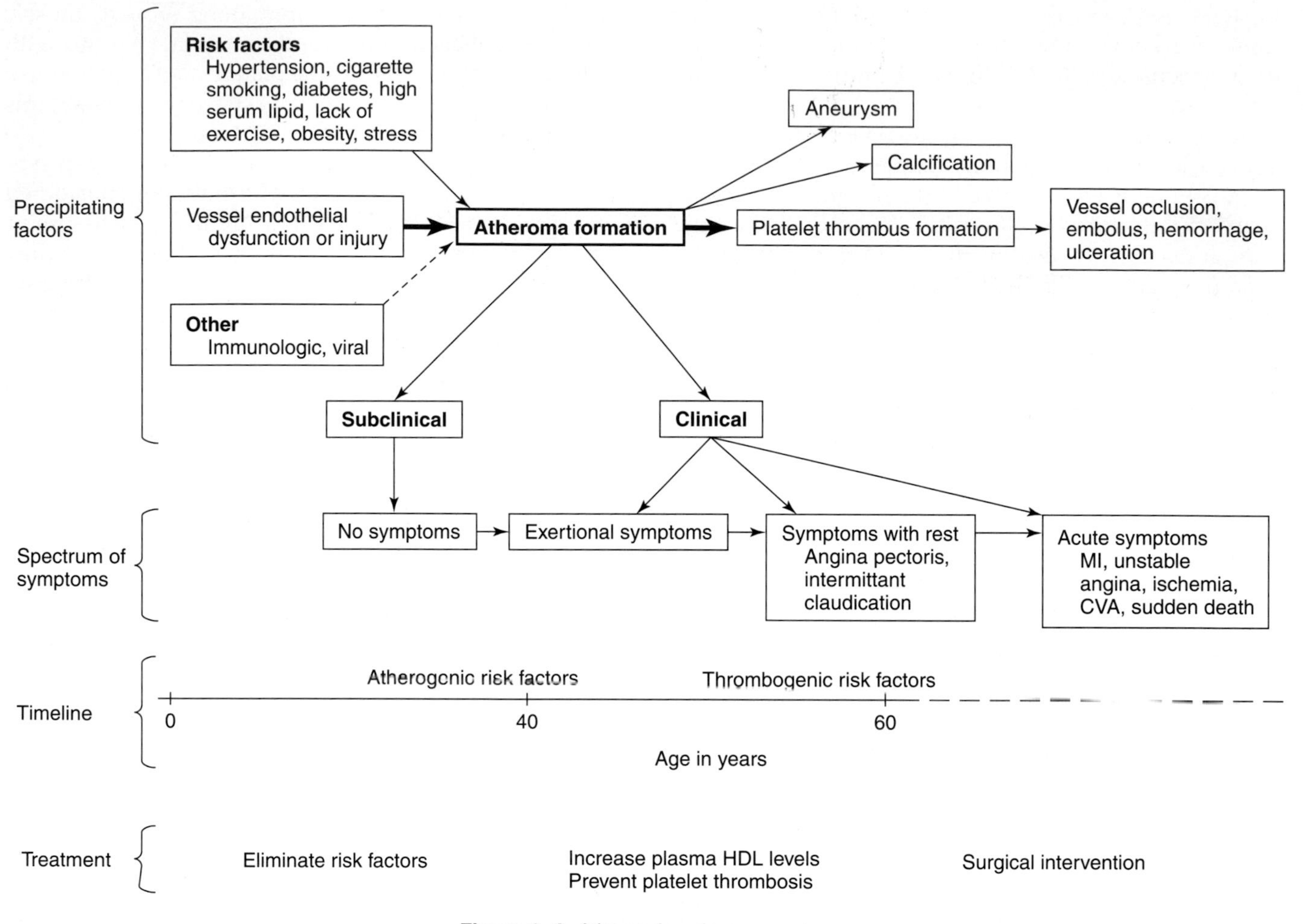

Figure 3–2. Atherosclerosis progression.

Since the progression of atherosclerosis is slow and chronic (Figure 3–2), patients may remain asymptomatic for a prolonged period of time. With continued progression, patients may be symptomatic only on exertion when the oxygen demands of the tissues surpass the supply of oxygenated blood being transported through narrowed vessels. Atherosclerotic plaques that progress to unstable forms are likely to fissure or rupture, leading to thrombosis. Plaques may undergo many cycles of rupture, thrombus formation, and sealing off of thrombus (healing) during the normal course of their natural history. This type of plaque (complicated) is known to be associated with unstable angina, acute myocardial infarction, and sudden ischemic death. Acute clinical symptoms generally are a consequence of plaque rupture with subsequent occlusive thrombus formation.

Arterial spasm also may play a role in acute ischemic events. Vasoactive mediators from endogenous and exogenous sources (e.g., cold exposure, emotional stress, cigarette smoking, vasoconstrictive drugs) are capable of producing vessel spasm sufficient to reduce blood flow. As the severity of the stenosis increases, the degree of vasomotor tone necessary to yield a clinically significant event decreases. Eccentric atherosclerotic plaques pose a greater risk in the presence of vasospasm than do concentric plaques in which the intimal disease causes more even scarring, atrophy, and thinning of the adjacent media. Eccentric plaques not only show a thinned media adjacent to the plaque but also a portion of the media adjacent to intima free of disease that is relatively normal and vasoactive (Figure 3–3). In patients who die as a direct result of coronary artery disease, approximately 70% of coronary arteries have eccentric atheromas. The extent of atherosclerotic disease may be underestimated angiographically when eccentric plaques are present.

The clinical manifestations of atherosclerotic disease vary with the degree of compromise in blood flow, the oxygen demands of the target organ(s), and the location of the plaque. Symptoms usually develop when the oxygen demands of a particular organ are not met. Patients with occlusive atherosclerotic disease of the aorta or the iliac, femoral, and popliteal arteries gen-

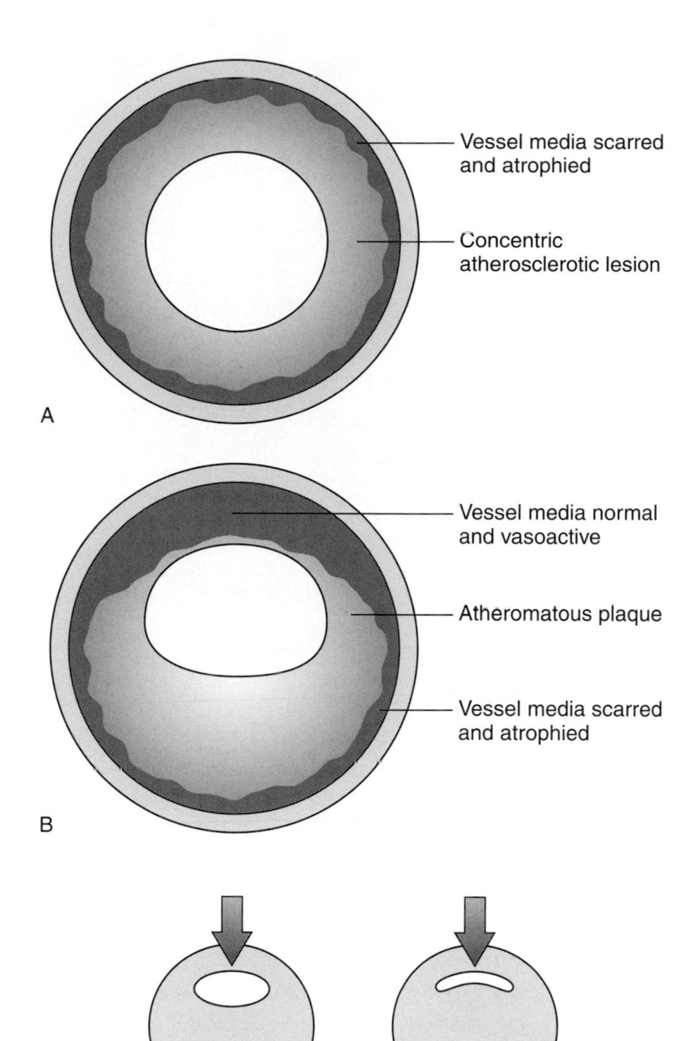

Figure 3–3. Concentric and eccentric atheroma. **A.** Concentric plaque. Concentric intimal disease; the adjacent media is thinned due to scarring and atrophy. **B.** Eccentric plaque. Eccentric intimal disease. The media adjacent to the plaque is similar to the media in concentric plaque. Media adjacent to normal intima is normal and vasoactive. **C.** Arterial spasm, particularly in the presence of eccentrically located plaques, is able to significantly reduce blood flow and may play a role in acute ischemic events. Vasoactive mediators are cold temperatures, emotional stress, cigarette smoking, and vasoconstrictive drugs.

erally present with complaints of intermittent claudication in the buttocks, thighs, knees, calves, or feet depending on the vessel occluded. The systemic and ocular manifestations of atherosclerosis are summarized in Table 3–1, and those of the cerebrovascular system are detailed in Chapter 5.

Atherosclerotic Heart Disease

The most common clinical consequences of atherosclerotic heart disease are angina pectoris (stable and unstable), acute myocardial infarction, and sudden death. Unfortunately, sudden death is the first clinical manifestation of atherosclerotic heart disease in approximately 25% of patients. Angina pectoris, defined as chest discomfort associated with myocardial ischemia, affects more than 5 million people in the United States. Although most cases are secondary to atherosclerotic heart disease, other causes of angina (literally "strangling" in the chest) include vasospasm, arteritis, and coronary dissection. Generally precipitated by emotional stress or physical exertion (especially lifting or fast-paced walking), angina often is described as a tightness or gripping sensation (as if someone were standing on the patient's chest), but not a sharp pain. It also has been described as indigestion, burning, or a vague discomfort. In the majority of cases (80 to 90%), the sensation is localized to the midsternum or immediately to the left of the sternum. Angina pain often radiates to the left shoulder and then down the arm, and it may radiate to the jaw and the back of

TABLE 3–1. SYSTEMIC AND OCULAR MANIFESTATIONS OF ARTERIOSCLEROSIS

Coronary Artery
- Location: Within first 6 cm
- Symptoms: Angina pectoris following stress or exertion, relieved by resting
- Signs: Significant elevation of both systolic and diastolic blood pressure; gallop rhythm; apical systolic murmur

Aorta/Iliac Artery
- Location: Just distal to the bifurcation (aorta), just proximal to the bifurcation of the common iliac
- Symptoms: Intermittent claudication (especially calf muscle)
- Signs: Possible bruit over aorta, iliac, or femoral artery

Femoral/Popliteal Artery
- Location: Distal portion of superficial femoral (common and deep generally patent)
- Symptoms: Intermittent claudication limited to calf/foot
- Signs: Affected area: hair loss, thinning of skin, decreased muscle mass, coolness to touch; good to fair femoral pulses (possible bruit); no popliteal or pedal pulse

Ocular
- Widening of the arterial reflex
- Copper-wire appearance of retinal arteries
- Silver-wire appearance of retinal arteries
- Loss of autoregulation of retinal arteries
- Contributing factor in ischemic retinal diseases
- Retinal vein or artery occlusion
- Atheromatous emboli (carotid) in retinal vasculature

> Sudden death is the first clinical manifestation of atherosclerotic heart disease in approximately 25% of all patients.

the neck. If the patient points to the source of pain with a single finger, the odds are it is not angina. Angina usually lasts only a few minutes and is alleviated by rest or sublingual nitroglycerin. Episodes of angina precipitated by anger or following a large meal may not resolve for 15 to 20 minutes.

A change in the usual pattern of angina (more frequent or severe, occurring at a lower level of exertion or at rest) is suggestive of unstable angina, which is less responsive to medication and of longer duration than stable angina. Unstable angina also is called *preinfarction angina* since it is associated with a high risk of subsequent myocardial infarction; within 3 months of onset, up to 20% of patients suffer an acute myocardial infarction with a mortality rate of 4 to 10%. In addition, approximately 50% of patients with unstable angina have multivessel disease and advanced or complicated atherosclerotic lesions. The most common cause of acute myocardial infarction is occlusive thrombosis of an atherosclerotic plaque. Chronic ischemic heart disease can lead to cardiac arrhythmias and congestive heart failure, which results in end-stage heart disease.

Many patients remain asymptomatic even when they have almost completely stenosed coronary arteries. These patients often have ischemic episodes known as *silent ischemia* that are undetected until a later time, such as after a symptomatic myocardial infarction or at autopsy following sudden death. Therefore, clinical symptoms, although providing some indication of the presence of atherosclerosis, may be a poor indicator of the extent of disease.

Ocular

The effects of arteriosclerosis on the eye are most significant when the disease affects the cerebral vascular system (producing a myriad of signs and symptoms, such as amaurosis fugax, retinal artery occlusion, and visual field loss).

Arteriolosclerosis results from a leakage of plasma components through the vessel endothelium. This process is presumably augmented by the chronic hemodynamic stresses of hypertension or the metabolic stresses of diabetes. The result is an irregular thickening of basement membrane with deposition of amorphous extracellular substances and smooth muscle cells within the vessel wall and collagenization of the intima and media. Histologically, the lesion appears homogeneous and pink with thickening of the arteriolar walls, loss of structural detail, and a narrowing of the vessel lumen. The descriptive term for this histologic presentation is *hyaline,* and the process is called *hyalinization* (Figures 3–4 and 3–5).

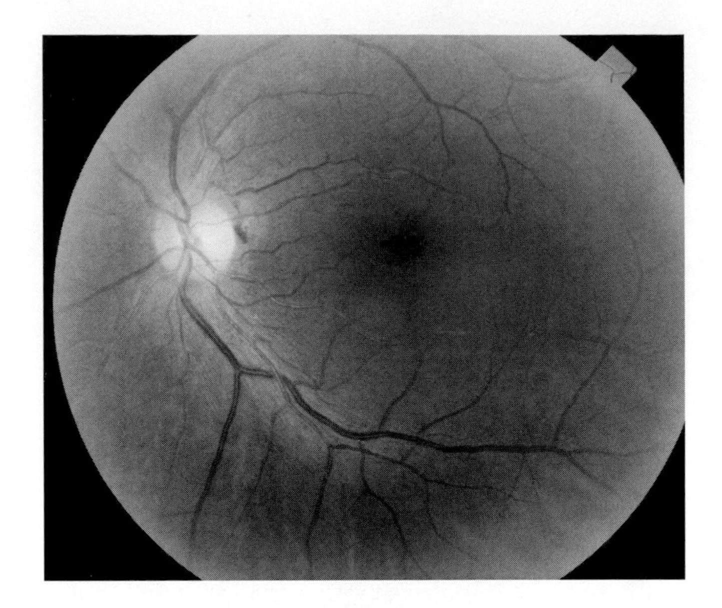

Figure 3–4. Hyalinization secondary to arteriolosclerosis.

The walls of normal retinal arteries are transparent, which allows the practitioner to view the column of blood within the vessel. The retinal arterial light reflex is produced by the reflection of light off this blood column that normally occupies the center one fifth of the width of the column. The progressive hyalinization of the vessel walls (as well as the normal deposition of basement membrane materials and other debris in the perivascular sheath) serves to make the vessel less transparent and the arterial light reflex appears to broaden. Previous clinical assessments of the degree of hyalinization in the retinal vasculature relied on estimations of the arterial reflex width. This approach offers poor

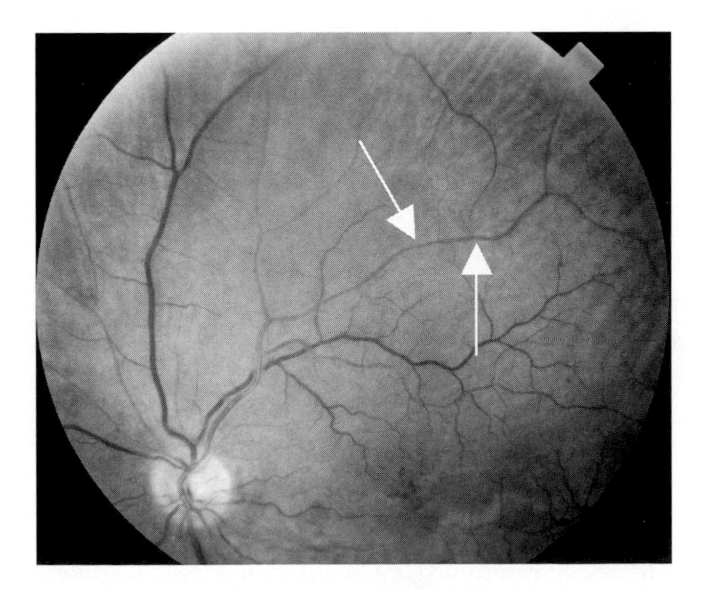

Figure 3–5. Hyalinization and sectorial sclerosis (arrows).

interobserver reliability, lacks specificity (because it includes normal age-related arterial changes), and provides little or no prognostic value. The blood column,

> Grading systems for arteriolosclerotic eye findings offer poor interobserver reliability, lack specificity (because it includes normal age-related changes), and provide little or no prognostic value.

viewed through the hyalinized vessel deposits, may appear copper in color (hence the term *copper-wire appearance*). Further hyalinization of the wall will cause a loss of vessel transparency and the appearance of a "silver wire," which is indicative of a severe loss in vessel transparency. Even so, fluorescein angiography may indicate that these vessels are patent. Complications associated with intraocular arteriolosclerosis include compromise of vessel autoregulation and vein occlusion (at arterial–venous crossings when the vessels share a common adventitial sheath), particularly if accompanied by high intraocular pressure. Intraocular arteriolosclerosis also may exacerbate retinal ischemic disease (hypoperfusion retinopathy).

> Complications of arteriolosclerotic eye disease include compromised vessel autoregulation and branch vein occlusion, and may exacerbate retinal ischemic disease.

Atheromas are rarely present in the intraocular retinal vessels. They may form where the artery enters into the optic nerve or at the lamina cribrosa, but this is relatively uncommon. Most of what could be confused for intraocular atheromas are actually emboli from either carotid or cardiac origins.

DIAGNOSIS

Systemic

The diagnosis of atherosclerosis is based on history, clinical presentation, physical examination, and laboratory test results (Table 3–2). For example, patients may relate during the history taking that they experience chest pain (angina) or leg cramps when walking (intermittent claudication), and during the physical examination, bruits may be heard over affected arteries and pulses may be weak or absent. Results of a blood chemistry may indicate elevated total cholesterol and triglyceride levels. The history, physical examination, and laboratory test results also may indicate the presence of other cardiovascular risk factors, such as hypertension, diabetes, and cigarette smoking, that may accelerate the progression of atherosclerosis. These evaluations are essential for making the diagnosis of atherosclerosis and for determining the need for additional testing.

TABLE 3–2. DIAGNOSIS OF ATHEROSCLEROSIS

History
Risk factor assessment
Clinical Presentation
Physical Examination
Laboratory Testing
Plasma lipid levels (including fasting LDL)
Electrocardiogram
Imaging Studies
Coronary
Exercise stress test (electrocardiogram, echocardiography)
Ultrasound (B-mode, Doppler)
Angiography (coronary, radionuclide, left ventricular)
Aorta/iliac
Ultrasound (Doppler)
Aortography
Femoral/popliteal
Ultrasound
Arteriogram

LDL = low density lipoprotein.

Specific imaging techniques are used to detect and assess atherosclerotic lesions and may be useful for developing a treatment strategy. Invasive imaging techniques include angiography, the standard by which other methods are measured, and thallium-201 perfusion testing. Noninvasive tests are exercise stress tests and ultrasound imaging techniques or echocardiography. Noninvasive tests provide beneficial diagnostic information, particularly in asymptomatic patients, and have the advantages of being generally available, not requiring the administration of contrast media, and not subjecting patients to radiation exposure.

Invasive Testing

Coronary angiography provides excellent resolution for defining coronary anatomy. However, it provides only a two-dimensional representation of the three-dimensional atherosclerotic process. Since it only visualizes the arterial lumen, not the vascular wall, angiography cannot detect early atherosclerotic lesions (types I, II, and III). It can detect type IV and V lesions since they change the contour of the lumen, and it can distinguish type IV and V lesions from type VI lesions. Angiography may underestimate the severity of stenosis if the atherosclerotic lesion is diffuse.

Therefore, angiography assists in determining the surgical procedure of choice (percutaneous transluminal coronary angioplasty [PTCA] or coronary artery bypass graft [CABG]) in presurgical patients. Coronary angiography has an overall mortality rate of 1 in 500 (Davis et al, 1979). As well as underestimating the degree of atherosclerotic disease, angiography provides a poor assessment of plaque fissuring, arterial dissections, composition of the plaque, depth of the plaque, presence of intracoronary thrombi, and degree of residual stenosis following surgical intervention. Eccentric plaques pose a particular problem, as angiography cannot localize the arterial lumen relative to the external arterial wall. The lumen may appear open on angiography (in two dimensions), but there may, in fact, be an atherosclerotic lesion at risk of rupturing or occluding the vessel. The limitations of angiography decrease its sensitivity and specificity for assessing intracoronary pathology.

The clinical utility of angiography is augmented by the use of invasive ultrasonography of the coronary arteries. Invasive or intravascular ultrasound, a relatively new procedure, differs from traditional ultrasound procedures in that the high-frequency transducer is placed internally close to the vessel wall rather than externally on the chest wall. Intravascular ultrasound can detect changes (from intimal thickening to atheroma) in arterial segments that are normal by angiography. The composition of a lesion can be determined by acoustic impedance rather than by histology. Intravascular ultrasound cannot study small or tortuous vessels.

Because of its limitations and the inherent risks associated with invasive procedures, angiography often is done after noninvasive tests have been performed to quantify disease severity and to determine whether the patient is a suitable candidate for surgery.

Noninvasive Testing

Exercise stress tests are beneficial in confirming the diagnosis of angina because the patient's symptoms and/or characteristic electrocardiographic patterns are elicited in a controlled environment. The test is less helpful in assessing asymptomatic patients because the rate of false-positives is high (often exceeding true-positives). Exercise stress testing is much more reliable when combined with the invasive procedure thallium-201 scintigraphy, as radionuclide uptake allows differentiation between hypoperfused and infarcted tissue. The combined test procedure generally identifies 75 to 90% of patients with significant coronary artery disease, and it provides insight into the subclinical limits of physical activity as well as the patient's response to therapeutic interventions (both medical and surgical).

Echocardiography, a group of ultrasound diagnostic procedures with the transducer placed externally on the chest wall, is used primarily to assess left ventricular function, which is an important prognostic indicator and a parameter for monitoring therapy. It records the structure of the heart and velocity of blood flow throughout a cardiac cycle, assessing patterns of cardiac chamber size and connection, wall thickness, wall motion, valve structure, and valve motion.

There are several types of echocardiography: B-mode, time-motion or M-mode, two-dimensional, and Doppler. M-mode echocardiography is the original type of ultrasound used for cardiac procedures, providing a one-dimensional view of target structures. Two-dimensional echocardiography is used with exercise to test myocardial performance because exercise is considered the best stress to the heart. Detection of a new or worsening wall motion abnormality is highly specific for determining the presence of coronary artery disease. B-mode ultrasound, which relies on differences in acoustic impedance in various tissues, images both the arterial wall and the lumen. The relatively high acoustic impedance of collagenous and calcified tissue provides for clear boundaries of the arterial collagenous tunica adventitia, collagenous atherosclerotic lesions, and the intima–lumen boundary. B-mode ultrasound may provide a means of assessing atherosclerotic plaques that are more likely to carry a high risk of an acute clinical event based on plaque morphology, location, or composition, and it may be helpful in assessing the effects of treatment. Doppler echocardiography, which adds sound to the echocardiographic picture, is similar to angiography in that it provides an image of the lumen of the vessel; however, it does not use an injected contrast medium, which may itself dilate an artery. Both B-mode and Doppler ultrasound are used to measure the severity of stenoses in peripheral vessels.

The limitations of echocardiography are that it is operator-dependent, images may be of poor quality in some patients, and complete quantitative data are not provided by all laboratories. It is, however, a safe, noninvasive procedure that does not place the patient at risk of an acute coronary event.

Ocular

The diagnosis of intraocular arteriolosclerosis is based on ophthalmoscopic findings (Table 3–1). The differential diagnosis of ocular findings is summarized in Table 3–3.

TABLE 3–3. DIFFERENTIAL DIAGNOSIS OF RETINAL ARTERIOLOSCLEROSIS

Normal age-related widening of the arterial reflex
Previous retinal inflammation (e.g., papillitis)
Previous retinal vascular ischemia (e.g., BRAO)
Congenital retinal vascular sheath
Lipemia retinalis

Reprinted with permission from Davies MJ. Atlas of Coronary Artery Disease. *Philadelphia: Lippincott-Raven; 1999:24–61.*

TREATMENT AND MANAGEMENT

Systemic

The treatment (Table 3–4) of atherosclerosis should address the control of associated risk factors, including lowering plasma lipid levels (particularly LDL cholesterol), cessation of cigarette smoking, and control of hypertension and diabetes if present, since modifying risk factors can prevent progression, and may promote regression, of atherosclerotic lesions. Treatment also is aimed at preventing a chronic disease process from precipitating acute events (antithrombotic therapy). The optimum approach to atherosclerosis, however, is prevention, rather than treatment, including lifestyle modifications, dietary intervention, and pharmacologic treatment of patients at increased risk of developing atherosclerosis.

Prevention

Epidemiologic evidence suggests that controlling risk factors such as smoking, elevated cholesterol levels, and elevated blood pressure and changes in lifestyle may retard progression of, and even reverse, atherosclerotic heart disease, as well as decrease the risk of mortality and morbidity. Epidemiologic studies indicate that each 1% reduction in serum cholesterol levels may lower the rate of coronary heart disease by as much as 3%. A program of stress management (eg, meditation, yoga), a purely vegetarian diet (with only 10% of calories from fat), moderate exercise, and support groups to assist in lifestyle changes has been advocated by Dean Ornish, Director of the Preventive Medicine Research Institute in Sausalito, California. This program was the first nonsurgical, nonpharmaceutical treatment for heart disease to qualify for insurance reimbursement.

> Each 1% reduction of serum cholesterol levels may lower the rate of coronary heart disease by as much as 3%.

The National Cholesterol Education Program (NCEP) guidelines (Table 3–5) recommend measuring fasting total serum cholesterol (and high-density

TABLE 3–4. PREVENTION AND TREATMENT OF ARTERIOSCLEROSIS

Prevention
Risk factor modification
- Lower total and LDL cholesterol
- Cigarette smoking cessation
- Control hypertension
- Control diabetes

Lifestyle modification
- Weight loss
- Modify diet (NCEP step I and II diets)
- Increase physical exercise

Treatment
Diet–pharmacologic therapy to lower total and LDL cholesterol
Acute coronary syndrome (angina, myocardial infarction)
- Angina
  - Sublingual nitroglycerin (acute episode)
  - Rest (acute episode)
  - Vasodilator (e.g., long-acting nitrate)
  - Beta-blocker
  - Calcium channel blocker
  - Aspirin (unstable angina)
  - Heparin (unstable angina)
  - Surgical procedure (PTCA, CABG)
- Myocardial infarction
  - Aspirin (acute and secondary prevention)
  - Reperfusion measures (acute: thrombolytic agent, PTCA)
  - Beta-blocker (acute and secondary prevention)
  - Nitroglycerin (acute)
  - ACE inhibitor (acute and secondary prevention)
  - Lipid-lowering therapy (secondary prevention)
  - Surgical procedure (PTCA, CABG)

Aorta/Iliac
- Endovascular
  - Balloon angioplasty
  - Atherectomy
- Prosthetic graft

Femoral/Popliteal
- Walking to develop collateral circulation
- Arterial graft
- Thromboendarterectomy
- Endovascular surgery

Ocular
- Monitor for secondary complications
- Maintain normal ocular pressure

Abbreviations: ACE = angiotensin-converting enzyme inhibitor; CABG = coronary artery bypass graft; LDL = Low-density lipoprotein; NCEP = National Cholesterol Education Program; PTCA = percutaneous transluminal coronary angiography.

TABLE 3–5. TREATMENT DECISIONS FOR LIPID-LOWERING THERAPY BASED ON LDL CHOLESTEROL LEVEL

Patient Characteristics	LDL Level for Therapy Initiation	Goal LDL Level
Dietary Therapy		
Without CHD and <2 risk factors	≥160 mg/dL (4.1 mmol/L)	<160 mg/dL (4.1 mmol/L)
Without CHD and ≥2 risk factors	≥130 mg/dL (3.4 mmol/L)	<130 mg/dL (3.4 mmol/L)
With CHD	>100 mg/dL (2.6 mmol/L)	≤100 mg/dL (2.6 mmol/L)
Drug Therapy		
Without CHD and <2 risk factors	≥190 mg/dL (4.9 mmol/L)	<160 mg/dL (4.1 mmol/L)
Without CHD and ≥2 risk factors	≥160 mg/dL (4.1 mmol/L)	<130 mg/dL (3.4 mmol/L)
With CHD	≥130 mg/dL (3.4 mmol/L)	≤100 mg/dL (2.6 mmol/L)

Abbreviations: CHD = coronary heart disease; LDL = low-density lipoprotein.

lipoprotein [HDL] cholesterol if accurate testing is available) in all adults 20 years of age and older at least once every 5 years. A total cholesterol level less than 200 mg/dL is considered desirable in adults without coronary heart disease; a level between 200 and 239 mg/dL is considered borderline high; and a level of more than 240 mg/dL is classified as high. An HDL cholesterol level less than 35 mg/dL increases the risk of coronary heart disease, whereas a level >60 mg/dL decreases the risk of coronary heart disease. Persons with a desirable or borderline high total cholesterol and HDL cholesterol <35 mg/dL are to be counseled on diet and risk factor modification and re-evaluated in 5 years (desirable total cholesterol level) or 1 to 2 years (borderline high level). Those with desirable or borderline high total cholesterol and HDL levels <35 mg/dL and those with high total cholesterol levels should have a lipoprotein analysis done.

Although epidemiologic reports from the National Institutes of Health suggest that the risk of coronary artery disease increases approximately 3% for every decrease of 1 mg/dL in HDL cholesterol less than 35 mg/dL independent of other risk factors, treatment recommendations are based on the LDL cholesterol level and coronary heart disease risk status because LDL cholesterol is more atherogenic (Table 3–4). For primary prevention (patients without evidence of coronary heart disease), dietary therapy (for at least 6 months) and increased exercise are recommended for patients at increased risk of coronary heart disease: those with an LDL cholesterol level of 130 to 159 mg/dL and who have two or more risk factors as well as those with an LDL cholesterol level >160 mg/dL. For secondary prevention (patients with clinical evidence of coronary or other atherosclerotic disease), the optimum LDL cholesterol level is 100 mg/dL, achieved either with dietary therapy (3 months) and exercise alone or combined with lipid-lowering therapy. The goal of both primary and secondary prevention is to lower LDL cholesterol to goal levels.

The major classes of lipid-lowering agents (Table 3–6) are bile acid sequestrants (cholestyramine, colestipol), nicotinic acid, 3-hydroxy-3-methylglutaryl-coenzyme A (HMG CoA) reductase inhibitors or statins (atorvastatin, lovastatin, pravastatin, simvastatin), fibric acid derivatives (clofibrate, gemfibrozil), probucol, and estrogen replacement (as adjunctive therapy in postmenopausal women). Bile acid sequestrants are both effective and safe for primary prevention in patients with moderately elevated levels of LDL cholesterol. Nicotinic acid lowers total cholesterol and triglyceride levels and raises HDL cholesterol levels, but side effects (e.g., flushing, itching, gastrointestinal disturbances, liver toxicity, hyperuricemia, hyperglycemia) limit its use in many patients. Fibric acid derivatives effectively lower triglyceride levels and, in some patients, modestly lower LDL cholesterol and raise HDL cholesterol levels. Probucol has only modest LDL cholesterol-lowering effects.

The statins have become the first-line treatment for lowering LDL cholesterol levels because they are more efficacious and have a more favorable safety profile than other classes of lipid-lowering agents. Since the publication of the NCEP guidelines, several large-scale clinical trials have demonstrated that statins substantially reduce both morbidity and mortality in patients with and without clinical evidence of coronary heart disease. These trials support the NCEP recommendations for adjusting cholesterol-lowering treatment based on the patient's absolute risk, and they confirm the benefit of cholesterol-lowering therapy for primary and secondary prevention of major cardiovascular events in high-risk patients. Based on these trials, the statins are indicated for treating hypercholesterolemia in patients with and without clinically evident coronary heart disease and in patients with prior myocardial infarction with normal cholesterol levels.

TABLE 3–6. OVERVIEW OF LIPID-LOWERING THERAPY

Parameter	Bile Acid Sequestrants	Nicotinic Acid	Statins	Fibric Acid Derivatives	Probucol
Lipid and lipoprotein effects	⇓ LDL 15–30% ⇑ HDL 3–5% ⇔/⇑ Triglycerides	⇓ LDL 10–25% ⇑ HDL 15–35% ⇓ Triglycerides 20–50%	⇓ LDL 20–40% ⇑ HDL 5–15% ⇓ Triglycerides 10–20%	⇓ LDL 10–15% ⇑ HDL 10–15% ⇓ Triglycerides 20–50%	⇓ LDL 5–15% ⇓ HDL 20–30% ⇔ Triglycerides
Major use	Lower LDL	Most lipid disorders	Lower LDL	Lower triglycerides	Lower CHD risk[a]
Reduce CHD risk	Yes	Yes	Yes	Yes (?)[b]	No data
Safe long term	Yes	Yes	Yes	Yes	No data
Major side effects	GI complaints, decrease absorption of other drugs	Flushing, hepatotoxicity, hyperglycemia, hyperuricemia, GI complaints	GI complaints	GI complaints, gallstones	GI complaints, QT interval prolongation

[a]No clearly defined role for probucol; reduction in CHD risk may be due to mechanisms other than cholesterol lowering.
[b]Data on reduction in mortality equivocal: some large studies show reduction in risk whereas others show increased mortality.
Abbreviations: CHD = coronary heart disease; GI = gastrointestinal; HDL = high-density lipoprotein; LDL = low-density lipoprotein.

Treatment

Medical. Diet, cholesterol-lowering therapy (primarily with a statin), and lifestyle modifications are the foundation for treating patients with atherosclerosis (Table 3–4). Other medical interventions are aimed at specific clinical manifestations of arteriosclerosis, particularly acute coronary syndrome. Because the goals of pharmacologic therapy for angina are to correct the imbalance between myocardial oxygen demand and supply by reducing oxygen demand and/or increasing coronary blood supply, therapy includes nitrates, beta-blockers, and calcium channel blockers. Nitrates reduce oxygen demand by relaxing vascular smooth muscle, causing peripheral venous pooling, which reduces systemic venous return, left ventricular end-diastolic pressure and volume, and left ventricular wall tension. They may improve coronary blood flow by causing vasodilation of coronary vessels, reversing or preventing coronary spasm, and enhancing collateral blood flow. Beta-blockers reduce oxygen demand by lowering heart rate, blood pressure, and myocardial contractility. Calcium channel blockers reduce oxygen demand and improve coronary blood flow by producing systemic arteriolar dilation, systemic venodilation, and reducing inotropism (muscle contractility), and they dilate coronary arteries and prevent spasm.

Aspirin and heparin are beneficial in patients with unstable angina to prevent progression to myocardial infarction and death. In addition, aspirin substantially reduces mortality in evolving acute myocardial infarction and protects against vascular events in patients with either acute or a history of myocardial infarction, patients with a history of stroke or transient cerebral ischemia, and patients with other vascular diseases. In acute myocardial infarction, the primary goal of early treatment is to limit the extent of infarction by instituting reperfusion therapy, either with a thrombolytic agent or percutaneous transluminal coronary angioplasty (PTCA). There is little evidence to support the use of heparin in patients who do not receive thrombolytic therapy. Patients with evolving acute myocardial infarction also receive a beta-blocker because beta-blockers reduce morbidity and mortality by limiting the extent of infarction, rate of reinfarction following thrombolytic therapy, and associated arrhythmias. Antiarrhythmics (except beta-blockers) are used acutely and long term only for severe, life-threatening arrhythmias. Calcium channel blockers have not been shown to reduce mortality in patients with acute myocardial infarction or as secondary prevention and may be harmful in some patients. Angiotensin-converting enzyme inhibitors administered early in the course of acute myocardial infarction reduce mortality, and long term, they reduce morbidity and mortality in patients with and without left ventricular dysfunction.

Surgical. In general, the indications for surgical intervention in otherwise healthy patients with coronary artery disease include the following: (1) failure of maximum medical therapy to relieve symptoms; (2) greater than 50% stenosis of the left main coronary artery (even in asymptomatic patients); (3) presence of three-vessel disease with moderate left ventricular dysfunction; (4) presence of unstable angina and continued ischemic episodes on exercise testing or monitoring despite medical therapy; and (5) previous heart attack and persistent symptoms or evidence of ischemia. The two most common surgical interventions in patients with coronary artery disease are PTCA and coronary artery bypass graft (CABG).

Percutaneous transluminal coronary angioplasty is a palliative procedure in which a balloon catheter, inserted via the femoral artery, is used to mechanically enlarge the lumen of a narrowed vessel by compressing plaque material remains. Approximately 30 to 40% of all patients with coronary artery disease are appropriate candidates for PTCA. Angioplasty is best suited for patients with single-vessel disease and angina pectoris of recent onset. It is less effective in patients with completely occluded arteries (approximately 50% success rate), diffuse disease, and restenosis, which may occur subsequent to PTCA (up to 40% of cases). The success rate with PTCA is influenced by many factors, including the extent of the patient's disease, the ability of the surgeon to obtain and accurately assess a presurgical image of the affected artery, and the experience of the surgeon. Angioplasty should be performed in a setting where open heart surgery is available should bypass surgery be immediately necessary (approximately 5% of cases).

Expansion of the balloon may cause a plaque to fracture at a weak point. If the fracture extends into the media of the artery, an arterial dissection may ensue, which is capable of occluding the vessel lumen. Catheters also may cause vasospasm by stimulating smooth muscle cells in the arterial media, an effect that may be minimized by administration of calcium channel blockers and intracoronary nitroglycerin. Vasovagal attacks (with bradycardia, hypotension, and possible loss of consciousness) also occur with enough regularity that intravenous atropine often is used as a routine presurgical medication. Although less invasive than coronary bypass surgery (and less expensive), the overall mortality rate with PTCA is approximately 1%. There are newer surgical catheter devices currently being used in the treatment of coronary atherosclerosis, but their success rates and long-term outcomes have yet to be determined.

CABG surgery involves grafting up to five segments of a vein (usually the saphenous vein) or preferably an artery from the aorta to a coronary artery past the locus of the obstruction. The internal mammary arteries generally are the vessels of choice due to the decreased long-term closure rate. Approximately 10 to 20% of grafts will close within the first 6 months, beyond which the annual failure rate is approximately 4%. If risk factors for atherosclerosis are not controlled following surgery, the risk of graft closure increases. Aspirin, used solely or in combination with dipyridamole, improves the overall failure rates of grafts.

Traditionally, the mortality rate associated with CABG in otherwise healthy patients was relatively low (1 to 3%). Mortality is higher in patients with preexisting left ventricular dysfunction, those over 70 years of age, and patients with significant concurrent noncardiac disease. In recent years, the mortality rate with CABG has increased to 5 to 10%, reflecting an increase in the numbers of high-risk and older patients who undergo a CABG procedure. If a repeat procedure is required, its success rate is generally less favorable.

Ocular

The treatment of intraocular arteriolosclerosis is limited to regular observation for complications of the disease (e.g., vein occlusion), proper monitoring, and maintenance of intraocular pressure. Concurrently, the patient should be treated systemically.

CONCLUSION

Arteriosclerosis, especially atherosclerosis, accounts for tremendous morbidity and mortality. In the United States, coronary heart disease is the leading cause of death in adults and accounts for 500,000 deaths each year. Patients with atherosclerosis may remain asymptomatic for decades or experience sudden death as the presenting sign. The goals of the practitioner are to identify patients at risk for atherosclerosis and to eliminate the risk factors before the onset of adverse clinical manifestations of the disease. In particular, each 1% reduction in serum cholesterol levels may lower the rate of coronary heart disease by as much as 3%. Although risk factor modification ideally should occur prior to the onset of symptoms, many patients do not seek medical care until such symptoms occur.

Atherosclerosis is a disease that is influenced, to a great extent, by the lifestyle of the patient. Poor dietary habits, high cholesterol levels, poor control of blood pressure, sedentary lifestyle, and cigarette smoking all contribute to atherosclerosis and its progression. Unless modified, risk factors continue to contribute to disease progression even with lipid-lowering therapy and/or surgical intervention. No amount of healthcare reform (or intervention) will be of benefit if patients do not contribute to their own health and well-being.

REFERENCES

Davies MJ. *Atlas of Coronary Artery Disease.* Philadelphia: Lippincott-Raven; 1999:24–61.

Davis K, Kennedy JW, Kemp HG, et al. Complications of coronary arteriography from the Collaborative Study of Coronary Artery Surgery (CASS). *Circulation.* 1979; 59:1105–1112.

Expert Panel on Detection, Evaluation, and Treatment of High Blood Cholesterol in Adults. Summary of the Second Report of the National Cholesterol Education Program (NCEP) Expert Panel on Detection, Evaluation, and Treatment of High Blood Cholesterol in Adults (Adult Treatment Panel II). *JAMA.* 1993;269:3015–3023.

Fuster V, ed. Progression-regression of atherogenesis: Molecular, cellular, and clinical bases. *Circulation.* 1992; 86(suppl):III-1–III-123.

Gomez CR. Carotid plaque morphology and risk for stroke. *Stroke.* 1990;21:148–151.

Grundy SM. Statin trials and goals of cholesterol-lowering therapy. *Circulation.* 1998;97:1436–1439.

National Cholesterol Education Program. Second Report of the Expert Panel on Detection, Evaluation, and Treatment of High Blood Cholesterol in Adults (Adult Treatment Panel II). *Circulation.* 1994;89:1329–1345.

Pearson TA, Heiss G, eds. Atherosclerosis: Quantitative imaging, risk factors, prevalence and change. *Circulation.* 1993;87(suppl):II-1–II-82.

Robbins SL, Cotran RS, Kumar V. *Pathologic Basis of Disease.* 3rd ed. Philadelphia: WB Saunders; 1984:506–518.

Ross R. The pathogenesis of atherosclerosis: A perspective for the 1990s. *Nature.* 1993;362:801–809.

Ryan TJ, Anderson JL, Antrman EM, et al. ACC/AHA Guidelines for the Management of Patients with Acute Myocardial Infarction: Executive summary. A report of the American College of Cardiology/American Heart Association Task Force on Practice Guidelines (Committee on Management of Acute Myocardial Infarction). *Circulation.* 1996;94:2341–2350.

Schroeder SA, Krupp MA, Tierney LM, McPhee SJ. *Current Medical Diagnosis and Treatment.* 30th ed. Norwalk, CT: Appleton and Lange; 1991:256–266, 316–320.

Sokolow M, McIlroy MB, Cheitlin MD. *Clinical Cardiology.* 5th ed. Norwalk, CT: Appleton and Lange; 1990:87–224, 333–436.

Stary HC, Chandler AB, Dinsmore RE, et al. A definition of advanced types of atherosclerotic lesions and a histological classification of atherosclerosis: A report from the Committee on Vascular Lesions of the Council of Arteriosclerosis, American Heart Association. *Circulation.* 1995; 92:1355–1374.

Stary HC, Chandler AB, Glagov S, et al. A definition of initial, fatty streak, and intermediate lesions of atherosclerosis: A report from the Committee on Vascular Lesions of the Council of Arteriosclerosis, American Heart Association. *Circulation.* 1994;89:2462–2478.

Tobis JM, Yock PG. *Intravascular Ultrasound Imaging.* New York: Churchill Livingstone; 1992.

Chapter 4

CARDIAC SOURCES OF RETINAL EMBOLI

Charles Haskes, Mitchell W. Dul

With improved diagnostic techniques, cardiogenic emboli have been increasingly recognized as a significant etiology of ischemic stroke and are clearly implicated in the genesis of retinal ocular disease. In recent years, atrial fibrillation has replaced disease of the mitral and aortic valves as the most common cause of emboli of cardiac origin. An increasing number of cardiac conditions have been identified as potential sources of cardiac embolism. Cardiac emboli, due to their relatively small size, often become lodged in the retinal and cerebral vasculature and are responsible for many cases of amaurosis fugax (transient monocular blindness), highly focal transient ischemic attacks, and retinal and cerebral arterial occlusions.

In the retinal vasculature, cardiogenic emboli can be symptomatic or asymptomatic and may sometimes be clinically differentiated from emboli of carotid origin. Clinical evidence suggesting their presence should prompt the eyecare practitioner to pursue a cardiovascular workup because prophylactic treatment with antithrombotic agents makes this one of the most preventable forms of ischemic cerebrovascular accidents.

EPIDEMIOLOGY

Systemic

Atrial fibrillation is the most common cause of emboli of cardiac origin. It accounts for nearly 50% of embolic phenomena originating from the heart. Approximately 20% of those patients have rheumatic valve disease as the cause of the atrial fibrillation, 70% have non-valvular atrial fibrillation (secondary to conditions such as hypertensive cardiovascular disease, chronic lung disease, congestive heart failure (CHF), and atrial septal defect), and the remaining 10% have no obvious structural heart disease (lone atrial fibrillation). The risk of emboli from atrial fibrillation increases with increasing patient age.

Valve disease is the second most common cause of cardiogenic emboli, accounting for approximately 20% of the cases. More than two-thirds of the patients are female. Until recently, it was believed that mitral and aortic valve disease most often occurred as a sequela of acute rheumatic fever. Recent widespread use of transesophageal echocardiography has led to the recognition of calcific valvular changes as a common cause of aortic valvular disease, namely aortic stenosis. When valvular disease is secondary to rheumatic fever, or its postinfectious sequela, the mitral valve is most often affected, followed by the aortic valve. Approximately 9 to 28% of patients with mitral valve stenosis produce emboli from calcific or thrombotic material. Approximately 30% of all cases of valvular infection result in embolization. Mitral valve prolapse occurs in up to 5% of the adult population. Patients with cardiogenic emboli have a worse prognosis than do patients with extracardiac sources of emboli.

Ocular

Ocular emboli of cardiac origin account for approximately 20% of all embolic retinal disease. In addition to atrial fibrillation and valve disease, other causes of emboli of cardiac origin are infectious endocarditis, cardiac tumors (myxomas), and acute myocardial infarction (MI) (emboli occur as a complication in 2 to 4% of these patients; Table 4–1). Another major source of retinal emboli is carotid artery disease. Less common sources of retinal emboli include tumor emboli from metastatic neoplasm, fat emboli from fractures of long bones, talc emboli from intravenous drug use, and air emboli from injections or trauma. Retinal emboli are even more likely to be of cardiac origin in younger patients, especially below the age of 50.

> Cardiac disease accounts for at least 20% of all retinal and cerebral emboli.

PATHOPHYSIOLOGY/DISEASE PROCESS

Systemic

Atrial Fibrillation

Atrial fibrillation is a common arrhythmia causing ineffective, irregular, and disorganized atrial contraction. The ventricular response is irregular and the first heart sound usually varies in intensity. It is found in 1% of people over the age of 65 and more than 5% of people over the age of 69. Atrial fibrillation may be caused by several cardiac diseases, but atrial fibrillation secondary to rheumatic heart disease is the most common cardiac disease associated with embolism (Table 4–2). Because of circulatory stasis and pooling of blood, a thrombus is formed in the left atrium or on the left atrial appendage. This thrombus then becomes a source for embolic material.

Valvular Disease

The heart valves function to prevent backflow of blood into the chambers or vessels of the heart. The tricuspid valve separates the right atrium and ventricle, the mitral valve separates the left atrium and ventricle,

TABLE 4–1. MAJOR SOURCES OF CARDIOGENIC EMBOLI

Mitral Valve
Mitral valve prolapse
Rheumatic mitral stenosis
Infectious endocarditis
Prosthetic valve

Aortic Valve
Infectious endocarditis
Calcific stenosis
Prosthetic valve

Left Atrium
Atrial fibrillation
Myxoma

Iatrogenic Emboli
Postcardiac catheterization
Prosthetic valves

Other Sources
Dilated cardiomyopathy (idiopathic, ischemic, valvular, toxic/crack cocaine use/alcohol use)
Paradoxical emboli (atrial septal defects, patent foramen ovale, ventricle septal defects)
Left ventricle (acute myocardial infarction)
Thrombus

TABLE 4–2. PATHOPHYSIOLOGY OF THE MAJOR DISEASES WHICH PRODUCE CARDIOGENIC EMBOLI

Atrial Fibrillation
Valvular atrial fibrillation
  Possible history of valvular heart disease, abnormal mitral or aortic valve function, or rheumatic heart disease
Nonvalvular Atrial Fibrillation
  Possible history of congestive heart failure, stroke, left atrial enlargement, treated systemic hypertension, or chronic lung disease

Mitral Stenosis
Thickened, less mobile valve
Increased atrial pressure
Atrial fibrillation (often develops)
Hyperplasia and hypertrophy of the pulmonary vessels
Pulmonary venous congestion
Right heart failure

Mitral Regurgitation
Left ventricular dilatation (chronic)
Increase in left ventricular wall thickness
Subsequent left atrial dilatation

Aortic Stenosis
Left ventricular hypertrophy
Increased left ventricular end-diastolic pressure
Decreased cardiac output
Pulmonary hypertension

Aortic Regurgitation
Left ventricular volume overload

Infectious Endocarditis
Infectious vegetations on the surface of damaged valves and local infection
Embolization of infected vegetation
Mitral regurgitation
Aortic regurgitation

Cardiac Tumors/Atrial Myxoma
Increased venous congestion
Right heart failure
Mitral valve blockage

and the aortic valve separates the left ventricle from the ascending aorta. Valve dysfunction may either be the result of failure of the valve to completely close, which results in the backflow of blood (regurgitation, insufficiency, or incompetence), or to completely open, which results in the impedance of blood flow (stenosis). These two disorders frequently occur concurrently in the same valve. Valvular stenosis or regurgitation generally occurs as a sequela of congenital anomalies (e.g., Marfan syndrome), infection or resultant post inflammatory scarring (e.g., acute rheumatic fever), autoimmune disease (e.g., systemic lupus erythematosus), or cardiac tumors (e.g., myxomas). Degenerative changes associated with aging (calcification) or infection (infectious endocarditis) may complicate the clinical appearance. Valvular disease is a source of emboli (e.g., calcific, platelet–fibrin, infectious, tumor) that may travel to the cerebrovascular or retinal vascular systems.

Rheumatic fever, an acute, recurrent inflammatory disease generally found in children, accounts for a significant percentage of valvular disease. Approximately 3% of patients having a pharyngeal infection with group A beta-hemolytic streptococci will develop rheumatic fever. Target tissues include cardiac smooth muscle, heart valves, and connective tissue. Postinflammatory scarring of valves (mainly mitral stenosis and/or regurgitation) occurs several decades after the resolution of the acute disease. Cardiac symptoms generally develop in the fourth and fifth decades. Many patients have no recollection of prior streptococcal infection.

Mitral stenosis is the resistance to flow through the mitral valve during diastolic filling of the left ventricle. The most common cause is rheumatic fever, where the leaflets and chordae tendineae are scarred and contracted. It can also result from congenital stenosis, thrombus formation, atrial myxoma, and calcification in the valve. Echocardiographic studies demonstrate thickened cusps and a narrowed opening into the left ventricle. The left atrial pressure must increase in order to maintain normal flow across the valve and normal cardiac output. This creates a pressure differential between the left atrium and ventricle during diastole. Predictable changes in cardiac structure and function ensue (Table 4–2). Fragmentation of calcific or thrombotic material introduces this embolic material to the systemic and retinal circulations.

Mitral regurgitation occurs when contraction of the left ventricle ejects blood into the left atrium as a result of abnormalities in the mitral valve apparatus. For many years, rheumatic fever was considered the most common etiology, but in recent years ischemic heart disease, degenerative changes, and mitral valve prolapse have become the predominant mechanisms and are probably the most common cause of mitral regurgitation in the adult population today. The compensatory mechanism of the left ventricle in chronic mitral regurgitation is dilatation to accommodate the increased left ventricular stroke volume necessary to maintain forward systemic stroke volume (Table 4–2).

In the mitral leaflet/valve prolapse syndrome, the abnormalities consist of thinning of the leaflet, elongation of the chordae, and dilatation of the mitral annulus. Abrupt deceleration of blood beneath the prolapsed mitral leaflet and the increased tension on the chordae produce a systolic click. Although many patients with mitral valve prolapse are asymptomatic, symptoms can develop, including palpatations, chest discomfort, fatigue, and anxiety. Sudden death is an extremely rare consequence.

Aortic stenosis is the obstruction of flow across the aortic valve during left ventricular systolic ejection. It is usually caused by degenerative calcification of the valve in the elderly or postinflammatory changes (e.g., following rheumatic fever). In general, aortic stenosis is either fibrous (causing fibrous contracture and shortening of the cusps) or calcific. Aortic valve stenosis increases the pressure inside the left ventricle because although the volume of the blood in the ventricles is essentially normal, it must pass through an impeded opening on the way to the aortic arch. This stimulates ventricular hypertrophy and other cardiac changes to meet the new demands (Table 4–2). A similar hypertrophy occurs when peripheral resistance is increased in atherosclerosis and hypertension. Angina pectoris is the most common clinical manifestation of aortic stenosis, occurring in 50 to 70% of affected individuals.

Aortic regurgitation is due to incompetence of the aortic valve, allowing the flow of blood from the systemic circulation into the left ventricle. It can result from intrinsic disease of the cusp or from diseases affecting the aorta. In the past, rheumatic fever and syphilis were major causes, but these diseases have diminished in frequency in recent years due to effective antimicrobials. Diseases of the connective tissue and anatomic abnormalities of the valve have become more frequent causes. Changes are also seen in longstanding vascular disorders such as hypertension and atherosclerosis and in other conditions such as rheumatoid arthritis, systemic lupus erythematosis, ankylosing spondylitis, and Reiter syndrome. The workload of the left ventricle is increased because of increased volume of blood in the chamber. Chronic aortic regurgitation gradually increases left ventricular end-diastolic volume because the chamber receives blood from the left atrium and the systemic circulation. This causes compensatory left ventricular wall hypertrophy (Table 4–2).

Infectious Endocarditis

Infectious endocarditis may be divided into two classifications: (1) subacute, which generally occurs in patients with pre-existing cardiac anomalies (e.g., degenerative heart disease, postrheumatic scarring, congenital anomaly), and (2) acute, which occurs primarily as a result of intravenous drug use, cardiovascular surgery, or very frequently prosthetic valve placement.

This potentially devastating infection is often associated with cardiac valvular disease. Incompetent valves cause blood flow regurgitation and stenotic valves cause jet streams of rapidly flowing blood. Hemodynamically, the blood surrounding the openings to these defective valves is relatively idle. This pooled blood provides an excellent medium for deposition of fibrin and aggregation of organisms. This promotes the development of infected vegetations on the surface of the damaged valve, which may then form embolic material. *Streptococcus viridans* (50%) and *Staphylococcus aureus* (20%) are the most common microbial agents implicated in the development of these infections (Table 4–2).

Despite advances in antibiotic treatment and surgical correction for valve lesions, there is an increase in the prevalence of foreign substances introduced to the systemic circulation (e.g., IV drug use, surgery). Replacement heart valves, catheters, pacemakers, and other devices all provide a potential port of entry for infectious agents. The vast majority of cases (90%) occur over the age of 20, with a peak incidence in the fourth to fifth decades. Nearly one quarter of new cases have had previous cardiovascular surgery.

Cardiac Tumors

Cardiac tumors can be a source of emboli to any part of the body. The most common benign primary tumor of the heart is a myxoma, which is usually found in the left atrium. Myxomas are generally slow growing, mobile, and surgically treatable. Signs and symptoms of cardiac myxoma correspond to their impact on normal heart and valve function (Table 4–2). Myxomas can form emboli and can result in sudden death from total obstruction of the mitral valve.

Ocular

Cardiac diseases produce several types of systemic and retinal emboli. The most common emboli that travel to the retinal arterial circulation are calcific emboli, platelet–fibrin emboli, and cholesterol emboli, all of which may be derived from the heart. The type of pathophysiologic change in the disease process will dictate which type of embolus will be observed. Atrial fibrillation, valvular disease, bacterial endocarditis, tumors, and ischemic lesions are the common sources of emboli from the heart. Cardiac emboli tend to lodge more frequently in the anterior circulation (i.e., carotid circulation) than the posterior circulation (i.e., vertebrobasilar circulation). The differential diagnosis of these emboli provides useful clinical information that assists in directing the clinician's attention to alternative origins (e.g., carotid, lungs).

> Atrial fibrillation is the most common cause of emboli of cardiac origin.

Ocular emboli of valvular origin are potentially sight-threatening because they can cause branch or central retinal artery occlusions. In general, emboli originating from the cardiac valves are relatively small in size. When introduced to the systemic circulation, these patients with these emboli often present with episodes of transient monocular blindness (amaurosis fugax) or with a highly focal transient ischemic attack. The left atrium and ventricle are sources for larger emboli (dislodged tumors, thrombus) that often produce branch artery syndromes. Therefore, oftentimes it will be noted that a patient with atrial fibrillation will present with a branch retinal artery occlusion or a cortical branch artery syndrome (i.e., especially homonymous hemianopsia and Wernicke aphasia).

DIAGNOSIS

Systemic

Patient History and Physical Examination

Patient history and physical examination may reveal signs and symptoms characteristic of heart diseases that yield emboli (Table 4–3). The patient should be questioned regarding past history of rheumatic fever, congenital disorders, infectious diseases, past drug use, myocardial infarction, and cardiac surgery. The most common symptoms of atrial fibrillation are syncope and fatigue. The most common symptom of mitral valve stenosis (in approximately 80% of all patients) is shortness of breath on exertion. Many patients with mitral regurgitation are asymptomatic. Detection of aortic stenosis in a patient under the age of 30 suggests a congenital stenotic aortic valve as the etiology; otherwise, degenerative calcification of the cusps of the aortic valve and rheumatic disease are the most common causes. The diagnosis of infectious endocarditis can be clinically challenging. The most common pre-

TABLE 4–3. DIAGNOSIS OF CARDIAC DISEASES WHICH PRODUCE RETINAL EMBOLI

Disease	Patient Signs/Symptoms	Physical Exam	Diagnostic Imaging (echo, ECG, x-ray)
Atrial fibrillation	Syncope; fatigue; angina; anxiety; palpitations; TIA	Excessive ventricular rate; first heart sound varies in intensity	Thrombus of left atrium or atrial appendage; aortic atherosclerotic plaque; left atrial enlargement; disorganized atrial activity
Mitral stenosis	Dyspnea on exertion most common; fatigue; palpitations; CVA from embolus	Distended neck veins; accentuated first heart sound or diastolic rumble	Thickened, less mobile valve; thickened chordae tendinae; narrowed orifice at tip of valve leaflets; often atrial fibrillation
Mitral regurgitation	Often asymptomatic for many years; chest pain; syncope; palpitations; fatigue; dyspnea; orthostatic hypotension	Peripheral edema; systolic click and apical murmur in mitral valve prolapse	Enlarged left atrium; excessive left atrial and ventricular wall motion; posterior motion of mitral leaflets; atrial arrhythmias develop, especially atrial fibrillation
Aortic stenosis	Symptoms usually occur late, when valve size reduced; angina; syncope; palpitations; fatigue	Delayed upstroke of peripheral pulse; systolic murmur; ejection click after first heart sound	Thickened aortic valve leaflets; less than normal leaflet separation; left ventricular hypertrophy; aortic valve often calcified
Aortic regurgitation	Fatigue; dyspnea; edema	Left ventricular volume overload	Echo from aortic valve leaflets noncontributory in diagnosis; left ventricular hypertrophy and dilatation; aortic dilatation; bundle block
Infective endocarditis	Fever of 1–2 weeks duration or longer; heart murmur; non-specific complaints of coughing, weight loss, diarrhea, malaise	Neurologic disturbances; fever; fatigue	Presence of vegetations; valve dysfunction secondary to vegetations
Cardiac tumors/ myxoma	Dyspnea; chest pain; fever	Mobility of tumor causes changes in the sound of murmur	Multiple dense echoes adjacent to mitral valve leaflet in diastole

senting sign is a fever of at least 1- to 2-week duration and a heart murmur (present in 90 to 95% of patients). In the elderly, fever may not be present. The longer the disease is left untreated, the greater the risk of embolization. Cardiac tumors often present with symptoms that may be confused with infectious endocarditis. The physical examination should include chest and heart auscultation and postural studies.

Diagnostic Imaging

Even though the patient history and physical exam yield the most important information on those with suspected cardiac disease, echocardiography also provides valuable information. Echocardiography is a noninvasive method of cardiac examination that provides direct information about cardiac anatomy and physiology. It provides useful diagnostic and functional information. Traditionally, transthoracic echocardiography (TTE) had been the most common form of echocardiography. In recent years, transesophageal echocardiography (TEE), through improved resolution, has elevated the role of echocardiography in diagnosing cardiac abnormalities. In contrast to TTE, the transesophageal approach frequently shows abnormalities even in the absence of clinical signs. Echocardiography, in general, is useful in detecting a direct source of emboli (e.g., thrombus from atrial fibrillation, myxoma, or vegetation), in detecting a condition with a known risk of producing emboli (e.g., mitral stenosis and other valvular diseases), and investigating the risk in a condition known to be associated with emboli (e.g., atrial fibrillation; Table 4–3). Further indications for echocardiography are ocular and/or ischemic events (e.g., transient weakness in arms or legs), chest pain, palpitations, dyspnea, and syncope. In addition, amaurosis fugax or retinal emboli in a patient under age 50 is also an indication for echocardiography (due to its increased probability of cardiac origins).

> Retinal emboli or amaurosis fugax in the younger patient (below age 50) is more likely to be of cardiac origin. These are indications for echocardiography in this age group.

Despite the diagnostic value of echocardiography in the assessment of valve disease, diagnosis generally should not be made based on abnormalities uncovered in a single test, especially if the patient is asymptomatic and otherwise normal. The electrocardiogram (ECG) and chest x-ray are two important procedures to consider in addition to echocardiography (Table 4–3).

Cardiac catheterization is generally reserved as a preoperative study, but provides useful information regarding the differential diagnosis of valve disease, including the extent to which the valves are damaged and the likelihood of a favorable surgical outcome. Blood culture and sensitivity studies provide the backbone for diagnosis and subsequent antibiotic treatment for infective endocarditis.

It is of extreme importance to rule out other conditions, which may produce signs and symptoms similar to cardiac diseases (Table 4–4). Some of these other conditions occur at least as frequently and a thorough history will often differentiate them. Occasionally, further blood work and/or imaging studies will be necessary for definitive diagnosis.

Ocular

In the eye, cardiogenic emboli may be difficult to differentiate from those of other origins (Tables 4–5 and 4–6). Emboli from the carotid artery (usually cholesterol) are most often mistaken for those of cardiac origin, especially from the valves. In general, however, carotid emboli are typically yellow-golden in color, refractile, smaller, often multiple, located at branch retinal artery bifurcations, and do not permanently affect blood flow. Cardiac emboli of valvular origin tend to be whiter and larger and are therefore more likely to be located in the central retinal artery prior to its branching. As such, these emboli are also more likely to cause a permanent retinal artery occlusion (Figures 4–1, 4–2, and 4–3). It is important to remember that certain types of emboli (ie, platelet–fibrin) are common to both sources, and it may therefore be more difficult to determine the source of the emboli on clinical examination alone. Of additional importance is the fact that emboli of thrombus material from atrial fibrillation will probably be noticed at least as frequently in the retina as the above-mentioned chalky-white calcific emboli.

> Without proper workup and referral, it may be difficult to determine whether a retinal embolus is of cardiac or carotid origin because they may both produce emboli of the same material.

TABLE 4–4. DIFFERENTIAL DIAGNOSIS OF CARDIAC DISEASES

Noncardiac Disorders That Must Be Ruled Out:
Chronic obstructive pulmonary disease (shortness of breath)
Exercise-induced asthma (shortness of breath on exertion)
Posterior circulation (vertebrobasilar) ischemia (generalized fatigue/weakness)
Positional vertigo (dizziness with change in posture)
Orthostatic hypotension (weakness with change in posture)
Central nervous system infiltration by inflammatory disorders (may produce similar neurologic disturbances as in infectious endocarditis)
Lymphoma (may produce persistent fever and fatigue as in infectious endocarditis)

Other Cardiac Disorders That Must Be Ruled Out:
Congestive heart failure
Myocardial infarction (can also produce emboli by causing cardiac damage)

TREATMENT AND MANAGEMENT

Systemic

Atrial Fibrillation

If atrial fibrillation is acute, a precipitaing factor such as fever, pneumonia, alcoholic intoxication, pulmonary emboli, congestive heart failure, or pericarditis should be sought. Treatment should be directed toward the primary abnormality. In addition, slowing of the ventricular rate becomes the initial treatment goal. This is done by slowing the conduction within the atrioventricular (AV) node (Table 4–7). Chronic treatment for atrial fibrillation with an anticoagulant is always needed to decrease the risk of embolization once sinus rhythm is restored.

Valvular Disease

Because medical management of *mitral stenosis* cannot reduce obstruction through the valve, efforts are directed at prevention of recurrent rheumatic fever and bacterial endocarditis. Rheumatic fever antibiotic prophylaxis should continue until 35 years of age (Table 4–7). Systemic embolization requires anticoagulation

TABLE 4–5. DIAGNOSIS OF RETINAL EMBOLI OF CARDIAC ORIGIN

Source/Cause of Embolus	Characteristics of Embolic Phenomena
Atrial fibrillation	Most common cause of cardiogenic emboli Source of embolus is thrombus within atrium Often a history of TIA Embolus often transported during activity More common in atrial fibrillation secondary to valvular disease Usually associated with atherosclerotic or rheumatic heart/valvular disease
Stenotic valves	Platelet–fibrin or calcific emboli noted in retina Usually secondary to mitral and aortic stenosis Often caused by rheumatic fever or calcific changes in the elderly The calcific embolus will usually be lodged in a branch or central retinal artery and be associated with a branch or central retinal artery occlusion
Incompetent valves	Often a calcific embolus Usually secondary to mitral and aortic regurgitation Often a history of ischemic heart disease and myocardial infarction, which may produce calcific valvular changes
Mitral valve/leaflet prolapse	Emboli may be from either a thrombus or of platelet–fibrin material
Infectious endocarditis	20–30% of these patients will produce emboli Aortic valve is most common source of emboli *Streptococcus* and *Staphylococcus* are the most common responsible organisms Embolus is often at the center of a retinal hemorrhage (Roth spot) Embolus is often composed of organisms mixed with inflammatory cells May cause branch or central retinal artery occlusion May be associated with conjunctival petechiae, cranial nerve III, IV, or VI dysfunction, or diplopia
Cardiac tumor/atrial myxoma	Rare, but treatable cause of emboli May be noted at any age Embolus is of platelet–fibrin material and/or tumor fragments Some myxomas are inherited May be family history of embolic phenomenon Usually arise from endocardium of left atrium Patient often has neurologic and visual symptoms May cause branch or central retinal artery occlusion, choroidal infarction, and anterior ischemic optic neuropathy
Iatrogenic causes of emboli	Retinal emboli noted after cardiac surgery, angioplasty, and coronary artery bypass grafting May be due to embolization of cholesterol, platelets, fibrin, foreign material, fragments of thrombus, or portions of a calcified valve Patients often complain of dimming of vision or fluctuating vision after heart surgery

for an indefinite period. Symtoms of dyspnea and fatigue due to pulmonary venous congestion and signs of fluid retention require evaluation for surgical valve replacement or reconstruction. Most patients will qualify for a porcine valve, but younger patients should have a mechanical valve. Atrial fibrillation in mitral stenosis should be treated with anticoagulation therapy to prevent coagulation and thrombus formation (potentiated by the pooling of blood in the atrium, which during fibrillation is no longer an effective pump).

Similarly, when rheumatic fever is the basis for *mitral regurgitation*, prophylaxis is recommended until 35 years of age (Table 4–7). Anticoagulation should be considered if atrial fibrillation exists. Surgical replacement of the valve should be performed before clinical evidence of impaired contractility of the ventricle becomes manifest. Most people with mitral leaf prolapse are asymptomatic and merely require assurance. Beta-blocking agents and calcium channel blocking drugs may be required in patients with chest pain even though coronary anatomy is normal. These patients

TABLE 4–6. DIFFERENTIAL DIAGNOSIS OF RETINAL EMBOLI

Embolus	Usual Source(s)/Cause(s)	Typical Appearance
Cholesterol	Carotid artery Aorta	Yellow-orange, refractile, glistening Usually lodged at retinal arteriolar bifurcation Usually do not obstruct blood flow May cause focal arteriolar opacification at embolus site
Platelet–fibrin	Carotid artery Heart valves Ischemic cardiac muscle after myocardial infarction Atrial myxoma	Dull, grey-white plugs Usually mobile Long, smooth shape before breaking up in the retinal arterioles Concave meniscus shape at ends of embolus
Calcium	Calcified heart valves Great vessels (usually calcified aorta)	Large, round or ovoid "chalk" white, nonrefractile Most often permanently lodge in first or second arterial bifurcation and may overlie optic disc
Tumor	Carcinoma Lymphoproliferative tumors Atrial myxoma Metastatic neoplasms	Usually white or grey Smooth
Fat	Fracture of long bones Autologous fat injection for facial wrinkles	Long, located at various points along the vessels, not just at bifurcations
Talc	Intravenous drug use	Yellow-white, glistening Numerous and tiny, bilateral Usually lodge at distal aspect of smallest retinal arterioles, often around macula
Infectious	Infectious endocarditis	Usually appear as Roth spots, with white center composed of organisms mixed with inflammatory cells
Air	Injected air into tissue organ or region of face or scalp during surgery	Glistening, silvery rods with convex meniscus at either end
Foreign body	Drug injections (usually corticosteroids) Prosthetic heart valves	White, flocculent material within several arteries Large, dull, and fluffy if secondary to prosthetic heart valve

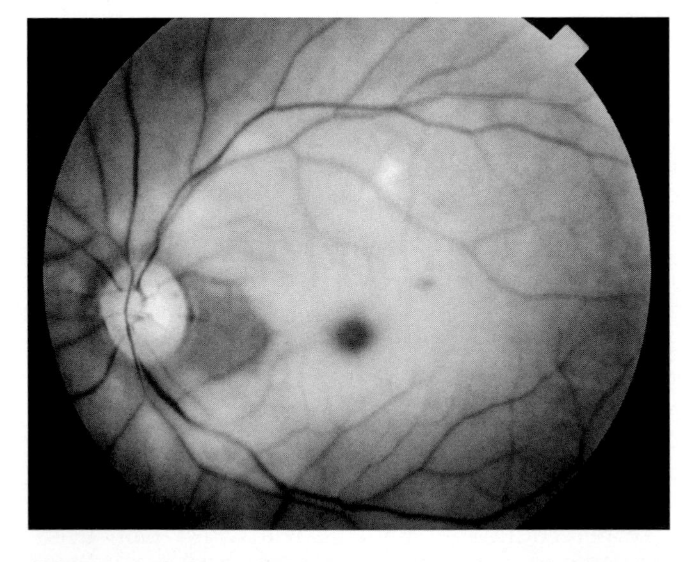

Figure 4–1. Central retinal artery occlusion, commonly secondary to an embolus of cardiac origin.

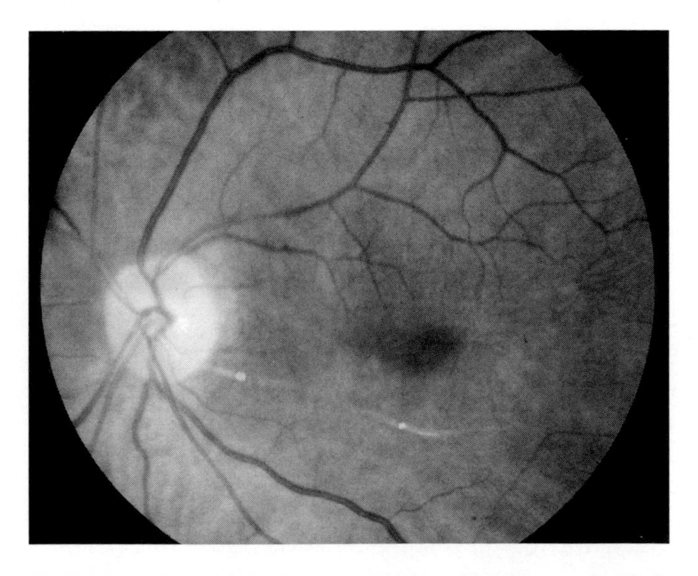

Figure 4–2. Branch retinal artery occlusion with evidence of emboli.

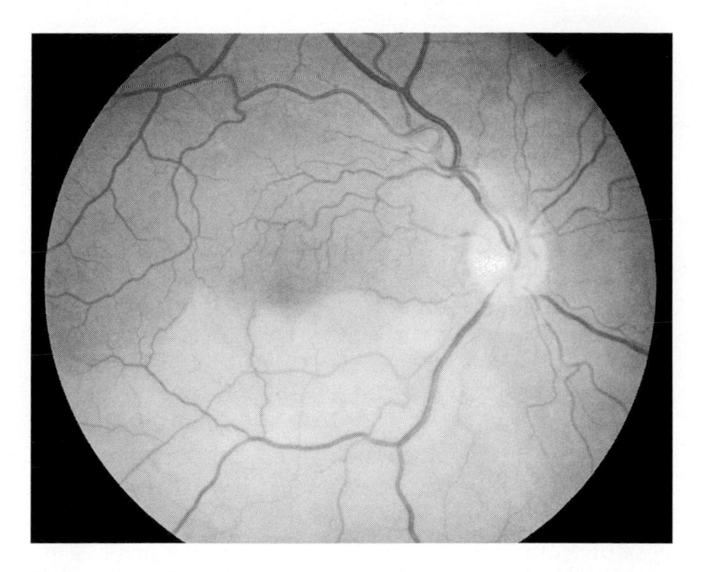

Figure 4–3. Retinal ischemia secondary to branch retinal artery occlusion.

should be advised of the need to prevent infectious endocarditis with antibiotics prior to dental work or other medical procedures in which bleeding may occur. In mitral regurgitation, calcification and immobility of the leaflets are indications for valve replacement. Beta-blockers, calcium channel blockers, and an anticoagulant are often required after surgery, as is antibiotic coverage for dental work.

In the asymptomatic state of *aortic stenosis,* prophylactic antibiotics are required to prevent bacterial endocarditis (Table 4–7). Small orifice size warrants serious consideration for valve replacement. With respect to potential surgery and valve disease, those with aortic stenosis have the poorest prognosis. Patients with congestive heart failure, angina, or exertional syncope should undergo aortic valve replacement promptly.

A primary concern in the care of the asymptomatic patient with *aortic regurgitation* is prophylaxis against bacterial endocarditis (Table 4–7). Heart failure can be treated with diuretics and vasodilating agents. However, the primary defect is mechanical, and medical therapy alone cannot modify the impaired or defective valve. Ideally, valve replacement should be proposed before clinical symptoms of heart failure develop or before dilatation of the ventricle has developed. Controversies persist regarding indications for surgery prior to symptoms. Chronic aortic regurgitation may be well tolerated for several years before causing evidence of left ventricular dysfunction and symptoms. In general, because of the increased likelihood of thrombogenesis, most mechanical prostheses require long-term anticoagulation; tissue prostheses do not, but these prostheses are less durable than most mechanical prostheses. Postoperative management is similar to aortic stenosis.

TABLE 4–7. TREATMENT AND MANAGEMENT OF CARDIAC DISEASES

Atrial Fibrillation
Acute treatment
- Slowing of ventricular rate with beta-adrenergic blockers and/or calcium channel blockers
- Electrical cardioversion if medical therapy fails within 24 hours

Chronic Treatment
- Quinidine or amiodarone to prevent recurrence
- Chronic anticoagulation with warfarin-like agents to reduce the risk of embolization

Mitral Stenosis
Prophylactic antibiotics
Anticoagulants
Surgery: valve replacement or reconstruction
Treatment for atrial fibrillation, if it exists

Mitral Regurgitation
Prophylactic antibiotics
Anticoagulants
Surgery: valve replacement
Treatment for atrial fibrillation, if it exists
Mitral valve prolapse: patient reassurance; may require beta-blockers or calcium channel blockers

Aortic Stenosis
Asymptomatic: prophylactic antibiotics
Symptomatic/severe: valve replacement

Aortic Regurgitation
Prophylactic antibiotics
Heart failure: diuretics, vasodilators
Surgery

Prophylaxis for Infectious Endocarditis
Adults: 2.0 g amoxicillin orally 1 hour before procedure
Children <60 lbs: 50 mg/kg amoxicillin orally 1 hour before procedure
If allergic to penicillin:
Adults: 600 mg clindamycin orally 1 hour before procedure
Children <60 lbs: 20 mg/kg clindamycin orally 1 hour before procedure

Cardiac Myxoma
Surgical removal of atrial myxoma

Anticoagulation is determined by the valve used. Prophylactic antibiotics are indicated during periods of increased susceptibility to bacteremia.

Infectious Endocarditis

Prophylaxis. The American Heart Association recommends pharmacologic prophylaxis for patients at high risk for infectious endocarditis (e.g., prosthetic heart valves; congenital cardiac conditions; acquired valvular dysfunction, especially due to rheumatic heart disease). Dental surgery (e.g., tooth extraction), genitourinary surgery, gastrointestinal tract surgery, and other similar procedures are strong indications for prophylaxis. *S. viridans* is the most common cause of endocarditis following such procedures; therefore, prophylaxis should be directed against these organisms.

Table 4–7 outlines the most recent recommendations by the American Heart Association.

Treatment for Active Infection. Treatment of active infectious endocarditis should begin once blood culture and sensitivity studies have been performed. The medication of choice is based upon the sensitivity studies and should be bactericidal. Treatment should continue until the infection is completely eliminated. Surgery may be required, especially in the case of fungal infections or when valvular function has been dramatically compromised. The benefits of anticoagulant therapy while treating the infection are not clear.

Cardiac Tumors

The only effective treatment for an atrial myxoma is surgical removal of the tumor (Table 4–7). The probable outcome is poor without treatment. Although a myxoma is a benign tumor, complications will occur because of growth and pendular movement of the tumor. Such complications may be atrial fibrillation, emboli, heart failure, and mitral valve obstruction.

Ocular

With retinal emboli of either cardiac or carotid origin, particularly in the presence of neurologic signs or symptoms (amaurosis fugax, hemianopsia, tingling or numbness of the extremities) or signs or symptoms suggestive of cardiac origins (angina, pulmonary edema), the most appropriate treatment is referral to a cardiologist and internist, and possibly a neurologist, for a comprehensive cardiovascular workup. Prior to referral there are certain procedures that may be done in the office and/or certain lab tests to request in order to appropriately direct the referral and eliminate other differential diagnoses (Table 4–8).

The management of the ocular manifestations of emboli of cardiac origin centers on treatment of the underlying systemic disease. Acute arterial occlusion secondary to emboli can be managed aggressively in an effort to dislodge the emboli (e.g., digital massage of the globe, paracentesis); however, this is rarely successful. Retinal emboli that are not causing arterial occlusions are best managed with the appropriate diagnostic tests and referrals.

CONCLUSION

It is important to remember that at least 20% of all retinal emboli are of cardiac origin. Of these, the most likely etiology is atrial fibrillation, although valvular

TABLE 4–8. MANAGEMENT OF RETINAL EMBOLI

Procedure / Lab Test / Referral	Purpose of Procedure / Lab Test / Referral
In-Office Procedures	
Ophthalmodynamometry	To rule out carotid artery as etiology of embolus
Carotid palpation	To rule out carotid artery as etiology of embolus
Carotid auscultation	To rule out carotid artery as etiology of embolus
Thorough case history (ask about fatigue, dyspnea, syncope, angina, amaurosis fugax, TIAs, diplopia, drop attack, slurred speech, jaw pain, headaches, lost weight	To investigate for and differentiate between cardiac, carotid, vertebrobasilar, and arteritic symptoms
Lab/Supplemental Tests	
ESR	Always rule out giant cell arteritis, especially in patients >55
Lipid profile	To look for a higher probability of carotid disease and/or ischemic heart disease
Carotid duplex	To look for carotid disease as the etiology of the embolus
Blood cultures	To look for bacteremia/infectious endocarditis if a persistent fever is present
Serum protein electrophoresis	In patients <55, to look for increased viscosity as a cause for arterial thrombus
Anticardiolipin antibodies	In patients <55, to look for increased viscosity as a cause for arterial thrombus
Referrals	
Cardiology	To perform echocardiography, electrocardiography, and/or chest x-ray and workup to investigate for cardiac source of embolus and need for antithrombotic/anticoagulant therapy
Internist/primary care	To complete cardiovascular workup
Neurology	To look for permanent deficits if history of TIAs, stroke, etc.

disease will produce a significant amount of retinal emboli. Therefore, a potential cardiac source should be considered in all patients presenting with both asymptomatic retinal emboli and ischemic neurologic deficits. Patients with cardiogenic emboli have a worse prognosis than do patients with extracardiac sources of emboli. Of critical importance is that retinal emboli are even more likely to be of cardiac origin in younger patients, especially below the age of 50. Fortunately, transesophageal echocardiography has improved the detection of cardiac sources of emboli.

Timely referral is essential because cerebrovascular accidents secondary to cardiogenic emboli are one of the most preventable forms of stroke. Patients with retinal emboli may appear otherwise healthy. This should not deter an appropriate workup and referral. Retinal emboli should be differentiated by their source in order to appropriately manage the patient. Emboli of carotid origin warrant a carotid workup as well as a comprehensive cardiovascular workup because the leading cause of mortality in patients with significant carotid stenosis is myocardial infarction. Care should be taken, particularly in patients with known valve replacement or other invasive cardiac procedures, to rule out ocular signs of infectious endocarditis.

REFERENCES

Abernathy WS, Willis PW. Thromboembolic complications of rheumatic heart disease. *Cardiovasc Clin.* 1973;5:131.

American College of Cardiology Task Force. ACC/AHA guidelines for the clinical application of echocardiography. *J Am Coll Cardiol.* 1997;4:862–879.

Bonow RO. Left ventricular structure and function in aortic valve disease. *Circulation.* 1989;79:966.

Braunwald E. Mitral regurgitation: Physiologic, clinical, and surgical consideration. *N Eng J Med.* 1969;281:425.

Braunwald E. Valvular heart disease. In: Braunwald E, ed. *Heart Disease.* 5th ed. Philadelphia: Saunders; 1997:1007.

Brickner ME. Cardioembolic stroke. *Am J Med.* 1996;100:465.

Chambers JB, de Belder MA, Moore D. Echocardiography in stroke and transient ischemic attack. *Heart.* 1997;2:(suppl) 78.

Chun PK, Gertz E, Davia JE, et al. Coronary atherosclerosis in mitral stenosis. *Chest.* 1982;81:36.

Cogan DG, Wray SH. Vascular occlusions in the eye from cardiac myxomas. *Am J Ophthalmol.* 1975;80:396–403.

Dajani AS, Taubert KA, Wilson W, et al. Prevention of bacterial endocarditis: Recommendations by the American Heart Association. *Circulation.* 1997;96(1):1069.

Davison ET, Friedman SA. Significance of systolic murmurs in the aged. *N Engl J Med.* 1968;279:225.

Eiden SB, Olivares G. Transient vision loss associated with Barlow's syndrome. *J Am Optom Assoc.* 1986;57:446–447.

Gallo I, Ruiz B, Duran CMG. Five to eight year follow-up of patients with the Hancock cardiac prosthesis. *J Thorac Cardiovasc Surg.* 1983;86:897.

Grayburn PA, Smith MD, Handshow R, et al. Detection of aortic insufficiency by standard echocardiography, pulsed Doppler echocardiography and auscultation. *Ann Intern Med.* 1986;104:599.

Hart RG. Cardiogenic embolism to the brain. *Lancet.* 1992; 339:589–594.

Jampol EM, Wong AS, Alber DM. Atrial myxoma and central retinal artery occlusion. *Am J Ophthalmol.* 1973;75: 242–249.

Karchmer AW. Infective endocarditis. In: Braunwald E, ed. *Heart Disease.* 5th ed. Philadelphia: Saunders; 1997:1077.

Marcus RH, Sareli P, Pocock WA, et al. Functional anatomy of severe mitral regurgitation in active rheumatic carditis. *Am J Cardiol.* 1989;63:577.

McNamara RL, Lima JAC, Whelton PK, Powe NR. Echocardiographic identification of cardiovascular sources of emboli to guide clinical management of stroke: A cost-effective analysis. *Ann Intern Med.* 1997;127:775–787.

Newman NJ. Cerebrovascular disease. In: Miller NR, Newman NJ, eds. *Walsh and Hoyt's Clinical Neuro-Ophthalmology.* 5th ed. Baltimore: Williams & Wilkins; 1998:3323.

Nutter DO, Wickliffe C, Gilbert CA, et al. The pathophysiology of idiopathic mitral valve prolapse. *Circulation.* 1975; 52:297.

Oh WMC, Taylor TR, Olsen EGJ. Aortic regurgitation in systemic lupus erythematosus requiring aortic valve replacement. *Br Heart J.* 1974;36:413.

Perloff JK, Roberts WC. The mitral apparatus: Functional anatomy of mitral regurgitation. *Circulation.* 1972;46:227.

Pomerance A. Pathogenesis of aortic stenosis and its relation to age. *Br Heart J.* 1972;34:569.

Rackley CE, Karp RB, Edwards JE. Mitral valve disease. In: Hurst JW, Schlant RC, eds. *The Heart.* 7th ed. New York: McGraw-Hill; 1990:820.

Rackley CE, Wallace RB, Edwards JE, et al. Aortic valve disease. In: Hurst JW, Schlant RC, eds. *The Heart.* 7th ed. New York: McGraw-Hill; 1990:795.

Selzer A. Changing aspects of the natural history of valvular aortic stenosis. *N Engl J Med.* 1987;317:91.

Sokolow M, McIlroy MB, Cheitlin MD. *Clinical Cardiology.* 5th ed. Norwalk, CT: Appleton and Lange; 1990:377–435.

Stollberger C, Chnupa P, Kronik G, et al. Transesophageal echocardiography to assess embolic risk in patients with atrial fibrillation. *Ann Intern Med.* 1998;128:630–638.

Stroke Prevention in Atrial Fibrillation Investigators Committee on Echocardiography. Transesophageal echocardiographic correlates of thromboembolism in high-risk patients with nonvalvular atrial fibrillation. *Ann Intern Med.* 1998;128:639–647.

Wrobleroski E, James F, Spann JF, et al. Right ventricular perfomance in mitral stenosis. *Am J Cardiol.* 1981;47:51.

Section III

NEUROLOGIC DISORDERS

Chapter 5

CEREBROVASCULAR DISEASE

Bernard H. Blaustein

Cerebrovascular disease defines any pathologic process affecting the blood vessels that supply blood to the brain. The underlying pathologic process may be an occlusive lesion of the vessel, such as a thrombus or embolus, or rupture of a vessel wall leading to hemorrhage. Of singular importance in cerebrovascular disease is the potential for cerebral ischemia.

The threat of stroke is the major concern regarding cerebrovascular disease. Stroke is frequently a devastating event. There is an initial mortality of 20 to 30%. Moreover, for survivors, the residual disability is often considerable. Results of the Framingham study (Greshan et al, 1975) indicate that 16% of the survivors remain institutionalized, 31% need long-term assistance in self-care, and 71% have a reduced capacity to earn a living.

Eyecare practitioners may play a vital role in the reduction of stroke, because many cases of cerebrovascular disease present with characteristic eye signs and symptoms. By identifying these patients and referring them to the appropriate healthcare practitioner, interventional therapy may be instituted, and stroke may be averted.

EPIDEMIOLOGY

Systemic

The incidence of cerebrovascular disease has declined significantly during the past 30 years. The public has acquired an increasing awareness of stroke risk factors: hypertension, smoking, elevated serum lipids, diabetes mellitus, and cardiac disease (Table 5–1). However, cerebrovascular disease is still the third leading cause of death in the United States after heart disease and cancer. About 70 to 80% of all strokes are due to thromboembolism, 10% to subarachnoid hemorrhage, and 4% to intracerebral hemorrhage. The American Heart Association estimates that there will be in excess of 500,000 new cases of stroke each year in the United States, with most cases occurring in persons over age 55.

The incidence of stroke is rare before the age of 55. However, it tends to double with each successive decade. Males are slightly more prone to stroke than females, with the male preponderance being greater in the younger age groups. In the United States, rates of cerebrovascular disease in African-Americans are higher than in Caucasians. Asians have higher rates of cerebral hemorrhage.

Ocular

Transient visual loss (TVL), or amaurosis fugax, is a sudden, transient, monocular alteration of vision. TVL is the most common symptom of transient ischemia within the carotid vascular system, occurring in about 40% of cases. The incidence of transient ischemia that results in TVLs has been reported at 31 in 100,000 among residents of Rochester, Minnesota, and 110 in 100,000 for the retirement community of Seal Beach,

TABLE 5–1. INCREASED RISK FACTORS FOR CEREBROVASCULAR DISEASE

Hypertension
Increased serum lipids
Diabetes mellitus
Cardiovascular disease
Atherosclerosis
Smoking
Oral contraceptives (?)
Increased age, male

California. The incidence of TVLs increases with each decade between 45 and 75 years, with the mean age of onset in the seventh decade. Between 40 and 80 years of age men experience more episodes of TVL than women by a 2.3 to 1.0 margin.

> Transient visual loss is the most common symptom of transient ischemia within the carotid vascular system.

Thromboembolic phenomena account for approximately 70 to 80% of all strokes. Most of the remainder are caused by intracerebral or subarachnoid hemorrhage.

The majority of this chapter is devoted to thromboembolic vascular disease. This entity may lead to ischemic stroke and is apt to present with ocular manifestations that herald its onset.

PATHOPHYSIOLOGY/DISEASE PROCESS

Systemic

Stroke is defined as a sudden, nonconvulsive, neurologic deficit caused by a reduction in blood flow below that which is necessary for the viability of brain cells. The term "cerebrovascular accident" (CVA) often is used interchangeably with the term "stroke." In its most severe form, the patient may become hemiplegic or comatose. In its mildest form, the stroke may cause a trivial neurologic disorder. All gradations exist between these two extremes. However, it is the abruptness with which the neurologic deficit develops—seconds, minutes, hours, or at most a few days—that marks the disorder as vascular. Embolic strokes characteristically begin suddenly, and the deficit reaches its peak almost at once. Thrombotic strokes also usually have an abrupt onset. However, in many the onset is somewhat slower, occurring over a period of several minutes, hours, or days in a step-like fashion.

In cerebral hemorrhage, the deficit may be sudden or may occur as a gradual, steadily progressive deterioration. Hemorrhage strokes are almost always caused by severe, uncontrolled hypertension. Blood leaks from the vessel directly into the brain, one of the ventricles, or the subarachnoid space. The subsequent compression and displacement of brain tissue within the narrow confines of the closed cranial vault almost always results in significant neurologic damage. Hemorrhagic strokes do not usually present with any warnings or prodromal symptoms.

Cerebral ischemia is a regional reduction in blood flow below that which is required for the normal function of brain tissue. It is usually caused by either a thrombus or an embolus. A thrombus may lead to cerebral ischemia by the obstruction of a larger vessel with an aggregation of platelets, fibrin, calcium, and other cellular elements. An embolus, a small portion of the clot, may break off from the parent thrombus and travel downstream to occlude a smaller vessel. If the reduction in blood flow is transitory or is not intense enough to result in cell death, neuronal function may return to normal.

Cerebral infarct is a histological term denoting the end result of sustained local ischemia to a particular part of the brain. The affected brain tissue undergoes irreversible ischemic necrosis and death. Lacunar infarctions are very small necrotic cavities and are caused by occlusions of small penetrating arterioles in the deeper, noncortical portions of the brain. In many instances the lacunae are so small that no clinically recognizable neurologic deficit manifests. Indeed, lacunar infarcts are often discovered incidentally on CT or MRI scans.

Atherosclerosis is the major pathologic process underlying ischemic cerebrovascular disease. It is characterized by the deposition of lipids in the innermost layer of medium and large arteries in areas of bifurcations and curves. Atherosclerotic lesions are found most frequently at the origin of the internal carotid artery (ICA). The next most common site is the proximal portion of the vertebral arteries just after they branch off the subclavian arteries.

> Atherosclerotic lesions are found most frequently at the origin of the internal carotid artery.

The pathophysiology of atherosclerosis has been under intense study for many years. It is felt that elevated levels of cholesterol, particularly with a concomitant elevation of low-density lipoproteins, encourage the deposition of lipids in the intima of medium and large arteries. Smooth muscle cells ultimately proliferate into the intimal layer, causing the formation of plaque. These plaques contain a central core of extracellular LDL, necrotic cell debris, and calcium salts. Subsequently, a narrowing of the arterial lumen occurs resulting in a relative stasis and turbulence of blood flow in that area.

The continual deposition of lipids into the intimal surface encourages the breakdown of the endothelial cells that make up the intima and leads to ulcer formation. The injured endothelium and turbulent blood flow encourage platelets to agglutinate and stick to the altered site.

The roughened ulcerative surface, presence of agglutinated platelets, and relative stasis of blood flow encourages the development of a thrombus. Subsequent bleeding into the thrombus from the vasa vasorum greatly enlarges the thrombus and can lead to occlusion of the parent vessel. In addition, small particles may break off and embolize to smaller vessels distally.

Hypertension, increased serum lipids, diabetes mellitus, and cardiac disease are risk factors known to increase the patient's liability for cerebrovascular disease. Some of these factors contribute to the development of atherosclerosis.

Hypertension is present in up to 30% of the American adult population over the age of 40 and is the major risk factor for stroke. It is strongly related to atherothrombotic brain infarction as well as intracerebral and subarachnoid hemorrhage.

It has been estimated that hypertensives have a stroke risk four times that of normotensives. The risk of stroke increases in direct relationship to both diastole and systole, but the strongest association is with systolic pressure. Furthermore, several studies have shown that effective treatment of hypertension will reduce stroke incidence and mortality.

> Hypertension is the major risk factor for stroke.

The major plasma lipids, including cholesterol and triglycerides, are transported in the form of lipoprotein complexes. The most important lipoproteins with regard to atherogenesis are the low-density lipoproteins (LDLs) and high-density lipoproteins (HDLs). LDL is thought to transport cholesterol to the tissues, and in particular, to the intimas of medium and large-sized arteries. HDL is thought to transport cholesterol to the liver for degradation.

Tell and colleagues (1988) reviewed the literature and concluded that there was a positive relationship between cerebral atherosclerosis and elevated LDL and triglyceride levels. However, it is not presently known whether the reduction of serum lipids will reduce the risk of cerebral infarction.

Several epidemiological studies have implicated cigarette smoking as a significant risk factor for stroke. Data from the Framingham study (Sacco et al, 1984) indicate that the relative risk for stroke in those who smoke more than 40 cigarettes per day is twice that of those who smoke less than 10 per day.

Diabetes mellitus is a specific risk factor for thromboembolic brain infarction. It is felt that the diabetes increases the LDL level within the serum and thus accelerates the production of atherosclerosis. When associated with hypertension, the risk is even stronger.

Impaired cardiac function, including coronary artery disease, congestive heart failure, left ventricular hypertrophy, valvular disease, and atrial fibrillation, is a major risk factor for stroke. At any level of blood pressure, persons with cardiac disease have more than twice the risk of stroke than those with normal function.

> Impaired cardiac function greatly increases the risk of stroke.

The role of oral contraceptives in stroke remains unclear. Some studies have suggested that oral contraceptives are associated with an increased risk of ischemic stroke. Others have revealed a significant risk for subarachnoid hemorrhage. Nevertheless, it seems that the risk of stroke is increased if users of oral contraceptives are older than 35 years, are smokers, are migraineurs, or are diabetics.

Anatomic Correlates

A review of the cerebral vascular supply explains the sequelae of compromised blood flow. The major blood supply to the brain arises from the aortic arch and involves two vascular systems: the anterior circulatory system, fed by the carotid artery system, and the posterior circulatory system, fed by the vertebrovascular artery system. Except for the origins and proximal portions of these systems, the blood supply is identical on each side (Figures 5–1 and 5–2).

The major derivative of the common carotid artery is the internal carotid artery. As it emerges from the cavernous sinus, the ICA gives off its first large branch, the ophthalmic artery, which supplies the ipsilateral globe and orbit. The ICA ends by dividing into the anterior and middle cerebral arteries. Most of the ipsilateral frontal, temporal, and parietal lobes are supplied by these arteries.

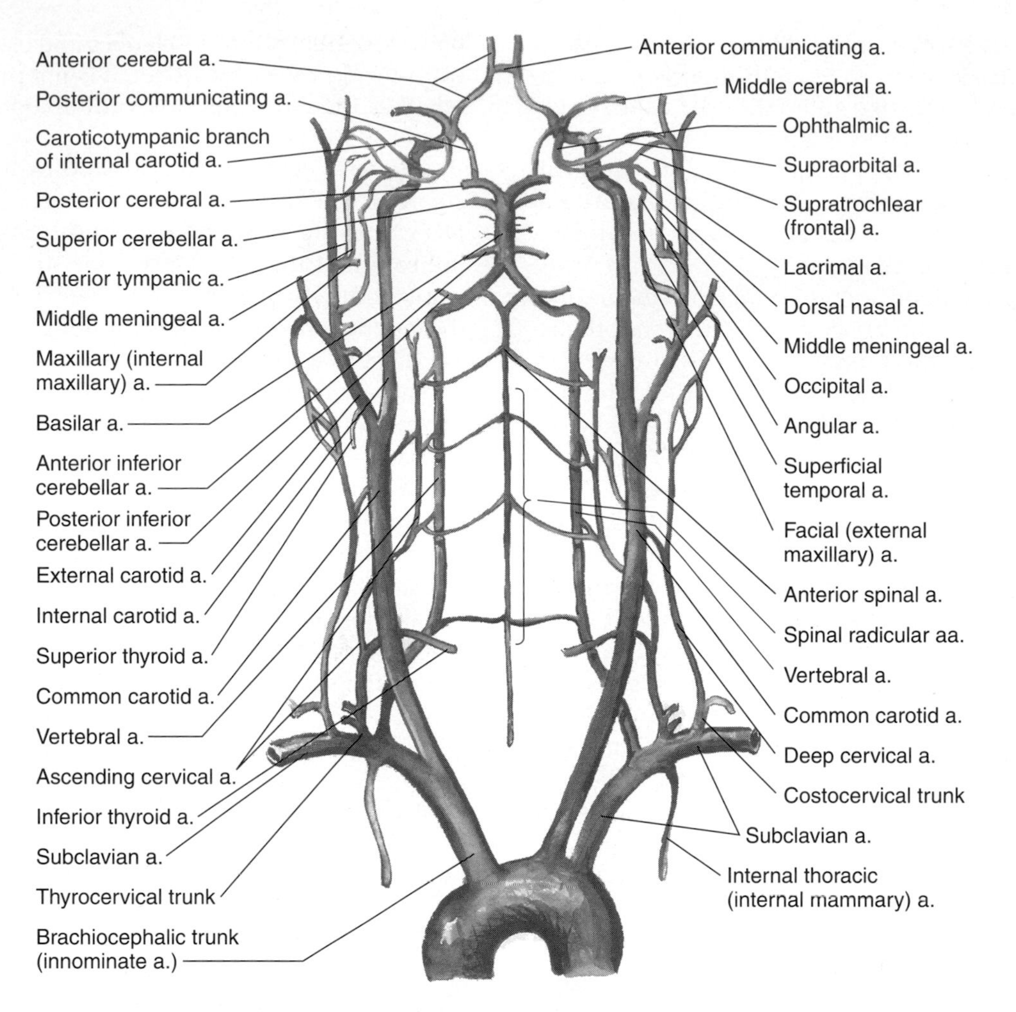

Figure 5–1. Cerebrovascular circulation.

Carotid artery disease or a decreased perfusion within the ICA may result in decreased ophthalmic artery pressure with a concomitant ipsilateral decrease in vision. When the middle cerebral artery or its branches are specifically involved, a contralateral hemiplegia results, with the motor deficit being more pronounced in the upper extremities. The hemiplegia is frequently associated with a hemisensory deficit and a homonymous hemianopsia. When the anterior cerebral artery is involved, a contralateral hemiplegia and an occasional hemisensory deficit result. The defect is greater in the lower extremity.

> Decreased perfusion within the internal carotid artery may result in ipsilateral vision deficit and contralateral body signs and symptoms.

Because the basilar artery is a single midline vessel with branches to both sides, the signs and symptoms that result from ischemia to the vertebrobasilar system may show considerable variation (Table 5–2). Unilateral, bilateral, or alternating involvement of cranial nerves III to VII may result in abnormal ocular motility, diplopia, or motor or sensory deficits in the face. Bilateral involvement of the medulla may impact on descending and ascending nerve tracts resulting in motor and sensory deficits in the limbs. If the descending sympathetic fibers that run along the lateral medulla are compromised, Horner's syndrome may result.

Cranial nerves housed in the medulla may be involved, resulting in dysphagia and dysphonia. Cerebellar defects may result in vertigo or ataxia. Ischemia to the occipital cortex may result in bilateral hemianopsia, which the patient often will interpret as a bilateral dimming of vision. Finally, headache, vomiting, and syncope may occur.

> Vertebrobasilar insufficiency may cause ischemia to the occipital cortex, a condition that will result in a bilateral dimming of vision.

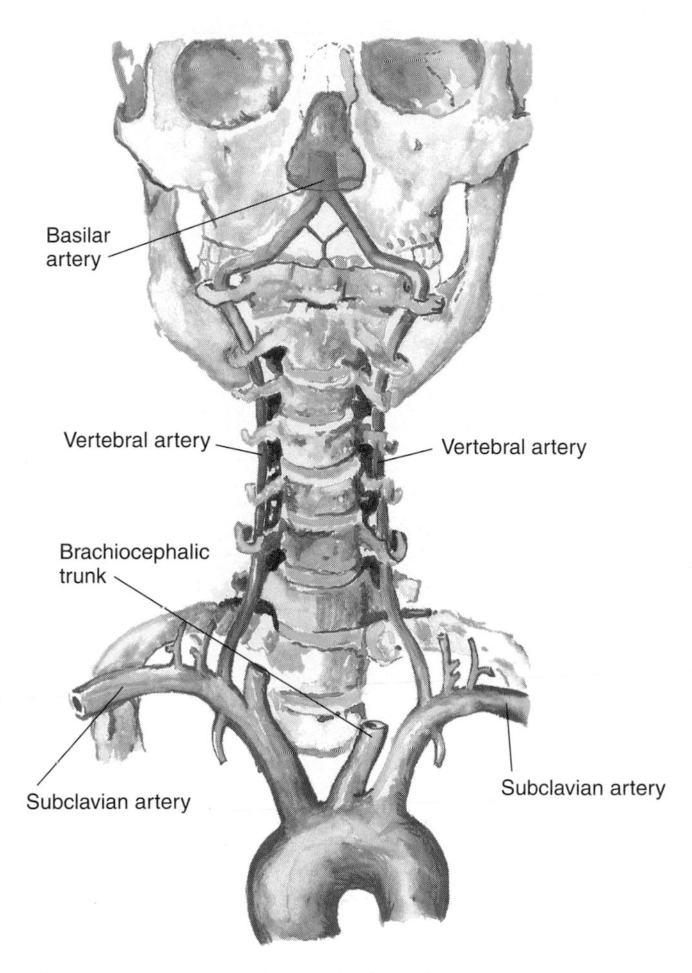

Figure 5–2. Course of the vertebral arteries.

Symptoms of vertebrobasilar insufficiency in conjunction with claudication of the exercised arm constitute the subclavian steal syndrome. This syndrome is most often caused by an atherosclerotic stenosis of the subclavian artery just proximal to the origin of the vertebral artery. As a pressure gradient develops between the exercised arm and the stenosed vessel, blood is diverted from the vertebrobasilar circulation to supply the arm.

Not all of the above signs and symptoms need occur with vertebrobasilar insufficiency. Moreover, vertigo and/or dizziness alone, without other symptoms, are often observed in older patients and do not necessarily indicate posterior circulation ischemia.

Transient ischemic attacks (TIAs) refer to temporary episodes of cerebral dysfunction of vascular origin. They are rapid in onset, variable in duration, and commonly last from 2 to 15 minutes but occasionally last for as long as one day. Signs and symptoms that last for 24 hours are called reversible ischemic neurologic deficits (RINDs). After the attack the patient returns to preattack status with no apparent clinical evidence of an infarct or permanent damage. Neuroimaging, however, may reveal evidence of minor cerebral infarct. The transient nature of the attack is explained by a temporary blockage of a vessel by a small embolus of fibrin–platelet material from a distant atherosclerotic site. The rapid fragmentation and dissolution of these microemboli preclude permanent neurologic dysfunction.

Carotid territory TIAs can be broadly divided into two categories: TVL and transient hemispheric attacks. TVL is the only feature distinguishing the extracranial carotid syndrome from that of an intracranial obstruction of the middle verebral artery.

TVL is a brief alteration of vision in one eye ipsilateral to the carotid disease. Patients will occasionally describe the phenomenon as a temporary mist or cloud before the eye. More frequently, the patient will describe the vision loss as altitudinal, as though a curtain had been pulled over one eye.

Occasionally, patients with carotid disease will report a prolonged dimunition of vision in the ipsilateral eye when they proceed from a dark environment to a very light environment, as for example when exiting a darkened movie theater on a bright day. Roberts and Sears (1992) describe this phenomenon as light-induced amaurosis and reason that the blood supply to the ophthalmic artery is compromised in carotid insufficiency. The short posterior ciliary arteries are derived from the ophthalmic artery, and hence perfusion to the choroid via the short posterior ciliary arteries is compromised. The reduced blood supply to the choroid slows the regeneration of bleached visual pigments in the photoreceptors when the eye is exposed to bright light.

The clinical manifestations of transient hemispheric attacks vary depending upon the location and severity of the cerebral ischemia. However, most symptoms are referable to the territory supplied by the middle cerebral artery. The most common symptoms include short-lived motor and sensory disturbances of the contralateral limbs. Depending on which hemisphere is involved, dysphasia and confusion due to spatial disorientation may occur. A less frequent occurrence is episodic limb shaking, a manifestation that may be mistaken for a focal seizure.

With vertebrobasilar TIAs, short-lived episodes of vertigo, unsteadiness, tunnel vision (bilateral hemianopsia), diplopia, dysarthria, nausea, headache, and vomiting are common.

The natural history of patients who experience TIAs is not precisely known. The general consensus is that persons who experience TIAs have a stroke risk of about 5 to 6% per year. The risk of subsequent infarction is greatest within the first month following a TIA; 36% of infarcts occur within this period. As a general rule, following a TIA about one-third of patients

TABLE 5–2. SYSTEMIC AND OCULAR MANIFESTATIONS OF CEREBROVASCULAR DISEASE

Vertebrobasilar Disease

Systemic

Transient ischemic attacks
Reversible ischemic neurologic deficits
Unilateral, bilateral, alternate cranial nerve III to VII deficits
Motor sensory deficits in limbs
Dysphagia, dysphonia
Vertigo/ataxia
Headache/vomiting/syncope
Claudication of exercised arm (subclavian steal syndrome)
Dizziness
Unsteadiness
Dysarthria

Ocular

Ocular motility disturbances
Diplopia
Horner's syndrome
Bilateral hemianopsia (bilateral dimming of vision/tunnel vision)

Carotid Artery Disease

Irregular pupil
Iris neovascularization
Hypotony (initial)
Orbital pain
Iris atrophy
Retina
- Plaques (Hollenhorst/calcific)
- Infarcts
- Cotton-wool spots
- Asymmetric retinopathy
- Hypoperfusion retinopathy (venous stasis retinopathy)

Intracranial Hemorrhage

Systemic

Severe headache
Coma
Death

Ruptured Saccular Aneurysm

Systemic

Transient ischemic attacks/transient hemispheric attacks (short-lived motor/sensory disturbances of the contralateral limbs)
Dysphasia
Spatial disorientation
Episodic limb shaking

Ocular

Transient visual loss (ipsilateral/one eye/temporary mist or cloud/altitudinal vision loss or curtain)
Ocular ischemic syndrome
- Engorged episcleral vessels
- Corneal edema
- Striate keratopathy
- Mild anterior uveitis
- Severe headache
- Transitory unilateral weakness, numbness, and tingling
- Speech disturbance
- Unconsciousness

AV Malformation

Systemic

Nondescript headache (may mimic migraine with visual aura)
Audible cranial bruit
Progressive neurologic impairment
Hemiparesis
Hemiplegia
Mental decline
Death

will have no further symptoms, one-third will have recurrent TIAs, and one third will go on to have a stroke. It is significant to note that 50% of patients suffering a cerebral infarction from occlusive carotid disease will have experienced a carotid territory TIA sometime beforehand.

Intracranial Hemorrhage

Spontaneous intracranial hemorrhage may involve bleeding into the parenchyma of the brain, the pituitary gland, the ventricular system, the subarachnoid space, or the epidural or dural spaces. In many instances the hemorrhage involves several of these compartments. A discussion of pituitary hemorrhage and isolated subdural or epidural hematomas is not included in this chapter.

Intracerebral hemorrhage (ICH), also known as primary hypertensive hemorrhage, almost always occurs as a result of sustained, elevated systolic blood pressure. The patient presents with an abrupt onset and rapid evolution of symptoms usually occurring over minutes or hours. Usually, there are no warnings or prodromal signs, although approximately 50% of patients report a severe headache as the stroke is evolving.

The hemorrhage occurs within brain tissue, forming an oval mass that disrupts the tissue and grows in volume as the bleeding continues. Adjacent brain tissue may be displaced and compressed. If the hemorrhage is very large, midline structures may be displaced to the opposite side, and vital centers may be compromised. Coma and death will usually result. The vessel involved is usually a small penetrating artery. The hemorrhage is thought to arise from an arterial wall that has become weakened from being impregnated with a hyalin–lipid material as a result of the sustained hypertension. In order of frequency, the most common sites of hypertensive hemorrhage are (1) the putamen and adjacent internal capsule; (2) various parts of the central white matter of the temporal, parietal, or frontal lobes; (3) the thalamus; (4) the cerebellar hemisphere; and (5) the pons.

Ruptured Saccular Aneurysm

Saccular aneurysms (berry aneurysms) take the form of small, thin-walled blisters protruding from the arteries of the circle of Willis or its major branches. As a rule, the aneurysms are located at bifurcations and branchings, and are presumed to result from developmental defects in the tunica media or internal elastic membrane. The resultant weakness in the arterial walls causes the intima to bulge outward, covered only by adventitia. The sac gradually enlarges and finally ruptures.

Prior to rupture, saccular aneurysms are usually asymptomatic. However, some patients will have had an episode of severe headache, or transitory unilateral weakness, numbness, and tingling, or speech disturbance in the days or weeks preceding the major event. These prodromal symptoms are generally attributed to minor leakage from the aneurysm. Rupture of the aneurysm usually occurs while the patient is active, and in many cases sexual intercourse or other exertion is the precipitant.

When the rupture occurs, blood under high pressure is forced into the subarachnoid space since the circle of Willis lies within this space. The resulting clinical events assume one of three patterns: (1) the patient may experience an excruciating headache and fall unconscious, (2) the patient may be stricken with a severe headache but remain relatively lucid, or (3) the patient may lose consciousness quickly without any preceding complaint.

Arteriovenous Malformation

An arteriovenous malformation (AVM) consists of a tangle of blood vessels that form an abnormal communication between the arterial and venous systems. AVMs may occur in all parts of the brain, brainstem, and spinal cord, but the larger ones are more frequently found in the posterior half of the cerebral hemispheres. AVMs are about one-tenth as common as saccular aneurysms and somewhat more common in males than in females.

The tangled blood vessels that are interposed between arteries and veins are abnormally thin, and their walls do not possess the structural integrity of normal arteries or veins. Although most AVMs are clinically silent for a long time, most will eventually bleed. When hemorrhage occurs, blood may enter the subarachnoid space but is more likely to be partly intracerebral, causing a hemiparesis, hemiplegia, or even death.

Before rupture, a chronic nondescript headache is a frequent complaint. Occasionally, these headaches mimic migraines, and if the AVM is located in the occipital cortex, visual auras may accompany the headache. Typically, the visual auras do not flicker as do the auras of classic migraine. Other symptoms of AVMs include audible bruit, convulsions, progressive neurological impairment, or mental decline.

Ocular

The nature of the ocular signs and symptoms that occur in cerebrovascular disease depends on whether the ischemia occurs in the carotid territory or the vertebrobasilar territory (see Table 5–2). It is important to ascertain the etiology of the ischemia, because the associated ocular findings and the subsequent treatment are different.

Ischemia of the anterior segment and the retina defines the carotid territory syndrome. If the patient experiences TVL, he or she often feels as though a shade has been pulled over one eye.

Prolonged generalized ischemia to the anterior portion of the eye presents a constellation of signs and symptoms known as the ocular ischemic syndrome. The anterior manifestations of this syndrome are characterized by engorged episcleral vessels, corneal edema and striate keratopathy secondary to poor oxygen perfusion, mild anterior uveitis with flare and cells, irregular pupil, and iris neovascularization around the pupil and in the anterior chamber angle. Initially, hypotony occurs because of impaired ciliary body function. Ultimately, neovascular glaucoma may occur secondary to the iris neovascularization. In addition, the patient reports deep orbital pain and photophobia. In time the iris atrophies and diffuse cataracts develop.

The presence of plaques, infarcts, or cotton-wool spots or evidence of venous stasis imply retinal ischemia. Retinal arteriolar plaques may appear as bright and glistening. These crystalline particles, known as Hollenhorst plaques, tend to lodge at arteriolar bifurcations (Figure 5–3). They are thought to originate from the inner layers of carotid atheromas and represent cholesterol deposits. They may rarely cause transient visual loss but more often will fragment and pass through the retinal circulation without incident. Solid, white nonrefractile plaques that lodge in the larger vessels around the optic nerve head originate from calcification of cardiac valves. These calcific emboli are often occlusive and may cause retinal infarcts.

Long dull-white plugs represent platelet emboli from the surface of atheromas. They are mobile and will undergo fragmentation and dissolution but can cause transient obstruction to retinal blood flow. TVL may occur. Linear white deposits within arterioles

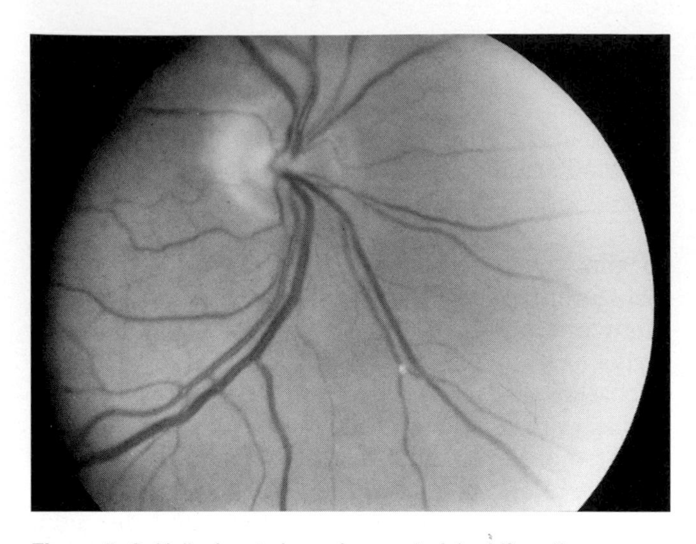

Figure 5–3. Hollenhorst plaque in an arteriolar bifurcation.

probably represent fibrin or thromboembolic material from the walls of the heart. They are less friable than platelets and may result in retinal artery occlusions and subsequent infarcts.

Asymmetric retinopathy may occur with carotid insufficiency to the eye. On the ipsilateral side there may be cotton-wool spots, indicating generalized retinal hypoxia, or frank retinal neovascularization. In addition, midperipheral blot and dot hemorrhages, microaneurysms, and dilated tortuous veins may be noted. This entity represents hypoperfusion retinopathy (venous stasis retinopathy, or nonischemic central vein occlusion), and is an important hallmark of carotid insufficiency. Gay and Rosenbaum (1966) implied that unilateral carotid artery disease with a resultant decrease in ocular perfusion led to less diabetic retinal neovascularization. However, studies by Browning (1988), Duker and associates (1990), were unable to confirm Gay and Rosenbaum's findings.

> Ischemia to the anterior segment and the retina defines the carotid territory syndrome. If the patient experiences TVL, he or she often feels as if a shade has been pulled over one eye.

The characteristic ocular symptomatology of vertebrobasilar insufficiency is associated with ischemia to the posterior portions of the brain: the occipital lobes, cerebellum, and brainstem. Bilateral disturbance of vision results from insufficiency of the posterior cerebral arteries that supply the visual cortex. Visual symptoms are described as being a bilateral dimming, graying, or blurring of vision. Total blindness may occur transiently. Attacks of vertigo and diplopia may also occur.

DIAGNOSIS

The diagnosis of cerebrovascular disease is often made by integrating ocular clinical data with systemic clinical data. Tables 5–3 and 5–4 delineate ancillary studies and testing procedures of cerebrovascular disease, and Table 5–5 provides a partial list for the differential diagnosis.

Systemic

After the appropriate workup by the ocular clinician, the patient may be referred to the vascular specialist for further evaluation and management. The physician will attempt to reduce the risk factors associated with cerebrovascular disease, particularly hypertension, hypercholesterolemia, and impaired cardiac function. Careful auscultation for bruits of the carotid arteries and their extracranial branches may add supportive evidence for a diagnosis of impending stroke.

Ancillary studies will be used to confirm or exclude other conditions that may be precipitating thromboemboic phenomena or intracranial hemorrhage (Table 5–3). Chest x-rays, urinalysis, complete blood count, erythrocyte sedimentation rate, serum electrolytes, blood urea nitrogen, blood sugar, serological

TABLE 5–3. ANCILLARY STUDIES FOR CEREBROVASCULAR DISEASE

Chest x-ray
Electrocardiogram

Brain Imaging
Computed tomography
Magnetic resonance imaging
Magnetic resonance angiography

Laboratory Tests
Urinalysis
Complete blood count
Erythrocyte sedimentation rate
Serum electrolytes
Blood urea nitrogen
Blood sugar
Serological tests for syphilis
Serum lipid profile
Serum uric acid
Blood clotting studies
Thyroid function studies

TABLE 5–4. DIAGNOSTIC TESTS FOR CAROTID ARTERY DISEASE

Systemic
Noninvasive assessment distal to the bifurcation
Oculoplethysmography
Periorbital directional Doppler
Noninvasive assessment at the bifurcation
B-scan ultrasonography
Doppler ultrasonography
Duplex scanning
Phonoangiography
Invasive
Arteriography
Digital venous subtraction angiography
Ocular
Ausculatate extracranial arteries
Palpate pulses (superficial temporal artery)
Ophthalmodynamometry
Blood pressure (difference in systolic right/left arm >20 mmHg)

TABLE 5–5. DIFFERENTIAL DIAGNOSIS OF CEREBROVASCULAR DISEASE (PARTIAL LIST)

Systemic
Migraine
Epilepsy
Vasospasm
AV malformation
Intracranial neoplasm
Multiple sclerosis
Intracranial infection/inflammation
Intracranial phakomatoses
Head trauma
Intracranial bleeds
Arterial vasculitides
Cervicocerebral artery dissections
Spinal cord ischemia
Hematologic disease
Ocular
Gaze Palsies and Pareses
Myasthenia gravis
Progressive supranuclear palsy
Chronic progressive external ophthalmoplegia
Parkinsons disease
Multiple sclerosis
Compressive cerebral, cerebellar, brainstem lesions, or orbital lesions
Oculomotor apraxias
Vasculopathic oculomotor neuropathy
Functional disturbances
Retina/Optic nerve
Proliferative diabetic retinopathy
Vasoocclusive disease
Hematologic disease
Radiation therapy vasculopathy
Compressive optic neuropathy
Infectious optic neuropathy
Ischemic optic neuropathy
Toxic optic neuropathy
Traumatic optic neuropathy
Granulomatous infiltration

tests for syphilis, serum lipid profile, serum uric acid, blood clotting studies, and thyroid function studies all may be helpful. An electrocardiogram may demonstrate conduction abnormalities and arrythmias.

Brain imaging is important in assessing the patient who has recently experienced a TIA or a stroke. Computed tomography (CT) and magnetic resonance imaging (MRI) scans will often demonstrate an area of infarction and will confirm or exclude the presence of an intracerebral, subdural, or epidural hemorrhage. Moreover, large aneurysms and AVMs as well as subarachnoid or intraventricular blood may be revealed, and mass lesions such as neoplasms, abscesses, and other conditions masquerading as cerebrovascular disease will be identified.

Magnetic resonance angiography (MRA) provides images of arterial flow in the extracranial circulation and in the large intracranial arteries. Flowing blood exhibits complex MR signals that range from bright to dark relative to background stationary tissue. Fast-flowing blood, such as arterial blood, shows no signal on routine MR images. Slower blood distal to arterial stenoses may appear high in signal. It is possible by varying the MR image parameters to assess blood flow either qualitatively or quantitatively.

Specific evaluation of the carotid and the vertebrobasilar vascular systems involves the utilization of noninvasive and/or invasive procedures. Whenever possible, noninvasive techniques are preferred because of the risks that attend invasive tests.

Noninvasive Tests

Noninvasive diagnostic techniques for the evaluation of carotid occlusive disease may be divided into those that indirectly assess the hemodynamics of the ICA distal to the bifurcation and those that directly assess the carotid bifurcation (Table 5–4).

Oculoplethysmography (OPG) combines some of the principles of ophthalmodynamometry and the old techniques of ocular plethysmography. The procedure is performed by applying small vacuum cups to both anesthesized sclerae. Intraocular pressure is increased in each eye simultaneously by the application of a vacuum. Subsequently, the ocular pulse disappears. The vacuum pressure is then reduced simultaneously until the pulsations just return. A delay in the pulse in one eye indicates decreased flow to that eye and implies obstruction in the ICA ipsilaterally. Gee and coworkers (1974) developed a conversion table relating the intracranial ICA pressure to the level of vacuum at which the first ocular pulse appears.

Periorbital directional Doppler ultrasonography uses high-frequency sound waves to ascertain the direction of blood flow in the periorbital arteries. The transducer is placed just below the supraorbital notch, and high-frequency sound waves are transmitted to the area. The frequency of the reflected sound waves is a function of the direction of blood flow relative to the source. If red blood cells are moving toward the transducer, the frequency is increased. A hemodynamically significant stenosis at any point along the ICA will cause a reversal of blood flow in the supraorbital and supratrochlear arteries (Figure 5–4).

Transcranial Doppler ultrasonography can assess blood flow in the middle cerebral and anterior cerebral arteries because stenotic lesions in these arteries increase systolic blood flow velocity. When there is an occlusion or a hemodynamically significant stenosis in the carotid siphon, transcranial Doppler assesses collateral flow across the anterior or posterior circle of Willis.

High-resolution B-scan ultrasonography provides a cross-sectional image of the carotid bifurcation by means of sound wave reflection from the interfaces of tissues of different acoustic impedances. Each point in the field being studied corresponds to a dot on the oscilloscope screen. The brightness of the dot is proportional to the amplitude of the reflected sound wave. This technique is capable of identifying subtle plaques and small ulcers as well as delineating the residual lumen diameter. Real-time ultrasonography has an accuracy approaching 90% when compared to carotid angiography. It is better than angiography for detecting small lesions, those with 1 to 25% luminal stenosis. However, with stenosis greater than 75%, B-mode images begin to suffer and become less reliable than angiograms. In addition, the presence of calcium within atheromatous plaques may degrade the image.

Doppler ultrasonography assesses carotid function by projecting high-frequency sound waves into the ICA at the bifurcation. The frequency of the reflected sound waves from the moving red blood cells is dependent upon the velocity of blood flow. When a stenosis is present, blood flow velocity increases in the stenotic portion of the vessel. The increased flow velocity results in an increase in the frequency of the reflected sound waves. The examiner may use an amplifier to audibly analyze the reflected signals as the probe is advanced along the carotid vessel. Additionally, the reflected waves may be displayed on an oscilloscope screen and plotted against time. Doppler ultrasonography has an accuracy of 90% when compared to carotid angiography.

Duplex ultrasonography is a combination of B-scan ultrasonography with Doppler flow studies. In this technique there is a rapid alternation of B-scan and Doppler signals. The result is an image of the bifurcation and a quantitative estimate of the blood flow. Studies using the duplex system followed by arteriography indicate a 95% agreement between the two methods in identifying carotid stenosis of greater than 50%.

Quantitative spectral phonoangiography analyzes the audible frequency–intensity components of a bruit via computer analysis. This technique provides an automatic auscultation of the bifurcation, and the sound is recorded and displayed on an oscilloscope. The residual lumen diameter is estimated from the intensity and frequency of the displayed bruit.

Atherothrombotic disease and patency of the vertebrobasilar system may be detected by MRA. Trans-

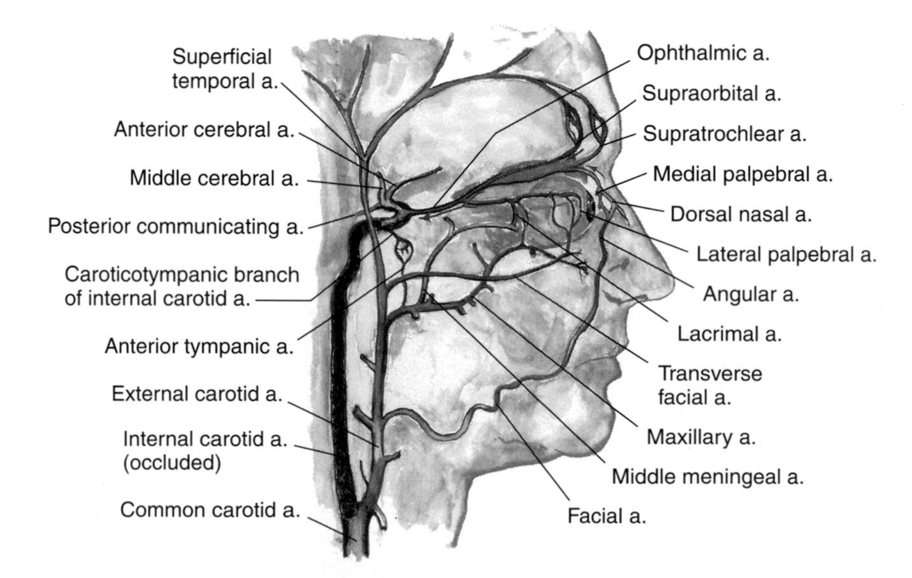

Figure 5–4. Retrograde blood flow from the superficial temporal artery to the ophthalmic artery.

cranial Doppler analysis of flow in the vertebral artery determines its patency, but its sensitivity in determining distal vertebral artery stenotic lesions is limited. MRA combined with transcranial Doppler ultrasound may eventually replace conventional angiography in documenting patency of the vertebrobasilar system.

A number of newer methods have recently become available for the noninvasive determination of cerebral blood flow. These include xenon clearance techniques, single photon emission computed tomography (SPECT), and positron emission tomography (PET).

Radioactive xenon may be administered into the general circulation by either intravenous injection or by inhalation of xenon gas. By an indicator dilution technique, regional cerebral blood flow can be determined. SPECT requires the use of iodine- , thallium- , or technetium-labeled tracers whose distribution is proportional to cerebral blood flow. PET has enabled study of both hemodynamic and metabolic changes in the brain by providing accurate quantitative measurements of regional blood flow for both deep and superficial structures.

Invasive Tests

Arteriography is the most definitive test for both the extracranial and intracranial vasculature, and has traditionally been considered the "gold standard" for evaluation of patients with cerebrovascular disease. It can detect atherosclerotic plaque stenosis and ulcers, intraluminal thrombi, arterial dissections, arteritis and vasospasm, collateral circulation around the circle of Willis and on the cortical surface, and occlusion of large and small arteries. The technique is performed by inserting a catheter transfemorally and advancing it into the aortic arch. From there, selective cannulization of the extracranial cerebral vessels can be achieved. An iodinated contrast agent is injected, and a fluoroscopic picture is taken.

Arteriography, like many other invasive procedures, is associated with certain risks. The principal risks are stroke, allergic reactions to the dye, and renal failure. In several large series, neurologic complications developed in 2.4 to 4.2% of patients with cerebrovascular disease. Most of the neurologic complications were transitory, but permanent neurologic defects occurred in 0.15 to 0.6% of the patients, and from 0.15 to 0.5% died. The neurological complications may develop from the embolization of fragile atheromatous material that becomes dislodged by the catheter. Because of the potential for neurologic complications, clinicians must be concerned about performing unnecessary angiographies. MRAs combined with carotid and transcranial ultrasound are supplanting it in many situations.

> Cerebral angiography, performed by injection of contrast dye into selected extracranial arteries, remains the most accurate method of assessing the cerebrovascular system. The advantages of this invasive technique must be balanced against the complications that may occur.

Digital venous subtraction angiography (DVSA) is a safer means of examining the extracranial and intracranial vasculature. Radiopaque contrast agent is injected into the brachial vein or superior vena cava. Before the arrival of contrast material at the region of interest, a fluoroscopic picture is taken, digitalized, and stored. The subsequent images with the dye are digitalized, and the original image is subtracted from them. The resultant images are viewed in real time.

DVSA is safer than conventional angiography because there is no catheter manipulation within the arterial system. The major limitations of DVSA are related to spatial resolution and motion artifacts. The spatial resolution is inferior to that of conventional arteriography, and the images are degraded if the patient moves or swallows during the extracranial studies.

Ocular

In addition to a careful history, biomicroscopy, ophthalmoscopy, and visual fields, the clinician can perform several clinical procedures in the office to further aid in the diagnosis of cerebrovascular disease.

Auscultating the extracranial arteries in the neck may reveal an abnormal sound associated with turbulent blood flow through the narrow vessels. The abnormal sound, known as a bruit, commonly is located over the carotid bifurcation, but may be heard in the supraclavicular fossa in vertebral insufficiency (Figure 5–5). These bruits suggest a hemodynamically significant arterial stenosis, that is, a narrowing of the lumen in excess of 50% of the original diameter. Placing the bell of the stethoscope over the closed lids may reveal an orbital bruit, indicating a carotid–cavernous fistula. Finally, auscultating over the occiptial cortex may reveal a bruit suggestive of an occipital cortical AVM.

Palpating the pulses through the superficial temporal arteries on each side and comparing their intensities may reveal reduced blood flow through one of the ICAs. Under normal circumstances, blood flows up the ICA into the ophthalmic artery. Flow then continues, via anastomotic channels, into the supraorbital and supratrochlear arteries and into the superficial temporal artery. If one of the ICAs is compromised, blood flow may be reversed. Blood may then flow retrograde from the superficial temporal artery to the

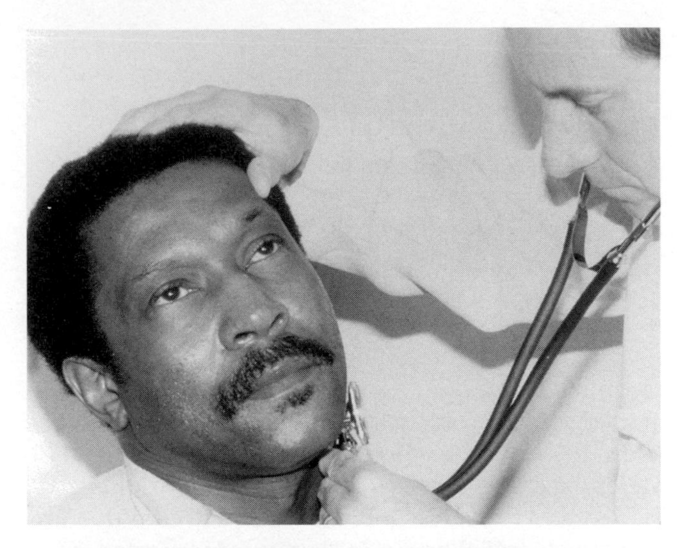

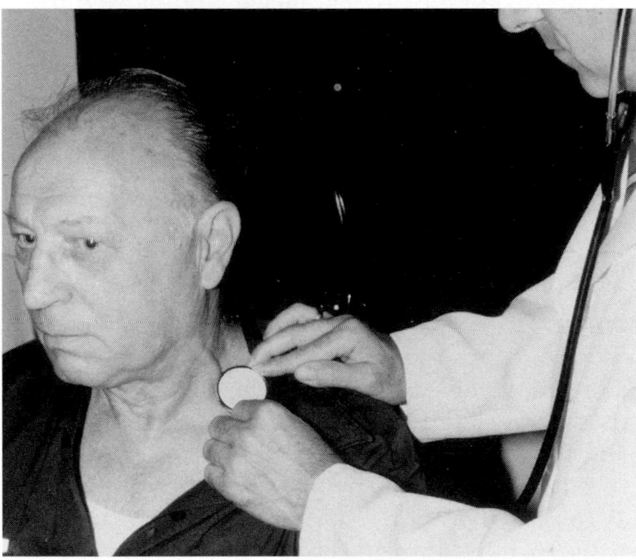

Figure 5–5. A. Auscultation of the carotid bifurcation. **B.** Auscultation of the vertebral artery in the supraclavicular fossa. (*Reprinted with permission from Blaustein BH. The subclavian steal syndrome.* Clin Eye Vision Care. *1991;3:25–28.*)

ophthalmic artery (see Figure 5–4). The pulse in the superficial temporal artery ipsilateral to the blocked ICA will be stronger than in its fellow ICA.

Ophthalmodynamometry (ODM) is performed by increasing the intraocular pressure through an external force on the sclera. The force is applied via a calibrated instrument known as an ophthalmodynamometer. The clinician notes the amount of pressure needed to induce arterial pulsations at the nerve head in one eye, and compares this finding with that in the other eye. A reduced ODM reading in one eye implies reduced perfusion through the central retinal artery. Because the central retinal artery is derived from the ophthalmic artery, which is the first branch of the ICA, a lower ODM implies occlusive disease in the ipsilateral ICA. A 20% difference in ODM between the two eyes is considered significant.

A difference in systolic blood pressure of greater than 20 mmHg between the arms suggests reduced flow in the subclavian artery to the arm with the lower blood pressure. Symptoms of claudication of the exercised arm accompanied by symptoms of vertebrobasilar insufficiency constitute the subclavian steal syndrome. Other significant findings in this syndrome include a diminished radial pulse and a supraclavicular bruit on the affected side.

TREATMENT AND MANAGEMENT

Table 5–6 gives an overview of treatment and management, which is discussed in the following sections.

Systemic

The medical approach to cerebrovascular disease concentrates on reducing the risk factors for stroke and administering specific prophylactic medications. If possible, all risk factors should be reduced or eliminated, but as the predominate precursor of stroke, hypertension control is particularly important. Indeed, prevention of atherosclerosis and its complications is the best management of ischemic brain disease. In addition, treating cardiac dysfunction is of major importance.

Platelet antiaggregation agents prevent atherothrombotic events by inhibiting the formation of thrombi that occlude arteries or embolize to distal circulation. Aspirin and ticlopidine are the antiplatelet agents in use today.

Aspirin results in a 25 to 30% reduction in the incidence of stroke after TIAs. The antiplatelet effect of aspirin is accomplished by acetylating the enzyme cyclooxygenase in platelets, thus inhibiting the formation of the aggregant thromboxane A_2. Paradoxically, aspirin also transiently inhibits the formation of the

TABLE 5–6 . TREATMENT AND MANAGEMENT OF CEREBROVASCULAR DISEASE

Systemic
Decrease the risk factors
Prophylactic medications
  Aspirin, 40 mg qd
  Ticlopidine
Intravenous tissue plasminogen activator
Carotid endarterectomy

Ocular
Treatment of systemic condition
Iris and/or retinal neovascularization, panretinal photocoagulation

antiaggregating and vasodilating prostaglandin, prostacyclin, in endothelial cells. As soon as aspirin is cleared from the blood, the endothelial cells again produce prostacyclin. The optimal dose of aspirin is debated, but one study indicated that low doses, such as 40 mg per day, may be as effective as larger doses and inhibits the formation of thromboxane A_2 without substantially inhibiting prostacyclin formation.

Ticlopidine produces a 12% greater reduction in stroke than aspirin. The antiplatelet effect occurs because ticlopidine blocks the adenosine diphosphate receptor on platelets. This blockade prevents the cascade resulting in the activation of the glycoprotein IIb/IIIa receptor that leads to fibrinogen binding to the platelets and consequent platelet aggregation. Ticlopidine has the disadvantage of causing neutropenia, diarrhea, and skin rash in many patients. In addition, it is costly compared to aspirin. Consequently, ticlopidine is recommended for use as an antiplatelet agent only if aspirin is contraindicated or fails.

The role of anticoagulation in atherothrombotic cerebral disease is uncertain. Four randomized prospective studies, using a small number of patients, comparing anticoagulant-treated patients with TIAs to controls showed no significant difference in the incidence of stroke or death in the two groups. Two large trials are currently in progress and should clarify the role of anticoagulation in the prevention of ischemic stroke.

The most common surgical procedure for the remediation of reduced perfusion through the carotid vasculature is carotid endarterectomy. Since 1971 there has been an increase of more than 500% in the use of this procedure in the United States.

In this procedure a longitudinal incision is made in the carotid artery and extended to the bifurcation to include the ICA. The atheromatous plaque is dissected and removed. The arterial incision is then closed with suture material. Often a patch graft can be made from either a leg vein or a polymer patch. Ott and coworkers (1990) have described a procedure using the argon laser to cleave the atheroma from the vessel wall.

In the past, carotid endarterectomy was fraught with considerable risk. Fields and associates (1970) reported on a large controlled prospective study between 1962 and 1968. The combined perioperative stroke and death rate varied from 2.5 to 24.4%. Brott and Thalinger (1984) indicated that the risks of carotid endarterectomy were a function of the surgeon's skill.

The North American Symptomatic Carotid Endarterectomy Trial (NASCET) and the European Carotid Surgery Trial (ECST) were conducted to evaluate the efficacy of carotid endarterectomy and medical treatment as compared to medical therapy alone in the prevention of stroke. The data indicated that carotid endarterectomy was highly beneficial in preventing stroke in patients who had recent cerebrovascular symptoms in the carotid territory and who had severe carotid stenosis (70 to 99%). The absolute risk of ischemic stroke at the end of 2 years after surgery was reduced by 17%. On the basis of the results of NASCET and ECST, the following recommendations can now be made: patients who have had recent symptoms within the carotid artery territory, have severe carotid stenosis, do not have cardiac disease or refractory hypertension, and who are otherwise fit for surgery should undergo carotid endarterectomy. Patients with mild stenosis, that is, less than 30%, should be treated medically. Patients with moderate stenosis (30 to 69%) should be randomized within ongoing carotid surgery trials.

The Asymptomatic Carotid Atherosclerosis Study (ACAS) demonstrated that asymptomatic patients with ICA stenosis greater than 60% are at low risk for stroke. The absolute risk reduction was 5.9% over 5 years, or 1.2% annually. Thus, patients with asymptomatic carotid stenosis should be treated medically.

The treatment for acute ischemic stroke in progress has concentrated on thrombolytic therapy. Optimally, the goal of thrombolytic therapy for the treatment of stroke is to achieve rapid lysis of the ischemic occlusion and restore cerebral perfusion in the area affected by the thrombus/embolus. If the occlusion remains, the loss of tissue perfusion leads to infarction and necrosis in the affected area. To date, alteplase tissue plasminogen activator (tPA) is the only medication approved for the treatment of acute ischemic stroke. This drug converts plasminogen to the enzyme plasmin. The fibrin clot is subsequently degraded by the plasmin.

> Carotid endarterectomy is highly beneficial in preventing stroke in patients who have had recent cerebrovascular symptoms in the carotid territory and who have severe carotid stenosis (70 to 99%).

A landmark randomized, placebo-controlled trial was completed in 1995 by the National Institute of Neurological Disorders and Stroke and Communicative (NINCDS). It demonstrated consistent and significant improvement in long-term clinical benefit for acute ischemic stroke patients treated with tPA within 3 hours of symptom onset. On the basis of this study and other clinical trials, the Food and Drug Administration approved the use of intravenous tPA for the treatment of acute ischemic stroke for patients who could be treated within 3 hours of stroke onset. Subsequently, the use of tPA was strongly endorsed by the American Academy of Neurology (AAN), the American Heart Association (AHA), and the American College of Chest Physicians (ACCP).

> Intravenous tissue plasminogen activator (tPA) is the first effective therapy approved for the treatment of acute ischemic stroke but must be used within 3 hours of stroke onset.

Ocular

The treatment of the ocular manifestations of cerebrovascular disease depends on the specific ocular stigmata that are present. Generalized ischemia to the anterior portion of the eye as well as emboli in the retinal artioles may be ameliorated by the successful recanalization of the carotid artery via endarterectomy.

If iris neovascularization and/or retinal neovascularization is present, panretinal photocoagulation is the treatment of choice. It consists of the application of several hundred burns 500 μm in diameter to each quadrant of the fundus. The treatment extends posteriorly to two disc diameters from the center of the macula in the temporal quadrants and one-half disc diameter from the border of the optic nerve nasally. The total number of burns may vary between 1200 and 1600. Additionally, focal treatment using moderate-intensity confluent burns may be applied directly to the new vessels on the retina.

Panretinal photocoagulation is often followed by regression of the retinal neovascularization and the rubeosis irides in several days. The beneficial effects of scatter photocoagulation stem from the ablation of retinal tissue sufficient to decrease retinal metabolic demands. It is believed that it is the decreased perfusion to the retina as a result of carotid artery disease that stimulates the formation of new vessels on the retina and on the iris.

Antiplatelet drugs are the current treatment of choice for vertebral insufficiency to the occipital cortex or brainstem. Treatment of the subclavian steal syndrome is aimed at restoring normal blood flow by various surgical anastomoses.

CONCLUSION

The very nature of cerebrovascular disease is apt to result in ocular manifestations. An understanding of the applied vascular anatomy and sequelae of impaired cerebrovascular blood flow will enable the eyecare practitioner to diagnose cerebrovascular disease and participate in its management.

REFERENCES

Abernathy M, Brandt NM, Robinson C. Noninvasive testing of the carotid system. *Am Fam Physician.* 1984;29:157–168.

Adams HP Jr, Brott TG, Furlan AJ, et al. Guidelines for thrombolytic therapy for acute stroke: A statement for healthcare professionals from a special writing group of the Stroke Council, American Heart Association. *Circulation.* 1996;94:1167–1174.

Adams HP Jr, Kassell NF, Wisoff HS, Drake CG. Intracranial saccular aneurysm and moyamoya disease. *Stroke.* 1979;10: 174–179.

Albers GW, Easton JD, Sacco RL, Teal P. Antithrombotic and thrombolytic therapy for ischemic stroke. *Chest.* 1998; 114(suppl):683S–698S.

American–Canadian Cooperative Study Group. Persantine aspirin trial in cerebral ischemia. 2. Endpoint results. *Stroke.* 1985;16:406–415.

Antiplatelet Trialists' Collaboration: Collaborative overview of randomized trials of antiplatelet therapy—I: Prevention of death, myocardial infarction, and stroke by prolonged antiplatelet therapy in various categories of patients. *BMJ.* 1994;308:81–98.

Beneficial effect of carotid endarterectomy in symptomatic patients with high-grade carotid stenosis. North American Symptomatic Carotid Endarterectomy Trial Collaborators. *N Engl J Med.* 1991;325:445–453.

Blackwood W, Hallpike JF, Kocen RS. Atheromatous disease of the carotid arterial system and embolism from the heart in cerebral infarction: A morbid anatomical study. *Brain.* 1969;92:897–908.

Blaustein BH. The subclavian steal syndrome. *Clin Eye Vision Care.* 1991;3:25–28.

Brott T, Thalinger K. The practice of carotid endarterectomy in a large metropolitan area. *Stroke.* 1984;15:950–955.

Brott T, Thalinger K, Hertzberg V. Hypertension as a risk factor for spontaneous intracerebral hemorrhage. *Stroke.* 1986;17:1078–1083.

Brown GC, Magargal LE. The ocular ischemic syndrome: Clinical, fluoroscein angiographic, and carotid angiographic features. *Int Ophthalmol.* 1998;11:239–251.

Brown MM, Humphrey PR. Carotid endarterectomy: Recommendations for management of transient ischaemic attack and ischaemic stroke. *BMJ.* 1992;305:1071–1074.

Browning DJ, Flynn HW, Blankenship GW. Asymmetric retinopathy in patients with diabetes mellitus. *Am J Ophthalmol.* 1988;105:584–589.

Cromwell RM, Ojemann R. Surgical management of extracranial occlusive disease. In: Barnett HJ, Stein B, Mohr JP, Yatsu F, eds. *Stroke: Pathophysiology, Diagnosis and Management.* New York: Churchill Livingstone; 1986:1014–1024.

Dorsch N. Cerebral aneurysms and subarachnoid hemorrhage. *Med J Aust.* 1966;1:651–657.

Duker JS, Brown GC, Bosley TM, et al. Asymmetric proliferative diabetic retinopathy and carotid artery disease. *Ophthalmology.* 1990;97:869–874.

Dyken ML, Wolf PA, Barnett HJM, et al. Risk Factors in stroke. A statement for physicians by the Subcommittee on Risk Factors and Stroke of the Stroke Council. *Stroke.* 1984;15:1105.

Earnest F, Forbes G, Sandok BA, et al. Complications of cerebral angiography: Prospective assessment of risk. *AJNR.* 1983;4:141–159.

Easton JD, Witterdink JL. Carotid endarterectomy: Trials and tribulations. *Ann Neurol.* 1994;35:5–12.

European Carotid Surgery Trialists' Collaboration Group: MRC European Carotid Surgery Trial: Interim results for symptomatic patients with severe (70–99%) or with mild (0–29%) carotid stenosis. *Lancet.* 1991;337:1235–1250.

Executive Committee for the Asymptomatic Carotid Atherosclerosis Study: Endarterectomy for asymptomatic carotid artery stenosis. *JAMA.* 1995;272:1421–1436.

Faught E, Trader SD, Hannah GR. Cerebral complications of angiography for transient ischemia and stroke: Prediction of risk. *Neurology.* 1979;29:4.

Feussner JR, Matchar DB. When and how to study the carotid arteries. *Ann Intern Med.* 1988:109–805.

Fields WJ, Maslenikov V, Meyer JS. Joint study of extracranial arterial occlusion, 5. Progress report of prognosis following surgery or nonsurgical treatment of transient ischemic cerebral attacks and cervical carotid artery lesions. *JAMA.* 1970;211:1993–2003.

Fisher CM. Clinical syndrome in cerebral thrombosis, hypertensive hemorrhage and ruptured saccular aneurysm. *Clin Neurosurg.* 1975;22:117–147.

Fisher CM, Robertson GH, Ojemann RG. Cerebral vasospasm with ruptured saccular aneurysm. The clinical manifestation. *Neurosurgery.* 1977;1:245–248.

Gautier JC. Clinical presentation and differential diagnosis of amaurosis fugax. In: Bernstein EF, ed. *Amaurosis Fugax.* New York: Springer-Verlag; 1988:24–42.

Gay AJ, Rosenbaum AL. Retinal artery pressure in asymmetric diabetic retinopathy. *Arch Ophthalmol.* 1966;75:758–762.

Gee W, Smith CA, Hinson CE, et al. Ocular pneumoplethysmography in carotid artery disease. *Med Instrument.* 1974;8:244–248.

Gresham GE, Fitzpatrick TE, Wolf PA, et al. Residual disability in survivors of stroke: The Framingham study. *N Engl J Med.* 1975;293:954.

Hijdra A, van Gijn J. Early death from rupture of an intracranial aneurysm. *J Neurosurg.* 1982;57:765–768.

Johnston ME, Gonder JR, Canny CLB. Successful treatment of the ocular ischemic syndrome with panretinal photocoagulation and cerebrovascular surgery. *Can J Ophthalmol.* 1988;23:114–121.

Kartchner MM, McRae LP, Morrison FD. Noninvasive detection and evaluation of carotid occlusive disease. *Arch Surg.* 1973;106:528.

Kearns TP, Hollenhorst RW. Venous stasis retinopathy of occlusive disease of the carotid artery. *Mayo Clin Proc.* 1963;38:304–312.

Kistler JP, Buonanno FS, De Witt LD, et al. Vertebral-basilar posterior cerebral territory stroke—delineation by proton nuclear magnetic resonance imaging. *Stroke.* 1984;15:417.

Kurtzke JF. Epidemiology and risk factors in thrombotic brain infarction. In: Harrison MJG, ed. *Cerebral Vascular Disease.* London: Butterworth; 1983:27–45.

Ljunggren B, Saveland H., Brandt L, Uski T. Aneurysmal subarachnoid hemorrhage. Total annual outcome in a 1.46 million population. *Surg Neurol.* 1984;22:435–438.

Moosey J. Cerebral atherosclerosis: Morphology and some relationships with coronary atherosclerosis. In: Zulch KJ, Kaufman W, Hossman KA, Hossman V, eds. *Brain and Heart Infarction.* New York: Springer-Verlag; 1977:253–260.

National Institute of Neurologic Disorders and Stroke rtPA study group. Tissue plasminogen activator for acute ischemic stroke. *N Engl J Med.* 1995;333:1581–1587.

North American Symptomatic Carotid Endarterectomy Trial Collaborators. Beneficial effect of carotid endarterectomy in symptomatic patients with high-grade carotid stenosis. *N Engl J Med.* 1991;325:445–453.

O'Donnell TF, Erdoes L, Mackey WC, et al. Correlation of B-mode ultrasound imaging and artereograph with pathologic findings at carotid endarterectomy. *Arch Surg.* 1985;120:443.

Ojemann RG, Heros RC. Spontaneous brain hemorrhage. *Stroke.* 1983;14:468–475.

Ott RA, Nudleman KL, Eugene J, et al. Initial clinical evaluation of carotid artery laser endarterectomy. *J Vasc Surg.* 1990;12:499–503.

Report of the Quality Standards Subcommittee of the American Academy of Neurology. Practice advisory: Thrombolytic therapy for acute ischemic stroke—summary statement. *Neurology.* 1996;47:835–839.

Riles TS, Lieberman A, Kopelman I, et al. Systems, stenosis, and bruit. Interrelationships in carotid artery disease. *Arch Surg.* 1981;116:218.

Roberts DK, Sears JM. Light-induced amaurosis associated with carotid occlusive disease. *Optom Vis Sci.* 1992;69:889–897.

Ross R, Glomset JA. The pathogenesis of atherosclerosis. *N Engl J Med.* 1976;295:369–377.

Sacco RL, Wolf PA, Bharucha NE, et al. Subarachnoid and intracerebral hemorrhage. Natural history, prognosis, and cursive factors in the Framingham study. *Neurology* (Cleveland). 1984;34:847–854.

Schroeder T. Hemodynamic significance of internal carotid artery disease. *Acta Neurol Scand.* 1988;77:353.

Sekhar LN, Heros RC. Origin, growth and rupture of saccular aneurysms. A review. *Neurosurgery.* 1981;8:248–260.

Stroke statistics from the American Heart Association. *Stroke.* 1988;19:547.

Tell GS, Crouse JR, Furberg D. Relation between blood lipids, lipoproteins and cerebrovascular atherosclerosis. *Stroke.* 1988;19:423.

Chapter 6

PRIMARY INTRACRANIAL TUMORS

Leonard V. Messner, Tricia L. Newman

Intracranial tumors include primary neoplasms, which arise from either the brain or meninges, and metastatic tumors to the brain from distant body sites. Tumors of the central nervous system (CNS) typically exhibit slow, insidious growth with a progression of clinically related signs and symptoms. Although 40% of all CNS tumors are benign, their growth and spread to adjacent structures may render them inoperable, and death may result from damage to vital brain centers. Ocular manifestations of intracranial tumors may result from increased intracranial pressure or damage to adjacent structures.

EPIDEMIOLOGY

Systemic

Tumors of the central nervous system constitute 1.6% of all cancers reported in the United States, with an annual incidence of 14,000 new cases. Of these, 10,000 are tumors of the brain. CNS tumors are responsible for 1.7% of all cancer-related deaths. There is a bimodal distribution of intracranial tumors, with one peak associated with children (3 to 12 years) and the other among older individuals (50 to 70 years). Regarding pediatric neoplasms, brain tumors are second only to leukemia among children younger than 10 years, and are approximately equal to leukemia between the ages of 10 and 14 years. Central nervous system neoplasms represent the third leading cause of cancer-related deaths in those between the ages of 15 and 34 years (Fueyo et al, 1999). Nearly two thirds of all pediatric central nervous system tumors are infratentorial in presentation, preferentially affecting the cerebellum, brainstem, midbrain, and thalamus.

Approximately 80% of all brain tumors are primary, while the remaining 20% develop elsewhere with intracranial metastases. Among primary tumors, gliomas are the most common, accounting for 50% of all intracranial tumors, followed by meningiomas (20%) (Bondy and Ligon, 1996), schwannomas (10%), and pituitary tumors (10%). The incidence of metastatic tumors increases proportionately according to patient age.

Intracranial tumors may present at any time. Embryonic tumors, such as medulloblastomas, typically develop early in life. Gliomas can occur at any age, with an increasing frequency of presentation up to age 65. Gender specificity reveals a slightly higher incidence of primary central nervous system tumors among males (6.3 per 100,000 population) versus that seen in females (4.4 per 100,000). Astrocytomas are more common among men, whereas meningiomas occur more frequently in women.

Ocular

Approximately 60% of patients with early developing brain tumors will manifest ocular signs or symptoms as the initial finding. Approximately 75% of all cases of papilledema are due to intracranial tumors. The prevalence of papilledema among individuals with brain tumors ranges from 59.9 to 80%.

PATHOPHYSIOLOGY/DISEASE PROCESS

Although a precise mechanism cannot be defined for most individuals, several etiologic factors have been reported within the literature regarding brain tumors. These include genetic factors, environmental factors, viral causes, radiation therapy, head trauma, and hormonal receptor binding sites (Black, 1993; Bondy and Ligon 1996).

There is no direct correlation between primary brain tumors and environmental factors. Nevertheless, chemical and radiation factors have been implicated in the development of both astrocytomas and meningiomas. Radiation is reported to be a definitive causative factor in the development of some meningiomas, including temporal, posterior fossa, and intracerebral lesions (Black, 1993). Radiation therapy may result in the chromosomal deletion of tumor suppressor sequences or genes that inhibit abnormal cell division (Black, 1993). Transplant recipients show a profound increase in the risk for the development of primary lymphoma of the brain.

A familial history of cancer may predispose some individuals toward the development of some primary brain tumors. Included among specific genetic disorders with intracranial complications are neurofibromatosis (type 2), von Hippel–Lindau disease, Turcot syndrome, and Li–Fraumeni syndrome.

The expression of certain chromosomal elements known as oncogenes has been shown to result in neoplastic cell proliferation with some primary tumors. Additionally, the loss of specific tumor suppressor genes has been implicated in the pathogenesis of retinoblastoma, osteosarcoma, meningiomas, acoustic neuromas, von Hippel–Lindau disease, and astrocytomas.

Angiogenic factors may also play a role in tumor development and progression. Many malignant tumors are capable of producing chemical mediators (e.g., acidic fibroblast growth factor [FGF], vascular endothelial growth factor [VEGF], transforming growth factor α [TGF-α] and β [TGF-β]) that allow for new vessel growth with subsequent tumor-cell proliferation and invasion (Fathallah-Shaykh, 1999).

Although no conclusive evidence exists linking brain tumors with a viral etiology, tumors have been produced in animals by viral inoculation. Hochberg and Miller (1988) have shown that patients with primary central nervous system lymphoma (PCNSL) exhibit a high incidence of seropositivity to Epstein–Barr virus. PCNSL and other primary intracranial tumors are reported at a higher incidence among HIV-infected patients. It is unclear whether HIV has oncogenic properties or if HIV-associated immunodeficiency places some individuals at greater risk for primary malignancy or infection-induced oncogenesis (Blumenthal et al, 1999).

Hormonal receptor binding sites, particularly for progesterone and estrogen, have been reported as potential etiologic factors in certain brain tumors. The precise role that these receptors play in the pathogenesis remains speculative; however, several clinical features (female predilection, increased tumor size during pregnancy) of some tumors suggest a possible hormonal linkage (Black, 1993).

Systemic

Intracranial tumors may present with a variety of signs and symptoms (Table 6–1). The clinical presentation is dependent on tumor size, location, effect on intracranial pressure, compression of cranial nerves, and invasion of adjacent structures. Patient signs and symptoms may be general or focal depending on the time course and position of the lesion. General signs and symptoms include headache, nausea and vomiting, vertigo, mental changes, dysphasia, circulatory and respiratory disturbances, papilledema, double vision, and seizures.

The clinical presentation of an intracranial tumor is determined by the following tumor-induced factors: increased intracranial pressure, irritation of electrically sensitive neural tissue, functional impairment or destruction of brain tissue, and endocrine effects. Increased intracranial pressure is most commonly induced by tumor-impaired cerebrospinal fluid (CSF) flow. Other causes of increased intracranial pressure are venous compression with reduced CSF absorption and increased CSF production.

The evolution of increased intracranial pressure is multifactorial. Tumors within the cranial vault act as space-occupying lesions leading to increased intracranial volume. This may be augmented by cerebral edema caused by the mass lesion. Brain tumors can

TABLE 6–1. SYSTEMIC MANIFESTATIONS OF PRIMARY INTRACRANIAL TUMORS

- Increased intracranial pressure
- Irritation of electrically sensitive neural tissue
- Functional impairment or destruction of brain tissue
- Endocrine changes
- Headache
- Nausea/vomiting
- Vertigo
- Mental changes
- Circulatory disturbances (tachycardia, arrhythmia)
- Respiratory disturbances (Cheyne–Stokes breathing)
- Seizures

block or impede the flow of CSF as well as stimulate production of CSF.

Headache

The most common symptom of increased intracranial pressure is headache. The pain is of notable intensity and may awaken the patient from sleep. It is continuous and typically diffuse in nature although some patients report a localized quality to the headache. The latter may be of some localizing value regarding tumor position, especially with dural tumors affecting the bone. The headache is often paroxysmal with the pain being most intense upon awakening with some remission as the patient assumes an upright position. Coughing, vomiting, defecation, and other Valsalva-like maneuvers also exacerbate the headache.

Nausea and Vomiting

Although both nausea and vomiting are associated with increased intracranial pressure, the presentation of vomiting alone is highly suggestive of acute pressure rise. Vomiting in conjunction with elevated intracranial pressure is due to compression of area postrema situated in the floor of the fourth ventricle.

Mental Changes

Changes in personality and mental ability may result from increased intracranial pressure. Patient symptomatology includes depression, irritability, indifference, loss of attention, and a dulling of intellectual function.

Circulatory and Respiratory Disturbances

Circulatory disturbances caused by increased intracranial pressure are tachycardia and arrhythmia with progression toward bradycardia. Increased respiration rate with altered respiration depth (Cheyne–Stokes breathing) may be coupled with circulatory deficits among individuals who exhibit a prolonged course of acute pressure rise. This is indicative of a poor prognosis.

Neuronal Irritation

Tumor invasion of cerebral cortex may irritate neurons, evoking seizure and related cortical disturbances. Seizures in an apparently healthy individual over the age of 20 years should alert the clinician to the possibility of a tumor. Seizures and convulsions are frequently associated with rapidly evolving tumors. The seizure pattern can be generalized or focal. Focal seizures that become generalized have a higher predictive value for an intracranial mass lesion.

Endocrine Effects

Endocrine disturbance is commonly associated with tumors affecting the pituitary gland and is discussed in Chapter 19.

Ocular

Careful ocular examination of a patient harboring an intracranial tumor is of paramount importance regarding the diagnosis and localization of the lesion. Given the extensive list of ocular manifestations (Table 6–2) associated with space-occupying lesions, this chapter limits discussion to those conditions most commonly encountered in clinical practice.

Papilledema

The term "papilledema" should be reserved for those cases of optic disc edema secondary to increased intracranial pressure. It is generally accepted that papilledema presents as a bilateral clinical entity, although some degree of asymmetry is common. Truly unilateral papilledema is exceedingly rare and may be caused by an ocular or orbital mass lesion. The presence of optic atrophy prohibits subsequent disc swelling from increased intracranial pressure. The presentation of papilledema in one eye with optic atrophy in the fellow eye is termed Foster–Kennedy syndrome and is typically associated with tumors of the frontal lobe. True Foster–Kennedy syndrome is quite rare and may be mimicked by acute anterior ischemic optic neuropathy in one eye and optic atrophy in the other.

Although the pathogenesis of papilledema remains a topic of debate, it appears likely that as intracranial pressure rises, this pressure elevation is transmitted throughout the subarachnoid space of the brain and optic nerve. The increased pressure within the vaginal sheaths of the optic nerve leads to axoplasmic stasis at the level of the lamina cribrosa. This produces leakage of water, protein, and other axoplasmic contents into the extracellular spaces of the prelaminar portion of the optic nerve. In addition to the mechanical disruption of axoplasmic flow, there is compression of the central retinal vein within the intraorbital portion of the optic nerve, further compounding the exudative response (Figure 6–1).

Many patients remain asymptomatic in the early stages of papilledema. Exceptions to this include individuals with profound disc leakage into the macula, resulting in macular edema. Chronic macular edema

TABLE 6–2. OCULAR MANIFESTATIONS OF INTRACRANIAL TUMORS

- Papilledema (increased blind spot)
- Ocular motility dysfunction (3rd, 4th, 6th cranial nerves; diplopia)
- Pupil abnormality (Horner, dilate pupil)
- Color vision defects
- Visual field defects

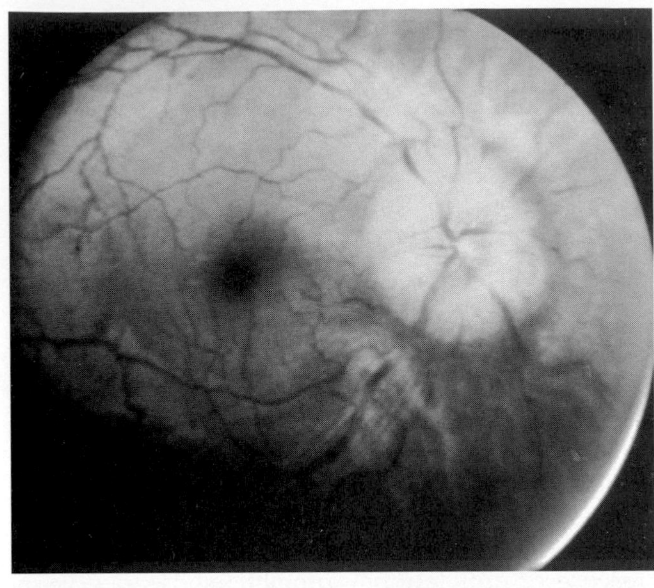

A

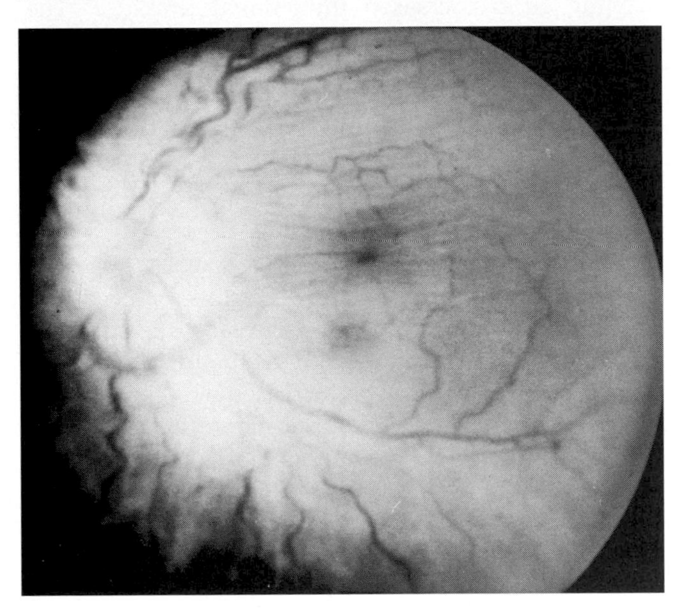

B

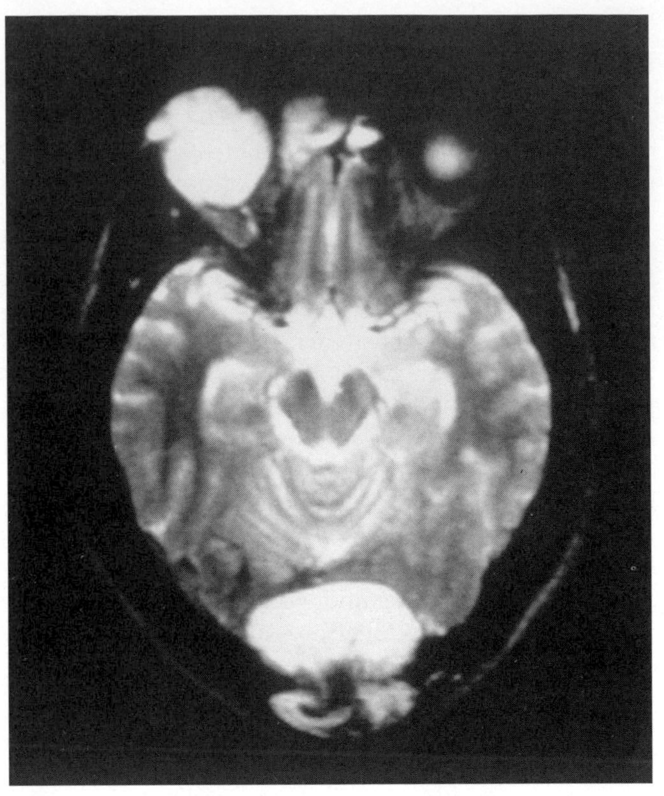

C

Figure 6–1. Funduscopic presentation of the right **(A)** and left **(B)** eyes of a patient with papilledema secondary to an intracranial soft tissue sarcoma. T_2 weighted MRI **(C)** demonstrates hyperdense signals, corresponding to sarcomatous lesions of the occipital lobe with extradural extension of the left orbit. (*Reprinted with permission from Conto JE. Soft tissue sarcoma metastatic to the orbit.* Clin Eye Vision Care *1991;3:126–134.*)

can progress toward further retinal disintegration with subsequent macular hole formation. Although most patients with papilledema demonstrate abnormal visual fields, the quality of the field loss is variable. Generalized depression, enlargement of the blind spot, contraction of the peripheral field, arcuate bundle defects, and other visual field abnormalities are reported. However, none of these field defects are diagnostically specific for papilledema.

Individuals with well-developed papilledema may report "gray-outs" or "black-outs" that are often precipitated by postural changes. These visual disruptions may be unilateral or bilateral, or may alternate between eyes. The episodes typically last for several minutes with complete visual recovery.

With prolonged axoplasmic stasis, the neurons of the optic nerve become atrophic resulting in permanent vision loss. The presence of an afferent pupillary defect is to be expected with asymmetric optic atrophy.

Dysfunction of Ocular Motility

In addition to papilledema, elevated intracranial pressure often leads to compression of the cranial nerves and nuclei that govern ocular movement. The possibility of an intracranial tumor must be considered in patients who present with acquired diplopia that is progressive in nature along with other neurologic symptoms.

> The possibility of an intracranial tumor must be considered in patients who present with acquired diplopia that is progressive in nature along with other neurologic symptoms.

Of the cranial nerves that control ocular motility, the abducens nerve is most susceptible to increased intracranial pressure. Sixth-nerve palsies associated with brain tumors are commonly unilateral and offer little localizing information regarding tumor position. Bilateral abducens palsies, although less frequent than unilateral palsies, are highly indicative of a neoplastic etiology and have been reported by Keane (1976) to have an associated tumor incidence of 25%. In children, tumors account for 33% of all cases of sixth-nerve palsies, with the majority of cases related to primary brainstem gliomas.

> An abduction deficit due to sixth-nerve paresis is suggestive only of increased intracranial pressure and has no localizing value with regard to tumor position.

From the point where the sixth nerve leaves the brainstem to its insertion within the lateral rectus, it is most vulnerable to insult from increased intracranial pressure where it crosses the petrous apex of the temporal bone. Downward displacement of the brainstem compresses the nerve between the petroclinoid ligament and bone, resulting in a sixth-nerve paresis with an abduction deficit of the ipsilateral eye.

In addition to the petrous ridge, the sixth nerve can also be compressed between the branches of the basilar artery as it emerges from the brainstem.

Elevated intracranial pressure frequently causes intermittent episodes of abducens impairment related to variances in intracranial pressure. Patients may or may not complain of diplopia depending on the magnitude and duration of sixth-nerve insult. It must be remembered that an abduction deficit due to sixth-nerve paresis is suggestive only of increased intracranial pressure and has no localizing value with regard to tumor position.

Tumor compression of the third nerve along its course produces progressive third-nerve palsy evidenced as a ptosis with a fixed and mid-dilated pupil associated with ipsilateral deficits of adduction, elevation, and depression. Tumors of the cavernous sinus are particularly unique in that combinations of third-, fourth-, and sixth-nerve palsies are common along with an ipsilateral Horner syndrome (Figure 6–2).

Primary Intracranial Tumors

Table 6–3 lists the primary intracranial tumors, which are described below.

Meningiomas

The most common form of benign intracranial tumor, meningiomas account for 10 to 20% of all primary brain tumors (Black, 1993; Bondy and Ligon, 1996). Meningiomas arise from mesodermal tissue and develop from the arachnoid layer of cells of the meninges. Intracranial meningiomas most commonly arise in the parasagittal region, sphenoid ridge, and falx cerebri (Figure 6–3). Sphenoid ridge meningiomas may invade the orbit via the optic canal or superior orbital fissure. Although they may be asymptomatic, their clinical presentation often includes seizures, hemiparesis, aphasia, and visual field cuts (Black, 1993). Middle-aged women are most commonly affected by these tumors.

Ocular meningiomas typically develop within the intraorbital portion of the optic nerve sheath. At this location, they can remain confined to the orbit or spread intracranially to occupy the middle cranial fossa. Patient signs and symptoms consistent with optic nerve sheath meningiomas include visual field cuts, reduced vision, disc edema, optic disc collaterals, proptosis, optic atrophy, afferent pupillary defects, and color desaturation. Disc edema may result from either direct compression of the optic nerve by the tumor or from increased intracranial pressure (papilledema). Intrapapillary refractile bodies may be observed in some cases of chronic disc congestion, although their precise composition remains speculative. Collateral vessels of the optic nerve head frequently evolve from meningiomas due to the compression of the central retinal vein producing obstructed venous outflow. These vessels are known to regress after surgical excision of the tumor. Ipsilateral proptosis may develop with some optic nerve sheath meningiomas and often precedes significant vision loss.

The presentation of optic atrophy with ipsilateral anosmia and contralateral papilledema has been termed the Foster–Kennedy syndrome. Although exceedingly rare, this constellation of findings is pathognomonic for a tumor growing at the base of the frontal lobes. Meningiomas occupying the olfactory grooves are the most common cause of the Foster–Kennedy syndrome. Although many maladies have been reported as "masquerades" of the true syndrome, it is

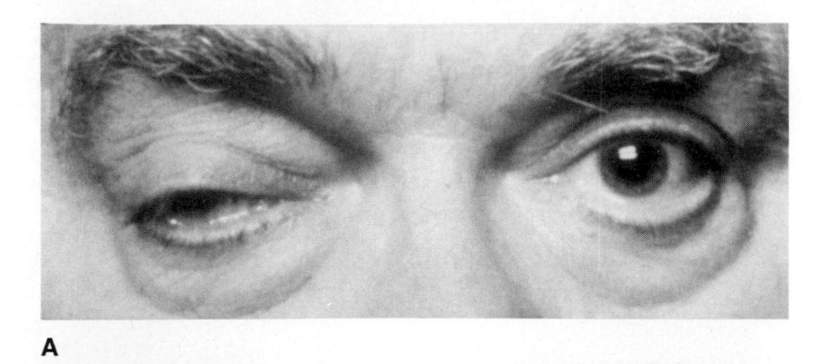

A

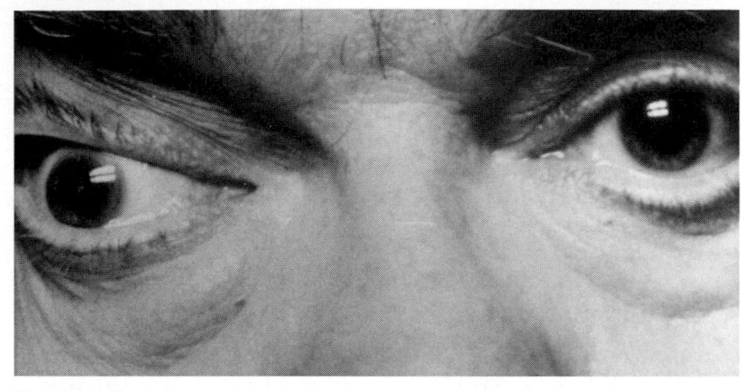

B

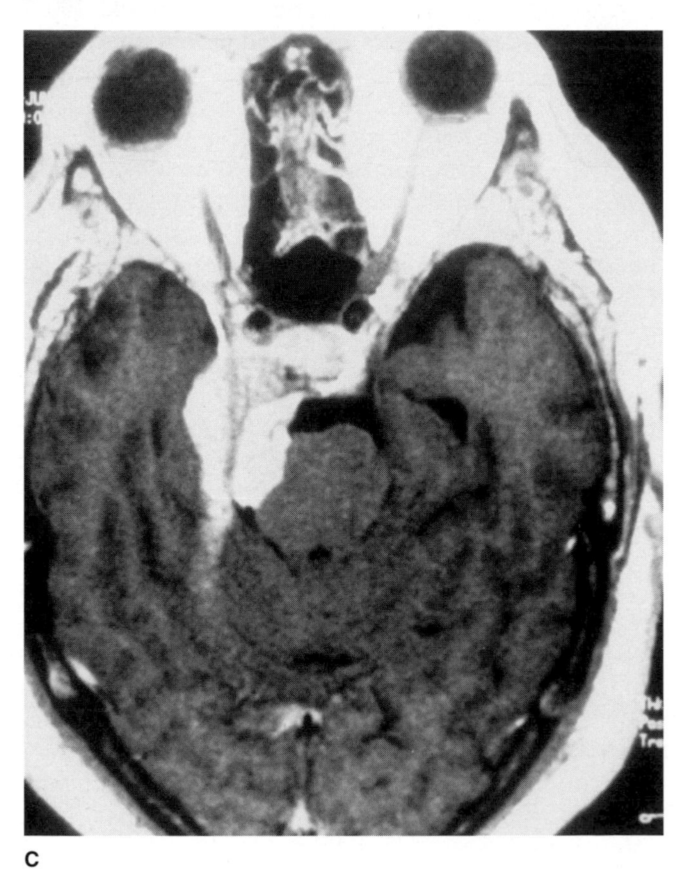

C

Figure 6–2. An incomplete right third-nerve palsy **(A, B)** caused by a meningioma of the cavernous sinus. MRI with enhancement **(C)** reveals a hyperintense lesion involving the right cavernous sinus. (*Courtesy of Dr. Jeffrey M. Augustine.*)

TABLE 6–3. PRIMARY INTRACRANIAL TUMORS

Meningiomas
Gliomas
Astroglial tumors: astrocytomas, anaplastic astrocytoma, glioblastoma
Oligodendroglioma
Ependymoma
Medulloblastoma
Ganglioglioma
Craniopharyngiomas
Pineal-area tumors
Primary CNS lymphomas
Hemangioblastomas
Schwannomas
Colloid cysts
Choristomas

most important to note that ischemic optic neuropathy is capable of producing similar ocular findings and must be considered in the differential diagnosis.

Treatment of meningiomas remains controversial. Patients with tumors of the optic nerve sheath with good vision and no evidence of intracranial extension are frequently followed. If vision is lost or if there is invasion of the middle cranial fossa, surgical excision is the treatment choice. Tumor resection is more difficult if the meningioma involves the cavernous sinus,

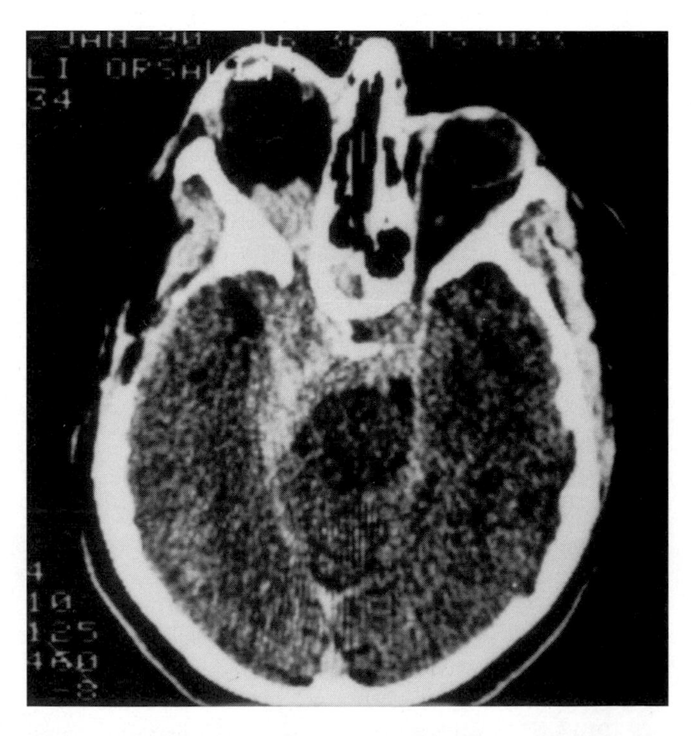

Figure 6–3. Axial CT scan of a sphenoid ridge meningioma that has spread to involve the left orbit and optic nerve. The left globe appears proptotic because of intraorbital tumor extension.

orbital apex, or superior orbital fissure. Radiotherapy holds promise as a lone therapeutic modality as well as an adjunct to surgery. Barbaro et al (1987) reported recurrent tumor growth in 60% of patients with subtotal tumor resection without adjuvant radiation therapy as compared to 32% of patients with adjuvant radiation. Recent studies have documented the presence of estrogen and progesterone receptors on meningioma cells. It has also been established that pregnancy can exacerbate tumor growth. Therefore, it is reasonable to assume that hormonal therapy may play a role in the future management of meningiomas.

Gliomas

Glial cells provide the supportive matrix for the central and peripheral nervous systems. Tumors of neuroglial origin are collectively termed "gliomas." Gliomas are of neuroectodermal origin and constitute the most common primary CNS tumors, accounting for 40 to 60% of these neoplasia. Gliomas display significant genetic tendencies and represent 60 to 90% of all childhood primary intracranial tumors. Adult-presenting gliomas generally involve the cerebral hemispheres, whereas the brainstem and cerebellum are most commonly affected in children. The classification of gliomas includes those tumors of astroglial origin (astrocytomas), tumors arising from oligodendrocytes (oligodendroglia), tumors derived from ependymal cells (ependymomas), tumors of cerebellar origin (medulloblastomas), and those tumors with glial and neuronal precursors (gangliogliomas).

Astroglial Tumors. The subclassification of astroglial tumors according to histologic composition and location has proven to be somewhat difficult with regard to ultimate prognosis. Consequently, a "three-tiered" system has been devised to classify these neoplasms.

1. *Astrocytomas* are relatively benign, slow-growing tumors that demonstrate mild hypercellularity and pleomorphism with no evidence of vascular proliferation or tissue necrosis. The term "low-grade astrocytomas" is commonly used to describe these tumors. They represent the most common primary brain tumors in both children and adults (Hill et al, 1999).
2. *Anaplastic astrocytomas* exhibit moderate hypercellularity and pleomorphism with vascular proliferation.
3. *Glioblastomas* demonstrate all of the characteristic features of anaplastic astrocytomas along with tissue necrosis and hemorrhage. Additionally, glioblastomas differ from other astroglial tumors in that they usually occur later in life, with peak incidence in the fifth and sixth decades. These are highly malignant neoplasms for which several genetic and chromosomal abnormalities have been implicated (Fueyo, 1999; Hill et al, 1999). Their multidimensional cellular organization has lead to the descriptive term glioblastoma multiforme in reference to these neoplasms.

Astrocytomas are considered to be fairly nonaggressive, whereas anaplastic astrocytomas and glioblastomas demonstrate increasing malignant tendencies.

The term "optic glioma" is used to describe astroglial tumors of the anterior visual pathways. Involved structures include the optic nerves, chiasm, and optic tracts. Optic gliomas are found almost exclusively among younger individuals, with 80% occurring before age 10 and over 90% occurring before age 20. They typically present as low-grade astrocytomas with malignant transformation occurring in only about 1% of affected patients. Rare cases of malignant optic nerve glioma in adults have been reported. These patients often exhibit early visually evoked potential (VEP) abnormalities that are followed by rapid visual deterioration. Optic nerve gliomas may be unilateral or bilateral with the latter often being associated with neurofibromatosis. The clinical presentation includes reduced vision, proptosis, and optic atrophy. Magnetic resonance imaging (MRI) has proven to be superior to computed tomography (CT) in the evaluation of optic gliomas because its high-resolution characteristics are relatively unaffected by surrounding bone.

Pontine gliomas can produce ocular motility abnormalities that mimic spasmus nutans (see Chapter 12). The triad of head tilt, head nod, and low-amplitude, high-frequency horizontal nystagmus is pathognomonic of spasmus nutans, and presents as a benign, self-limiting disorder of young children. Deviations from this constellation of signs should alert the clinician to the possibility of a brainstem tumor, necessitating prompt neuroradiologic evaluation. It is generally recommended that acquired nystagmus in childhood be investigated by neuroimaging techniques, especially if the criterion for spasmus nutans are not met with precision.

The management of optic glioma remains a topic of debate. Many optic nerve gliomas remain relatively stable and do not merit treatment. In the event of progressive vision loss or intracranial tumor extension, surgical resection or radiation treatment may be warranted. If the tumor is confined to one optic nerve and vision is severely reduced, total resection of the tumor and nerve is recommended. The preservation of a nerve stump connected to the eye will also preserve the globe due to collateral anastomoses between the short posterior ciliary arteries and the central retinal artery. Radiation for optic nerve and chiasmal gliomas has proven effective with regard to the stabilization or improvement of vision in many cases.

Newer surgical resection techniques (eg, gamma knife stereotactic external beam radiotherapy), radiation, chemotherapy, and brachytherapy (the stereotactic implantation of radioactive seed or plaques with or without subsequent removal) have improved the overall survival rate for intracranial gliomas. Younger patients tend to fare better after surgery and radiation treatment. The Brain Tumor Cooperative Group (Shapiro et al, 1989) reported that individuals under the age of 40 had a 64% survival rate after 18 months compared to only 8% over age 60, after surgery and radiation/chemotherapy.

Interferon and other methods of immunotherapy have not proven successful in the management of malignant astrocytomas. There is optimism that monoclonal antibodies directed against tumor-specific antigens may hold promise in the treatment of some patients with these tumors.

Oligodendrogliomas. Oligodendrocytes are the myelin-producing cells of the central nervous system. Histologically, the cells have a "halo" or "fried-egg" appearance. Oligodendrogliomas are uncommon gliomas representing less than 10% of all intracranial tumors (Hill et al, 1999). They are typically slow-growing tumors with varying degrees of calcification that appear as hypodense lesions with CT and MRI. The frontal and parietal lobes represent the most common tumor locations with the presenting signs and symptoms consistent with lesions of these areas.

Although usually benign, oligodendrogliomas may be malignant and can present in conjunction with astrocytomas. Surgical resection is the most common form of treatment; however, concomitant radiation and chemotherapy are also indicated in the management of malignant oligodendrogliomas (Perry et al, 1999).

Ependymomas. Ependymal cells line the ventricular cavities and canals of the central nervous system. Ependymomas arise from these cells, and are deeply situated within the spinal cord and brain. Children are most frequently affected, with the spinal cord being the most common site of tumor growth. The cerebral hemispheres are rarely affected by ependymomas. Ependymomas appear as round hyperintense lesions with gadolinium-enhanced MRI and exhibit a circular growth pattern.

The treatment of choice for ependymomas is surgical resection followed by radiation unless obviated by tumor location.

Medulloblastomas. Medulloblastomas are rare tumors arising from primitive neuroepithelial cells of the roof of the fourth ventricle that grow to involve the cerebellum. The exact cellular origin of these tumors remains unknown. These are malignant tumors of childhood with very aggressive growth patterns. They account for up to 20% of all intracranial tumors in children and less than 5% in adults (Hildebrand et al, 1997). The tumor is appreciated as a hyperintense lesion with MRI that is enhanced with gadolinium.

Although invasive in nature, medulloblastomas are amenable to surgical resection followed by radiation. Radiation therapy results in a 50 to 70% cure rate at 5 years and greater than 40% at 10 years (Hildebrand et al, 1997).

Gangliogliomas. Gangliogliomas are unique tumors of both astrocytic and neuronal origin (ganglion cells). These are tumors that afflict children and young adults, usually involving the temporal and frontal lobes. The most common clinical presentation is seizure. Rarely, gangliogliomas can manifest as intrinsic tumors of the optic nerve or chiasm, and as such can mimic optic gliomas. CT and MRI demonstrate low-density lesions that enhance with contrast. However, as is true for all intracranial tumors, histologic evaluation is required for definitive diagnosis. Surgery remains the most acceptable mode of treatment.

Craniopharyngiomas

Craniopharyngiomas are tumors derived from the colloid–cystic remnants of the Rathke pouch, and constitute 3% of all intracranial tumors and up to 13.5% of all CNS tumors found in children. Craniopharyngiomas generally occur during childhood and account for approximately 50% of all sellar and parasellar tumors of childhood and infancy. A second smaller peak occurs from the fourth to sixth decades of life (Banna, 1976). Most craniopharyngiomas arise within the sellar and suprasellar region. They typically develop as lobulated tumors that have both cystic and solid components. The solid portion of the tumor appears iso to hypointense on T_1-weighted MRI and iso to hyperintense with T_2 weighting. The cystic components appear hyperintense owing to protein and methemoglobin fluid constituents. Internal calcification of cholesterol/keratin/iron aggregates appears as hypointense granulations on both T_1 and T_2 weighting (Figure 6–4) (Faerber, 1995).

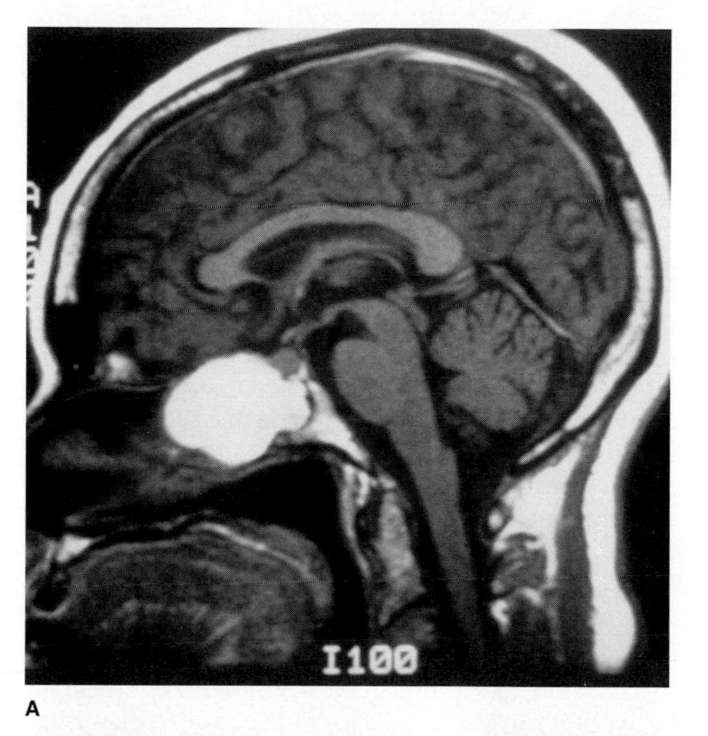

A

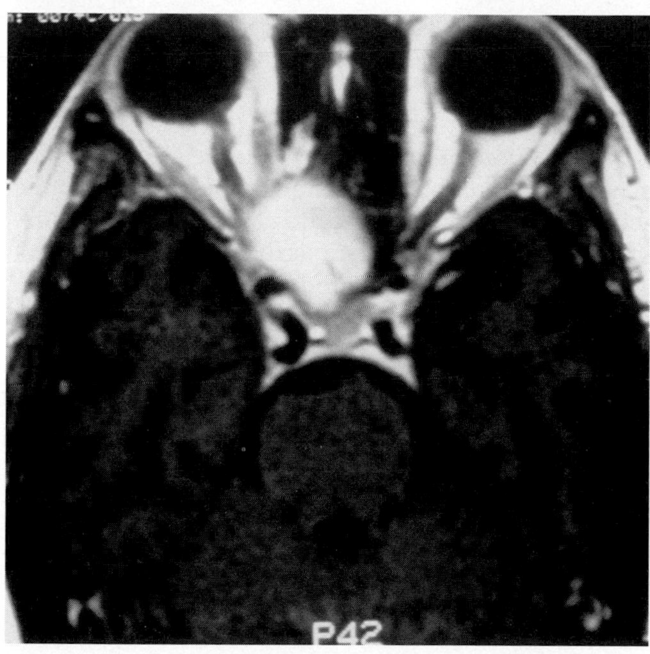

B

Figure 6–4. T_1-weighted coronal **(A)** and axial **(B)** MRI sections with gadolinium enhancement showing a hyperintense right-sided sphenoid mass with compression of the right optic nerve. Histologic examination of the lesion revealed cholesterol clefts and giant cells with fibrous tissue consistent with a craniopharyngioma. (*Courtesy of Dr. Ruth Trachimowicz.*)

Craniopharyngiomas liberate a viscous fluid of cholesterol composition that is highly irritating to the CNS. Although craniopharyngiomas are represented histologically as benign lesions, they nevertheless are associated with a higher-than-expected morbidity and mortality due to their high rate of recurrence. Because of their sellar location and relationship to the visual pathways, progressive vision loss is the most frequent presenting symptom of these tumors. Unless treated, continued compression of the anterior visual pathway structures leads to permanent vision loss.

If vision is affected, surgical resection followed by radiation therapy is the treatment of choice. Postoperative visual prognosis is not as good for craniopharyngiomas as for pituitary adenomas or suprasellar meningiomas. This is probably because craniopharyngiomas are more tightly adherent to visual structures and are located more posteriorly, making removal more difficult. Complete tumor resection is imperative for optimal postoperative success. Concomitant radiation therapy has proven to be effective for increased patient survival as opposed to surgery alone. If treated effectively, vision loss can often be stabilized and in some case improved. Progressive vision loss after treatment frequently denotes tumor recurrence.

Pineal-Area Tumors

Tumors of the pineal region include neoplasms of germ-cell origin (germinoma, teratoma, embryonal carcinoma, choriocarcinoma, and endodermal sinus tumor) as well as pinealomas, astrocytomas, cysts, and vascular lesions. Pinealomas can be subdivided into the poorly differentiated pinealoblastomas and pineocytomas, which are composed of mature pineal gland cells. There is a high incidence of retinoblastoma among patients with pinealomas.

Although rare, pineal-area tumors often present with ocular consequences. In addition to the general pressure effects caused by obstructive hydrocephalus, these tumors compress the dorsal midbrain structures and posterior commissure, producing the constellation of pupillary and ocular motility abnormalities referred to as Parinaud syndrome.

Parinaud syndrome (dorsal midbrain syndrome, sylvian aqueduct syndrome) is characterized by a vertical-gaze palsy that is evident on attempted upgaze caused by compression of the rostral interstitial nucleus of the medial longitudinal fasciculus (riMLF) fibers in the vicinity of the posterior commissure. Associated with the gaze palsy is convergence and (rarely) divergence retraction movements of the eyes into the orbits due to co-firing of extraocular muscle fibers. These unusual eye movements are most evident when upward saccadic movements are attempted. Additionally, lid retraction (Collier sign) is produced with attempted supraduction. Pupillary manifestations of mesencephalic compression include bilateral middilated pupils that do not react to light but become miotic when presented with a near target (light-near dissociation). With progressive compression of the Edinger–Westphal subnucleus, the pupils become fixed to both light and near stimuli. Also, convergence and downgaze pareses can develop. Along with oculomotor dysfunction, tumor of the pineal region may compress the trochlear nerve as it decussates within the superior medullary velum, resulting in a contralateral superior oblique palsy.

The presentation of a dorsal midbrain syndrome is often accompanied by headache and papilledema, and warrants immediate investigation by MRI. Germ-cell tumors respond nicely to radiation, whereas resection along with radiation is the treatment of choice for most other pineal-area tumors.

Primary CNS Lymphomas

Lymphoma is a malignant, nonencapsulated neoplasm that originates from the precursor cells of B and T lymphocytes. There are two categorical divisions of lymphoma: (1) Hodgkin disease and (2) the non-Hodgkin lymphomas. Non-Hodgkin lymphoma is also referred to as reticulum cell sarcoma, diffuse histiocytic lymphoma, microgliomatosis, and diffuse large-cell lymphoma. It is the non-Hodgkin variant that is responsible for primary brain and eye involvement. See Chapter 57, Non-Hodgkin Lymphoma and Intraocular Lymphoma.

Hemangioblastomas

Vascular tumors of the brain include hemagiomas, hemangioblastomas, and arteriovenous malformation. Of particular interest to the eyecare practitioner are hemangioblastomas, which present along with retinal angiomatosis as the syndrome of von Hippel–Lindau (see Chapter 37).

Schwannomas (Neuromas, Neurinomas, Neurilemomas)

Along with oligodendrocytes, Schwann cells are responsible for the production of myelin. Schwann cells cover cranial nerves III through XII, the spinal roots, and most peripheral nerves.

As the name implies, schwannomas arise directly from Schwann cells and represent 8 to 10% of all intracranial tumors. They are almost always benign, but can coexist along with neurofibromatosis, often in association with meningiomas and gliomas. The vast majority of these tumors involve the eighth cranial nerve and are termed "acoustic schwannomas." The peak incidence for acoustic schwannomas is the fourth to fifth decade of life. There is a slight female predilection.

Acoustic schwannomas typically arise within the internal auditory canal and spread to occupy the cerebellopontine angle. The initial presentation is progressive or sudden hearing loss, along with vestibular dysfunction and vertigo. Concomitant compression of cranial nerve VII (facial) results in a progressive facial paralysis that includes difficulty of attempted lid closure and loss of taste sensation to the anterior two thirds of the tongue. Involvement of the trigeminal nerve is common with these tumors, and results in the loss of corneal and facial sensation and weakening to the muscles of mastication. It is important to note that the triad of (1) unilateral deafness, (2) corneal hypoesthesia, and (3) incomplete facial palsy is highly indicative of a cerebellopontine angle mass lesion that is usually an acoustic schwannoma. As neoplasia of this region enlarge, there is further compression of brainstem structures and cerebellum, with associated neurologic dysfunction. Neuro-ophthalmic manifestations include skew deviations and nystagmus.

> The triad of (1) unilateral deafness, (2) corneal hypoesthesia, and (3) incomplete facial palsy is highly indicative of a cerebellopontine angle mass lesion that is usually an acoustic schwannoma.

Abduction deficits from acoustic schwannomas may be due to either direct tumor compression of the abducens nerve or from elevated intracranial pressure. Exceptionally large acoustic schwannomas can compress the trochlear nerve, producing a superior oblique palsy with vertical diplopia. Oculomotor involvement by these tumors is exceedingly rare.

Progressive unilateral deafness should be considered to be highly suggestive of acoustic schwannoma, necessitating appropriate auditory and vestibular investigation. CT and MRI with contrast enhancement are both useful in the identification of cerebellopontine angle mass lesions. MRI is relatively unaffected by surrounding bone, and is particularly useful for the visualization of small tumors that are located in the internal auditory canal.

Surgical resection is extremely effective in the management of these tumors. Early tumor detection and removal is essential for postoperative preservation of hearing and facial nerve function. Care must be taken to ensure removal of the entire tumor to minimize the chance of recurrence.

Colloid Cysts

Colloid cysts are rare (representing less than 1% of all intracranial tumors) neoplasms of neuroepithelial origin that invariably arise within the third ventricle.

These circular tumors are attached to the ventricular wall by a fibrous stalk. Most cysts exhibit some degree of motility that is affected by body position and movement. This allows the tumor to function in a "valve-like" fashion, producing intermittent occlusion of the foramen of Monro, resulting in the obstruction of cerebrospinal fluid flow between the third and fourth ventricles. The ultimate consequence of this action is a paroxysmal rise in intracranial pressure with subsequent headache, hydrocephalus, and (rarely) sudden death.

Neuro-ophthalmic manifestations of colloid cysts are compatible with pressure-related signs and symptoms, and may include papilledema, optic atrophy, abduction deficits, and variants of the dorsal midbrain syndrome.

The diagnosis of a colloid cyst is readily obtained with the use of neuroimaging studies. CT scanning and MR imaging reveal a well-delineated, circular mass lesion within the midline of the third ventricle.

The treatment of choice is surgical resection. Because of the risk of sudden death, these tumors always require immediate removal even in the absence of profound symptomatology or hydrocephalus. The use of CT-guided stereotactic cyst aspiration is the treatment of choice beacause of the relatively low risk associated with the procedure. Shunting procedures are reserved only for those cases where hydrocephalus persists following surgery.

Choristomas

Choristomas are congenital, usually benign tumors that are composed of normal tissues that develop in abnormal locations. These tumors can develop in many anatomical regions including the brain, eye, and orbit. The most common types of intracranial choristomas are epidermoids and dermoids. Both are cyst-like tumors of ectodermal origin.

Epidermoids usually develop within the cisterns at the base of the brain as well as on the tela choroidae of the ventricles. As opposed to colloid cysts, epidermoids tend to exhibit a more lateral position away from the midline. The most common anatomic substrate for these tumors is the cerebellopontine angle. Histologically, they are encapsulated, cystic tumors that contain an amorphous, granular material that is laden with cholesterol crystal. The latter has lead to the rubric "cholesteatomas" to describe these types of tumors.

Although congenital, epidermoids are extremely slow growing and may remain asymptomatic for many years. Seizure is the most commonly reported presenting symptom. Other nonspecific neurologic signs include dementia, cranial nerve abnormalities, and hydrocephalus. The neuro-ophthalmic signs and symptoms of epidermoids are dependent on tumor location. Suprasellar epidermoids can produce visual field defects often associated with hypothalamic dysfunction. Parasellar tumors can invade the cavernous sinus producing a painful ophthalmoplegia along with other aspects of cavernous sinus syndromes. Epidermoid tumors of the cerebellopontine angle can produce ipsilateral deafness, facial paralysis, and trigeminal dysfunction, and mimic acoustic schwannomas.

Intracranial dermoids demonstrate a gross and histologic composition similar to epidermoids, with the inclusion of hair follicles and secretory glands within the capsular wall. As with epidermoids, the clinical signs and symptoms are slow to evolve, and depend on tumor location and involvement of associated structures.

The diagnosis of intracranial choristomas is best achieved by CT or MRI. Both epidermoids and dermoids exhibit a hypodense internal core surrounded by an enhanced capsular rim. Treatment is surgical removal of the entire tumor, with care taken not to rupture the tumor wall, as spillage of the internal contents can result in aseptic meningitis.

Metastatic Tumors

Approximately 20 to 30% of all systemic cancers result in intracranial metastases. Primary systemic cancers with reported brain metastases include melanoma, breast carcinoma, lung carcinoma, pelvic–abdominal tumors, renal-cell carcinoma, and non-Hodgkin lymphoma. These extracranial tumors metastasize to the brain usually as arterial emboli that most commonly lodge within the cerebral cortex of the frontal and parietal lobes. Among individuals with cerebral metastases, one half exhibit CNS involvement as the only metastatic site. External irradiation of the whole brain remains the mainstay of treatment for brain metastases. Radiosurgery may be used as an adjuvant therapy for small brain metastases that are not amenable to surgical excision (Hildebrand et al, 1997). Chapter 56 discusses metastasis of systemic malignancies to the eye and orbit.

DIAGNOSIS

There is no substitute for a careful case history and physical examination of the patient who is suspected of harboring an intracranial tumor. The ocular examination of these patients is particularly critical given the plethora of ophthalmic signs and symptomatology associated with brain tumors. Once a tumor is suspected, it is imperative to order the correct test to ensure

TABLE 6–4. DIAGNOSTIC STUDIES

Neuroimaging
Computed tomography (CT)
Magnetic resonance imaging (MRI)

Angiography
Arteriography
Magnetic resonance angiography (MRA/MRV)

Metabolic Studies
Positron emission tomography (PET)
Single photon emission computed tomography (SPECT)

Serology
Antiphospholipid antibodies (APAs)
FTA–Abs
ACE/serum lysozyme
ANA
Lyme titers
CBC with differential

Lumbar Puncture

proper diagnosis (see Table 6–4 and 6–5) and management (see Table 6–6).

Systemic

Neuroimaging

The advent of CT and MRI has eliminated the need for conventional brain scanning and pneumoencephalography in the investigation of suspected intracranial mass lesions. In addition to specific neuroradiologic characteristics, the differential diagnosis of intracranial tumors is established based on the statistical prevalence of certain tumors for anatomical regions and tissue substrates. It is important to be aware of the salient attributes and drawbacks of specific neuroimaging techniques so as to maximize the diagnostic potential for the case at hand while at the same time minimizing the expense and trouble incurred by the patient for unnecessary studies.

CT employs an x-ray technique to image the cranial vault and its contents. The intensity and resolution of the scan is dependent upon the relative tissue densities being studied, with high-density structures displaying a high degree of appreciation. This feature makes CT particularly effective for visualization of the skull and bony defects (Figure 6–5). Because of the low tissue density of cortex and other brain structures, an intravenous contrast agent is required to elicit anatomic detail, tumor structure, hemorrhage, infarction, and abscess. CT scanning is the preferred technique for patients with acute stroke and bone-related lesions and for patients who are obese or claustrophobic or cannot remain still for an MRI.

MRI uses a high-intensity magnetic field to align the free protons of hydrogen atoms throughout the body. A pulsed electromagnetic field is then applied to

TABLE 6–5. DIFFERENTIAL DIAGNOSIS OF PRIMARY INTRACRANIAL TUMORS

Systemic
Idiopathic intracranial hypertension (pseudotumor cerebri)
Primary seizure disorder
Cerebral vascular accident
Dementia
Migraine
Cardiac arrhythmia
Intracranial vascular abnormalities (arteriovenous malformation)
Demyelinating disease
Intracranial infectious/inflammatory disease (eg, syphilis, systemic lupus erythematosus, giant-cell arteritis, herpes simplex, herpes zoster, toxoplasmosis)

Ocular
Optic nerve
- Papillitis
- AION
- Perioptic neuritis
- Primary central vein occlusion
- Hyaline bodies (buried drusen)

Compressive/restrictive orbitopathies
- Dysthyroid orbitopathy
- Orbital pseudotumor

Cavernous sinus syndromes
- Cavernous sinus fistula
- Inflammatory disease (Tolosa–Hunt syndrome)
- Aneurysm
- Metastatic neoplasia

Ocular motilities
- Ischemic vascular cranial neuropathies
- Non-neoplastic compressive cranial neuropathies (eg, aneurysm)
- Vertebrobasilar insufficiency
- Congenital oculomotor palsies

disrupt this alignment, and the resultant energy changes are detected as the protons are permitted to relax their alignment. The relaxation times incurred during realignment are termed T_1- and T_2-weighted images. Because most hydrogen atoms are confined to water molecules, MRI, simply put, images the water content of a particular structure. This property makes MRI the method of choice for soft tissue investigation, and results in greater sensitivity and accuracy in the detection of many tumors when compared to CT. Bone, because of its low water content, appears dark with MRI, thus affording greater resolution of tumors in close proximity to bone as well as lesions of the posterior fossa. Vascularized tumors may be readily enhanced by employing the contrast agent gadolinium-DTPA. Because of the breakdown of the blood–brain barrier, hyperintense enhancement is associated with these lesions (Figure 6–6).

Angiography

Vascularized intracranial tumors and intracranial vascular abnormalities (eg, arteriovenous malformations, cerebral venous thrombosis, and intracranial aneurysms)

TABLE 6–6. SYSTEMIC AND OCULAR MANAGEMENT OF PRIMARY INTRACRANIAL TUMORS

Systemic
Surgery
Microneurosurgery
ISG viewing wand
Laser therapy
Radiation
Focal
Limited-field
Interstitial brachytherapy
Radiosurgery
Gamma knife
Linac
Chemotherapy
Carnustine (BCNU)
Lomustine (CCNU)
Cisplatin (CDDP)
Procarbazine
Methotrexate (MTX)
Vincristine (VCR)
Gene therapy
Suicide gene therapy
Antiangiogenesis
Immunogene therapy
Oncolytic viruses
Corticosteroids
Hyperthermia
Ocular
Prismatic correction
Muscle surgery

can be appreciated with angiographic techniques. Although digital subtraction intravenous angiography has shown much value for visualization of the major extracranial vessels of the neck, intracranial vascular resolution is markedly affected and degraded by bone-hardening artifacts of the skull. Consequently, direct arteriography is the procedure of choice for intracranial angiography. Because of the inherent risk associated with arteriography, magnetic resonance angiography (MRA) holds great promise as a safe and effective alternative.

Metabolic Studies

Many tumors display an increased rate of protein synthesis and uptake of glucose and amino acids, making them amenable to identification by positron emission tomography (PET). Particularly effective in the imaging of astroglial tumors, PET can be used preoperatively to determine the degree of malignancy associated with these neoplasms. The implementation of radiotracer elements like *L*-3-iodo-alpha-methyl tyrosine (IMT) and thallium-201 T_1 coupled with single photon emission computed tomography (SPECT) is extremely useful for the identification of high-grade malignant gliomas because of the increased metabolic activity and growth rate associated with these tumors. Black and associates (1989) reported an 89% accuracy

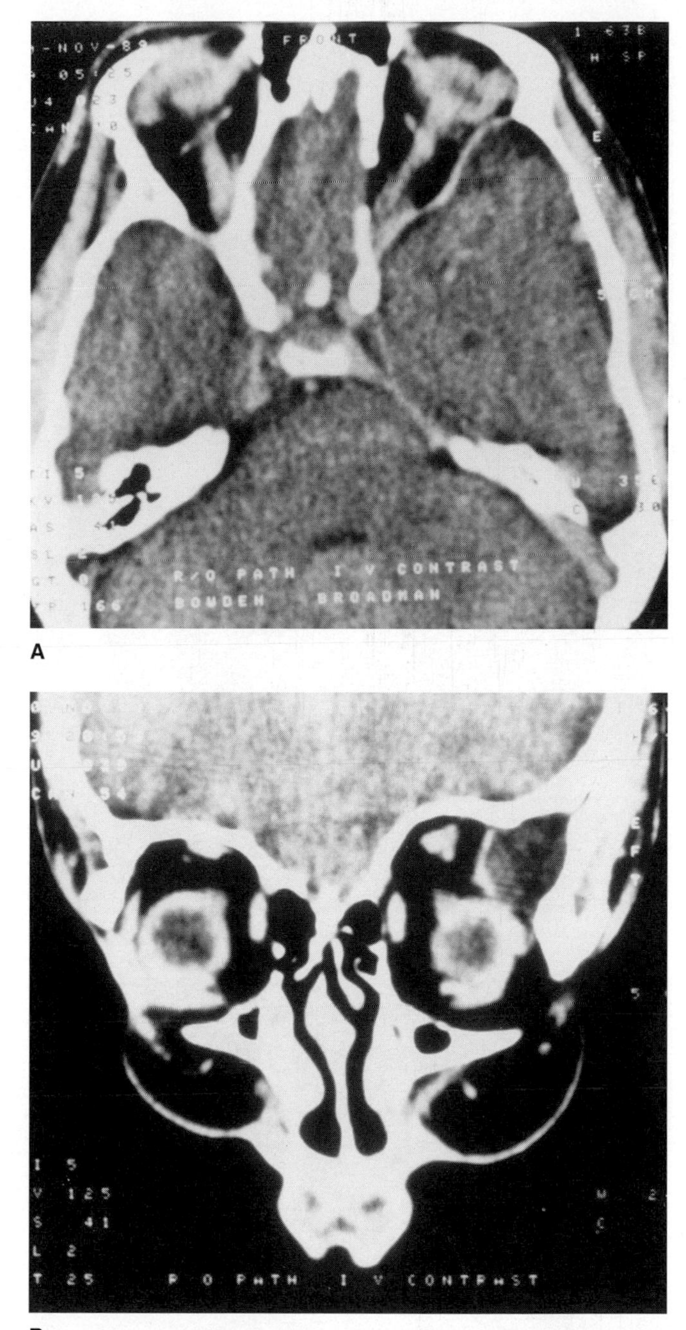

Figure 6–5. Axial **(A)** and coronal **(B)** sections of a meningoencephalocele produced by sphenoid wing defects. Note the total absence of the greater wing of the left sphenoid, allowing for herniation of the frontal lobe into the orbit and resulting in direct apposition with the globe. Such bony defects are commonly associated with neurofibromatosis.

in the prediction of low-grade versus high-grade malignant gliomas using T_1-SPECT.

Ocular

Ocular testing includes evaluation of motilities, pupils, color vision, and visual fields. When papilledema is

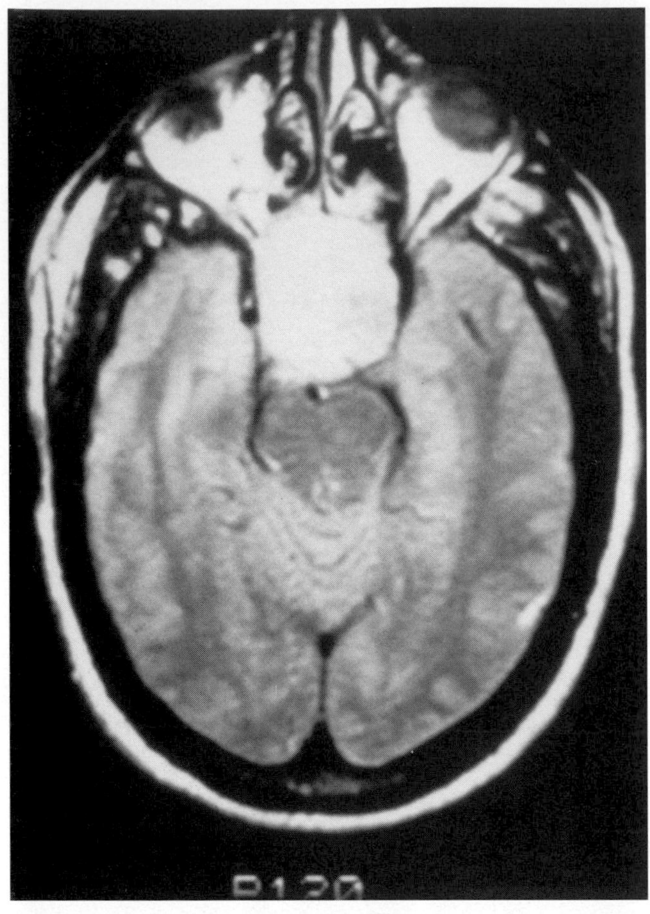

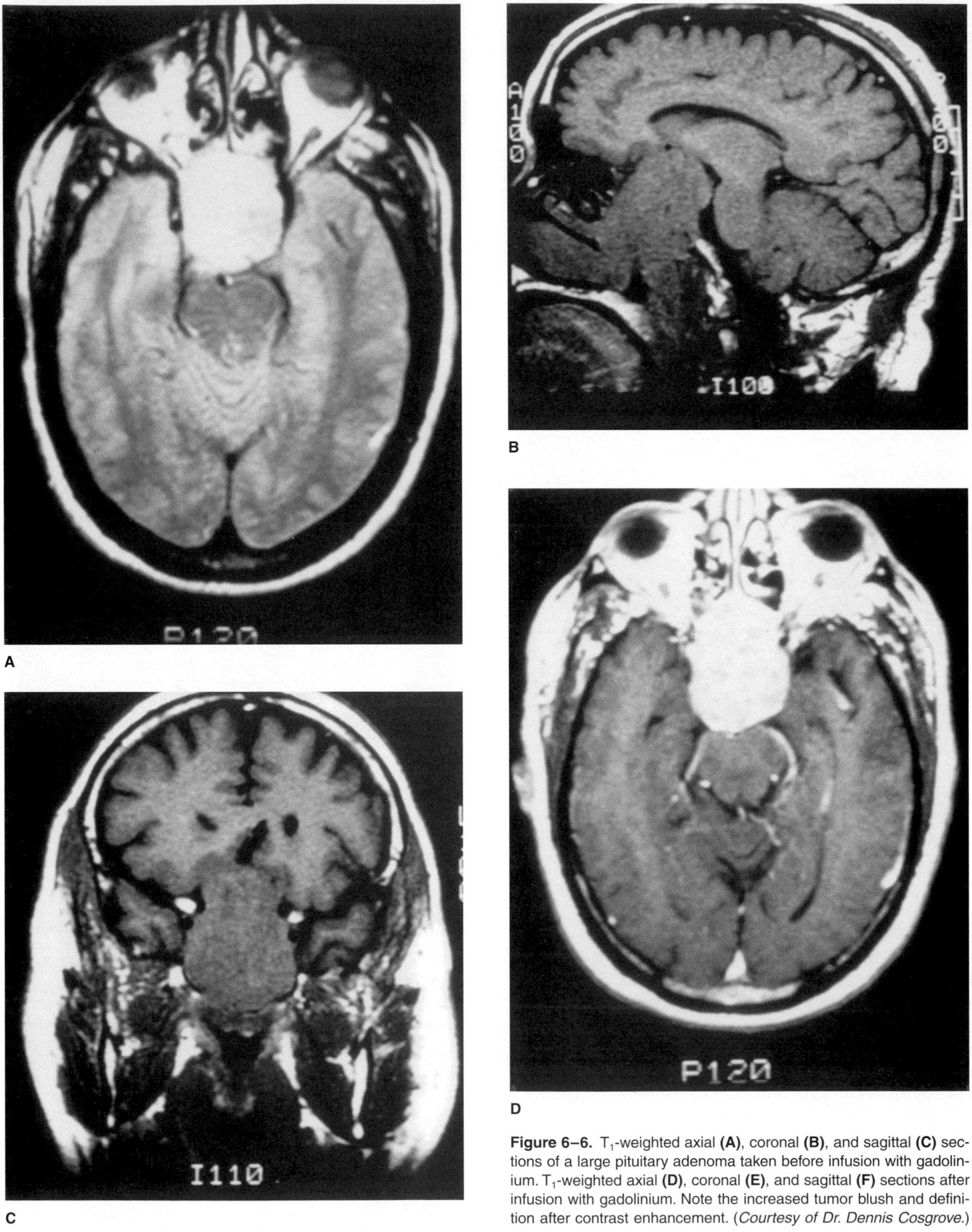

A

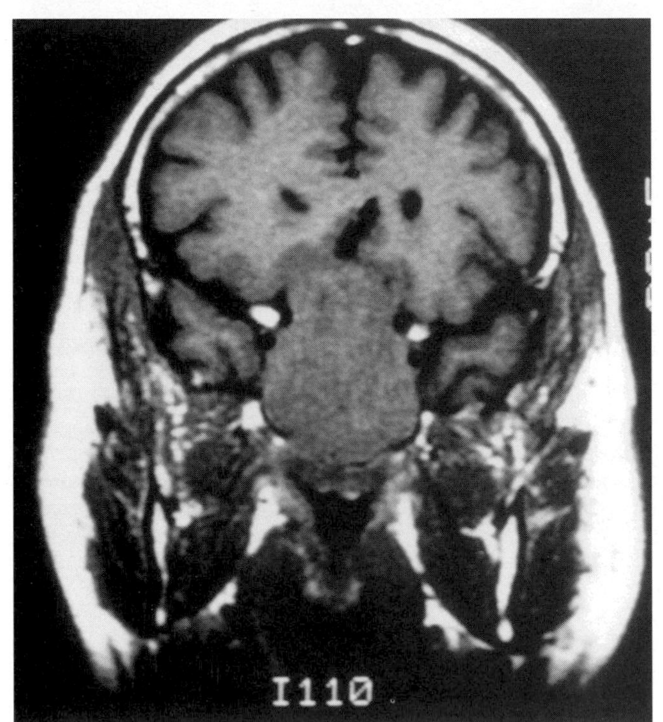

C

B

D

Figure 6–6. T_1-weighted axial **(A)**, coronal **(B)**, and sagittal **(C)** sections of a large pituitary adenoma taken before infusion with gadolinium. T_1-weighted axial **(D)**, coronal **(E)**, and sagittal **(F)** sections after infusion with gadolinium. Note the increased tumor blush and definition after contrast enhancement. (*Courtesy of Dr. Dennis Cosgrove.*)

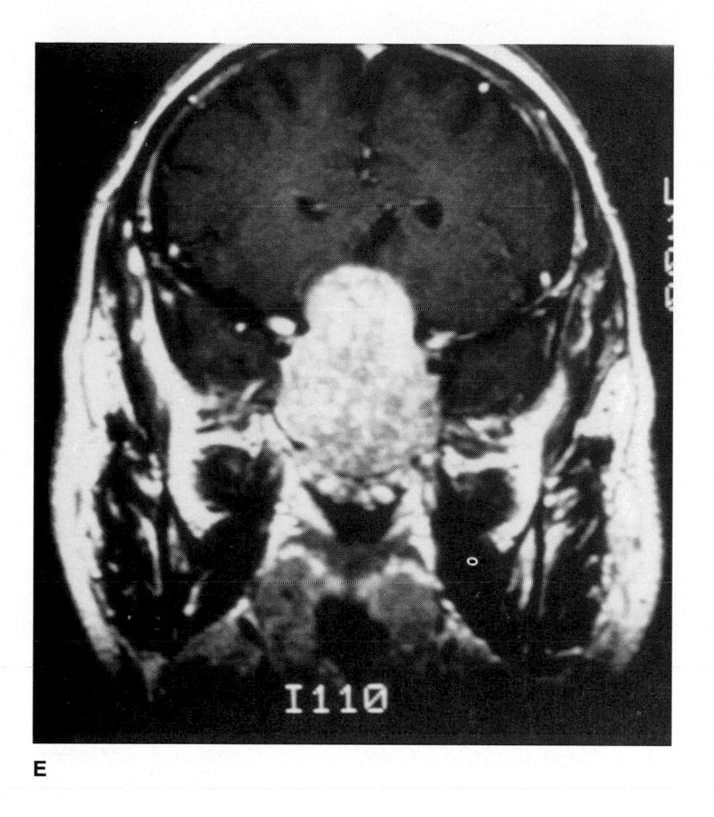

E

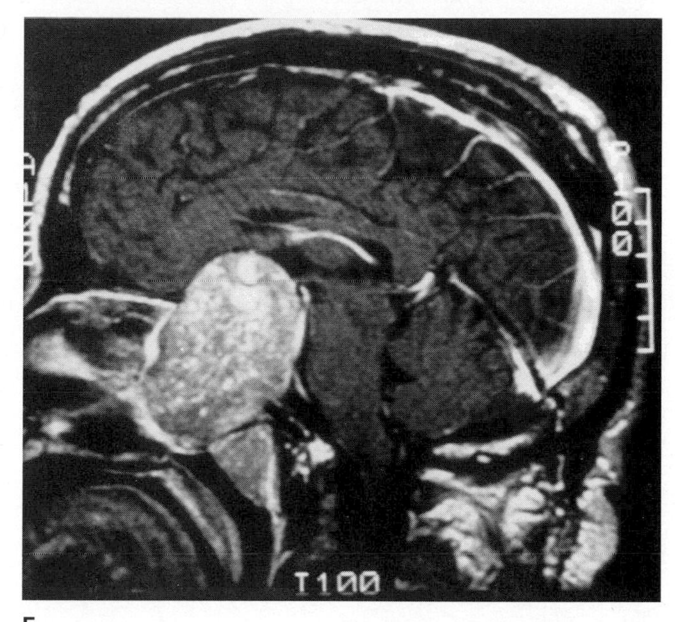

F

present, it should be considered as a sign of increased intracranial pressure secondary to a mass lesion until proven otherwise. Neuroradiologic evaluation should be ordered immediately to rule out a space-occupying intracranial process. If there is no evidence of a mass lesion, lumbar puncture is indicated to exclude idiopathic intracranial hypertension (pseudotumor cerebri) and meningitis as the cause of papilledema. Lumbar puncture serves both as a measure of intracranial pressure as well as analysis of CSF. Ultrasonic examination of the optic nerve is useful both to measure nerve diameter and to detect the presence of hyaline bodies (buried drusen) that can mimic true papilledema. The 30-degree test, as described by Galetta and associates (1989), is a reliable procedure used to detect the presence of fluid engorgement of the intervaginal space of the optic nerve. The 30-degree test relies on the premise that the intraorbital portion of the optic nerve is somewhat sinusoidal in primary position and tends to straighten when the eye is abducted 30 degrees. Therefore, conditions that result in the accumulation of fluid within the subarachnoid space of the optic nerve (papilledema, optic neuritis, ischemic optic neuropathy) will produce maximal distention to the optic nerve in primary position, as measured through A-scan echography with regression of nerve sheath diameter as the eye is abducted, allowing for a more even distribution of subarachnoid fluid with reduction of the optic nerve diameter. The "compression" of the optic nerve is termed a positive 30-degree test, and is pathognomonic for fluid engorgement within the subarachnoid space of the optic nerve.

TREATMENT AND MANAGEMENT

Systemic

Surgery

Surgery is the primary method of treatment for most benign, as well as malignant, brain tumors. Advances in surgical techniques, equipment, and imaging systems have led to the successful resection of tumors that were previously considered to be inoperable. The rate of success is determined largely by the location of the tumor and invasion of adjacent structures.

The evolution of microneurosurgery has greatly contributed to the effectiveness of tumor removal. The use of stereoscopic magnification allows for precise tumor dissection, with relative sparing of associated neuroanatomical structures. The advent of new lasers as well as computer-assisted navigational aides allows for the precise resection of malignant gliomas (Demianczak and Antonyshyn, 1999; Shapiro, 1999; Sipos et al, 1996). The ISG viewing wand is one of the frameless stereotactic systems that assists in the preoperative surgical planning and intraoperative neuronavigation for intracranial tumors. This technology adds minimal additional intraoperative time, while increasing the precision of tumoral resection. Microneurosurgery is particularly effective for tumors of the sellar and parasellar regions, cerebellopontine angle, ventricles, cavernous sinus, brainstem, odontoid process of the vertebral column, clivus, foramen magnum, and pineal region.

The use of CT- or MRI-guided surgery coupled with three-dimensional coordinates (stereotactic surgery) allows for the precise localization and manipulation of intracranial lesions. In addition to a more controlled surgery, stereotaxis allows for the relatively safe biopsy of tumorous lesions. Approximately 10 to 12% of previously undiagnosed lesions have been accurately identified by this technique.

Intraoperative monitoring of evoked potentials (brainstem auditory, visual, and somatosensory) has enhanced the precision and safety involved with tumor resection and has resulted in improved postoperative neurologic function.

Laser

Laser therapy is beneficial for some brain neoplasms. The photocoagulation, vaporization, and tissue ablation features of various laser wavelengths can be coupled with stereotaxis for the treatment of certain tumors. The use of photosensitizing agents combined with laser therapy appears promising, in that this method allows for greater accuracy in the treatment of neoplastic tissue while preserving normal structures.

Radiation

Radiation therapy is useful both as a primary form of treatment as well as combined with surgical removal. Many malignant neoplasms are particularly sensitive to radiotherapy. Focal and limited-field radiation techniques allow for a more directed approach to tumor treatment and reduce the amount of radiation exposure to uninvolved brain areas. Because of the reported complications of developmental delays, pituitary dysfunction, and secondary tumor growth associated with radiation, this form of treatment is generally not recommended for children under the age of 2 years.

Interstitial brachytherapy employs the stereotactic implantation of either temporary high-activity or permanent low-activity radioactive seeds that are placed within the tumoral bed after surgical resection of the tumor. The technique has been used previously as adjuvant treatment for malignant brain tumors; however, recent studies have shown that some newly diagnosed tumors (glioblastoma multiforme, recurrent malignant glioma, brain metastases, and low-grade gliomas) seem to benefit from this treatment modality (McDermott et al, 1998; Prados et al, 1992). Brachytherapy is useful in the treatment of highly malignant gliomas, particularly large tumors not suitable for radiosurgery, or when combined therapy is planned.

As has been described with laser treatment, the use of tissue-sensitizing agents (metronidazole, misonidazole, and etanidazole) can be used with stereotactic radiotherapy in the treatment of hypoxic tumor cells. The use of these agents is somewhat limited due to their neurotoxic side effects.

Radiosurgery

Radiosurgery is an adjunctive form of treatment for both malignant primary and metastatic cerebral tumors. This modality allows for the stereotactic delivery of high-dose radiation to a single target on a single exposure (Hildebrand et al, 1997; Young, 1998). Currently, two methods of delivery are available: gamma knife and linear accelerator (linac). Both systems are limited to the treatment of small intracranial tumors. Lesions larger than 3.5 to 4.0 cm in diameter are not yet amenable to radiosurgery.

Two types of complications from gamma knife radiosurgery include radiation reactions and radiation necrosis. Radiation reactions appear as hyperintense perilesional signal areas on a T_2-weighted MRI. Although it has the appearance of edema, it is thought that this is actually a type of glial inflammation. Corticosteroids may be used to treat symptomatic reactions, although response to treatment is variable (Young, 1998).

Radiation necrosis results from destruction of tumor cells with associated damage to surrounding normal brain tissue. This reaction is commonly seen with the treatment of larger lesions, and patients are often symptomatic. Failure to respond to corticosteroid treatment may require surgical resection of necrotic tissue (Young, 1998).

Chemotherapy

Chemotherapeutic (antineoplastic) agents are widely used in the treatment of many cancers. Categorically, these drugs work by suppression of tumor-cell growth or through the inhibition of cellular reproduction. The mode of action is dependent on the mechanism by which these agents affect cell growth, and they are most effective in the treatment of actively mitotic tumors.

The alkylating agents carnustine (BCNU), lomustine (CCNU), and cisplatin (CDDP) replace hydrogen atoms with an alkyl group, resulting in abnormal DNA synthesis. The abnormal DNA molecules are unable to perform their normal function related to cellular reproduction. Alkylating agents are somewhat effective in the treatment of adult malignant gliomas.

Procarbazine is a chemotherapeutic agent whose exact mechanism remains speculative. It is thought that procarbazine inhibits both RNA and DNA synthesis, with positive results reported in the treatment of Hodgkin disease and gliomas.

Methotrexate (MTX) is an antimetabolite that competitively inhibits the enzyme dihydrofolic acid reductase required for DNA synthesis and cellular reproduction. MTX is particularly useful in the treatment of rapidly dividing tumors such as lymphomas and medulloblastomas.

Vincristine (VCR) is a mitotic inhibitor that is derived from the periwinkle plant. Its mode of action is related to interference with intracellular tubulin (protein) function. Non-Hodgkin lymphomas are among the tumors most sensitive to vincristine.

A major complication of all antineoplastic agents is cytotoxicity. Normal tissues that are most adversely affected include bone marrow, hair follicles, and mucous membranes of the GI tract. Conservatively, 30% of all individuals committed to chemotherapy experience some degree of GI distress.

Due to the associated complications of radiation, chemotherapy is generally recommended as an alternative to primary or adjuvant radiotherapy for children under the age of 2 years.

Gene Therapy

Recent advances in the field of molecular genetics have improved the understanding of events leading to tumorigenesis and from that, new treatment modalities are being tested in both animal and clinical trials. Gene therapy involves the transfer of genetic material into host cells in an attempt to elicit a therapeutic response. This technology encompasses the replacement of defective genes, antiangiogenesis, immunotherapy, and suppression of harmful genes (Fathallah-Shaykh, 1999; Youle, 1996).

Other Treatment Regimens

Corticosteroids have been shown to suppress lymphocyte production and have been used in the treatment of some lymphomas. They are also helpful in reducing the cerebral edema associated with many tumors. Antiprogesterone therapy has shown some benefit in the treatment of meningiomas and may become an adjunctive treatment for residual or recurrent tumors (Black, 1993).

Hyperthermia has the effect of "sterilizing" tumor cells and has been used as an adjunct to enucleation or the treatment of malignant uveal melanomas. Microwave-induced hyperthermia has been employed coupled with surgical debulking in the management of certain brain tumors.

Ocular

Management of the ocular manifestations of intracranial tumors is primarily directed toward the treatment of the tumor itself, as delineated above. As needed, residual ocular motility dysfunctions may be managed with prismatic correction or muscle surgery.

CONCLUSION

The ocular practitioner is frequently the first clinician consulted by a patient with an intracranial tumor. The recognition of associated ophthalmic signs and symptoms is paramount for early diagnosis and successful treatment. The evolution of neuroimaging technology along with other diagnostic studies permits earlier and more accurate diagnoses of intracranial lesions.

Advances in microneurosurgery and radiosurgery have lead to more favorable postoperative outcomes with fewer associated complications among many individuals with tumors that were once considered to be inoperable. Radiation and chemotherapy used alone or in combination with surgery have resulted in higher treatment success rates, often with improved patient quality of life. Immunotherapy and gene therapy hold great promise as future methods of tumor management. As the understanding of the pathogenesis of tumor growth is expanded, the role of genetic, microbial, and environmental triggering mechanisms may significantly identify those individuals who are at risk for developing certain neoplasms, and allow for prophylaxis or early treatment.

REFERENCES

Ainbinder DJ, Faulkner AR, Haik BG. Review of orbital tumors. *Curr Opin Ophthalmol.* 1991;2:281–287.

Ammirati M, Vick N, Liao YL, et al. Effect of the extent of surgical resection on survival and quality of life in patients with supratentorial glioblastomas and anaplastic astrocytomas. *Neurosurgery.* 1987;21:201–206.

Anderson DR, Trobe JD, Taren JA, Gebarski SS. Visual outcome in cystic craniopharyngiomas treated with intracavitary phosphorus-32. *Ophthalmology.* 1989;96:1786–1792.

Apuzzo ML, Chandrasoma PT, Cohen D, et al. Computed imaging stereotaxy: Experience and perspective related to 500 procedures applied to brain masses. *Neurosurgery.* 1987;20:930–937.

Atta HR. Imaging of the optic nerve with standardized echography. *Eye.* 1988;2:358–366.

Bailey P, Cushing H. *A Classification of the Tumors of the Glioma Group on Histogenetic Basis with a Correlated Study of Prognosis.* Philadelphia: Lippincott; 1926.

Banna M. Craniopharyngioma: Based on 160 cases. *Br J Radiology.* 1976;49:206–23.

Barbaro NM, Gutin PH, Wilson CB, et al. Radiation therapy in the treatment of partially resected meningiomas. *Neurosurgery.* 1987;20:525–528.

Benedict WF, Murphree AL, Banerjee A, et al. Patient with 13 chromosome deletion: Evidence that the retinoblastoma gene is a recessive cancer gene. *Science.* 1983;219:973–975.

Biersack HJ, Coenen HH, Stocklin G, et al. Imaging of brain tumors with *L*-3-[^{123}I]iodo-alpha-methyl tyrosine and SPECT. *J Nucl Med.* 1989;30:110–112.

Bigner SH, Mark J, Burger PC, et al. Specific chromosomal abnormalities in malignant human gliomas. *Cancer Res.* 1988;48:405–411.

Black KL, Hawkins RA, Kim KT, et al. Use of thallium-201 SPECT to quantitate malignancy grade of gliomas. *J Neurosurg.* 1989;71:342–346.

Black PMcL. Medical progress: Brain tumors. *N Engl J Med.* 1991;324:1471–1476,1555–1564.

Black PMcL. Meningiomas. *Neurosurgery.* 1993;32:643–657.

Blumenthal DT, Raizer JJ, Rosenblum MK, et al. Primary intracranial neoplasms in patients with HIV. *Neurology.* 1999;52:1648–1651.

Bondy M, Ligon BL. Epidemiology and etiology of intracranial meningiomas: A review. *J Neurooncol.* 1996;29: 197–205.

Bowman CB, Farris BK. Primary chiasmal germinoma. *J Clin Neuro-ophthalmol.* 1990; 10:9–17.

Brant-Zawadzki M, Norman D. *Magnetic Resonance Imaging of the Central Nervous System.* New York: Raven; 1987.

Brem S. The role of vascular proliferation in the growth of brain tumors. *Clin Neurosurg.* 1976;23:440–453.

Bullard DE, Rawlings CE III, Philips B, et al. Oligodendroglioma: An analysis of the value of radiation therapy. *Cancer.* 1987; 60:2179–2188.

Burde RM, Savino PJ, Trobe JD. *Clinical Decisions in Neuro-ophthalmology.* St. Louis: Mosby; 1985.

Burger PC, Vogel FS, Green SB, Strike TA. Glioblastoma multiforme and anaplastic astrocytoma: Pathologic criteria and prognostic implications. *Cancer.* 1985;56:1106–1111.

Cairncross JG, MacDonald DR. Successful chemotherapy for recurrent malignant oligodendroglioma. *Ann Neurol.* 1988;23:360–364.

Camel PW. Tumors of the third ventricle. *Acta Neurochir* (Wien). 1985;75:136–146.

Carr WA, Baumann RJ, Baker RS. Nuclear magnetic resonance imaging in neuro-ophthalmology. Demonstration of a pontine glioma. *Surv Ophthalmol.* 1984;29:79–83.

Castillo M, Davis PC, Takei Y, Hoffman JC Jr. Intracranial ganglioglioma: MR, CT, and clinical findings in 18 patients. *AJR.* 1990;154:607–612.

Chang CH, Horton J, Schoenfeld D, et al. Comparison of postoperative radiotherapy and combined postoperative radiotherapy and chemotherapy in the multidisciplinary management of malignant gliomas. *Cancer.* 1983;52: 997–1007.

Cherninkova S, Tzekov H, Karakostov V. Comparative ophthamologic studies on children and adults with craniopharyngioma. *Ophthalmologica.* 1990;201:201–205.

Chowdury CR, Wood CM, Samuel PR, Richardson J. Frontal bone epidermoid—A rare cause of proptosis. *Br J Ophthalmol.* 1990;74:445–446.

Chutorian AM. Optic gliomas in children. *Int Pediatr.* 1988; 3:115–119.

Coleman DJ, Silverman RH, Iwamoto T, et al. Histopathologic effects of ultrasonically induced hyperthermia in intraocular malignant melanoma. *Ophthalmology.* 1988; 95:970–981.

Coppeto JR, Monteiro MLR, Uphoff DF. Exophytic suprasellar glioma: A rare cause of chiasmic compression. *Arch Ophthalmol.* 1987;105:28.

DeAngelis LM, Yahalom J, Heinemann MH, et al. Primary CNS lymphoma: Combined treatment with chemotherapy and radiotherapy. *Neurology.* 1990;40:80–86.

Delattre JY, Krol G, Thaler HT, Posner JB. Distribution of brain metastases. *Arch Neurol.* 1988;45:741–744.

Del Regato JA, Harlan JS, Cox JD, eds. *Ackerman and del Regato's Cancer: Tumors of the Central Nervous System.* 6th ed. St. Louis: Mosby; 1985:119–154.

Demianczuk AN, Antonyshyn OM. Application of a three-dimensional intraoperative navigational system in craniofacial surgery. *J Craniofac Surg.* 1997;8(4):290–297.

Doyle WK, Budinger TF, Valk PE, et al. Differentiation of cerebral radiation necrosis from tumor recurrence by [^{18}F]FDG and ^{82}Rb positron emission tomography. *J Comput Assist Tomogr.* 1987;11:563–570.

Dumanski JP, Caribom E, Collins VP, Nordenskjold M. Deletion mapping of a locus on human chromosome 22 involved in the oncogenesis of meningioma. *Proc Natl Acad Sci USA.* 1987;84:9275–9279.

Eijpe AA, Koornneef L, Verbeeten B Jr, et al. Intradiploic epidermoid cysts of the bony orbit. *Ophthalmology.* 1991;98: 1737–1743.

Faerber EN, Roman NV. Central nervous system tumors of childhood. *Radiol Clin North Am.* 1997;35:1301–1328.

Fathallah-Shaykh H. New molecular strategies to cure brain tumors. *Arch Neurol.* 1999;56:449–453.

Fine HA, Dear KBG, Loeffler JS, et al. Meta-analysis of radiation therapy with and without adjuvant chemotherapy for malignant gliomas in adults. *Proc Am Soc Clin Oncol.* 1991;10:125.

Folkman J, Klagsbrun M. Angiogenic factors. *Science.* 1987; 235:442–447.

Frenkel REP, Spoor TC. Visual loss and intoxication. *Surv Ophthalmol.* 1986;30:391–396.

Friedman WA, Sceats JR, Nestok BR, Ballinger WE Jr. The incidence of unexpected pathological findings in an image-guided biopsy series: A review of 100 consecutive cases. *Neurosurgery.* 1989;25:180–184.

Fueyo J, Gomez-Manzano C, Yung WKA, et al. Targeting in gene therapy for gliomas. *Arch Neurol.* 1999;56:445–448.

Fukuyama J, Hayasaka S, Setogawa T, et al. Foster–Kennedy syndrome and optociliary shunt vessels in a patient with an olfactory groove meningioma. *Ophthalmologica.* 1991; 202:125–131.

Galetta S, Byrne SF, Smith JL. Echographic correlation of optic nerve sheath size and cerebrospinal fluid pressure. *J Clin Neuro-ophthalmol.* 1989;9:79–82.

Gans MS, Byrne SF, Glaser JS. Standardized A-scan echography in optic nerve disease. *Arch Ophthalmol.* 1987; 105:1232–1236.

Garner A. Orbital lymphoproliferative disorders. *Br J Ophthalmol.* 1992;76:47–48.

Gelwan MJ, Seidman M, Kupersmith MJ. Pseudo-pseudo-Foster–Kennedy syndrome. *J Clin Neuro-ophthalmol.* 1988; 8:49–52.

Gilroy J. *Basic Neurology.* 2nd ed. New York: Pergamon; 1990:223–250.

Gittinger JW. To image or not to image. *Surv Ophthalmol.* 1988;32:350–356.

Glaser JS. Topical diagnosis: Prechiasmal visual pathways. In: Glaser JS, ed. *Neuro-ophthalmology.* 2nd ed. Philadelphia: Lippincott; 1990:83–170.

Gonzalez CF, Becker MH, Flanagan JC, eds. *Diagnostic Imaging in Ophthalmology.* New York: Springer-Verlag; 1986.

Greig NH, Ries LG, Yancik R, Rapoport SI. Increasing annual incidence of primary malignant brain tumors in the elderly. *JNCI.* 1990;82:1621–1624.

Guidetti B, Gagliardi FM. Epidermoid and dermoid cysts: Clinical evaluation and late surgical results. *J Neurosurg.* 1977;47: 12–18.

Gum KB, Frueh BR. Transantral orbital decompression for compressive optic neuropathy due to sphenoid ridge meningioma. *Ophthalmic Plast Reconstr Surg.* 1989;5:196–198.

Haik BG, Saint Louis L, Bierly J, et al. Magnetic resonance imaging in the evaluation of optic nerve gliomas. *Ophthalmology.* 1987;94:709–717.

Hall WA, Lunsford LD. Changing concepts in the treatment of colloid cysts: An 11-year experience in the CT era. *J Neurosurg.* 1987;66:186–191.

Hardwig P, Robertson DM. Von Hippel-Lindau disease: A familial, often lethal, multi-system phakomatosis. *Ophthalmology.* 1984;91:263–270.

Hildebrand J, Dewitte O, Dietrich PY, et al. Management of malignant brain tumors. *Eur Neurol.* 1997;38:238–253.

Hill JR, Kuriyama N, Kuuiyama H, et al. Molecular genetics of brain tumors. *Arch Neurol.* 1999;56:439–441.

Hochberg FH, Miller DC. Primary central nervous system lymphoma. *J Neurosurg.* 1988;68:835–853.

Holman RE, Grimson BS, Drayer BP, et al. Magnetic resonance imaging of optic gliomas. *Am J Ophthalmol.* 1985; 100:596–601.

Hoyt WF, Beeston D. *The Ocular Fundus in Neurologic Disease.* St. Louis: Mosby; 1966.

Huber A; Blodi FC, trans. *Eye Signs and Symptoms in Brain Tumors.* 3rd ed. St. Louis: Mosby; 1976.

Imes RK, Hoyt WF. Magnetic resonance imaging signs of optic nerve gliomas in neurofibromatosis, 1. *Am J Ophthalmol.* 1991; 111:729–734.

Imes RK, Schatz H, Hoyt WF, et al. Evolution of optociliary veins in optic nerve sheath meningioma. *Arch Ophtholmol.* 1985;103:59–60.

Jakobiec FA, Depot MJ, Kennerdell JS, et al. Combined clinical and computed tomographic diagnosis of orbital glioma and meningioma. *Ophthalmology.* 1984;91:137–155.

Johnson LN, Hepler RS, Yee RD, et al. Magnetic resonance imaging of craniopharyngioma. *Am J Ophthalmol.* 1986; 102:242–244.

Kalofonos HP, Pawlikowska TR, Hemingway A, et al. Antibody guided diagnosis and therapy of brain gliomas using radiolabeled monoclonal antibodies against epidermal growth factor receptor and placental alkaline phosphatase. *J Nucl Med.* 1989;30:1636–1645.

Kalyan-Raman UP, Olivero WC. Ganglioglioma: A correlative clinicopathological and radiological study of ten surgically treated cases with follow-up. *Neurosurgery.* 1987;20:428–433.

Keane JR. Bilateral 6th-nerve palsy. Analysis of 125 cases. *Arch Neurol.* 1976;33:681–683.

Kennerdell JS, Maroon JC, Malton M, Warren FA. The management of optic nerve sheath meningiomas. *Am J Ophthalmol.* 1988;106:450–457.

Kepes JJ. *Meningiomas: Biology, Pathology, and Differential Diagnosis.* New York: Masson; 1982.

Kernohan JW, Mabon RF, Svien HJ, Adson AW. A simplified classification of gliomas. *Proc Staff Meet Mayo Clin.* 1949; 24:71–75.

King RA, Nelson LB, Wagner RS. Spasmus nutans: A benign clinical entity? *Arch Ophthalmol.* 1986;104:1501–1504.

Klein G. The approaching era of tumor suppressor genes. *Science.* 1987;238:1539–1545.

Kornblith PL, Walker MD, Cassady JR. Neoplasms of the central nervous system. In: DeVita VT Jr, Hellman S, Rosenberg SA, eds. *Cancer: Principles and Practice of Oncology.* 2nd ed. Philadelphia: Lippincott; 1985:1437–1510.

Kupersmith MJ, Warren FA, Newall J, Ransohoff J. Irradiation of meningiomas of the intracranial anterior visual pathway. *Ann Neurol.* 1987;21:131–137.

Larson DA, Gutin PH, Leibel SA, et al. Stereotaxic irradiation of brain tumors. *Cancer.* 1990;65:792–799.

Lashford LS, Davies AG, Richardson RB, et al. A pilot study of ^{131}I monoclonal antibodies in the therapy of leptomeningeal tumors. *Cancer.* 1988;61:857–868.

Lavery MA, O'Neill JF, Chu FC, Martyn LJ. Acquired nystagmus in early childhood: A presenting sign of intracranial tumor. *Ophthalmology.* 1984;91:425–435.

Leibel SA, Sheline GE. Radiation therapy for neoplasms of the brain. *J Neurosurg.* 1987;66:1–22.

Lesch KP, Schott W, Engl HG, et al. Gonadal steroid receptors in meningiomas. *J Neurol.* 1987;234:328–333.

Linden RD, Tator CH, Benedict C, et al. Electrophysiological monitoring during acoustic neuroma and other posterior fossa surgery. *Can J Neurol Sci.* 1988;15:73–81.

Lueder GT, Judisch GF, Wen BC. Heritable retinoblastoma and pinealoma. *Arch Ophthalmol.* 1991;109:1707–1709.

MacCarty CS, Leavens ME, Love JG, Kernohan JW. Dermoid and epidermoid tumors in the central nervous system of adults. *Surg Gynecol Obstet.* 1959;108:191–198.

Mahaley MS Jr, Mettlin C, Natarajan N, et al. National survey of patterns of care for brain-tumor patients. *J Neurosurg.* 1989;71:826–836.

Mahaley MS Jr, Urso MB, Whaley RA, et al. Immunobiology of primary intracranial tumors, 10. Therapeutic efficacy of interferon in the treatment of recurrent gliomas. *J Neurosurg.* 1985;63:719–725.

Mansour AM, Barber JC, Reineeke RD, Wang FM. Ocular choristomas. *Surv Ophthalmol.* 1989;33:339–358.

Masuyama Y, Kodama Y, Matsuura Y, et al. Clinical studies on the occurrence and the pathogenesis of optociliary veins. *J Clin Neuro-ophthalmol.* 1990; 10:1–8.

Maxwell M, Black PMcL. Oncogenes, growth factors and brain tumors. In: Komblith PL, Walker MD, eds. *Advances in Neuro-oncology.* Mount Kisco, NY: Futura; 1988:159–176.

McDermott MW, Sneed PK, Gutin PH. Interstitial brachytherapy for malignant brain tumors. *Semin Surg Oncol.* 1998;14:79–87.

McFadzean RM. Visual prognosis in craniopharyngioma. *Neuro-ophthalmology.* 1989;9:337–341.

McFadzean RM, McIlwaine GG, McLellan D. Hodgkin's disease at the optic chiasm. *J Clin Neuro-opthalmol.* 1990;10: 248–254.

McNab AA, Wright JE. Cysts of the optic nerve: Three cases associated with meningioma. *Eye.* 1989;3:355–359.

Mindel JS, Fetell MR. A pituitary adenoma with dilated ventricles. *Surv Ophthalmol.* 1985;30:59–61.

Mulvihill J, Parry DM, Sherman JL, et al. Neurofibromatosis I (Recklinghausen disease) and neurofibromatosis 2 (bilateral acoustic neurofibromatosis): An update. *Ann Intern Med.* 1990;113:39–52.

Munden PM, Sobol WM, Weingeist TA. Ocular findings in Turcot syndrome (gliomapolyposis). *Ophthalmology.* 1991; 98:111–114.

Nerad JA, Kersten RC, Anderson RL. Hemangioblastoma of the optic nerve: Report of a case and review of the literature. *Ophthalmology.* 1988;95:398-402.

Neumann HP, Eggert HR, Weigel K, et al. Hemangioblastomas of the central nervous system: A 10-year study with special reference to von Hippel–Lindau syndrome. *J Neurosurg.* 1989;70:24–30.

Neville RG, Greenblatt SH, Kollarits CR. Foster–Kennedy syndrome and an optociliary vein in a patient with a falx meningioma. *J Clin Neuro-ophthalmol.* 1984;4:97–101.

O'Neill BP, Illig JJ. Primary central nervous system lymphoma. *Mayo Clin Proc.* 1989;64:1005–1020.

Patchell RA, Tibbs PA, Walsh JW, et al. A randomized trial of surgery in the treatment of single metastases to the brain. *N Engl J Med.* 1990;322:494–500.

Patronas NJ, Di Chiro G, Kufta C, et al. Prediction of survival in glioma patients by means of positron emission tomography. *J Neurosurg.* 1985;62:816–822.

Perry JR, Louis DN, Cairncross G. Current treatment of oligodendrogliomas. *Arch Neurol.* 1999;56:434–436.

Prados MD, Gutin PH, Phillips TL, et al. Interstitial brachytherapy for newly diagnosed patients with malignant gliomas: The UCSF experience. *J Rad Oncol Biol Phys.* 1992;24:593–597.

Probst C, Gessaga E, Leuenberger AE. Primary meningioma of the optic nerve sheaths: Case report. *Ophthalmologica.* 1985;190:83–90.

Reifler DM, Holtzman JN, Ringel DM. Sphenoid ridge meningioma masquerading as Grave's orbitopathy. *Arch Ophthalmol.* 1986;104:1591.

Repka MX, Miller NR. Optic atrophy in children. *Am J Ophthalmol.* 1988;106:191–193.

Repka MX, Miller NR. Papilledema and dural sinus obstruction. *J Clin Neuro-ophthalmol.* 1984;4:247–250.

Repka MX, Miller NR, Miller M. Visual outcome after surgical removal of craniopharyngiomas. *Ophthalmology.* 1989;96:195–199.

Ridley M, Green J, Johnson G. Retinal angiomatosis: The ocular manifestations of von Hippel–Lindau disease. *Can J Ophthalmol.* 1986;21:276–283.

Rudd A, Rees JE, Kennedy P, et al. Malignant optic nerve gliomas in adults. *J Clin Neuro-ophthalmol.* 1985;5:238–243.

Russell DC, Rubinstein LJ. *Pathology of Tumors of the Nervous System.* 4th ed. Baltimore: Williams & Wilkins; 1977.

Ryder JW, Kleinschmidt-DeMasters BK, Keller TS. Sudden deterioration and death in patients with benign tumors of the third ventricle area. *J Neurosurg.* 1986;64:216–223.

Salcman M, Samaras GM. Interstitial microwave hyperthermia for brain tumors: Results of a phase-1 clinical trial. *J Neurooncol.* 1983;1:225–236.

Schanzer MC, Font PL, O'Malley RE. Primary ocular malignant lymphoma associated with the acquired immune deficiency syndrome. *Ophthalmology.* 1991;98:88–91.

Schatz H, Green WR, Talamo JH, et al. Clinicopathologic correlation of retinal to choroidal venous collaterals of the optic nerve head. *Ophthalmology.* 1991;98:1287–1293.

Schoenberg BS. Epidemiology of primary intracranial neoplasms: Disease distribution and risk factors. In: Salcman M, ed. *Neurobiology of Brain Tumors.* Vol 4 of *Concepts in Neurosurgery.* Baltimore: Williams & Wilkins; 1991:3–18.

Schrell UMH, Fahlbusch R. Hormonal manipulation of cerebral meningiomas. In: Al-Mefty O, ed. *Meningiomas.* New York: Raven; 1991:273–283.

Schwartz RB, Carvalho PA, Alexander E III, et al. Radiation necrosis vs high-grade recurrent glioma: Differentiation by using dual-isotope SPECT with ^{201}Tl and ^{99}mTc-HMPAO. *AJNR.* 1991;12:1187–1192.

Seiff SR, Brodsky MC, MacDonald G, et al. Orbital optic glioma in neurofibromatosis: Magnetic resonance diagnosis of perineural arachnoidal gliomatosis. *Arch Ophthalmol.* 1987;105:1689–1692.

Seizinger BR, Rouleau GA, Ozelius LJ, et al. Common pathogenetic mechanism for three tumor types in bilateral acoustic neurofibromatosis. *Science.* 1987;236:317–319.

Shapiro WR. Current therapy for brain tumors. *Arch Neurol.* 1999;56:429–432.

Shapiro WR, Green SB, Burger PC, et al. Randomized trial of three chemotherapy regimens and two radiotherapy regimens in postoperative treatment of malignant glioma. Brain Tumor Cooperative Group trial 8001. *J Neurosurg.* 1989;71:1–9.

Sibony PA, Kennerdell JS, Slamovits TL, et al. Intrapapillary refractile bodies in optic nerve sheath meningioma. *Arch Ophthalmol.* 1985;10:383–385.

Sibony PA, Krauss HR, Kennerdell JS, et al. Optic nerve sheath meningiomas: Clinical manifestations. *Ophthalmology.* 1984;91:1313–1326.

Sipos EP, Tebo SA, Zinreich SJ, et al. In vivo accuracy testing and clinical experience with the ISG viewing wand. *Neurosurgery.* 1996;39:194–202.

Slavin ML. Isolated trochlear nerve palsy secondary to cavernous sinus meningioma. *Am J Ophthalmol.* 1987;104: 433–434.

Smith RW. Tumors. In: Wiederholt WC, ed. *Neurology for the Non-neurologist.* Philadelphia: Grune & Stratton; 1988: 320–327.

Tan TJ. Epidermoids and dermoids of the central nervous system. *Acta Neurochir.* 1972;26:13–24.

Tator CH, Nedzelski JM. Preservation of hearing in patients undergoing excision of acoustic neuromas and other cerebellopontine angle tumors. *J Neurosurg.* 1985;63:168–174.

Tomita T, McLone DG. Medulloblastoma in childhood: Results of radical resection and low-dose neuraxis radiation therapy. *J Neurosurg.* 1986;64:238–242.

Vander JF, Kincaid MC, Hegarty TJ, et al. The ocular effects of intracarotid bromodeoxyuridine and radiation therapy in the treatment of malignant glioma. *Ophthalmology.* 1990; 97:352–357.

Walker AE, Robins M, Weinfeld FD. Epidemiology of brain tumors: The national survey of intracranial neoplasms. *Neurology.* 1985;35:219–226.

Walker MD, Green SB, Byar DP, et al. Randomized comparisons of radiotherapy and nitrosoureas for the treatment of malignant glioma after surgery. *N Engl J Med.* 1980; 303:1323–1329.

Waliner KE, Wara WM, Sheline GE, Davis RL. Intracranial ependymomas: Results of treatment with partial or whole brain irradiation without spinal irradiation. *Int J Radiat Oncol Biol Phys.* 1986;12:1937–1941.

Walsh FB, Hoyt WF: In: Miller NR, ed. *Clinical Neuro-ophthalmology.* 4th ed. Baltimore: Williams & Wilkins; 1988:3.

Walsh TJ, Garden J, Gallagher B. Obliteration of retinal venous pulsations. *Am J Ophthalmol.* 1969;67:954.

Wan WL, Geller JL, Feldon SE, Sadun AA. Visual loss caused by rapidly progressive intracranial meningiomas during pregnancy. *Ophthalmology.* 1990;97:18–21.

Wara WM. Radiation therapy for brain tumors. *Cancer.* 1985;55:2291–2295.

Weir B. The relative significance of factors affecting postoperative survival in astrocytomas, grades 3 and 4. *J Neurosurg.* 1973;38:448–452.

Weir B, Grace M. The relative significance of factors affecting postoperative survival in astrocytomas, grades one and two. *Can J Neurol Sci.* 1976;3:47–50.

Wilson WB, Lloyd LA, Buncic JR. Tumor spread in unilateral optic glioma. *Neuro-ophthalmology.* 1987;7:179–184.

Wright JE, McNab AA, McDonald WI. Primary optic nerve sheath meningioma. *Br J Ophthalmol.* 1989;73:960–966.

Youle RJ. Immunotoxins for central nervous system malignancy. *Semin Cancer Biol.* 1996;7:65–70.

Young IL, Percy CL, Asire AJ, eds. *Surveillance, Epidemiology and End Results: Incidence and Mortality Data, 1973–77.* National Cancer Institute. Monograph 57. Washington, DC: U.S. Government Printing Office; 1981.

Young RF. The role of the gamma knife in the treatment of malignant primary and metastatic brain tumors. *CA Cancer J Clin.* 1998;48:177–188.

Zhou XP, Zhao MY, Ma YJ. Blindness from intracranial tumors: A clinical analysis of 60 cases. *Am J Optom Physiol Optics.* 1987;64:329–332.

Zimmerman CF, Schatz NJ, Glaser JS. Magnetic resonance imaging of optic nerve meningiomas: Enhancement with gadolinium-DTPA. *Ophthalmology.* 1990;97:585–591.

Chapter 7

PSEUDOTUMOR CEREBRI

Kelly H. Thomann

Pseudotumor cerebri (PTC), also known as idiopathic intracranial hypertension, is a disease characterized by increased intracranial pressure in the absence of a mass lesion or infection. Ocular involvement is a prominent component of PTC. Permanent visual loss is the most serious possible sequela of this disease, which is sometimes erroneously called benign intracranial hypertension. Patients with PTC must be followed closely through monitoring of their visual acuity, visual field, and optic nerve appearance.

EPIDEMIOLOGY

Systemic

Durcan and co-workers (1988) reported the annual incidence of PTC to be 0.9 per 100,000 in the general population. The incidence rises to 14 in 100,000 in women between the ages of 20 and 44 who are 10% over ideal weight, and almost 15 per 100,000 in those females who are 20% over ideal weight. Obesity is the most commonly associated condition, found in 50% of PTC patients.

Female-to-male ratio in PTC is 8 to 1, and men who are affected fall into the same age group as women. Digre and Corbett (1988) reported that men may be at a greater risk for visual loss, especially African-American males. Male and female children are affected equally, and also may be especially vulnerable to vision loss. When present in a child, obesity is less common, compared to the adult population with PTC. Approximately one half of pediatric cases of PTC have other/associated conditions or secondary causes.

Among the initial symptoms of PTC, headache is the most common, found in 75 to 80% of patients. Nausea and vomiting are initially present in 21% of patients with PTC. Five percent of patients have no symptoms when the disease is diagnosed.

Ocular

Disturbances of visual acuity (VA) occur as initial symptoms in 68%, transient visual obscurations occur in up to 72%, diplopia is reported in 35%, and 22% have other visual complaints. Papilledema is the most prominent sign in PTC and is found in almost every case. Visual loss is the major morbidity associated with this disorder as a sequela to papilledema. Visual acuity better than 20/25 was found initially in 89% of patients by Rush (1980) and abnormal visual fields (VFs) in 93%. Final visual acuity worse than 20/30 was found in 11% of Rush's patients, and 46% of the patients had permanent visual field defects after resolution of the disease. According to Corbett and associates (1982), an enlarged blind spot is the most common type of visual field loss, followed by inferior nasal field loss. It was previously believed that duration of symptoms, degree of papilledema, and transient visual obscurations were indicative of a more severe visual outcome. However, many recent studies have found no relationship of these findings to the final visual outcome.

PATHOPHYSIOLOGY/DISEASE PROCESS

Systemic

Intracranial pressure (ICP) is created by the cerebrospinal fluid (CSF), blood, and brain tissue, which are housed within the skull. The normal range of intracranial pressure is between 50 and 200 mm H_2O. The volume of each component can vary slightly without causing increased ICP, due to an internal mechanism that compensates for any changes. However, in PTC the ICP is above that which can be compensated for by this mechanism. The cause of the raised ICP in PTC remains unknown in about 90% of the cases.

Various mechanisms have been proposed to explain the etiology of the increased ICP. Dandy (1937) originally discussed 22 cases of PTC and thought it was due to increased cerebral blood volume. Diffuse cerebral edema (Sahs & Joynt, 1956) and abnormal CSF circulation (Symonds, 1931; Bercaw & Greer, 1970) have also been proposed. More recently, Johnston and Paterson (1974), and others have postulated an obstruction to the outflow of CSF within the venous sinus due to increased resistance of the arachnoid villi. Most speculate this to be the primary cause or it may be a mixed mechanism. Researchers felt current imaging techniques would prove the etiology, but to date they have not.

Many associated conditions have been proposed and studied as causes of PTC. Although a definite correlation has been found with some, the majority have not been proven with scientific documentation (Table 7–1). Endocrine abnormalities, menstrual irregularities, pregnancy, and the use of oral contraceptives have all been linked with PTC, although studies consistently have found no causal relationship. It is true that obesity is a common factor; however, endocrine and menstrual abnormalities are frequently found in obese women. Also, a relationship to hypertension and diabetes mellitus has been discussed, but these too are more common in obese persons.

Intracranial hypertension may be caused by any factor that causes a decrease in flow through the arachnoid villi or obstructs the venous pathway to the heart. Examples of conditions that can cause a state that resembles PTC are dural sinus thrombosis, which may occur following head trauma or secondary to radical neck dissection, or venous sinus thrombosis due to middle ear infection. Whether these are true cases of PTC or conditions resembling the idiopathic type is a semantic issue. However, PTC due to venous sinus thrombosis can only be diagnosed by visualization of venous sinus drainage. In cases where it is suspected, angiography is necessary.

Exogenous agents such as excessive doses of vitamin A, tetracyclines, lithium, and nalidixic acid all have a longstanding association with PTC in the literature. Although the causal relationship is not clear, a careful drug history may be important in those patients

TABLE 7–1. PSEUDOTUMOR CEREBRI AND POSSIBLE ASSOCIATED CAUSES

Highly Likely
Decreased flow through arachnoid granulations
  Scarring from previous inflammation (eg, meningitis, sequel to subarachnoid hemorrhage)
Obstruction to venous drainage
  Venous sinus thromboses (hypercoagulable states, or contiguous infection such as middle ear or mastoid–otitic hydrocephalus)
  Bilateral radical neck dissection
  Superior vena cava syndrome
  Increased right heart pressure
Endocrine disorders
  Addison disease
  Hypoparathyroidism
  Obesity
  Steroid withdrawal
Nutritional disorders
  Hypervitaminosis A (vitamin, liver, or isotretinoin intake)
  Hyperalimentation in deprivation dwarfism
Arteriovenous malformations

Probable Causes
Anabolic steroids (may cause venous sinus thrombosis)
Chlordecone (Kepone)
Ketoprofen or indomethacin in Bartter syndrome
Minocycline
Systemic lupus erythematosus
Thyroid replacement therapy in hypothyroid children
Uremia

Possible Causes
Amiodarone
Diphenylhydantoin
Iron deficiency anemia
Lithium carbonate
Nalidixic acid
Sarcoidosis
Sulfa antibiotics

Causes Frequently Cited That Are Unproven
Corticosteroid intake
Hyperthyroidism
Hypovitaminosis A
Menarche
Menstrual irregularities
Multivitamin intake
Oral contraceptive use
Pregnancy
Tetracycline use

Reprinted with permission from Wall, M: Differential diagnosis of idiopathic intracranial hypertension. Neurol Clin *1991;9:76.*

suspected of having PTC. It is unclear if steroids play a role in the pathogenesis of PTC, although there are reports of this disorder following steroid use and its resolution after discontinuation.

> Headache is the most frequent presenting symptom in pseudotumor cerebri and papilledema is the most prominent finding.

The most frequent presenting symptom in PTC is headache. The headache is described as severe, throbbing, nonlocalizable, episodic pain that occurs daily, usually lasting hours. It may be worse in the morning, exacerbated with head movement and the Valsalva maneuver. Patients may also complain of blurred vision, transient visual obscurations, diplopia, neck stiffness, or pulsatile intracranial noises (Table 7–2). Minor symptoms include paresthesias, back and leg pain, arthralgia, and unsteady gait.

Cerebral function remains normal in PTC. There is no change in consciousness or mentation. If focal neurologic deficits are found, the diagnosis of PTC may be incorrect.

The increased intracranial pressure found in PTC causes papilledema, and occasionally sixth (abducens) cranial nerve palsies. These are the only clinical signs found with this disease (see the "Ocular" section below for discussion).

The course of PTC varies considerably from patient to patient. It is never fatal, and in many cases it will resolve on its own without treatment and leave no permanent damage. Most cases resolve in 3 to 9 months; however, in some cases, even with the most aggressive surgical treatment, vision loss may still ensue. Up to 37% of patients have recurrence of the disease, with the interval from onset to recurrence about 4 years.

Ocular

Papilledema (Figure 7–1) is the most prominent finding in PTC, although it may occasionally be absent. Visual symptoms secondary to papilledema vary considerably. They include transient visual obscurations (monocular or binocular) and blurred vision. Papilledema initially does not cause any visual symptoms or noticeable field defects unless it causes macula edema or hemorrhage. It is difficult to judge by the appearance of the papilledema the duration of the disease. The discs may remain elevated and unchanged for a number of years even after resolution of the disease. Signs that may be helpful in a gross estimate of duration include the presence of resolving hemorrhages, cotton-wool spots, vascular tortuosity, presence of optociliary shunt vessels, nerve fiber layer defects, horizontal choroidal folds, or gliosis of the discs. Prolonged or severe papilledema may cause optic atrophy and circumpapillary rings (Paton's folds) (which indicate the amount the disc had previously been elevated). It may also cause the disc margins to become more indistinct with time, creating a circumpapillary haze. Differential diagnosis includes other causes of papilledema, disc edema, or pseudopapilledema (such as disc drusen or oblique optic nerve insertion).

Visual loss may seem to occur quickly; however, the disease may go undiagnosed for some time without any subjective visual disturbance. Some patients experience gradual visual loss months to years after diagnosis; the rate and symptoms vary greatly in each case. Factors that appear to be related to a greater risk

TABLE 7–2. SYSTEMIC MANIFESTATIONS OF PSEUDOTUMOR CEREBRI

- Headache[a]
- Nauseousness and vomiting[b]
- Vertigo[b]
- Pulsatile intracranial noises[c]
- Shoulder, arm, leg, or neck pain[c]
- Tinnitus[c]
- Paresthesias[c]
- Arthralgia[c]
- Unsteady gait[c]

[a]Very common.
[b]Common.
[c]Rare, but reported in the literature.

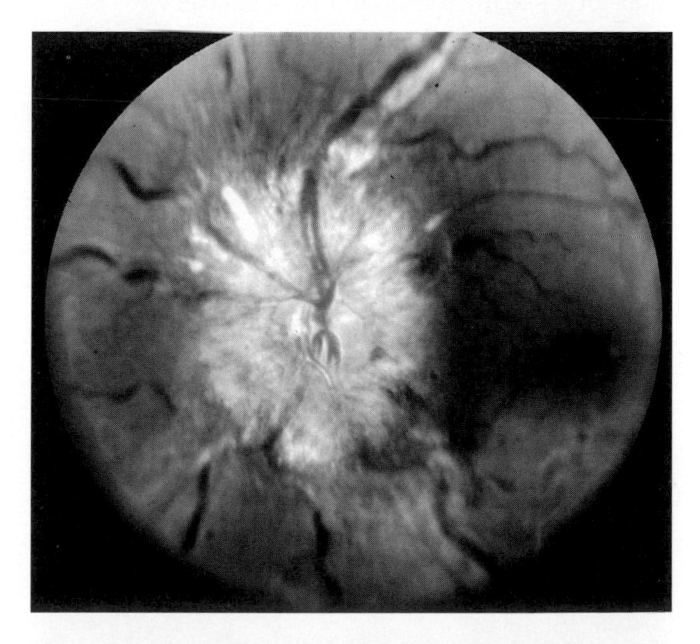

Figure 7–1. Papilledema in a 30-year-old female with intracranial pressure of 280 with normal imaging and laboratory studies. *(Courtesy of Dr. Scott Richter.)*

of visual loss are systemic hypertension, anemia, peripapillary subretinal neovascularization, older age, and high myopia. Patients with any of these factors should be watched more carefully and treated more aggressively to avoid visual loss.

Papilledema causes characteristic visual field defects, which are disc related (Table 7–3). An enlarged blind spot, seldom noticed by the patient, is almost always found. This defect may remain following resolution of the disease, and therefore is not used to evaluate the success of therapy. The enlarged blind spot is due to the displacement of the peripapillary nerve fibers as they exit the optic disc. Inferior nasal visual field deficits are second most commonly found, and are due to destruction of peripheral nerve fibers by progressive gliosis. The fibers subserving the inferior nasal visual field seem to be most at risk to mechanical compression and ischemic damage at the disc as in other causes of ischemia to the optic nerve (eg, anterior ischemic optic neuropathy). Glaucoma-like nerve fiber bundle defects and arcuate scotomas may also occur suggesting a similar mechanism at the level of the lamina cribrosa.

Patients may complain of diplopia, and motility disturbances in the form of sixth cranial nerve palsies may be found. The long intracranial course of the abducens nerve makes it vulnerable to any shifts in the brain, and one or both nerves are especially susceptible as they course over the clivus (the bone that forms the foramen magnum in the skull). Paralysis of the other ocular motor nerves is not likely, and if found, a cause other than PTC should be suspected.

DIAGNOSIS

Systemic

PTC may be diagnosed by a practitioner during routine examination on an asymptomatic individual or on a patient who complains of headaches or visual symptoms. There are no systemic findings used to corroborate the diagnosis of PTC other than imaging studies and lumbar puncture. PTC is purely a diagnosis of exclusion made following ocular and neurologic examination, and rarely after the complaint of headaches alone. It should be emphasized that cerebral function remains intact in PTC. If neurologic findings other than papilledema and sixth-nerve palsy are found, another diagnosis should be considered. Table 7–4 outlines Dandy's criteria for the diagnosis of PTC.

Indicated tests include lumbar puncture and brain scan by computed tomography (CT) or magnetic resonance imaging (MRI) (Table 7–5). Imaging studies must be performed before lumbar puncture. The CT or MRI will be "normal" in PTC, although small ventricles and an empty sella turcica are sometimes found. Brodsky and Vaphiades (1998) studied abnormal MRI findings in PTC and found flattening of the posterior sclera on MRI in 80% of patients with PTC. The T_2-weighted fast spin-echo sequence with fat suppression can increase the sensitivity of the orbital image, thus making the flattened sclera more evident. This may be a useful tool in the diagnosis of PTC; however, this finding may be overlooked by a radiologist reviewing the film.

Lumbar puncture will reveal an opening pressure greater than 200 mm H_2O in PTC. The cerebral spinal fluid must show normal cell count, glucose, and protein, and negative Venereal Disease Research Laboratory (VDRL) for the diagnosis. The CSF protein concentration will typically be low in PTC.

Ultrasonography of the optic nerve has been recommended as a useful nonnivasive test in the diagnosis of PTC in children, along with its role in ruling out tumors or drusen of the optic nerve. A-scan can allow an accurate measurement of optic nerve width and with the addition of the 30-degree tilt test, it can also allow for the detection of increased intracranial pressure. Ultrasonography does not replace the necessity for an initial lumbar puncture in the diagnosis of PTC; however, in cases in which lumbar puncture is difficult, it may reduce the need for subsequent lumbar puncture.

Differential diagnosis of PTC (Table 7–6) includes brain lesions such as primary or secondary tumors that may cause increased ICP with or without other neu-

TABLE 7–3. OCULAR MANIFESTATIONS OF PSEUDOTUMOR CEREBRI

Papilledema
- Vision disturbances
  - Decreased vision
  - Transient visual obscurations
  - Alterations of vision
- Visual field defects
  - Enlarged blind spot
  - Inferior nasal loss
  - Nerve fiber layer defects
- Retro-ocular pain

Sixth (Abducens) Cranial Nerve Palsy
- Diplopia

TABLE 7–4. DANDY'S CRITERIA FOR DIAGNOSIS OF PSEUDOTUMOR CEREBRI

1. Signs/symptoms of increased intracranial pressure
2. Absence of localized findings on neurologic examination
3. Normal neuroradiologic studies
4. Patient awake and alert
5. No other causes for increased intracranial pressure

TABLE 7–5. DIAGNOSTIC TESTS UTILIZED IN THE DIAGNOSIS OF PSEUDOTUMOR CEREBRI

Test	Diagnostic Criteria
CT/MRI	Must be normal; exceptions: small ventricles or empty sella turcica
Lumbar puncture	Opening pressure >200 mm H_2O, normal cell count, protein, glucose, (−) VDRL
Orbital ultrasound[a]	Increased width of optic nerve may be found
Blood tests[a]: CBC, ESR, ANA, FTA-ABS, T_4, TSH, Lyme titer	Normal values

[a]Adjunct tests; not necessary for diagnosis, but may be utilized to rule out other etiologies.

TABLE 7–6. DIFFERENTIAL DIAGNOSIS OF PSEUDOTUMOR CEREBRI

Headache Syndromes
Migraine
Tension headache
Sinusitis
Giant cell arteritis
Intracranial mass
Trigeminal neuralgia
Postherpetic neuralgia
Hypertension
Meningitis
Encephalitis
Subarachnoid hemorrhage

Papilledema
Primary or secondary tumors
Hydrocephalus
Infection:
  Encephalitis
  Meningitis
  Brain abscess
Trauma:
  Subarachnoid hemorrhage
  Subdural/epidural hematoma
Vascular:
  AV malformation
  Subarachnoid hemorrhage
Malignant hypertension
Toxic conditions

Congenital Disc Elevation
Buried disc drusen
Hypoplastic disc
Malinsertion of disc
Tilted disc

Other Causes of Acquired Bilateral Disc Edema
Hypertensive retinopathy
Infiltrative optic neuropathy (sarcoidosis, leukemia, non-Hodgkin lymphoma)
Inflammatory optic neuropathy
Toxic/hereditary optic neuropathy
Diabetic papillopathy

rologic localizing signs, hydrocephalus, and encephalopathies. Enlargement of the ventricles will be found in hydrocephalus, usually along with other neurologic signs. Infections, toxins, and malignant hypertension all may cause encephalopathy, and should be ruled out during the examination and by lumbar puncture. Blood tests to rule out systemic etiologies of swollen discs should include CBC, ESR, ANA, FTA-ABS, T_4, TSH, and Lyme titer.

Ocular

The ocular findings of papilledema and, less frequently, sixth-nerve palsy are the hallmarks in the diagnosis of PTC. Visual acuity will be reduced or normal. Automated perimetry is the preferred type of visual field test because of the ability to quantify defects for future follow-up of the patient. Full threshold 30-2 is the preferred automated field test. Defects range from mild loss to severe constriction of the visual field. Enlargement of the blind spot is almost always found, and will also vary with the patient's refractive error. Other visual field losses are similar to those found in any case of papilledema, and include decreased inferior nasal field, peripheral constriction, scotomas, and nerve fiber bundle defects.

Contrast sensitivity testing will show defects over all spatial frequencies. Color vision testing and pupil evaluation will not generally add helpful information unless the disc swelling is asymmetric. Visual evoked responses have limited use in the diagnosis and management of PTC.

TREATMENT AND MANAGEMENT

Systemic

Management of PTC ranges from monitoring the patient carefully to surgery (Table 7–7). A patient who has no vision loss and is not bothered by headaches or other symptoms is monitored monthly for any worsening of vision or new visual field loss and every 3 months if no change is found after the first 3 months. Many cases will resolve with no treatment, and patient follow-up is then tapered accordingly. Weight loss should be encouraged in all nonpregnant patients with PTC, although this alone is usually not sufficient to cure the disease. Johnston and co-workers (1998) reported improvement in PTC with as little as 3.3% weight loss and complete resolution of some cases with 6% weight loss. They correlated the amount of improvement to the percentage of weight loss. Standard analgesics, migraine medication, or beta-blockers are used initially to control headaches.

TABLE 7–7. TREATMENT AND MANAGEMENT OF PSEUDOTUMOR CEREBRI

Manifestation(s)	Treatment/Management
• No decrease in visual acuity • No visual field loss (except enlarged blind spot)	• Follow monthly for at least 6 months (must measure VA, VF, binocular optic nerve assessment with stereo photos, IOP) and if improvement, or no new symptoms, taper to every 3 months • Manage headaches with analgesics, beta-blockers, migraine medications • Weight-reduction program
• Early (minimal) decrease in visual acuity or loss of visual field • Headaches not managed or relieved by above medications	• Oral acetazolamide (Diamox) 500 mg bid • If Diamox contraindicated or not tolerated, consider furosemide (Lasix) 40–160 mg bid
• Medical treatment not effective • Recent loss of acuity not secondary to macular edema • Progression of a pre-existing visual field defect • Persistent, intractible headache not relieved by oral medications • Anticipation of oral therapy likely to cause hypotension	• Manage as above • Lumbar peritoneal shunt • Optic nerve sheath fenestration (primarily used to treat vision loss, may be done if lumbar peritoneal shunt not efficacious)

Severe headaches and progression of visual loss are the primary reasons to initiate medical and surgical treatment. Options include dehydrating agents, corticosteroids, serial lumbar puncture, and surgery.

Carbonic anhydrase inhibitors (CAIs) have been shown to play a large role in the management of this disorder and are recommended as the initial means to control PTC. These medications cause a decrease in CSF production by inhibiting carbonic anhydrase. Acetazolamide (Diamox) has been suggested (Tomsak, 1988) as the initial drug of choice in the treatment of PTC. However, maximum doses of CAIs are often necessary to decrease CSF effectively, and this frequently leads to adverse side effects and poor patient compliance. Side effects include nauseousness, gastrointestinal upset, perioral and digital tingling, loss of appetite, tin-like taste in the mouth, electrolyte imbalance, renal stones, fatigue, and depression. Diamox Sequel (the long-acting form) may cause fewer side effects and be more efficacious.

Corticosteroids are used frequently in the management of the patient with PTC. However, today most advocate only a short dose in cases of progressive vision loss or debilitating symptoms. Long-term steroid use can increase intraocular pressure (IOP) and aggravate vision loss. When steroids are discontinued, patients may also experience recurrence of PTC.

Repeated lumbar punctures were once used to treat PTC but they are no longer advocated, because lumbar punctures are difficult to perform on obese individuals and become more painful each time one is done. Also, their effect is short-lived, as the CSF pressure can return to its previous level within 2 hours of the procedure.

Indications for surgery include recent or progressive visual loss not responding to medical treatment and not secondary to macula edema, debilitating headaches not responding to medications, and the anticipation of medical treatment that may lead to a hypotensive event and cause further damage to the disc (eg, the initiation of systemic antihypertensive medications).

Subtemporal decompression was the first form of surgery used in the treatment of PTC. However, it is rarely done today because it has a high incidence of complications such as strokes or seizures. It has been replaced by lumbar peritoneal shunt and optic nerve sheath decompression.

Lumbar peritoneal (LP) shunt remains the most common surgical technique used in the management of PTC. In this procedure, a catheter is placed in the subarachnoid space of the lumbar vertebrae and the tubing is passed to the abdominal region, where it empties into the abdominal cavity. Burgett, Purivin, and Kawasaki (1997) found LP shunt effective in the acute reduction of ICP. In this study, 82% with headaches improved, and papilledema resolved completely or almost completely in 96% with 68% improvement in visual function. It acts like a constant lumbar puncture. Problems include infection, blockage, or movement of the tube. Signs and symptoms of PTC can improve within 1 month of this procedure; however, over 50% of cases require shunt revision. There appear to be two types of lumbar peritoneal shunt patients—one group in which the initial shunt works very well, and another group where reshunting is required, often more than once. The use of stereotactic technique to place the ventricular end of a ventriculoperitoneal shunt has proved promising and may result in less shunt failure.

Ocular

Ocular management (Table 7–7) includes visual acuity measurement, quantitative perimetry, stereo optic nerve photographs, and intraocular pressure measurement. Contrast sensitivity and color vision offer some assistance in following these patients, and visual evoked potentials (VEPs) are generally not useful. Follow-up is monthly for at least 6 months, and if no changes are noted, every 3 months thereafter as long as the edema persists.

Optic nerve sheath decompression is the second form of surgery used in the management of patients with severe vision loss from the papilledema. It was first performed by DeWecker in 1872, but did not gain widespread acceptance until 1964 when Hayreh revived the procedure. There are two approaches used to fenestrate the optic nerve and each has its proponents. One involves a medial approach to the optic nerve and the other a lateral approach. If medially done, the medial rectus is disinserted and the globe is retracted. The exposed optic nerve sheath is incised. Some remove a single square-shaped portion (like a window) while others make multiple incisions to fenestrate the meninges. The lateral approach entails an incision from the lateral canthus toward the ear. The temporalis muscle is retracted, the orbital rim cut and removed, and the lateral rectus muscle retracted. The nerve is then exposed and fenestrated.

Proposed theories regarding the mechanism of optic nerve sheath decompression include local decompression of the optic nerve by filtration from the creation of a permanent fistula to drain CSF. Another theory proposes that scarring in the subarachnoid space around the optic nerve causes a shift of the pressure gradient from the back of the lamina cribrosa to the myelinated portion of the optic nerve, thus relieving the pressure on the anterior portion of the optic nerve.

Optic nerve sheath decompression is done unilaterally. The second eye may be operated on if worsening occurs in that eye. Most studies show improvement of papilledema in half of cases in the eye not operated on. Headaches are usually relieved, but should not be an indication for this type of surgery. Most advocate standard medical treatment of headache with analgesics and migraine medications and then lumbar peritoneal shunt for treatment of headache.

Several studies have shown improvement of visual acuity and visual field after surgery despite optic nerve pallor preoperatively. Therefore optic nerve pallor is not a contraindication to surgery, but vision may not return to 20/20. Pallor may indicate the need for more prompt, aggressive treatment to preserve the remaining visual fibers.

Results from optic nerve sheath fenestration surgery have shown sustained improvement of visual acuity and visual field along with frequent improvement of the opposite eye and headaches. There is less need for repeat surgery, and less intraoperative and postoperative complications when compared to lumbar peritoneal shunt. Some patients who have undergone optic nerve sheath decompression have shown vision improvement following unsuccessful lumbar peritoneal shunt. Postoperative complications include disturbances of ocular motility and irregular pupils.

CONCLUSION

The eyecare practitioner plays a major role in the diagnosis and management of the patient with PTC. Headaches, blurred vision, and loss of vision are frequent causes for patients to seek eyecare, and these are the most common symptoms of PTC. The eyecare practitioner must understand this disorder and be able to recognize it in the patient who may or may not fit the typical clinical picture (a young, obese female). Thus, when a patient presents with headaches or visual symptoms, and papilledema is found on examination, timely referral must be made to a neurologist, and lumbar puncture and brain imaging should be ordered. Careful monitoring of ocular health, visual acuity, and visual fields by an eyecare practitioner is the mainstay for long-term follow-up in patients with PTC.

REFERENCES

Ahlskog JE, O'Neill BP. Pseudotumor cerebri. *Ann Intern Med.* 1982;97:249–256.

Baker RS, Carter D, Hendrick EB, Buncic JR. Visual loss in pseudotumor cerebri of childhood: A follow-up study. *Arch Ophthalmol.* 1985;103:1681–1686.

Bercaw BL, Greer M. Transport of intrathecal 13 1T RISA in benign intracranial hypertension. *Neurology.* 1970;20:787–790.

Brodsky MC, Vaphiades M. Magnetic resonance imaging in pseudotumor cerebri. *Ophthalmology.* 1998;105:1686–1693.

Brourman ND, Spoor TC, Ramocki JM. Optic nerve sheath decompression for pseudotumor cerebri. *Arch Ophthalmol.* 1988;106:1378–1383.

Bulens C, DeVries WA, Van Crevel H. Benign intracranial hypertension: A retrospective and follow-up study. *J Neuro Sci.* 1979;40:147–157.

Burgett RA, Purivin VA, Kawasaki A. Lumboperitoneal shunting for pseudotumor cerebri. *Neurology.* 1997;49:734–739.

Chiu AM, Chuenkongkaew WL, Cornblath WT, et al. Minocycline treatment and pseudotumor cerebri syndrome. *Am J Ophthalmol.* 1998;126:116–121.

Cody CM. Benign intracranial hypertension. *Am Fam Physician.* 1992;45:1671–1678.

Corbett JJ, Nerard JA, Tse DT, Anderson RL. Results of optic nerve sheath fenestration for pseudotumor cerebri. *Arch Ophthalmol.* 1988;106:1391–1397.

Corbett JJ, Savino PJ, Thompson HS, et al. Visual loss in pseudotumor cerebri: Follow-up of 57 patients from 5 to 41 years and a profile of 14 patients with permanent severe visual loss. *Arch Neurol.* 1982;39:461–474.

Corbett JJ, Thompson S. The rational management of idiopathic intracranial hypertension. *Arch Neurol.* 1989; 46:1049–1051.

Dandy WE. Intracranial pressure without brain tumor. *Ann Surg.* 1937;106:492–513.

Digre KB, Corbett JJ. Pseudotumor cerebri in men. *Arch Neurol.* 1988;45:866–872.

Durcan FJ, Corbett JJ, Wall M. The incidence of pseudotumor cerebri—Population studies in Iowa and Louisiana. *Arch Neurol.* 1988;45:875–877.

Goh KY, Schatz NJ, Glaser JS. Optic nerve sheath fenestration for pseudotumor cerebri. *J Neuro Ophthalmol.* 1997; 17:86–91.

Hupp SL, Glaser JS, Frazier-Byrne S. Optic nerve sheath decompression: Review of 17 cases. *Arch Ophthalmol.* 1987; 105:386–389.

Ireland B, Corbett JJ, Wallace RB. The search for causes of idiopathic intracranial hypertension—a preliminary case-control study. *Arch Neurol.* 1990;47:315–320.

Johnson LN, Krohel GB, Madsen RW, et al. The role of weight loss and acetazolamide in treatment of idiopathic intracranial hypertension. *Ophthalmology.* 1998;105:2313–2317.

Johnston I, Paterson A. Benign intracranial hypertension—cerebral spinal fluid pressure and circulation. *Brain.* 1974;97:308–312.

Kelman SE, Sergott RC, Cioffi GA, et al. Modified optic nerve decompression in patients with functioning lumboperitoneal shunts and progressive visual loss. *Ophthalmology.* 1991;98:1449–1453.

Keltner JL. Optic nerve sheath decompression—How does it work? Has its time come? *Arch Ophthalmol.* 1988; 106:1365–1369. Editorial.

Orcutt JC, Page NGR, Sanders MD. Factors affecting visual loss in benign intracranial hypertension. *Ophthalmology.* 1984;91:1303–1312.

Park S. Primo SA. Pseudotumor cerebri: Diagnosis and treatment. *Clin Eye Vision Care.* 1992;4:70–79.

Rowe FJ, Sarkies NJ. Assessment of visual function in idiopathic intracranial hypertension: A prospective study. *Eye.* 1998;12(pt 1):111–118.

Rush JA. Pseudotumor cerebri—clinical profile and visual outcome in 63 patients. *Mayo Clinic Proc.* 1980;55:541–546.

Sahs AL, Joynt RJ. Brain swelling of unknown cause. *Neurology.* 1956;6:791–803.

Scott IU, et al. Idiopathic intracranial hypertension in children and adolescents. *Am J Ophthalmol.* 1997;124:253–255.

Sergott RC. Modified optic nerve sheath decompression provides long-term visual improvement for pseudotumor cerebri. *Arch Ophthalmol.* 1988;106:1391–1397.

Shuper A, Snir M, Barash D, et al. Ultrasonography of the optic nerves: Clinical application in children with pseudotumor cerebri. *J Pediatr.* 1997;131:734–740.

Smith CH, Orcutt JC. Surgical treatment of pseudotumor cerebri. *Int Ophthalmol Clin.* 1986;26:265–275.

Sullivan JC. Diagnosis and management of pseudotumor cerebri. *J Natl Med Assoc.* 1991;83:916–918.

Susman JL. Benign intracranial hypertension. *J Fam Practice.* 1990;30:290–292.

Symonds CP. Otitic hydrocephalus. *Brain.* 1931;54:55–71.

Tomsak R. Treatment of pseudotumor cerebri with Diamox (acetazolamide). *J Clin Neuro-ophthalmol.* 1988;8:93–98.

Tulipan N, Lavin PJ, Copeland M. Stereotactic ventriculoperitoneal shunt for idiopathic hypertension: Technical note. *Neurosurgery.* 1998;43:175–176.

Wall M. Idiopathic intracranial hypertension. *Neuro Clin.* 1991;9:73–95.

Wall M, George D. Visual loss in pseudotumor cerebri—incidence and defects related to visual field strategy. *Arch Neurol.* 1987;44:170–175.

Wall M, Hart WM, Burde RM. Visual field defects in idiopathic intracranial hypertension (pseudotumor cerebri). *Am J Ophthalmol.* 1983;92:654–669.

Chapter 8

MULTIPLE SCLEROSIS

Susan C. Oleszewski

Multiple sclerosis (MS) is one of the most common acquired neurological diseases of young adults in the temperate zones. The disease probably accounts for more disability, more cost in care, and more lost income than any other neurological disease in this age group in Western Europe and in North America. Despite extensive research, the etiology remains unknown, treatment remains unsatisfactory, and the pathogenesis of the lesions is poorly understood. Neuro-ophthalmic signs and symptoms occur in virtually all patients some time during the course of the disease and are often critical in establishing a diagnosis.

EPIDEMIOLOGY

Systemic

Many aspects of the epidemiology of MS are controversial. However, a number of features, such as the overall geographic pattern, are clear and unequivocal. It is rare in the tropics and increases in frequency at higher latitudes north and probably also south of the equator. The prevalence in the United States is reported at 57.8 per 100,000, but increases in a somewhat continuous fashion with increasing latitude. Below the 37th parallel, the prevalence is reported at 35.5 per 100,000; above it, 68.8 per 100,000 (thus forming what is known as an "MS belt").

The risk of acquiring MS appears to be established around the time of puberty. Migration studies have found that persons less than 15 years of age migrating from high- to low-risk areas had a decrease in their risk of developing MS. Conversely, migration from low- to high-risk areas before age 15 resulted in an increased risk of acquiring MS. Presenting symptoms in MS vary according to what part of the brain or spinal cord is involved (Table 8–1).

Studies strongly suggest that there is a major genetic influence on susceptibility to MS (Sadovnick, 1988). The calculated risk for children and siblings of patients with MS of developing the disease is 3 to 5%, about 30 to 50 times the 0.1% rate for the general population. Although there is a definite genetic predisposition to MS, there is also strong evidence that having the prerequisite genetic background does not automatically lead to development of the disease and that exogenous or environmental factors are required to produce MS.

Given the genetic factors that are at least partially responsible for the development of MS and the immunologic aspects of the disease, it follows that patients with MS seem to have a higher incidence of other autoimmune diseases. Autoimmune diseases believed to occur with increased frequency in patients with MS compared to normal persons include diabetes mellitus, systemic lupus erythematosus, ankylosing spondylitis, and myasthenia gravis.

TABLE 8–1. INITIAL SYMPTOMS IN MULTIPLE SCLEROSIS PATIENTS

Symptom	Percent[a]
Sensory disturbance in one or more limbs	33
Disturbance of balance and gait	18
Visual loss in one eye	17
Diplopia	13
Progressive weakness	10
Acute myelitis	6
Lhermitte symptom	3
Sensory disturbance in face	3
Pain	2

[a]Total is more than 100% because some patients presented with more than one major symptom.

Reprinted with permission from Poser S. The Diagnosis of Multiple Sclerosis. *New York: Thieme; 1984:30.*

Ocular

Neuro-ophthalmic signs and symptoms occur in virtually all MS patients some time during the course of the disease. Poser and co-workers (1979) reported that 60% of the 1271 cases retrospectively studied during an 11-year period had an episode of optic neuritis, and 34% experienced diplopia. Poser also reported that optic neuritis was the initial symptom in 35% of the 1271 cases and diplopia the initial symptom in 13% of cases.

PATHOPHYSIOLOGY/DISEASE PROCESS

The pathogenesis of MS is complex and at present poorly understood. Association between susceptibility and specific major histocompatibility complex (MHC) genes suggests a genetic predisposition. A widely considered hypothesis is that MS is the result of an immune reaction directed against self-myelin antigens. Another important hypothesis under consideration is that in MS the myelin is an "innocent bystander" that is destroyed as a consequence of an immune response triggered by a viral infection. To date, attempts to identify a single infectious agent as the cause of MS have been unsuccessful.

MS affects scattered areas of the central nervous system in the form of plaques, with a predilection for periventricular white matter, brainstem, spinal cord, and optic nerves. The plaques are characterized by primary demyelination (destruction of myelin sheaths with preservation of axons) and death of oligodendrocytes (myelin-producing cells) within the center of the lesion. During the early evolution of the plaque, perivascular inflammatory cells (lymphocytes, plasma cells, macrophages) invade the substance of the white matter and are thought to play a critical role in myelin destruction. This process is followed by extensive gliosis by astrocytes and aberrant attempts at remyelination, with oligodendrocytes proliferating at the edges of the plaque. In addition, immunoglobulins are deposited within each plaque.

The neurologic deficits that occur in patients with MS are caused primarily by the effects of inflammation and demyelination on nerve conduction. Demyelinated fibers may experience a complete block of conduction, intermittent conduction block, or slowed conduction. Demyelinated fibers are also thermolabile. This phenomenon likely accounts for the production or exacerbation of neurologic symptoms, visual symptoms, or both, in patients with MS when their body temperature is raised through a hot shower or exercise (Uhtoff sign). Demyelinated nerve fibers demonstrate abnormal excitability. This may provide an explanation for symptoms and signs that commonly occur in MS patients, such as focal or generalized paresthesias, sudden electric-like sensations that radiate down the spine or extremities when the neck is flexed (Lhermitte sign), facial myokymia, and the phosphenes and photopsias that may be induced by eye movements and optic neuritis.

Demyelination is not the only cause for the clinical manifestations of MS. Secondary degeneration of axons that occurs with time after demyelination is probably responsible for the slowly progressive manifestations and visual deterioration that occur in patients with chronic MS.

The clinical course of MS can be classified as exacerbating–remitting, acute progressive, or chronic progressive. Exacerbating–remitting MS is the most common form in persons under age 40. It usually begins with the acute or subacute onset of focal neurologic signs and symptoms. The symptoms vary from mild to severe, and can result from involvement of any part of the brain or spinal cord.

Common presentations include blurred vision, diplopia, vertigo, weakness, and sensory symptoms. The focal symptoms and accompanying signs may come on rapidly over a few minutes, but more commonly progress gradually over several days. Symptoms typically evolve over 24 to 72 hours, stabilize for a few days, and then improve spontaneously. They may be followed months or years later by new focal symptoms or signs, which again may remit either partially or completely. Patients commonly experience a recurrence of old symptoms with or without new ones.

Acute progressive MS, a rarer form of MS, has a relatively acute onset with a rapidly downhill course. This type involves multiple areas of the nervous system simultaneously and leads to severe impairment and death within a few weeks or months.

Chronic progressive MS advances in most patients with disease onset after age 35. The disease most often begins insidiously with slowly or intermittently progressive monoparesis, paraparesis, hemiparesis, or axial instability. A slowly progressive pattern is rare in patients below age 35 and usually indicates another etiology.

The long-term outcome of patients with MS is variable; some patients apparently remain asymptomatic throughout the course, and others (a minority) have a fulminant, rapid progression to death. Most patients have a course somewhere between these two extremes. At least 20% of the patients have a benign course for 15 years or more.

Several studies have attempted to determine the factors that have predictive value for the long-term outcome. Not all studies have reached the same conclusions, but there seems to be consensus about certain factors (Table 8–2). The relapse rate does not seem to be a predictive value. The search for markers that have predictive value for the future course in MS patients continues.

Systemic

Multiple sclerosis is characterized by a myriad of neurological symptoms and signs (Table 8–3). The disease usually presents in patients under age 35 with the subacute onset of focal neurologic symptoms and signs indicative of disease in the optic nerve, pyramidal tract, posterior column, cerebellum, central vestibular system, or medial longitudinal fasciculus. Patients in the older age group more commonly present with an insidiously progressive myelopathy, manifesting as some combination of progressive spastic paraparesis, axial instability, and bladder impairment.

One of the most common clinical features in MS is the upper motor neuron syndrome. This consists of loss of motor control, spastic weakness, exaggerated tendon stretch reflexes, and extensor plantar responses (positive Babinski sign). Early in the course of the disease the patient complains of heaviness, stiffness, or clumsiness in one or both legs and a tendency to stumble. These symptoms are more prominent late in the day.

Fatigue, depression, and emotional lability are common symptoms of MS. Fatigue may be the most common single complaint of MS patients, and is often disabling. It usually comes on late in the afternoon, with strenuous activity, or in the heat. The etiology and mechanisms of depression in MS are unknown, but it appears to be more common in those with cerebral involvement than in those with predominantly spinal cord disease. Emotional lability may also be found in MS patients, ranging from a barely noticeable tendency to giggle or tear readily, to a very distressing and less common syndrome of powerful paroxysmal emotional outbursts.

Sensory symptoms in one or more extremities are common as initial symptoms and nearly universal in advanced stages of MS. These are most often described as "pins and needles" and less commonly as sensory loss. The paresthesias may be described as burning or hot. Defective postural, vibratory, and cutaneous sensations are common sensory signs in MS.

Cerebellar involvement may occur concurrently, resulting in severe gait disturbance, a decreased facility of fine finger movements, and intention tremor.

Lower back, hip, and leg pain are common, are usually associated with significant gait disturbance or weakness, and may be caused in part by spasticity. Compensation for this weakness can further exacerbate the pain. Typical tic douloureux (usually bilateral) and atypical facial pain may be caused by disease in the pontine tegmentum.

On occasion, with plaque involvement of the cervical cord, flexing the neck gives rise to a sensation resembling an electric shock, which radiates through the neck and may extend to the trunk (Lhermitte sign). This is not specific for MS; other types of cervical cord lesions can also be associated with this sign.

Elevation in ambient temperature or endogenous temperature (eg, fever or exercise) can be associated with marked increases in symptoms and signs. These may include ataxia and weakness.

Bladder dysfunction, an autonomic nervous system disorder, is extremely common, occurring in two thirds of MS patients as a later manifestation. Patients may fail to empty urine adequately, leading to high urinary residual volumes and at times to frank urinary retention. MS may also be accompanied by severe

TABLE 8–2. FACTORS WITH PREDICTIVE VALUE IN MULTIPLE SCLEROSIS PATIENTS

Feature	Relatively Favorable	Relatively Unfavorable
Sex	Female	Male
Age at onset (years)	< 40	> 40
Initial signs or symptoms	Optic nerve and sensory dysfunction	Motor dysfunction (cerebellar, corticospinal)
Disability	None after 5 years	Rapidly progressive disease

Reprinted with permission from Swanson I. Update in diagnosis and review of prognostic factors. Mayo Clinic Proc. *1989;64:578.*

TABLE 8–3. PRESENTING SYMPTOMS IN MULTIPLE SCLEROSIS BASED ON A STUDY OF 144 PATIENTS

Symptom	Patients	
	Number	Percentage[a]
Paresthesia	53	37
Gait difficulty	50	35
Weakness or incoordination of one or both lower extremities	25	17
Visual loss (retrobulbar neuritis)	22	15
Weakness or incoordination of one or both upper extremities	15	10
Diplopia	14	10
Urinary difficulty	9	6
Dysarthria	8	6
Hemiparesis	7	5
Severe fatigue	5	3
Vertigo	4	3
Impotence	4	3
Convulsion	3	2
Severe emotionality	3	2
Lhermitte sign	2	1
Muscle cramps (legs)	2	1
Fecal incontinence	2	1
Dysphagia	1	<1
Severe movement tremor	1	<1
Hearing loss	1	<1

[a]Total is more than 100% because some patients presented with more than one major symptom.

Reprinted with permission from Swanson I. Update in diagnosis and review of prognostic factors. Mayo Clinic Proc. *1989;64:585.*

constipation. Vascular congestion in the feet, or alternating pallor and congestion, are other autonomic nervous system dysfunctions, which occur most commonly in patients with moderate to severe paraparesis. Patients report a "hot and cold foot syndrome" in which their feet are either pale and cold or hot and flushed, but rarely comfortable.

Memory and learning impairment may occur frequently and early in MS. On rare occasions, MS appears to cause a progressive dementing illness, while at the other extreme it may have little if any cognitive or memory impairment, even in late stages of the disease.

Dysarthria, imperfect articulation, is a late occurrence in MS. This may present as a scanning speech pattern in which the words are measured or scanned with a pause after every slowly pronounced syllable. Dysarthria is reported to be present in approximately 6% of MS patients.

Sexual dysfunction was reported in 56% of women and 75% of men with MS in a population survey. This included fatigue, decreased sensation, decreased libido, erectile dysfunction, and a myriad of other symptoms. The sexual problems do not appear to be closely associated with motor system impairment.

Ocular

The neuro-ophthalmic manifestations of MS can be divided into two main categories: those that affect the visual sensory system and those that affect the ocular motor system (Table 8–4).

Visual sensory disturbances in the MS patient may result from disease of the retina, the optic nerve, the optic chiasm, the postchiasmal visual pathway, or a combination of these locations. Visual disturbances may precede, occur coincidently with, or follow the development of neurologic or psychiatric manifestations. Visual impairment eventually occurs in at least 80% of patients with MS and may be the presenting symptom in up to 50% of patients with MS.

Uthoff sign is defined by a reduction or diminution of vision following exercise or any other cause of increased body temperature. This symptom is usually found in patients with chronic, rather than acute, optic nerve disease. It has been reported that the patients with a pre-existing scotoma can get an enlargement of that scotoma following exercise. Other ocular manifestations of MS, such as diplopia, also can be exacerbated by heat. Uhtoff sign typically resolves rapidly once a patient ceases exercise or finishes bathing or showering.

An "inverse" Uthoff sign has been reported in MS patients (Honan et al, 1987). In these patients cold produced a temporary exacerbation of symptoms and signs, including paresthesias or deteriorating motor function. Patients have reported their vision to worsen in cold weather, when they were in an air-conditioned room, or when they drank an iced liquid. Improvement in function seemed to occur if their body temperature was raised through exercise or hot shower.

TABLE 8–4. OCULAR MANIFESTATIONS OF MULTIPLE SCLEROSIS

- Optic neuritis
  - Visual loss
  - Visual field defect (central scotoma)
  - Afferent pupillary defect
  - Color desaturation
  - Nerve fiber layer defects
- Ocular motility dysfunction
  - INO/BINO (diplopia)
  - Impaired smooth pursuit
  - Impaired saccades
  - Ocular dysmetria
  - Conjugate gaze palsy
  - Nystagmus
- Other
  - Granulomatous uveitis
  - Uhtoff sign

BINO, bilateral internuclear ophthalmoplegia; INO, internuclear ophthalmoplegia.

Sheathing of retinal veins (periphlebitis) is often seen in MS patients. The sheathing may present as focal, hazy gray patches that obscure the blood column in the vein. In other patients, the sheathing may appear as fine, white, linear streaks that parallel the blood column.

Uveitis, though not a common finding in MS, is found about 10 times more frequently in an MS patient than in the general population. The uveitis may be posterior, anterior, or both. In a retrospective study (Biousse, Trichet, Block-Michel, 1999) drawing from 1098 consecutive patients seen in a multiple sclerosis clinic, as well as 1530 consecutive patients seen in a uveitis clinic, only 28 patients (1%) had "definite multiple sclerosis" and uveitis. Pars planitis and panuveitis were the most commonly encountered types.

There is a well-established association of acute optic neuritis with demyelinating disease. Acute optic neuritis usually presents with the patient experiencing monocular loss of central vision, commonly associated with pain in, around, or behind the eye. The pain usually increases with movement of the eyes. Acute optic neuritis occurs most often in women between 15 and 45 years of age, although it may occur in both younger and older individuals. The degree of visual acuity loss varies considerably and may be associated with phosphenes that may be precipitated by eye movement.

The onset of visual loss typically varies from a few hours to 7 days, with some cases progressing for weeks or months. The severity may range from mild impairment to complete blindness, more typically with peripheral vision preserved. The visual loss stabilizes, and then usually improves slowly over a period of weeks. Less commonly, visual loss occurs abruptly or the patient may awaken with a maximal deficit. The Optic Neuritis Study Group (1997a) found that the mean visual acuity 5 years after an attack of acute demyelinating optic neuritis was 20/16. Even patients who lose all perception of light may regain vision to a 20/20 level.

Both retrospective and prospective studies have been performed to determine the prognosis for the development of MS in patients who have experienced an attack of acute optic neuritis. The Optic Neuritis Study Group (1997b) found that the risk of developing MS in a patient who experienced an attack of acute optic neuritis was about 30% after 5 to 7 years. The average time interval from an initial attack of optic neuritis until other symptoms and signs of MS develop varies considerably. Most agree that the majority of persons who develop MS after an attack of optic neuritis do so within 7 years of the onset of the visual symptoms.

A central visual field defect is common in patients with acute optic neuritis. The central scotoma has been heralded as the hallmark in optic neuritis. However, the central scotoma occurs in a minority of patients. A variety of patterns of visual field loss have been reported in patients with acute optic neuritis, including altitudinal, arcuate, cecocentral, diffuse, and even unilateral hemianopic visual field defects.

> Visual impairment eventually occurs in at least 80% of patients with MS and may be the presenting symptom in up to 50% of patients with MS.

Patients with unilateral acute optic neuritis invariably have a relative afferent pupillary defect (RAPD), as well as reduced sensation of brightness in the affected eye. The optic disc is normal in appearance in approximately two-thirds of patients. There may be an occasional cell in the vitreous overlying the optic nerve head, but there rarely is a significant cellular reaction associated with the optic neuritis of MS.

> The majority of persons who develop MS after an attack of optic neuritis do so within 7 years of the onset of visual symptoms.

The ocular motor system is often affected in MS. Patients with MS develop disorders of fixation, ocular motility, and ocular alignment, and such disorders are often the initial sign of the disease. The most common disorder of fixation associated with MS is nystagmus. Demyelinating lesions in the cerebellum and brainstem may result in saccadic intrusions, that is, inappropriate saccades that interfere with fixation.

Disturbances of ocular motility and alignment may develop during the course of MS, or occur as the first presenting sign weeks, months, or years before other neurologic symptoms and signs. These disturbances usually result from demyelinating lesions in the brainstem that affect supranuclear, internuclear, or fascicular pathways.

One of the neuro-ophthalmic hallmarks of MS is internuclear ophthalmoplegia (INO). INO is caused by damage to a portion of the medial longitudinal fasiculus (MLF), the fiber tract that connects the abducens nerve nucleus on one side of the brainstem and the medial rectus subnucleus on the contralateral side. INO, when unilateral, is characterized by weakness or absence of adduction in the eye on the side of the lesion combined with nystagmus of the contralateral abducting eye. Convergence is usually preserved. Although there are causes of INO other than demyelinating disease, the development of this condition in a young adult, particularly when it is bilateral, should be taken as a sign of MS until proven otherwise.

Patients with MS may develop ocular motor nerve pareses. The pareses may be single or multiple and unilateral or bilateral. Abducens nerve paresis is the most common ocular motor nerve paresis that occurs in patients with MS.

DIAGNOSIS

Systemic

The diagnosis of MS is based primarily on the neurological history, findings on neurological examination, and to a lesser extent, results of special testing (Table 8–5). The diagnosis is based on symptoms and objective evidence of white matter lesions of the central nervous system disseminated both temporally and spatially. Disturbances of sensation and gait and monocular loss of vision are the most common symptoms at the time of initial examination.

Clinicians have long used spinal fluid changes to support the diagnosis of MS. However, it should be recognized that CSF abnormalities are not diagnostic, as they are also present in other neurological and inflammatory diseases (Table 8–6). The cardinal features of the MS CSF profile include increased IgG levels, qualitative abnormalities in CSF IgG (IgG oligoclonal bands), mild pleocytosis, and occasionally an elevation of myelin breakdown products such as myelin basic protein (MBP).

Although computed tomography (CT) is not as sensitive as magnetic resonance imaging (MRI) in the detection of abnormalities in MS, it nevertheless may demonstrate a wide variety of findings. Cerebral atrophy is the most common and least specific abnormality. It usually is seen in patients with long-standing MS, although sometimes it is observed early and probably is related to widespread cerebral lesions. Increased size of ventricles, cisterns, and sulci are seen commonly in MS, particularly in later stages of the disease, and suggest loss of brain tissue.

MRI is currently the preferred imaging technique for obtaining diagnostic support of MS. The typical abnormalities on MRI are most commonly located in the supratentorial white matter, especially in the periventricular region. They may appear as multiple discrete lesions, or they may coalesce to form more homogeneous borders surrounding the ventricles. Less commonly, lesions can be detected in the cerebellum and brainstem (Figure 8–1).

TABLE 8–5. DIAGNOSTIC TESTS IN MULTIPLE SCLEROSIS

- CSF (cerebrospinal fluid)
- PET (positron emission tomography)
- CT (computed tomography)
- MRI (magnetic resonance imaging)
- MRSI (proton magnetic resonance spectroscopy imaging)

TABLE 8–6. DIFFERENTIAL DIAGNOSIS OF MULTIPLE SCLEROSIS

- Neuromyelitis optica (Devic disease)
- Myelinoclastic diffuse sclerosis (Schilder disease)
- Encephalitis periaxialis concentrica (concentric sclerosis of Balo)
- Acute disseminated encephalomyelitis (ADEM, postinfectious encephalomyelitis)

MRI is positive in 70 to 95% of patients with clinically definite MS. Of more importance, MRI has been found to support a diagnosis of MS in a high percentage of patients in whom the diagnosis was suspected. With isolated optic neuritis at initial examination, MRI detects disseminated lesions in 61% of the patients. The lesions were primarily found in the periventricular white matter of the cerebral hemispheres, brainstem, and cerebellum.

MRI techniques provide an objective, sensitive, and quantitative assessment of the evolving pathology in MS. Not only is MRI irreplaceable in the diagnosis of MS, but the importance of MRI as a tool in monitoring current therapies is becoming firmly established.

Positron emission tomographic (PET) scanning has demonstrated reduced cerebral blood flow and reduced oxygen utilization in MS patients. These findings may reflect decreased neuronal activity caused by large demyelinating lesions. At present, PET is used primarily as a research tool and not diagnostically.

Ocular

Ophthalmic testing that will delineate ocular involvement (optic neuritis) in MS includes visual acuity testing, visual field testing, pupillary reflex testing, color vision assessment, contrast sensitivity testing, and visual evoked potential (VEP) assessment. Common eye movement abnormalities (INO, BINO, nystagmus) will be evident on external evaluation.

The pattern shift VEP is currently the most useful evoked potential test in diagnosing optic nerve involvement of MS. VEPs can provide objective evidence of an optic nerve lesion, with or without associated visual symptomatology. However, VEP testing is not specific for MS; therefore the data from VEP testing should be placed in the context of the overall clinical picture. Differential diagnoses of MS optic neuritis are listed in Table 8–7.

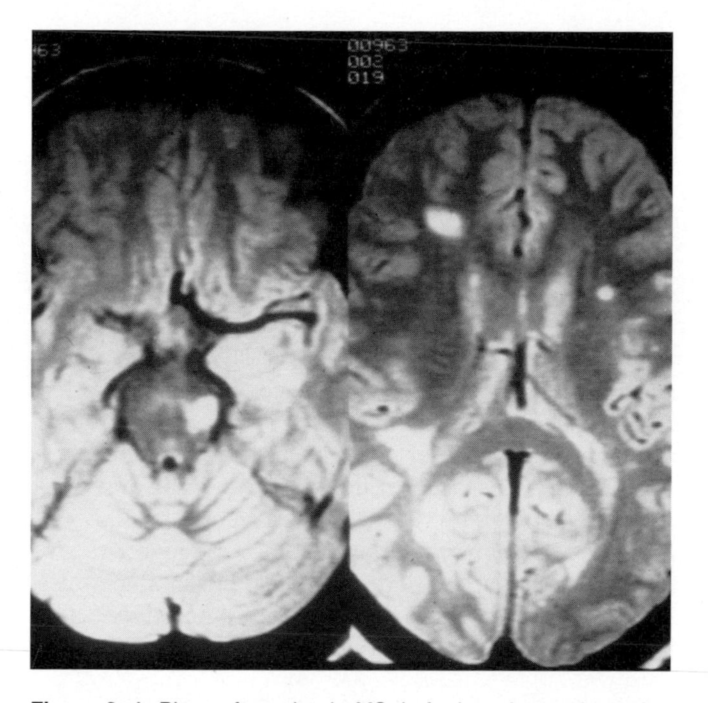

Figure 8–1. Plaque formation in MS. Left view shows plaque formation at the junction between the pons and midbrain; the right view shows a larger plaque in the white matter of the frontal lobe and a smaller plaque at the junction of the frontal and temporal lobes. *(Courtesy of Dr. Lawrence Gray.)*

Slit-like defects (Figure 8–2) in the peripapillary nerve fiber layer and corollary defects in the field of vision occur frequently in MS, often before there is a change in the patient's visual acuity, color perception, or optic disc. Nerve fiber defects have been observed in two thirds of MS patients. These defects indicate retrograde degeneration of scattered axon bundles from disease somewhere in the pregeniculate pathways.

TREATMENT AND MANAGEMENT

Because MS is thought by many to be an immunologically mediated illness, immunosuppressive therapy may play a role in its management (Table 8–8). The goals of immunosuppressive therapy in MS vary in accordance with the clinical stage of disease. The goals of therapy include (1) improving recovery from each exacerbation, (2) decreasing the number of future exacerbations, (3) decreasing the accumulation of additional disability, and (4) preventing the development of chronic progressive disease.

Systemic

Beck and associates (1993) reported the results of a 2-year study examining the risks of developing new demyelinating events following the treatment of acute optic neuritis with IV methylprednisolone followed by oral prednisone, or oral prednisone alone, or placebo. The results of this study have shown that those treated with IV methylprednisolone followed by oral prednisone had a reduction in new clinical manifestations of MS over the next 2 years compared to the other two groups. This treatment strategy was most beneficial to those patients with multiple signal abnormalities on MRI at the time of diagnosis of optic neuritis. The value of treatment in those with normal MRI scans could not be adequately assessed.

TABLE 8–7. DIFFERENTIAL DIAGNOSIS OF OPTIC NEURITIS

- Unknown etiology
- Multiple sclerosis
- Granulomatous inflammation (eg, syphilis, sarcoidosis, tuberculosis)
- Inflammation of the meninges, orbit, or sinuses
- Viral encephalitides
- Herpes zoster
- Intraocular inflammations
- Viral infections of childhood (measles, mumps, or chicken pox)

Immunosuppressive therapy for MS has involved the use of azathioprine, cyclophosphamide, cladribine, and cyclosporine. Evidence of modest efficacy has been tempered by significant side effects associated with these agents. Azathioprine has been shown to decrease the relapse rate in MS. It may possibly slow the

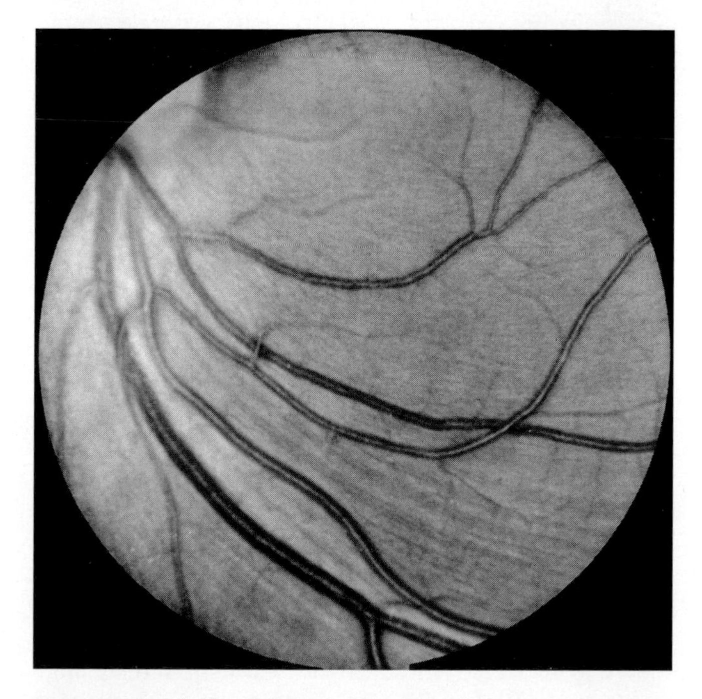

Figure 8–2. Slit-like defects in the peripapillary nerve fiber layer (NFL dropout).

TABLE 8–8. TREATMENT AND MANAGEMENT OF MULTIPLE SCLEROSIS

Systemic
- Corticosteroids
- Azathioprine
- Cladribine
- Glatiramer acetate (copolymer 1)
- Beta interferons
- Intravenous immunoglobulin
- Anticholinergic drugs (bladder dysfunction)
- Muscle relaxants (spasticity)
- Tricyclic antidepressants (depression)
- Physical and occupational therapy
- Psychotherapeutic support

Ocular
- Optic neuritis: no treatment or IV methylprednisolone followed by oral prednisone

progress of disability. However, azathioprine is not as widely prescribed because of side effects that include leukopenia, anorexia, diarrhea and vomiting, abdominal pain and other gastrointestinal disturbances, abnormal liver function, and skin rashes. Cladribine treatment has shown highly significant improvements in the neurological ratings of patients with chronic progressive MS.

Glatiramer acetate (Copaxone), previously called copolymer 1, has been shown to significantly reduce the relapse rate and tends to slow progressive disability in patients with relapsing-remitting MS, while having an excellent history of patient tolerance. Glatiramer acetate has been considered a first-line drug for the prevention of relapses and as replacement treatment for patients who fail with other therapies.

Interferon B-1b and interferon B-1a have been approved by the U.S. Food and Drug Administration for use in relapsing forms of MS. Interferon B-1a has reduced exacerbations in patients with relapse-remitting MS, as well as delayed progression of disability. There is also evidence that interferon B-1b delays sustained neurological deterioration in patients with secondary progressive MS.

Interferon B-1b and B-1a and glatiramer acetate have become widely prescribed in North America to patients with relapsing MS. However, these drugs do have limitations, including cost (approximately $11,000 per year), inconvenience (parenteral administration), and frequency of adverse effects (flu-like symptoms for several hours after each injection).

Intravenous immunoglobulin (IVIg) has been shown to also have efficacy in the treatment of relapsing-remitting multiple sclerosis. Monthly administration of IVIg seems to be as effective as interferon-B or glatiramer acetate in improving clinical disability and reducing the rate of relapses.

Other drug therapies in MS include anticholinergic drugs such as propantheline bromide for bladder function. Treatment for spasticity includes dantrolene, which acts at the level of the muscle, and diazepam and baclofen, which act centrally. Of all these therapies, baclofen is the drug of choice for symptomatic spasticity in MS.

Patients with mild or transient depression may be managed with supportive measures. However, more severe depression is best managed with the addition of a tricyclic antidepressant such as amitriptyline.

A multidisciplinary approach to the care in MS is most effective because of the many systemic and neurological problems present. Physical and occupational therapy are often part of the comprehensive care required for the MS patient. A clinical psychologist also can play an important role in helping the patient deal with the depression that often accompanies this disease.

Ocular

The efficacy of corticosteroids and corticotropin as treatments for optic neuritis had been debated for many years. The results of a multicenter, randomized clinical trial were reported in 1992 by Beck and associates. The results of this trial indicated that patients who received IV methylprednisolone followed by oral prednisone recovered vision faster than patients given placebo, but their visual outcome at the end of a 6-month follow-up period was only slightly better than that in the placebo group. Oral prednisone alone provided no benefit in terms of either the rate of recovery or the outcome at 6 months. However, Beck and associates (1993) reported the results of a study that found IV methylprednisone followed by oral prednisone as treatment for acute optic neuritis resulted in the reduction of subsequent new manifestations of MS. The authors report that these results justify the consideration of treatment of acute optic neuritis with IV methylprednisone followed by oral prednisone, even though the Optic Neuritis Treatment Trial results showed that this had only a marginal effect on visual recovery.

Five-year follow-up of patients in the Optic Neuritis Treatment Trial has revealed valuable information regarding the risk of developing clinically definite MS (CDMS) following an initial acute episode of optic neuritis. The 5-year risk of development of CDMS was 30%. When CDMS did develop, neurologic disability was mild in most patients. The 5-year study further revealed that brain MRI performed at study entry was a strong predictor of CDMS. The 5-year risk of CDMS ranged from 16% in those patients who had no MRI lesions at study entry to 51% in patients with three or more MRI lesions.

Five-year follow-up of this cohort of patients has also provided important conclusions regarding the visual function 5 years after the initial diagnosis of optic neuritis. Visual test results (as measured with visual acuity, contrast sensitivity, visual field, and color vision) 5 years after enrollment in the study were normal or only slightly abnormal in the eyes with optic neuritis at the time of study enrollment. This study has also suggested that the cumulative probability of having a new episode of optic neuritis during the 5 years of follow-up was 19% for the affected eye, 17% for the fellow eye, and 30% for either eye.

Counseling a patient who develops an acute unilateral idiopathic optic neuritis can be a complicated clinical dilemma. There may be a relatively long symptom-free interval between optic neuritis and the possible development of clinical MS. Therefore, some believe that it is not appropriate to inform the patient of this association. Speculating on the likelihood of developing MS is of no apparent benefit to the patient; however, the patient's right to know is a compelling argument in favor of disclosure. A varying spectrum of disclosure should be individually determined.

CONCLUSION

MS is a common neurological disorder whose ocular complications may be frequently encountered by the eyecare practitioner. With technological advances, the diagnosis of MS has become more definitive. However, this has done little to simplify management, patient apprehension, and prognosis. Rehabilitative and counseling services can provide improvement in quality of life for the MS patient. Ocular manifestations are common in MS; therefore, the eyecare practitioner is an integral part of the care and management of these patients.

REFERENCES

Anderson DW, Ellenberg JH, Leventhal CM, et al. Revised estimate of the prevalence of multiple sclerosis in the United States. *Ann Neurol.* 1992;31:333–336.

Archambean PL, Hollenhorst RW, Rucler CW. Posterior uveitis a manifestation of multiple sclerosis. *Mayo Clin Proc.* 1965;40:544.

Arnold AC, Pepose JS, Hepler RS, et al. Retinal periphlebitis and retinitis I multiple sclerosis. I. Pathologic characteristics. *Ophthalmology.* 1984;91:255–262.

Bachman DM, Rosenthal AR, Beckingsale AF. Granulomatous uveitis in neurological disease. *Br J Ophthalmol.* 1985; 69:192.

Bamford CR, Ganley JP, Sibley WA, Laguna JF. Uveitis, perivenous sheathing and multiple sclerosis. *Neurology.* 1978;28:119.

Baum HM, Rothschild BB. The incidence and prevalence of reported multiple sclerosis in the United States. *Ann Neurol.* 1981;10:42.

Beck RW, Cleary PA, Anderson MM, et al. A randomized, controlled trial of corticosteroids in the treatment of acute optic neuritis. *N Engl J Med.* 1992;326:581–588.

Beck RW, Cleary PA, Trobe JD, et al. The effect of corticosteroids for acute optic neuritis on the subsequent development of multiple sclerosis. *New Engl J Med.* 1993;329: 1764–1769.

Biousse V, Trichet C, Block-Michel E. Multiple sclerosis associated with uveitis in two large clinic-based series. *Neurology.* 1999;52:179.

Bornstein MB, Miller A, Slagle S, Weitzman M. A pilot trial of Cop 1 in exacerbating–remitting multiple sclerosis. *N Engl J Med.* 1987;317:408.

Caroscio JT, Kochwa S, Sacks H, et al. Quantitative CSF IgG measurements in multiple sclerosis and other neurologic diseases. *Arch Neurol.* 1983;40:409.

Chiappa KG. Pattern-shift visual, brainstem auditory and short-latency somatosensory evoked potential in multiple sclerosis. *Ann NY Acad Sci.* 1984;436:315.

Chiappa KH. Evoked potentials in clinical medicine. In: Joynt RJ, ed. *Clinical Neurology.* Philadelphia: Lippincott; 1988; 2:1–55.

Clifford DB, Trotter JL. Pain in multiple sclerosis. *Arch Neurol.* 1984;41:1270.

Cohen SR, Herndon RM, McKhann GM. Radioimmunoassay of myelin basic protein in spinal fluid: An index of active demyelination. *N Engl J Med.* 1976;295:1455.

Cox TA, Thompson HS, Clorbett JJ. Relative afferent pupillary defects in optic neuritis. *Am J Ophthalmol.* 1981;92:685.

Dailey FL, Brown JR, Goldstein F. Dysarthria in multiple sclerosis. *J Speech Hear Res.* 1972;15:229–245.

Duquette P, Girard M. Hormonal factors in susceptibility to multiple sclerosis. *Curr Opin Neurol Neurosurg.* 1993;6: 195–201.

Durelli L, Cocito D, Riccio A, et al. High-dose intravenous methylpredisolone in the treatment of multiple sclerosis: Clinical–immunologic correlations. *Neurology.* 1986;36:238.

European Study Group on Inteferon B-1b in Secondary Progressive MS. Placebo-controlled multicentre randomized trial of interferon B-1b in treatment of secondary progressive multiple sclerosis. *Lancet.* 1998;352:1491–1497.

Farlow MR, Markand ON, Edwards MK, et al. Multiple sclerosis: Magnetic resonance imaging, evoked responses, and spinal fluid electrophoresis. *Neurology.* 1986;36:828.

Fazekas F, Deisenhammer F, Strasser-Fuchs S, et al. Randomised placebo-controlled trial of monthly intravenous immunoglobulin therapy in relapsing-remitting multiple sclerosis. *Lancet.* 1997;349:589–593.

Feinsod M, Hoyt WF. Subclinical optic neuropathy in multiple sclerosis. *J Neurol Neurosurg Psychiatr.* 1975;38:1190.

Filippi M, Silver NC, Yousry TA, et al. Newer magnetic resonance techniques and disease activity in multiple sclerosis: New concepts and new concerns. *Multiple Sclerosis.* 1998;4:469–470.

Frisen L, Hoyt WF. Insidious atrophy of retinal nerve fibers in multiple sclerosis. *Arch Ophthalmol.* 1974;92:91.

Ganley JP. Uveitis and multiple sclerosis: An overview. In: Saari KM, ed. *Uveitis Update.* Amsterdam: Excerpta Medica; 1984:345–349.

Gebarski SS, Gabrielson TO, Gilman S, Knake JE. The initial diagnosis of multiple sclerosis: Clinical impact of magnetic resonance imaging. *Ann Neurol.* 1985;17:469.

Grant I, McDonald WI, Trimble MR, et al. Deficient learning and memory in early and middle phases of multiple sclerosis. *J Neurol Neurosurg Psychiatr.* 1984;47:250.

Griffin JF, Wray SH. Acquired color vision defects in retrobulbar neuritis. *Am J Ophthalmol.* 1978;86:193.

Gyldensted C. Computer tomography of the cerebrum in multiple sclerosis. *Neuroradiology.* 1976;12:33.

Hauser SL, Bhan AK, Gilles F, et al. Immunohistochemical analysis of the cellular infiltrate in multiple sclerosis lesions. *Ann Neurol.* 1986;19:578.

Honan WP, Heron JR, Foster DH, et al. Paradoxical effects of temperature in multiple sclerosis. *J Neurol Neurosurg Psychiatry.* 1997;50:1160–1164.

INFB Multiple Sclerosis Study Group. Interferon beta-1b is effective in relapsing-remitting multiple sclerosis. I. Clinical results of a multicenter, randomized, double-blind, placebo-controlled trial. *Neurology.* 1993;43:655–661,

Jacobs LD, Cookfair DL, Rudnick RA, et al. Intramuscular inteferon beta-1a for disease progression in relapsing multiple sclerosis. *Ann Neurol.* 1996;39:285–294.

Jensen TS, Rasmussen P, Reske-Nelsen E. Association of trigeminal neuralgia with multiple sclerosis: Clinical and pathological features. *Acta Neurol Scand.* 1982;65:182.

Johnson KP, Brooks BR, Cohen JA, et al. Extended use of glatiramer acetate (Copaxone) is well tolerated and maintains its clinical effect on multiple sclerosis relapse rate and degree of disability. *J Am Acad Neurol.* 1998; 50:701–708.

Kurtze JF, Beebe GW, Norman JE. Epidemiology of multiple sclerosis in U.S. veterans, 3. Migration and the risk of MS. *Neurology.* 1985;35:672.

Link H, Laurenze MA. Immunoglobulin class and light chain type of oligoclonal bands in CSF in multiple sclerosis determined by agarose gel electrophoresis and immunofixation. *Ann Neurol.* 1979;6:107.

Lukes SA, Crooks LE, Aminoff MJ, et al. Nuclear magnetic resonance imaging in multiple sclerosis. *Ann Neurol.* 1983;13:592.

Mastaglia FL, Black JL, Collins DWK. Quantitative studies of saccadic and pursuit eye movements in multiple sclerosis. *Brain.* 1979;102:817.

Mastaglia FL, Black JL, Thickbroom G, Collins DWK. Saccadic eye movements in multiple sclerosis. *Neuro-ophthalmol.* 1982;4:225.

Miller AE. Cessation of stuttering with progressive multiple sclerosis. *Neurology.* 1985;35:1341–1343.

Miller DG. Multiple sclerosis: Use of MRI in evaluating new therapies. *Sem Neurol.* 1998;18:317–325.

Muri RM, Meienberg O. The clinical spectrum of internuclear ophthalmoplegia in multiple sclerosis. *Arch Neurol.* 1885;42:851.

Optic Neuritis Study Group. The clinical profile of optic neuritis: Experience of the Optic Neuritis Treatment Trial. *Arch Ophthalmol.* 1991;109:1673–1678.

Optic Neuritis Study Group. Visual function five years after optic neuritis: Experience of the Optic Neuritis Treatment Trial. *Arch Ophthalmol.* 1997a;115:1545–1552.

Optic Neuritis Study Group. The 5-year risk of multiple sclerosis after optic neuritis: Experience of the Optic Neuritis Treatment Trial. *Neurology.* 1997b;49:1404–1413.

Ormerod IEC, McDonald WI, duBoulay GH, et al. Disseminated lesions at presentation in patients with optic neuritis. *J Neurol Neurosurg Psychiatr.* 1986;49:124–127.

Palace J, Rothwell P. New treatments and azathioprine in multiple sclerosis. *Lancet.* 1997;350:261.

Paty DW, Oger JJF, Kastrukoff LF, et al. MRI in the diagnosis of MS: A prospective study with comparison of clinical evaluation, evoked potentials, oligoclonal banding, and CT. *Neurology.* 1988;38:180.

Paty DW, Poser CM. Clinical symptoms and signs of multiple sclerosis. In: Poser CM, ed. *The Diagnosis of Multiple Sclerosis.* New York: Thieme & Stratton; 1984:37.

Poser S. *The Diagnosis of Multiple Sclerosis.* New York: Thieme; 1984.

Poser S, Wikstrom J, Bauer HJ. Clinical data and the identification of special forms of multiple sclerosis in 1271 cases studied with a standardized documentation system. *J Neurolog Sci.* 1979;40:159–168.

Prineas JW. The neuropathology of multiple sclerosis. In: Vinken PG, Bruyn GW, Klawans HL, eds. *Handbook of Clinical Neurology.* Vol 47: *Demyelinating Diseases.* New York: Elsevier; 1985:213–257.

PRISMS (Prevention of Relapses and Disability by Interferon B-1a Subcutaneously in Multiple Sclerosis Study Group). Randomized double-blind placebo-controlled study of interferon B-1a in relapsing/remitting multiple sclerosis. *Lancet.* 1998;352:1498–1504.

Rizzo JF III, Lessell S. Risk of developing multiple sclerosis after uncomplicated optic neuritis: A long-term prospective study. *Neurology.* 1988;38:185–190.

Rose AS, Kuzma JW, Kurtzke JF, et al. Cooperative study in the evaluation of therapy in multiple sclerosis: ACTH vs placebo; final report. *Neurology.* 1970;29:1–59.

Sadovnick AD, Baird PA. The familial nature of multiple sclerosis: Age-corrected empiric recurrence risks for children and siblings of patients. *Neurology.* 1988;38: 990–991.

Schiffer RB, Babigian HM. Behavior disorders in multiple sclerosis, temporal lobe epilepsy, and amyotropiclateral sclerosis. An epidemiologic study. *Arch Neurol.* 1984; 41:1067.

Schiffer RB, Herndon RM, Rudick RA. Treatment of pathologic laughing and weeping with amitriptyline. *N Engl J Med.* 1985;312:1480.

Sipe JC, Romine JS, Koziol JA, et al. Cladribine in treatment of chronic progressive multiple sclerosis. *Lancet.* 1994;344:9–13.

Swanson J. M.S.: Update in diagnosis and review of prognostic factors. *Mayo Clinic Proc.* 1989;64:578–585.

Szasz G, Paty D, Maurice WL. Sexual dysfunctions in multiple sclerosis. *Ann NY Acad Sci.* 1984;436:443.

Thompson HS, Corbett JJ, Cox TA. How to measure the afferent pupillary defect. *Surg Ophthalmol.* 1981;26:39.

Tourtellotte WW, Baumhefner RW, Rotvin AR, et al. Multiple sclerosis de novo CNS IgG synthesis: Effect of ACTH and corticosteroids. *Neurology.* 1980;30:1155.

Troiano R, Hafstein M, Ruderman M, et al. Effect of high-dose intravenous steroid administration on contrast-enhancing computed tomographic scan lesions in multiple sclerosis. *Ann Neurol.* 1984;15:257.

Valleroy ML, Kraft GH. Sexual dysfunction in multiple sclerosis. *Arch Phys Med Rehabil.* 1984;65:125.

Weinshenker BG, Ebers GC. The natural history of multiple sclerosis. *Can J Neurol Sci.* 1987;14:255.

Whitaker JN, Gupta M, Smith OF. Epitopes of immunoreactive myelin basic protein in human cerebrospinal fluid. *Ann Neurol.* 1986;20:329.

Yudkin PL, Ellison GW, Ghezzi, A, et al. Overview of azathioprine treatment in multiple sclerosis. *Lancet.* 1991;338: 1051–1055.

Chapter 9

ALZHEIMER DISEASE

Susan C. Oleszewski

Alzheimer disease (AD), which becomes more prevalent with age, is a major cause of dementia in the older population. It is characterized by a progressive loss of memory, orientation, and other cognitive functions. As the population continues to become older, its incidence will increase further. Ocular manifestations of AD are not prominent and are usually the result of degeneration of the visual association areas of the cortex.

EPIDEMIOLOGY

Systemic

Alzheimer disease is a major cause of dementia; however, exact data on the prevalence of dementia or AD is not available. It is estimated that 4 to 5% of the U.S. population over age 65 has severe dementia, and that an additional 10% has mild to moderate impairment. In the 65- to 70-year age group, the prevalence of severe dementia is only 1% or less, but in those over 85, the fastest-growing segment of the population, the prevalence rises to over 15%. At this rate of increase, and as life expectancy extends into the late 90s (as anticipated by about the year 2040), an astonishing 45% of the population is likely to develop dementia.

Few studies exist on the incidence of AD in the general population. The most reliable data suggest an incidence rate of 0.7 and 0.5% for men and women, respectively, aged 70 to 79; and 1.9 and 2.5% for men and women aged 80 years and older.

Ocular

Although there is a broad range of visual system disorders in AD, data are not available on the percentages of patients who suffer from these disorders. At present it is known that AD patients vary considerably in extent of their visual system pathology. Most of the abnormalities are associated with the visual association cortex, rather than the retina and visual pathway.

PATHOPHYSIOLOGY/DISEASE PROCESS

Systemic

Consistent changes are found in the brains of the AD patients. These include atrophy, especially a loss of synapses in the cortex; the presence of abnormally stained neurons, called neurofibrillary tangles; and the presence of numerous, neuritic plaques (focal collections of degenerating nerve terminals that surround a core of an abnormal fibrillar protein, B-amyloid). Additionally, the cholinergic projection system to the neocortex is altered in AD, as indicated by decreased levels of choline acetyltransferase, a marker of cholinergic neurons. The decreased cholinergic function in the neocortex has been found to correlate well with the degree of dementia associated with AD. Many of the changes in the neocortex are part of the normal aging process; however, they seem to be markedly exaggerated in Alzheimer patients.

Neuritic plaques are spherical, multicellular lesions that are usually found in moderate or large numbers in limbic structures and the association neocortex in the AD patient. Neuritic plaques contain extracellular deposits of amyloid-B protein (AB) that include abundant amyloid fibrils intermixed with nonfibrillar forms of the peptide. Neuritic plaques have degenerating axons and dendrites (neurites) within and surrounding the amyloid deposits.

Neurofibrillary tangles generally occur in large numbers in the Alzheimer brain. Neurofibrillary tangles are intraneuronal cytoplasmic lesions consisting of non-membrane-bound bundles of paired, helically wound filaments. The subunit protein of the tangle is the microtubule-associated tau protein. The hyperphosphorylated, insoluble form of the tau protein in tangles is often conjugated with ubiquitin, a characteristic feature shared with other disorders such as Parkinson disease and diffuse Lewy body disease.

It appears that the earlier the onset and the more severe the disease, the higher the risk to relatives. Genetic and molecular research has accumulated evidence that AD has a multifactorial etiology: genetic and environmental factors may interact in a complex manner controlling the risk for developing the disease. Genetic variants and mutations have been found to be associated with an increased likelihood or younger age at onset of the disease. Mutations in several genes, amyloid precursor protein (APP), apolipoprotein 4 allele, presenilin-1 (PS1), and presenilin-2 (PS2), are related to autosomal dominantly inherited AD. Defects in these genes have been associated with increased amyloid production or accumulation, and with enhanced susceptibility to apoptosis.

Common population polymorphisms (CPPs) in the interleukin 1 genes (IL-1A and IL-1B) are reported to be associated with increased risk of AD, as well as early onset of AD. IL-1 is a proinflammatory cytokine that is markedly expressed in the microglia of brains of AD patients. It is speculated that CPPs in the interleukin genes may instigate a substantial cytokine-mediated inflammatory cascade in regions of the brain in AD patients. Research data suggest that perhaps anti-inflammatory therapies, especially therapies aimed at countering cytokine-mediated inflammation, could be useful in treating and preventing AD.

The course of AD is characterized by progressive cognitive and functional decline. It is important to stress that the course of the disease is quite variable. This may range from an individual with mild forgetfulness for a number of years, to a rapid decline.

> Visual acuity is often difficult to assess in Alzheimer patients because of the underlying dementia. Nonetheless, acuity of patients with AD appears to be normal in the early stages of the disease.

The onset and details of the early course of the disease are often difficult to establish. The demented patient may be an unreliable witness, and the early symptoms are often so subtle as to escape the notice of even the most attentive family member or associate. Most often the initial symptoms are impaired memory, difficulty with problem solving, failure to respond to the environment with customary speed and accuracy, and easy distractibility. As the patient becomes more aware of the loss of mental efficiency, depression frequently occurs, taking a toll on mental function (Table 9–1).

Inability to recall acquired material of an impersonal nature is the most apparent memory defect in AD. Environmental disorientation is also common. Patients are unable to find their way around familiar surroundings, including their own homes. They may have a tendency to wander and may become agitated, especially at night ("sundowning").

Language dysfunction is evident in AD patients, with dysnomia (incorrect naming of objects) usually the initial manifestation. This may lead to some form of dysphasia, which is encountered in almost every AD patient. This speech disorder usually progresses to a fluent aphasia, where there may be remarkable preservation of grammar and prose but the conversation is often devoid of ideas and can be called "empty speech." Alexia (inability to read), as well as agraphia (inability to write), is also common in AD patients.

TABLE 9–1. COMMON SYSTEMIC MANIFESTATIONS OF ALZHEIMER DISEASE

- Aphasia
- Impaired memory
- Difficulty with problem solving
- Dysphagia
- Alexia
- Agraphia
- Extrapyramidal signs (rigidity and hypokinesia)
- Prosopagnosia
- Environmental disorientation

Extrapyramidal signs, particularly rigidity and hypokinesia (decreased movements), frequently occur in patients with AD, especially those with severe dementia. Tremor is less prominent than in other degenerative disorders, as are other dyskinesias. Disorders of gait, limb paralysis, seizures, and urinary incontinence are less prominent and appear later than the dementia.

AD has three phases. In the initial phase, the patient becomes aware of intellectual or memory impairment, but the mild symptoms are not noticed by family and friends. As the disease progresses into the second phase, close family and friends begin to notice the patient's difficulties with memory, intellect, and judgment. Finally, in the third stage the patient loses awareness of the illness, but the symptoms are so advanced as not to be missed by those around the patient. The clinical and behavioral observations of patients in these three stages are further delineated in Table 9–2. The progression of AD is a relentless process that occurs over 2 to 10 years or longer. The expected survival, following a diagnosis of AD, is between 5 and 15 years.

AD alone does not cause death. Rather, death usually results from a concurrent infection that is exacerbated by extreme weight loss, weakness, decreased metabolism, and dehydration. Bronchopneumonia is one of the major infections responsible for the death of AD patients. Stroke and myocardial infarction have also been identified as complications that may be associated with morbidity.

TABLE 9–2. STAGES OF ALZHEIMER DISEASE

Stage 1
Memory loss
Lack of spontaneity
Subtle personality changes
Disorientation to time and date

Stage 2
Impaired cognition and abstract thinking
Restlessness and agitation
Wandering, "sundowning"
Inability to carry out activities of daily living
Impaired judgment
Inappropriate social behavior
Lack of insight, abstract thinking
Repetitive behavior
Voracious appetite

Stage 3
Emaciation, indifference to food
Inability to communciate
Urinary and fecal incontinence
Seizures

Reprinted with permission from Matterson MA, McConnell ES. Gerontological Nursing: Concepts and Practice. *Philadelphia: Saunders; 1988:251.*

Ocular

Ocular manifestations of AD are not prominent. Findings consist of subtle disturbances of function that may or may not be noticed by the patient or family members. A broad range of visual disorders in AD may result from the involvement of the visual association cortex and optic nerves (Table 9–3).

> The initial symptoms of the AD patient include impaired memory, disorientation of his or her environment, and language dysfunction, most commonly incorrect naming of objects (dysnomia).

Visuospatial difficulties are common. Agnosia, the inability to recognize familiar objects, is common, and is present in almost half of AD patients, resulting in a major source of disability. It may manifest as visuospatial agnosia (loss of visuospatial orientation), prosopagnosia (difficulty in facial recognition), simultanagnosia (inability to attend to more than one visual object at the same time), and topographagnosia (inability to follow a route).

Difficulties locating objects in space occur frequently, along with loss of the sense of "whereness" and clumsiness in attempts to reach for objects or avoiding bumping into them. This "spatial agnosia" is responsible for visual localization difficulties, a common complaint in AD. Spatial agnosia may also cause abnormalities in scanning, searching, and hand-eye coordination severe enough to constitute Balint syndrome in up to 20% of AD patients. Balint syndrome consists of simultanagnosia, oculomotor apraxia (inaccurate eye movements), and optic ataxia (inability to

TABLE 9–3. OCULAR MANIFESTATIONS OF ALZHEIMER DISEASE

- Optic nerve degeneration
- Dyschromatopsia
- Depressed contrast sensitivity
- Impaired ocular motility/reading difficulty
- Visuospatial disorientation
- Agnosia
  - Visual: visuospatial, prosopagnosia, simultanagnosia
  - Spatial: Balint syndrome (simultanagnosia, oculomotor apraxia, optic ataxia)
- Apraxia, constructional
  - Oculomotor
- Hallucinations
- Impaired saccades, pursuits, tracking, and scanning

direct hand or other movements by visuospatial guidance). Constructional apraxia (inability to draw a design such as a circle, triangle, or clock face) may also occur in AD patients.

An early symptom of AD is the complaint of reading difficulty; specifically, losing one's place on the line or page, dancing of print, and blurred vision. Hallucinations may occur in up to 20% of patients with AD, and 80 to 90% of these are visual hallucinations.

Acuity is often difficult to confidently assess in Alzheimer patients because of their underlying dementia. Nonetheless, acuity of patients with AD appears to be normal, at least in the earlier stages of the disease.

There is both histological and clinical evidence that AD damages the retina and optic nerve. Degeneration has been noted in both the optic nerves and the retinas of mild and severe AD patients. Specific histological findings include widespread axonal degeneration, preferential loss of large-diameter axons, loss of retinal ganglion cells, and thinning of the nerve fiber layer. Optic nerve head pallor has been observed in AD patients.

Abnormal color vision has been reported and a significant percentage of errors fall in the tritan (blue) category. Dyschromatopsia may be one manifestation of the optic neuropathy of AD. Examination of the visual system in AD may reveal visual field defects, prolonged visual evoked potentials, abnormal eye movement recordings, and decreased contrast sensitivity. Contrast sensitivity studies have yielded contradictory results that may reflect differences in patient selection.

Saccadic velocity, latency, and accuracy have been found to be abnormal with a higher frequency of ocular velocity arrests during smooth pursuits. Additionally, a significant correlation between the severity of the dementia and the frequency of velocity arrests during smooth pursuit has been found. Eye tracking (slow eye movements) and visual scanning have also been found to be abnormal in AD patients.

DIAGNOSIS

Systemic

Alzheimer disease is a clinical diagnosis of exclusion. The physical exam, including the detailed neurological examination, is usually normal. The definitive diagnosis is histopathologic. Nonetheless, there are several diagnostic tests that are helpful. The clinician must rule out other systemic diseases, organic or psychogenic brain disorders that might account for the impairment in memory and cognitive function (Table 9–4). Clinical analysis must also include a detailed inventory of all medications that the patient may be taking, along with a study of their interactions and side effects. Any medications suspected of affecting memory and cognitive function should be discontinued if possible, and the patient observed without medication before the final diagnosis.

TABLE 9–4. DIFFERENTIAL DIAGNOSIS OF DEMENTIA

- Alzheimer disease
- Vascular dementia (eg, multi-infarct dementia)
- Drugs and toxins (eg, chronic alcoholic dementia)
- Intracranial masses
- Anoxia
- Head trauma (eg, dementia pugilistica)
- Neurodegenerative disorders (eg, Parkinson disease, Huntington chorea)
- Infections (eg, AIDS, cryptococcal meningitis, viral encephalitis)
- Nutritional disorders (eg, Wernicke–Korsakoff syndrome, vitamin B_{12} deficiency)
- Metabolic disorders (eg, Cushing syndrome, hypo- and hyperthyroidism)
- Chronic inflammation (eg, MS, systemic lupus erythematosus and other collagen–vascular disorders)

The following criteria support a clinical diagnosis of *probable AD.* The onset of cognitive and memory disturbances must occur between ages 40 and 90. There must be no systemic disorders or other neurologic disease that could account for the cognitive and memory deficits. Dementia must be established and documented through neuropsychologic testing. There must be deficits in two or more areas of cognition, and no disturbances of consciousness.

The diagnosis of *probable AD* is supported if there is progressive deterioration of specific cognitive functions such as language (aphasia), motor skills (apraxia), and perception (agnosia). Family history of similar disorders further assists an AD diagnosis. A diagnosis of AD will be further supported by impaired activities of daily living, as well as altered patterns of behavior.

Standard diagnostic testing is often used to rule out other disorders, rather than to definitively diagnose AD (Table 9–5). Electroencephalography (EEG) will

TABLE 9–5. DIAGNOSTIC INVESTIGATIONS UTILIZED IN ALZHEIMER DISEASE

Routine hematologic studies (to rule out potentially treatable or reversible causes)
- Complete blood count and erythrocyte sedimentation rate
- Concentration of electrolytes and calcium
- Renal, liver, and thryroid function tests
- Serum vitamin B_{12}
- Syphilis serology

CSF cell count, protein, and sugar concentrations
EEG (electroencephalogram)
CT (computed tomography)
MRI (magnetic resonance imaging)

either show normal patterns or nonspecific changes. Computerized tomography (CT) studies are essential to exclude intracranial structural disorders. CT also provides evidence of cerebral atrophy with progression documented by serial observation. Magnetic resonance imaging (MRI) has not been applied in a systematic way to aid in the diagnosis of AD. More recently, positron emission tomography (PET) has found significant reductions in glucose metabolism in both cerebral hemispheres of Alzheimer patients.

After excluding other causes of dementia, clinical features consistent with the diagnosis of *probable AD* include associated symptoms of depression; insomnia; incontinence; delusions; hallucinations; verbal, emotional, or physical outbursts; sexual disorders; and weight loss. Other neurological abnormalities that occur in advanced disease include motor signs such as increased muscle tone, myoclonus, or gait disorder. Seizures are rare, but may be present in advanced disease.

Advancing age and family history of AD are significant risk factors. There is some clinical evidence that prior head trauma may be a potential risk factor for AD. Identifying aluminum compounds in association with the neurofibrillary tangles and the core plaques that occur in the brains of AD patients has caused speculation that exposure to high levels of aluminum may be an additional risk in developing AD. Down syndrome or a family history of Down syndrome, and thyroid disease, are considered additional risk factors.

Ocular

Of special interest to eyecare practitioners is the prominence of visual symptoms at a time when the diagnosis is still uncertain. While there is nothing pathognomonic about visual symptoms of patients with AD, clinicians ought to be aware that early symptoms of patients with AD may be visual in nature.

TREATMENT AND MANAGEMENT

Drug treatment and other intervention strategies (Table 9–6) to prevent or delay progression of AD have been limited, primarily because so little is known about the cause or risk factors for the disease. Ideally, treatment would involve either replacement therapy or drugs that prevent or delay the pathologic changes that occur in AD.

There are two main objectives in the treatment and management of AD. The primary objective is to achieve some improvement in cognitive symptoms or to at least stabilize the dementia associated with AD. A second objective is to treat noncognitive manifestations of the disease such as agitation, paranoia, uncooperativeness, and depression.

TABLE 9–6. TREATMENT AND MANAGEMENT OF ALZHEIMER DISEASE

Neurotransmission-enhancing agents
• Cholinesterase inhibitors
• Nicotine[a]
• *Ginkgo biloba*[a]
• Neurotrophic factors[a]
Vitamin E
Selegiline (a selective MAO-B inhibitor)
NSAIDs
Neuroprotective agents
• Estrogen[a]
• Nerve growth factor
• Beta-amyloid
Antipsychotics (eg, haloperidol)
Sedatives (eg, chloral hydrate)
Counseling
• Family counseling
• Genetic counseling
• Support groups
Daycare

[a]Still under investigation.

The drugs available that theoretically improve the cognitive symptoms in AD or drugs for stabilizing the dementia associated with AD can be divided into those whose actions enhance the effect of neurotransmitters and those thought to protect neurons. The best known neurotransmission-enhancing drugs are the cholinesterase inhibitors. Cholinesterase inhibitors block acetylcholinesterase and therefore preserve acetylcholine for a longer period of time. The two available agents in the United States are tacrine and donepezil, with the latter compound being more commonly prescribed today. Therapy with cholinesterase inhibitors may result in symptomatic improvement in mild to moderate AD. Presently, there is no evidence that cholinesterase inhibitors modify the course of the disease. There are three additional cholinesterase inhibitors in the development phase being evaluated by the Food and Drug Administration (FDA): rivastigmine, metrifonate, and galanthamine.

Other neurotransmission-enhancing drugs under investigation include nicotine, *Ginkgo biloba,* and neurotrophic factors. Nicotine is known to stimulate acetylcholine receptors. The results of a small pilot study suggest that nicotine might improve the cognition in some patients with AD. Still under investigation, it is premature to recommend nicotine as an efficacious treatment for AD. *Ginkgo biloba* has been approved in Germany for treatment of dementia. Results of European studies suggest that *Ginkgo biloba* may benefit patients with AD, possibly through its ability to enhance neurotransmission by activating presynaptic cholinergic receptors.

Vitamin E (alpha-tocopherol) and selegiline, a selective monoamine oxidase type B (MAO-B) inhibitor, have been reported to delay functional deterioration, particularly as reflected by the need for institutionalization. The American Psychiatric Association recommends the use of vitamin E in the treatment of AD patients with moderate dementia.

It has been suggested that there may be a role for nonsteroidal anti-inflammatory drugs (NSAIDs) in the treatment of AD. NSAIDs decrease the inflammatory changes in the brains of patients with AD.

Several neuroprotective therapies are currently under investigation and may prove to be useful in the treatment of AD. Animal studies have shown that administration of estrogen to estrogen-deficient laboratory animals restores the number of neural synapses, causes beta-amyloid to be more soluble, and has an antioxidant effect. This protective effect of estrogen has also been demonstrated in cultured hippocampal neurons exposed to the toxic effects of beta-amyloid.

Nerve growth factor (NGF) in rats is known to protect the cortical cholinergic system following experimental injury. Additionally, NGF improves the maze learning performance of impaired elderly rats. NGF is viewed by some as a potential treatment that may play a role in future management modalities for AD patients.

Schenk and colleagues (1999) reported that when mice were injected with the protein beta-amyloid, antibodies were generated that prevented further accumulation of beta-amyloid, as well as clearing existing amyloid plaques. This report provides cautious optimism that a vaccine for AD may be in the future treatment armamentarium.

An additional objective in the managment of patients with AD is treating the depression, agitation, or sleep disorders often associated with AD. Agitated or aggressive behavior may require administration of a neuroleptic agent (haloperidol) to allow the patient to remain within his or her family or social situation.

The most meaningful aspect of the care and management of AD should involve the maintenance of the patient's socialization and support for the family. Self-help groups that provide both educational and psychological support have proliferated during recent years. Daycare and respite centers can provide needed relief for the caregivers.

CONCLUSION

Alzheimer disease is the major cause of admission to nursing homes, and it is an important cause of chronic disability in the elderly. The emotional and socioeconomic price that society must pay for longevity is the tragic reality of caring for the AD patient. The visual system abnormalities contribute to the disability caused by AD, and may magnify the effects of other cognitive deficits.

The future challenges for those committed to research in AD are to understand its cause and to intervene to prevent the disease or halt its progression. Better diagnostic capabilities must be developed, along with improved treatment modalities.

REFERENCES

Barclay LL, Zemov A, Blass JP, Sansome J. Survival in Alzheimer's disease and vascular dementias. *Neurology.* 1985;35:834–840.

Cogan DG. Visual disturbances with focal progressive dementing disease. *Am J Ophthalmol.* 1985;100:68.

Corkin SH, Growdon JH, Nissen MJ, et al. Recent advances in the neuropsychological study of Alzheimer's disease. In: Wurtman J, Corkin SH, Growdon JH, eds. *Alzheimer Disease: Advances in Basic Research and Therapies.* Proceedings of the third meeting of the International Study Group on the Treatment of Memory Disorders Associated with Aging. Zurich: Center for Brain Sciences and Metabolism Charitable Trust; 1984:75.

Cronin-Golomb A, Corkin S, Rizzo JF, et al. Visual dysfunction in Alzheimer's disease: Relation to normal aging. *Ann Neurol.* 1991;29:41.

Eagger SA, Levy R, Sahakian BJ. Tacrine in Alzheimer disease. *Lancet.* 1991;337:989–992.

Evans DA, Scherr PA, Cook NR, et al. Impact of Alzheimer's disease in the United States population. In: Suzman R, Willis DP, eds. *The Oldest Old.* London: Oxford; 1992.

Fletcher WA, Sharpe JA. Saccadic eye movements dysfunction in Alzheimer disease. *Ann Neurol.* 1986;20:464.

Foster NL, Chase TN, Mansi L, et al: Cortical abnormalities in AD. *Ann Neurol.* 1984;16:649.

Goedert M. Tau mutations cause frontotemporal dementias. *Neuron.* 1998;21:955–958.

Goodman Y, Annadora BJ, Bheng B, et al. Estrogens attenuate and corticosterone exacerbates excitotoxicity, oxidative injury, and amyloid B-peptide toxicity in hippocampal neurons. *J Neurochem.* 1996;66:1836–1844.

Grimaldi LME, Casadei VM, Ferri C, et al. Association of early-onset Alzheimer's disease with an interleukin-1A gene polymorphism. *Ann Neurol.* 2000;47:361.

Henderson AS. The epidemiology of Alzheimer's disease. *Br Med Bull.* 1986;42:3.

Hershey LA, Whicker L, Abel LA, et al. Saccadic latency measurements in dementia. *Arch Neurol.* 1983;40:592.

Heyman A, Wilkinson WE, Hurwitz BJ, et al. Alzheimer's disease: A study of epidemiology aspects. *Ann Neurol.* 1984;15:335.

Hinton, DR, Sadun AA, Blanks JC, Miller CA. Optic nerve degeneration in Alzheimer's disease. *N Engl J Med.* 1986; 315:485.

Hutton JT. Eye movements and Alzheimer disease: Significance and relationship to visuospatial confusion. In: Hutton JT, Kennedy AD, eds. *Senile Dementia of the Alzheimer Type.* New York: Liss; 1985:3–33.

Hutton JT, Nagel JA, Loewenson RB. Eye tracking dysfunction in Alzheimer-type dementia. *Neurology.* 1984;34:99.

Katz B, Rimmer S, Iragui V, Katzman R. Abnormal pattern ERG in AD: Evidence for retinal ganglion cell degeneration. *Ann Neurol.* 1989;26:221.

Katzman R. Alzheimer disease. *N. Engl J Med.* 1986;314:964.

Kristofikova Z, Klasachka J. In vitro effect of *Ginkgo biloba* extract (EGb 761) on the activity of presynaptic cholinergic nerve terminals in rat hippocampus. *Dement Geriatr Cogn Disord.* 1997;8:43–48.

Larson EB, Kukull WA, Katzman RL. Cognitive impairment: dementia and Alzheimer's disease. *Ann Rev Pub Health.* 1992;13:431–449.

Lewis DA, Campbell MJ, Terry RD, Morrison JH. Laminar and regional distributions of neurofibrillary tangles and neuritic plaques in Alzheimer's disease: A quantitative study of visual and auditory cortices. *J Neurosci.* 1987;7:1799.

Matteson MA, McConnell ES. *Gerontological Nursing: Concepts and Practice.* Philadelphia: Saunders; 1988.

Mayeux M, Sano M. Treatment of Alzheimer's disease. *N Engl J Med.* 1999;341:1670–1679.

McKhann G, Drachman D. Folstein M, et al. Clinical diagnosis of the NINCDS-ADRDA Work Group under the auspices of Department of Health and Human Services Task Force on Alzheimer's Disease. *Neurology.* 1984;34:939.

Mendes MD, Mendez MA, Martin R, et al. Complex visual disturbances in Alzheimer's disease. *Neurology.* 1990;40:439.

Nicoll JAR, Mrak RE, Grahm DI, et al. Association of interleukin-1 gene polymorphisms with Alzheimer's disease. *Ann Neurol.* 2000;47:365.

Pearson RCA, Esiri MM, Hiorn RW, et al. Anatomical correlates of the distribution of the pathological changes in the neocortex in Alzheimer's disease. *Proc Natl Acad Sci USA.* 1985;82:4531.

Rabins P, et al. Practice guideline for the treatment of patients with Alzheimer's disease and other dementias of late life. *Am J Psychiatry.* 1997;5(suppl):1–38.

Sadun AA. The optic neuropathy of Alzheimer's disease. *Metab Pediatr Syst Opthalmol.* 1989;12:64.

Sadun AA, Miao M, Johnson BM. Morphometric analysis of optic nerve axons in patients with Alzheimer's disease. *Invest Opthamol Vis Sci.* 1986;27(suppl):198. Abstract.

Sano, S, Ernesto C, Thomas RG, et al. A controlled trial of selegiline, alpha-tocopherol, or both as treatment for Alzheimer's disease. *N Engl J Med.* 1997;336:1216–1222.

Schenk D, Barbour R, Whitney D, et al. Immunization with amyloid-B attenuates Alzheimer-disease-like pathology in the PDAPP mouse. *Nature.* 1999;400:173.

Spillantini MG. Mutation in the tau gene in familial multiple system taupathy with presenile dementia. *Proc Natl Acad Sci USA.* 1998;95:7737–7741.

Stewart WF, Kawas C, Corrada M, et al. Risk of Alzheimer's disease and duration of NSAID use. *Neurology.* 1997;48: 626–632.

Terry RD, Katzman R. Senile dementia of the Alzheimer type. *Ann Neurol.* 1983;14:497.

Terry RD, Peck A, DeTeresa R, et al. Some morphometric aspects of the brain in senile dementia of Alzheimer type. *Ann Neurol.* 1981;10:184.

Trick GL, Barris ML, Bickler-Bluth M. Abnormal-pattern ERG in patients with senile dementia of ADT. *Ann Neurol.* 1989;26:226.

Wright CE, Drasdo N, Harding GF. Pathology of the optic nerve and visual association areas. Information given by the flash and pattern visual evoked potential and the temporal and spatial contrast sensitivity function. *Brain.* 1987;110:107.

Xia W, Zhang J, Perez R, et al. Interaction between amyloid precursor protein and presenilins in mammalian cells: Implications for the pathogenesis of Alzheimer's disease. *Proc Natl Acad Sci USA.* 1997;94:8208–8213.

Chapter 10

PARKINSON DISEASE

Susan C. Oleszewski

Parkinson disease (PD), also known as parkinsonism or Parkinson syndrome, is a disorder consisting of tremor, rigidity, postural changes, and a decrease in spontaneous movement. This disorder is associated with several pathologic processes that damage the extrapyramidal system. It is considered Parkinson syndrome when etiologic causes such as infection, intoxication, vascular disease, and degenerative disease can be identified. However, this disorder is most commonly the degenerative or idiopathic type, in which case it is called Parkinson disease.

Although visual disturbances are not a major component of PD, a number of ocular motor abnormalities may be present, as well as loss in contrast sensitivity.

EPIDEMIOLOGY

Systemic

The worldwide prevalence of PD is between 90 and 100 per 100,000 population. There are approximately 40,000 new cases in the United States each year. The prevalence is similar in other countries. PD affects all ethnic groups and socioeconomic classes, with no sex predilection. Familial cases of PD are rare. It is estimated that PD makes up 1 to 2% of all neurological disorders.

PD usually begins in persons between 40 and 70 years of age, with the peak age of onset in the sixth decade. In the United States, about 1% of the population over 50 years of age is affected. It is infrequent before 30 years of age.

Ocular

Although ocular and visual disturbances associated with PD are commonly seen, prevalence and incidence data are not available.

PATHOPHYSIOLOGY/DISEASE PROCESS

The most common degenerative condition affecting the extrapyramidal system is idiopathic Parkinson disease (PD or IPD). Most patients with PD have the degenerative or idiopathic type, and no clear cause can be demonstrated through diagnostic testing. However, PD can be secondarily caused by infections (eg, encephalitis), intoxication (eg, carbon monoxide poisoning), vascular or arteriosclerotic disease, and brain tumors.

The two main histopathologic findings in PD are a pattern of depigmentation and cell loss in the substantia nigra and the presence of Lewy bodies. Neurons in the substantia nigra are a specialized population of nerve cells that contain neuromelanin and manufacture the neurotransmitter dopamine. The motor dysfunction of PD patients is linked to the decreased levels of dopamine in the substantia nigra. The clinical signs associated with PD develop when the levels of dopamine are reduced to about 70% of normal. In addition to dopamine, noradrenaline, serotonin, gamma-aminobutyric acid (GABA), and other neuropeptides are also depleted in the substantia nigra.

Lewy bodies represent another defining pathological characteristic of PD. Lewy bodies are spherical inclusions 5 to 25 μm in diameter, seen as a dense eosinophilic core with a pale surrounding halo in the cytoplasm of affected neurons. A-synuclein is a prominent constituent of Lewy bodies in idiopathic PD. A-synuclein is normally a soluble unfolded protein. In PD, this protein is seen to aggregate into insoluble fibrils that help to form Lewy bodies.

Diffuse cortical atrophy may also be found in patients with idiopathic PD. These patients have more cortical degeneration and more dementia than other patients of similar age without PD, suggesting a diffuse degenerative brain disease. When dementia is marked, the changes in the brain outside the substantia nigra are similar to those found in Alzheimer disease, suggesting that some cases of PD may be variants of senile dementia.

The cause of the death of dopaminergic neurons in the substantia nigra is unknown, but both genetic and environmental factors have been postulated. Familial PD is common, representing up to 40% of patients. Furthermore, the risk of idiopathic PD in first-degree relatives is 3.5 times greater than in relatives of control subjects. The discovery of gene linkage in rare families with strong patterns of inheritance of PD-like disease, and the identification of individual genes involved, has provided new insight into the involvement of specific genes and molecules, in particular a-synuclein.

Other factors have been implicated in causing the degeneration of dopaminergic neurons in the substantia nigra of PD patients, including mitochondrial dysfunction, oxidative stress, exogenous toxins, the intracellular accumulation of toxic metabolites, viral infections, excitotoxicity, and immune mechanisms.

Systemic

Parkinson disease is characterized by tremor, rigidity, and dyskinesia or difficulty with voluntary movement (Table 10–1). Any one of these signs may predominate. In the majority of patients, PD develops insidiously and progresses slowly. Initial symptoms may consist of aching pains in the neck, back, or limbs. Such pain may precede the appearance of motility disturbances by months or years. Although absent in about 30% of patients, tremor is usually the first feature that makes the patient aware of the disorder. This begins most commonly in one of the upper extremities. As the disorder progresses, the tremor worsens and spreads to other limbs.

TABLE 10–1. SYSTEMIC MANIFESTATIONS OF PARKINSON DISEASE

- Tremor
- Rigidity
- Bradykinesia
- Gait disturbances
- Postural changes
- Loss of facial expression (mask-like face)
- Infrequent blinking (reptilian stare)
- Micrographia
- Sialorrhea
- Dementia
- Sleep disturbances
- Depression

> Although absent in 30% of PD patients, tremor is usually the first feature that alerts the patient to the disorder. The tremor of PD is often noticeably worse in stressful situations, and may be dampened when the patient is more relaxed.

The tremor of PD is characteristically regular and rhythmic. It is made noticeably worse with attention or in stressful situations. It may become so marked that patients are nearly disabled by it. The tremor is less severe or absent when relaxed. As rigidity increases, it may be dampened or even abolished. "Pill rolling" is a characteristic PD hand tremor that many patients with the disease manifest. In general, tremor is not as disabling as the rigidity and bradykinesia (sluggishness of movement).

When bradykinesia and rigidity are the initial manifestations, patients report difficulty in walking, attempting to stand, getting in and out of bed, and turning in bed. Patients feel as if they are walking or moving against great resistance. As rigidity becomes more prominent, postural changes become apparent. Patients develop a simian-like posture, with slight flexion of all joints, such as ankles, hips, back, and neck.

These patients often feel insecure walking in crowds, because they may lose their balance easily and fall forward. In an effort to restore balance, they may break into a small-stepped run or propulsive gait. Lack of postural reflexes thus leads to frequent falls due to the inability to correct the imbalance by appropriate arm or leg movements. Ambulatory patterns therefore may include difficulty starting to walk (start hesitation), shuffling, or taking many tiny steps and then walking faster and faster (festination). Decreased arm swing excursion typically accompanies the stride.

An early manifestation of hypokinesia is the loss of facial expression, which results in a mask-like face. Infrequent eye blinking also contributes to the staring look of PD (reptilian stare).

> The loss of facial expression (hypokinesia) resulting in a mask-like face, along with infrequent blinking, contributes to the "staring look" (reptilian stare) of the PD patient.

Changes in handwriting may be an early manifestation of PD. Writing is agonizingly slow and the script is often small (micrographia), letters are tightly bunched together, and the ends of lines tend to veer downward or upward.

Sialorrhea, or drooling, may be found in patients with PD. This is a loss of the autonomic process of clearing the throat and swallowing, rather than an excess production of saliva.

The speech patterns of PD patients are distinctive. Their voices lack volume and force. Their speech is monotonous and has a rapid, staccato quality. Enunciation is often impaired.

Dementia has been recognized as part of PD, with a prevalence of about 30 to 50%. The etiology of the dementia has yet to be determined. Sleep disturbances and depression may also be found in PD.

Characteristically, a gradual increase in all of the manifestations of PD occurs. Before L-dopa treatment was available, 25% of patients with symptoms of less than 5 years duration were severely disabled, while 75% of the patients with symptoms of 10 to 15 years duration who survived, were completely disabled. Patients with bradykinesia and rigidity have a poorer prognosis than those with tremor as their main manifestation. PD in itself does not lead to death, but increased mortality occurs because of debility, aspiration pneumonia, urinary tract infections, and decubitus ulcers.

Ocular

Ocular motor and visual abnormalities can occur at any stage of the disease process (Table 10–2). Blepharospasm occurs without apparent cause and it may be the earliest evidence of PD. It may be severe enough to impair vision. Blepharoplegia, real or apparent weakness of eyelid closure, may also be observed, and many patients show infrequency of blinking. Paradoxically, it has been observed that frequent blinking movements occur when quick thrusts are made toward the eyes with a finger. A more useful test is to tap on the glabella. This glabellar tap results in a blink that cannot be suppressed in a PD patient (Myerson sign) as it can in normals.

TABLE 10–2. OCULAR MANIFESTATIONS OF PARKINSON DISEASE

- Blepharospasm
- Blepharoplegia
- Myerson sign
- Wilson sign
- Abnormal saccades and pursuits
- Convergence insufficiency
- Decreased contrast sensitivity
- Abnormal VEPs

VEPs, visually evoked potentials.

Patients with PD may manifest abnormalities in saccadic and pursuit movements. Saccades are characteristically hypometric, particularly in the vertical plane. Some patients cannot move their eyes laterally unless there is a preceding eyelid blink (Wilson sign).

Ocular motor abnormalities result in defective eye–head coordination. Patients may tend to move their head much later than normal individuals, in response to visual targets. Also, full lateral movements of the eyes may be obtained only in association with parallel movement of the head (doll's-head phenomenon).

Convergence insufficiency is another physical finding in PD. Defective convergence or accommodation in PD patients can result in part from medication.

Although motor manifestations are the main PD sequelae, the generalized dopaminergic deficiency is also responsible for visual dysfunction. These include loss of contrast sensitivity and abnormal visually evoked potentials (VEPs). The site of the altered visual function in PD is still unknown.

DIAGNOSIS

Systemic

Diagnosis of PD is generally made on the basis of findings in the physical and neurological examinations, as well as general observation of the patient. The major motor signs such as tremor, rigidity, hypokinesia, bradykinesia, and abnormalities in gait are usually quite evident on neurologic examination, and help distinguish PD from other sources of akinesia (Table 10–3.)

Electroencephalography (EEG), computed tomography (CT), and magnetic resonance imaging (MRI) (Table 10–4) do not provide diagnostic information specific to PD, other than to rule out diseases that

TABLE 10–3. DIFFERENTIAL DIAGNOSIS OF AKINESIA

- Parkinson disease
- Essential tremor
- Arteriosclerotic (or vascular) Parkinson disease
- Drug-induced parkinsonism
- Multiple system atrophy (MSA)
- Progressive supranuclear palsy (PSP)
- Diffuse Lewy body disease (DLB)
- Corticobasal ganglionic degeneration (CBGD)

may mimic it, such as tumors affecting basal ganglia function.

Ocular

There are several ocular motor signs that present in PD. Although these signs are supportive of a diagnosis of PD, they are not generally diagnostic.

TREATMENT AND MANAGEMENT

Systemic

There is no known cure for PD. Most treatments have been directed toward relieving symptoms and signs rather than altering the course of the disease (Table 10–5).

The earliest effective treatment for PD was with belladonna derivatives. These anticholinergic agents appear to relieve tremor and lessen rigidity. They provide only a modest improvement in symptoms, which progress despite medical therapy. The most commonly used anticholinergic drugs are trihexyphenidyl hydrochloride (Artane), procyclidine (Kemadrin), benztropine mesylate (Cogentin), and ethopropazone (Parsidol).

Since the introduction of L-dopa (levo-dopa) treatment, the course of PD has changed dramatically. L-Dopa is clearly the most effective medication available. L-Dopa greatly decreases hypokinesia, bradykinesia, rigidity, and tremor, even though postural instability may persist. In addition, some patients become more alert and have improved mental function. Administration of anticholinergic drugs may provide an additive effect when taken with L-dopa.

TABLE 10–4. DIAGNOSTIC TESTS UTILIZED IN PARKINSON DISEASE

- CSF (usually normal in PD)
- CT (computed tomography)
- MRI (magnetic resonance imaging)
- PET (positron emission tomography)

TABLE 10–5. TREATMENT AND MANAGEMENT OF PARKINSON DISEASE

- L-Dopa in conjunction with dopa-decarboxylase inhibitors (eg, carbidopa)
- Amantidine hydrochloride (eg, Symmetrel)
- Dopamine agonists (eg, ropinirole, pramipexole, cabergoline)
- COMT inhibitors (eg, tolcapone)
- Monoamine oxidase inhibitors (eg, selegiline)
- Neurosurgical therapies (eg, pallidotomy, thalamotomy)
- Deep brain stimulation
- Tissue implantation
- In the future: neurotrophic factors, gene therapy

The side effects of L-dopa are common and may be quite distressing. Nausea is the most common adverse effect encountered soon after initiating L-dopa therapy. Nausea tends to decrease during long-term therapy and is seldom a problem when L-dopa is given in conjunction with a decarboxylase inhibitor. Abnormal involuntary movements (dyskinesia) are the most striking side effect of L-dopa. At least 80% of patients develop these movements at some time during treatment. The dyskinetic movements include lip smacking, tongue movements, grimacing, dystonic twisting of the trunk and the extremities, and motor restlessness. These abnormal movements are dose-related side effects, and can be relieved by reducing the dose; but they may reappear.

The mortality rate has been reduced by half since the introduction of L-dopa. Despite the potential for troublesome adverse effects with chronic L-dopa therapy, many patients continue to have a substantial response to the drug for a decade or more.

The use of dopa-decarboxylase inhibitors (eg, carbidopa) in conjunction with L-dopa has become the preferred therapy for PD patients. This combination (L-dopa/carbidopa) lowers the required total daily dose of L-dopa, which in turn markedly reduces or eliminates its side effects.

The levodopa–carbidopa combination is often effective in relieving the symptoms associated with PD. However, in addition to the side effects associated with levodopa–carbidopa treatment, doses typically need to be increased over time, and the disease manifests an "on-off" syndrome in which the drug simply does not work for unpredictable durations. Fortunately, alternative drug treatments are available.

Amantadine hydrochloride (Symmetrel), an antiviral agent, also relieves symtoms. Amantadine is effective in approximately 60% of patients and partially relieves rigidity, akinesia, and to a lesser extent, tremor.

In patients who are responding to L-dopa, amantadine may potentiate the effect of L-lopa, prolonging the period of therapeutic benefit.

Dopamine agonists are a class of drugs that act directly on postsynaptic dopamine receptors. Pergolide and bromocriptine are two dopamine agonists that are traditionally used as adjunctive therapy with levodopa. Three new dopamine agonists (ropinirole, pramipexole, and cabergoline) are all effective in de novo patients. Use of dopamine agonists results in a lower incidence of motor complications. It remains to be seen whether the long-term use of these drugs results in fewer complications and more effective delay in the need for levodopa therapy than previously available dopamine agonists.

Catechol *O*-methyltransferase (COMT) inhibitors are another important class of drugs with important treatment implications for PD patients. The COMT inhibitors have no clinical effect unless combined with levodopa. Tolcapone, a recently FDA-approved COMT inhibitor, blocks the degradative enzyme catechol *O*-methyltransferase and slows clearance of levodopa from plasma, thereby increasing the fraction of drug crossing the blood–brain barrier for conversion to dopamine.

Selegiline, a selective monoamine oxidase inhibitor, has been shown to delay the need for levodopa in patients with PD. In current clinical practice, selegiline is more commonly used in patients early in the disease and withdrawn later in the disease course when patients are on multiple antiparkinsonian drugs.

Improved understanding of the functional organization of the basal ganglia and thalamus and the pathophysiology of movement disorders has revived neurosurgical procedures for PD patients. Pallidotomy is currently the most widely used surgical procedure for advanced PD. Through the use of a microelectrode probe, a small portion of globus pallidus on one side is destroyed; this is an area believed to be overactive in PD. Severe dyskinesia is the major indication for the procedure.

Thalamotomy, destruction of selected cells in the thalamus, has been successful in alleviating disabling tremor in PD patients. Unilateral thalamotomies alleviate or greatly reduce contralateral tremor, but do not affect the other parkinsonian signs of rigidity and bradykinesia. Bilateral procedures are associated with a high incidence of dysarthria, dysphagia, and disequilibrium, and therefore are reluctantly used in severely affected patients.

Deep brain electrode stimulation of areas of the thalamus offers a safer, reversible alternative to thalamotomy. High-frequency stimulation will inactivate neurons in the vicinity of the electrode tip. Adverse side effects can be minimized by altering the stimulation parameters, and bilateral procedures can be done without the concern of irreversible dysarthria, dysphagia, and disequilibrium.

Clinical trials have shown that mesencephalic dopamine neurons obtained from human embryo cadavers can survive and function when transplanted into the brains of patients with PD. The demonstration that embryonic dopamine neurons can survive and function in the human brain represents a first important step toward a cell replacement therapy in PD. Current research is aimed at improving the survival and growth of transplanted dopamine neurons, and finding alternative sources of cells for grafting.

In addition to the promising results from fetal brain cell transplants for PD, many other promising experimental approaches in the treatment of PD are ongoing. Clinical trials using intraventricular injections of neurotrophic factor have begun. Recombinant glial cell line–derived neurotrophic factor (GDNF) has been shown to promote axon sprouting of dopamine neurons in lesioned animals. GDNF also stimulates dopamine turnover and function in lesioned animals and possibly in intact nigral neurons.

In the future gene transfer in PD could be used in two ways. It could be used to replace dopamine in the affected striatum by introducing the enzymes responsible for L-dopa or dopamine synthesis. Gene transfer might also be used to introduce potential neuroprotective molecules that may either prevent the dopamine neurons from dying or stimulate regeneration and functional recovery in the damaged nigrostriatal system.

Ocular

The eyelid and ocular motility deficits of PD patients are challenging problems that are rarely successfully addressed in isolation. In general, the nonocular problems in PD are considered much more serious, with management directed at alleviating them. Some of the ocular manifestations may be decreased with the use of systemic therapy.

CONCLUSION

The diagnosis of PD is usually based on the cardinal manifestations of bradykinesia, rigidity, tremor, and the characteristic disorder of posture and gait. Ocular motor disturbances are also frequent manifestations that reflect the affected extrapyramidal system in PD.

Recognition of these signs, understanding the course of the disease, and medical co-management challenges the primary eyecare practitioner.

REFERENCES

Adams RD, Victor M. *Principles of Neurology.* 2nd ed. New York: McGraw-Hill; 1981;807–813.

Agid Y, Jovoy-Agid F. Peptides and Parkinson's disease. *Trends Neurol Sci.* 1985;8:30–35.

Bodis-Wollner I, Marx MS, Mitra S, et al. Visual dysfunction in Parkinson's disease. *Brain.* 1987;110:1675–1698.

Bodis-Wollner I, Yahr MD. Measurements of visual evoked potentials in Parkinson's disease. *Brain.* 1978;101:661–671.

Bulens C, Meerwaldt JD, van der Wildt GJ, Keemink CJ. Contrast sensitivity in Parkinson's disease. *Neurology.* 1986;36:1121–1125.

Corin MS, Elizan TS, Bender MB. Oculomotor function in patients with Parkinson's disease. *J Neurol Sci.* 1972;15: 251–265.

Corin MS, Mones RJ, Elizan TS, Bender MB. Paresis of vertical gaze in basal ganglia disease. *Mt Sinai J Med.* 1972;39:330–342.

de Bie RMA, de Haan RJ, Nijssen PCG, et al. Unilateral pallidotomy in Parkinson's disease: A randomized, single blind, multicentre trial. *Lancet.* 1999;354:1665–1669.

Dunnett SB, Bjorklund A. Prospects for new restorative and neuroprotective treatments in Parkinson's disease. *Nature.* 1999;399:32–39.

Fernadez HH, Friedman JH. New anti-parkinsonian drugs. *Med Health RI.* 1998;81:237–238.

Gasser T. A susceptibility locus for Parkinson's disease maps to chromosome 2p13. *Nat Genet.* 1998;18:262–265.

Goedert M, Jakes R, Spillantini M. a-Synuclein and the Lewy body. *Neurosci News.* 1998;1;47–52.

Hirsch EC, Faucheux BA. Iron metabolism and Parkinson's disease. *Mov Disord.* 1998;13(suppl 1):39–45.

Hoehn MM, Yahr MD. Parkinsonism: Onset, progression, and mortality. *Neurology.* 1967;17:427–442.

Itakura T, Nakai E, Naoyuki N, et al. Transplantation of neural tissue into the brain. *Neurol Med Chir (Tokyo).* 1998; 38:756–762.

Jenner P. Oxidative mechanisms in nigral cell death in Parkinson's disease. *Mov Disord.* 1998;13(suppl):24–34.

Kruger R. Ala30Pro mutation in the gene encoding a-synuclein in Parkinson's disease. *Ann Neurol.* 1998;18:106–108.

Kurth MC, Adler CH. COMT inhibition: A new treatment strategy for Parkinson's disease. *Neurology.* 1998;50 (suppl 5):S3–S14.

Langston JW. Aging, neurotoxins, and neurodegenerative disease. In: Terry RD, ed. *Aging and the Brain.* New York: Raven; 1988:149–164.

Lees AJ, Smith E. Cognitive deficits in the early stages of Parkinson's disease. *Brain.* 1983;106:257–270.

Lieberman A, Dziatolowski M, Kupersmith M, et al. Dementia in Parkinson's disease. *Ann Neurol.* 1979;6:355–359.

Lloyd K, Hornykiewicz O. Parkinson's disease: Activity of L-dopa decarboxylase in discrete brain regions. *Science.* 1970;170:1212–1213.

Lozano AM, Lang AE, Hutchinson WD, et al. New development in understanding the etiology of Parkinson's disease and in its treatment. *Curr Opin Neurobiol.* 1998;8: 783–790.

Lukes SA, Aminoff MJ, Crooks L, et al. Nuclear magnetic resonance imaging in movement disorders. *Ann Neurol.* 1983;13:690–691.

Mars H. Modification of levodopa effect by systemic decarboxylase inhibition. *Arch Neurol.* 1973;28:91–95.

Marsden CD, Parkes JD. Success and problems of long-term levodopa therapy in Parkinson's disease. *Lancet.* 1977; 1:345–349.

Martin WR, Beckman JH, Calne DB, et al. Cerebral glucose metabolism in Parkinson's disease. *Can J Neurol Sci.* 1984;11:169–173.

McDowell FH, Cedarbaum JM. The extrapyramidal system and disorders of movement. In: Joynt RJ, ed. *Clinical Neurology.* Philadelphia: Lippincott; 1988;3.

Nutt JG. New pharmacological and surgical therapies for Parkinson's disease. *West J Med.* 1998:168:267–268.

Pleet AB. Newly diagnosed Parkinson's disease: A therapeutic update. *Geriatrics.* 1992;417:24–29.

Quinn N. Progress in functional neurosurgery for Parkinson's disease. *Lancet.* 1999;354:1658–1659.

Rajput AH, Offord KP, Beard CM, Kurl LT. Epidemiology of parkinsonism: Incidence, classification and mortality. *Ann Neurol.* 1984;16:278–282.

Schapira AH. Pathogenesis of Parkinson's disease. *Baillieres Clin Neurol.* 1997;6:15–36.

Slatt B, Loeffler JD, Hoyt WF. Ocular motor disturbances in Parkinson's disease: Electromyographic observation. *Can J Ophthalmol.* 1966;1:267–273.

Villardita C, Smirni P, Zappala G. Visual neglect in Parkinson's disease. *Arch Neurol.* 1983;40:737–739.

White OB, Saint-Cyr JA, Sharpe JA. Ocular motor deficits in Parkinson's disease, 1. The horizontal vertibulo-ocular reflex and its regulation. *Brain.* 1983;106:555–570.

White OB, Saint-Cyr JA, Tomlinson RD, Sharpe JA. Ocular motor deficits in Parkinson's disease, 2. Control of the saccadic and smooth pursuit systems. *Brain.* 1983;106: 571–587.

Chapter 11

GUILLAIN–BARRÉ SYNDROME

John E. Conto, Janice M. McMahon

Guillain–Barré syndrome (GBS) is an acute, relatively symmetrical, and progressive inflammatory neuropathy characterized by the loss of motor function of the limbs and areflexia. It has a transient course with spontaneous recovery in the majority of patients. Although the etiology and pathogenesis of GBS remain in debate, the disease is currently thought to be an autoimmunopathy that initiates a demyelination of the peripheral nerves. Both humoral and cellular mechanisms presumably contribute to the immune response. GBS often follows a preceding event, such as a viral or bacterial infection, a surgical procedure, trauma, or exhaustion. The most common variant, Miller–Fisher syndrome (MFS), presents with acute ophthalmoplegia, ataxia, and areflexia.

The ocular findings in GBS are secondary to cranial nerve dysfunction. Paresis of the oculomotor, trochlear, or abducens nerves causes extraocular motility disturbances. Involvement of the trigeminal and facial nerves can lead to ocular surface abnormalities, such as keratoconjunctivitis sicca or exposure keratopathy.

EPIDEMIOLOGY

Systemic

- Estimated reported incidence 1.7 cases per 100,000.
- Most common cause of acute generalized paralysis.
- Greater incidence in males than females.
- Incidence increases with age.
- Largest predominance in Caucasians.
- Preceded by illness in one half to two thirds of cases, typically viral.
- Miller–Fisher variant comprises 5% of GBS.
- Males affected two times as often as females.
- Mean age of onset is 44 years.
- Children represent 14% of cases.

Ocular

- Involvement of one or both facial nerves in 40% of patients.
- Solitary or combined paresis of third, fourth, and sixth cranial nerves in 10%.
- Papilledema is rare in adults, but occurs in 4 to 6% of children.
- Most common ocular finding in MFS is complete ophthalmoplegia (49%).
- Isolated external ophthalmoplegia in 32% of patients.
- Ptosis, unilateral or bilateral, is present in 47% of cases.

PATHOPHYSIOLOGY/DISEASE PROCESS

Systemic (Table 11–1)

- GBS is characteristically termed an acute inflammatory demyelinating polyneuropathy.
- A viral infection can precipitate an autoimmune response in which lymphocytes attack the myelin sheath of nerves.
- Destruction of the myelin, and progressively, the underlying axon, impedes neural transmission and leads to loss of muscle control.
- GBS may be separated into three phases: progressive, plateau, and recovery.
- The progression from onset of symptoms to stable state is typically 8 to 12 days but may range from 3 days to several weeks.
- The plateau phase occurs when symptoms do not worsen.
- Recovery can span weeks to years, but 80% of patients recover fully within 1 year.
- In 50% of cases, acute onset presents as paresthesias and back or extremity pain.
- Weakness spreads throughout arms and legs, usually symmetrically, and can involve respiratory paralysis as well.
- Deficits include:
  - 60% of patients are unable to independently walk.
  - 15 to 20% require ventilation.
  - 40 to 50% have involvement of the facial nerve.
  - Other affected cranial nerves control tongue (speech), swallowing, and extraocular muscles.
- Residual deficits after recovery are extremely variable:
  - 15% of patients have no lasting effects.
  - 65% have minor disabilities, mainly noted as loss of power, which may impact their psychosocial status more so than any daily activities.
  - 5 to 10% suffer permanent damage such as facial and limb weakness, urinary retention, and impotence.
- Risk factors for poor recovery are: age (over 50 years), long-term assisted ventilation, and a rapid progressive phase.
- Common complications noted during the disease process are pulmonary infection, urinary tract infection, decubitus ulceration, cardiac arrhythmias, postural hypotension, and impaired sweating.
- Mortality rate has dropped from 33 to 5% with advent of modern artificial respiration; death may occur due to pneumonia, respiratory failure, cardiac arrest, or pulmonary emboli.

Ocular (Table 11–2)

- Painless and rapidly progressive ophthalmoplegia is the hallmark sign of GBS, usually appearing after development of peripheral neuropathy; it is typically bilateral.
- Diplopia is also a common presenting complaint.
- Weakness of the orbicularis oculi muscle and levator result in lagophthalmos, ectropion, or ptosis, with subsequent exposure of the globe.
- Paralysis of the seventh nerve can reduce lacrimation.
- Increased risk of keratoconjunctivitis sicca and exposure keratitis with greater risk of subsequent infection.
- Pupils rarely involved, but may show anisocoria or a sluggish response to light and near targets.

TABLE 11–1. SYSTEMIC MANIFESTATIONS OF GUILLAIN–BARRÉ SYNDROME

Symptoms
• Pain and burning of back and extremities
• Loss of touch sensation
• Weakness of limbs
• Difficulty swallowing
• Diplopia
• Difficulty breathing
Signs
• Impaired vital capacity
• Areflexia
• Reduced motor amplitude
• Ataxia (in MFS)
• Mild pleocytosis
• Elevated CSF protein (in MFS)

TABLE 11–2. OCULAR MANIFESTATIONS OF GUILLAIN–BARRÉ SYNDROME

Symptoms
• Diplopia
• Increased tearing
• Irritation and foreign body sensation
• Burning
• Intermittent blurred vision
Signs
• Keratoconjunctivitis sicca
• Exposure keratitis
• Neurotrophic corneal ulceration
• Ectropion
• Ptosis
• Lagophthalmos
• External ophthalmoplegia
• Papilledema

- Elevated protein levels may cause decreased cerebrospinal fluid (CSF) absorption and papilledema; slightly more common in children (4 to 6%) than adults.
- Patients with severe disease may retain residual eyelid weakness or diplopia, but complete recovery from ocular involvement is the typical outcome.

DIAGNOSIS

Systemic (Tables 11–3 and 11–4)

- Clinical definition is progressive motor weakness in more than one limb and areflexia.
- Other supportive diagnostic features are rapid progression to plateau within 4 weeks, relative symmetry, mild sensory signs, involvement of cranial nerves, recovery beginning 2 to 4 weeks after plateau, presence of autonomic disturbances, and absence of fever at onset.
- Examination of CSF shows elevated protein level in 80% of cases; CSF pressure and mononuclear cell count are normal.
- Slowing or blockage of nerve conduction by serial electromyography also seen in 80% of patients; demonstrates that segmental demyelination and axonal degeneration has taken place.
- Serological testing may reveal IgG and IgM antibodies to cytomegalovirus (CMV) or herpes simplex virus (HSV); respiratory syncytial virus (RSV) and *Mycoplasma* can be discovered by complement fixation; and bacterial stool cultures may show strains of *Camphylobacter jejuni/coli.*
- MFS variant requires triad of ophthalmoplegia, areflexia, and ataxia with no other severe neurological signs and elevated CSF protein.
- Radiological testing with computed tomography (CT) or magnetic resonance imaging (MRI) should be performed to rule out intracranial disease.

TABLE 11–3. DIAGNOSTIC TESTS FOR GUILLAIN–BARRÉ SYNDROME

- Total CSF protein (>15–45 mg/dL)
- Serological testing for CMV, HSV, RSV, and *Mycoplasma*
- Urinalysis (e.g., toxicology screen)
- Stool culture (e.g., to rule out poliomyelitis)
- Serial EMG showing slow or blocked nerve conduction
- CT/MRI (to rule out brain infarctions or spinal cord lesions)

TABLE 11–4. DIFFERENTIAL DIAGNOSES FOR GUILLAIN–BARRÉ SYNDROME

- Ischemic brain damage
- Brainstem/spinal cord lesions
- Poliomyelitis
- Myasthenia gravis
- Botulism
- Acute thiamine deficiency
- Acute drugs/substance intoxication including arsenic, lead, and organic phosphates

Ocular

- Many patients are incapacitated by muscular weakness and unable to respond to subjective questioning.
- Objective ocular assessment should include, if possible, visual acuities, external appearance, and anterior and posterior segment evaluation.

TREATMENT AND MANAGEMENT

Systemic (Table 11–5)

- Respiratory failure treated promptly by intratracheal tube or tracheostomy.
- Frequent repositioning to prevent ulceration and careful attention to pressure areas such as eyes, mouth, bowel, and bladder since paralysis may be prolonged.

TABLE 11–5. TREATMENT AND MANAGEMENT OF GUILLAIN–BARRÉ SYNDROME

Systemic
- Assisted ventilation to maintain airway and monitor vital lung capacity
- Increase fluid intake to maintain urinary output
- ECG to monitor for cardiac arrhythmias
- Aggressive treatment of lung or urinary tract infections
- Protection of extremities and pressure points
- IV heparin to prevent deep venous thromboses and pulmonary emboli
- Plasmapheresis
- Immune gammaglobulin (IV 400 mg/kg/day given during first 2 weeks)
- Physical therapy and exercise during entire course of the disease
- Heat therapy for pain relief
- Counseling for depression if indicated

Ocular
- Artificial tear supplements (e.g., 2% methylcellulose q2h to qid)
- Temporary lid patching
- Diplopia occlusion
- Levator resection for residual ptosis
- Muscle surgery for residual deviation

- Increased fluid intake to maintain urinary output.
- Aggressive treatment of lung and urinary tract infections.
- Prophylactic intravenous (IV) heparin to prevent deep venous thromboses and pulmonary emboli.
- Electrocardiogram (ECG) monitoring for potential cardiac arrhythmias.
- Plasmapheresis reduces the severity and shortens the duration of GBS, but is only effective if started no later than 2 weeks after disease onset.
- Current preferred treatment is IV gammaglobulin early in the course of the disease, which has equivalent efficacy to plasmapheresis but easier execution.
- Corticosteroids are no longer considered appropriate treatment.
- Physical and occupational therapy to overcome residual defects.
- Counseling for depression if indicated.

Ocular (Table 11–5)

- Combat exposure through use of lubricants and ointment, as well as temporary patching as needed in severe cases.

> The management of exposure keratitis is the main focus of treatment in the acute phase of GBS, with surgical correction of residual extraocular muscle deficits once stable and irreversible.

- Occlusion may also be utilized to relieve diplopic complaints.
- Muscle surgery not recommended until deviation is stable and irreversible.
- Residual ptosis corrected by levator resection.
- Monitor papilledema, but it should spontaneously resolve.

CONCLUSION

Guillain–Barré syndrome is thought to be an autoimmune disease that is characterized by paralysis of the extremities, impaired respiratory function, and cranial nerve dysfunction. Recovery of function is usually complete, although in severe cases residual deficits may persist. Diplopia and ocular surface drying are the most common ocular complications. The Miller–Fisher syndrome, the most common variant, is typified by ophthalmoplegia and loss of reflexes and muscle coordination.

REFERENCES

Alter M. The epidemiology of Guillain–Barré syndrome. *Ann Neurol.* 1990;27:S7–S12.

Asbury AK, Cornblath DR. Assessment of current diagnostic criteria for Guillain–Barré syndrome. *Ann Neurol.* 1990;27:S21–S24.

Berlit P, Rakicky J. The Miller–Fisher syndrome: A review of the literature. *J Neuroophthalmol.* 1992;12:57–63.

Bernsen RAJAM, de Jager AEJ, et al. Residual physical outcome and daily living 3 to 6 years after Guillain–Barré syndrome. *Neurology.* 1999;53:409–410.

Boucquey D, Sindic CJM, Lamy M, et al. Clinical and serological studies in a series of 45 patients with Guillain–Barré syndrome. *J Neurol Sci.* 1991;104:56–63.

De Jager AEJ, Minderhoud JM. Residual signs in severe Guillain–Barré syndrome: Analysis of 57 patients. *J Neurol Sci.* 1991;104:151–156.

De Jager AEJ, Sluiter HJ. Clinical signs in severe Guillain–Barré syndrome: Analysis of 63 patients. *J Neurol Sci.* 1991;104:143–150.

Farrell K, Hill A, Chuang S. Papilledema in Guillain–Barré syndrome. *Arch Neurol.* 1981;38:55–57.

Giroud M, Mousson C, Chalopin JM, et al. Miller–Fisher syndrome and pontine abnormalities on MRI. *J Neurol.* 1990;237:489–490.

Hadden RD, Hughes RA. Guillain–Barré syndrome: Recent advances. *Hosp Med.* 1998;59:55–60.

Hahn AF. Guillain–Barré syndrome. *Lancet.* 1998:352:635–641.

Haymaker W, Kernohan JW. The Landry-Guillain–Barré syndrome: A clinical pathological report of 50 fatal cases and a review of the literature. *Medicine.* 1949;28:59–141.

Hughes RA, Hadden RD, Gregson NA, Smith KJ. Pathogenesis of Guillain–Barré syndrome. *J Neuroimmunol.* 1999; 100(1–2):74–97.

McFarlin DE. Immunological parameters in Guillain–Barré syndrome. *Ann Neurol.* 1990;27:S25–S29.

McKhann GM, Griffen FW, Cornblath DR, et al. Plasmapheresis and Guillain–Barré syndrome: Analysis of prognostic factors and the effect of plasmapheresis. *Ann Neurol.* 1988;23:347–353.

McLeod JG, Polland JD. Inflammatory neuropathies. In: Swash M, Oxbury J, eds. *Clinical Neurology.* Edinburgh: Churchill Livingstone; 1991:1189–1201.

Ropper AH. The Guillain–Barré syndrome. *N Engl J Med.* 1992;326:1130–1135.

Visser LH, Schmitz PIM, et al. Prognostic factors of Guillain–Barré syndrome after intravenous immunoglobulin or plasma exchange. *Neurology.* 1999;53:598–604.

Willison HJ, O'Hanlon GM. The immunopathogenesis of Miller–Fisher syndrome. *J Neuroimmunol.* 1999;100(1–2): 3–12.

Chapter 12

SPASMUS NUTANS

John E. Conto

Spasmus nutans is an infantile syndrome characterized by the triad of nystagmus, head nodding, and abnormal head position. The etiology remains unknown, but is thought to be due to either an anatomic or developmental lesion of the ocular motor system. It is generally considered to be a benign condition, but can be difficult to distinguish from more serious disorders such as visual pathway gliomas or infantile nystagmus. Spasmus nutans usually presents before the age of 1 year and resolves by the age of 3, but abnormal eye movements may persist beyond age 7.

EPIDEMIOLOGY

Hoyt and Aicardi (1979) reported that spasmus nutans has an incidence of 2 to 3 cases per 1000 infants. It affects males and females equally and does not occur with increased frequency in any racial group. Familial cases are occasionally seen.

PATHOPHYSIOLOGY/DISEASE PROCESS

Spasmus nutans was once thought to be caused by a variety of conditions, including epilepsy, malnutrition, and light deprivation. However, the etiology of spasmus nutans is still unclear. Gresty and associates (1982) suggested that a yoking abnormality of the ocular motor system, caused either by a distinct anatomic lesion of the oculomotor nuclei or a delayed development of the conduction relays to the system, causes pendular nystagmus. Other studies have demonstrated that the nystagmus is not the result of an aberrant vergence or pursuit system (Weissman et al, 1987).

Spasmus nutans usually presents between 4 and 12 months of age. Although the majority of cases arise within the first year of life, onset may occur as late as 3 years of age. Recovery typically occurs over a period of several months to 1 or 2 years. However, subclinical abnormal eye movements, such as nystagmus, may persist beyond the age of 7 (Gottlob et al, 1995).

> The clinical triad of nystagmus, head nodding, and head tilting in an infant is highly suggestive of spasmus nutans.

The classic features of spasmus nutans (Table 12–1) are nystagmus, head nodding, and abnormal head position. When all three signs are present, the diagnosis is straightforward, but it is more difficult if only one or two components exist. Nystagmus appears to be the most frequent finding, and is usually the last to resolve. Head nodding also occurs in most cases,

TABLE 12–1. SYSTEMIC AND OCULAR MANIFESTATIONS OF SPASMUS NUTANS

- Head nodding
- Head turn or tilt
- Pendular nystagmus
- Strabismus
- Amblyopia

whereas abnormal head position, such as head turns and tilts, is the least seen of the three.

Arnoldi and Tychsen (1995) noted that nystagmus is the most common feature of spasmus nutans to prompt examination or referral. Nystagmus is the first to develop and the most consistent feature of the syndrome. The oscillations are pendular and typically horizontal, although a vertical or rotary component may also be present. Horizontal convergence nystagmus has also been reported in association with spasmus nutans (Massry et al, 1996). The nystagmus can be constant or intermittent. It tends to be bilateral, but asymmetric. Gresty and associates (1976) found that the nystagmus had a frequency between 6 and 11 cycles/second, and an amplitude of 2 degrees. Because the amplitude is small and the frequency is high, the eye appears to flutter. Persistent subclinical nystagmus, as measured by electro-oculogram (EOG), has been described as fine, intermittent, asymmetric, horizontal, and/or vertical pendular in character.

Head nodding, like the nystagmus, is variable in appearance and presentation. The direction of the head movement may be horizontal, vertical, or a combination of both. It has a frequency of 2 to 4 cycles/second, and an amplitude of 3 degrees. Head nodding is believed to be a compensatory response to the nystagmus, because the eye movements decrease or disappear when the head motion occurs. Head nodding increases with visually related tasks, and ceases with eyelid closure or sleep.

Abnormal head position, or torticollis, is never seen in isolation with spasmus nutans, and is the most variable of the signs. About 50 to 60% of patients with spasmus nutans have a head tilt or turn. The head position is thought to stimulate the vestibular otoliths in an effort to lessen the nystagmus. The head turn or tilt is absent during periods of sleep.

Strabismus is another frequent finding in spasmus nutans, occurring in 55% of cases. It tends to appear following the onset of the other signs, and often persists beyond recovery. Esotropia is the most common associated deviation. Young and co-workers (1997) noted a higher incidence of strabismus in the eye with the greater amplitude of nystagmus. Amblyopia may develop as a result of strabismus or from manifest latent nystagmus.

DIAGNOSIS

Although the triad of nystagmus, head nodding, and torticollis is distinctive for spasmus nutans, the diagnosis of spasmus nutans only requires that nystagmus and head nodding be present. If other neurological signs are evident—such as lethargy, see-saw nystagmus, headache, or visual field defects—the diagnosis becomes less certain, and other intracranial disorders must be considered, especially gliomas. When the diagnosis of spasmus nutans is suspected, further radiological assessment, with either computed tomography (CT) or magnetic resonance imaging (MRI), is indicated (Table 12–2). Other conditions that have a similar clinical appearance include acquired pendular nystagmus and infantile nystagmus (Table 12–3).

Spasmus nutans may be distinguished from acquired pendular nystagmus by the absence of oscillopsia. Unlike patients with acquired pendular nystagmus, children with spasmus nutans do not appear to suffer from oscillopsia.

Infantile nystagmus can be difficult to differentiate from spasmus nutans, but Gottlob and colleagues (1990) provided diagnostic criteria that assist in discriminating between the two conditions. Infantile nystagmus is present at birth, whereas in spasmus nutans the nystagmus appears later, when the child is at least several months of age. Strabismus is more frequently found in spasmus nutans than infantile nystagmus. In spasmus nutans, the head nodding occurs more commonly, and is larger in amplitude. However, the nystagmus is smaller in amplitude and higher in frequency in spasmus nutans than in infantile nystagmus. The nystagmus can be intermittent in spasmus nutans, but is constant in infantile nystagmus. If bilateral, the nystagmus is asymmetric in spasmus nutans and symmetrical in infantile nystagmus. The nystagmus is characteristically pendular in spasmus nutans, but in infantile nystagmus it is a mixture of jerk and pendular waveforms.

Intracranial gliomas of the optic nerve and chiasm often present with clinical signs similar to those seen with spasmus nutans. Fifty percent of optic nerve and chiasmal gliomas are initially diagnosed as spasmus nutans, causing a mean delay of 15 months in the di-

TABLE 12–2. DIAGNOSTIC TESTS FOR SPASMUS NUTANS

- CT/MRI (to exclude other intracranial etiologies)

TABLE 12–3. DIFFERENTIAL DIAGNOSIS OF SPASMUS NUTANS

- Infantile nystagmus
- Visual pathway gliomas
- Arachnoid cysts
- Empty sella syndrome

agnosis of glioma. Because gliomas are life-threatening, any child presenting with the nystagmus without head nodding must be further evaluated.

The presenting sign of optic nerve and chiasmal gliomas is often pendular nystagmus, which is bilateral in 50% of the cases. Like spasmus nutans, the nystagmus usually develops before 10 months of age. Head nodding and torticollis arise in 60% of patients. Features that are not found in spasmus nutans but are seen in intracranial gliomas include optic atrophy, increased intracranial pressure, and diencephalic syndrome.

Optic atrophy results from the direct compression of the optic nerve and chiasm from the glioma, or from chronic increased intracranial pressure. This may cause decreased visual acuities, afferent pupillary defects, and visual field deficits. Obstruction of the ventricles by the tumor may cause an increase in intracranial pressure, which produces papilledema, headaches, and hydrocephalus. The presence of diencephalic syndrome, failure to thrive, hyperactivity, and hyperhydrosis is highly characteristic of optic nerve and chiasmal gliomas, and occurs in 50% of cases.

TREATMENT AND MANAGEMENT

Spasmus nutans is generally a self-limiting condition; therefore, no current effective medical treatment is suggested. Concurrent strabismus and amblyopia can be managed with visual therapy or surgery when appropriate (Table 12–4).

CONCLUSION

Nystagmus, head nodding, and abnormal head position are the characteristic findings of spasmus nutans. Because it is self-limiting, there is no specific treatment for this condition. Since the presenting signs of optic nerve and chiasmal gliomas are similar to those in spasmus nutans, radiological assessment should be performed if the diagnosis of spasmus nutans is questionable.

TABLE 12–4. TREATMENT AND MANAGEMENT OF SPASMUS NUTANS

- Monitor
- Rule out other etiologies
- Vision therapy and/or strabismus surgery as needed

REFERENCES

Antony JH, Ouvrier RA, Wise G. Spasmus nutans, a mistaken identity. *Arch Neurol.* 1980;37:373–375.

Arnoldi KA, Tychsen L. Prevalence of intracranial lesions in children initially diagnosed with disconjugate nystagmus (spasmus nutans). *J Pediatr Ophthalmol Strabismus.* 1995;32:296–301.

Chrousos GA, Reingold DR, Chu FC, Cogan DG. Habitual head turning in spasmus nutans: An oculographic study. *J Pediatr Ophthalmol Strabismus.* 1985;22:113–116.

Doummar D, Roussat B, Beauvais P, et al. Spasmus nutans: Apropos of 16 cases. *Arch Pediatr.* 1998;5:264–268.

Farmer J, Hoyt CS. Monocular nystagmus in infancy and early childhood. *Am J Ophthalmol.* 1984;98:504–509.

Gottlob I, Wizov SS, Reinecke RD. Spasmus nutans: A long-term follow-up. *Invest Ophthalmol Vis Sci.* 1995;36:2768–2771.

Gottlob I, Zubcov A, Catalano RA, et al. Signs distinguishing spasmus nutans (with and without central nervous system lesions) from infantile nystagmus. *Ophthalmology* 1990;97:1166–1175.

Gresty M, Leech J, Sanders M, Eggars H. A study of head and eye movements in spasmus nutans. *Br J Ophthalmol.* 1976;60:652–654.

Gresty MA, Ell JJ, Findley LJ. Acquired pendular nystagmus: Characteristics, localizing value and pathophysiology. *J Neurol Neurosurg Psychiatry.* 1982;45:431–439.

Hertle RW, Zhu X. Oculographic and clinical characterization of thirty-seven children with anomalous head postures, nystagmus and strabismus: The basis of a clinical algorithm. *J AAPOS.* 2000;4:25–32.

Hoyt CS, Aicardi E. Acquired monocular nystagmus in monozygous twins. *J Pediatr Ophthalmol Strabismus.* 1979; 16:115–118.

King RA, Nelson LB, Wagner RS. Spasmus nutans: A benign clinical entity? *Arch Ophthalmol.* 1986;104:1501–1504.

Lavery MA, O'Niell JF, Chu FC, Martyn LJ. Acquired nystagmus in early childhood. *Ophthalmology.* 1984;91: 425–435.

Massry GG, Bloom JN, Cruz OA. Convergence nystagmus associated with spasmus nutans. *J Neuroophthalmol.* 1996; 16:196–198.

Newman SA. Spasmus nutans—Or is it? *Surv Ophthalmol.* 1990;34:453–456.

Norton EWD, Cogan DG. Spasmus nutans. *Arch Ophthalmol.* 1954;52:442–446.

Weissman BM, Dell'Osso LF, Abel LA, Leight RJ. Spasmus nutans: A qualitative study. *Arch Ophthalmol.* 1987;105: 525–528.

Young TL, Weis JR, Summers CG, Egbert JE. The association of strabismus, amblyopia, and refractive errors in spasmus nutans. *Opthalmology.* 1997;104:112–117.

Chapter 13

MYASTHENIA GRAVIS

Diane T. Adamczyk

Myasthenia gravis (MG) is an immunologic disorder that affects the neuromuscular junction and transmission. Myasthenia (mys, Greek for "muscle," plus "asthenia," Greek for "weakness," and gravis, Latin for "heavy") manifests in the voluntary muscles, with the clinical characteristics of weakness and fatigability brought on by sustained or repeated muscle activity. Ocular involvement may occur in isolation or in association with generalized disease. It frequently occurs at some time during the course of the disease, often as the presenting sign.

Understanding of the pathophysiology of MG has grown over the past few decades. This, along with advances in treatment and management, have greatly improved both prognosis and quality of life.

EPIDEMIOLOGY

Systemic

MG occurs with an incidence between 1 in 20,000 and 1 in 40,000. The actual number of cases may be higher, because many go undiagnosed. These include mild cases, severe cases that result in sudden death, and paradoxical cases.

MG shows no racial preference and may be found at any age and in either sex. However, it occurs more commonly in females between the ages of 20 and 40 years, at a ratio of approximately 2 to 3 females to every male. It occurs equally in both sexes between 40 and 50 years and more commonly in males older than 50 years. The median age of onset is 20 years, with an overall mean age of 33 years. Onset in females is earlier, at the age of 28, versus the male onset of 42 years.

The mortality rate of MG is approximately 1 per million. This increases with age, reaching a peak of 6.4 per million in those between 75 and 84 years (Cohen, 1987). A decrease in the last 20 years in the mortality rate to 5% has occurred (Pourmand, 1997).

Ocular

Ocular involvement occurs at some time during the course of the disease in up to 90% (Osserman, 1967). It is the initial presentation, along with other symptoms, in up to 84%, and is the sole presentation in approximately 50% of cases (Bever et al, 1983). Of those patients presenting with ocular involvement, 86% go on to develop generalized disease (Grob et al, 1987). A later study shows this trend to generalize to be much less, with 31% of ocular MG patients developing generalized disease (Sommer et al, 1997). Ocular MG, affects older males more frequently. The mean age of onset is 38 years.

PATHOPHYSIOLOGY/DISEASE PROCESS

In looking at the natural history of MG, the advancements in diagnosis and treatment must be considered, because both are now integral to the course of the disease. Prior to the use of anticholinesterase drugs for diagnosis, only severe cases of MG, which had a high mortality, were recognized. With the advent of anticholinesterase drugs in 1934, less severe forms have been recognized and subsequently treated, altering the course of the disease.

MG is divided into ocular and generalized disease. It may be further categorized according to sex; age of onset (neonatal, congenital, adolescent, or acquired); or according to the presence or absence of a thymoma (a tumor of the thymus, particularly the thymic epithelial cells). Osserman, in 1967, described a clinical classification of MG. Although this was prior to the increased understanding of the pathophysiology of the disease, it still provides a frequently used delineation of the natural history of the disease (Table 13–1). Compston and associates, in 1980, examined the relationship of various clinical, pathological, and immunologic characteristics found in MG. This subsequently led to a different categorization of patients, along with providing support for a multi-etiologic mechanism in MG (Table 13–2).

Neonatal, congenital, Lambert–Eaton myasthenic syndrome, and drug-induced MG all have a different pathophysiological basis than acquired MG. These will be briefly described, with the remainder of the chapter devoted to the more classic autoimmune-based MG.

Neonatal MG results from a transfer of maternal acetylcholine receptor antibodies through the placenta to the fetus. This occurs in 20% of infants born to MG mothers. Difficulty in sucking, ptosis, and extraocular muscle (EOM) involvement may occur. These transient symptoms, lasting 1 to 6 weeks, appear to coincide with decreasing antibody titers.

Congenital MG may be a genetically transmitted disease, characterized by weakness and abnormal fatigability. These rare congenital myasthenic syndromes may be the result of a defect in neuromuscular transmission, which differs from that found in acquired MG (Engel, 1984).

Lambert–Eaton myasthenic syndrome is characterized by weakness and fatigability of the proximal limb muscles, particularly the lower limbs, usually without ocular involvement. It affects males more frequently, and is often associated with carcinomas, particularly oat cell carcinoma of the lung. Other clinical features include a brief initial increase in strength after voluntary muscle contraction, followed by fatiguing, hyporeflexia, dry mouth, and impotence. Lambert–Eaton syndrome is believed to result from a defect in neuromuscular transmission, probably secondary to decreased acetylcholine release, at the presynaptic terminal (as opposed to true MG, in which the defect is postsynaptic). The pre- and postsynaptic mechanism appears to be normal. As compared to those with adult MG, these patients respond poorly to Tensilon testing. Lambert–Eaton syndrome is suggestive of an autoimmune disorder. Therapies include tu-

TABLE 13–1. CLINICAL CLASSIFICATION OF MYASTHENIA GRAVIS (MG)

I. Pediatric Group
A. Neonatal: infants of mothers with MG
  Self-limited, lasting no more than 6 weeks
B. Juvenile: develops birth to puberty
  Siblings, close relatives (not mother) may have MG

II. Adult Group
Group I: Ocular myasthenia
  Excellent prognosis
Group IIA: Mild generalized MG
  Ocular involvement gradually generalizes
  Good prognosis
Group IIB: Moderate generalized MG
  Ocular involvement progresses to more severe generalized involvement, with dysarthria, dysphagia
Group III: Acute fulminating MG
  Rapid onset with severe ocular and skeletal weakness
  Progression of disease is complete within 6 months
  Involvement of respiratory muscles, thymomas
Group IV: Late severe MG
  Severe, with progression gradual or sudden
  Thymomas
  Poor prognosis

Adapted from Osserman KE. Ocular myasthenia gravis. Invest Ophthalmol. *1967;6:277–287.*

TABLE 13–2. CATEGORIZATION OF MYASTHENIA GRAVIS BASED ON ASSOCIATED FINDINGS

Group 1
No HLA antigen association
High antibody titers
Thymoma
Males = females

Group 2
HLA association (A1, B8, and/or DRw3)
Intermediate antibody titers
No thymoma
Female patients younger than 40

Group 3
HLA association (A3, B7, and/or DRw2)
Low levels of antibodies
No thymoma
Males older than 40

Adapted from Compston DAS, et al. Clinical, pathological, HLA antigen and immunological evidence for disease heterogeneity in myasthenia gravis. Brain. *1980;103:579–601.*

mor removal if present, steroids, other immunosuppressants, and plasmapheresis.

Drug-induced MG can result from a wide variety of medications. Some examples include D-penicillamine, β-blockers, antibiotics, lithium, steroids, and a few isolated cases of ophthalmic medications (eg, timolol, tropicamide, proparacaine) (Coppeto, 1984; Meyer et al, 1992). D-Penicillamine, used to treat rheumatoid arthritis and Wilson disease, may produce a presentation similar to acquired MG. This includes comparable antibody titers, electromyography results, and symptoms of muscle fatigue, which are usually mild and localized to the ocular muscles. These present after months of D-penicillamine treatment. Remission usually occurs within 1 year of discontinuing the drug. However, there are some cases that will continue on with the clinical presentation of acquired MG.

Systemic

MG is an autoimmune disease that affects the postsynaptic neuromuscular junction. Specifically, there is an autoimmune attack against the receptors at the postsynaptic neuromuscular junction, resulting in a decrease in acetylcholine receptors that subsequently alters neuromuscular transmission. Normally, acetylcholine is released from the presynaptic nerve terminal. It binds to the acetylcholine receptor (AChR) at the postsynaptic muscle fiber. This initiates a series of events that result in an action potential, with subsequent muscle fiber contraction. The acetylcholine then dissociates from the receptor and is degraded by acetylcholine esterase. The receptors degrade and rebuild in a normal cycle of 7 days.

In up to 90% of MG patients, antibodies to AChR, mostly IgG, are present. These appear to cause a decrease in the number of AChR. This decrease may result from decreased receptor cycle time, AChR being blocked from acetylcholine, and/or a damaged postsynaptic membrane. A defect in neuromuscular transmission then results.

Although the AChR antibody level does not always coincide with clinical severity or improvement, it may be higher in generalized MG and patients with thymomas, while being lower in ocular MG or in cases showing remission. In addition, 10 to 15% of MG patients are antibody negative. This inconsistency in antibody level may result from limitations in testing, such as the inability to test for bound antibodies or the presence of antibody variation.

Continued research will provide an even better understanding of the pathophysiology of myasthenia gravis. For example, in both ocular and general myasthenia gravis patients who test negative for acetylcholine receptor antibody, an immune reaction against skeletal muscle proteins other than acetylcholine receptors is speculated to play a role in muscle weakness (Gunji et al, 1998).

A genetic predisposition for MG has been suggested, although it has not been substantiated. Support for a genetic factor includes the rare familial instances of MG, occasional EMG, and AChR antibody results suggestive of MG in asymptomatic relatives, and a possible HLA association.

The exact role of the thymus (an organ actively involved in immunologic functions, particularly in producing T cells) in MG has not been established, but its influence cannot be denied. This is substantiated by the clinical improvement and remission found after its removal. Thymic abnormalities may be present clinically in 70% of MG patients, and possibly all patients subclinically. Thymic changes include hyperplasia and thymoma. Thymomas may occur in 10 to 15% of patients with MG and one third of the patients with a thymoma have MG. Thymomas are present more commonly in 40- to 60-year-olds, and are associated with a more severe clinical presentation and higher mortality rate.

In addition to thymomas, MG may be associated with other autoimmune diseases. These most commonly include Graves disease, hyperthyroidism, rheumatoid arthritis, systemic lupus erythematosus, and sarcoidosis. Based on a number of associated findings, including the absence or presence of HLA, MG may be categorized into three groups (see Table 13–2).

> Myasthenia gravis is often associated with thymomas and other autoimmune diseases, such as Graves disease.

A variety of triggering factors may precede the initial onset of MG. These may include childbirth, use of certain muscle relaxants with general anesthesia, or an infection that results in respiratory failure.

The clinical presentation of MG (Table 13–3) includes muscle fatigue after repeated use of the muscle, with improvement seen after a period of rest. Signs and symptoms include muscle weakness (particularly limb, facial, and neck regions), slurred or nasal speech, and pharyngeal weakness. The severity usually peaks between 1 and 3 years after the onset of symptoms. This may be followed by a chronic form of the disease that has episodes of milder exacerbations and remissions. Usually clinical improvement occurs with spontaneous remission taking place in approximately 10%. Spontaneous remission is more likely to occur in patients with mild or localized muscle weakness. In one

TABLE 13–3. SYSTEMIC MANIFESTATIONS OF MYASTHENIA GRAVIS

- Difficulty swallowing or chewing
- Weakness of limb, neck, or facial muscles (myasthenic facies or "snarl")
- General fatigue
- Dysphagia
- Tingling and numbness (paresthesias)
- Slurred or nasal speech (dysarthria)
- Weight loss
- Pharyngeal weakness
- Nasal regurgitation
- Respiratory distress or failure
- Myasthenic tongue (longitudinal furrowing)
- Muscle atrophy
- Myasthenic crisis (loss of strength; difficulty talking, breathing, swallowing)

TABLE 13–4. OCULAR MANIFESTATIONS OF MYASTHENIA GRAVIS (MG)

- Ptosis
- Ophthalmoplegia
- Diplopia
- Blurred vision
- Lid twitch
- Orbicularis weakness
- Incomplete lid closure
- Nystagmus
- Pseudo-internuclear ophthalmoplegia (internuclear-ophthalmoplegia-like ocular motility disturbances secondary to MG)
- Convergence difficulties
- Saccadic quiver
- Anisocoria; sluggish and fatigable pupillary responses
- Decreased corneal sensitivity
- Decreased accommodation

study of patients who began with ocular MG that generalized, 46% went into remission (Sommer et al, 1997). Clinical manifestations of MG may be exacerbated with pregnancy, infection, emotional problems, menses, excessive heat, sun exposure, and medications (Pourmand, 1997).

Patients older than 50 years, with generalized MG, and with a greater risk for respiratory failure, have a poorer prognosis. Respiratory failure may develop after surgery, an upper respiratory tract infection, emotional stress, pregnancy, or certain drug use. The myasthenic crisis may occur, and is characterized by loss of strength and difficulty talking, breathing, and swallowing that may be severe. Myasthenic crisis and respiratory failure have a good prognosis if appropriate medical intervention is available.

Prior to the advancements in diagnosis and treatment, mortality was as high as 70%, with death resulting from respiratory failure or dysphagia. Medical therapy and intervention has decreased mortality for generalized disease to 7% (Grob et al, 1987) and a 5% mortality rate for myasthenic crisis (Pourmand, 1997). Today, morbidity and mortality usually result from an infection, a complicating illness, or therapy.

Ocular

Ocular involvement in MG (Table 13–4) may present as a clinically distinct entity, associated with generalized disease, or as a precursor to generalized disease.

Generalization of ocular myasthenia is less likely to develop as time continues on. Those that will develop generalized myasthenia will usually do so within 2 to 3 years of the initial onset of ocular symptoms. Earlier studies show that within the first year of ocular myasthenia, 87% will develop generalized disease, and by the third year 94% will progress to general disease (Grob et al, 1987). More recent studies show that 31% of patients with ocular myasthenia develop generalized disease, usually within an average of 24.5 months after the first ocular symptoms. The overall positive outcome in patients with ocular myasthenia may reflect current treatment modalities used in autoimmune disease (Sommer et al, 1997).

Although it may be questioned whether ocular MG has a distinct pathophysiology from general MG, clearly some clinical findings are similar. Additionally, electromyography and drug testing may show the same changes seen in generalized disease in patients with only clinical ocular involvement.

The levator palpebrae is the most commonly involved ocular structure, with either a monocular or asymmetric bilateral ptosis. It characteristically worsens with fatigue, sustained action, or in bright lights.

> Myasthenia gravis often presents initially with ocular manifestations, with ptosis the most common presentation, followed by diplopia (EOM involvement).

Extraocular muscle involvement is also common, with a variety of presentations. Diplopia follows ptosis as a common presentation. Diplopia, sometimes described as blurred vision, results from ophthalmoplegia secondary to MG. Often more than one muscle is involved. However, if only one muscle is involved, it is most commonly the medial rectus. Convergence difficulties resulting from EOM involvement have also been noted. Additionally, a quiver movement of the eye may occur during a rapid saccade of small excursion. The orbicularis oculi may also show signs of fatiguing, with a resultant incomplete lid closure. The EOMs may be more commonly affected in MG than other muscles because of fewer AChRs and lower acetylcholine concentrations, as well as a higher operating frequency of the motor unit (Kaminski et al, 1990).

Pupillary involvement in MG has not been firmly established. It is probably rare, but may include anisocoria, along with sluggish and fatigable pupil responses. It has been speculated that pupillary involvement in MG is related to cholinergic innervation. Other clinical findings that may relate to cholinergic innervation include an increased corneal sensitivity threshold and accommodative dysfunction. Accommodative fatigue may be an early sign of MG in prepresbyopic patients (Cooper et al, 2000).

Ocular MG generally has a good prognosis. Although severity of the disease may vary, peak severity is reached between 1 to 3 years (Grob et al, 1987). Most patients with ocular MG remain ocular (69%). Of those with ocular disease, 54% go into remission, 33% improve, and 13% remain unchanged. Prognosis varies based on severity of symptoms, and electrophysiologic and serum acetylcholine receptor antibody findings. The patients that do not progress to general disease have mild versus severe symptoms; more typically have normal electrophysiology testing, and have a negative serum AchR antibody test (Sommer et al, 1997).

DIAGNOSIS

Systemic

The diagnosis of MG may be made based on its clinical presentation, specific test results, and differentiation from Lambert–Eaton syndrome, chronic progressive external ophthalmoplegia, and other neurologic disorders (Table 13–5). A pattern suggestive of MG can be established through the history. This includes muscle weakness that varies with physical activity, rest, or time of day, and precipitating factors such as emotional stress, medications, or infection. A cranial nerve workup should be done to differentiate MG from other neurologic diseases. Specific testing includes the Tensilon test, determining the presence and level of acetylcholine receptor antibody, and electromyography (Table 13–6). Other testing procedures previously utilized include curare and quinine. Both of these drugs increased myasthenic manifestations and the potential for respiratory or myasthenic crisis. Although quinine is no longer used in testing, precautions must be given to patients who drink tonic water, which contains quinine, or who use quinine to treat leg cramps.

The Tensilon (edrophonium) test is often the first diagnostic test used in MG. Tensilon acts by inhibiting acetylcholine esterase. This results in an increase of acetylcholine available to stimulate the receptors at the neuromuscular junction. The patient is observed in a quantitative and qualitative way before and after intravenous injection of Tensilon. Improvement in ptosis, diplopia, or ease of arm use is noted following injection of 2 mg of Tensilon. If there is no effect after 45 seconds, an additional 8 mg is injected. When a positive response occurs, it usually lasts a few minutes, but may last as long as 30 minutes. Adverse reactions to

TABLE 13–5. DIFFERENTIAL DIAGNOSIS OF MYASTHENIA GRAVIS: GENERAL AND OCULAR[a]

Chronic progressive external ophthalmoplegia
Cavernous sinus lesions
Amyotrophic lateral sclerosis
Multiple sclerosis
Myotonic dystrophy
Guillain–Barré syndrome
Polymyositis
Lambert—Eaton myasthenic syndrome
Intracranial mass/lesion
Drug-induced myasthenia
Graves disease, thyroid disease

[a]In addition to the above, consider conditions associated with ptosis and diplopia, internuclear ophthalmoplegia, horizontal or vertical gaze palsy, and third, fourth, and sixth cranial nerve palsies.

TABLE 13–6. DIAGNOSTIC TESTING (GENERAL AND OCULAR MYASTHENIA GRAVIS)

Overview
Anticholinesterase test: edrophonium (Tensilon)
Electrophysiologic/myographic studies
  Repetitive nerve stimulation
  Single-fiber electromyography
Acetylcholine receptor antibody titers
Muscle biopsy

Specific for Ocular
Sustained upgaze
Lid twitch
Ice pack
Peak sign
Sleep test

Other Testing
MRI or CT of mediastinum
Chest radiography
ANA, RF, antithyroid antibodies
Thyroid function test
Pulmonary function test

Tensilon include a cholinergic crisis, consisting of bradycardia, tearing, salivation, flushing, sweating, abdominal cramps, nausea, hypotension, and cardiopulmonary arrest. Atropine sulfate (5 mg or more) should be available for intravenous injection, to counteract an adverse reaction. The test should be performed in a clinical setting in which appropriate emergency care can be provided.

The Tensilon test has a sensitivity and specificity of 95% for generalized MG (Phillips & Melnick, 1990). False-positive results are possible. Although false-negatives do occur, which on retesting may be positive, a negative result usually strongly indicates another diagnosis.

Various immunologic tests are used in the diagnosis of MG. These include AChR antibody titers, serum IgG concentrations, ELISA for AChR antibody detection, and measurement of the degradation rate of acetylcholine receptors. The most widely used test, AChR antibody testing, has a sensitivity of 89% and a specificity of 99% in generalized MG (Phillips & Melnick, 1990).

Electromyography (EMG) is used in questionable cases of MG. EMG measures the action potential generated by a muscle. In MG, the amplitude of the response declines over time. The sensitivity of the test is 76%, with a specificity of 90% (Phillips & Melnick, 1990). Single-fiber EMG is slightly more sensitive than regular EMG testing; however, it is more time consuming and often reserved for specific study purposes.

Ocular

When a patient presents with ocular signs and symptoms of MG, the eyecare practitioner can perform a number of in-office tests to assist in the diagnosis. These include the lid twitch sign, the sustained upgaze test, repeated lid opening and closure, the ice pack test, the peek sign, and the sleep test. A cranial nerve workup to assist in ruling out other etiologies should be performed.

The lid twitch sign, sustained upgaze test, and repeated lid opening and closure specifically evaluate the function of the levator palpebrae muscle. It is the most commonly affected muscle, and these tests will show the characteristic sequelae of fatigue.

The lid twitch sign or irritable lid phenomenon was first described by Cogan in 1965. It may be observed in the ptotic lid when the patient is instructed to look from the down position to primary gaze, or to blink. The lid shows an overshoot or upward twitch movement. This results as the levator, relaxing or recovering in the down position (or with the blink), elevates to the primary position, and then rapidly fatigues or falls, giving a flutter or twitch-like appearance.

In the sustained upgaze test, the lid position in primary gaze is observed before and after the test. The patient is instructed to look up, without blinking (which simulates a rest period), for approximately 1 minute, or until a normal fatigue onset is expected, and then back to primary gaze. If the lid position is lower than initially observed, a positive test is present. When the patient is instructed to repeatedly open and close their eyes, a fatiguing of the levator occurs. A positive result shows increased ptosis.

Other EOMs, like the levator, may show signs of fatigue. EOM fatigue may be seen when the position of the globe is observed as the patient looks in a sustained extreme lateral gaze. As the medial rectus fatigues, the eye slowly drifts toward primary position (Osher & Glaser, 1980).

In addition to the levator and EOMs, the orbicularis oculi may also be affected in MG. The resulting "peek" sign occurs when the patient's eyes are gently closed. Initially there will be no visible sclera because the lids are in apposition. However, after a couple of seconds, the orbicularis begins to weaken, with a separation of the lids, allowing the white sclera to "peek" through (Osher & Griggs, 1979).

Muscle function in MG can be improved by both rest and cold. Two tests that utilize rest and cold respectively are the sleep test and the ice pack test. The sleep test (Figure 13–1) may be used in cases of ptosis or ophthalmoplegia. The patient's palpebral apertures and EOMs are initially evaluated. The patient is then instructed to close the eyes in a dark, quiet room for 30 minutes and rest with an attempt to sleep. The palpebral apertures and EOMs are again evaluated for improvement. Improvement usually lasts for 2 to 5 minutes. The results of the sleep test are comparable to the Tensilon test in both time and magnitude. It therefore provides a safe, noninvasive alternative to the Tensilon test (Odel et al, 1991).

The ice pack test uses the improvement MG patients experience after muscle cooling. The initial lid position is evaluated. An ice pack, wrapped in either a towel or a surgical glove, is applied to the lightly closed, more ptotic lid for a period of 2 minutes, with the other eye serving as a control. The patient is then reevaluated for any improvement in lid position. Improvement in ptosis is usually greater with the cooling from ice than rest alone. The ice pack test is a good indicator of MG, with a positive response the result of decreased acetylcholinesterase activity and increased transmitter release (Sethi et al, 1987).

In addition to the tests an eyecare practitioner can perform in the office, confirmation of ocular MG can be made utilizing the same tests used for generalized disease. These include the Tensilon test, antibody titer

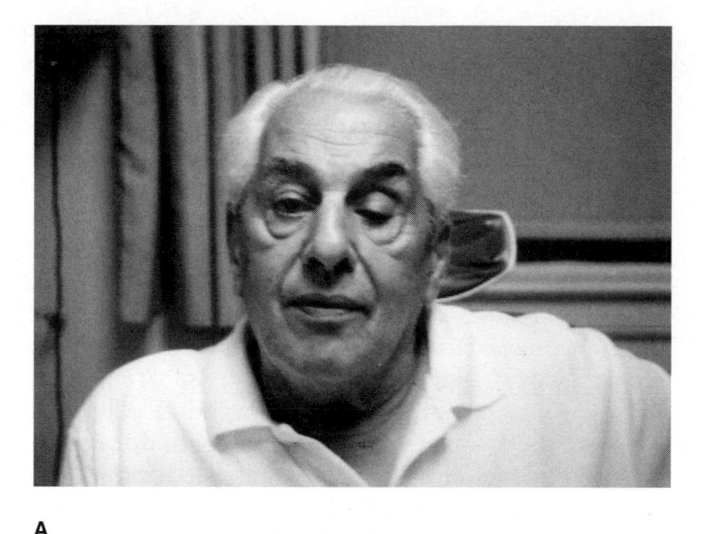

A

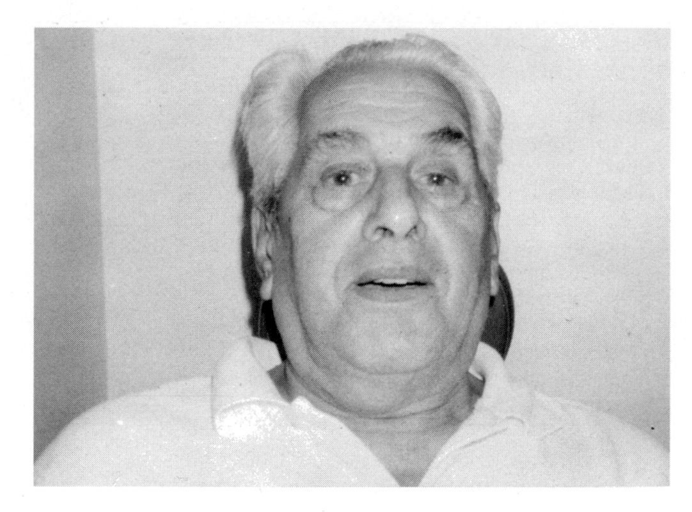

B

Figure 13–1. A. 70-year-old patient with ocular MG. **B.** The sleep test shows improvement in left ptosis following 30 minutes of sleep. *(Courtesy of Optometry Service, FDR VA Hospital, Montrose, NY.)*

determination, and EMG. However, in ocular MG, the sensitivity and specificity of these tests are often less than that found in generalized disease.

When using the Tensilon test to determine improvement of EOM function and diplopia, it is important to evaluate both subjective responses and objective findings (eg, use of prisms or Hess Lancaster screen). A patient may still report diplopia after the test, even if the EOMs show a measured improvement. The sensitivity of the Tensilon test in ocular MG is 86% and the specificity is 80% (Phillips & Melnick, 1990). The Tensilon test was found to be positive in 97% of those with ocular MG (Sommer et al, 1997). A negative Tensilon test in ocular MG usually indicates another etiology, with further testing only indicated if there is a high suspicion of MG.

Many patients with ocular MG have a lower level or lack of AChR antibodies as compared to generalized MG. This may be the result of different antibodies present in ocular MG compared to generalized MG, which may not be detectable by present testing methods. AChR antibody testing has been found to have a sensitivity of 64%, but a specificity of 99% (Phillips & Melnick, 1990). Because antibody testing has a relatively low cost and a high specificity, it is a good choice of testing methods.

TREATMENT AND MANAGEMENT

With the advancements in treatment and management, the morbidity and mortality rates of patients with MG have tremendously improved, particularly in the last 30 years (Table 13–7). Neurological consultation and co-management with the eyecare practitioner will provide optimal care. The goal of treatment in MG is to improve neuromuscular transmission and/or control the autoimmune involvement in MG with minimal side effects. Presently, however, the treatments are nonspecific and have side effects. Treatment may result in improvement in over 95% of patients (Drachman et al, 1988).

Systemic

Once the diagnosis of MG is made, management should include chest x-rays or computed tomography (CT) scan to rule out a thymoma, respiratory function tests, and appropriate testing to rule out associated diseases such as thyroid and collagen vascular disease (e.g., rheumatoid arthritis and systemic lupus erythematosa).

Treatment in MG does not follow a specific protocol. In generalized disease it may include use of cholinesterase drugs, immunosuppressive drugs, thymectomy, and plasmapheresis.

Cholinesterase inhibitor (CHEI) improves transmission at the neuromuscular junction by increasing acetylcholine. Dosage must be controlled because once patients reach a peak improvement, increased dosage may lead to muscle weakness and cholinergic crisis. Cholinergic crisis is similar to the manifestations of myasthenic crisis, and may include diarrhea, nausea, salivation, and lacrimation. Oral neostigmine and pyrodostigmine (Mestinon) are the CHEI drugs of choice, with pyrodostigmine preferred. Tensilon is used diagnostically, but is not used in treatment because of its

TABLE 13–7. TREATMENT AND MANAGEMENT OF MYASTHENIA GRAVIS

Systemic
- Co-management with neurologist
- Chest x-ray or CT scan (rule out thymoma)
- Respiratory function tests (lung volume and capacity)
- Testing to rule out associated diseases (eg, thyroid, collagen vascular—rheumatoid arthritis, systemic lupus)
- Cholinesterase Inhibitors:
  - Neostigmine 15 mg q4h, increased to 30 mg q3h if needed
  - Pyridostigmine 60 mg q6h, increased to 120 mg q4h if needed
- Immunosuppressive Drugs:
  - Steroid: prednisone 60–80 mg initial, 30–40 mg daily (taper, may have to continue on alternate-day schedule for several years)
  - Azathioprine: 2–3.5 mg/kg per day (slow taper, continue 1–2 years)
  - Cyclosporin: 3–6 mg/kg per day (12-hour divided dose)
  - Cyclophosphamide: 3–5 mg/kg
- Thymectomy
- Plasmapheresis (4–8 exchanges, over 1–2 weeks)
- Intravenous immune globulin

Ocular
- Cholinesterase inhibitors
- Steroids
- Azathioprine
- Thymectomy
- Ptosis tape/crutch
- Dark tinted glasses
- Fresnel prism
- Patching
- Monitor decreased corneal sensitivity
- Lubricants for exposure keratitis
- Vision training for convergence problems

potency and short half-life. CHEIs were formerly a major treatment modality for generalized disease. They have been used less because they provide only symptomatic relief, usually in mild cases, with some residual disability remaining.

Immunosuppressant therapy includes steroids, azathioprine, plasmapheresis, and cyclosporin. Immunosuppressant therapy is nonspecific, consequently it can affect the entire immune system.

Steroids may be used alone or in conjunction with other therapies for MG. The action of steroids is to lower acetylcholine receptor antibodies. Steroids are often the first choice of therapy, causing a rapid improvement. However, side effects may occur in up to 67% of treated patients (Johns, 1987). These may include, but are not limited to, weight gain, cataracts, diabetes mellitus, gastric ulcer, and hypertension. Steroid therapy may be administered by oral or intravenous routes. Treatment schedules may vary, utilizing incremental dosage or alternate day administration. When improvement is noted, the dosage is slowly decreased; however, the patient may need to be on a maintenance dose. Once the patient begins treatment, it should continue for a minimum of 2 years. Improvement or remission may be seen in up to 80% of treated patients (Johns, 1987). It usually occurs within a few weeks to 6 months.

Azathioprine, another immunosuppressant drug, may be used alone or with other treatment modalities. Azathioprine is best used in difficult to treat, severe, late-onset MG patients, who have high AChR antibody titers. It is usually not the first drug of choice. Although the exact mechanism is not known, azathioprine decreases the level of acetylcholine receptor antibodies. Improvement or remission often occurs between 3 and 12 months. Treatment should be continued for 1 to 2 years and slowly reduced.

Side effects of azathioprine may be seen in up to 33% of the patients (Genkins et al, 1987), thus precluding its use as a drug of first choice. These include but are not limited to bone marrow dysfunction, hepatic dysfunction, and gastrointestinal disturbances. The patient must be followed with complete blood counts and liver function/enzyme tests.

Thymectomy may be done alone or in conjunction with other treatment modalities. Thymectomy is used to remove a thymoma, or with the intent to provide remission or improvement to the condition (Drachman, 1994). Removal of the thymus is most often recommended to patients with generalized disease who have moderate to severe symptomatology or have a thymoma. It is not the preferred treatment in the older or younger population.

Clinical improvement may be found up to 96% of those treated by thymectomy (Younger et al, 1987). Extended thymectomy shows good results in patients with MG, especially in those with no thymoma, younger than 34 years, and having a shorter disease duration. Remission in nonthymomatous patients at 1 year is 22.4% (versus 27.5% in thymoma patients), at 5 years is 45.8% (versus 23%), and at 10 years is 67.2% (versus 30%) (Masaoka et al, 1996).

Although the reason for improvement is not completely understood, removal of the thymus may result in the elimination of the source of antibodies and antigens. The removal of the thymus may also decrease the occurrence of or improve the course of any associated autoimmune diseases. Evidence of improvement may not be seen for months or possibly years after treatment, but when it does occur, it may last for years. It is difficult to determine if the improvement is a result of the thymectomy or the normal course of the disease.

Plasmapheresis or plasma exchange may be used in severe cases of MG, along with other treatment modalities. Plasmapheresis removes toxins, metabolic substances, and plasma constituents (antibodies) from the blood. The blood is removed, with plasma separated from the formed elements. The formed elements and replaced plasma are then reinfused. It is not used as an initial treatment in MG because it is a complicated procedure with risks and high costs. Its mode of action in MG is thought to be related to the removal of acetylcholine receptor antibodies (Consensus Conference, 1986).

Improvement from plasmapheresis is usually rapid, transient, reaching a temporary peak, and then declining. It may occur after one exchange, but usually requires a few exchanges. Improvement may be seen in approximately 75% of treated patients, lasting days to months. Complications may include hypotension, hypocalcemia, sepsis, embolism, chest pain, and death (Seybold, 1987). An alternative to plasma exchange is intravenous immune globulin (Pourmand, 1997).

Ocular

Treatment and management of ocular MG may take a variety of forms. Dependent on the severity of the ocular disease, systemic treatment may be warranted, along with specific ocular management. Management may also include observation alone.

Treatment of ocular myasthenia may include those mentioned for systemic disease; however, the responses may differ greatly from those found in generalized disease.

In ocular MG, pyridostigmine may be tried, and then followed by steroids or used in conjunction with steroids. Azathioprine may be used for long-term treatment, in cases that are not adequately controlled by steroids or cases that show no remission. In ocular disease, thymectomy, once thought to not to have a role in ocular MG, may be another treatment option (Sommer et al, 1997) in ocular MG (Masaoka et al, 1996).

Patients who suffer from ptosis may benefit from lid supports such as lid tape and ptosis crutches, along with darkly tinted glasses. Ptosis surgery should be considered only after a stable lid position is present for 3 to 4 years.

In cases of diplopia, occlusion of one eye (e.g., via a patch or opaque lenses) or Fresnel prisms may used. Since the symptoms of diplopia may fluctuate, ground in prism should not be used. Vision therapy has been found to improve convergence dysfunction (Vogel & Soden, 1981).

Other considerations in ocular MG include decreased corneal sensitivity and exposure keratitis. If corneal sensitivity is affected, special attention should be given to those wearing contact lenses or those at risk for injury or infection. If exposure keratitis results from fatigue of the orbicularis oculi and incomplete lid closure, appropriate treatment with lubricating ointment and/or taping the lids should be considered.

CONCLUSION

Myasthenia gravis is an autoimmune disease that affects the neuromuscular junction, resulting in weakness and fatigue of voluntary muscles. A better understanding of the pathophysiology of MG has resulted in improved management. Ocular manifestations commonly occur during the course of the disease, often as the presenting sign, underscoring the importance of the eyecare practitioner's role in the diagnosis and subsequent management of this disorder.

REFERENCES

Berrih-Aknin S, Morel E, Raimond F, et al. The role of the thymus in myasthenia gravis: Immunohistological and immunological studies in 115 cases. *Ann NY Acad Sci.* 1987;505:50–70.

Bever CT, Aquino AV, Penn S, et al. Prognosis of ocular myasthenia. *Ann Neurol.* 1983;14:516–519.

Bryant RC. Asymmetrical pupillary slowing and degree of severity in myasthenia gravis. *Ann Neurol.* 1980;7:288–289.

Castronuovo S, Krohel GB, Kristan RW. Blepharoptosis in myasthenia gravis. *Ann Ophthalmol.* 1983;15:751–754.

Cogan DG. Myasthenia gravis. *Arch Ophthalmol.* 1965;74:217–221.

Cogan DG, Yee RD, Gittinger J. Rapid eye movements in myasthenia gravis, 1. Clinical observations. *Arch Ophthalmol.* 1976;94:1083–1085.

Cohen MS. Epidemiology of myasthenia gravis. *Monogr Allergy.* 1987;21:246–251.

Compston DAS, Newsom-Davis VJ, Batchelor JR. Clinical, pathological, HLA antigen and immunological evidence for disease heterogeneity in myasthenia gravis. *Brain.* 1980;103:579–601.

Consensus Conference. The utility of therapeutic plasmapheresis in neurologic disorders. *JAMA.* 1986;256:1333–1337.

Cooper J, Pollak GJ, Ciuffreda KJ, et al. Accommodative and vergence findings in ocular myasthenia: A case analysis. *J Neuro-ophthalmol.* 2000;20:5–11.

Coppeto JR. Timolol-associated myasthenia gravis. *Am J Ophthalmol.* 1984;98:244–245. Letter.

Cornelio F, Peluchetti D, Mantegazza R, et al. The course of myasthenia gravis in patients treated with corticosteroids, azathioprine, and plasmapheresis. *Ann NY Acad Sci.* 1987;505:517–525.

Daroff R. The office Tensilon test for ocular myasthenia gravis. *Arch Neurol.* 1986;43:843–844.

Drachman DB. Myasthenia gravis. *N Eng J Med.* 1994:330: 1797–1810.

Drachman DB, De Silva S, Ramsay D, Pestronk A. Humoral pathogenesis of myasthenia gravis. *Ann NY Acad Sci.* 1987;505:90–105.

Drachman DB, McIntosh KR, De Silva S, et al. Strategies for the treatment of myasthenia gravis. *Ann NY Acad Sci.* 1988;540:176–186.

Ellenhorn N, Lucchese N, Greenwald M. Juvenile myasthenia gravis and amblyopia. *Am J Ophthalmol.* 1986;101: 214–217.

Engel AG. Myasthenia gravis and myasthenic syndromes. *Ann Neurol.* 1984;16:519–534.

Genkins G, Kornfeld P, Papatestas AE, et al. Clinical experience in more than 2000 patients with myasthenia gravis. *Ann NY Acad Sci.* 1987;505:500–513.

Giese AC. *Cell Physiology.* Philadelphia: Saunders; 1979: Chapter 21.

Gorelick PB. Office Tensilon test. *Arch Neurol.* 1987; 44: 689–690.

Grob D, Arsura EL, Brunner NG, Namba T. The course of myasthenia gravis and therapies affecting outcome. *Ann NY Acad Sci.* 1987;505:472–499.

Gunji K, Skolnick C, Bednarczuk T, et al. Eye muscle antibodies in patients with ocular myasthenia gravis: Possible mechanism for eye muscle inflammation in acetylcholine-receptor antibody-negative patients. *Clin Immunol Immunopathal.* 1998;87:276–281.

Havard CWH, Fonseca V. New treatment approaches to myasthenia gravis. *Drugs.* 1990;39:66–73.

Herishanu Y, Lavy S. Internal "ophthalmoplegia" in myasthenia gravis. *Ophthalmologica.* 1971;163:302–305.

Honeybourne D, Dyer PA, Mohr PD, et al. Familial myasthenia gravis. *J Neurol Neurosurg Psychiatr.* 1982;45: 854–856.

Howard FM, Lennon VA, Finley J, et al. Clinical correlations of antibodies that bind, block or modulate human acetylcholine receptors in myasthenia gravis. *Ann NY Acad Sci.* 1987;505:526–537.

Jay WM, Nazarian SM, Underwood DW. Pseudo-internuclear ophthalmoplegia with downshoot in myasthenia gravis. *J Clin Neuro-ophthalmol.* 1987;7:74–76.

Johns TR. Long-term corticosteroid treatment of myasthenia gravis. *Ann NY Acad Sci.* 1987;505:568–583.

Kaminski HJ, Maas E, Spiegel P, Ruff L. Why are the eye muscles frequently involved in myasthenia gravis? *Neurology.* 1990;40:1663–1669.

Lanska DJ. Indications for thymectomy in myasthenia gravis. *Neurology.* 1990;40:1828–1829.

Lepore FE, Sanborn GE, Slevin JT. Pupillary dysfunction in myasthenia gravis. *Ann Neurol.* 1979;6:29–33.

Linton DM, Philcox D. Myasthenia gravis. *Disease-a-Month.* November 1990;595–637.

Masaoka A, Yamakawa Y, Niwa H, et al. Extended thymectomy for myasthenia gravis patients: A 20 year review. *Ann Thorac Surg.* 1996;62:853–859.

Matell G. Immunosuppressive drugs: Azathioprine in the treatment of myasthenia gravis. *Ann NY Acad Sci.* 1987; 505:589–594.

Meyer D, Hamilton RC, Gimbel HV. Myasthenia gravis-like syndrome induced by topical ophthalmic preparations. *J Clin Neuro-ophthalmol.* 1992;12:210–212.

Miller NR, Morris JE, Maquire M. Combined use of neostigmine and ocular motility measurements in the diagnosis of myasthenia gravis. *Arch Ophthalmol.* 1982;100:761–763.

Monden Y, Fujii Y, Masaoka A. Clinical characteristics of myasthenia gravis with other autoimmune diseases. *Ann NY Acad Sci.* 1987;505:876–878.

Morel E, Eymard B. Immunological and clinical aspects of neonatal myasthenia gravis. *Ann NY Acad Sci.* 1987; 505:879–880.

Nazarian J, O'Leary DJ. Corneal sensitivity in myasthenia gravis. *Br J Ophthalmol.* 1985;69:519–521.

Oda K. Ocular myasthenia gravis: Antibodies to endplates of human extraocular muscle. *Ann NY Acad Sci.* 1987; 505:861–863.

Odel JG, Winterkorn JMS, Behrens MM. The sleep test for myasthenia gravis. A safe alternative to Tensilon. *J Clin Neuro-ophthalmol.* 1991;11:288–292.

Olanow CW, Wechsler AS, Sirotkin-Roses M, et al. Thymectomy as primary therapy in myasthenia gravis. *Ann NY Acad Sci.* 1985;505:595–606.

Osher RH, Glaser JS. Myasthenic sustained gaze fatigue. *Am J Ophthalmol.* 1980;89:443–445.

Osher RH, Griggs RC. Orbicularis fatigue. The "peek" sign of myasthenia gravis. *Arch Ophthalmol.* 1979;97:677–679.

Osher RH, Smith JL. Ocular myasthenia gravis and Hashimoto's thyroiditis. *Am J Ophthalmol.* 1975;79: 1038–1043.

Osserman KE. Ocular myasthenia gravis. *Invest Ophthalmol.* 1967;6:277–287.

Osterman PO. Current treatment of myasthenia gravis. *Prog Brain Res.* 1990;84:151–161.

Pascuzzi RM, Phillips LH, Johns TR, Lennon VA. The prevalence of eletrophysiological and immunological abnormalities in asymptomatic relatives of patients with myasthenia gravis. *Ann NY Acad Sci.* 1987;505:407–415.

Perlo VP, Poskanzer DC, Schwab RS, et al. Myasthenia gravis: Evaluation of treatment in 1355 patients. *Neurology.* 1966;16:431–439.

Phillips LH, Melnick PA. Diagnosis of myasthenia gravis in the 1990s. *Sem Neurol.* 1990;10:62–69.

Pourmand R. Myasthenia gravis. *Disease-a-Month.* February 1997:67–109.

Rodgin SG. Ocular and systemic myasthenia gravis. *Am Optom Assoc.* 1990;61:384–389.

Rodriguez M, Gomez MR, Howard FM, Taylor WF. Myasthenia gravis in children: Long-term follow-up. *Ann Neurol.* 1983;13:504–510.

Romano PE, Stark WJ. Pseudomyopia as a presenting sign in ocular myasthenia gravis. *Am J Ophthalmol.* 1973;75: 872–875.

Rowland LP. General discussion on therapy in myasthenia gravis. *Ann NY Acad Sci.* 1987;505:607–609.

Rowland LP. Therapy in myasthenia gravis: Introduction. *Ann NY Acad Sci.* 1987;505:566–567.

Sanders DB. The electrodiagnosis of myasthenia gravis. *Ann NY Acad Sci.* 1987;505:539–556.

Sethi KD, Rivner MH, Swift TR. Ice pack test for myasthenia gravis. *Neurology.* 1987;37:1383–1385.

Seybold ME. Plasmapheresis in myasthenia gravis. *Ann NY Acad Sci.* 1987;505:584–587.

Seybold ME. The office Tensilon test for ocular myasthenia gravis. *Arch Neurol.* 1986;43:842–844.

Sobocinsky-Olsson B, Sandström I, Pirskanen R, Matell G. Evaluation of press-on prisms for diplopia correction in myasthenia gravis. *Ann NY Acad Sci.* 1987;505:836–837.

Sommer N, Sigg B, Melms A, et al. Ocular myasthenia gravis: Response to long-term immunosuppressive treatment. *J Neurol Neurosurg Psychiatry.* 1997;62:156–162.

Vogel MS, Soden R. The functional management of ocular myasthenia gravis. *J Am Optom Assoc.* 1981;52:829–831.

Walsh FB, Hoyt WF. *Clinical Neuro-ophthalmology.* Baltimore: Williams & Wilkins; 1969:1277–1297.

Walsh TJ. *Neuro-ophthalmology: Clinical Signs and Symptoms.* Philadelphia: Lea & Febiger; 1985:77–88, 110–126.

Yamazaki A, Ishikawa S. Abnormal pupillary responses in myasthenia gravis, a pupillographic study. *Br J Ophthalmol.* 1976;60:575–580.

Yee RD, Cogan DG, Zee DS, et al. Rapid eye movements in myasthenia gravis, 2. Electro-oculographic analysis. *Arch Ophthalmol.* 1976;94:1465–1472.

Younger DS, Jaretzki A, Penn AS, et al. Maximum thymectomy for myasthenia gravis. *Ann NY Acad Sci.* 1987;505:832–835.

Zweiman B, Arnason BGW. Immunologic aspects of neurological and neuromuscular diseases. *JAMA.* 1987;258:2970–2973.

Chapter 14

MYOTONIC DYSTROPHY

Diane T. Adamczyk

Myotonic dystrophy (MD) is a disease that is characterized by myotonia (increased muscle contraction and slow relaxation), muscle weakness, and atrophy. It affects many systems, including the cardiac, endocrine, and respiratory. Ocular manifestations are numerous, including cataracts, hypotony, and retinal pigmentary changes.

EPIDEMIOLOGY

Systemic

- Myotonic dystrophy is a familial disease, inherited in an autosomal dominant fashion, with variable penetrance.
- It affects all races and sexes equally.
- Incidence is approximately 1 in 5000 to 8000.
- MD may affect infants and children, but it occurs more commonly in those in their 20s to 30s.

Ocular

- Cataracts or lenticular changes probably affect all MD patients, with one third showing clinically significant changes.
- Almost half the patients have pigmentary changes in the peripheral retina and 20% have macular changes.
- Fifty to 84% have ptosis.

(Burian & Burns, 1966)

> Lens changes are typical of MD patients, including polychromatic cataracts.

PATHOPHYSIOLOGY/DISEASE PROCESS

Systemic

- A genetic defect affects chromosome 19 (19q13.3), involving an expanded trinucleotide (CTG) repeat in the myotonic protein kinase gene. A greater number of repeats results in the patient being more severely affected.
  - The disease is more severe with each generation affected (anticipation).
  - The genetic defect may not be the sole cause for the multisystem, clinical presentation of MD (Winchester et al, 1999).
- Multiple systems are affected in MD that include the endocrine, respiratory, and cardiovascular systems (Table 14–1).
- Myotonic dystrophy often presents insidiously, at any age.
  - Infants with myotonic dystrophy may show signs of difficulty sucking.
  - More commonly patients in their 20s and 30s are affected.

TABLE 14–1. SYSTEMIC MANIFESTATIONS OF MYOTONIC DYSTROPHY

Muscular Manifestations
- Myotonia
- Myopathic facies
- Affected muscles
  - Muscles of facial expression
  - Small muscles of the hand
  - Muscles of mastication (difficulty chewing)
  - Sternocleidomastoid (difficulty raising head)
  - Muscles of arms
  - Muscles of feet (affected gait)
  - Quadriceps
  - Deep muscles of the neck
  - Palatal muscle (nasal voice)
  - Tongue
  - Deep tendon reflex (may be weak or absent)

Systemic Manifestations
- **Endocrine**
  Pituitary, adrenal, thyroid involvement; insulin changes (high fasting serum insulin levels, hypersecretion of insulin), irregular menses, abnormal carbohydrate metabolism
- **Cardiovascular**
  Conduction involvement, left and right ventricular blocks, premature beats, atrial fibrillation, prolapsed mitral valve, heart enlargement, hypotension, systolic murmurs, electrocardiographic abnormalities
- **Respiratory**
  Weakness of respiratory muscles (chest and diaphragm), weak pharyngeal and laryngeal muscles, hypoventilation syndrome, pulmonary infection
- **Gastrointestinal**
  Pharyngeal and esophageal abnormalities (contraction/paresis), dysphagia, constipation
- **Genitourinary**
  Gonadal atrophy (sterility), incontinence, urinary retention
- **Skeletal**
  High palate, cleft palate, scoliosis

Other Manifestations
- Scanty body hair (with frontal baldness)
- Psychological disturbances (e.g., depression)
- Skin dryness
- Loss of high-tone hearing
- Weight loss
- Mental retardation
- Deficient immunoglobulin IgG
- Increased creatine in plasma concentration and urinary excretion

- First generations may have only subtle signs present, with subsequent generations expressing more severe disease.
  - Decreasing intelligence or mental retardation may manifest after three or four generations.
- Myotonic dystrophy is classically characterized with myotonia.
  - Myotonia may occur with use of a muscle, or with mechanical or electrical stimulation.
  - Myotonia is often exacerbated by emotional excitement, cold, and menstruation.
  - Myotonia is relieved with increased or repetitive use of the muscle.
- Other muscle manifestations include weakness and atrophy.
  - This generally affects the distal muscles of the limbs, face, and neck.
  - Muscle atrophy may follow a slowly progressive course over years, or may take a rapidly declining course within a year, possibly resulting in paralysis.
    - When the facial muscles atrophy, a characteristic myopathic facies is seen (Figure 14–1).

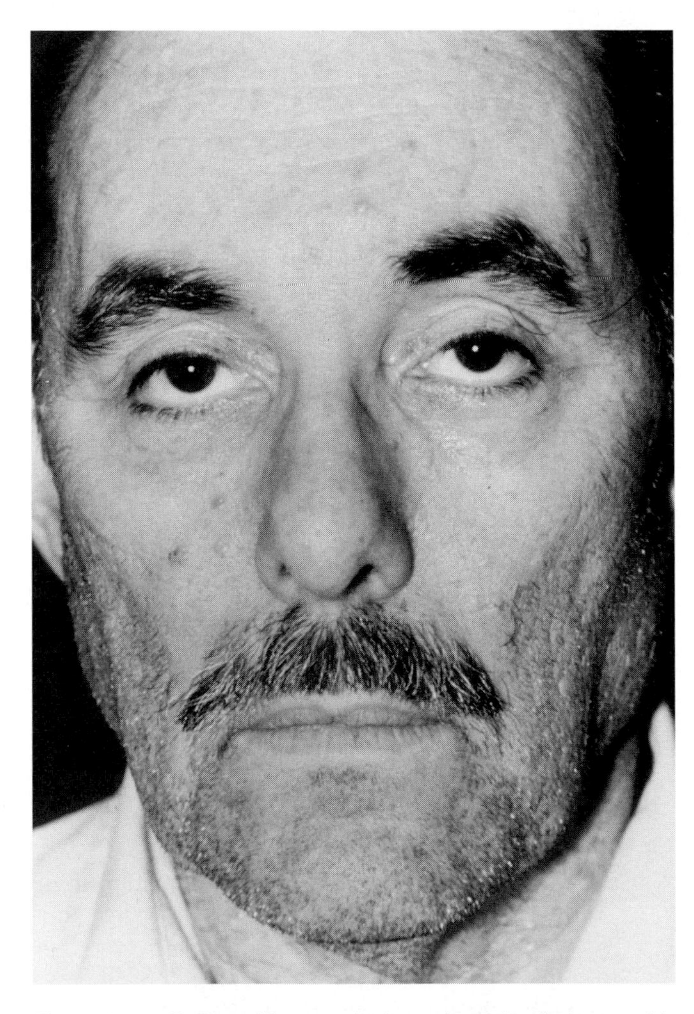

Figure 14–1. Patient with myotonic dystrophy and typical myopathic facies. Note the lean, narrowed, lengthened, expressionless face and ptosis. (*Reproduced with permission from Adamczyk DT.* J Am Optom Assoc. 1987;58:408–412.)

- Later involvement of MD includes the larynx, vocal cords, and pharynx, with resultant nasal voice and difficulty swallowing.
- MD patients may have a shorter life expectancy, with death resulting from pulmonary or cardiac complications (Longstaff et al, 1991).

Ocular

- A second gene, overlapping the gene described above, may be involved in the ocular manifestations of MD (Winchester et al, 1999).
- Manifestations include cataracts; external ocular muscle involvement, particularly the orbicularis oculi and levator (ptosis); hypotony; and retinal changes (Table 14–2).
- Cataracts occur in almost all patients with MD.
  - Cataracts may occur before overt disease.
  - Later MD generations develop lens changes at a younger age.
  - Lens changes may affect the cortex, suture lines, or subcapsular area or form a star at the lens poles (Figure 14–2).

TABLE 14–2. OCULAR MANIFESTATIONS OF MYOTONIC DYSTROPHY

More Common
• Lens opacity
• Hypotony
• Extraocular muscle involvement
Ptosis
Orbicularis oculi: weakness (lagophthalmus, infrequent blink) and myotonia
Motility disturbances
Exotropia, exophoria, convergence insufficiency
Poor Bell phenomenon
• Retinal changes: macular pigmentary changes, peripheral pigment changes, epiretinal membranes
Less Common
• Enophthalmus
• Microphthalmos
• Low-amplitude ERG (abnormal)
• Abnormal dark adaptation curves
• Choroidal coloboma
• Cornea: exposure keratitis, keratopathy, decreased corneal sensation, vascularization, keratitis sicca/dry eye, filamentary keratitis
• Anterior segment: loss of iris pigment, pigment deposited on lens, angle, corneal endothelium
• Blepharoconjunctivitis/blepharitis
• Pupil dysfunction: miosis/weak pupil reflex (react sluggishly to light and near; with pupillograph)
• Optic atrophy
• Ectropion
• Loss of orbital fat

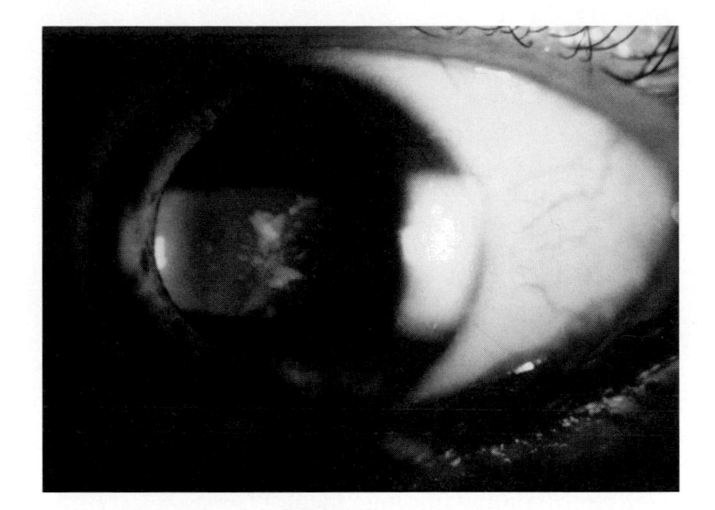

Figure 14–2. Myotonic cataract; note the classic star formation. (*Courtesy Optometry Service*, FDR VA Hospital, Montrose, NY.)

  - Lens changes may be punctate, dust-like, globular, iridescent, white, red, green, or blue. The polychromatic lens changes are pathognomonic of MD.
  - The cataracts may remain stable or progress.
- External ophthalmoplegia includes:
  - Levator weakness/ptosis (common)
  - Orbicularis oculi weakness
  - Ocular motility disturbances (uncommon)—decreased saccadic velocity, gaze restrictions.
    - Rarely: diplopia.
  - A myotonic response may be found with Bell phenomenon.
- Hypotony:
  - May result from degenerative or atrophic changes in the ciliary processes and/or increased outflow facility.
  - Intraocular pressure may range from 4 to 17 mm Hg (average of 10 mmHg).
  - The average pressure decreases with age, with 8.5 mmHg in patients 50 to 57 years old.
- Retinal involvement:
  - Clusters of pigment in the peripheral retina may occur, along with yellow flecks.
  - Macular changes include:
    - Granular pigmentary changes that follow a streak or stellate pattern, with occasional gray-white or yellow spots. This may resemble macular degeneration.
    - A variant of retinal pigment epithelial patterned dystrophy may occur in MD as butterfly or reticular lesions (Hayasaka et al, 1984).

DIAGNOSIS

Table 14–3 lists the various diagnostic tests used in MD, and Table 14–4 provides the differential diagnosis.

Systemic

- Diagnosis of MD is typically based on family history, clinical presentation, and electromyographic (EMG) findings.
  - Additionally, a DNA probe (p5B1.4) can detect the genetic mutation (Shelbourne et al, 1993).
  - DNA analysis may also include southern blot and polymerase chain reaction.
  - Myotonic findings include:
    - Percussion myotonia where a prolonged contraction results from a blow, for example, to the thenar muscle of the thumb.
    - Poor release of hand grasp, e.g., after shaking hands. The warm-up phenomenon decreases the myotonia by repeated opening and closing of the hand, making the release of the hand grasp easier.

  (Kuhn & Fiehn, 1981)

Ocular

- Ocular manifestations of MD are diagnosed through routine eye evaluation, including anterior and posterior segment examination.
- Extraocular muscle involvement is determined through pursuits, observation of lid position for ptosis, and a myotonic response of the orbicularis oculi on forced lid closure.
- In addition, myotonia can be elicited from a flash of bright light, which produces prolonged lid closure (Walsh & Hoyt, 1969).
- Electrodiagnostic testing shows an abnormal electroretinogram (ERG) and decreased dark adaptation findings. ERG findings are affected, in almost all patients, even in the absence of ophthalmoscopic findings.

TABLE 14–3. DIAGNOSTIC TESTING FOR MYOTONIC DYSTROPHY

Electromyographic testing
DNA related:
DNA probe
Polymerase chain reaction
Southern blot analysis
Electrodiagnostic testing (if retinal changes warrant)

TABLE 14–4. DIFFERENTIAL DIAGNOSIS OF MYOTONIC DYSTROPHY (SYSTEMIC/OCULAR)

Overview:
Oculopharyngeal muscular dystrophy
Myasthenia gravis
Other types of myotonia:
Hyperkalemic periodic paralysis
Paramyotonia congenital
Myotonia fluctuans
Thomsen myotonia congenita
Becker myotonia congenita
Ocular differential includes various causes related to:
Early-onset cataracts
Ptosis
Retinal pigment changes, e.g., retinitis pigmentosa
Macular degeneration, Stargardt disease

TREATMENT AND MANAGEMENT

Systemic

- Treatment (Table 14–5):
  - Palliative (eg, heat, cold avoidance, or quinine).
  - Antimyotonic drugs, if needed, such as procainamide and diphenlyhydantoin.
- Comanagement with:
  - Neurologist.
  - Appropriate specialist dependent on the systemic manifestations.
- Pharyngeal and esophageal testing if there is difficulty in swallowing.
- Any surgical procedure done with general anesthesia requires caution and testing for respiratory function because of the potential for respiratory depression and exacerbation of myotonia.

TABLE 14–5. TREATMENT AND MANAGEMENT OF MYOTONIC DYSTROPHY

Systemic
- Palliative
- Heat
- Cold avoidance
- Quinine
- Antimyotonic drugs (e.g., procainamide, diphenylhydantoin)
- Comanagement with neurologist, and specialist per systemic involvement
- Pharyngeal and esophageal testing if difficulty swallowing
- Caution with general anesthesia
- Genetic counseling

Ocular
- Lubricants
- Surgery as needed: cataract, removal, tarsorrhaphy (exposure keratitis), ptosis

- Education and counseling include genetic counseling.

Ocular

- Routine ocular care is necessary in the management of MD patients.
- Cataract extraction as needed.
- Surgical treatment as needed for exposure keratitis (tarsorrhaphy) and ptosis.

CONCLUSION

Myotonic dystrophy is a multisystemic disease, classically characterized by myotonia, ptosis, and facial weakness. Ocular manifestations are common, and may be a presenting sign in asymptomatic patients. Although the genetic findings associated with MD are important to understanding the disease, much still needs to be learned.

REFERENCES

Allen JH, Barer CG. Cataract of dystrophia myotonica. *Arch Ophthalmol.* 1940;24:867–884.

Babel J. Ophthalmological aspects of myotonic dystrophy. In: Huber A, Klein D, eds. *Neurogenetics and Neuro-ophthalmology.* New York: North-Holland Biomedical; 1981: 19–30.

Betten MG, Bilchik RC, Smith ME. Pigmentary retinopathy of myotonic dystrophy. *Am J Ophthalmol.* 1971;72:720–723.

Blanksma LJ, Kooijman AC, Sier Tsema JV, Roze JH. Fluorophotometry in myotonic dystrophy. *Documenta Ophthalmologica.* 1983;56:111–114.

Bollen E, Den Heyer JC, Tolsma MHJ, et al. Eye movements in myotonic dystrophy. *Brain.* 1992;115:445–450.

Bruggen JP Ter, Bastiaensen LAK, Tyssen CC, Gielen G. Disorders of eye movement in myotonic dystrophy. *Brain.* 1990;113:463–473.

Burian HM, Burns CA. Ocular changes in myotonic dystrophy. *Am J Ophthalmol.* 1967;63:22–34.

Burian HM, Burns CA. Ocular changes in myotonic dystrophy. *Trans Am Ophthalmol Soc.* 1966;69:250–273.

Eustace P. Corneal lesions in myotonic dystrophy. *Br J Ophthalmol.* 969;53:633–637.

Garla PE. Cataracts in myotonic dystrophy. *J Am Optom Assoc.* 1983;54:1067–1068.

Hayasaka S, Kiyosawa M, Kastumata S, et al. Ciliary and retinal changes in myotonic dystrophy. *Arch Ophthalmol.* 1984;102:88–93.

Huff TA, Horton ES, Lebovitz HE. Abnormal insulin secretion in myotonic dystrophy. *N Engl J Med.* 1967;277: 837–841.

Kuhn E, Fiehn W. Adult form of myotonic dystrophy. In: Huber A, Klein D, eds. *Neurogenetics and Neuro-ophthalmology.* New York: North-Holland Biomedical; 1981:31–43.

Longstaff S, Curtis D, Quick J, Talbot J. Genetic counselling for myotonic dystrophy: A comparison of lens examination and DNA linkage studies. *Eye.* 1991;5:93–98.

Mausolf FA, Burns CA, Burian HM. Morphologic and functional retinal changes in myotonic dystrophy unrelated to quinine therapy. *Am J Ophthalmol.* 1972;74:1141–1143.

Meyer E, Navon D, Auslender L, Zoni SS. Myotonic dystrophy: Pathological study of the eyes. *Ophthalmologica.* 1980;181:215–220.

Pizzuti A, Friedman DL, Caskey T. The myotonic dystrophy gene. *Arch Neurol.* 1993;50:1173–1179.

Ptacek LJ, Johnson KJ, Griggs RC. Genetics and physiology of the myotonic muscle disorders. *N Eng J Med.* 1993; 328:482–489.

Raitta C, Karli P. Ocular findings in myotonic dystrophy. *Ann Ophthalmol.* 1982;14:647–650.

Shelbourne P, Davies J, Buxton J, et al. Direct diagnosis of myotonic dystrophy with a disease-specific DNA marker. *N Engl J Med* 1993;328:471–475.

Thompson HS, Van Allen MW, von Noorden GK. The pupil in myotonic dystrophy. *Invest Ophthalmol.* 1964;3:325–338.

Walker SD, Brubaker RF, Nagataki S. Hypotony and aqueous humor dynamics in myotonic dystrophy. *Invest Ophthalmol Vis Sci.* 1982;22:744–751.

Walsh FB, Hoyt WF. *Clinical Neuro-ophthalmology.* Baltimore: Williams & Wilkins; 1969:1266–1277.

Winchester CL, Ferrier RK, Sermoni A, et al. Characterization of the expression of DMPK and SIX5 in the human eye and implications for pathogenesis in myotonic dystrophy. *Hum Mol Genet.* 1999;8:481–492.

Chapter 15

SELECTED MUSCLE DISORDERS

Diane T. Adamczyk

There are a number of rare muscle disorders involving the extraocular muscles that fall under the all-encompassing term "chronic progressive external ophthalmoplegia (CPEO)." These diseases have the underlying feature of external ophthalmoplegia, without intrinsic muscle or pupillary involvement. Other characteristic features may include weakness of the skeletal muscles, pigmentary retinopathy, or cardiac abnormalities. Myopathic or neurogenic etiologies have been considered, with mitochondrial DNA changes more recently shown to play a major role in many of these disorders.

The following disorders will be discussed: CPEO and the specific entities of oculopharyngeal muscular dystrophy (ptosis and dysphagia) and Kearns–Sayre syndrome (progressive external ophthalmoplegia, retinal pigmentary changes, and heart abnormalities).

CHRONIC PROGRESSIVE EXTERNAL OPHTHALMOPLEGIA

CPEO is a disorder of slowly progressive external ophthalmoplegia that may occur alone or often associated with other clinical manifestations that are specific to a particular disorder.

Epidemiology

Systemic

- CPEO may have a family tendency, inherited in an autosomal dominant fashion, although recessive and sporadic cases also occur.
- Males and females are affected equally.
- The exact incidence is not known.
- The age of onset is usually in the second decade; however, any age may be affected.
- Initial symptoms in mitochondrial myopathies include (Petty et al, 1986):
  - Fatigue (42.4%)
  - Limb weakness (27.3%)
  - Dysphagia (6.1%)
- Other findings include:
  - Normal intelligence: 80.3%
  - Dementia: 19.7%
  - Cerebellar ataxia: 40.9%
  - Other muscle involvement (facial and limb): approximately 25% (Drachman, 1968)

Ocular

- The most common ocular manifestation of CPEO is ptosis.
  - In mitochondrial myopathies ptosis is the initial symptom in 59.1% of cases.

- Ptosis and/or extraocular muscle involvement: 78.8%.
- Pigmentary retinopathy: 36%.

Pathophysiology/Disease Process

Systemic

- Mitochondrial DNA deletions have been found (Moraes et al, 1989).
  - Mitochondria, the powerhouses of the muscle cell, have been found to be abnormal, subsequently affecting muscle function and performance.
    - High-energy requirements occur particularly in the muscle, as well as the brain and heart, which subsequently may be affected by these disorders.
  - On histologic stain these abnormal mitochondria appear as ragged red fibers.
- The characteristic feature of CPEO is slowly progressive muscle involvement (Table 15–1).
  - In addition to the external ocular muscles, muscle weakness may affect the face, neck, and limbs.
  - Manifestations may vary from mild to severe, some having the potential to lead to death (e.g., heart block).
- Ophthalmoplegia plus involves progressive external ophthalmoplegia (PEO) and other clinical associations.

Ocular

- CPEO is characterized by a slowly progressive ptosis and ophthalmoplegia, in the absence of pupillary involvement (Table 15–2).
- The external ocular muscles (EOMs) may be involved more frequently and earlier in CPEO because of:
  - Morphologic differences from other muscles (eg, smaller fibers, richer blood supply) (Scully et al, 1985).
  - EOMs' greater dependence on mitochondrial function, which results in greater adverse affect from mitochondrial abnormalities than other muscle groups (Mitsumoto et al, 1983).
- Ptosis is often the presenting symptom and is usually bilateral and relatively symmetric. In order to compensate for the ptosis, patients may raise their eyebrows and tilt their head back to see under the lids (Hutchinson facies).

TABLE 15–1. SYSTEMIC MANIFESTATIONS

Chronic Progressive External Ophthalmoplegia
- Weakness of muscles of the face, neck, limb (especially proximal), pharynx (causing dysphagia), larynx (causing nasal speech), skeleton
- Cardiac involvement (heart block)
- Central nervous system involvement: seizure, ataxia, deafness, dementia, cerebellum and corticospinal pathway disorders, increased CSF protein, dysmetria
- Endocrine dysfunction: growth and development, short stature
- Mental changes (lower IQ)

Oculopharyngeal Muscular Dystrophy
- Dysphagia (pharyngeal muscle weakness): pharyngeal oral/nasal regurgitation, tracheal aspiration, pulmonary infection, weight loss, choking
- Rasping to nasal voice
- Other muscle weakness: facial, neck, shoulder, hip, limbs (especially proximal), masseter, tongue
- Esophageal carcinoma

Kearns–Sayre Syndrome
- Cardiac involvement (heart block, bradycardia)
- Neurologic involvement: cerebellar involvement (ataxia), deafness, mental retardation/dementia, elevated CSF protein, corticospinal dysfunction, vestibular system dysfunction, abnormal MRI findings (cerebral, cerebellar, brainstem, thalamus, and/or basal ganglia)
- Respiratory failure
- Endocrine involvement: diabetes, growth hormone deficiency, delayed puberty, amenorrhea, hypogonadism, hypoparathyroid, short stature

TABLE 15–2. OCULAR MANIFESTATIONS

Chronic Progressive External Ophthalmoplegia
- Ptosis (Hutchinson facies)
- Ophthalmoplegia (restricted extraocular muscles, diplopia [rare], poor Bell phenomenon, proptosis—possibly from lax ocular muscles)
- Orbicularis oculi weakness (lagophthalmos, secondary corneal exposure)
- Pigmentary retinopathy
  - Salt-and-pepper pigment, in equatorial region, bilateral, may have macular mottling; vision generally good unless associated optic atrophy
  - Bone spicule pigment, optic atrophy, attenuated blood vessels, and macular pigment clumping, severe vision loss (to hand motion or light perception)
  - RPE and choriocapillaris atrophy, vision good
- Reduced saccadic velocity
- Abnormal corneal endothelium (rare)

Oculopharyngeal Muscular Dystrophy
- Ptosis (Hutchinson facies)
- Ophthalmoplegia (infrequent)

Kearns–Sayre Syndrome
- Ptosis
- Ophthalmoplegia
- Salt-and-pepper retinopathy
- Visible choroidal vessels
- Peripapillary changes (metallic sheen, mottling)
- Corneal endothelium affected (corneal clouding)

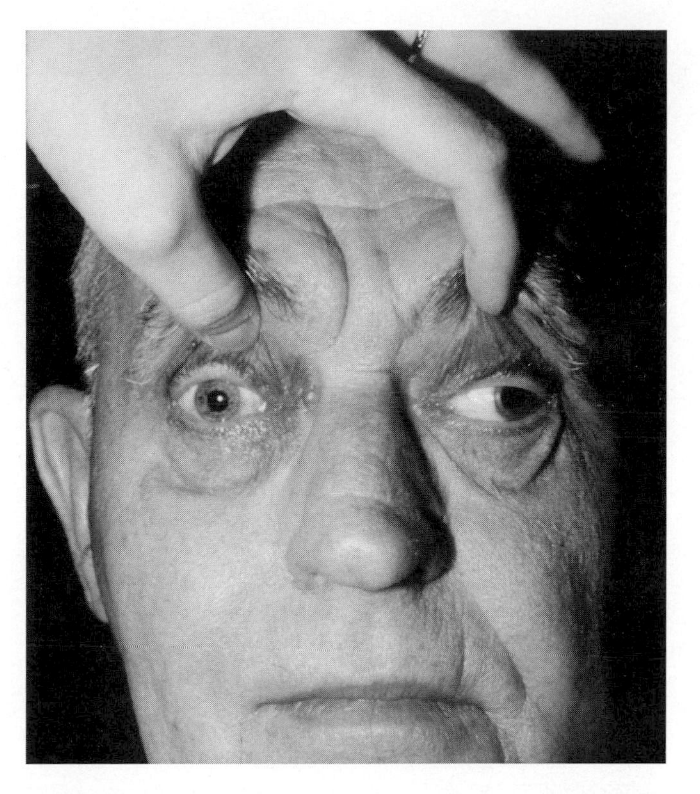

Figure 15–1. Patient with CPEO. Note the position of the eyes as lids are held open. (*Reprinted with permission from Adamczyk DT, Oshinkie L. Oculopharyngeal muscular dystrophy.* J Am Optom Assoc. *1987;58:408–412.*)

- Extraocular muscle involvement often presents insidiously, following the ptosis.
  - Elevation of the eyes is usually affected initially, with progression to complete inability to move the eyes (Figure 15–1).
  - Diplopia rarely is a symptom because of the symmetric, bilateral progression of the disease, in addition to the ptosis occasionally occluding one eye.
    - However, diplopia may still may occur (Sorkin et al, 1997; Wallace et al, 1997).
  - Eso-, exo-, or hypertropia may occur.
  - The orbicularis oculi, along with other facial muscles, also may be involved.
- Retinal pigmentary retinopathy may occur and include (see Table 15–2):
  - Bilateral salt and pepper retinopathy located in the equatorial region, usually with good vision.
  - Bone spicule pigmentation, optic atrophy, and attenuated blood vessels, with poor vision.
  - Atrophy of the retinal pigment epithelium and choriocapillaris, with good vision.

Diagnosis

Systemic

- Diagnosis is based on clinical presentation, family history, neurologic evaluation, and a negative Tensilon test (Table 15–3).
- Associated systemic involvement diagnosis is based on:
  - Complete physical examination
  - Specific testing (eg, electromyography, blood workup).
- Differential diagnosis (Table 15–4) is based on:
  - Clinical presentation, neurologic evaluation, Tensilon test, serum acetylcholine receptor antibody, and thyroid function tests.

Ocular

- Diagnosis at first may be elusive, but is based on:
  - Ptosis, ophthalmoplegia, and lack of pupil involvement (see Table 15–4).
  - Family history, complete physical, neurologic results, and associated clinical manifestations.
  - Cranial nerve workup, EOM testing procedures (eg, sustained upgaze and forced duction), and fundus evaluation (see Table 15–3).

Treatment and Management

Table 15–5 gives an overview of the treatment and management of CPEO.

Systemic

- Neurology consult
- Comanagement for systemic involvement

TABLE 15–3. DIAGNOSTIC TESTS

Chronic Progressive External Ophthalmoplegia
Electromyography
Skeletal muscle histochemistry
Oxidative phosphorylation enzymology
Southern blot testing (skeletal muscle mitochondrial DNA)
Tensilon test
Serum acetylcholine receptor antibody
Thyroid function tests
Oculopharyngeal Muscular Dystrophy
Additional to CPEO:
Barium swallow
Esophagram
Polymerase chain reaction (gene/DNA assessment)
Kearns–Sayre Syndrome
Additional to CPEO:
PCR test on blood DNA
Electrocardiogram
Ocular Considerations
Electrodiagnostic tests

TABLE 15-4. DIFFERENTIAL DIAGNOSIS (SYSTEMIC/OCULAR)

CPEO/OPMD/KSS
Myasthenia gravis
Thyroid disease
Cranial nerve pareses
Orbital myositis
Progressive supranuclear palsy
Myotonic dystrophy
Other mitochondrial diseases
Amyotrophic lateral sclerosis (dysphagia)

Ocular Considerations
Ptosis
- Congenital
- Trauma related
- Third-nerve involvement (and its various etiologies)
- Horner syndrome
- Myotonic dystrophy
- Myasthenia gravis

Ophthalmoplegia
- Trauma
- Myathenia gravis
- Opthalmoplegic migraine
- Aneurysm
- Cranial nerve (various etiologies)
- Amyotrophic lateral sclerosis
- Others

Retinal changes (Kearns–Sayre syndrome)
- Retinitis pigmentosa

TABLE 15–5. TREATMENT AND MANAGEMENT

Systemic
Chronic Progressive External Ophthalmoplegia
- Complete physical exam
- Neurologic workup
- Comanagement with specialist dependent on systemic involvement

Oculopharyngeal Muscular Dystrophy
- Include above for CPEO
- Comanagement with ENT
- Cricopharyngeal myotomy
- Sphincter dilation
- Esophagram

Kearns–Sayre syndrome
- Include above for CPEO
- Comanagement with cardiologist
- Pacemaker
- Vitamins
- Special considerations for potential respiratory involvement (e.g., use of steroids, general anesthesia, high-altitude travel)

Ocular
Chronic Progressive External Ophthalmoplegia
Oculopharyngeal Muscular Dystrophy
- Ptosis: tape, crutch, surgery
- Lagophthalmos: lubricants, moisture chamber
- Diplopia: prism, surgery

Kearns–Sayre syndrome
- Include above for CPEO
- Special consideration for contact lens wear
- Special consideration for glaucoma treatment with beta-blocker or adrenergic agents

Ocular

- Monitor
- Advanced ptosis:
  - Ptosis tape, lid crutches (Figure 15–2), crutch and moisture chamber (Cohen & Waiss, 1997), or surgery (caution of the progressive nature of ptosis).
  - Weak orbicularis function/lagophthalmos: lubricant therapy, moisture chamber.
  - Diplopia: prism, surgery.

OCULOPHARYNGEAL MUSCULAR DYSTROPHY

Oculopharyngeal muscular dystrophy (OPMD) is a slowly progressive disease characterized by ptosis and dysphagia.

> OPMD is distinguished from the other CPEO disorders by having a later age of onset and dysphagia.

Epidemiology

Systemic

- OPMD occurs most commonly in French Canadians.
  - The disease has been traced back to a couple who migrated from France to Canada in the 1600s, with subsequent generations affected.
- OPMD may also occur in other ethnic groups.
- Age of onset is the 40s or 50s.

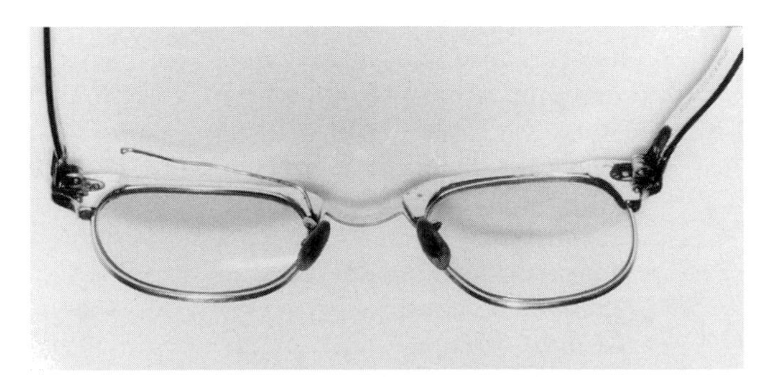

Figure 15–2. Ptosis crutch used by patient shown in Figure 16–1.

- Inheritance is usually autosomal dominant, but autosomal-recessive and sporadic cases may occur.
- Males and females are equally affected.
- Pharyngeal muscles:
  - Second most commonly affected muscle group.
  - Pulmonary infection reported in 25% of cases (Duranceau et al, 1983).
- Other muscle involvement includes facial, limb, and neck in 25% of the cases (Dayal & Freeman, 1976).

Ocular

- The levator is the most commonly affected muscle in OPMD.

Pathophysiology/Disease Process

Systemic

- Chromosome 14Q11.2-q13 has been identified with OPMD (Brais et al, 1995).
- Table 15–1 delineates the systemic manifestations of OPMD.
- Dysphagia:
  - Typically follows ptosis, but may occur at the same time or prior to ptosis.
  - Swallowing difficulties begin with solid foods and progress to liquids.
  - More pronounced when the patient is anxious or drinks cold fluids.
  - Results from food not moving into the esophagus, secondary to poorly functioning pharyngeal muscles and lack of relaxation of the cricopharyngeal muscle.
  - May vary from mild to severe, with the potential of regurgitation, aspiration pneumonia, and loss of weight.
    - Although unlikely today, starvation and death have resulted.
- Other muscle groups (those of the neck, shoulder, hip, and limbs) are inconsistently involved.
- A nasal voice often accompanies the other symptoms.
- Esophageal cancer is found more frequently with these patients.

Ocular

- Levator/ptosis:
  - Levator is the most commonly affected muscle in OPMD.
  - Bilateral, progressive ptosis may be asymmetric (Figure 15–3).
  - Ophthalmoplegia is not typical in OPMD, and if present, has minimal involvement (see Table 15–2).

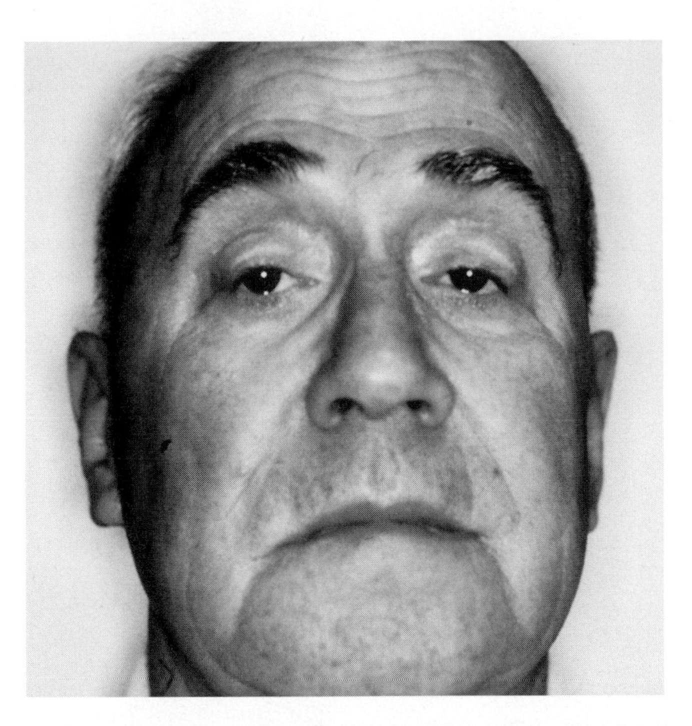

Figure 15–3. Patient with OPMD. Note Hutchinson facies. (*Reprinted with permission from Adamczyk DT, Oshinskie L. Oculopharyngeal muscular dystrophy.* J Am Optom Assoc. *1987;58:408–412.*)

Diagnosis

Systemic

- Based on family history and clinical presentation.
  - Specifically: later age of onset, slow progressive ptosis and dysphagia.
  - Barium swallow testing to assess the swallowing mechanism.
  - Workup to rule out other etiologies (as delineated under CPEO) (see Tables 15–3 and 15–4).

Ocular

- Based on clinical presentation.
  - Distinguishing feature is lack of EOM and pupillary involvement.
  - Workup as delineated under ocular diagnosis for CPEO (see Table 15–4).

Treatment and Management

See Table 15–5 for an overview of the treatment and management of OPMD.

Systemic

- Comanagement with throat specialist for dysphagia.

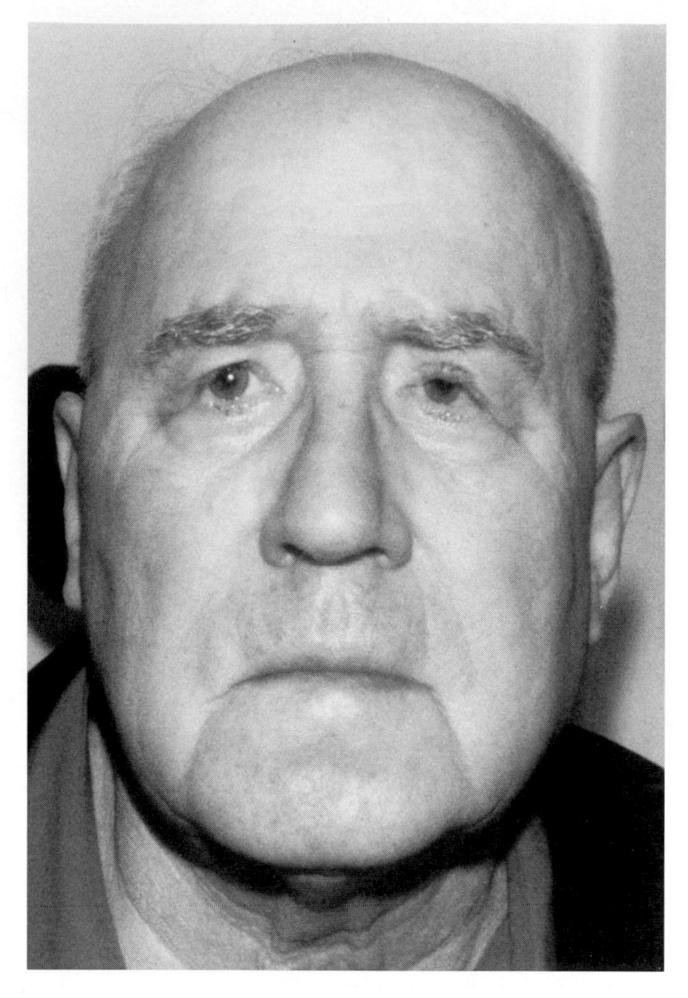

Figure 15–4. Patient in Figure 15–3 after ptosis surgery.

- If dysphagia becomes severe: cricopharyngeal myotomy or sphincter dilatation.
- Esophagram: rule out esophageal carcinoma.

Ocular

- Monitoring.
- Ptosis advancement: ptosis tape, lid crutches, or surgery.
  - Ptosis recurs after surgery in 13% with OPMD (Molgat & Rodrigue, 1993).
  - Lagophthalmos: lubricant therapy used (Figure 15–4).

KEARNS–SAYRE SYNDROME

Kearns–Sayre syndrome (KSS) (oculocraniosomatic neuromuscular disease) is a rare disease that afflicts the young. It consists of external ophthalmoplegia, pigmentary retinopathy (salt and pepper fundus), and cardiac involvement (heart block or conduction defects). The initial presentation is usually ptosis or ophthalmoplegia, usually followed by retinal and cardiac involvement.

> Kearns–Sayre syndrome consists of external ophthalmoplegia, pigmentary retinopathy (salt and pepper fundus), and cardiac involvement (heart block or conduction defects).

Epidemiology

Systemic

- Affects those under 20 years of age.
- Occurs sporadically.
- Systemic manifestations in addition to cardiac involvement include (Berenberg et al, 1977):
  - Short stature (63%)
  - Cerebellar signs (69%)
  - Hearing loss (54%)
  - Mental retardation (40%)
  - Vestibular dysfunction (33%)
  - Mortality secondary to heart block (20%)

Ocular

- Ptosis or ophthalmoplegia initially presents in 88.6% of patients.
- Pigmentary degeneration may occur either alone or with ophthalmoplegia in 23% of patients (Berenberg et al, 1977).

Pathophysiology/Disease Process

Systemic

- Mitochondrial DNA deletions may occur in KSS.
- KSS may occur in infantile, juvenile, and adult forms, each progressive but varied in severity.
  - Age of onset appears related to severity, with the infantile form being the most severe (McKechnie et al, 1985).
- The patient may remain symptom-free for up to 33 years.
- Systemic manifestations (see Table 15–1) may involve:
  - Cardiac abnormalities.
  - Neurologic abnormalities.
  - Endocrine abnormalities.
  - When cerebrospinal fluid protein is increased in patients with ophthalmoplegia and retinal changes, the potential for heart block is increased (Berenberg et al, 1977).
  - Vital functions may be affected, such as those of the heart and breathing, which may ultimately result in death.

Ocular

- Characterized by extraocular muscle and retinal involvement, usually with preservation of vision (see Table 15–2).
- Ptosis is most commonly the first sign, with ophthalmoplegia usually the presenting sign.
  - Retinal and cardiac involvement often is not present until 5 years after the ophthalmoplegia.
- Retinal abnormalities may be related to disturbances in the mitochondria and its affect on the photoreceptors (McKechnie et al, 1985).
  - Retinal manifestations:
    - Usually in the posterior pole
    - Salt and pepper retinopathy
    - Visible choroidal vessels
    - In advanced cases, peripapillary changes

Diagnosis

Systemic

- Based on clinical presentation with cardiac involvement.
  - Complete physical and a cardiac evaluation with electrocardiogram.
  - Southern blot and PCR test on blood DNA (De Coo et al, 1997) (see Table 15–3).

Refer to Table 15–4 for differential diagnosis (systemic/ocular).

Ocular

- Based on clinical presentation.
- Pigmentary changes: electrodiagnostic testing may assist in the differential diagnosis with retinitis pigmentosa.
- EOM involvement is as delineated under CPEO.
- Corneal endothelium may be affected.

Treatment and Management

See Table 15–5 for an overview of the treatment and management of Kearns–Sayre syndrome.

Systemic

- Comanagement with a cardiologist.
  - Pacemaker, if necessary.
- Caution with use of certain drugs (e.g., sedatives and steroids), general anesthesia, and high-altitude travel because of potential respiratory involvement.
- Role of vitamins?

Ocular

- As delineated under CPEO.
- Caution with contact lens wear because of corneal endothelial abnormalities.
- Caution with use of beta-blockers or adrenergic agents in glaucoma because of cardiac involvement.

CONCLUSION

Chronic progressive external ophthalmoplegia represents a general grouping of rare ocular myopathies, which include specific entities with associated clinical features, such as oculopharyngeal muscular dystrophy and Kearns–Sayre syndrome. A slowly progressive ptosis and ophthalmoplegia are characteristic of these diseases. Diagnosis may be initially difficult, because these disorders often mimic myasthenia gravis. The correct diagnosis is important not only for the potential of ocular intervention, but also for appropriate referral and comanagement of systemic involvement, which may be life-saving.

REFERENCES

Chronic Progressive External Ophthalmopathy

Cohen JM, Waiss B. Combination ptosis crutch and moisture chamber for management of progressive external ophthalmoplegia. *J Am Optom Assoc.* 1997;68:663–667.

Danta G, Hilton RC, Lynch PG. Chronic progressive external ophthalmoplegia. *Brain.* 1975;98:473–492.

Daroff RB. Chronic progressive external ophthalmoplegia. A critical review. *Arch Ophthalmol.* 1969;82:845–850.

Eshaghian J, Anderson RL, Weingeist TA, et al. Orbicularis oculi muscle in chronic progressive external ophthalmoplegia. *Arch Ophthalmol.* 1980;98:1070–1073.

Lane CM, Collin JRO. Treatment of ptosis in chronic progressive external ophthalmoplegia. *Br J Ophthalmol.* 1987;71:290–294.

Lowes M. Chronic progressive external ophthalmoplegia, pigmentary retinopathy and heart block (Kearns–Sayre syndrome). *Acta Ophthalmol.* 1975;53:610–619.

Metz HS, Meshel L. Ocular saccades in progressive external ophthalmoplegia. *Ann Ophthalmol.* 1974;6:623–628.

Mills PV, Bowen DI, Thompson DS. Chronic progressive external ophthalmoplegia and pigmentary degeneration of the retina. *Br J Ophthalmol.* 1971;55:302–311.

Mitsumoto H, Aprille JR, Wray SH, et al. Chronic progressive external ophthalmoplegia: Clinical, morphologic, and biochemical studies. *Neurology.* 1983;33:452–461.

Mullie MA, Harding AE, Petty RKH, et al. The retinal manifestations of mitochondrial myopathy. *Arch Ophthalmol.* 1985;103:1825–1830.

Petty RK, Harding AE, Morgan-Hughes JA. The clinical features of mitochondrial myopathy. *Brain.* 1986;109:915–938.

Scully RE, Mark EJ, McNeely BV. Case records of the Massachusetts General Hospital. *N Engl J Med.* 1985;312:171–177.

Sorkin JA, Shoffner JM, Grossniklaus HE, et al. Strabismus and mitochondrial defects in chronic progressive external ophthalmoplegia. *Am J Ophthalmol.* 1997;123:235–242.

Stanescu B, Ferriere G. Electroretinographic alterations in progressive external ophthalmoplegia, Kearns Sayres syndrome. In: Huber A, Klein K, eds. *Neurogenetics and Neuro-ophthalmology.* New York: Elsevier/North-Holland Biomedical; 1981:215–221.

Wallace DK, Sprunger DT, Helveston EM, Ellis FD. Surgical management of strabismus associated with chronic progressive external ophthalmoplegia. *Ophthalmology.* 1997; 104:695–700.

Walsh FB (ed), Hoyt WR. *Clinical Neuro-ophthalmology.* Baltimore: Williams & Wilkins; 1969;2:1254–1265.

Oculopharyngeal Muscular Dystrophy

Adamczyk DT, Oshinskie L. Oculopharyngeal muscular dystrophy. *J Am Optom Assoc.* 1987;58:408–412.

Brais B, Rouleau GA, Bouchard JP, et al. Oculopharyngeal muscular dystrophy. *Semin Neurol.* 1999;19(1):59–66.

Brais B, Xie YG, Sanson M, et al. The oculopharngeal muscular dystrophy locus maps to the region of the cardiac alpha- and beta-myosin heavy chain genes on chromosome 14q11.2-q13. *Hum Mol Genet.* 1995;4:429–434.

Dayal VS, Freeman J. Cricopharyngeal myotomy for dysphagia in oculopharyngeal muscular dystrophy. *Arch Otolaryngol.* 1976;102:115–116.

Duranceau AC, Beauchamp G, Jamieson GG, Barbeau A. Oropharyngeal dysphagia and oculopharyngeal muscular dystrophy. *Surg Clin North Am.* 1983;63:825–832.

Duranceau A, Forand MD, Fauteux JP. Surgery in oculopharyngeal muscular dystrophy. *Am J Surg.* 1980;139:33–39.

Ford LH, Holinger PH. Hereditary dysphagia: The oculopharyngeal syndrome. *Laryngoscope.* 1971;81:373–378.

Fried K, et al. Autosomal recessive oculopharyngeal muscular dystrophy. *J Med Genet.* 1975;12:416–418.

Hardiman O, Halperin JJ, Farrell MA, et al. Neuropathic findings in oculopharyngeal muscular dystrophy. *Arch Neurol.* 1993;50:481–488.

Johnson CC, Kuwabara T. Oculopharyngeal muscular dystrophy. *Am J Ophthalmol.* 1974;77:872–879.

Molgat YM, Rodrigue D. Correction of blepharoptosis in oculopharyngeal muscular dystrophy: Review of 91 cases. *Can J Ophthalmol.* 1993;28:11–14.

Probst A, Tackmann W, Stoeckli HR, et al. Evidence for chronic axonal atrophy in oculopharyngeal "muscular dystrophy." *Acta Neuropathologica.* 1982;57:209–216.

Rare muscular dystrophy: Tracking disease through 300 years. *JAMA.* 1967;199:40–41.

Victor M, Hayes R, Adams RD. Oculopharyngeal muscular dystrophy. *N Engl J Med.* 1962;267:1267–1272.

Kearns–Sayre Syndrome

Bachynski BN, Flynn JT, Rodrigues MM, et al. Hyperglycemic acidotic coma and death in Kearns–Sayre syndrome. *Ophthalmology.* 1986;93:391–396.

Bastiaensen I, Stadhovders A, Trijbels J, et al. Kearns syndrome. Concept of a disease. In: Huber A, Klein K, eds. *Neurogenetics and Neuro-ophthalmology.* New York: Elsevier/North-Holland Biomedical; 1981;205–210.

Berenberg RA, Pellock JM, DiMauro S, et al. Lumping or splitting? "Ophthalmoplegia-plus" or Kearns–Sayre syndrome. *Ann Neurol.* 1977;1:37–54.

Chu BC, Terae S, Takahashi C. MRI of the brain in the Kearns–Sayre syndrome: Report of four cases and a review. *Neuroradiology.* 1999;41:759–764.

De Coo IFM, Gussinklo T, Arts PJW, et al. A PCR test for progressive external ophthalmoplegia and Kearns–Sayre syndrome on DNA from blood samples. *J Neurol Sci.* 1997; 149:37–40.

Drachman DA. Ophthalmoplegia plus. *Arch Neurol.* 1968; 18:654–674.

Eagle RC, Hedges TR, Yanoff M. The atypical pigmentary retinopathy of Kearns–Sayre syndrome. A light and electron microscopic study. *Ophthalmology.* 1982;89: 1433–1440.

Kalenak JW, Kolker AE. Kearns–Sayre syndrome and primary open-angle glaucoma. *Am J Ophthalmol.* 1989; 108:335–336.

Kosmorsky GS, Meister DM, Sheeler LR, et al. Familial ophthalmoplegia-plus syndrome with corneal endothelial disorder. *Neuro-ophthalmology.* 1989;9:271–277.

McKechnie NM, King M, Lee WR. Retinal pathology in the Kearns–Sayre syndrome. *Br J Ophthalmol.* 1985;69:63–75.

Moraes CT, DiMauro S, Zeviani M, et al. Mitochondrial DNA deletions in progressive external ophthalmoplegia and Kearns–Sayre syndrome. *N Engl J Med.* 1989;320: 1293–1299.

Ohkoshi K, Ishida N, Yamaguchi T, Kani K. Corneal endothelium in a case of mitochondrial encephalomyopathy (Kearns–Sayre syndrome). *Cornea.* 1989;8:210–214.

Phillips CI, Gosden CM. Leber's hereditary optic neuropathy and Kearns–Sayre syndrome: Mitochondrial DNA mutations. *Surv Ophthalmol.* 1991;35:463–472.

Section V

ENDOCRINE DISORDERS

Chapter 16

DIABETES MELLITUS

Elliot Sternthal, Anthony Cavallerano,
Jerry Cavallerano

Diabetes mellitus (DM) has been recognized for thousands of years, but the pathogenesis of the condition is only now being elucidated through advances in molecular biology, immunology, and genetics. The ancient Greeks named the disease "diabetes," meaning "to run through," reflecting common symptoms of the condition—excessive thirst and frequent urination. In the 19th century it was noted that the urine of persons with diabetes was sweet, and the Latin adjective *mellitus* (sweet) was added to the disease name.

Today, diabetes mellitus is recognized as a chronic syndrome of hyperglycemia and disordered metabolism of fat and protein. Undoubtedly, a more sophisticated classification of the diabetic subgroups will evolve through an ever-increasing understanding of pancreatic beta-cell function and insulin signaling pathways.

EPIDEMIOLOGY

Systemic

Diabetes is a worldwide medical problem. The disease afflicts approximately 16 million Americans, one third of whom have not been diagnosed and are unaware of their condition. Of those with DM in the United States, approximately 5 to 10% have type 1 DM and 90% have type 2 DM. The various types of DM encompass the most common endocrine disorder in the United States. Each year there are 725,000 newly diagnosed cases, and the demographics of the American population suggest that the incidence will continue to rise as the population ages. There is a higher prevalence of type 2 DM among select cultural and ethnic groups, including Native American, African-American, and Latino populations. There is evidence of an increasing incidence of type 2 DM in these populations within the past 20 years.

Diabetes is a significant cause of morbidity and mortality in the United States and worldwide. The disease is the seventh leading cause of death overall in the United States, and the American Diabetes Association estimates that the total cost of DM in the United States exceeds $100 billion each year. DM remains the leading cause of acquired blindness and renal failure for working-aged Americans, and the leading cause of peripheral neuropathy in the world. DM is also a significant risk factor for coronary artery disease (CAD) and stroke, and a leading cause of nontraumatic lower extremity amputation.

Ocular

DM is a leading cause of blindness and visual impairment in the United States. Despite advances in treating diabetic retinopathy and diabetic macular edema, the risk of blindness is 25 times greater for a person with DM. Diabetes results in 8000 new cases of blindness annually, representing 12% of newly diagnosed cases.

> There has been a dramatic increase in the prevalence of diabetes mellitus in the United States over the past 40 years.

Approximately 25% of persons with type 1 DM have some level of diabetic retinopathy within 5 years of diagnosis; after 10 years, 60% have some level of retinopathy; and after 15 years, more than 80%. Proliferative diabetic retinopathy is present in 25% of the type 1 population within 15 years of diagnosis, and ultimately 70% of those with type 1 DM can expect to develop proliferative retinopathy. Diabetic macular edema develops in 40% of the type 1 population during a lifetime.

> There has been an increased incidence of type 2 diabetes mellitus in children, in the elderly, and in high-risk ethnic groups.

Presently, there are 700,000 Americans with proliferative diabetic retinopathy. Furthermore, there are 500,000 with diabetic macular edema, and 325,000 with clinically significant macular edema. There are 63,000 new cases of proliferative diabetic retinopathy each year and 29,000 cases of high-risk proliferative diabetic retinopathy. The annual incidence of diabetic macular edema in the US is 75,000, including 50,000 cases of clinically significant macular edema.

> Diabetes is the leading cause of morbidity and mortality in the United States today, consuming 1/7 of all U.S. healthcare dollars.

PATHOPHYSIOLOGY/DISEASE PROCESS

In normal human metabolism, the digestive process breaks down ingested carbohydrates into glucose, a simple sugar. This glucose then enters the blood circulation and is delivered to other cells as the most important source of energy for the human body. Excess glucose is changed either to glycogen and stored in the liver or skeletal muscles, or to fat and stored in fatty tissue. Stored liver glycogen can be converted into glucose when the body requires extra energy; however, without insulin this glucose cannot enter and be used by most human cells. Insulin permits the entry and metabolism of glucose in liver, muscle, and fat cells.

> Diabetes is the leading cause of acquired blindness in the United States.

Insulin is produced, stored, and released into the bloodstream by the beta cells of the islets of Langerhans of the pancreas. Glucose is the major stimulus for regulating insulin secretion. Once released into the bloodstream, insulin binds to hepatic and peripheral cell membrane insulin receptors. This binding inhibits hepatic glucose production and enhances peripheral glucose uptake, resulting in a reduction of plasma glucose.

In type 1 DM, beta cells of the pancreas are destroyed and little or no insulin is produced. In type 2 DM, these beta cells produce a relatively inadequate amount of insulin to overcome the insulin resistance of the target tissues.

Classification of Diabetes Mellitus

The Expert Committee of the American Diabetes Association (ADA) defines four major categories of DM (Table 16–1). Type 1 DM, formerly called insulin-dependent or juvenile onset diabetes, can be diagnosed at any age, but the age of onset is usually prior to age 40 years. Only approximately 5 to 10% of the diabetic population has type 1 DM. The condition is caused by reduced or absent insulin production, resulting from autoimmune destruction of pancreatic beta cells, and insulin injections are required to sustain life. There is a high incidence of islet-cell antibodies at the time of diagnosis. Affected persons are usually moderately to severely ill at the time of diagnosis, manifesting the classic symptoms of polyuria, polydipsia, and polyphagia. Other symptoms may include nausea, vomiting, abdominal pain, lethargy, or coma. Onset is usually rapid, and treatment includes daily insulin injections, appropriate diet and meal planning, and exercise.

In general, persons with type 1 DM:

- May be of any age, are usually thin, and usually have abrupt onset of signs and symptoms before age 40 years.
- Have strongly positive urine glucose and ketone tests.
- Are dependent upon exogenous insulin replacement to prevent ketoacidosis and to sustain life.

TABLE 16–1. CLASSIFICATION OF DIABETES MELLITUS (DM)

Type	Characteristics
Type 1 DM	Onset at any age, but usually prior to age 40 years; usually thin; abrupt onset of symptoms; immune-mediated or idiopathic beta-cell destruction; strongly positive urine glucose and ketone tests; dependent upon exogenous insulin to prevent ketoacidosis and sustain life
Type 2 DM	Usually older than 40 years at diagnosis; usually obese; few classic symptoms; insulin resistance and beta-cell secretory defect both present; not prone to ketoacidosis except during periods of stress; not dependent upon exogenous insulin for survival, but may require insulin for stress-induced hyperglycemia and hyperglycemia that does not respond to other therapy
Gestational DM	Onset or discovery during pregnancy; may or may not require insulin
Other types	• Secondary to exocrine pancreatic disease (eg, pancreatectomy, cystic fibrosis, chronic pancreatitis, hemochromatosis) • Secondary to endocrinopathies (eg, Cushing syndrome, acromegaly, pheochromocytoma, primary aldosteronism, glucagonoma) • Secondary to drugs and chemical agents (eg, certain antihypertensive drugs, thiazide diuretics, glucocorticoids, beta-adrenergic agonists, dilantin, alpha-interferon, psychoactive agents, catecholamines) • Associated with genetic syndromes (eg, Down syndrome, Klinefelter syndrome, Turner syndrome, Wolfram syndrome, Huntington chorea)

Report of the Expert Committee on the Diagnosis and Classification of Diabetes Mellitus. Modified from Diabetes Care. *2000;23(suppl 1):S6.*

Multiple factors are involved in the development of type 1 DM. Environmental and genetic factors have been implicated, with specific HLA groups conferring increased risk. Acute stress and viral infection are suspected in the development of type 1 DM in a genetically predisposed or susceptible person. The 50% concordance rate of type 1 DM in identical twins strongly supports the role of environmental and other factors in the onset of the disease. Type 1 DM is frequently associated with other autoimmune disorders such as chronic lymphocytic (Hashimoto) thyroiditis and may be a component of a polyglandular endocrine autoimmune syndrome.

The risk of developing type 1 DM is approximately 5% for a person with a sibling with the condition. If two siblings have type 1 DM, the risk rises to 10%. The risk of type 1 DM before the age of 20 years is 5 to 10% if a person's father has type 1 DM, and 3 to 5% if the mother has type 1 DM. If an aunt or uncle has type 1 DM, the risk is approximately 1 to 2%.

In type 2 DM, patients are usually over 40 years of age at diagnosis; therefore, type 2 DM was formerly called adult onset or noninsulin-dependent DM. Over the last decade, however, there has been a dramatic increase in type 2 DM in obese children as young as 8 to 10 years old who are members of high-risk ethnic groups. Type 2 DM is by far the most prevalent form of DM. Onset is frequently insidious, and the classic symptoms may be absent. Hence, the diagnosis is frequently not made for 7 to 10 years after the onset of hyperglycemia. The risk of developing type 2 DM increases with age and obesity. At the time of diagnosis of type 2 DM, a person may experience only minor symptoms or none at all. The cause of type 2 DM is insulin resistance and relative or absolute insulin deficiency. Three factors seem to contribute to the development of type 2 DM:

1. Insulin resistance, defined as a subnormal biological response to a given amount of insulin, is often present in a silent preclinical phase for 15 to 20 years before the onset of recognized hyperglycemia. Although largely genetically determined, its expression is enhanced by environmental, lifestyle (inactivity, obesity), and metabolic (elevated free fatty acid levels, hyperglycemia) factors. The insulin resistance is due to reduced insulin-binding receptors on the target cell surface, and, more importantly, its postreceptor defects. These defects are due to impaired internalization of the receptor after binding and subsequent reduced insulin signal transduction within the cell.
2. A defect in the insulin-producing beta cells of the pancreas prevents the necessary hyperinsulinemic response to the insulin resistance. This defect may be due to interplay of genetic defects of the beta cell, "pancreatic exhaustion," and "toxicity" to the beta cell due to elevated glucose and free fatty acid levels. Only later in the course of established type 2 DM is a reduction in the number of beta cells felt to be of clinical importance.

3. Unrestrained overproduction of glucose from the liver is the last occurring defect in type 2 DM. Initially due to hepatic insulin resistance, it accelerates because of inadequate insulinization of the liver and is primarily responsible for the fasting hyperglycemia seen in type 2 DM.

> Some level of diabetic retinopathy is present in over 80% of the type 1 and type 2 diabetic population 20 years after the initial diagnosis of diabetes.

Patients with type 2 DM are frequently overweight, but proper diet and exercise are most often insufficient to control type 2 DM. Medical treatment includes oral hypoglycemic and/or insulin-sensitizing agents, insulin, or both insulin and oral agents. These patients are not prone to ketoacidosis and are not dependent upon exogenous insulin for survival, although they may require insulin for stress-induced hyperglycemia and hyperglycemia that persists despite other therapy. The risk of type 2 DM increases with age and obesity. The etiology seems to be related to both environmental and genetic factors, although no specific HLA associations have been recognized.

Persons with type 2 DM have both insulin resistance and a progressive insulin deficiency. Insulin levels range from hyperinsulinemic in the very early stages with only postprandial hyperglycemia, to normoinsulinemic at the onset of mild fasting hyperglycemia, to hypoinsulinemic in those with well-established fasting and postprandial hyperglycemia. Multiple factors are involved in the development of type 2 DM. If both parents have type 2 DM, the risk of a person developing type 2 DM is as high as 75%. The risk is reduced to 25 to 30% if only one parent has type 2 DM. Obesity is present in 60 to 80% of the type 2 population. Studies of identical twins show a 90% concordance in the development of type 2 DM, and over 30% of the siblings of patients with type 2 DM show abnormal glucose tolerance.

Gestational diabetes mellitus (GDM) has its onset or discovery of glucose intolerance during pregnancy. GDM does *not* include diabetic women who become pregnant, and women with GDM may or may not require insulin. Elevated blood glucose levels or GDM is present in about 4% of pregnancies, resulting in 135,000 cases annually in the United States. Diagnostic criteria specific for pregnancy have been developed. The ADA recommends that higher-risk pregnant women be screened for GDM during the 24th to 28th week of pregnancy. Women with GDM have a 25 to 30% risk of developing DM within 10 years postpartum.

Other types of DM are listed in Table 16–1 for completeness but are not discussed further in this chapter. These types include diabetes secondary to pancreatic exocrine disease, endocrinopathies, or drugs and chemical agents; and diabetes associated with insulin-receptor abnormalities or genetic syndromes; and miscellaneous conditions.

Impaired glucose tolerance (IGT) refers to the metabolic stage when plasma glucose levels are higher than normal but are not diagnostic for DM after a 75-g glucose challenge. Patients with IGT have a 1 to 7% risk per year of developing type 2 DM. Most patients with IGT have normal blood glucose levels, except when challenged with a glucose load, and have normal or near-normal glycosylated hemoglobin (HbA_{1c}) levels.

Impaired fasting glucose (IFG) is a recently introduced metabolic stage that includes individuals with fasting plasma levels that are higher than normal but are not diagnostic of DM. IFG is considered to represent a similar intermediate stage of glucose tolerance as IGT, and like IGT is a risk factor for type 2 DM. IFG and IGT are also associated with the cardiovascular risk factors of the insulin resistance syndrome (syndrome X) and thus appear to be risk factors for cardiovascular disease.

Designating the type of DM is not always a straightforward task. The phenotypic appearance of a milder-onset type 1 patient may be very similar to that of a nonobese type 2 patient. In fact, as many as 50% nonobese type 2 patients may have latent autoimmune (type 1) diabetes in adults (LADA). Unfortunately, the absence of islet cell antibodies does not exclude the possibility of type 1 DM. A clinical estimation and an understanding that future reclassification might be necessary are frequently required.

DIAGNOSIS

The Expert Committee of the American Diabetes Association recently revised the specific criteria for the diagnosis of DM in adults and children (Table 16–2). DM can be diagnosed in three different ways and requires confirmation on another day. If the diagnosis cannot be made based on the casual or fasting plasma glucose, then a 75-g glucose load is given and only the 2-hour glucose level reading is required. Diagnosis of DM cannot be made by testing capillary (finger-stick) blood glucose. Rather, individuals with fasting capil-

TABLE 16–2. DIAGNOSIS OF DIABETES MELLITUS

Criteria for the Diagnosis of Diabetes Mellitus

1. Symptoms of diabetes plus casual plasma glucose concentration ≥ 200 mg/dL (11.1 mmol/L). Casual is defined as any time of day without regard to time of last meal. The classic symptoms of diabetes include polyuria, polydipsia, and unexplained weight loss.

OR

2. Fasting plasma glucose (FPG) ≥ 126 mg/dL (7.0 mmol/L). Fasting is defined as no caloric intake for at least 8 hours.

OR

3. Two-hour plasma glucose ≥ 200 mg/dL (11.1 mmol/L) during an oral glucose tolerance test (OGGT). The test should be performed using a glucose load containing the equivalent of 75 g of anhydrous glucose dissolved in water.

Report of the Expert Committee on the Diagnosis and Classification of Diabetes Mellitus. Modified from Diabetes Care. *2000;23(suppl 1):S11.*

lary blood glucose of 110 mg/dL or greater or a random capillary glucose level of 140 mg/dL or greater should be referred for formal plasma glucose screening. Diagnosis of GDM remains unchanged and based on an oral glucose challenge. In pregnant women, a 50-g oral glucose challenge test is used (without regard to last meal) for screening for GDM. A glucose level greater than 140 mg/dL 1 hour later is an indication for a complete 100-g oral glucose tolerance test.

Screening for type 1 DM is unnecessary since the acute clinical syndrome is readily detected. Due to theoretical and pragmatic considerations, screening of asymptomatic individuals for the presence of islet cell antibodies is not recommended. In contrast, type 2 DM is often clinically silent in its early stages and as many as 5.4 million Americans may be undiagnosed. Screening for type 2 DM is indicated if one or more risk factors are present: family history of DM, obesity, at-risk ethnicity, age 45 years or greater, previous IFG or IGT, hypertension, hyperlipidemia, and history of GDM or babies with birth weight over 9 pounds. All pregnant women at high risk for DM should be screened as early as possible in the pregnancy. Testing is done at 24 to 28 weeks for women negative for GDM at the first screening and for women at average risk for GDM. Very-low-risk women need not be screened.

> Screening is essential to diagnose the estimated 5 to 6 million Americans with clinically silent type 2 diabetes, many of whom are already affected by microvascular and macrovascular disease.

TREATMENT AND MANAGEMENT

Type 1 Diabetes Mellitus

Insulin is an endogenous hormone secreted directly into the blood circulation by the pancreas. When this hormone is absent, exogenous insulin must be injected to sustain life. Persons with type 1 DM require exogenous insulin in order to survive. The treatment of type 1 DM, however, is more complicated than merely injecting insulin and requires a careful balance of meal planning (diet), exercise, blood glucose monitoring, and medical management.

Banting and Best first used insulin in 1922. The goal of insulin therapy is to restore near-normal glucose patterns, correct disordered fat and protein metabolism, and foster normal growth and development. Insulin overdose lowers blood glucose levels, causing hypoglycemic reactions. Insufficient insulin dosage results in hyperglycemia, which can result in ketoacidosis or diabetic coma. Consequently, insulin dosage needs to be tailored to the specific metabolic needs of each individual, considering not only dietary habits, but personal activity, lifestyle, and age.

Four characteristics of commercially available insulin have clinical significance: concentration, type, purity, and species of the insulin. Insulin *concentration* is measured in units (one U equals 36 μg of insulin), and this measurement is consistent for all commercially available insulin worldwide. These units are labeled on the insulin bottles. For example, insulin marked U-100 has 100 units of insulin in 1 cc. U-100 insulin is the standard in the United States and worldwide. U-500 insulin is required for rare cases of severe insulin resistance.

The *type* of insulin reflects the speed of onset of insulin action, its period of peak action, and the duration of action (Table 16–3). Short-acting insulin includes regular and lispro insulin, whose onset of action varies from 1/4 to 1 hour after injection. The peak action occurs at 1 to 4 hours and the duration of action is relatively brief, lasting an average of 3 to 6

TABLE 16–3. INSULIN PREPARATION

Preparation	Onset (Hours)	Peak Activity (Hours)	Duration (Hours)
Rapid acting			
Lispro	0.25	1	3–4
Regular	0.5–1	2–5	4–6
Intermediate acting			
NPH/lente	2–4	6–12	16–24
Long acting			
Ultralente	4–6	8–20	24–28

hours. Intermediate-acting insulin includes NPH (neutral protamine Hagedorn) and lente insulin, with an onset of action after injection of 3 to 4 hours. Peak action is 6 to 14 hours after injection, and the duration of action ranges from 18 to 26 hours. The only long-acting insulin is ultralente, which acts 4 to 6 hours after injection, and its peak action is 14 to 20 hours after injection. Its duration of action may last up to 32 hours. Manipulation of the molecular structure of insulin has resulted in the development of novel rapid-acting and extended-duration (or basal) insulin analogues. These new forms of insulin should be available within the next few years.

The choice of insulin or combination of insulin types, and the mode of delivery (single daily injection, multiple daily injections, or insulin pump) should be determined by the patient and diabetologist or primary physician depending on the patient's lifestyle, dietary habits, mode of glucose monitoring, compliance, social needs, and numerous other factors. Insulin types are frequently mixed for injection to take advantage of the peak action time of each insulin.

A third characteristic of insulin describes its *purity*. For many years insulin was available only from the pancreases of animals, particularly cattle and pigs. Animal pancreases also contain elements in addition to insulin, such as other hormones and cell fragments, and these impurities were present in the insulin. Methods were developed to extract these impurities from the final insulin product because antibodies can develop in response to their presence. At present, the only animal species insulins produced in the United States are purified pork regular and NPH, which are 99.99% pure (proinsulin contaminants less than 10 parts per million). Recombinant DNA technology to produce human insulin has been developed to overcome the problems of insulin impurities and to ensure against shortages of animal pancreases needed. The source of insulin (human or pork) defines the *species* of the insulin. Insulin from animal sources has amino acids linked in slightly different sequences. Although pork insulin is effective in humans, the difference can cause antibodies to the insulin to form, making the injected insulin less effective. The advent and use of human insulin reduces the risk of this complication.

The goal of insulin therapy is to maintain circulating blood glucose levels as close to normal as possible; however, the autoregualtion of the healthy human system to circulating levels of blood glucose cannot be duplicated by subcutaneous insulin injections. Therefore, strategies have been devised to mimic the natural autoregualtion of blood glucose levels. Daily multiple injections of insulin are the norm for most type 1 DM patients, and the use of programmable continuous subcutaneous insulin infusion pumps has proliferated in recent years. Frequency of insulin injections depends on a person's motivation and the severity of the diabetic condition, among other factors.

Regular exercise and appropriate meal planning to adjust the daily caloric intake and types of food are significant components of diabetes control. Patients with diabetes need to work closely with their doctors, dieticians, and other members of their healthcare team. Dietary considerations are not limited merely to the total daily caloric intake. The timing and source of caloric intake are also significant factors.

The Diabetes Control and Complications Trial (DCCT), a 10-year study sponsored by the National Institutes of Health, enrolled 1441 patients with type 1 DM and investigated two questions:

1. *Primary Prevention:* Does intensive therapy of diabetes prevent development of retinopathy and other long-term complications compared with conventional therapy?
2. *Secondary Intervention:* Does intensive therapy affect the progression of diabetic retinopathy and other chronic complications compared with conventional therapy?

The DCCT showed that intensive therapy reduced clinically meaningful diabetic retinopathy by 35 to 74%. Intensive therapy also reduced severe nonproliferative diabetic retinopathy, proliferative diabetic retinopathy, and a need for laser surgery by 45%. First appearance of any retinopathy was reduced by 27%. Furthermore, intensive therapy reduced the development of microalbuminuria by 35%, clinical proteinuria by 56%, and clinical neuropathy by 60%. Adverse effects of intensive therapy included hypoglycemia, catheter complication, weight gain, and ketoacidosis. This prospective landmark study demonstrated that intensive glycemic control slows or prevents diabetic microvascular complication. It is now the standard of care to maintain as good control as possible of any diabetic condition based on the DCCT findings.

> Glycemic control has been repeatedly shown to reduce the incidence and progression of microvascular disease.

Type 2 Diabetes Mellitus

Diet, exercise, and weight loss in obese persons may be sufficient to control type 2 DM; however, in most cases pharmacological treatment is needed. Approximately 15% of persons with type 2 DM control their condition by diet alone, and 25% are essentially on "no therapy." Patients with type 2 DM may medically control their diabetes with oral agents (35%), insulin (25%), or both insulin and oral agents. Many type 2 patients require insulin if oral agents fail to achieve proper blood glucose control. Also, high doses of injected insulin sometimes may not be effective without oral agents; conversely, oral agents may not be effective without injected insulin. These individuals are still considered to have type 2 DM because they can sustain life without insulin injections, but the insulin is crucial to maintain good health.

Recent advances in the treatment of type 1 diabetes include intense insulin administration by multiple injection or continuous subcutaneous infusion pump and novel insulin analogues, which enhance pre- and postmeal glycemic control.

The current available oral pharmacologic agents can be mechanistically categorized as insulin secretagogues, insulin sensitizers, and agents that delay glucose absorption (Table 16–4). Insulin secretagogues (oral hypoglycemic agents) potentiate the release of insulin from the beta cell in response to the prandial increase in blood glucose. Most widely used in this category are the sulfonylureas, which act by depolarizing the beta cell. Hepatic gluconeogenesis and glucagon levels are suppressed. Some agents in this class might also potentiate insulin action in target tissue. First- and second-generation agents differ in drug potency, binding, drug interaction, and metabolism. The maximum biological response, however, is similar for both generations. Because of the possibility of sustained hyperinsulinemia, hypoglycemia, although uncommon, can be severe and require hospitalization. Repaglinide stimulates a brief surge in insulin response, akin to the insulin profile seen after lispro insulin injection. This agent needs to be taken 15 to 30 minutes before a meal and is omitted if a meal is skipped. Generally, less hypoglycemia is observed.

TABLE 16–4. ORAL AGENTS FOR TYPE 2 DIABETES

Class	Drugs
Insulin Secretagogues	
Sulfonylurea	First generation
	Tolbutamide (Orinase)
	Chlorpropamide (Diabinese)
	Tolazamide (Tolinase)
	Second generation
	Glyburide (DiaBeta, Micronase, Glynase)
	Glipizide (Glucotrol, Glucotrol XL)
	Glimepiride (Amaryl)
Metiglinide	Repaglinide (Prandin)
Insulin Sensitizers	
Biguanide	Metformin (Glucophage)
Thiazolidinedione	Rosiglitazone (Avandia)
	Pioglitazone (Actos)
Alpha-glucosidase inhibitors	
	Acarbose (Precose)
	Miglitol (Glyset)

Therapeutic progress for type 2 diabetes includes oral rapid-acting insulin secretagogues and insulin sensitizers.

Insulin sensitizers (antihyperglycemic agents) enhance the action of insulin on hepatic, muscle, and fatty tissue, and reduce ambient plasma insulin levels. Metformin, a biguanide in worldwide clinical use for over 30 years, most effectively inhibits hepatic gluconeogenesis in addition to its more modest potentiation of peripheral glucose disposal. Gastrointestinal side effects can be minimalized by taking metformin with food. Lactic acidosis is extremely uncommon if this medication is avoided in patients with renal or hepatic insufficiency, heart failure, and alcohol abuse.

The thiazolidinediones (or glitazones) are recently developed insulin-sparing agents that act by binding to a receptor in the target cell nucleus. The result is an enhancement of the insulin signal in insulin response genes leading to improved glucose transport into muscle tissue and reduced free fatty acid levels. Thus, glucose disposal is increased and insulin resistance is reduced. Additionally, an improvement in lipid and coagulation profiles, as well as endothelial function, may translate into reduction of cardiovascular risk. Side effects include rare hepatotoxicity (necessitating regular liver enzyme monitoring), weight gain, edema, and anemia. Toglitazone, the first available glitazone in the United States, was withdrawn from the market in March 2000 after a review of safety data suggested that the two newer glitazones, rosiglitazone and pioglitazone, offered similar benefits with less liver toxicity.

Acorbose and miglitol, drugs that delay glucose absorption, do so by a reversible competitive inhibition of hydrolytic enzymes of the small intestine. As a result, sucrose and starches are incompletely digested to glucose and there is a blunting of the postprandial glucose excretion. There is minimal effect on the fasting glucose level. Insulin levels tend to decrease after a meal, and hypoglycemia does not occur with monotherapy. However, if hypoglycemia occurs due to a concurrently administered insulin secretagogue or insulin, this must be treated with simple glucose rather than complex carbohydrates or sucrose. The side effects of abdominal cramping, flatulence, and diarrhea can be mitigated by a very gradual dosage titration.

All oral agents require functioning beta cells to be effective and are therefore contraindicated in patients with type 1 DM. Monotherapy may be successful initially, but because of the progressive nature of beta-cell decline in type 2 DM, a combination of different categories of agents is usually required after 3 to 4 years of treatment. The choice of medical therapy for type 2 DM must be made carefully by the patient's diabetologist or primary physician. Consideration is given to the person's dietary habits, weight, physical activity, and the consistency of the day-to-day eating habits and dietary control. An oral agent that may be effective when a person is controlling dietary intake and exercising regularly may cause serious hypoglycemia when that person cuts back on meals, further increases physical activity, or otherwise modifies lifestyle.

Recently, the United Kingdom Prospective Diabetes Study (UKPDS) Group released data from a 20-year study of 5102 newly diagnosed type 2 diabetic patients. This study addressed the question of whether intense glycemic control would reduce microvascular and cardiovascular complications and whether sulfonylureas, metformin, or insulin offered any specific advantages or disadvantages. The results mirrored those of the DCCT, with a 25% reduction in risk of retinal and renal complications seen in the intensively treated patients, regardless of the type of pharmacologic treatment. Although there was a trend to reduced cardiovascular events with improved glycemic control, this benefit did not reach statistical significance. There were no adverse effects of sulfonylureas, insulin, or metformin on cardiovascular events. The DCCT and UKPDS provide incontrovertible evidence that rigorous glycemic control in type 1 and type 2 DM reduces microvascular complications.

ASSOCIATED ACUTE COMPLICATIONS OF DIABETES MELLITUS

Systemic

Three major acute complications of DM are diabetic ketoacidosis, nonketotic hyperosmolar syndrome, and hypoglycemia. Each of these conditions is a medical emergency.

Diabetic Ketoacidosis

Diabetic ketoacidosis (DKA) is a potentially life-threatening catabolic condition that results from insulin deficiency. The diagnostic triad comprises metabolic acidosis, hyperglycemia, and ketogenesis. DKA is unlikely in type 2 DM except during periods of significant stress induced by trauma, intercurrent infection, or disease. Despite modern treatment strategies and insulin availability, DKA is still relatively common, accounting for 10% of hospital admissions that list DM as the primary cause of hospitalization. Although DKA may be an initial presentation of type 1 DM, only 20% of cases of DKA occur in new-onset type 1 DM. The diagnosis of DKA may be difficult. Typically, polyuria and polydipsia are present for several days prior to onset. Gastric stasis and distension, nausea, vomiting, and anorexia are frequently present. Dehydration may result in tachycardia, disorientation, tremulousness, and decreased renal elimination of glucose and ketoacids.

An excess of counterregulatory hormones such as glucagon, catecholamines, cortisol, and growth hormone accompanies the insulin deficiency. Glucagon directly stimulates hepatic gluconeogenesis and ketogenesis in the absence of insulin. The degree of ketone body production correlates with the plasma glucagon concentration. Excess catecholamine, cortisol, and growth hormone further increase hepatic glucose production. These hormones and the acidemic state further inhibit peripheral glucose utilization, already severely compromised by insulin deficiency. Accelerated lipolysis of adipose tissue, due to hypoinsulinemia and excess counterregulatory hormones, provides the substrate (free fatty acids) for unrestrained production of ketoacids in the liver.

Deficiencies in diabetes management skills, in conjunction with infection or coexistent illness, are the most common precipitating factors for DKA. Malfunction of insulin pumps and omission of insulin injections also may lead to DKA. Prompt treatment is essential, with the goal being to increase glucose utilization, correct acidosis and ketonemia, and return normal hydration and electrolyte composition. However, there may be serious complications due to treatment, including hypokalemia, hypoglycemia, and central nervous system deterioration. Meticulous diabetes management reduces the risk of complications, but DKA has been shown to cause nearly 10% of deaths associated with DM.

Alcoholic ketoacidosis is considered in the differential diagnosis of diabetic ketoacidosis. Hyperketonemia, acidosis, and dehydration characterize this condition, although hyperglycemia is uncommon. The condition follows heavy and prolonged drinking, and is characterized by anorexia, nausea, vomiting, and alcohol abstinence during the previous day.

Nonketotic Hyperosmolar Syndrome

Nonketotic hyperosmolar syndrome is an acute diabetic complication that most commonly affects the elderly with type 2 DM who suffer from insidious hyperglycemia. Diuresis and subsequent dehydration leading to marked elevation in blood glucose and osmolarity result. Impaired thirst perception and impaired renal function predispose to extreme hyperglycemia without ketoacidosis—the hallmark of this condition. Undiagnosed type 2 DM or type 2 DM stressed by infection, stroke, or steroid or diuretic therapy may precipitate nonketotic hyperosmolar syndrome. Treatment includes fluid replacement, insulin and electrolyte replacement, and identification of precipitating factors such as infection or cerebral vascular accident. The disorder can be fatal, and early recognition is essential in successful management. In many instances, diet and/or oral agents can maintain adequate glycemic control after the volume and metabolic perturbations are corrected.

Hypoglycemia

Hypoglycemia is the most common and potentially most serious acute complication of DM. Insulin, oral agents, and alcohol are the most frequent causes of exogenous hypoglycemia. Insulin therapy results in monthly episodes of mild hypoglycemia in more than 50% of patients with type 1 DM. Attempts at tight metabolic control, such as in systems of continuous subcutaneous insulin infusion or with multiple daily injections, can result in profound hypoglycemia and a threefold increased risk of severe hypoglycemia, as was found in the DCCT. Hypoglycemic unawareness can be due to either a maladaptive response to prior hypoglycemic episodes or an autonomic neuropathy in type 1 diabetic patients. Frequent blood sugar monitoring and blood glucose awareness training can be beneficial.

Several commonly used drugs can increase the hypoglycemic effect of insulin and oral agents. These drugs include alcohol, sulfonylureas, biguanides, glitazones, nonselective beta-blockers, monoamine oxidase inhibitors, salicylates, and tetracycline. Certain antibiotics such as chloramphenicol, sulfonamides, and doxycycline increase the risk of hypoglycemia by inhibiting the excretion or metabolism of sulfonylureas. This same effect is observed with ethanol, phenylbutazone, coumadin, allopurinol, and phenyramidol. Competition for albumin-binding sites increases first-generation sulfonylurea action when used in combination with salicylates, sulfonamides, and phenylbutazone. Beta-adrenergic receptor blocking agents increase the risk of hypoglycemia by reducing gluconeogenesis.

ASSOCIATED CHRONIC COMPLICATIONS OF DIABETES MELLITUS

Persons with type 1 and type 2 DM are susceptible to the chronic complications of DM (Table 16–5). Several pathogenic mechanisms by which sustained hyperglycemia results in tissue damage have been described. These include (1) nonenzymatic glycosylation of proteins (Amadori products), (2) irreversible cross-linking of Amadori products to form advanced glycosylation endproducts (AGEs), (3) accumulation of sorbitol and depletion of myoinositol in tissues by activating the polyol pathway, and (4) hemodynamic alterations affecting tissue perfusion. Although the exact pathophysiology of diabetic complications has not been established, the above mechanisms appear to be particularly involved in the causation of microvascular disease, as well as exacerbating the traditional atherosclerotic risk factors of macrovascular disease.

Systemic

Microvascular Disease

Microvascular diseases represent the pathogenic signature of DM. Microvascular diseases result from basement membrane disorders in the vessels, disorders of blood flow, increased vascular permeability, and abnormalities of blood platelets. Diabetic retinopathy, nephropathy, and neuropathy are categorized as microvascular diseases.

Antiplatelet agents such as aspirin have been tested to determine their value in reducing diabetic vascular complications. Studies to date have been equivocal, although the Early Treatment Diabetic

TABLE 16–5. COMPLICATIONS OF DIABETES MELLITUS

Acute complications	Diabetic ketoacidosis (DKA)
	Nonketotic hyperosmolar syndrome
	Hypoglycemia
Chronic complications	Microvascular disease
	Retinopathy
	Nephropathy
	Neuropathy
	Macrovascular disease
	Cardiovascular disease
	Cerebrovascular disease
	Peripheral vascular disease

Retinopathy Study (ETDRS) demonstrated neither any advantage nor disadvantage to the daily use of 650 mg of aspirin in relation to diabetic retinopathy.

Retinal ischemia is a precursor of diabetic retinopathy. Dilation and increased capillary permeability, thickening of the capillary basement membrane, capillary occlusion due to increased aggregation of red blood cells and platelets, loss of endothelial cells and pericytes, and formation of arteriovenous shunts are early findings. The clinical manifestations of diabetic retinopathy range from various levels of nonproliferative to proliferative retinopathy and include diabetic macular edema. The prevalence of nonproliferative diabetic retinopathy increases with duration of DM, exceeding 80% at 20 years. Over a lifetime, the prevalence of proliferative diabetic retinopathy may approach 70% in patients with type 1 DM. In newly diagnosed type 2 DM, 15 to 20% of patients already have some degree of nonproliferative diabetic retinopathy, and 2% may have proliferative diabetic retinopathy or macular edema. This is likely a result of the prolonged period of undiagnosed and silent hyperglycemia that typifies type 2 DM. Although diabetic retinopathy may pursue a more aggressive course in type 1 DM, demographics confer the majority of retinal complications upon the type 2 diabetic population.

Nephropathy. Diabetic nephropathy is thought to result from an interplay of hyperglycemia-induced renal hyperperfusion, damaging AGEs, and genetic susceptibility for this complication. Early changes include increased kidney size and glomerular filtration, thickening of glomerular and tubular capillary basement membranes, and increased mesangial matrix volume. The hallmark microscopic changes are diffuse or nodular glomerulosclerosis (Kimmelstiel–Wilson syndrome). After an asymptomatic period of 7 to 15 years in type 1 DM, microalbuminuria (30 to 300 μg/24 hours) and hypertension appear. Generally, once clinical albuminuria exceeds 300 μg per 24 hours, overt nephropathy is present and follows a progressive course to renal failure.

Diabetes is the leading cause of end-stage renal disease (ESRD) in the United States. The risk of renal disease for a diabetic person is 20 times that of a person without diabetes, and diabetic nephropathy is responsible for one half the deaths of type 1 patients under age 40 years. Approximately 30 to 40% of type 1 patients and 25 to 30% of type 2 patients develop nephropathy. Although a greater percentage of type 1 patients advance to ESRD, more than 50% of diabetic patients on dialysis have type 2 DM because of its overwhelming prevalence. Certain minority groups, hypertension, and smoking are added risk factors for ESRD. Both the DCCT and UKPDS showed that near-euglycemic control can prevent or delay progression of diabetic nephropathy in patients with either type 1 or type 2 DM. However, when advanced renal complications are present, the benefits of intensive glycemic control are negligible. At this stage, diet modification and reduction of dietary protein are important management strategies. Treatment of concomitant systolic and/or diastolic hypertension decreases the rate of decline in renal function. Angiotensin-converting enzyme (ACE) inhibitor medications appear to be particularly effective in decreasing microalbuminuria and slowing the progression of diabetic nephropathy. Dialysis or kidney transplantation becomes necessary in ESRD.

The most frequent cause of death for persons with diabetic nephropathy is cardiovascular disease. Nephropathy may be implicated because of the presence of atherogenic AGEs and the exacerbation of dyslipidemia and hypertension frequently present in type 2 patients. Therefore, all comorbid risk factors must be identified and aggressively treated.

Neuropathy. Diabetic neuropathy is a common microvascular complication of diabetes, affecting approximately 40% of diabetic individuals. Diabetic neuropathies are generally considered in three categories: (1) distal symmetric polyneuropathy (chronic), (2) asymmetric neuropathy, such as cranial and truncal mononeuropathy (acute and showing resolution), and (3) autonomic neuropathy (chronic).

There is evidence of demyelination and remyelination of nerve fibers, loss of endothelial cell tight junctions, and basement membrane thickening in patients with distal symmetric and autonomic neuropathy. The underlying etiology for distal symmetric neuropathy is a general metabolic abnormality involving neurons and Schwann cells. Activation of the polyol pathway and disturbances in myoinosital levels may be causative. Distal symmetric neuropathy can be either asymptomatic or symptomatic. Loss of vibration sense and light touch in the feet and loss of ankle reflexes characterize the asymptomatic type. The symptomatic type is characterized by numbness and parethesia of the feet, often worse at night, and may progress to dull aches or severe, knife-like, or burning pain. Neuropathic ulcers are frequent in the foot because of decreased proprioception and sensation and abnormal pressure distribution caused by weakness of the intrinsic muscles of the foot.

Microvascular occlusion or ischemia is considered the underlying cause of asymmetrical or focal mononeuropathy, such as cranial or peripheral mononeuropathy. Focal neuropathies are more common among older patients with type 2 DM, whereas the incidence of symmetric neuropathies is approximately equal for those with type 1 and type 2 DM.

Cranial mononeuropathy usually involves nerves III, IV, VI, or VII. The sixth and third nerves are most frequently affected, and there is pupillary sparing in approximately 80% of diabetes-related third-nerve palsy. Mononeuropathies of peripheral nerves usually involve nerves predisposed to pressure or entrapment, such as the median nerve (carpal tunnel syndrome). Visceral (autonomic) neuropathy impairs both parasympathetic and sympathetic nerves and can result in gastroparesis, diabetic diarrhea, neurogenic bladder, impotence in men, and impaired cardiovascular reflexes.

Treatment for diabetic neuropathy and its complications varies. Aldose reductase inhibitors have been suggested as a means to prevent diabetic neuropathy. Many complications of neuropathy can be prevented by prudent and judicious care, such as foot self-examination and appropriate choice of shoes. As with other microvascular complications, achievement of near euglycemia can provide symptomatic relief and reduce pathologic changes of the diabetic neuropathies. However, due to the state of the art, most treatment is symptomatic, and often involves a trial-and-error approach utilizing anticonvulsants, tricyclic antidepressants, nonsteroidal anti-inflammatory drugs, analgesics, gamma-linolenic acid, B vitamins, and topical capsaicin, often in various combinations. Measures to lessen postural hypotension and improve gastric emptying are moderately successful.

Macrovascular Disease

Cardiovascular disease is the most frequent cause of death in diabetic patients. Coronary artery disease (CAD) is four to six times more prevalent in a diabetic population than in a nondiabetic population. Moreover, diabetes robs women of their natural protection from cardiovascular disease. The presence of traditional risk factors such as age, obesity, smoking, hypertension, and hyperlipidemia confers even greater morbidity and mortality in diabetic persons. However, diabetes by itself predisposes to increased cardiovascular risk. Diabetic individuals have increased platelet aggregation, decreased red blood cell deformability, reduced fibrinolytic activity, glycosylated (more atherogenic) lipoproteins, vascular endothelial abnormalities, and AGEs. Insulin resistance, present in IGT and type 2 DM, has recently been recognized as a nontraditional cardiovascular risk factor. It cosegregates with a constellation of other CAD risk factors, such as central obesity, hypertension, elevated triglycerides, low HDL-cholesterol, increased small dense LDL-cholesterol, and increased plasminogen activator inhibitor-1 (insulin resistance or cardiac dymetabolic syndrome). Recently, cross-sectional data from the Framingham Offspring Study showed an association between elevated endogenous fasting insulin levels (presumably a surrogate for increased insulin resistance) and impaired fibrinolysis in persons with IFG/IGT and type 2 DM. This linkage of thrombotic potential and insulin resistance may explain the increased risk of cardiovascular disease in IGT and type 2 DM. Measures that decrease insulin resistance might prove useful in improving fibrinolysis and reducing macrovascular disease. Duration of DM does not seem to be an independent risk factor for CAD in type 2 patients, but the risk of CAD for type 1 DM patients rises from less than 10% after 25 years duration to over 60% after 40 years of type 1 DM.

Patients with DM also have a higher incidence of silent ischemia, congestive heart failure, cardiomyopathy, cardiogenic shock, and recurrent myocardial infarction. The risk of stroke is two to four times greater for a diabetic person than for a nondiabetic person, and the risk of peripheral vascular disease is increased fourfold. Diabetes is the leading cause of nontraumatic lower extremity amputation in the United States. Treatment of macrovascular disease is similar for those without diabetes. More stringent reduction of hypertension (130/85) and LDL-cholesterol (<100 mg/dL) is required. Reduced HDL-cholesterol, elevated triglycerides, obesity, inactivity, and smoking are also addressed. Angiotensin-converting enzyme inhibitors and statins are favored for treatment of hypertension and hypercholesterolemia, respectively. Recent evidence suggests that agents that reduce insulin resistance (glitazones) have a beneficial effect on vascular endothelial function. Further studies are underway to determine if this effect translates into a meaningful reduction of the cardiovascular risk profile.

Ocular

Ocular complications of DM are common, and all structures of the eye are susceptible to the deleterious effects of DM (Table 16–6). Diabetic retinopathy is the leading cause of new blindness in Americans of working age. Vision loss from DM results from nonresolving vitreous hemorrhage, fibrovascular tissue resulting in traction retinal detachment, and diabetic macular edema and macular nonperfusion (Table 16–7; Figures 16–1 to 16–4) Presently, there is no complete protection from or cure for diabetic retinopathy or diabetic macular edema, although the management of these conditions and their complications have been defined by the Diabetic Retinopathy Study, Early Treatment Diabetic Retinopathy Study, and Diabetic Retinopathy Vitrectomy Study. Briefly, these studies show that:

TABLE 16–6. OCULAR COMPLICATIONS OF DIABETES MELLITUS

Visual function
- Reduced accommodation
- Fluctuating vision and refraction
- Tritan color defect

Increased incidence of primary open-angle glaucoma
Extraocular muscle palsy (III, IV, VI cranial nerve mononeuropathy)
Decreased tear production
Periorbital edema
Cornea
- Reduced corneal sensitivity
- Corneal abrasion and recurrent corneal erosion
- Slow, defective corneal re-epithelialization

Iris
- Neovascularization of the iris (rubeosis iridis)
- Ectropion uveae
- Neovascular glaucoma

Lens
- Premature cataract
- Diabetic cataract

Retina
- Nonproliferative diabetic retinopathy
- Proliferative diabetic retinopathy
- Diabetic macular edema

- Appropriate and properly timed scatter (panretinal) laser photocoagulation surgery can reduce the risk of severe vision loss (best corrected visual acuity of 5/200 or worse) from proliferative diabetic retinopathy to 4% or less.
- Appropriate and properly timed focal laser photocoagulation surgery can reduce the risk of moderate vision loss (a doubling of the visual angle, such as a reduction from 20/40 to 20/80) from diabetic macular edema by 50% or more.
- Early vitrectomy may be valuable in restoring useful vision in patients with severe vitreous hemorrhage, particularly in those with type 1 DM, compared to delaying vitrectomy.

Diabetic retinopathy is a highly specific microvascular complication that affects persons with either type 1 or type 2 DM. After 20 years of DM, almost all patients with type 1 DM and over 60% of patients with type 2 DM have some degree of diabetic retinopathy. Laser surgery and other surgical modalities help reduce the risk of moderate and severe vision loss from DM, and in some cases can restore useful vision for those who have suffered vision loss. These surgical modalities, particularly laser surgery, are most effective if initiated when a person approaches or just reaches high-risk proliferative diabetic retinopathy, or before a person has symptoms of reduced vision.

The 5-year risk of severe vision loss from high-risk proliferative diabetic retinopathy may be as high as 60%, and the risk of moderate vision loss from clinically significant diabetic macular edema may be as high as 25 to 30% over a 3-year period. Because these conditions may cause no ocular or visual symptoms when they are most amenable to treatment, the responsibility is to identify eyes at risk of vision loss and direct patients to appropriate laser surgery. Significantly, diabetic macular edema can be present with any level of nonproliferative or proliferative diabetic retinopathy. Both macular edema and diabetic retinopathy are exacerbated by hypertension. Serum lipid levels are associated with hard exudates in the retina and vision loss. As previously noted, the DCCT and the UKPDS demonstrated that near-euglycemic control can prevent or delay the progression of diabetic retinopathy. Recent

TABLE 16–7. CLINICAL LEVELS OF DIABETIC RETINOPATHY WITH RESPECT TO ETDRS RETINOPATHY SEVERITY LEVELS

Nonproliferative Diabetic Retinopathy (NPDR)

A. Mild NPDR (ETDRS Level 20–35)
At least one microaneurysm
Definition not met for B, C, D, E, F

B. Moderate NPDR (ETDRS Level 43–47)
H/Ma ≥ standard photograph No. 2A
OR
Soft exudates, VB, and IRMAS definitely present
Definition not met for C, D, E, F

C. Severe NPDR (ETDRS Level 53 A–D)
H/Ma ≥ standard photograph No. 2A in all 4 quadrants
OR
VB in 2 or more quadrants
OR
IRMA ≥ standard photograph No. 8A in at least 1 quadrant

D. Very Severe NPDR (ETDRS Level 53 E)
Any two or more of C
Definition not met for E, F

Proliferative Diabetic Retinopathy (PDR)

E. Mild (Early) PDR (< High Risk) (ETDRS Level 61)
New Vessels
Definition not met for F

F. High-Risk PDR (ETDRS Level 71)
NVD ≥ 1/3–1/2 disc area
OR
NVD and vitreous or preretinal or vitreous hemorrhage
OR
NVE and vitreous or preretinal or vitreous hemorrhage

Clinically Significant Macular Edema (CSME)
Thickening of the retina located ≤ 500 microns from the center of the macula
OR
Hard exudates ≤ 500 microns from the center of the macula with thickening of the adjacent retina
OR
A zone of retinal thickening, 1 disc area or larger in size, any portion of which is ≤ 1 disc diameter from the center of the macula

From Early Treatment Diabetic Retinopathy Study Research Group. Grading diabetic retinopathy from stereoscopic color fundus photographs—An extension of the modified Airlie House classification: ETDRS report 10. Ophthalmology. *1991;98:786–806.*

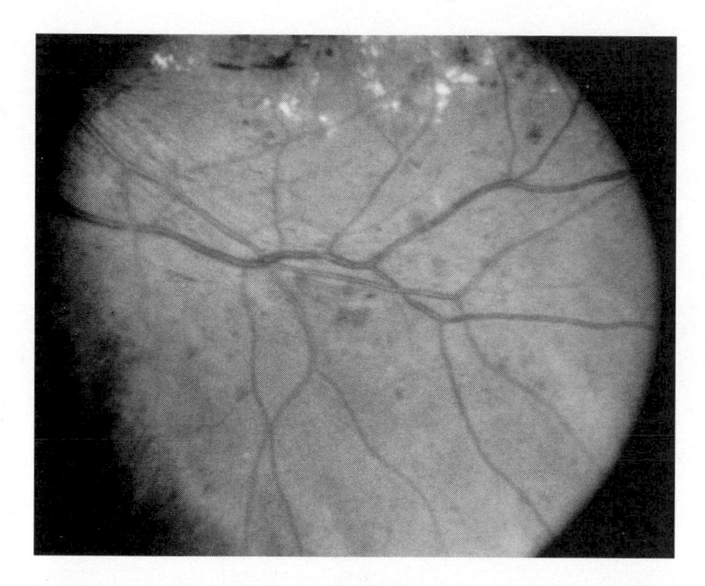

Figure 16–1. Severe nonproliferative diabetic retinopathy (NPDR). The various lesions of NPDR are shown, including cotton-wool spots, venous caliber abnormality, and hemorrhages and microaneurysms.

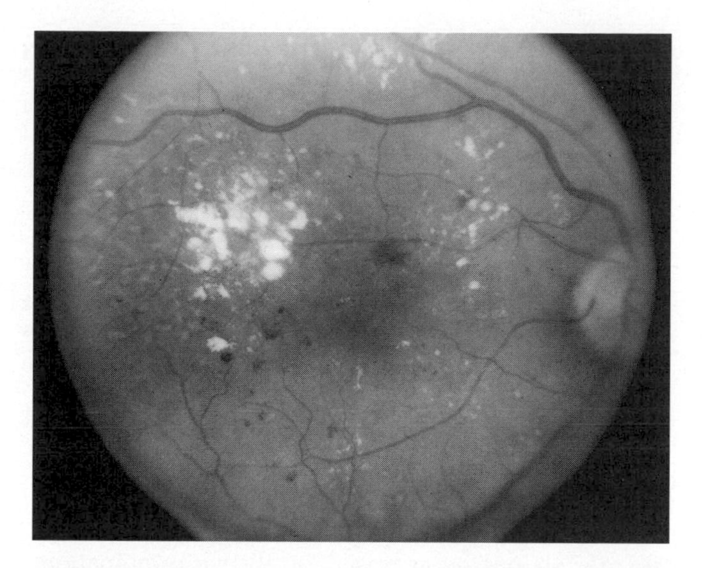

Figure 16–3. Diabetic macular edema. This eye has clinically significant macular edema with hard exudates <500 microns from the center of the macula with an adjacent area of retinal thickening (thickening not appreciated without stereoscopic viewing).

work showing the involvement of vascular endothelial growth factor and protein kinase C in the development of diabetic retinopathy and diabetic macular edema has fostered hope that inhibition of these proteins will be clinically efficacious.

Proper ocular examination of the diabetic patient requires careful attention to visual acuity measurement and refraction, pupillary responses, extraocular muscle movements, the presence or absence of new vessels on the iris, cataracts, and careful fundus examination through dilated pupils annually. The presence of ocular or other medical abnormalities requires more frequent examination (Table 16–8).

CONCLUSION

Diabetes mellitus is a complex syndrome with the potential for devastating systemic and ocular complications. Eyecare providers and other healthcare

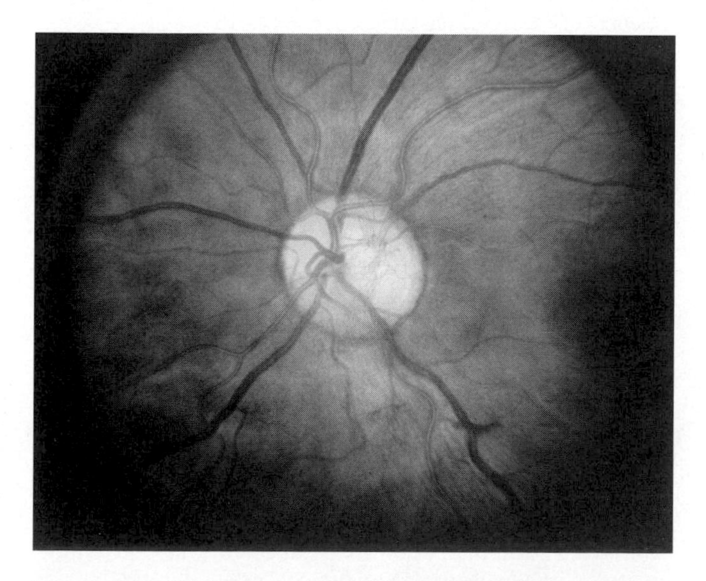

Figure 16–2. Proliferative diabetic retinopathy (PDR). There are new vessels on the optic nerve head greater than 1/4 of disc area. This patient has high-risk PDR and should be referred for prompt scatter (panretinal) laser photocoagulation surgery.

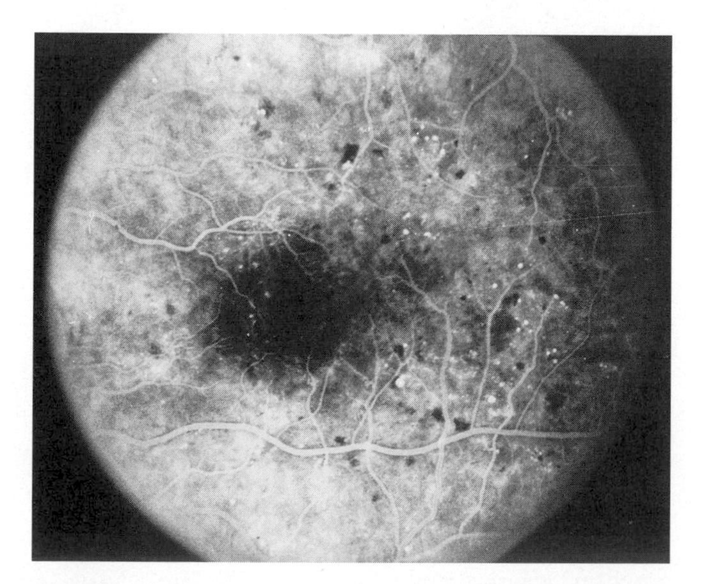

Figure 16–4. Fluorescein angiogram showing nonperfusion in the macular area.

TABLE 16–8. SUGGESTED FREQUENCY OF EYE EXAMINATION

Patient Group	Recommended First Examination	Minimum Routine Follow-Up (Abnormal Findings Necessitate More Frequent Follow-Up)
29 years or younger (type 1 DM)	Within 3–5 years of diagnosis once person is age 10 years or older	Yearly
30 years or older (type 2 DM)	Upon diagnosis of DM	Yearly
Pregnancy in pre-existing DM	• Prior to conception for counseling • Early in first trimester	Physician discretion pending results of first trimester examination

providers caring for patients with diabetes need to pay constant attention to all potential ocular complications of diabetes. A patient's diabetologist or primary provider should be apprised of all eye examination findings, and patients should be encouraged to maintain an active role in the care of their diabetes in conjunction with the other members of the healthcare team. Aggressive control of blood sugar, blood pressure, and serum lipids translates into preservation of eyesight and a reduced need for laser and other surgical treatment.

> Our current understanding and classification of the diabetic syndromes is in a continuous state of evolution.

REFERENCES

American Diabetes Association. Clinical practice recommendations 2000. *Diabetes Care.* 2000;23 (suppl 1):1–112.

Kahn CR, Weir GC, (eds). *Joslin's Diabetes Mellitus.* 13th ed. Philadelphia: Lea & Febiger; 1994:771–793.

Klein R, Klein BEK, Moss SE, et al. The Wisconsin Epidemiologic Study of Diabetic Retinopathy, 2. Prevalence and risk of diabetic retinopathy when age at diagnosis is less than 30 years. *Arch Ophthalmol.* 1984;102:520–526.

Klein R, Klein BEK, Moss SE et al. The Wisconsin Epidemiologic Study of Diabetic Retinopathy, 3. Prevalence and risk of diabetic retinopathy when age at diagnosis is 30 or more years. *Arch Ophthalmol.* 1984;102:527–532.

McDermott M, ed. *Endocrine Secrets.* Philadelphia: Hanley and Belfus; 1995.

Meigs JB, Mittleman MA, Nathan DM, et al. Hyperinsulinemia, hyperglycemia, and impaired hemostasis: The Framingham Offspring Study. *JAMA.* 2000;283:221–228.

White JR Jr. The pharmacologic reduction of blood glucose in patients with type 2 diabetes mellitus. *Clin Diabetes.* 1998;16:58–67.

Zimmer P, Turner R, McCarty D, et al. Crucial points at diagnosis. Type 2 diabetes or slow type 1 diabetes. *Diabetes Care.* 1999;22 (suppl 2):B59–64.

Diabetic Retinopathy Study (DRS)

Diabetic Retinopathy Study report 1: Preliminary report on effects of photocoagulation therapy. *Am J Ophthalmol.* 1976; 81:1–14.

Diabetic Retinopathy Study report 2: Photocoagulation of proliferative diabetic retinopathy. *Ophthalmology.* 1978; 85:82.

Diabetic Retinopathy Study report 3: Four risk factors for severe visual loss in diabetic retinopathy. *Arch Ophthalmol.* 1979;97:658.

Diabetic Retinopathy Study report 4: A short report of long range results. Proceedings of the 10th Congress of International Diabetes Federation. *Excerpta Medica.* 1980.

Diabetic Retinopathy Study report 5: Photocoagulation treatment of proliferative diabetic retinopathy. Relationship of adverse treatment effects to retinopathy severity. *Dev Ophthalmol.* (S. Karger, Basel). 1981;2(39):1–15.

Diabetic Retinopathy Study report 6: Design, methods, and baseline results. *Invest Ophthalmol.* 1981;21:149–209.

Diabetic Retinopathy Study report 7: A modification of the Airlie House Classification of Diabetic Retinopathy. *Invest Ophthalmol.* 1981;21:210–226.

Diabetic Retinopathy Study report 8: Photocoagulation treatment of proliferative diabetic retinopathy. Clinical application of Diabetic Retinopathy Study (DRS) findings. *Ophthalmology.* 1981;88:583–600.

Diabetic Retinopathy Study report 9: Assessing possible late treatment effects in stopping clinical trials early: A case study by F Ederer, MJ Podgor. *Control Clin Trials.* 1984; 5:373–381.

Diabetic Retinopathy Study report 10: Factors influencing the development of visual loss in advanced diabetic retinopathy. *Invest Ophthalmol.* 1985;26:983–991.

Diabetic Retinopathy Study report 11: Intraocular pressure following panretinal photocoagulation for diabetic retinopathy. *Arch Ophthalmol.* 1987;105:807–809.

Diabetic Retinopathy Study report 12: Macular edema in Diabetic Retinopathy Study patients. *Ophthalmology.* 1987; 94:754–760.

Diabetic Retinopathy Study report 13: Factors associated with visual outcome after photocoagulation for diabetic retinopathy. *Invest Ophthalmol.* 1989;30:23–28.

Diabetic Retinopathy Study report 14: Indications for photocoagulation treatment of diabetic retinopathy. *Int Ophthalmol Clin.* 1987;27:239–253.

Early Treatment Diabetic Retinopathy Study (ETDRS)

Chew EY, Klein ML, Ferris FL III, et al. Early Treatment Diabetic Retinopathy Study report 22. Association of elevated serum lipid levels with retinal hard exudates in diabetic retinopathy. *Arch Ophthalmol.* 1996;114:1079–1084.

Chew EY, Klein ML, Murphy RP, et al. Early Treatment Diabetic Retinopathy Study report 20. Effects of aspirin on vitreous/preretinal hemorrhage in patients with diabetes mellitus. *Arch Ophthalmol.* 1995;13:52–55.

Diabetic Retinopathy Study Research Group. Macular edema in diabetic retinopathy study patients. DRS report 12. *Ophthalmology.* 1987;94:754–760.

Diabetic Retinopathy Study report 13: Factors associated with visual outcome after photocoagulation for diabetic retinopathy. *Invest Ophthalmol.* 1989;30:23–28.

Diabetic Retinopathy Study Research Group. Indications for photocoagulation treatment of diabetic retinopathy. DRS report 14. *Int Ophthalmol Clin.* 1987;27:239–253.

Early Treatment Diabetic Retinopathy Study Research Group. Photocoagulation for diabetic macular edema. ETDRS report 1. *Arch Ophthalmol.* 1985;103:1796–1806.

Early Treatment Diabetic Retinopathy Study Research Group. Treatment techniques and clinical guidelines for photocoagulation of diabetic macular edema. ETDRS report 2. *Ophthalmology.* 1987;96:761–774.

Early Treatment Diabetic Retinopathy Study Research Group. Techniques for scatter and local photocoagulation treatment of diabetic retinopathy. ETDRS report 3. *Int Ophthalmol Clin.* 1987;27:254–264.

Early Treatment Diabetic Retinopathy Study Research Group. Photocoagulation for diabetic macular edema. ETDRS report 4. *Int Ophthalmol Clin.* 1987;27:265–272.

Early Treatment Diabetic Retinopathy Study Research Group. Case reports to accompany early treatment diabetic retinopathy study reports 3 and 4. *Int Ophthalmol Clin.* 1987;27:273–333.

Early Treatment Diabetic Retinopathy Study Research Group. Detection of diabetic macular edema: Ophthalmoscopy versus photography. ETDRS report 5. *Ophthalmology.* 1989;96:746–751.

Early Treatment Diabetic Retinopathy Study Research Group. C-peptide and the classification of diabetes patients in the Early Treatment Diabetic Retinopathy Study. ETDRS report 6. *Ann Epidemiol.* 1993;3:9–17.

Early Treatment Diabetic Retinopathy Study Research Group. Design and baseline patient characteristics. ETDRS report 7. *Ophthalmology.* 1991;98:741–756.

Early Treatment Diabetic Retinopathy Study Research Group. Effects of aspirin treatment on diabetic retinopathy. ETDRS report 8. *Ophthalmology.* 1991;98:757–765.

Early Treatment Diabetic Retinopathy Study Research Group. Early photocoagulation for diabetic retinopathy. ETDRS report 9. *Ophthalmology.* 1991;98:766–785.

Early Treatment Diabetic Retinopathy Study Research Group. Grading diabetic retinopathy from stereoscopic color fundus photographs: An extension of the modified Airlie House classification. ETDRS report 10. *Ophthalmology.* 1991;98:786–806.

Early Treatment Diabetic Retinopathy Study Research Group. Classification of diabetic retinopathy from fluorescein angiograms. ETDRS report 11. *Ophthalmology.* 1991; 98:807–822.

Early Treatment Diabetic Retinopathy Study Research Group. Fundus photographic risk factors for progression of diabetic retinopathy. ETDRS report 12. *Ophthalmology.* 1991;98:823–833.

Early Treatment Diabetic Retinopathy Study Research Group. Fluorescein angiographic risk factors for progression of diabetic retinopathy. ETDRS report 13. *Ophthalmology.* 1991;98:834–840.

Early Treatment Diabetic Retinopathy Study Research Group. Aspirin effects on mortality and morbidity in patients with diabetes mellitus. ETDRS report 14. *JAMA.* 1992;268:1292–1300.

Early Treatment Diabetic Retinopathy Study Research Group. Aspirin effects on the development of cataracts in patients with diabetes mellitus. ETDRS report 16. *Arch Ophthalmol.* 1992;110:339–342.

Early Treatment Diabetic Retinopathy Study Research Group. Pars plana vitrectomy in the Early Treatment Diabetic Retinopathy Study. ETDRS report 17. *Ophthalmology.* 1992;99:1351–1357.

Early Treatment Diabetic Retinopathy Study report 19. Focal photocoagulation treatment of diabetic macular edema: Relationship of treatment effect to fluorescein angiographic and other retinal characteristics at baseline. *Arch Ophthalmol.* 1995;113:1144–1155.

Diabetic Retinopathy Vitrectomy Study (DRVS)

Diabetic Retinopathy Vitrectomy Study report 1: Two-year course of visual acuity in severe proliferative diabetic retinopathy with conventional management. *Ophthalmology.* 1985;92:492–502.

Diabetic Retinopathy Vitrectomy Study report 2: Early vitrectomy for severe vitreous hemorrhage in diabetic retinopathy. Two-year results of a randomized trial. *Arch Ophthalmol.* 1985;103:1644–1652.

Diabetic Retinopathy Vitrectomy Study report 3: Early vitrectomy for severe proliferative diabetic retinopathy in eyes with useful vision. Results of a randomized trial. *Ophthalmology.* 1988;95:1307–1320.

Diabetic Retinopathy Vitrectomy Study report 4: Early vitrectomy for severe proliferative diabetic retinopathy in eyes with useful vision. Clinical application of results of a randomized trial. *Ophthalmology.* 1988;95:1331–1334.

Diabetic Retinopathy Vitrectomy Study report 5: Early vitrectomy for severe vitreous hemorrhage in diabetic retinopathy. Four-year results of a randomized trial. *Arch Ophthalmol.* 1990;108:958–964.

Diabetes Control and Complications Trial (DCCT)

Diabetes Control and Complications Trial Research Group. Are continuing studies of metabolic control and microvascular complications in insulin-dependent diabetes mellitus justified? *N Engl J Med.* 1988;318:246–250.

Diabetes Control and Complications Trial Resesearch Group. The relationship of glycemic exposure (HbA_{1c}) to the risk of development and progression of retinopathy in the Diabetes Control and Complications Trial. *Diabetes.* 1995; 44:968–983.

Diabetes Control and Complications Trial Research Group. Progression of retinopathy with intensive versus conventional treatment in the Diabetes Control and Complications Trial. *Ophthalmology.* 1995;102:647–661.

Diabetes Control and Complications Trial Research Group. Hypoglycemia in the Diabetes Control and Complications Trial. *Diabetes.* 1997;46:271–286.

Diabetes Control and Complications Trial Research Group. Lifetime benefits and costs of intensive therapy as practiced in the Diabetes Control and Complications Trial. *JAMA.* 1996;276:1409–1415.

Diabetes Control and Complications Trial Research Group The effect of intensive treatment of diabetes on the development and progression of long term complications in insulin-dependent diabetes mellitus. *N Engl J Med.* 1993; 329:977–986.

United Kingdom Prospective Diabetes Study (UKPDS)

UK Prospective Diabetes Study Group. Effect of intensive blood-glucose control with metformin on complications in overweight patients with type 2 diabetes. *Lancet.* 1998; 352:854–865.

UK Prospective Diabetes Study Group. Intensive blood-glucose control with sulphonylureas or insulin compared with conventional treatments and risk of complications in patients with diabetes. *Lancet.* 1998;352:837–853.

UK Prospective Diabetes Study Group. Tight blood pressure control and the risk of macrovascular and microvascular complications in type 2 diabetes: UKPDS 38. *BMJ.* 1998; 703–713.

UK Prospective Diabetes Study Group. Cost-effectiveness analysis of improved blood pressure control in hypertensive patients with type 2 diabetes: UKPDS 40. *BMJ.* 1998; 317:720–726.

Chapter 17

THYROID DYSFUNCTION

Bernard J. Dolan

The thyroid gland secretes hormones that maintain the normal metabolic function of the body. The production and release of excess thyroid hormones results in increased metabolic activity, and is referred to as hyperthyroidism. The most common form of hyperthyroidism is Graves' disease, an autoimmune condition of the thyroid. A decrease in the production and release of thyroid hormones results in decreased metabolic activity and is called hypothyroidism. The most common cause of noniatrogenic thyroid failure in the United States is chronic autoimmune thyroiditis (Hashimoto's disease). Normal production and release of thyroid hormones is called the euthyroid state. Goiter is a diffuse or nodular enlargement of the thyroid that can occur in the hyperthyroid, hypothyroid, or euthyroid states. The most common thyroid disorder is iodine deficiency, which leads to goiter and hypothyroidism. This discussion will emphasize those thyroid disorders that are associated with the ocular findings of Graves' ophthalmopathy.

EPIDEMIOLOGY

Systemic

Hyperthyroidism

Graves' disease most commonly presents in adults 20 to 50 years old. It occurs about eight times more often in females than males. It is much less common in the elderly and is unusual in children under 10 years of age (Volpé, 1991). Prevalence in the United States is unknown, but a well-designed population study in England reported a past and present prevalence of 2.7% in women and 0.3% in men (Vanderpump et al, 1998).

Hypothyroidism

There are a variety of causes of hypothyroidism, with the epidemiology varying with the specific disorder. Factors that influence the incidence of hypothyroidism include population, age, and genetic characteristics, as well as geography and dietary iodine intake. Hypothyroidism affects approximately 2% of females and 0.1 to 0.2% of males in North America (Larsen et al, 1998). The most common cause of goiterous hypothyroidism in iodine-sufficient areas occurs in the presence of thyroid antibodies which lead to the term autoimmune thyroiditis (Hashimoto's disease). It occurs four times more often in women than men with an approximate incidence of 3.5 cases per 1000 individuals per year in women and 0.8 cases per individual per year in men (Vanderpump et al, 1998). Sporadic congenital hypothyroidism arrests normal development and results in the physical and mental retardation. It occurs in about 1 in every 5000 births in the white population and 1 in every 32,000 births in the African-American population (Greenspan, 1997).

Ocular

Hyperthyroidism

Graves' ophthalmopathy most commonly presents in 30- to 50-year-old females. The female to male ratio is 4 to 1. The severe form of the disease represents only 3 to 5% of cases (Burch & Wartofsky, 1993). Elderly patients with Graves' disease are less likely to develop eye findings. However, elderly patients tend to have more severe eye disease, and men seem to be more severely affected than are women (Kendler et al, 1993). Incidence in this country is 16 cases per 100,000 individuals per year for women and 2.9 cases per 100,000 individuals per year for men (Bartley, 1994). Smoking appears to be a risk factor for development and severity of ocular findings (Bartalena et al, 2000). Approximately 50% of patients with Graves' ophthalmopathy have some component of clinically evident ophthalmopathy, and it occurs in some patients with Hashimoto's thyroiditis.

Hypothyroidism

No information is available in the literature concerning the epidemiology of the ocular involvement, which is more an ocular manifestation of systemic hypothyroidism.

PATHOPHYSIOLOGY/DISEASE PROCESS

Anatomy and Physiology

The thyroid is the largest endocrine gland in the normal adult. Located in the anterior portion of the lower neck, it consists of a right and left lobe that are lateral to the trachea and connected by a small isthmus. An embryologic remnant of the thyroglossal duct is sometimes present in the form of a pyramidal lobe. Due to the migration of the thyroglossal duct from the second pharyngeal pouch during embryonic development, thyroid tissue may be found throughout the neck region.

The thyroid is composed of numerous microscopic closed vesicles, called follicles, lined by a simple cuboidal epithelium and filled with a proteinaceous colloidal material. This colloidal material is composed of thyroglobulin, a high-molecular-weight iodinated glycoprotein that stores the thyroid hormones.

Iodine, an essential component of thyroid hormones, is a somewhat rare element. Therefore, proper dietary intake is necessary to ensure an adequate iodine supply. Iodized salt, sea fish, milk, and eggs are good dietary sources of this element. The epithelial cells lining the thyroid follicle act as a very efficient trap to concentrate the iodide available in the body. The presence of thyroid-stimulating hormone (TSH), or thyrotropin, from the pituitary acts to stimulate thyroid iodide transport, while its absence results in markedly decreased iodide transport.

Iodide trapped by the thyroid is rapidly oxidized to iodine and through a series of complex reactions is incorporated into the tyrosine molecule to form the basic building blocks of the thyroid hormones triiodothyronine (T_3) and thyroxine (T_4). Thyroglobulin acts as a substrate for the iodination and coupling of the tyrosines. The T_3 and T_4 hormones are stored in the follicular lumen attached to thyroglobulin until they are released.

Both the production and release of the thyroid hormones are stimulated by TSH. The secretion of TSH is under control of thyroid-releasing hormone (TRH), which is synthesized in the hypothalamus. TRH binds to the thyrotrope cells of the anterior pituitary and stimulates the release of TSH. This hormone then binds to specific receptors of the thyroid follicular cell, stimulating the production and release of thyroid hormones (Figure 17–1).

The normal thyroid gland does not produce equal amounts of the thyroid hormones. The extrathyroidal pool of T_4 is approximately 20 times greater than the pool of T_3 and the half-life of T_4 is 7 days versus 1 day for T_3. Although T_3 is the more potent thyroid hormone, only a small amount of the peripheral concentration comes from direct thyroidal secretion. The major component of thyroid secretion is T_4, which is converted by deiodination in the peripheral tissues to produce active T_3. The effects of T_4 in the peripheral tissues may rely on its conversion to T_3. This has lead to the suggestion that T_4 is a T_3 prohormone. In addition, the conversion

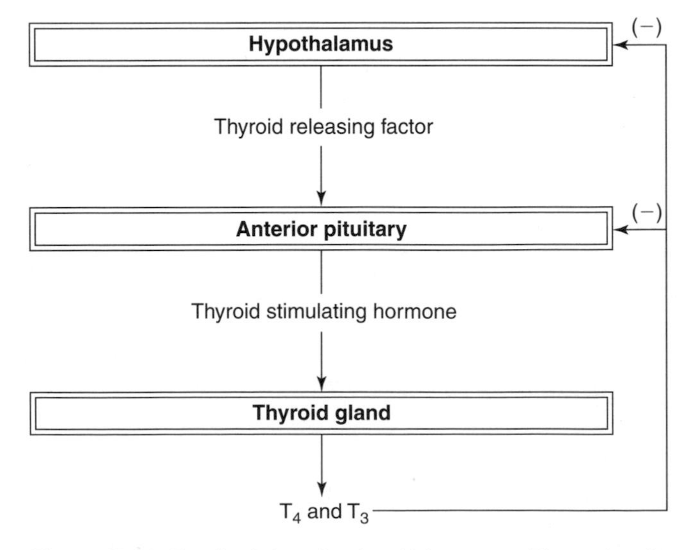

Figure 17–1. Feedback loop for thyroid hormones. The major site of the inhibition is at the pituitary level, with the inhibitory effect of T_4 primarily mediated through its conversion to T_4 within the gland.

of T_4 to T_3 is controlled by different enzymes of various tissue types, which may provide additional regulation of thyroid hormone function.

Thyroid hormones in the blood are bound to specific serum proteins, thyroxine-binding globulins (TBG), thyroxine-binding prealbumin (TBPA), and albumin. These proteins have a higher affinity for T_4, which normally has only 0.03% of the hormone circulating in the free unbound state. T_3 is less tightly bound, with about 0.3% of the hormone in the unbound state. Serum-binding proteins act as a metabolic storage compartment for the thyroid hormones, protecting this reservoir from excretion and metabolic degradation. The metabolic effects of the thyroid hormones appear to be related to the amount of hormone circulating in the free state.

In order to prevent the excess production and secretion of thyroid hormones, a negative feedback loop is required. An increase in the serum concentration of the thyroid hormones is effective in inhibiting the pituitary production and secretion of TSH. In addition, thyroid hormones influence the inhibition of TSH when injected into the hypothalamus; however, the role they play in affecting TRH concentration is uncertain.

Thyroid hormones act to stimulate the cellular metabolic reactions of tissues throughout the body. By enhancing oxygen consumption, stimulating protein synthesis, stimulating lipolysis, and activating hepatic glyconeogenesis, the thyroid hormones enhance the generation of body heat. It has been estimated that thyroid hormones regulate 40% of the body's resting oxygen consumption. Normal growth and sexual development of the body will not occur in the absence of thyroid hormones. Skin and connective tissue depend on these hormones for the integrity of normal collagen and hair growth. Myocardial proteins regulating cardiac contractibility are affected by thyroid hormones. The nervous system requires these hormones for the normal production of neurons, dendrite and myelin formation, and normal nerve conduction. In addition, the thyroid hormones affect gastrointestinal motility, endocrine gland functions, and red blood cell production.

TABLE 17–1. SYSTEMIC MANIFESTATIONS OF THYROID DISORDERS

Hyperthyroidism	Hypothyroidism
• **Symptoms**	• **Symptoms**
Nervousness	Cold intolerance
Heat intolerance	Weakness
Sweating	Reduced energy
Fatigue	Lethargy
Palpitation	Muscle cramps
Insomnia	Constipation
Early waking	Increased sleeping
Alopecia	Weight gain
Vitiligo	Reduced appetite
Brittle nails	Joint stiffness
• **Signs**	• **Signs**
Sweating	Cool, scaling skin
Proximal muscle weakness	Puffy hands and face
Emotionally labile	Deep voice
Tremor	Myotonia
Tachycardia	Delirium
Arrhythmia (atrial fibrillation)	Bradycardia
Hypertension (systolic)	Slow reflexes
Brisk deep-tendon reflexes	Obesity
Diabetes	Hypothermia
Increased triglycerides and calcium	Myxedema
Decreased cholesterol	• **Signs in children (cretinism)**
Microcytic anemia	Growth failure
	Delayed puberty
	Mental retardation
	Sparse hair
	Large abdomen
	Flat nose
	Poor muscle tone

Systemic

Table 17–1 summarizes the systemic manifestations of thyroid disorders.

Thyrotoxicosis

Thyrotoxicosis refers to a clinical syndrome comprising many physiologic and biochemical changes. These are produced by the alterations in cellular metabolism due to increased amounts of thyroid hormones. The signs and symptoms of thyrotoxicosis involve many organ systems, because thyroid hormone receptors are present on all cells of the body. Thyrotoxicosis has a number of etiologies, including primary hyperthyroidism (Graves' disease), excess thyroid medication in the treatment of hypothyroidism or goiter, a toxic multinodular goiter, toxic adenoma, excess iodine, inflammatory induced leakage of thyroid hormones, excess hormone produced by ectopic thyroid tissue, and thyroid carcinoma or choriocarcinoma. Thus, *thyrotoxicosis* refers to disorders of elevated thyroid hormones without regard for the source, while *hyperthyroidism* is reserved for those cases where excess thyroid hormones are a product of thyroid hypersecretion. The clinical presentation of thyrotoxicosis in these various disorders has many similar components; however, these will vary with the age of the patient, severity of the disorder, and pathophysiology of the specific syndrome.

The clinical manifestations of thyrotoxicosis are usually dramatic and involve virtually every body system. The mechanism of the thyroid hormone action on different body tissues varies, and the sum total of these actions results in the clinical findings of this disorder. These clinical characteristics are modulated through thyroid hormone interaction with the plasma membrane in some tissues and the mitochondria in other tissues, but more commonly the cell nucleus is the target. When the hormone target is the cell nucleus, the mode of action is classified as genomic. The nongenomic mode of action includes the plasma membrane, mitochondria, or any other cell structure outside the nucleus. Genomic action involves only T_3 and takes several hours for the modification of gene transcription. Nongenomic action involves T_3 and T_4 and occurs rapidly. Some thyroid-mediated processes seem to involve both genomic and nongenomic action.

Some details in the genomic action of thyroid hormone have been identified. T_3 and T_4 enter the cytoplasm of the target tissue cell. In some tissues T_4 is convert into T_3, the active form of hormone. T_3 enters the nucleus and binds to high-affinity thyroid hormone receptors. These complexes then bind with DNA nucleotide sequences in the regulatory region of specific genes. A wide variety of these thyroid receptor elements in the DNA have been identified. The thyroid receptor–DNA interaction is a complex process that involves the thyroid hormone nuclear receptors interacting with various receptor partner molecules. These partners may bind with a specific thyroid receptor forming a heterodimer, which will bind to a specific DNA sequence. The binding to the DNA sequence modulates gene transcription and is further influenced by cofactors that may act to stimulate or inhibit gene expression.

Nongenomic actions of thyroid hormone often involve the interaction with part of the cellular transduction pathways such as protein kinase and cAMP. Hormone targets include the plasma membrane, mitochondria, sarcoplasmic reticulum, and vascular smooth muscle contractile elements. They may modulate cellular respiration, cell morphology, vascular tone, or ion homeostasis. In these nongenomic actions of thyroid hormone, the response of the tissues is seen within minutes of stimulation. Examples include inactivation of the Na^+ channel in myocardium cells, increased red blood cell Ca^{++} ATPase activity, and relaxation of vascular smooth muscle.

Thyrotoxicosis affects the metabolism and removal of numerous drugs from the body. This usually results in requiring an increased medication dosage to maintain the therapeutic effect. However, the therapeutic activity of some drugs, including the anticoagulants heparin and coumadin, are enhanced by increased thyroid hormone levels.

Thyrotoxicosis varies in its clinical presentation from a syndrome with few clinical features to a life-threatening alteration of metabolic functions called thyroid storm. This is a rapidly progressing decompensation of hyperthyroidism with marked delirium, severe tachycardia, vomiting, diarrhea, and often very high fever. If not promptly identified and properly treated, it often results in death due to cardiovascular collapse. Thyroid storm is rarely seen today, but may occur in patients with additional stress from surgery or illness.

Hyperthyroidism

Graves' disease is an autoimmune-induced thyrotoxicosis characterized by a diffuse goiter. About one half of cases have some clinically evident component of the associated infiltrative orbitopathy. This is due to cellular infiltration and mucopolysaccharide deposition in the extraocular muscle and cellular infiltration of the orbit. The associated dermopathy is an uncommon manifestation characterized by a localized nonpitting edema (myxedema) occurring in 0.5 to 4%. Also less commonly associated is clubbing of the fingers, called thyroid acropachy (1%). Stress or hormone change have been implicated as contributing to the onset, although this remains controversial.

In Graves' disease, as in other autoimmune disorders, the immune system fails to recognize self from non-self. Antibodies are produced by lymphocytes that bind to the TSH receptor in the plasma membrane of the thyroid follicular cell. These antibodies mimic the action of TSH and stimulate the receptor. This activates the metabolic processes in the production and secretion of the thyroid hormones. The resulting high concentrations of thyroid hormones act on the pituitary to inhibit the release of TSH and the thyrotropes' response to TRH. Since there is no negative feedback to the lymphocytes producing the antibodies, the result is an uncontrolled production and release of the thyroid hormones. This leads to thyroid growth, increased vascularity, and excess thyroid function, which are manifested clinically as goiter and thyrotoxicosis. Improved assays have demonstrated TSH-receptor antibodies in the peripheral blood of 95% of untreated patients, and their presence in all patients with Graves' disease is widely accepted (McIver & Morris, 1998). Antibodies to other thyroid antigens including thyroid peroxidase and thyroglobulin appear to play no role in the pathogenesis of this disorder; however, they are markers of widespread thyroid autoimmunity and immune system dysfunction in Graves' disease. Lymphocyte infiltration of the thyroid is a characteristic of this disorder with T cell infiltration greater than B cell and plasma-cell infiltration (Wiersinga, 1997). Activated T cells secrete cytokines with interleukins in a Th2 profile, stimulating B cells and antibody production in the thyroid. This is in contrast to a Th1 pattern of interleukin secretion in the retroorbital tissues that promote a cell-mediated response.

With constant stimulation by thyroid receptor antibodies, the production of thyroid hormones increases many times the normal rate. This excess stimulation of the thyroid hormones biosynthetic pathway results in a relative increase in the production of T_3 as compared to T_4. The amount of T_3 in the blood derived from thyroidal secretion has been estimated to increase from less than 20% in normals to more than 40% in hyperthyroidism.

The presence of excess thyroid hormones produces abnormalities in the biochemical pathways and has a marked effect on almost every tissue of the body. Numerous enzymes and proteins are synthesized, while others are broken down. The complex interaction of these tissues and their metabolic response cannot be explained by a single mechanism.

The natural history of Graves' disease is unclear. It is evident that some patients can recover normal thyroid function spontaneously without treatment, sometimes even becoming hypothyroid. However, other untreated patients will remain chronically hyperthyroid, with cyclic periods of exacerbation and remission, and only after months or years will the thyrotoxic component burn itself out; still other patients will progress and die from the complications of thyroid storm. It has been estimated that one third of the patients with Graves' disease would fall into each category; however, other forms of hyperthyroidism could not easily be distinguished at the time these observations were made. Although it is clear that some patients can improve without therapy, presently there is no reliable way to identify them. Therefore, until the clinical or laboratory testing characteristics of these patients who spontaneously return to normal are clearly identified, treatment is recommended for all symptomatic patients.

The signs and symptoms of Graves' disease are a gradual onset of thyrotoxicosis, with or without the signs of ophthalmopathy. Symptoms of thyrotoxicosis can include heat intolerance, weight loss, increased appetite, palpitation, fatigue, muscular weakness, nervousness, irritability, depression, and increased bowel motility. Difficulty sleeping and early-morning wakening are common findings. The apparent need to be constantly active contrasts with the concurrent symptoms of fatigue and muscle weakness. Difficulty concentrating on tasks and a decreased tolerance to emotional stress may also be present. Increased bowel motility often results in more frequent and softer bowel movements, but rarely in frank diarrhea. Skin may be smooth, soft, warm, oily, and moist. Hair may also be oily. Alteration of libido or menstrual cycle—with decrease in flow or oligomenorrhea may also be noted.

Often the symptoms may be vague, or the significance of an isolated complaint may be difficult to recognize. Heat intolerance may contribute to strain on the living situation, as the patient is constantly lowering the thermostat, opening windows, or removing covers from the bed. Climbing stairs leads to weakness, fatigue, and shortness of breath. Chronic muscular fatigue in the proximal muscle groups more than the distal may result in complaints of shoulder weakness and difficulty raising from a low chair. Although weight loss with increased appetite is most common, a few patients may gain weight. Loss of ability to concentrate or to withstand emotional stress, or increased irritability, emotional lability, or depression may underlie complaints of difficulty with interpersonal relationships.

An increased basal metabolic rate and moderately elevated respiratory rate are also evident. Microcytic anemia and weak contraction of skeletal muscle may be seen in some cases. Changes in the skin include alopecia, vitiligo, and brittle nails. Thyrotoxicosis alters the carbohydrate, lipid, and calcium metabolism. This can result in abnormal glucose tolerance curves, diabetes, or the exacerbation of existing diabetes. Serum calcium, fasting free fatty acids, and triglyceride levels can increase, while cholesterol is reduced. In addition, there are brisk deep-tendon reflexes.

The cardiovascular signs can be among the most prominent, with increased demand due to elevated metabolic rate and the need to dissipate excess heat. Tachycardia is often present, with a pulse rate of greater than 90, even at rest. The increased force of contraction can be felt as palpitation, which increases in frequency with exercise. Some 10% of thyrotoxic patients may develop an arrhythmia, most often atrial fibrillation. The increased demand does not commonly lead to cardiac disorders unless underlying heart disease is present. Elevation of the systolic, but not the diastolic, blood pressure is common.

Thus, the classic thyrotoxicosis patient is a sweaty, tremulous, fidgety individual with a short attention span. Most often this complex of symptoms develops slowly over a period of months or years; however, it can occur within a few weeks or less. More acute development may be associated with emotional stress at the time symptoms appeared.

Hypothyroidism

Hypothyroidism is the clinical syndrome characterized by the deficiency of thyroid hormones and the resultant cellular responses. It is classified as primary hypothyroidism when alteration in the thyroid gland is responsible for the decrease in thyroid hormones. This occurs due to chronic autoimmune thyroiditis (Hashimoto's disease), surgical or radioiodine treatment for Graves' disease, irradiation of neck neoplasm, subacute thyroiditis, dietary deficiency of iodine (endemic goiter), drugs (eg, lithium), or congenital biosynthetic defect. Secondary hypothyroidism is the deficiency of thyroid hormones due to pituitary TSH deficit, which can occur in pituitary adenoma or ablative therapy. Tertiary hypothyroidism is due to deficiency of hypothalamic TRH, and is rare. Finally, hypothyroidism can be due to peripheral tissue resistance to the action of the thyroid hormones, an extremely rare condition.

Chronic autoimmune thyroiditis (Hashimoto's disease) is the most common type of hypothyroidism in this country. This disorder frequently occurs in individuals with a positive family history or with family members but no clinical manifestations, who have antithyroidal antibodies. It may be associated with a goiter in younger patients, but the gland is often destroyed by the immune processes in the adult. It is characterized by thyroid destruction as the thyroid is infiltrated primarily with T cells that produce lymphokines, resulting in a cell-mediated destructive mechanism. Autoantibodies to thyroglobulin and thyroid peroxidase are common. Infrequently, patients with this disorder will develop Graves' ophthalmopathy.

Because the thyroid hormones are necessary for normal development, the clinical manifestations of hypothyroidism depend more on the age of onset than the specific cause of the disorder. Hypothyroidism in infants (cretinism) leads to interruption of bone growth, sparse hair, large abdomen, flat nose, poor muscle tone, and mental retardation. In children, the interruption of bone growth is seen, with retarded sexual development. In adults, hypothyroidism is characterized by myxedema.

In addition to myxedema, adult hypothyroidism is characterized by symptoms that include lethargy, chronic fatigue, weakness, muscle cramps, inability to concentrate, cold intolerance, decreased sweating, weight gain, amenorrhea, and chronic constipation. Clinical signs include bradycardia, with cardiac enlargement, occasionally hypertension, shallow respirations, cool skin, dry skin and hair, puffy hands and face, and slow reflexes.

Ocular

Table 17–2 summarizes the ocular manifestations of thyroid disorders.

TABLE 17–2. OCULAR MANIFESTATIONS OF THYROID DISORDERS

Hyperthyroidism

- Lids
  - Lid retraction
  - Lid lag
  - Lagophthalmos
- Cornea
  - Exposure keratitis
  - Photophobia
- Conjunctiva
  - Conjunctival or periorbital edema
- Extraocular muscles
  - Restriction
  - Diplopia
  - Increased IOP
  - Proptosis
  - Wide-eyed stare
- Optic nerve
  - Decreased vision
  - Visual field loss
  - Afferent pupillary defect
  - Decreased color vision
  - Blurred disc margins

Hypothyroidism

- Madarosis
- Periorbital myxedema
- Loss of lateral third of eyebrow
- Thyroid orbitopathy (rare)

Hyperthyroidism

Graves' ophthalmopathy is the most frequent extrathyroidal manifestation of Graves' disease (Figure 17–2). Its pathogenesis is not completely understood; however, the primary role of an autoimmune process is increasingly supported. The leading hypothesis suggests that there is a shared antigen between the thyroid and the orbital tissues, with the TSH receptor the leading candidate, which autoreactive T cell recognize (Bahn & Heufelder, 1993). Antigen recognition stimulates CD4+ T lymphocytes to secrete cytokines with interleukins that activate either CD8+ T lymphocytes or antibody-producing B cells. In addition, cytokines stimulate the synthesis and secretion of glycoaminoglycans by the fibroblasts. Present evidence suggest the fibroblasts and adipocytes are most likely the primary target of the autoimmune response in Graves' ophthalmopathy, with the muscle cells involved in a secondary response to the ongoing autoimmune reactions. The clinical complications are due to increased orbital volume caused by edematous expansion of the extraocular muscles and orbital connective tissues caused by the increased production of the hydrophilic glycosaminoglycans and proliferation of fibroblasts.

> Graves' ophthalmopathy is the leading cause of unilateral or bilateral exophthalmos in adults.

The natural history of Graves' ophthalmopathy is not well documented. In addition, its relationship to Graves' disease is confusing since the eye findings can occur before the onset, concomitantly, or after the on-

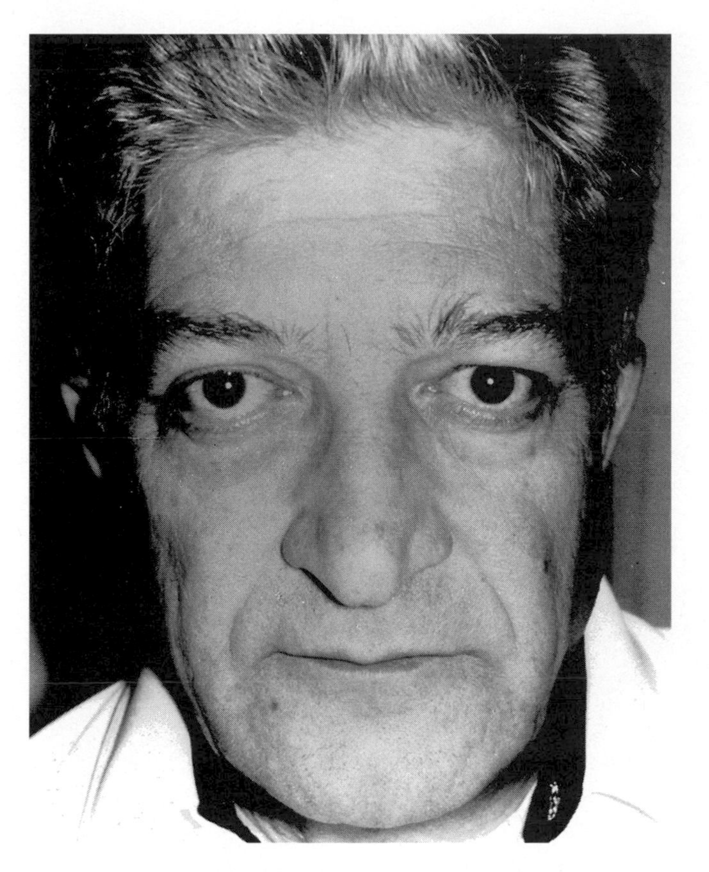

Figure 17–2. Patient with Graves' disease. Note proptosis and assymetric inferior lid retraction as evidenced by scleral show. (*Photo courtesy of Dr. Diane T. Adamczyk.*)

set of hyperthyroidism. The majority of patients develop hyperthyroidism prior to the ocular findings. Although in some cases the eye findings present prior to the development of hyperthyroidism, in 80% of cases they both develop within 18 months of each other (Gorman, 1983). In a few cases, their presentations may be separated by years. Most patients with Graves' disease develop some degree of ocular involvement. When findings are not clinically evident, enlargement of extraocular muscles is detectable by CT scan, MR imaging, or orbital ultrasound (Gorman, 1994). A more detailed analysis of the 10% of patients with apparent euthyroid ophthalmopathy reveals evidence of thyroid autoimmune disease when evaluated for thyroid antibodies, TSH regulation, and thyroid hormone production (Salvi et al, 1990). Recent studies suggest that 66% of Graves' ophthalmopathy cases spontaneously regress over 5 years, whereas only 15% become more severe (Bartley et al, 1996; Perros et al, 1996). Thus ophthalmopathy initially appears to undergo an active phase of progressive exacerbation, is followed by a slight regression, and finally reaches a stable, inactive phase where the ocular findings are unlikely to show further progression. The eye signs associated with Graves' disease are generally self-limiting and mild, yet in some cases become severe and threaten vision (Wiersinga, 1997).

The incidence of eye findings was recently reported with eyelid retraction as the most frequent sign (91%), followed by proptosis (62%), extraocular muscle dysfunction (42%), conjunctival injection (34%), eyelid edema (32%), chemosis (23%), and optic neuropathy (6%). Ocular symptoms in this series showed diplopia as the most frequent complaint (33%), followed by discomfort of pain (30%), lacrimation (21%), photophobia (16%), and blurred vision (7%) (Bartley et al, 1996).

Lids. Retraction of the upper or lower lid, and upper lid lag, are the ocular signs of thyrotoxicosis without regard to the specific cause. The normal position of the upper eyelid is 2 mm below the limbus, and the lower eyelid is at the limbus. Lid retraction is noted when the upper lid is positioned at the limbus or above with visible scleral tissue (Dalrymple sign) or the lower lid is 1 to 2 mm below the limbus. Widening of the palpebral fissure causes a characteristic stare. Closer observation is required to notice the upper lid lagging behind the globe as the eye is depressed (von Graffe sign). Elimination of thyrotoxicosis leads to the resolution of lid retraction and stare in one half to two thirds of patients.

The eye signs of infiltrative orbitopathy are due to the increased volume of the extraocular muscles or orbital tissue. These can include puffy, swollen lids; unilateral or bilateral proptosis; restriction of extraocular muscle; increased introcular pressure (IOP) upon upgaze; conjunctival injection; corneal exposure; decreased vision; blurred optic disc margins; or chorioretinal striae.

Conjunctiva/Periorbital Edema. Conjunctival or periorbital edema is a common early sign of thyroid eye disease. The swelling is most noticeable in the morning and decreases throughout the day. Inflammation of subcutaneous connective tissue and anterior displacement of orbital fat due to orbitopathy can lead to periorbital edema.

Extraocular Muscle Involvement/Proptosis. Enlargement of the extraocular muscles (EOM) is the prominent anatomical abnormality in infiltrative orbitopathy, which causes proptosis (Figure 17–3). Histologic studies have indicated lymphocytic infiltration, proliferation of fibroblasts, and edema within the interstitial tissue of the muscles. The muscle fibers appear normal. It is clear that both the extraocular muscle cells and the fibroblast play important roles in the patho-

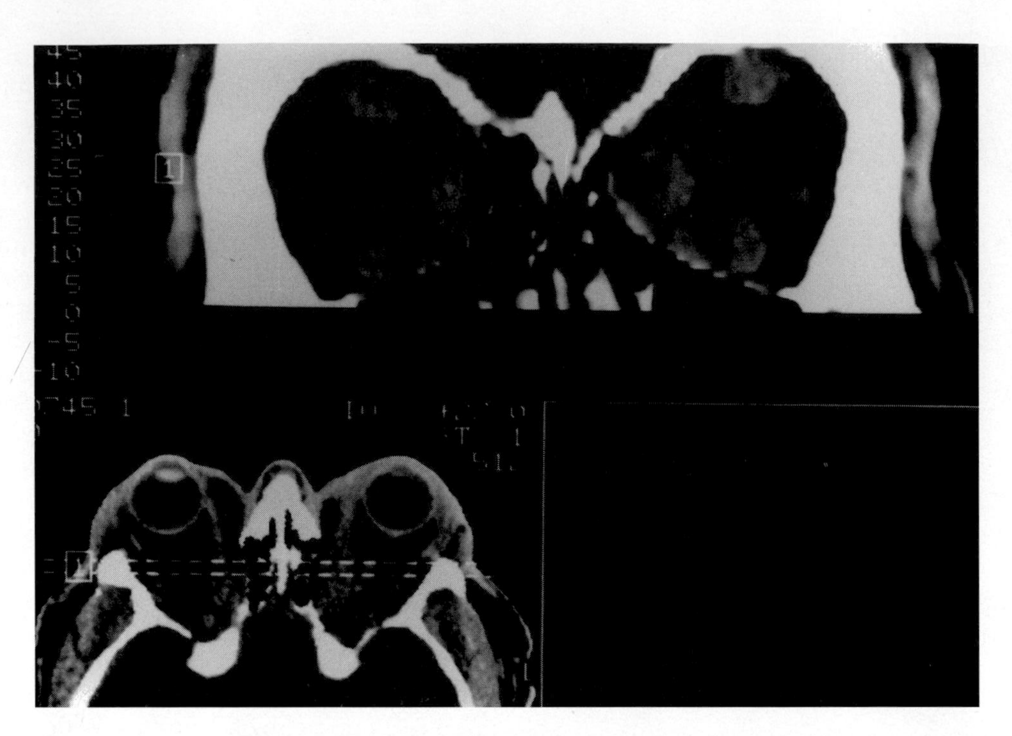

Figure 17–3. CT scan of the orbit demonstrating the enlargement of the extraocular muscles. Note that the inferior rectus and medial rectus are the two muscles most involved, with minimal involvement of the lateral rectus.

genesis of this disorder, and that the autoimmune basis for Graves' ophthalmopathy is directed against one or both of these tissues. Orbital fibroblasts have also been implicated in the production of glycoaminoglycans and collagenous connective tissue to replace orbital fat. This may occur by direct fibroblast stimulation, by antibodies, or due to interaction with lymphocytes within the inflammatory response. Despite the large body of clinical and experimental evidence regarding the role EOM cells and fibroblasts play in this disorder, the exact relationship between the orbital infiltration and hyperthyroidism remains unclear.

Proptosis may be unilateral or bilateral, with about 50% of patients having a difference of less than 5 mm between eyes, 89% having less than 7 mm of difference, and none with over 11 mm. A complaint of lashes touching the back of spectacle lenses may occur in advanced proptosis. Proptosis most often remains stable after reaching its maximum, usually within the first 2 years.

Abnormalities in extraocular muscle function can lead to restriction of movements. Initial complaints are of diplopia in upgaze, because the inferior rectus muscle is most commonly involved, followed by the medial, superior, and lateral recti muscles. These complaints are most common upon wakening, when very tired, or after one alcoholic beverage. An abnormal head position with an elevated chin may be necessary for driving to relieve the diplopia in upgaze. However, symmetric restriction from enlarged muscles does not always cause symptoms. Increased vascularity over the medial or lateral rectus insertion is found both with thyroid eye disease and myositis.

Cornea. When proptosis is severe enough to prevent lid closure, chronic corneal exposure can result. Ocular symptoms due to exposure keratopathy include gritty, irritable eyes and tearing. Proptosis can lead to complaints of corneal foreign body or reduced contact lens tolerance. This can be further complicated by the common loss of a Bell phenomenon due to significant involvement of the inferior rectus. Corneal scarring and ulceration can result with associated loss of vision. Occasionally this results in corneal perforation.

Optic Nerve Involvement. Only 2 to 7% develop severe, vision-threatening orbitopathy from optic nerve involvement. Patients with compressive optic neuropathy have gradual onset of visual loss, or visual field loss. The scotomas can be central, arcuate, altitudinal, paracentral, or a generalized constriction. Decreased vision associated with reduced brightness of colors is suggestive of optic nerve compression. Associated signs include afferent pupillary defect, color vision loss, disc edema, chorioretinal striae, and visual evoked potential abnormalities. The vast majority have an extraocular muscle disorder. Imaging studies have revealed apical compression of the optic nerve by enlarged muscle bodies as the underlying cause of this finding. Unilateral compression occurs in approximately 30% of cases.

Although many patients with extraocular myopathy may have only transient problems, the course of compressive neuropathy is difficult to predict. The majority of patients that develop eye findings associated with Graves' disease have mild disorders that are subject to exacerbations and remissions during the course of the disease.

NOSPECS. Historically, a detailed classification of the eye signs associated with Graves disease was devised, abbreviated NOSPECS. NOSPECS stands for class 0, *N*o signs or symptoms; class 1, *O*nly signs; class 2, *S*oft tissue involvement; class 3, *P*roptosis; class 4, *E*OM involvement; class 5, *C*orneal involvement; and class 6, *S*ight loss from optic nerve involvement. It is of little use in the clinical setting because it provides no prognostic value, contributes little assistance in management decisions, and does not present a logical progressive sequence of the disorder, with patients skipping over several steps in the progression.

Hypothyroidism

Ocular findings in hypothyroidism are usually the systemic manifestations of the disease expressed within the ocular tissues and adnexa. The ocular tissues most commonly involved are the skin of the eyelid and the eyebrows. Myxedema is sometimes especially prominent in the eyelids as a boggy, nonpitted edema. Another ocular sign is loss of the outer third of the eyebrow. In addition, a few patients with chronic autoimmune thyroiditis may develop Graves' ophthalmopathy and keratitis sicca.

DIAGNOSIS

Systemic

Table 17–3 provides the diagnostic testing for thyroid disease.

TABLE 17–3. DIAGNOSTIC TESTING IN DIAGNOSIS OF THYROID DISEASE

Graves' disease	Serum TSH—suppressed Free T_4—elevated
Primary hypothyroidism	Serum TSH—elevated Free T_4—may be low/low normal
Hashimoto's disease	Thyroid peroxidase antibody—elevated Thyroglobulin antibody—elevated

Hyperthyroidism

Diagnostic investigation of hyperthyroidism is critically linked to the history and findings on physical examination. Therefore, the patient presenting with findings of thyrotoxicosis is best served by referral to an endocrinologist who can evaluate the diagnostic findings within the context of the overall systemic health. With suspected Graves' disease, the initial step would be to demonstrate the hyperthyroid state, with an elevated free T_4 level and a decreased thyrotropin (TSH) level with a sensitive immunometric assay. If the free T_4 level is normal and the TSH level is reduced, a T_3 level or free T_3 will usually be elevated. Serum TSH receptor antibodies, as well as antithyroglobulin and antimicrobial antibodies, are usually elevated but not ordinarily needed to make the diagnosis. See Table 17–4 for the differential diagnosis of thyrotoxicosis.

Hypothyroidism

The diagnosis of hypothyroidism is based on the history and physical examination, along with laboratory studies used to differentiate between disorders with similar or confusing presentations. The classic presentation of myxedema leaves little doubt about the diagnosis. A history of radioiodine or surgical treatment of hyperthyroidism is also significant. Elevated TSH levels confirm the diagnosis of primary hypothyroidism with the appropriate clinical findings. Eventually T_4 levels and free T_4 will be depressed, and this will occur prior to decrease in T_3 levels. Serum antimicrosomal and antithyroglobulin tests are useful to confirm the presence of autoimmune disease.

Ocular

Table 17–5 delineates the differential diagnosis of Graves' ophthalmopathy.

Hyperthyroidism

The diagnosis of Graves' ophthalmopathy may or may not coincide with systemic thyroid disease. Differentiation from other orbital disorders may include history and physical findings, diagnostic evaluation, ultrasonography, and imaging studies of the orbit. The ocular examination places emphasis on observation of lid position and function, corneal and conjunctival signs, position of the globe, and function of the extraocular muscles and optic nerve.

> The diagnosis of Graves' ophthalmopathy may or may not coincide with systemic thyroid disease.

TABLE 17–4. DIFFERENTIAL DIAGNOSIS OF THYROTOXICOSIS

Graves' disease	Most common form of thyrotoxicosis Diffuse enlargement of the gland Infiltrative orbitopathy and pretibial myxedema Antibodies to TSH receptor
Toxic adenoma (single nodule)	Thyroid nodules present
Toxic multinodular goiter	Radioactive iodine scan localized to nodules Autonomous production of thyroid hormone
Subacute thyroiditis	Moderately enlarged, tender thyroid Increased ESR Destruction of follicles
Iodine-induced hyperthyroidism	Transient thyrotoxicosis with endemic goiter Nonendemic suggests autonomy with large dietary intake, contrast dyes, or amiodarone
Thyrotoxicosis factitia	Ingestion of excessive exogenous thyroid hormone
Struma ovaril	Ovarian tumor composed of thyroid tissue
Hashimoto's thyroiditis	Transient hyperthyroidism in initial destructive stage
Pituitary hypersecretion of TSH	TSH-secreting adenoma

TABLE 17–5. DIFFERENTIAL DIAGNOSIS OF OCULAR FINDINGS IN GRAVES' OPHTHALMOPATHY

Clinical Finding	Associated Findings	Differential Diagnosis
Exophthalmos	May be unilateral or bilateral Forward displacement due to increased retro-orbital soft tissue	Pseudotumor Lymphoma Wegner granulomatosis Orbital cellulitis Carotid–cavernous sinus fistula Mucormycosis Cavernous hemangioma Rhabdomyosarcoma (children) Optic nerve tumor
Exposure keratopathy	Incomplete blink Altered tear distribution Inadequate eye closure	Ectropion Floppy lid syndrome Bell palsy Eyelid trauma
Eyelid retraction	Adrenergic stimulation of Mueller muscle Levator contraction from thickened muscle Levator adhesions to orbicularis muscle Overaction of levator–superior rectus due to fibrosis/retraction of inferior rectus Fibrosis of inferior rectus	Progressive supranuclear palsy Aberrant third-nerve regeneration Unilateral ptosis Dorsal midbrain (Parinaud) syndrome Hyperkalemic periodic paralysis Chronic systemic corticosteroids
Periorbital edema	Ranges from mild to severe Forward displacement of orbital fat Increased interstitial fluids	Preseptal cellulitis Carotid–cavernous sinus fistula
Strabismus	Restrictive myopathy Loss of elasticity and fibrotic contracture Unilateral elevator palsy—fibrotic inferior rectus Reduced lateral gaze—medial rectus fibrosis Limited downgaze—superior rectus fibrosis CT—enlarged EOM with anterior tendon sparing	Orbital myositis Pseudotumor Lymphoma Orbital mass Sixth-nerve palsy Myasthenia gravis
Compressive optic neuropathy	Gradual vision loss, usually bilateral Reduced color vision Afferent pupillary defect (35% of cases) Various visual field defects (66% of cases)	Anterior ischemic optic neuropathy Optic neuritis Retrobital mass Carotid–cavernous sinus fistula Pseudotumor

Lid lag may be an uncommon first presentation. It is best evaluated by instructing the patient to follow a target that is slowly moved downward while carefully observing the position of the lid relative to the globe. Lid movements may be spasmodic or jerky, and a fine tremor may be detected in a lightly closed lid. Increased adrenergic activity is presumed to be the basis for these findings. In addition, position of the lids should be evaluated and any retraction noted.

Proptosis of more than 22 mm, or a difference of more than 2 mm as measured by exophthalmometry between eyes, is considered suspicious for orbital disease. When proptosis is seen in combination with lid retraction and lid lag, diagnostic possibilities other than Graves' opthalmopathy are limited. However, proptosis greater than 23 mm is unusual as an isolated presenting sign for Graves' ophthalmopathy, and other orbital disorders must be considered. The proptosis of Graves' ophthalmopathy is straight out and protrusion of the eye in any other direction suggests another diagnosis. Graves' ophthalmopathy can present with unilateral proptosis; however, imaging studies often show subtle abnormalities in the other orbit. The most common cause of both bilateral and unilateral proptosis in the adult is Graves' ophthalmopathy.

The normal eye should be able to elevate and depress 5.5 mm or the approximate distance from limbus to pupil. Horizontal limitation secondary to extraocular muscle involvement is best noted as an inability to "bury the limbus" on full abduction or adduction and the amount of sclera showing can be measured. Due to EOM restriction, especially of the inferior rectus muscle, vertical diplopia and/or increased IOP may be elicited on attempted upgaze. Binocular fields of fusion and diplopia measured on a Goldmann perimeter are helpful in evaluation and following the EOM dysfunction. Forced duction tests can distinguish nonrestrictive ophthalmoplegias.

Special attention should be given to the evaluation of optic nerve function every time a patient with Graves' ophthalmopathy is examined. This should include pupils, brightness comparison, and color vision screening. Baseline threshold visual fields should be obtained and repeated if there is any symptom or sign that indicates an optic neuropathy may be present.

Because orbitopathy is occasionally the presenting sign of Graves' disease, it must be considered as a diagnosis in patients presenting with proptosis, lid retraction, or impaired eye movement. When it presents with goiter and thyrotoxicosis, there is no difficulty making the diagnosis. Differentiating Graves' ophthalmopathy in an otherwise asymptomatic patient may require diagnostic testing. A depressed TSH level by a very sensitive immunometric assay is highly suggestive of hyperthyroidism. Obtaining thyroid receptor antibody levels can be helpful. High antibody levels can be supportive but not conclusive in making a diagnosis. Orbital ultrasound studies can detect muscle enlargement and demonstrate it in patients with minimal thyroid orbitopathy. With unilateral proptosis or an atypical presentation, a CT scan of the orbit is indicated due to the possibility of orbital tumor.

Hypothyroidism

The ocular disorders in association with hypothyroidism are part of the systemic condition; therefore, the diagnosis is made on the systemic basis. External evaluation may reveal periorbital edema and loss of the lateral one third of the eyebrow.

TREATMENT AND MANAGEMENT

Systemic

Hyperthyroidism

Table 17–6 delineates the treatment and management of hyperthyroidism. The treatment of Graves' hyperthyroidism can involve medical therapy, radioactive iodine, surgery, or a combination of these modalities. Medical therapy has the advantage of potentially avoiding life-long medication; however, the chance for long-term remission is low. Radioactive iodine provides definitive therapy with a high remission rate, yet usually involves life-long therapy with replacement levothyroxine (Synthroid). Surgery provides rapid definitive therapy, but is associated with risk of recurrent nerve or parathyroid damage; life-long levothyroxine therapy is usually required, and the outcome is dependent on the surgeon's skill. The selection of treatment should include the clinical considerations (age, pregnancy, breast-feeding, goiter size, severity of the disease), physician preferences, and patients' choice.

The thioamide antithyroidal drugs used in the treatment of Graves' hyperthyroidism are propylthiouracil (PTU) and methimazole (Tapazole). Both are derivatives of thiourea. Acting as preferred substrates for the iodinating intermediary of thyroid peroxidase, they reduce the available oxidized iodine in the follicular cell, which results in decreased production of T_3 and T_4. They do not interfere with the release of thyroid hormone. PTU inhibits the formation of T_3 from T_4 in the peripheral tissues. Antithyroidal drugs are used in short-term therapy to reduce hyperthyroidism prior to definitive radiotherapy or surgery. They can also be used as a primary treatment of hyperthyroidism.

The goal of long-term antithyroidal drug therapy is to control the hyperthyroidism with the hope that there will be remission from the disease during the

TABLE 17–6. TREATMENT/MANAGEMENT OF HYPERTHYROIDISM

Treatment	Dosage	Indications	Side Effects
Propylthiouracil	Initial 100 mg tid; decrease to 50 mg bid or qd for 1 to 2 years	Initial treatment; prior to RAI; presurgical	Rash, fever, urticaria, joint pain, hepatitis, agranulocytosis
Methimazole	Initial 10 to 30 mg qd; decrease to 5 to 2.5 mg qd for 1 to 2 years	Initial treatment; prior to RAI; presurgical	Rash, fever, urticaria, joint pain, agranulocytosis
Propranolol	Initial 10 mg qd; then increased 20 mg qid or more	Symptomatic relief prior to RAI or surgery	Bradycardia, bronchospasm, congestive heart failure, mental depression, electrolyte imbalance, arrhythmias, agranulocytosis, confusion (in elderly), hepatotoxicity, thrombocytopenia
Radioiodine (RAI)	^{131}I varies with goiter size	Initial treatment	Hypothyroidism; may aggravate severe Graves' ophthalmopathy
Subtotal thyroidectomy		Pregnant and failure of antithyroidal drug therapy; large goiter and poor response to RAI; children	Recurrent laryngeal nerve damage; hypoparathyroidism

course of therapy. Antithyroidal drugs are usually administered for 12 to 24 months. Although almost all patients on antithyroidal drug therapy become euthyroid, only 40 to 50% achieve remission. Remission is defined as 1 year of biochemical euthyroidism following discontinuation of the drug. Unfortunately, the ability to predict those patients who will achieve remission is difficult. Although many factors have been examined to predict the risk of relapse and the results between studies are conflicting, elevated pretreatment levels of T_3 and T_4 seem to correlate with higher risk of relapse. Adolescents or children with mild disease and small goiter are probably the best candidates.

Initial dosage is 100 mg tid for PTU and 10 to 30 mg daily for methimazole. Most patients become euthyroid in 6 to 12 weeks. Serum T_3 and serum T_4 levels should be closely monitored. The utility of serum TSH levels is limited because they can remain suppressed for several months even with biochemical hypothyroidism. Dosage of the medication can be reduced with time. At some point the medication is withdrawn, with tapering recommended. Although relapse can occur at any time, it most commonly occurs within the first 6 months and remission reaches a plateau at 5 years. Ultimately 50 to 60% of patients are destined to relapse. A therapeutic plan should be in place if relapse occurs, which is generally a second trial of medical therapy in children while radioactive iodine treatment is often recommended to adults. Some clinics put patients on a long-term low dose of antithyroidal drugs. Spontaneous hypothyroidism develops in 5 to 20% of patients in remission; thus life-long follow-up of patients is required.

Radioactive iodine treatment results in ablation of the thyroid and correction of hyperthyroidism; however, life-long levothyroxine treatment is usually required. It is contraindicated with pregnancy or breastfeeding, and many clinicians hesitate to treat younger patients because of concerns about possible long-term effects of radiation exposure. Patients at increased risk for complicated thyrotoxicosis should be pretreated with antithyroidal drugs or beta-blockers prior to radioactive iodine, whereas some practitioners pretreat all patients. Thyroid radioactive iodine uptake is measured prior to treatment. Patients are monitored closely for the resolution of thyrotoxicosis and symptoms of hypothyroidism. Alteration in thyroid function is slow to occur, and is usually seen 1 to 2 months after therapy. Those who remain hyperthyroid at 12 weeks should consider a second treatment of radioactive iodine. Most patients will require life-long treatment with levothyroxine (Peden & Hart, 1984). A few patients recover thyroid function and can stop levothyroxine therapy. Although there is some concern that radioactive iodine may cause pre-existing ophthalmopathy to worsen, this has not been clearly demonstrated (Tallstedt et al, 1992). Nevertheless, it is probably prudent to diligently avoid post treatment hypothyroidism with early replacement therapy and consider concomitant treatment with oral prednisone in cases of moderate or severe ophthalmopathy to reduce any potential risk (Bartalena et al, 1989).

Subtotal thyroidectomy is infrequently used as a treatment of Graves' disease in this country. Indications include children and pregnant women allergic to or noncompliant with antithyroidal drugs, a poor response to radioiodine with large goiters, and those emotionally resistant to radioiodine who desire definitive therapy. With a skilled surgeon risk of damage to recurrent laryngeal nerve is 1 to 2% of cases and hypocalcemia develops in less than 1% of cases. Approximately 6% of cases relapse and less than 10% develop overt hypothyroidism (Kuma et al, 1991; Sugino et al, 1993).

Preoperative management usually includes the use of antithyroidal therapy to render the patient euthyroid prior to the procedure. When this is achieved, potassium iodine solution is added for 5 or 6 days to reduce vascularity and the potential for interoperative bleeding. To reduce the risk of goiter enlargement, levothyroxine is advocated. The goal is to reduce hormone stores in the gland and return metabolic function to normal prior to the operation.

Hypothyroidism

Levothyroxine is used in the treatment of hypothyroidism. Levothyroxine is converted to T_3 peripherally in the body; thus both thyroid hormones are available to the tissues despite only one being administered. Table 17–7 delineates the treatment of hypothyroidism.

Ocular

Hyperthyroidism

Table 17–8 summarizes the treatment of Graves ophthalmopathy. Most patients with Graves' ophthalmopathy have mild manifestations that require only supportive therapy. Mild irritation and gritty sensation that is related to poor tear film can be treated with artificial tears. Lid retraction often responds to the treatment of the underlying thyrotoxicosis. Prior to and during treatment it can be treated with guanethidine or beta-blocker eye drops although guanethidine side effects of ptosis, miosis, and punctate keratitis limit its effectiveness. Corneal exposure caused by lagophthalmos should be treated aggressively with ocular lubricant ointments and if necessary, taping eyelids at night. Photophobia can be helped with tinted lenses. Mild diplopia can be corrected with prisms, and press-on prisms provide flexibility. Elimination of smoking as a potential risk factor for the progression of ophthalmopathy is prudent despite the lack of evidence from controlled trials. Patients with mild ophthalmopathy can be reassured that the chance for regression in nonsevere ophthalmopathy is high and the chance of progression to more severe forms is unlikely. Thus, the majority of patients with Graves' ophthalmopathy can be managed in the primary eyecare setting.

Management of patients with severe Graves' ophthalmopathy is challenging and can be associated with unfavorable outcomes. Complications include marked proptosis with potential corneal exposure, constant diplopia in primary or reading gaze position, or compressive optic neuropathy. Glucocorticoid therapy, orbital radiotherapy, and orbital decompression are the established treatments for severe Graves' ophthalmopathy. The choice of therapy involves many factors including the availability of a skilled orbital surgeon or experienced radiotherapist, contraindications to glucocorticoid therapy, and lack of prompt response to sight-threatening disease. In addition, since glucocorticoids and radiotherapy are directed against the inflammatory process, they are likely to be more effective during the active phase of the disease. The goals of therapy are to preserve vision, maintain patient comfort, and minimize oculomotor disorders.

TABLE 17–8. TREATMENT OF GRAVES' OPHTHALMOPATHY

Lid retraction	Guanethidine 2%; topical beta-blocker
Stable post muscle surgery	Eyelid surgery
Corneal exposure	Artificial tears q2h; lubricating ointment qhs or as needed
Severe	Orbital decompression
Lagophthalmos	Tape lids hs
Photophobia	Tint in spectacles
Periorbital edema	Elevate head hs
Diplopia	Head position; prism in spectacles or press-on; orbital radiotherapy
Stable for 6 months	Muscle surgery
Optic neuropathy	Prednisone 60–100 mg qd; orbital radiotherapy; orbital decompression

TABLE 17–7. TREATMENT OF HYPOTHYROIDISM (SYSTEMIC AND OCULAR FINDINGS)

Drug	Initial Dosage	Adjustment of Dosage	Side Effects
Levothyroxine (T_4)	50–100 μg qd; over 60 or coronary disease, 25–50 μg qd	Increase 25 μg qd every 1–3 weeks until patient euthyriod	Allergic reaction (rare); hyperthyroidism in overdosage; pseudotumor cerebri (children); hypothyroidism in underdosage

High-dose prednisone (60 to 100 mg/day) for a period of several months has been demonstrated to be effective on the active inflammatory soft tissue changes and optic neuropathy. Improvement in ocular motility is less responsive, and decrease in proptosis is not impressive. Prednisone has anti-inflammatory and immunosuppressive actions that interfere with T cell and B cell functions, reduce the recruitment of other white blood cells to the involved area, inhibit the release of cytokines and other mediators, and decrease the production and secretion of glycosaminoglycans. Oral prednisone is reported to be effective in about 60% of cases. Withdrawal and tapering of dosage frequently involve recurrence of active ophthalmopathy. Intravenous methylprednisolone acetate has been tried with a similar result to oral therapy, although it may be more effective in severe ophthalmopathy. Systemic glucocorticoid therapy has many side effects. Local therapy has been attempted to avoid these side effects, but it is less effective than systemic treatment.

Orbital radiotherapy has been demonstrated to be as effective in about 60% of cases, particularly in treating active soft tissue inflammatory changes and optic neuropathy. Proptosis is not responsive. A recent report indicates improvement of motility in patients with moderately severe ophthalmopathy (Mourits et al, 2000). Radiotherapy has nonspecific anti-inflammatory effects and suppression of the infiltrating T lymphocytes. A dosage of 20 Gy is considered optimal, and it takes several days to weeks to be effective. Transient exacerbation of eye inflammatory signs can occur, but can be prevented by concomitant glucocorticoid therapy (Bartalena et al, 1983). No carcinogenic complication has been reported, but avoiding radiotherapy in patients under 30 is recommended.

Orbital decompression is effective in treating proptosis with severe corneal exposure, optic nerve compression, and the manifestations of venous congestion. Typically, the approach is subciliary or transconjunctival, with removal of the orbital floor and the medial wall. Sometimes the lateral wall is also removed. Although not attacking the pathogenesis of the disorder, this allows increased space for the orbital content to decompress into the ethmoid sinus, maxillary antrum, and temporalis fossa. This technique has been reported to be effective in patients with optic nerve compression by maintaining or increasing visual acuity, reducing papilledema, improving visual field defects, reducing exposure keratitis, and reducing proptosis. A transantral approach is sometimes preferred but has the major complication of postoperative diplopia, which can occur in two thirds of patients without preoperative diplopia.

Extraocular muscle surgery should be deferred until the ophthalmopathy has been inactive and muscle deviations stable for 4 to 6 months. The goal of extraocular muscle surgery is to reduce the diplopia. It is often difficult to get fusion in all fields of gaze, so elimination of diplopia in primary and reading gaze is often considered a success. Recession of the most restricted muscle is often performed with the inferior rectus the most common muscle involved, followed by the medial and superior rectus. Rarely is the lateral rectus operated upon. Approximately 40% of cases require two or more operations.

Eyelid surgery for persistent lid retraction should be delayed until ophthalmopathy is controlled and stable for 4 to 6 months and the diplopia has been addressed. Upper lid techniques can involve removal of Muller's muscle, recession of levator aponeurosis, or levator myotomy. Lower lid procedure is frequently a recession of the lid retractors with insertion of a cartilage graft or scleral spacer. Indications for eyelid surgery include protection of the cornea and improvement of appearance.

Hypothyroidism

Because the eye findings in hypothyroidism are manifestations of the systemic disease, most clear with the treatment of the systemic disease (Table 17–7).

CONCLUSION

Thyroid disease is a challenging disorder for the clinician to treat and manage. Uncertainty regarding the pathogenesis of these autoimmune disorders, coupled with a clinical course of Graves' disease that is characterized by exacerbations and remissions of varying duration, leads to difficulty in evaluating the effectiveness of therapy. In addition, Graves' ophthalmopathy often does not correlate with systemic severity or course, and it is difficult to predict which patients will develop sight-threatening complications. Nevertheless, ocular signs such as lid retraction and proptosis may lead to the diagnosis of this complex disorder.

REFERENCES

Bahn R, Heufelder A. Pathogenesis of Graves' ophthalmopathy. *N Engl J Med.* 1993;329:1468–1475.

Bartalena L, Marcocci C, Bogazzi F, et al. Use of corticosteroids to prevent progression of Graves' ophthalmopathy after radioiodine therapy for hyperthyroidism. *N Engl J Med.* 1989;321:1349–1359.

Bartalena L, Marcocci C, Laddaga M, et al. Orbital cobalt irradiation combined with systemic corticosteroids for Graves' ophthalmopathy: Comparison with system corticosteroids alone. *J Clin Endocrinol Metab.* 1983;56:1139–1144.

Bartalena L, Pinchera A, Marcocci A. Management of Graves' ophthalmopathy: Reality and perspectives. *Endocr Rev.* 2000;21:168–199.

Bartley GB. The epidemiologic characteristics and clinical course of ophthalmopathy associated with autoimmune thyroid disease in Olmsted County, Minnesota. *Trans Am Ophthalmol Soc.* 1994;92:477–588.

Bartley GB, Fatourechi V, Kadrmas EF, et al. The treatment of Graves' ophthalmopathy in an incidence cohort. *Am J Ophthalmol.* 1996;121:200–206.

Bartley GB, Fatourechi V, Kadrmas EF, et al. Clinical features of Graves' ophthalmopathy in an incidence cohort. *Am J Ophthalmol.* 1996;121:284–290.

Burch HB, Wartofsky L. Graves' ophthalmopathy: Current concepts regarding pathogenesis and management. *Endocr Rev.* 1993;14:747–793.

Dabon-Almirate CLM, Surks MI. Clinical and laboratory diagnosis of thyrotoxicosis. *Endocrinol Metab Clin North Am.* 1998;27:25–35.

Gorman C. Pathogenesis of Graves' ophthalmopathy. *Thyroid.* 1994;4:379–383.

Gorman CA. Temporal relationship between onset of Graves' ophthalmopathy and diagnosis of thyrotoxicosis. *Mayo Clin Proc.* 1983;58:515–519.

Greenspan FS. The thyroid gland. In: Greenspan FS, Strewler GJ, eds. *Basic & Clinical Endocrinology.* 5th ed. Stamford, CT: Appleton & Lange; 1997:226.

Heufelder AE. Pathogenesis of Graves' ophthalmopathy: Recent controversies and progress. *Eur J Endocrinol.* 1995; 132:532–541

Kendler DL, Lippa J, Rootman J. The initial clinical characteristics of Graves' orbitopathy vary with age and sex. *Arch Ophthalmol.* 1993;111:197–201.

Kuma K, Fukata S, Sugawara M. Hypothyroidism. In: Clark OH, Duh QY, eds. *Textbook of Endocrine Surgery.* Philadelphia: WB Saunders; 1997:39–46.

Kuma K, Matsuzuka F, Kobayashi A, et al. Natural course of Graves' disease after subtotal thyroidectomy and management of patients with postoperative thyroid dysfunction. *Am J Med Sci.* 1991;302:8–12.

Larsen PR, Davies TF, Hay ID. The thyroid gland. In: Wilson JD, Foster DW, Kronenberg Hm, Larsen PR, eds. *Williams' Textbook of Endocrinology.* 9th ed. Philadelphia: WB Saunders; 1998:460.

McIver B, Morris JC. The pathogenesis of Graves' disease. *Endorinol Metab Clin North Am.* 1998;27:73–89.

Mourits M, van Kempen-Harteveld M, García M, et al. Radiotherapy for Graves' orbitopathy: Randomised placebo-controlled study. *Lancet.* 2000;355:1505–1509.

Peden NR, Hart IR. The early development of transient and permanent hypothyroidism following radioiodine therapy for Graves' disease. *Can Med Assoc J.* 1984;130: 1141–1144.

Perros P, Crombie AL, Kendall-Taylor P. Natural history of thyroid-associated ophthalmopathy. *Clin Endocrinol (Oxf).* 1996;121:284–290.

Salvi M, Zhang ZG, Haegert D, et al. Patients with endocrine ophthalmopathy not associated with overt thyroid disease have multiple thyroid immunological abnormalities. *J Clin Endocrinol Metab.* 1990;70:89–94.

Sugino K, Mimura T, Toshima K, et al. Follow-up evaluation of patients with Graves' disease treated by subtotal thyroidectomy and risk factor analysis for post-operative thyroid dysfunction. *J Endocrinol Invest.* 1993;16:195–199.

Tallstedt L, Lundell G, Torring O, et al. Occurrence of ophthalmopathy after treatment of Graves' hyperthyroidism. *N Eng J Med.* 1992;231:205–211.

Vanderpump MP, French JM, Appleton D, et al. The prevalence of hyperprolactinenemia and association with markers of autoimmune thyroid disease in survivors of the Whickham Survey cohort. *Clin Endocrinol.* 1998;48:39–44.

Volpé R. Autoimmune thyroiditis. In: Braverman LE, Utiger RD, eds. *The Thyroid.* 6th ed. Philadelphia: JB Lippincott; 1991:921.

Wiersinga WM. Graves' ophthalmopathy. *Thyroid.* 1997; 3:1–15.

Chapter 18

DISORDERS OF THE PARATHYROID GLANDS

Bernard J. Dolan

The parathyroid glands are located on the posterior aspect of the thyroid gland. There are usually four parathyroid glands, but they can vary in number and location. The main secretion of the parathyroid glands is parathyroid hormone (PTH), a polypeptide that plays an important role in maintaining serum calcium levels within normal range. Disorders of the parathyroid glands lead to the disruption of calcium regulation. The resulting clinical syndromes can be broadly classified into hyperparathyroidism (primary and secondary) and hypoparathyroidism, with pesudohypoparathyroidism a rare disorder of PTH resistance. Secondary hyperparathyroidism occurs when external factors, such as chronic renal failure, result in the stimulation of the parathyroid glands to increased PTH production. This condition is not associated with hypercalcemia or its ocular complications and is not included in this discussion.

Ocular findings in parathyroid disorders are associated with the physiological responses of ocular tissues to the long-term alteration of calcium levels in the body. Chronic primary hyperparathyroidism can result in calcium deposition in the cornea, conjunctiva, and sclera. Chronic hypoparathyroidism can cause ocular surface disease, cataracts, and, rarely, papilledema. Pseudohypoparathyroidism can display lens opacities and is occasionally associated with papilledema.

EPIDEMIOLOGY

Hyperparathyroidism

- Primary hyperparathyroidism is a relatively common disorder.
- Prevalence is 1 in 2000 in males over 40, 1 in 500 in females over 40, and 2% in postmenopausal women (Clark, 1997).
- Parathyroid carcinoma is found in 0.5 to 2% of cases of hyperthyroidism (Herrera & Gamboa-Dominguez, 1997).

Hypoparathyroidism

- The idiopathic form is rare.
- Most common occurence is secondary to parathyroid removal during total thyroidectomy or interruption of blood supply to parathyroid glands during surgery (8 to 32%).

PATHOPHYSIOLOGY/DISEASE PROCESS

Systemic

Table 18–1 delineates the systemic manifestations of parathyroid disease.

TABLE 18–1. SYSTEMIC MANIFESTATIONS OF PARATHYROID DISORDERS

Hyperparathyroidism
- Proximal muscle weakness
- Fatigue
- Headache
- Weight loss
- Malaise
- Constipation
- Mild depression
- Hypercalcemia
- Renal calculi
- Pseudo-gout (calcium-crystal-induced arthropathy)
- Peptic ulcer
- Hyperactive reflexes
- Osteoporosis
- Weak, easily fractured bones

Hypoparathyroidism
- Mild paresthesias
- Muscle cramps
- Carpopedal spasms
- Convulsions
- Mental status changes
- Irritability
- Hypocalcemia
- Hyperphosphatemia
- Normal renal function
- Dental problems
- Basal ganglia calcifications
- Brittle nails
- Cardiac arrhythmias

Hyperparathyroidism

- Primary hyperparathyroidism, a condition of excess secretion of PTH, is due to adenoma of the parathyroid gland in 80 to 90% of cases (usually a single gland) and primary parathyroid hyperplasia in other cases (Herrera & Gamboa-Dominguez, 1997).
- Multiple endocrine neoplasm (MEN) is a classification of several distinct syndromes in which parathyroid tumors are associated with other endocrine disorders.
- Excess PTH results in dysfunction of calcium, phosphate, and bone metabolism, leading to hypercalcemia and hypophosphatemia.
- Once considered a rare disorder, with increased screening of serum calcium the diagnosis is made most often in asymptomatic patients with minimal signs or with vague symptoms of fatigue, abdominal complaint, or mental changes (Heath, 1992).
- Primary hyperparathyroidism can be normocalcemic due to vitamin D deficiency, low serum albumin, pancreatitis, increased phosphate intake, or excessive hydration.
- The clinical manifestations of primary hyperparathyroidism are often subtle (see Table 18–1).
- Although few patients have dramatic symptoms, the classic symptoms are painful bones, kidney stones, abdominal groans, psychic moans, and fatigue overtones.

Hypoparathyroidism

- Hypoparathyroidism is an uncommon disorder.
- Complications of head and neck surgery and idiopathic autoimmune destruction of the parathyroid glands in a sporadic or familial pattern are the most common causes.
- Hypomagnesemia, genetic defects in PTH synthesis, and infiltration of the parathyroid glands are uncommon causes of hypoparathyroidism.
- Symptoms of hypoparathyroidism are increased nerve and muscle activity due to decreased calcium levels (see Table 18–1).

Ocular

Table 18–2 delineates the ocular manifestations of parathyroid disorders.

Hyperparathyroidism

- It is associated with deposition of calcium in the cornea, called band keratopathy, and conjunctiva (Blake, 1976).

> Hyperparathyroidism is associated with calcium deposits in the cornea or band keratopathy.

- Band keratopathy is usually asymptomatic, but can progress into the visual axis, causing decreased vision, or disrupt the epithelium, causing irritation or pain (Cogan et al, 1948).

TABLE 18–2. OCULAR MANIFESTATIONS IN PARATHYROID DISORDERS

Hyperparathyroidism	
• **Disorder**	• **Manifestation**
Band keratopathy	Decreased vision, surface irritation
Pannus formation	
Conjunctival calcification	Asymptomatic
Hypoparathyroidism	
• **Disorder**	• **Manifestation**
Keratoconjunctivitis	Foreign body sensation, photophobia
Cataract (polychromatic)	Normal to decreased vision
Papilledema (rare)	Normal to transient vision loss (seconds)

Hypoparathyroidism

- Ocular surface disease is due to keratoconjunctivitis; severe corneal involvement is associated with blepharospasm and photophobia with candidiasis or adrenal insufficiency.
- Bilateral polychromatic lens opacities in cortical and subcapsular regions become visually significant only if the disease goes unrecognized because progression is arrested with systemic therapy.
- Rarely, papilledema is found, caused by a reduction in cerebrospinal fluid reabsorption.

> Polychromatic lens opacities are associated with hypoparathyroidism.

DIAGNOSIS

Table 18–3 lists the diagnostic tests for parathyroid disorders and Table 18–4 provides a differential diagnosis of hypercalcemia.

Systemic

Hyperparathyroidism

- Hypercalcemia with an unremarkable history, elevated serum PTH, and hypercalcemia is diagnostic of primary hyperthyroidism.
- Normocalcemic primary hyperthyroidism is diagnosed by recurrent nephrolithiasis or osteoporosis.

Hypoparathyroidism

- Hypocalcemia, hyperphosphatemia, and normal renal function are diagnostic of hypoparathyroidism.

TABLE 18–3. DIAGNOSTIC TESTING IN PARATHYROID DISORDERS

Disorder	Tests
Primary hyperparathyroidism	Serum calcium elevated Serum PTH elevated Urinary calcium normal or elevated
Hypoparathyroidism	Serum calcium decreased Serum phosphate elevated Urinary calcium decreased Serum PTH decreased

Ocular

Diagnosis of the ocular findings associated with parathyroid disorders is made by their clinical appearance.

Hyperparathyroidism

- Band keratopathy appears as a white, opaque material in the superficial corneal stroma (see Figure 18–1).
  - It has a frosted or ground glass appearance.
  - It is characteristically located at 3- and 9- o'clock positions within the palpebral aperture.
  - The peripheral edge is separated from limbus by a sharp clear margin.
  - The central edge is diffuse and gradually fades into the cornea.
- Conjunctival calcium deposits are small, hard, white flecks or glass crystals in palpebral conjunctiva.

Hypoparathyroidism

- Photophobia and blepharospasm can be associated with keratoconjunctivitis.
- Recognition of polychromatic lens opacities may lead to systemic diagnosis.
- Papilledema is sometimes associated with convulsions and may mimic an intracranial mass; a neuro-ophthalmologic consultation is advised.

TREATMENT AND MANAGEMENT

Systemic

Table 18–5 delineates the systemic treatment and management of parathyroid disorders.

Hyperparathyroidism

- Parathyroidectomy is the definitive treatment for hyperparathyroidism with 95% of patients cured by this technique (Clark, 1996).
- Mild hyperparathyroidism in asymptomatic patients may be treated medically with large fluid intake; however, reports indicate that less than 5% are truly asymptomatic because many have nonspecific symptoms that improve with parathyroidectomy (Clark, 1995).
- Pamidronate and alendronate are used in hypercalcemia associated with neoplasms to inhibit bone resorption, but efficacy and safety in long-term use with hyperparathyroidism has not been established.
- Older asymptomatic patients may be followed with serum calcium, renal function, bone density, and clinical manifestations (Heath, 1992).

TABLE 18–4. DIFFERENTIAL DIAGNOSIS OF HYPERCALCEMIA

Disorder	Mechanism	Associated Findings
Artifact	Laboratory error	Excess tourniquet time; high serum protein concentrations; dehydration
Primary hyperparathyroidism	Parathyroid adenoma/hyperplasia	Elevated serum PTH; hypercalcemia; normal or elevated urinary calcium
Malignant neoplasms of breast, lung, pancreas, uterus, hypernephroma	Tumors secrete proteins with homologies to PTH	Serum phosphate is often low, but plasma PTH low by immunometric assay
Multiple myeloma	Renal dysfunction with increased carboxyl terminal PTH	Elevated PTH with carboxyl terminal assay
Granulomatous disorders such as tuberculosis, sarcoidosis, berylliosis, histoplasmosis, coccidioidomycosis, leprosy, or foreign body	Granulomatous tissue synthesizes 1,25 dihydroxycholecalciferol	Serum 1,25 dihydroxycholecalciferol is elevated
Exogenous calcium or vitamin D	Excess ingestion calcium, usually antacids	Reversible with cessation
Benign familial hypocalciuric hypercalcemia	Autosomal dominant inheritance	Family history; low urinary calcium
Adrenal insufficiency	Disinhibition of GI and renal calcium uptake	Dehydration; hyperproteinemia
Hyperthyroidism	Increased bone turnover	Clinical features of thyrotoxicosis
Other causes	Various	Thiazide diuretics or lithium; prolonged immobility; acute illness in intensive care units

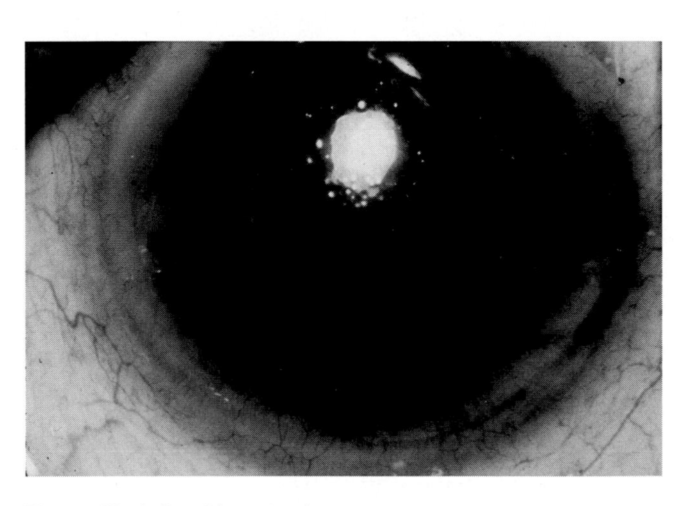

Figure 18–1. Band keratopathy.

Hypoparathyroidism

- Use calcium and vitamin D supplements with dosage varying with the specific preparation (Rude, 1997).
- Monitor serum calcium level every 3 months and "spot" calcium urine level.

Ocular

Table 18–6 delineates the ocular treatment and management of parathyroid disorders.

Hyperparathyroidism

- Band keratopathy is only treated with decreased vision or symptomatic irritation.
- Ethylenediamine tetraacetic acid (EDTA) 0.5% is irrigated on Bowman's membrane after the

TABLE 18–5. MANAGEMENT/TREATMENT OF PARATHYROID DISORDERS

Disorder	Treatment	Dosage/Type	Side Effects/Complications
Primary hyperthyroidism	Surgical	Parathyroidectomy	Hypoparathyroidism; recurrent hyperparathyroidism
	Medical	Large fluid intake	
Hypoparathyroidism	Calcium with vitamin D	Calcium 1–2 g/day; calcitriol 0.50–2.0 μg/day	Excess dosage: hypercalcemia

TABLE 18–6. MANAGEMENT/TREATMENT OF OCULAR FINDINGS ASSOCIATED WITH PARATHYROID DISORDERS

Condition	Treatment	Indication
Hyperparathyroidism		
Band keratopathy	Observation	Peripheral location
	EDTA	Decreased vision
	Excimer laser	Decreased vision
Hypoparathyroidism		
Cataract	Observation, surgical removal	Visual symptoms
Keratoconjunctivitis	Topical lubricants	Presence of finding
Papilledema	Correction of hypocalcemia	Presence of finding

corneal epithelium has been removed (Grant, 1952).

- The excimer laser has been reported to successfully remove band keratopathy (O'Brart et al, 1993).

Hypoparathyroidism

- Keratoconjunctivitis is treated with supportive therapy and ocular lubricants; a corneal specialist consultation is advised with superficial stromal or extensive peripheral neovascularization.
- Cataract extraction is indicated with visually significant cataract from long-term disease.
- Papilledema should resolve as the systemic disorder is treated.

CONCLUSION

The disruption of normal function of the parathyroid glands leads to alterations in calcium and phosphate blood levels, which manifests systemically as disruption in the normal function of nerve, muscle, bones, kidney, and gastrointestinal system. The ocular manifestations of parathyroid disorders include corneal and conjunctival changes, as well as cataracts. These ocular findings usually present as part of the clinical picture of chronic parathyroid dysfunction. Detection of polychromatic lenticular opacities may assist in the diagnosis of hypoparathyroidism.

REFERENCES

Blake J. Eye signs in idiopathic hypoparathyroidism. *Trans Ophthalmol Soc UK.* 1976;46:488 – 451.

Chan AK, Duh QY, Katz MH, et al. Clinical manifestations of primary hyperparathyroidism before and after parathyroidectomy. A case-control study. *Ann Surgery.* 1995; 222:402–412.

Clark OH. "Asymptomatic" primary hyperthyroidism: Is parathyroidectomy indicated? *Surgery.* 1994;116: 947–953.

Clark OH. Current management of patients with hyperparathyroidism. *Adv Surg,* 1996;30:179–187.

Clark OH. Diagnosis of primary hyperparathyroidism. Clark OH, Duh QY, eds. In: *Textbook of Endocrine Surgery.* Philadelphia: WB Saunders: 1997;297–301.

Clark OH. Surgical treatment of primary hyperparathyroidism. *Adv Endocrinol Metab.* 1995;6:1–16.

Cogan DG, Albright F, Batter FC. Hypercalemia and band keratopathy. Report of nineteen cases. *Arch Ophthalmol.* 1948;40:624–638.

Davies M. Primary hyperthyroidism: Aggressive or conservative treatment? *Clin Endocrinol.* 1992;36:325–332.

Grant WM. New treatment for calcific corneal opacities. *Arch Ophthalmol.* 1952;48:681–685.

Heath DA, Heath E. Conservative management of primary hyperthyroidism. *J Bone Miner Res.* 1991;6:S121–124.

Heath H III. Primary hyperparathyroidism: Recent advances in pathogenesis, diagnosis, and treatment. *Adv Intern Med.* 1992;37:275–293.

Herrara MR, Gamboa-Dominguez A. Parathyroid embryology, anatomy and pathology. Clark OH, Duh QY, eds. In: *Textbook of Endocrine Surgery.* Philadelphia: WB Saunders: 1997;277–283.

Ledger GA. Hypocalcemia and hypoparathyroidism. *Curr Ther Endocrinol Metab.* 1994;5:508–510.

Loh KC, Duh QY, Shoback D, et al. Clinical profile of primary hyperparathyroidism in adolescents and young adults. *Clin Endocrinol.* 1998;48:435–443.

O'Brart DP, Gartry DS, Lohmann CP, et al. Treatment of band keratopathy by excimer laser phototherapeutic keratectomy: Surgical techniques and long term follow up. *Br J Ophthalmol.* 1993;77:702–708.

Rude RK. Hypocalcemia and hypoparathyroidism. *Cur Ther Endocrinol Metab.* 1997, 6:546–551.

Sambrook AB, Sherwood LM. Pathogenesis and management of hypoparathyroidism and other hypocalcemic disorders. *Metabolism.* 1975;24:871–898.

Chapter 19

DYSFUNCTION OF THE PITUITARY GLAND

Bernard J. Dolan

The primary dysfunction of the pituitary gland that affects the visual system is the pituitary adenoma, a nonmetastasizing neoplasm of adenohypophysial glandular cells. Because of the proximity of the optic chiasm, the pituitary adenoma can cause visual loss when it compresses the adjacent optic pathways. The widespread availability and use of imaging systems, as well as advances in imaging systems, have altered the clinical presentation of this disorder. High-resolution magnetic resonance imaging (MRI) scans commonly result in an incidental finding of a small lesion consistent with a pituitary adenoma. These lesions have no visual signs or symptoms. The vast majority of individuals with these lesions have neither hypersecretion of a pituitary hormone nor clinical evidence of hypopituitarism. These incidental adenomas challenge endocrinologists to define the appropriate clinical evaluation of these otherwise normal patients. Pituitary adenomas may produce a clinical syndrome caused by the hypersecretion of an anterior pituitary hormone, such as Cushing's syndrome or acromegaly. Other adenomas are clinically nonfunctioning and may go undetected until the mass effects of the expanding tumor, hypopituitarism, headache, or visual complaints, are recognized. The ophthalmic practitioner must be vigilant and have an appropriate degree of suspicion when evaluating patients with unexplained visual loss or visual field defects that suggest a bitemporal flavor. The clinical diagnosis of the pituitary adenoma continues to be challenging and can be missed without a thoughtful evaluation of the patient.

EPIDEMIOLOGY

Systemic

The true incidence of pituitary adenomas is not clearly established. Epidemiologic data suggest a prevalence of 20 cases per 100,000 and an incidence of 2 cases per 100,000 (Gold, 1981). Autopsy studies utilizing careful histological assessment have prevalence rates of 22.5 to 27% with equal sex distribution (Burrow et al, 1981). Less than 1% have multiple adenomas. High-resolution imaging studies report lesions consistent with pituitary adenoma in 10 to 20% of asymptomatic individuals (Elster, 1993). Clinically diagnosed pituitary adenomas account for 10 to 15% of all intracranial neoplasms. Pituitary adenomas are infrequent in children, with only 3.5 to 8.5% being diagnosed before 20 years of age, and adenomas are seen in imaging studies in only 3% of individuals less than age 18 (Kane et al, 1994).

Pituitary adenomas are classified clinically by their hormonal activity. Prolactin-secreting adenomas are the most common, with a frequency of 40 to 50% (Terada et al, 1995). Clinically nonfunctioning adenomas comprise 25 to 30% of pituitary adenomas. About 90% of these clinically nonfunctioning adenomas show evidence of gonadotropin production when tumor tissue is studied with sensitive immunohistochemical techniques. Growth hormone–secreting adenomas are found in 10 to 15% of patients with pituitary tumors. ACTH-producing adenomas also comprise 10 to 15% of pituitary adenomas (Minderman et al, 1994). TSH-secreting adenomas are rare, representing less than 1% of pituitary adenomas (Beck-Peccoz et al, 1996).

Ocular

The prevalence of visual symptoms and signs associated with pituitary adenomas is decreasing because of early diagnosis due to recognition of endocrine complaints and imaging studies for unrelated causes. Decreased visual acuity was noted in 4% and visual field loss in 9% of pituitary adenoma patients at a neuroendocrine service between 1976 and 1981 (Anderson et al, 1983). Progressive deterioration of vision, however, was the leading initial major complaint in 42% of patients with clinically nonfunctioning adenomas with 73% having visual field defects (Arafah, 1986.) In these patients, the lack of hormonal hypersecretion, with its recognizable clinical effects, often delays the diagnosis until the tumor compresses the optic chiasm and patients present with an ocular complaint.

TABLE 19–1. HORMONE FUNCTIONS OF THE ANTERIOR PITUITARY GLAND

Polypeptides
Adrenocorticotropin hormone (ACTH)
- Synthesis and secretion of glucocorticoids
- Release of mineralocorticoids and adrenal androgens (minor influence)

Growth hormone (GH)
- Promote metabolism and growth

Prolactin
- Development of mammary gland and lactation
- Physiological function of liver, ovary, testes, and prostate

Glycoproteins
Thyroid-stimulating hormone (TSH)
- Production and release of thyroxine (T_4) and triiodothyronine (T_3), which increases metabolic activity

Follicle-stimulating hormone (FSH)
- Gonadotropin
- Gametogenesis; with LH produces sex hormones
- Follicular maturation
- Production of mature sperm

Luteinizing hormone (LH)
- Gonadotropin
- With FSH produces sex hormones
- Ovulation
- Maintains corpus luteum; production of estrogen and progesterone
- Testosterone production

PATHOPHYSIOLOGY/DISEASE PROCESS

The pituitary gland extends from the median eminence at the base of the hypothalamus into a bony projection of the sphenoid bone, the sella turcica. Dura mater lining the sella surrounds the gland, separating it laterally from the cavernous sinus and superiorly from the brain with a dural fold called the diaphragma sellae. Important anatomical relationships to the pituitary gland include the internal carotid arteries and cavernous sinus laterally, the sphenoid air sinus inferiorly and anteriorly, and the optic chiasm and the optic tracts superiorly.

Six major hormones have been identified as being produced and secreted in the anterior pituitary gland. These include glycoproteins and polypeptides. The polypeptides include prolactin, growth hormone (GH), and adenocorticotropin hormone (ACTH), which is derived from pro-opiomelanocortin (POMC). The glycoproteins are thyroid-stimulating hormone (TSH), and the gonadotropins, luteinizing hormone (LH) and follicle-stimulating hormone (FSH). The glycoprotein hormones are made up of an identical alpha subunit and a slightly different beta subunit that appears to delineate the specific hormone function. Table 19–1 delineates each hormone's function.

Most anterior pituitary hormones are secreted in bursts that result in sharp peaks in the systemic blood levels of the hormone. Between these bursts of hormone release, the blood levels may be low. Therefore, a single random measurement of hormonal levels may not provide a clear indication of hormonal secretion.

Pituitary secretions are regulated by the hypothalamus, which is influenced by input from the autonomic nervous system and cerebral cortex, such as breast–suckling–stimulating prolactin secretion (Figure 19–1). The hypothalamus produces specific polypeptides called releasing factors that act on the corresponding cells of the anterior pituitary to control hormone secretion. These factors are released into the capillaries of the hypothalamus and are made available to the glandular cell receptors of the anterior pituitary by the hypothalamic–hypophysial portal system. These polypeptides stimulate or inhibit the pituitary hormone by regulating gene expression and secretion. Although the predominant releasing factor of most hormones is stimulatory, dopamine is the major physiologic regulator of prolactin secretion and has an inhibitory effect. Various prolactin-stimulating agents that play a minor role in prolactin control have been identified, but the physiologic role of these factors is presently unclear. GH has a stimulatory releasing factor, and somatostatin inhibits GH. ACTH and TSH secretion are each primarily controlled by a specific stimulatory releasing factor. LH and FSH have a

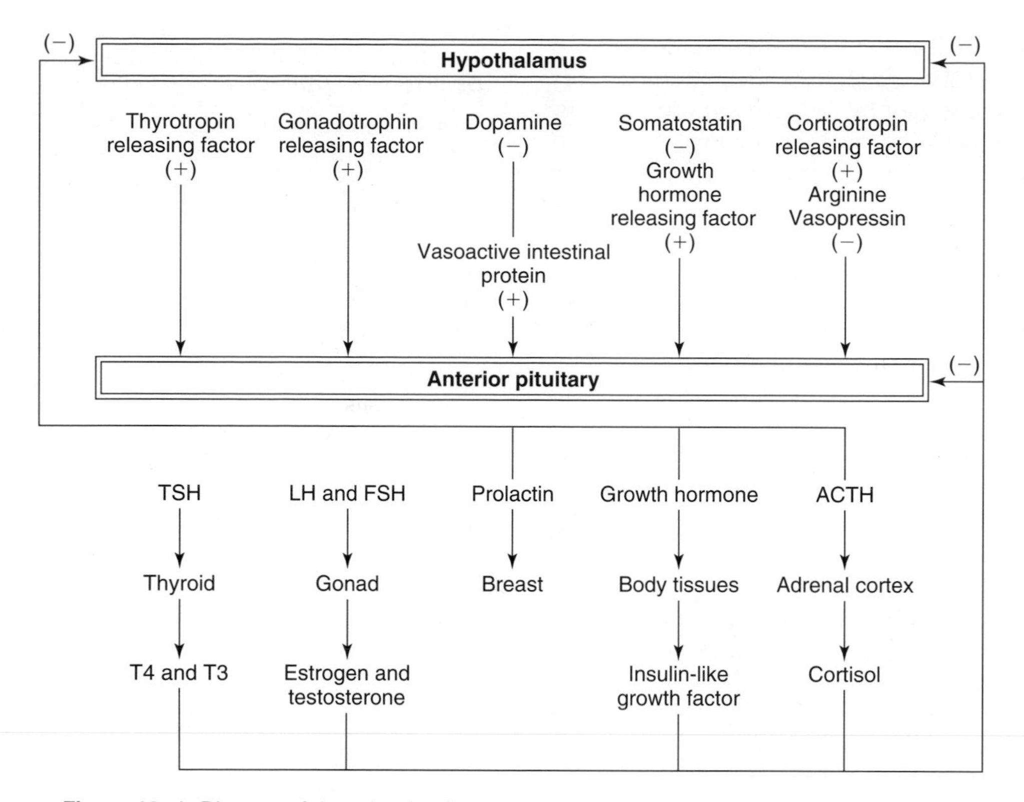

Figure 19–1. Diagram of the releasing factors and feedback loops for the pituitary hormones.

common stimulating factor. The hypothalamus also receives negative feedback from the hormones secreted by target organs or other metabolic products. Disruption of this balance may result in the selective overstimulation of one target gland or tissue, or deficiency of one of more of the pituitary hormones.

In addition to regulation by the hypothalamus, the anterior pituitary is influenced by the circulating levels of hormone from the target organ (see Figure 19–1). This provides a negative feedback loop for regulation in the levels of pituitary hormones. The thyroid hormones, cortisol, peptide growth factors, and sex hormones all act to inhibit the release of the corresponding pituitary hormone. Furthermore the hormones from the target organs provide a feedback control upon the secretion of the hypothalamic-releasing hormones by influencing neuroregulators and other central neurotransmissions. These additional neural and endocrine influences act to maintain a homeostatic balance for each individual hormone.

Systemic

Although the precise pathogenesis of pituitary adenomas is yet to be elucidated, recent observations suggest that virtually all pituitary tumors arise from a single cell (Herman et al, 1990). This implies that initiating events in the formation of pituitary adenomas are intrinsic molecular genetic alterations, which lead to cell transformation and the release of the cell from growth inhibition. The responsible gene or genes have not been identified. The ultimate manifestation of these genetic alterations is determined by their interaction with multifactorial mechanisms including hypothalamic hormone regulatory signals, local pituitary cell growth factors, and altered cell cycle regulation (Asa & Ezzat, 1998). It is likely that these factors play a role in the progression of tumor development. This results in monoclonal anterior pituitary cell proliferation and autonomous hormone production, which are the characteristics of pituitary adenoma. Investigations into the subcellular mechanisms that are responsible for dysregulated cell growth and hormone hypersecretion are ongoing and may provide strategies to develop more specific and potent treatments for pituitary adenoma.

Clinically diagnosed pituitary adenomas are functionally classified based on the systemic manifestations they produce and most are associated with hormone hypersecretion. However, some clinically detectable hypersecreting adenomas may not produce clinical symptoms depending on the hormone being secreted, size and shape of the tumor, and age and sex of the patient. In addition, many pituitary adenomas present without clinical evidence of hormone hypersecretion and are classified as clinically nonfunctioning adenomas. Other adenomas may hypersecrete more than one hormone but with the clinical manifestations of only one hormone. A few may hypersecrete more than one hormone and produce no clinical signs or symptoms. Plurihormonal adenomas are explained by common cellular differentiation with one cell type producing two hormones, although a few tumors appear to be composed of more than one cell type. Despite this variation, most tumors can be classified as a specific secretory type using clinical manifestations, serum hormone levels, and tumor tissue immunohistochemistry. These include prolactinomas, GH-secreting adenomas, ACTH-secreting adenomas, and TSH-secreting adenomas. Clinically nonfunctioning adenomas produce no clinically detectable endocrine hypersecretion, but the majority of these tumors show evidence of gonadotropin secretion when tested with sensitive immunohistochemical techniques.

The signs and symptoms of pituitary adenoma are secondary to either the mass effects of the expanding tumor or excess hormone secretion. The clinical manifestations of a pituitary adenoma vary with age, gender, cell type, and the extent of compression on the gland and surrounding structures (Table 19–2). The size of the adenoma is a major factor in determining the extent of the signs and symptoms associated with mass effects, but has no correlation with the effects of hormonal hypersecretion. When the tumor is an encapsulated lesion, 10 mm or less in diameter, but distinguished from the gland, it is classified as a microadenoma. Microadenomas located within the sella turcica can cause marked hormonal imbalances in Cushing's disease, but rarely produce the mass effects of hypopituitarism and do not compress the optic pathways. Tumors greater than 10 mm in diameter are macroadenomas. Most commonly, these tumors expand superiorly through the diaphragma sellae, which offers little resistance. All suprasellar extensions have the potential for the tumor to impinge on the optic chiasm, optic tracts, or optic nerves. Some continue to grow and compress the hypothalamus. Macroadenomas may also grow down through the thin layer of bone into the sphenoid sinus, laterally into the cavernous sinus, or into the orbital surface of the frontal bone. Rarely does the tumor grow posteriorly and compress the basilar artery and brainstem.

The shape of the tumor is dependent on the resistance of the diaphragma sellae and the size of the pituitary stalk opening. Some tumors may pass easily through the opening; others take a dumbbell shape due to more resistance in the opening, and still others may expand with the diaphragma. A common presentation of a slow-growing adenoma is the mass effect on the surrounding structures. Mass effects include headache, hypopituitarism, and compression of the optic pathways. Headache, although not always a component of the symptoms of pituitary adenoma, can vary in location, but may be localized to the retro-orbital or bitemporal areas. Persistent headaches, particularly those that present in the morning or wake the patient at night always cause concern for the potential of an intracranial lesion. Hypopituitarism can be caused by local compression of the normal pituitary gland or the hypophysial–portal system.

The most common presenting symptom for pituitary adenomas has changed from visual loss to endocrine dysfunction. This change in the presenting symptoms and signs is related to the development of

TABLE 19–2. SYSTEMIC MANIFESTATIONS OF PITUITARY ADENOMA

Prolactin-secreting Adenoma
Females: galactorrhea, amenorrhea
Males: impotence, decreased libido
Both: infertility, headache, weight gain
GH-secreting Adenoma
Gigantism (Child)
Acromegaly (Adult)
Large jaw/nose, growth of hands/feet, thickened skin, increased metabolic rate, enlargement of body organs, impaired glucose tolerance, headache, peripheral neuropathy, fibrous thickening of joint capsule, fatigue, recurrent sinusitis, deepening voice, increased spacing of teeth, menstrual disturbance
ACTH-secreting Adenoma
"Moon face"
Centripetal obesity
"Buffalo hump"
Bruising easily
TSH-secreting Adenoma
Heat intolerance
Weight loss
Nervousness
Tremor
Increased appetite
Clinically Nonfunctioning Adenoma
Headache
Hypopituitarism
Visual loss
Hypopituitarism
Hypogonadism
Hypothyroidism
Adrenal insufficiency
Pituitary Apoplexy
Sudden decrease in vision
Ophthalmoplegia
Headache
Sensory perception changes
Nausea/vomiting
Seizures
Hemiplegia

sensitive radioimmunoassays to clinically measure anterior pituitary hormone levels and the increased sensitivity and clinical use of computed tomography (CT) scanning and MRI. The detection of adenomas on CT scanning and MRI in patients being evaluated for trauma or other unrelated conditions is increasing. With improved techniques and sensitivity these findings often are incidental microadenomas in individuals without endocrine signs or symptoms. This is challenging endocrinologists to provide an appropriate, yet cost-effective workup.

> The most common presenting symptom for pituitary adenomas has changed from visual loss to endocrine dysfunction.

The three most common endocrine disorders due to excess hormone secretion from pituitary adenomas are hyperprolactinemia with amenorrhea and galactorrhea, acromegaly with the clinical manifestations of growth hormone hypersecretion, and Cushing's disease with the clinical manifestations of excess cortisol due to ACTH hypersecretion. Other endocrine dysfunctions associated with pituitary adenomas include impotence, decreased libido, gigantism, dysthyroidism, and hypogonadism. Some of these endocrine manifestations result from anterior pituitary deficiency from the mass effect causing destruction of normal pituitary tissues. The mass effect of an expanding adenoma can also result in compression of the pituitary stalk or hypothalamus, resulting in endocrine dysfunction of the anterior or posterior pituitary.

Prolactinomas

The most common secreting pituitary adenomas are prolactinomas. The presence of endocrine symptoms varies with gender and age, as well as the size of the tumor. Prolactinomas are a common cause of reproductive and sexual dysfunction. The hypogonadism seen with prolactinomas is probably mediated by prolactin inhibiting the release of hypothalamic gonadotropin-releasing factor and the resulting decreased gonadotropin secretion by the pituitary.

Prolactinomas are most frequently found in women 20 to 50 years old. Common presenting symptoms in women of childbearing age are galactorrhea, amenorrhea, or infertility. Other symptoms include weight gain, decreased libido, fatigue, acne, oily skin, vaginal dryness, and constipation. The presence of these additional symptoms does not appear to increase the probability of finding an adenoma. Postmenopausal women commonly only complain of headache. Women tend to present at an earlier age with microadenomas.

Men may present with decreased libido, impotence, infertility, and in some cases galactorrhea. Poor development of acini in the male breast is responsible for the low frequency of this presentation. Vigorous manipulation of the breast, however, may demonstrate the presence of this finding. Partial or complete impotence, decreased libido, and infertility may be ignored for years and only be recognized after successful treatment. Hypogonadism can also manifest as decreased body hair or beard. Decreased frequency of shaving may be a contributory diagnostic sign. Increased appetite with resultant obesity and apathy may be present. Headache may be the only complaint. Prolactinomas in men are more likely to be macroadenomas with associated visual field defects and hypopituitarism, diagnosed at 60 to 70 years of age.

Although the natural history of prolactinoma is not completely understood, it appears that there is slow growth of the tumor in some cases. In autopsy studies of microadenomas where the majority of patients had no clinical evidence of endocrine dysfunction, 40% of the tumors tested positive for prolactin with immunohistochemical stain. Studies following untreated prolactin-secreting microadenomas reveal that most tumors are unchanged over the 3- to 6-year observation period with a minority showing a significant increase in tumor size so that the risk of progression from microadenoma to macroadenoma is only 7% (Schlechte et al, 1989). Factors responsible for tumor enlargement in these cases have not been identified. In a series of patients with microprolactinomas and careful observation for as long as 15 years, one third of the patients who were untreated or received intermittent medical treatment with dopamine agonists returned to normal prolactin levels after all therapy was removed. Pregnancy increased this remission rate, 35% compared to 14% in those who did not become pregnant (Jeffcoate et al, 1996).

GH-secreting Adenomas

The hypersecretion of growth hormone most often is due to pituitary adenoma. This results in gigantism in a child or young adolescent in which the epiphyseal plates have not closed. Growth of the long bones is stimulated and an individual can reach the height of 8 to 9 feet if untreated. In the adult, GH hypersecretion results in acromegaly. This condition most commonly presents between 20 and 40 years of age. The well-developed case of acromegaly may be easily identified; however, early signs are subtle, gradual changes that are often not recognized. This lack of recognition is why most GH-secreting adenomas are macroadenomas at clinical diagnosis. The gradual nature of the hormonal effects are why GH-secreting adenomas are an exception to the rule that hormonal hypersecretion associated with a recognizable clinical syndrome is detected early and associated with a microadenoma. Growth hormone levels often correlate with tumor size.

Acromegalics have characteristic growth changes in the soft tissues and bones of the face, hands, and feet. These patients may complain of increased shoe, glove, or ring size. Growth occurs in the mandible, nasal, mallar, and frontal bones, changing facial appearance. Marked jaw projection and exaggerated nasolabial folds develop slowly over the years and may elicit no complaint from the patient; however, those who do not see the patient frequently may comment on the changes. Proliferation of the connective tissues leads to increased subcutaneous tissue and thickened oily skin. This can contribute to nerve entrapment as in carpal tunnel syndrome. The enlargement of body organs may occur, including the viscera, heart, kidney, pancreas, and liver. Metabolic rate may increase with normal thyroid hormone levels. Impaired glucose tolerance is common due to insulin resistance actions of GH, and may put the patient at risk for development of diabetes mellitus. Long-standing disease can lead to fatigue, weakness, and muscle abnormalities with electromyogram (EMG) changes. Peripheral neuropathy with paresthesias of the hands and feet may develop. Fibrous thickening of the joint capsule with joint pain may be confused with arthritis. Hypertrophy of pharyngeal and laryngeal tissue cause deepening of the voice, and obstructive sleep apnea may occur. Other manifestations include headache, increased spacing of teeth, recurrent sinusitis, otitis media, and hyperhydrosis of the skin. Women may complain of menstrual disturbances, whereas men may experience decreased libido and impotence.

Acromegalics are at risk for hypertension (50%), cardiomegaly, and associated cardiovascular morbidity. Population studies have identified that active acromegalic patients have a twofold greater mortality than the general population for cerebrovascular, cardiovascular, and respiratory diseases and malignancies. There is some evidence that in acromegalics a reduction of GH levels below 2.5 ng/mL is protective for this increased mortality. Thus, acromegaly needs to be managed aggressively; to reduce the associated mortality risk, GH levels of less that 2 ng/mL are desired.

ACTH-secreting Adenomas

Cushing's disease refers to the clinical manifestations of hypercortisolism caused by pituitary hypersecretion of ACTH. This almost always is due to an ACTH-secreting adenoma. Microadenomas of less than 5 mm are common with this disorder; macroadenomas are rare. In fact, only 40 to 50% of surgically cured Cushing's disease patients demonstrated an adenoma on imaging preoperatively (Findling & Doppman, 1994). The sensitivity of microadenoma detection on MRI has been reported to be as high as 71% (Buchfelder, et al 1993).

Clinical recognition is relatively easy when the disease is fully developed; however, early in its course there may be difficulty in establishing the clinical diagnosis. Cushing's disease has been described most frequently in women between 20 and 40 years of age, because it is five times more frequent in women than men. It can occur at any age, in either sex, or in any race. There is loss of the diurnal rhythm of ACTH secretion by the pituitary gland; however, many patients who are ill, under stress, or hospitalized demonstrate this loss of diurnal rhythm.

Cushing's syndrome is characterized by increased weight due to adipose tissue deposition in the face, back of the neck, and trunk, with thin arms and legs. Prominent cheek fat pads produce a "moon face" appearance, and deposition of fat pads in the supraclavicular fossae and back of the neck ("buffalo hump") occur frequently. Sexual dysfunction is a common complaint with amenorrhea or oligomeorrhea in women and decreased libido or impotence in men. Protein loss leads to abnormalities of the skin, and muscle wasting. Common skin findings include thinning of the epidermis, purple striae from subcutaneous vasculature, slow repair, and easy bruising. Other skin changes include acne, skin pigmentation, or rash. Generalized osteoporosis caused by loss of bone matrix can lead to vertebral compression fractures and resultant back pain. Occasionally, pathological fractures of extremities may occur. Headache, increased body hair, and ankle edema may also be found. Impaired glucose tolerance without overt diabetes mellitus and hypertension associated with left ventricular hypertrophy are common associated findings. Mental disturbances range from mild anxiety to severe depression.

If untreated, Cushing's disease produces serious morbidity and can even lead to death. Complications of hypertension, diabetes, osteoporotic spine, and aseptic necrosis of the femoral head may lead to significant disabilities. Increased susceptibility to infections, nephrolithiasis, and psychosis may occur.

Clinically Nonfunctioning Adenomas

Clinically nonfunctioning adenomas are pituitary tumors that do not produce clinically detectable hormone hypersecretion and thus have no specific endocrine abnormality. Without a recognizably clinical syndrome, these tumors are diagnosed late in the disease course and are commonly macroadenomas at diagnosis. The initial major complaint of patients with clinically nonfunctioning adenomas was progressive visual loss (42%), persistent headaches (23%), impotence or decreased libido (23%), and fatigue or weakness (12%) (Arafah, 1986).

Clinically nonfunctioning adenomas are often recognized by the signs and symptoms associated with the mass effect of the tumor such as headaches, visual field defects, and hypopituitarism. Large tumors may cause other cranial nerve dysfunction due to invasion of the cavernous sinus. In addition, a study of clinically nonfunctioning adenomas revealed a high frequency of hypopituitarism including 100% with GH deficiency, 96% with hypogonadism, 81% with hypothyroidism, and 61% with adrenal insufficiency (Arafah, 1986). Large tumors may compress the pituitary stalk and interfere with the delivery of dopamine, the hypothalamic prolactin inhibitory factor, to the lactotrophs of the anterior pituitary, resulting in mild hyperprolactinemia.

Most clinically nonfunctioning adenomas are gonadotropic in origin. When tested with sensitive immunohistochemical techniques the production of LH, FSH, or their subunits can be detected. There are a few reports of FSH-secreting adenomas producing testicular enlargement in men.

TSH-secreting Adenomas

TSH-secreting adenomas are rare and associated with mass effect and hyperthyroidism. The majority only hypersecrete TSH, but 31% are associated with the hypersecretion of other hormones including GH (16%), prolactin (11%), and gonadotropins (1.4%) (Beck-Peccoz et al, 1996). Goiter is found in 95% of cases. The majority of TSH-secreting adenomas are macroadenomas with extrasellar extension (71%), whereas intrasellar macroadenomas and microadenomas are seen less frequently (29%). Thus, secondary mass effects are common with these tumors since 42% present with visual field defects and 17% with headache complaints. Bilateral exophthalmos is rare, with unilateral exophthalmos occurring only with orbital invasion of the tumor.

Hypopituitarism

Hypopituitarism is the loss of or reduction in function of the anterior pituitary. Total or selective loss may occur with pituitary adenoma because of the compromise of the normal cells from the tumor expansion. This occurs more commonly with macroadenomas such as prolactin-secreting, GH-secreting, or clinically nonfunctioning adenomas.

The clinical features of hypopituitarism will depend on the age, gender, and the types of hormones that lose function. One or more hormone functions may be affected as the adenoma expands. The symptoms of loss of function due to tumor compression may be masked by the signs and symptoms of the pituitary tumor hypersecretion. Hypopituitarism is also seen in patients with head injury or parasellar disease who have undergone a surgical procedure or radiation treatment for pituitary adenomas.

The most common symptom of hypopituitarism is gonadal dysfunction in both men and women. Loss of pituitary hormonal secretion with systemic deficiency of hormone is progressive and often occurs initially with gonadotropins, followed by GH, TSH, and ACTH. Variations occur so that adrenal dysfunction and hypothyroidism may be the initial presentation. Deficiency of the gonadotropins causes delayed or arrested puberty in adolescents, infertility, amenorrhea or menstrual disorders in women, and slow reduction of libido and impotence in men that may be attributed to aging. GH hyposecretion leads to interruption of normal growth and delayed puberty in children; however, there is no recognized pathologic syndrome in adults (Schmidt & Wallace, 1998).

Secondary hypothyroidism usually occurs late in the development of hypopituitarism and is usually more mild than primary hyperthyroidism. ACTH deficiency leads to a secondary adrenal deficiency with malaise, loss of energy, and postural hypotension. Adrenal insufficiency can lead to a medical emergency.

Pituitary Apoplexy

Pituitary apoplexy describes a spontaneous hemorrhage within the tumor, with or without tumor infarction. This results in a rapid, acute expansion of the gland with sudden compression and compromise of the surrounding structures. The resulting clinical syndrome may include sudden changes in visual function ophthalmoplegia, headache, or sensory perception, often associated with nausea and vomiting. Occasionally, compression of the carotid artery against the anterior clinoid process can result in cerebral hemispheric disorders including seizures and hemiplegia.

Ocular

The ocular disorders associated with pituitary adenomas are secondary to the expansion of the tumor and the compression of nerves that serve the ocular structures (Table 19–3). Because of the proximity of the optic chiasm, pituitary tumors can lead to compression of the optic pathway and result in visual loss. In addition, expansion laterally into the cavernous sinus may compress the oculomotor nerve (III), trochlear nerve (IV), abducens nerve (VI), and the ophthalmic and maxillary divisions of the trigeminal nerve (V).

TABLE 19–3. OCULAR MANIFESTATIONS OF DYSFUNCTIONS OF THE PITUITARY GLAND

Compression of Optic Nerve, Chiasm, or Pathway
- Visual field loss: central and/or peripheral (classically bitemporal)
- Decreased visual acuity
- Decreased color vision
- Optic atrophy

Compression of Cranial Nerves III, IV, or VI
- Ophthalmoplegia
- Diplopia
- Ptosis

Compression of Cranial Nerves V_1 or V_2
- Facial pain

Retro-orbital Venous Congestion
- Proptosis (rare)

With the advancement of neuroimaging techniques, visual loss as the presenting sign of a pituitary tumor is less common.

Ocular findings are absent in microadenomas, because the tumor is too small to compress the adjacent nerves. Macroadenomas most commonly expand superiorly, and extrasellar extension often results in the compression of the optic chiasm. The type of visual field defect produced is dependent on the anatomic relationship between the chiasm and the pituitary gland. The chiasm is normally directly above the pituitary; however, the chiasm is anterior in about 15% of cases (prefixed chiasm) and posterior in about 5% of cases (postfixed chiasm). Lateral expansion of the tumor into the cavernous sinus occurs less frequently, but can result in complaints of diplopia, ptosis, and alteration of facial sensation.

The bitemporal hemianopic field defect is the classic sign of chiasmal disorder and the visual abnormality most commonly observed in a patient with a pituitary macroadenoma (Figure 19–2). It is a common presenting finding in prolactinomas and GH-secreting and clinically nonfunctioning adenomas. The superior temporal quadrants are usually the first to be affected, with the inferior temporal quadrants following. The inferior nasal quadrants are the next to become involved, followed by the superior nasal quadrants and blindness. This correlates with the compression coming from directly below the chiasm and causing damage to the crossed fibers first and later involving the uncrossed fibers.

Visual field defects other than the classic bitemporal distribution are possible due to alterations in the relationship between the chiasm and the sella. Rarely, the compression is anterior on the intracranial portion of an optic nerve, with unilateral decreased vision and central or arcuate scotoma. With a postfixed chiasm, compression of one optic nerve just anterior to the chiasm can result in an ipsilateral visual loss, relative afferent pupillary defect, decreased color vision, and a visual field defect that may have a suggestion of temporal loss. The contralateral eye has a superior temporal defect that may be missed unless careful perimetry is performed. This is due to compression of inferior nasal fibers of the contralateral eye that project forward into the optic nerve of the ipsilateral eye just anterior to the chiasm (Wilbrand knee). With a prefixed chiasm, the field defect can be a bitemporal scotomatous pattern with normal vision from pressure on the posterior aspect of the chiasm. Incongruous homonymous hemianopic defects are possible if the adenoma compresses the optic tract on one side. Rarely, growth of the tumor between the optic nerves may produce binasal defects as the nerve is pushed laterally against the internal carotid arteries.

The visual field defects may be relative or absolute. The use of a red target may elicit a defect in a field that appears normal to a white target. The visual acuity may be normal in patients with early bitemporal field defects; therefore, these patients may be visually asymptomatic. However, a number of patients develop decreased visual acuity in one or both eyes as the bitemporal defects progress. This may be associated with other clinical signs of optic neuropathy such as color vision defects. Thus, the symptomatic patient may complain of central vision loss or peripheral field loss.

The visual loss associated with pituitary tumors is slowly progressive and gradual so that it can be well established prior to its detection. Continuous expansion of the tumor leads to progressive visual field loss and can result in blindness if no treatment is instituted. Damage from compression of the pituitary adenoma eventually produces optic atrophy. This may be appreciated after 6 weeks of nerve compression. The atrophy caused by pituitary adenomas is usually diffuse.

Paresis of the nerves controlling the extraocular muscles is associated with the complaint of diplopia. This finding can be caused by compression on the cavernous sinus wall or by invasion of the sinus. This occurs in about 15% of patients, usually without signs or symptoms. Both large tumors with lateral extension, possibly due to a small diaphragma opening, and smaller tumors, often associated with Cushing's disease, may grow laterally into the cavernous sinus. With significant invasion of the cavernous sinus, the trigeminal nerve may also be affected, and venous stasis rarely may produce moderate proptosis.

A few patients with complete bitemporal hemianopia may complain of horizontal or vertical diplopia and difficulty reading in the absence of extraocular

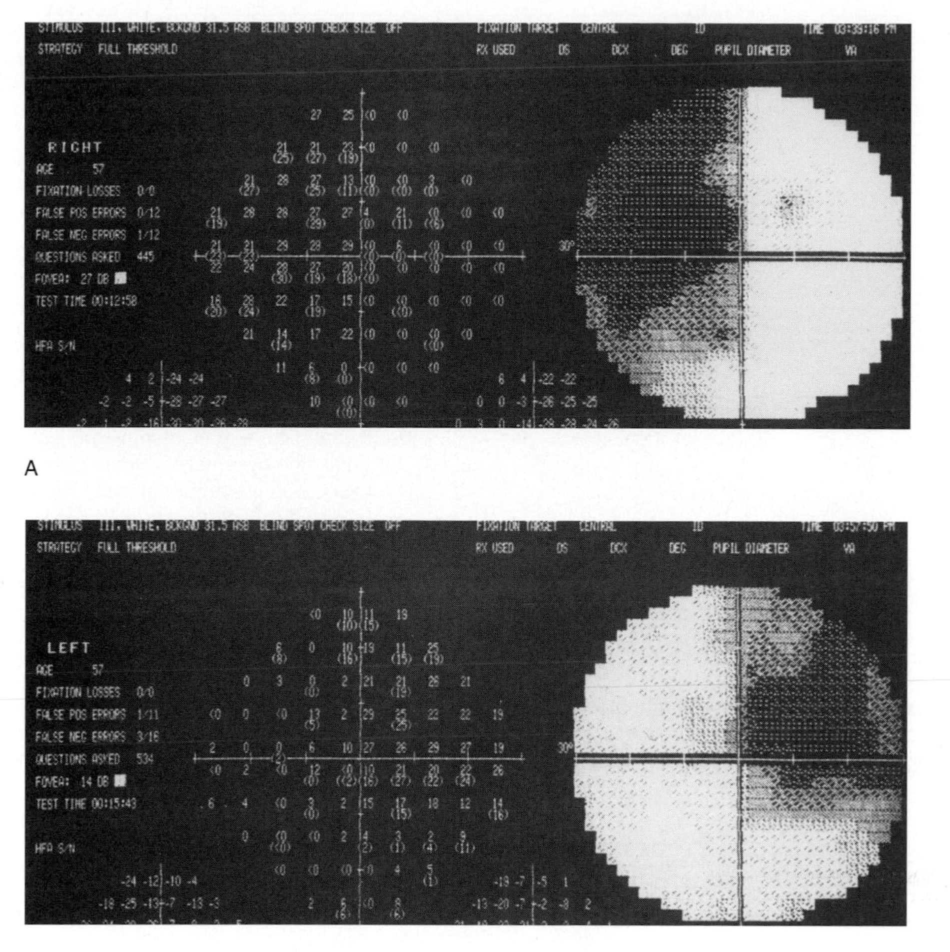

Figure 19–2. Visual fields, examination (right eye **[A]** and left eye **[B]**) demonstrating a bitemporal hemianopsia in a patient with a pituitary adenoma. Note the slight assymetry with more involvement of the left inferior nasal quadrant.

muscle nerve paresis. This may result from loss of the normal overlap of ganglion-receptive fields in the nasotemporal fusional areas, causing the breakdown of pre-existing phoria. The remaining nasal fields may overlap or separate, causing diplopia and reading disturbances.

DIAGNOSIS

Table 19–4 delineates the differential diagnosis of sellar masses.

Systemic

The clinical characteristics of a patient with a pituitary adenoma will vary with the size and cell type of the tumor. Microadenomas are associated with complaints suggesting an endocrine disorder, or they may be detected with imaging studies for an unrelated disorder. Young women with galactorrhea–amenorrhea syndrome, patients with acromegaly, and patients with Cushing's disease are usually diagnosed because of complaints regarding their endocrine disorders. On the other hand, macroadenomas are often associated visual system abnormalities as the tumor compresses the surrounding nerves. This most commonly occurs in prolactinomas in males, with clinically nonfunctional adenomas, and often in acromegaly. However, many patients with clinically nonfunctioning adenomas are diagnosed due to CT scans or MRI studies performed for reasons unrelated to the tumor. In addition, these large tumors can be associated with hypopituitarism as the function of the other secreting cells is compromised by the tumor expansion. The sequence of the diagnostic workup in pituitary adenomas will vary depending on the presenting signs or symptoms.

History and physical examination of the patient with a suspected or documented pituitary adenoma

TABLE 19–4. DIFFERENTIAL DIAGNOSIS OF SELLAR MASSES

Cysts of the Sellar and Parasellar Regions	Craniopharyngioma	Children (5–10 years): headache, nausea, vomiting, papilledema, visual loss; adults: 80% vision loss
	Rathe's cleft cysts	Adults (38 years mean): 2:1 female:male; typically small, asymptomatic; rarely compress optic chiasm
	Arachnoid cysts	Rare; can compress optic pathway; hydrocephalus
	Epidermal cysts	Rare (30–50 years); endocrine and visual disturbances
Other Parasellar Lesions	Chordomas	Rare (30–50 years); more in males; diplopia, cranial neuropathy
	Germinoma	10–30 years; endocrine abnormalities, diabetes insipidus, visual dysfunction, visual field defects, precocious puberty
	Dermoid	Rare, children; recurrent meningitis
	Optic nerve glioma	Rare in children: slow-growing, vision loss, headaches, proptosis Adults: retrobulbar pain; rapidly progresses to blindness
	Hypothalamic glioma	Rare, hypothalamic dysfunction, diabetes insipidus, visual loss
	Parasellar meningioma	40–50 years; more in women; vision loss with field defect, no endocrine dysfunction, headaches common
	Pituitary metastases	>50 years; women, breast primary; men, lung primary; endocrine dysfunction with diabetes insipidus, visual field loss, cranial nerve palsies
Aneurysms	Internal carotid	Bitemporal field defects, ocular motor palsies, supraorbital pain, intense headache, hyperprolactinemia, hypopituitarism
Granulomatous, Inflammatory, and Infectious Processes	Tuberculosis	Tuberculoma—visual field defects, hypopituitarism
	Sarcoid	Neurosarcoidosis—diabetes insipidus, hyperprolactinemia
	Giant cell granuloma	Rare; hypopituitarism, hyperprolactinemia
	Pituitary abscess	Rare; visual defects, hypopituitarism, hyperprolactinemia
	Lymphocytic hypophysitis	Rare; women (60–70%); late pregnancy or early postpartum; associated with other autoimmune disorders (thyroiditis); headache, visual impairment, hypopituitarism, hyperprolactinemia, diabetes Insipidus
Mucoceles	Sphenoid sinus	Optic neuropathy, proptosis, paresis of III or IV, diplopia

should include evaluation of growth curve, sexual development or dysfunction, presence of galactorrhea, diabetes insipidus, or acromegaly, thyroid function, and adrenal function. Clinical evidence of acromegaly, hyperprolactinemia, or Cushing's syndrome should focus the type of investigation. Because detecting the hypersecretion of one or more anterior pituitary hormones and documenting the normal function of other pituitary systems can lead to extensive and expensive testing, laboratory investigation should always be directed by the clinical findings and interpreted within the context of the physical examination and patient history. In addition, interpretation of the laboratory investigation relies upon understanding the limitations of each type of assay, the relationship between the levels of pituitary and target hormones, and the pulsatile hormonal secretion of the anterior pituitary. Other factors influencing hormone levels can include the time of day, developmental stage, stress level, fasting state, concurrent pharmaceutical use, and level of patient activity. This evaluation is best performed by an endocrinologist or experienced internist (Table 19–5).

TABLE 19–5. SYSTEMIC DIAGNOSTIC TESTING

Overview
Blood chemistries
Glucose testing
Thyroid function (serum free thyroxine and TSH)
Adrenal function
Pregnancy tests
Imaging studies: CT, MRI
Prolactinoma
Analysis of serum prolactin levels
Blood chemistries
Thyroid function
Pregnancy tests
Acromegaly
GH levels
Prolactin level
IGF-1
Glucose
Thyroid function
Cushing's Syndrome
Dexamethasone suppression test
24-hour urine cortisol and creatine
Salivary cortisol

In patients with suspected prolactinoma, the analysis of serum prolactin levels and the diagnosis of hyperprolactinemia is difficult due to the pulsatile secretion of this hormone and its response to stress and breast manipulation. Serum prolactin levels of 20 to 60 ng/mL represent mild elevations and are difficult to interpret. They must be repeated several times prior to concluding that pathologic hyperprolactinemia is present. A careful history and physical with normal screening blood chemistries, thyroid functions (serum free thyroxine and TSH), and pregnancy tests (serum hCG) excludes the most common causes of hyperprolactinemia. With normal laboratory results and a negative history for concurrent phenothiazine derivatives, tricyclic antidepressants, or oral contraceptives, MRI with gadolinium enhancement is indicated. Serum prolactin levels of less than 150 to 200 ng/mL indicate the presence of a macroadenoma that most likely represents a secondary hyperprolactinemia. This is due to pituitary stalk compression from a non-prolactin-secreting tumor and the interruption of dopamine delivery from the hypothalamus. This might involve a different treatment. The diagnosis of a sellar lesion with moderately elevated prolactin levels is further complicated by the potential of a false-positive imaging result, as these techniques now detect cysts, infarcts, and incidental clinically nonfunctional tumors. However, a single value of 200 ng/mL or greater in a patient with a documented macroadenoma is likely to be due to a prolactinoma.

Postmenopausal women and men with prolactinomas are commonly identified on radiologic imaging for an unrelated problem or complaint of headache. In addition, a history of combined galactorrhea and amenorrhea with elevated prolactin levels increases the probability of a pituitary adenoma being found with high-resolution imaging techniques.

The measurement of GH levels is complicated by the numerous factors that can influence an abnormally high serum GH. Recent eating or exercise, agitation or acute illness, renal or hepatic failure, diabetes mellitus, malnourishment, and concurrent estrogens, beta-blockers, or clonidine can influence GH levels. Suspected acromegalics should have an overnight fasting serum sample tested for prolactin levels (GH tumors may cosecrete), IGF-1, glucose (diabetes is a common comorbidity), serum free thyroxine, and TSH (secondary hypothyroidism is common). IGF-1 is a somatomedin, which reflects growth hormone levels over the past 24 hours and is elevated five times over normal in acromegaly. Elevated serum IGF-1 indicates excess GH secretion except during pregnancy and puberty, when IGF-1 is normally increased. A serum GH measurement 1 hour after oral glucose is the definitive test for acromegaly. After ingestion of glucose, serum GH levels will normally decrease to less than 2 ng/mL. In acromegaly, serum GH fails to drop below this level. MRI on acromegalics detects adenomas in 90% of cases.

Macroadenomas are rare in Cushing's disease, and only about 50% of the microadenomas are detectable with imaging studies. This adds to the complexity of distinguishing between primary tumors of the adrenal glands, ectopic ACTH-secreting tumors, and ACTH-secreting pituitary tumors. After ruling out an iatrogenic source of cortisol, the most common biochemical testing in the diagnosis of Cushing's syndrome includes the dexamethasone suppression test and 24-hour urine cortisol and creatinine. In the absence of overt pituitary adenoma on MRI, a corticotropin-releasing factor test is being recommended to confirm a pituitary source of ACTH hypersecretion. Recent studies have also recommended two or three late-night (11 P.M.) salivary cortisol measurements and a 24-hour urine free cortisol as the most accurate and simplest tests to evaluate Cushing's disease.

The diagnosis of clinically nonfunctioning adenomas is often based on visual disturbances, headache evaluation, particularly significant changes in headaches pattern, or symptoms of hypopituitarism. Hypopituitarism should be evaluated by investigating the hormonal levels of the anterior and posterior pituitary. History and physical findings may suggest deficient hormones.

Appropriate imaging studies are essential for the diagnosis of pituitary tumor. CT scans and MRIs (Figures 19–3 and 19–4) have replaced plain skull x-rays, cerebral angiography, and pneumoencephalography in the evaluation of pituitary adenoma. These earlier techniques provided poor visualization of the gland and the surrounding structures. CT scans will provide direct imaging of the gland, identify large tumors, and delineate early hemorrhage. High-resolution and contrast CT scans, with 1-mm images in the axial and transverse planes, are recommended for detection of pituitary tumors. Sagittal reconstructions can be performed from the data of these scan sequences.

MRI provides the best method for direct imaging of the gland and its surrounding structures (optic chiasm, diaphragma sellae, and vascular structures), along with identifying large and small tumors (Wu & Thomas, 1995). Standard protocol is for 1- to 2-mm slices through the sella in both sagittal and coronal planes using T_1 images. An intravenous gadolinium-based medium is infused and these images are repeated. T_2 images are not part of the routine pituitary evaluation but can be useful in the detection of cystic

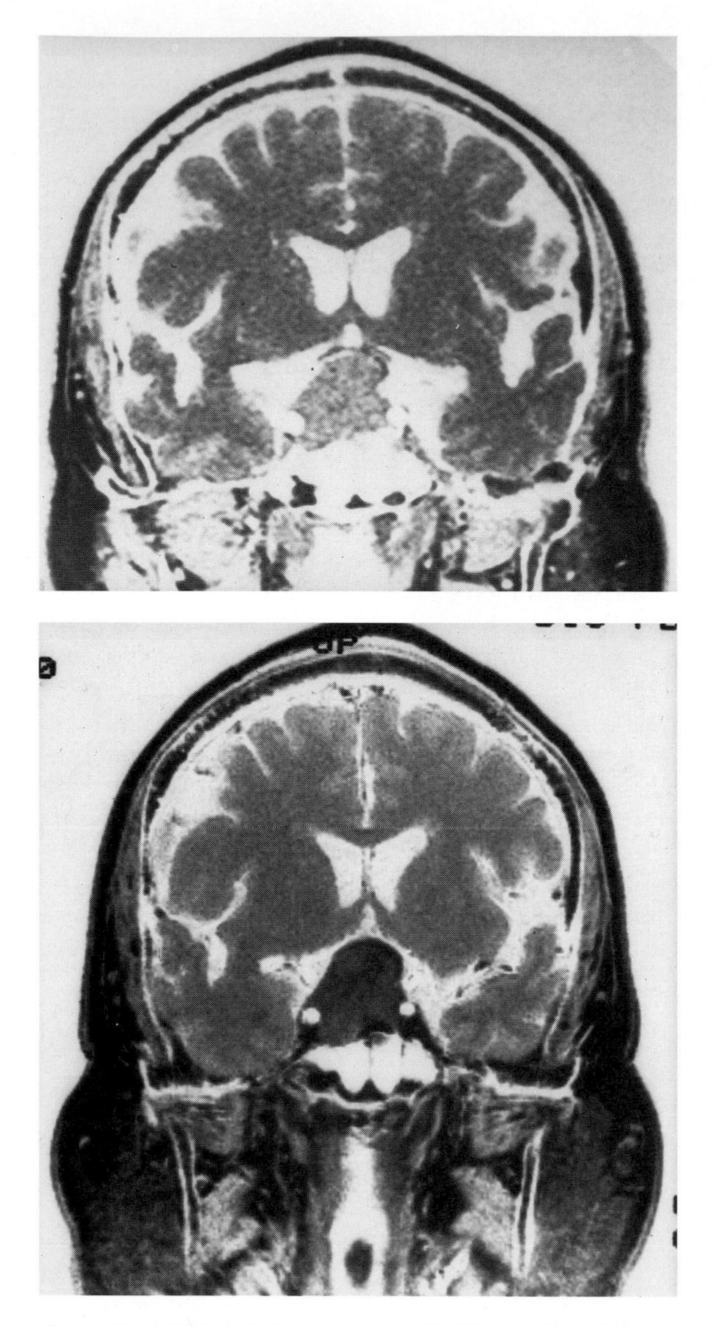

Figure 19–3. MRI of pituitary adenoma with (A) and without (B) contrast. Note the compression of the chiasm just above the adenoma.

change and hemorrhage. Recent advances in MRI include enhancement, recognizing that the peak enhancement with contrast of the adenoma occurs after the peak enhancement of the gland. This has improved MRI detection of adenomas to about the 65 to 85% rate. Dynamic imaging acquires images on a faster time scale in concert with microcirculation and may provide an overall sensitivity of 90% (Elster, 1994). However, the cost of dynamic imaging may not be justified in most clinical settings.

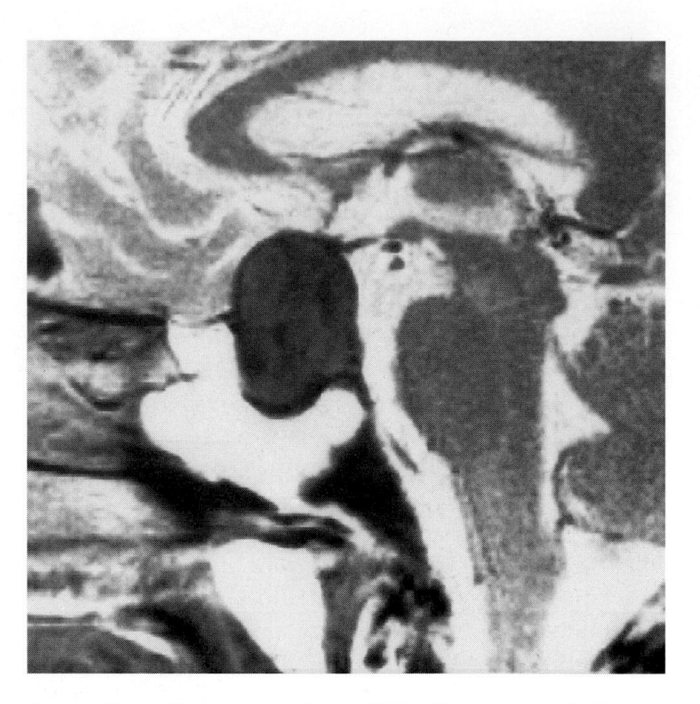

Figure 19–4. Midsagittal section of MRI with contrast, with the optic chiasm stretched over the pituitary adenoma.

Ocular

Although pituitary adenomas without endocrine symptoms were traditionally diagnosed in response to dysfunction of the visual system, the frequency of this method of detection has been reduced by the common use of high-quality imaging studies. However, patients still present to ophthalmic practitioners with and without complaints of visual loss who harbor pituitary tumors compressing the optic pathway. A patient without endocrine or visual symptoms may have early visual signs that are missed due to lack of testing visual fields or poor technique in testing visual fields (Table 19–6). When visual field defects are detected, the recognition of a bitemporal defect may lead to the proper diagnosis. However, if central arcuate, centrocecal, or nasal defects are revealed, the proper diagnosis may be missed. Some rare cases may mimic retrobulbar neuritis. Therefore, any suggestion of a temporal defect that respects the vertical meridian or an asymptomatic defect in the other eye should raise the suspicion that the cause of visual loss is in the region of the chiasm. A pituitary mass should be considered as a potential etiology of unexplained visual loss. The classic pattern of "bow tie" atrophy can be seen in patients with long-standing temporal field defects. The loss of the nasal retinal fibers leads to atrophy at the 3 to 9 o'clock margins of the disc. In the clinical setting of a known adenoma, visual field testing is indicated only if the imaging studies show optic nerve compression.

TABLE 19–6. DIAGNOSTIC TESTING OF OCULAR FINDINGS

Ocular Findings	Mechanism	Diagnostic Testing
Unexplained decreased vision ± pallor of optic nerve	Compression of optic chiasm or optic nerve	Visual field testing
Bitemporal visual field defects	Compression of optic chiasm or optic nerve	MR scan with contrast; CT scan with contrast
Diplopia, ophthalmoplegia, ptosis (III, IV, VI palsy)	Compression of more than one nerve suggests cavernous sinus lesion	MR scan with contrast; CT scan with contrast

> Pituitary adenoma should be included in the differential diagnosis of any patient with unexplained vision loss.

Disorders of eye movements are less common than visual loss. In most cases, eye movement findings are associated with visual loss, field defect, or trigeminal deficit, suggesting the presence of a tumor; nevertheless, these are sometimes isolated findings. Most commonly, the oculomotor nerve is partially affected with or without pupillary involvement. This normally occurs without pain; however, painful recurrent oculomotor palsy has been reported with prolactin-secreting adenoma. Damage to the oculosympathetic pathway may occur, resulting in a smaller, less reactive pupil. The trochlear and abducens nerves are less frequently involved and seldom in isolation. Complete ophthalmoplegia occurs most often with pituitary apoplexy but is extremely rare.

TREATMENT AND MANAGEMENT

Systemic

The management of pituitary adenomas (Table 19–7) varies with the size of the tumor, functional type, age and health of the patient, and in women, any future desire for pregnancy. Present management may include observation, medical therapy, surgical excision, radiation, or a combination of these modalities. The goals of treatment are to return the hormonal hypersecretion to normal, decrease tumor size, return the pituitary to normal function, recover any visual loss (Figure 19–5), and resolve any cranial nerve impairment. Ideally, this is achieved without chronic hormonal replacement therapy. Only partial achievement of these goals is often possible with very large tumors.

Prolactin-secreting Adenomas

When hyperprolactinemia is present in an asymptomatic patient, with a small or nonvisible lesion on CT scan or MRI, appropriate management may be observation. This is based on the potential of long-term change of microprolactinomas. Almost 95% of patients show no enlargement over a 4- to 6-year observation (Schlechte et al, 1989). Since prolactinomas rarely grow without change in serum prolactin levels, patients can be followed with serial prolactin levels and one or two follow-up scans. Elevation of serum prolactin levels would indicate a repeat scan. Any growth should be an indication for treatment. Other indications for treatment would be any clinical effects of hormone hypersecretion. In a series of endocrine asymptomatic

TABLE 19–7. SYSTEMIC AND OCULAR TREATMENT AND MANAGEMENT OF PITUITARY ADENOMA

Prolactin-secreting Adenoma

Asymptomatic microadenoma

- Observation (serum prolactin levels, MRI)

Symptomatic microadenoma and macroadenoma

- Cabergoline (increasing dosage to 0.5 mg twice weekly orally)
- Bromocriptine (1.25–7.5 mg/day orally)
- Transsphenoidal excision with medical failure
- Adjunctive radiotherapy

GH-secreting Adenoma

- Transsphenoidal excision
- Octreotide 50μg injection tid
- Cabergoline 1–1.75 mg/week orally
- Adjunctive radiotherapy

ACTH-secreting Adenoma

- Transsphenoidal excision
- Radiotherapy
- Adjunctive medical therapy
- Replacement therapy

TSH-secreting Adenoma

- Transsphenoidal excision
- Adjunctive radiotherapy
- Adjunctive octreotide 50μg injection tid

Clinically Nonfunctioning Adenoma

- Transsphenoidal excision
- Adjunctive radiotherapy
- Replacement therapy

Ocular

- Reduction in adenoma size
- Visual field examination

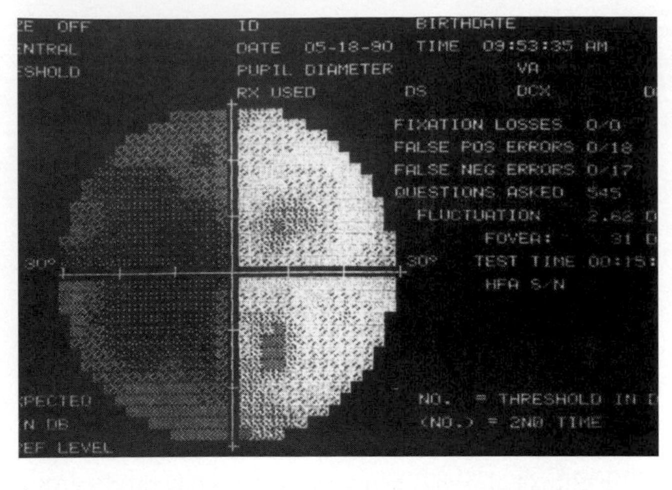

A

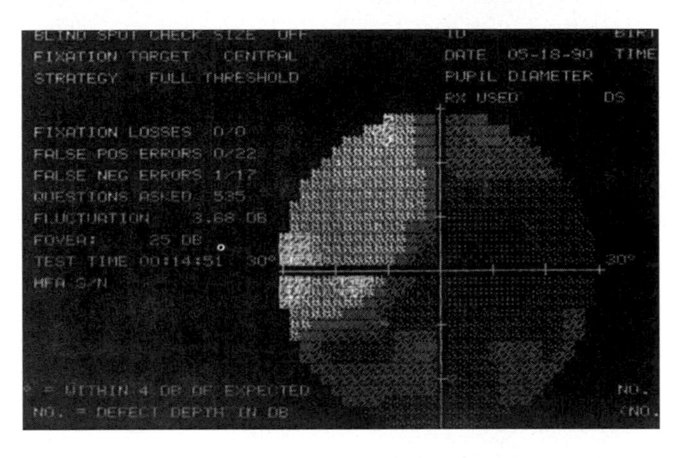

B

Figure 19–5. Visual fields examination of the patient in Figure 19–2 (right eye **[A]** and left eye **[B]**) 3 days after transsphenoidal resection of the tumor. Note the rapid recovery of the left eye.

women, except for nonbothersome galactorrhea, prolactin levels return to normal in about one third of cases (Jeffcoate et al, 1996).

Medical therapy is the initial treatment of choice. Bromocriptine (Parlodel), a dopamine agonist, is very effective and its long safety record make it the preferred choice in hyperprolactinemic women with infertility as the primary treatment indication. Treatment results in 70 to 80% normalized prolactin levels, during therapy, and return to menses and improved galactorrhea (Molitch, 1995). Bromocriptine therapy in men results in increased testosterone levels with improvement of libido and potency. Effectiveness of bromocriptine therapy is correlated with the number and binding affinity of dopamine receptors on the tumor. Side effects of nausea, orthostatic hypotension, and headache cause 3 to 5% to discontinue therapy. Medical therapy for macroadenomas may involve a longer treatment period to get prolactin levels within the normal range. As this medical therapy is not tumoricidal, withdrawal of the medication usually leads to increased prolactin levels, re-expansion of the tumor, and return of symptoms. Continued therapy is required even after normal prolactin levels are achieved. Medically treated patients are followed with CT or MRI every 1 to 2 years. Patients with fewer receptors may respond partially or not at all to medical therapy; this represents 5 to 10% of patients put on therapy. Surgical resection of the tumor should be considered when medical therapy fails.

Cabergoline is better tolerated in most patients with prolactinoma. It is a longer-acting dopamine agonist that can be given orally once or twice a week. Initial studies indicate that it might be more efficacious and better tolerated than bromocriptine (Webster et al, 1994).

Surgical removal of the tumor by the transsphenoidal approach was the most effective treatment prior to development of medical therapy. Surgical results vary with the skill and experience of the surgeon, size of the tumor, and the presurgical prolactin levels. Surgery is effective in resecting microadenomas, with a reversal of symptoms in 71% of cases and 32% with macroadenomas. However, due to recurrence, about 50 to 60% of patients with microadenomas and 25% with macroadenomas have long-term success as defined by normal prolactin levels (Molitch, 1995). Nevertheless, surgical resection is effective in reducing the size of macroadenomas. Residual therapy is often required with large tumors because of partial resection.

Radiotherapy is effective in arresting tumor growth but less effective in reducing serum prolactin levels. It is not the treatment of choice in prolactinoma, but is used in postoperative patients or in combination with bromocriptine in more rapidly growing tumors. Hypopituitarism and damage to optic pathways are complications seen with pituitary radiation therapy.

Growth-hormone-secreting Adenomas

Transsphenoidal surgical removal has been the preferred initial treatment of GH-secreting adenomas. Results depend on the skill of the surgeon and the size of the tumor, with tumor extension beyond the sella decreasing the chances of a surgical cure (Abosch et al, 1998). Experienced surgeons have reported cure rates of 80 to 90% for GH microadenomas; however, macroadenoma cure rates are often less than 50% (Ahmed et al. 1999).

Medical therapy of GH macroadenomas is receiving more attention because of lack of a surgical cure. Medical treatment of GH macroadenomas in the postsurgical patient has the goals of maintaining GH less than 2 ng/mL and normal IGF-1. Octreotide, a somatostatin analogue, has been used and restores IGF-1 levels to normal in 55 to 65% of patients, yet it demonstrates tumor shrinkage in only 40% of patients (Newman et al, 1998). It also has the disadvantage of administration by injection. A long-acting form has been developed, Octreotide-LAR, which requires a dose every 4 weeks (Davies et al, 1998). Dopamine agonists have been used in the treatment of GH-secreting tumors. Cabergoline appears to be more effective than bromocriptine and has the advantage of oral administration (Abs et al, 1998). The efficacy of these medical treatments as a primary treatment awaits confirmation in randomized masked placebo-controlled studies.

Postoperative radiotherapy is useful with persistent tumor to prevent tumor growth and control hypersecretion. Radiotherapy alone is less useful, because the time interval to reach normal levels is often 10 years and it has a high risk of causing hypopituitarism (Landolt et al, 1998).

ACTH-secreting Adenomas

Transsphenoidal surgical excision of localized adenomas is the preferred treatment in Cushing's disease and hemihypophysectomy or total hypophysectomy in cases where the tumor is not localized. The cure rate is approximately 80% with an identified microadenoma and experienced surgical team (Sonino et al, 1996). Radiation is an option, with 80% of children responding to therapy, but it is disappointing in adults, with only about 20% being successful. The potential development of pituitary dysfunction and other long-term effects of radiation must be considered. Medical treatment includes ketoconazole, metyrapone, and aminoglutemide, which blocks or inhibits cortisol synthesis. These medications have limited usefulness due to side effects and ineffectiveness. Their main role is adjunctive use in preparing extremely ill patients for surgery or while waiting for the full effects to occur after radiation treatment.

Clinically Nonfunctioning Adenomas

Surgical excision, via the transsphenoidal approach, is the recommended therapy for macroadenomas, although pituitary hypofunction is a frequent side effect of surgery. Radiation therapy is an alternative for poor surgical candidates or those with residual tumor following surgery. Medical therapy with somatostatin analogues has limited indications and octreotide may be of benefit in poor surgical candidates with aggressive tumors who failed control with radiotherapy. Microadenomas that are clinically nonfunctioning can be viewed as "incidentalomas" and since they have no mass effect or hormone hypersecretion, they may be followed with observation. Postoperative management includes evaluation for replacement therapy.

TSH-secreting Adenomas

For these rare adenomas, transsphenoidal surgery is the primary treatment. Medical control of hyperthyroidism prior to surgery is important. Radiation is used to treat patients with large tumors who do not have normal thyroid hormone levels postoperatively. Medical therapy in the form of octreotide has been efficacious with normal TSH in 79% of patients, tumor shrinkage in 52%, and vision improvement in 75% of patients (Beck-Peccoz et al, 1996).

Ocular

When successful, surgical resection, radiation therapy, or medical therapy results in reduction in the size of an adenoma with decompression of the chiasm and optic nerves. This results in improvement of visual acuity and the visual field. Eyes with preoperative visual acuity of at least 20/100 almost always improve postsurgically, as do 60% of eyes with a preoperative acuity of less than 20/100. Surgical removal has resulted in improvement of visual function in 75 to 95% of patients. Improvement may start hours after the surgery and continue for months and occasionally years. Transsphenoidal surgical resection of macroadenomas has resulted in improved visual fields in 81%, unchanged in 15%, and deterioration in 4% of patients (Laws & Thapar, 1995). Improvement in visual field defects with medical therapy can occur prior to detection of tumor regression on imaging studies. Prolactinomas treated with bromocriptine in a small series showed improvement in visual fields in 90% of cases (Molitch et al, 1985). The improvement started 24 to 72 hours after initiation of therapy and slowly improved over several weeks. Complications of radiation therapy include damage to the optic chiasm or optic nerves.

Ocular examination prior to and after surgical or medical treatment, including visual field examination, is needed to document effectiveness of therapy and monitor tumor recurrence. This should be done in conjunction with imaging studies. In some cases, changes in visual field or visual acuity may indicate tumor recurrence that is not seen on imaging studies.

CONCLUSION

A pituitary adenoma can present with abnormal levels of hormone secretion in a recognized clinical syndrome such as prolactinoma in women, Cushing's disease, or acromegaly. Incidental adenomas without hormonal activity are discovered on imaging studies in increasing number of patients evaluated for trauma or nasal sinus problems. Occasionally, an adenoma presents with the clinical manifestations of hypopituitarism due to mass effect. More commonly, the mass effect of a pituitary macroadenoma presents with the complaint of decreased vision. The classic textbook sign, the bitemporal hemianopia, may not be as clear as the textbook stated. More often it is masked by other ocular presentations that may provide diagnostic difficulty, or the decreased vision has been attributed to another cause. The astute clinician remembers to consider a pituitary adenoma as a potential cause when faced with unexplained vision loss. Consequently, an understanding of both the ocular and systemic manifestations of pituitary adenomas may lead to the appropriate diagnosis and subsequent management.

REFERENCES

Abosch A, Tyrrell JB, Lamborn KR, et al. Transsphenoidal microsurgery for growth hormone-secreting pituitary adenomas: Initial outcome and long-term results. *J Clin Endocrinol Metab.* 1998;83:3411–3418.

Abs R, Verhelst J, Maiter D, et al. Cabergoline in the treatment of acromegaly: A study in 64 patients. *J Clin Endocrinol Metab.* 1998;83:374–378.

Ahmed S, Elsheikh M, Stratton IM, et al. Outcome of transsphenoidal surgery for acromegaly and its relationship to surgical experience. *Clin Endocrinol.* 1999;50:561–567.

Anderson D, Faber P, Marcovitz S, et al. Pituitary tumors and the ophthalmologist. *Ophthalmology.* 1983;90:1265–1270.

Arafah BM. Reversible hypopituitarism in patients with large nonfunctioning pituitary adenomas. *J Clin Endocrinol Metab.* 1986;62:1173–1179.

Asa SL, Ezzat S. The cytogenesis and pathogenesis of pituitary adenomas. *Endocr Rev.* 1998;19:798–827.

Beck-Peccoz P, Brucker-Davis F, Perdani L, et al. Thyrotropin-secreting pituitary tumors. *Endocr Rev.* 1996;17:610–638.

Buchfelder M, Nistor R, Fahlbusch R, et al. The accuracy of CT and MR evaluation of the sella turcica for detection of adrenocorticotropic hormone-secreting adenomas in Cushing disease. *Am J Neuroradiol.* 1993;14:1183–1190.

Burrow GN, Wortzman G, Rewcastle NB, et al. Microadenomas of the pituitary and abnormal sellar tomograms in an unselected autopsy series. *N Engl J Med.* 1981;304:156–158.

Colao A, Ferone D, Maezullo P, et al. Effect of dopaminergic agents in the treatment of acromegaly. *J Clin Endocrinol Metab.* 1997;82:518–523.

Davies PH, Stewart SE, Lancranjan I, et al. Long-term therapy with long-acting octreotide (Sandostatin-LAR) for the management of acromegaly. *Clin Endocrinol.* 1998;48:311–136.

Elster A. Commentary—High resolution, dynamic pituitary MR imaging: Standard or academic pastime. *Am J Roentgenol.* 1994;163:680–682.

Elster AD. Modern imaging of the pituitary. *Radiology.* 1993;187:1–14.

Findling JW, Doppman JL. Biochemical and radiologic diagnosis of Cushing's syndrome. *Endocrinol Metab Clin North Am.* 1994;23:511–537.

Gold EB. Epidemiology of pituitary adenomas. *Epidemiol Rev.* 1981;3:163–183.

Herman V, Fagin J, Gonsky R, et al. Monoclonal origin of pituitary adenomas. *J Clin Endocrinol Metab.* 1990;71:1427–1433.

Jeffcoate WJ, Pound N, Sturrock ND, et al. Long-term follow-up of patients with hyperprolactinaemia. *Clin Endocrinol.* 1996;45:299–303.

Kane LA, Leinung MC, Scheithauer BW, et al. Pituitary adenomas in childhood and adolescence. *J Clin Endocrinol Metab.* 1994;79:1135–1140.

Landolt AM, Haller D, Lomax N, et al. Stereotactic radiosurgery for recurrent surgically-treated acromegaly: Comparison with fractionated radiotherapy. *J Neurosurg.* 1998;88:1002–1008.

Laws ER Jr, Thapar K. Surgical management of pituitary adenoma. *J Clin Endocrinol Metab.* 1995;9:391–406.

Mindermann T, Wilson CB. Age-related and gender-related occurrence of pituitary adenomas. *Clin Endocrinol (Oxf).* 1994;41:359–364.

Molitch ME. Prolactinomas. In: Medmed S, ed. *The Pituitary* Cambridge, MA: Blackwell Science, 1995:136–186.

Molitch ME, Elton RL, Blackwell RE, et al. Bromocriptine as primary therapy for prolactin-secreting macroadenomas: Results of a prospective multicenter study. *J Clin Endocrinol Metab.* 1985;60:698–705.

Newman CB, Melmed S, George A, et al. Octreotide as primary therapy for acromegaly. *J Clin Endocrinol Metab.* 1998;83:3034–3040.

Orrego JJ, Barkan AL. Pituitary disorders. Drug treatment options. *Drugs.* 2000; 59:93–106.

Ortiz JM, Stein SC, Nelson P, et al. Pituitary adenoma presenting as unilateral proptosis. *Arch Opththalmol.* 1992; 110:282–283.

Schlechte J, Dolan K, Sherman B, et al. The natural history of untreated hyperprolactinemia: A prospective analysis. *J Clin Endocrinol Metab.* 1989;68:412–418.

Schmidt DN, Wallace K. How to diagnose hypopituitarism. Learning the features of secondary hormonal deficiencies. *Postgrad Med.* 1998;104:77.

Shimon I, Melmed S. Management of pituitary tumors. *Ann Intern Med.* 1998;129:472.

Sonino N, Zielezny M, Fava GA, et al. Risk factors and long-term outcome in pituitary-dependent Cushing's disease. *J Clin Endocrinol Metab.* 1996;81:2647–2652.

Terada T, Kovacs K, Scheihauer BW, et al. Incidence, pathology, and recurrence of pituitary adenomas: Study of 647 unselected surgical cases. *Endocr Pathol.* 1995;6:301–310.

Webster J, Piscitelli G, Polli A, et al. A comparison of cabergoline and bromocriptine in the treatment of hyperprolactinemic amenorrhea. Cabergoline Comparative Study Group. *N Engl J Med.* 1994;331:904–909.

Wu W, Thuomas K. Pituitary microadenomas: MR appearance and correlation with CT. *Acta Radiol.* 1995;36:529–535.

Section VI

RHEUMATOLOGIC AND INFLAMMATORY DISORDERS

Chapter 20

RHEUMATOID ARTHRITIS

Teresa A. Lowe

Rheumatoid arthritis (RA) is a chronic systemic inflammatory disease of unknown etiology. Although there is a wide spectrum of clinical findings, the characteristic feature of RA is inflammatory synovitis, usually affecting the peripheral joints in a symmetric pattern. The inflammation causes the destruction of cartilage and results in bony deformities. Physical impairment results from progressive joint disease and can have a major impact on the quality of life for most patients. Ocular manifestations include anterior and posterior segment inflammation as well as ocular side effects from systemic medications.

EPIDEMIOLOGY

Systemic

Rheumatoid arthritis affects approximately 1% of the general population of the United States, with women being affected three times more frequently than men (Hochberg, 1981). RA occurs worldwide and affects all ethnic groups. A higher prevalence rate of 3.5 to 5.3% has been found in certain Native American tribes (Beasley et al, 1973). In 1994, there were an estimated 5 million cases of RA in the United States, with about 170,000 new cases being reported for that year (Harris, 1997b). Other studies have found annual figures between 2.9 to 9 cases per 10,000 people (Wollheim, 1998). The age of onset is 25 to 50 years, with the peak incidence occurring during the fourth and fifth decades of life (Lipsky, 1998). However, RA can occur at any age. Patients with RA may have a genetic predisposition for this disease.

Ocular

Keratoconjunctivitis sicca (KCS) is the most common ocular manifestation of RA and occurs in 15 to 25% of patients (Harper & Foster, 1998; Mody et al, 1988; Lamberts, 1983). Episcleritis and scleritis occur less often. In an extensive study of RA patients, McGavin and colleagues (1976) found a 0.17% incidence of episcleritis and a 0.67% incidence of scleritis. RA is the most common systemic condition associated with scleritis and accounts for 20 to 33% of all scleritis cases (Benson, 1988; McGavin et al, 1976; Narsing et al, 1985). There is approximately a 5.7% incidence of RA in patients with episcleritis (McGavin et al, 1976).

PATHOPHYSIOLOGY/DISEASE PROCESS

Systemic

The exact cause of the immune responses and inflammation seen in RA is unknown. Genetic factors may play a role in the development as well as the severity of the disease. The HLA-DR4 haplotype can be found in approximately 65% of patients with RA (Stastny, 1978). Patients with severe disease have an increased frequency of the DQw7 allele, whereas patients with milder or nonprogressive RA have a higher incidence of the DR1 allele (Harper & Foster, 1998). Therefore, patients who carry certain genes may have a higher risk of developing RA, possibly in its more severe forms (Harper & Foster, 1998; MacGregor et al, 1995). Other genes may protect against the development of RA (Larsen et al, 1989).

Theoretically, there may be an environmental factor, such as a virus or bacteria, that initiates the disease process in susceptible individuals. The antigenic trigger causes the lymphocytes to produce an abnormal IgG, which results in the production of autoantibodies or rheumatoid factors directed against the abnormal IgG. Rheumatoid factors are most commonly of the IgM type but also may be of the IgG, IgA, or IgE type. The production of rheumatoid factor-containing immune complexes activates complement and attracts inflammatory cells. The inflammatory process is amplified by various mediators, which include prostaglandins and cytokines released by synovial and infiltrating cells (Wigley, 1995).

Synovial inflammation causes cartilage destruction and bone erosions that result in damage to the joints. Lymphocytes, primarily T helper cells, infiltrate the synovial tissue and produce proinflammatory cytokines. Polymorphonuclear leukocytes and macrophages and their cytokines also are found in the synovium. The synovial membrane becomes thickened and edematous from the cellular infiltration. The lining cells produce collagenase, interleukin-1, and prostaglandins, which all contribute to cartilage destruction. Fibrin deposition, fibrosis, and necrosis also occur. Infiltration granulation tissue (pannus) erodes cartilage, bone, and ligaments. The bones in the affected joints become osteoporotic. Periarticular tendons and muscles become edematous and infiltrated with cells. The destruction of joint cartilage, capsule, and ligaments results in joint deformity.

An overview of the systemic findings in RA is listed in Table 20–1. The clinical findings of RA may be highly variable. The onset of joint inflammation is usually insidious over a period of weeks or months, and may be accompanied by symptoms of malaise, weight loss, fever, and joint pain or stiffness. Less commonly, there is an acute onset that may have been triggered by infection, surgery, trauma, emotional strain, or the postpartum period (Tierny et al, 1999). This acute onset over a period of hours or days occurs in about 10 to 20% of patients (Calabro, 1971; Harris, 1997a; Kanski & Thomas, 1990). Symmetric joint swelling is associated with stiffness, warmth, tenderness, and pain. Stiffness is worse in the morning and gradually improves during the day. Duration of the stiffness may correlate with the severity of the disease. It may recur with inactivity and can worsen after strenuous activity.

TABLE 20–1. SYSTEMIC MANIFESTATIONS OF RHEUMATOID ARTHRITIS

Symptoms
- Malaise
- Fever
- Weight loss
- Morning stiffness

Signs

Articular
- Early
  - Small joints of hands and feet affected
  - Warm, swollen, tender joints (symmetric involvement)
  - Joint stiffness decreases during the day and with activity
- Progressive
  - Larger joints (elbows, shoulders, knees) involved
  - Joint deformity: swan neck
    - boutonniére deformity
    - ulnar deviation

Extra-Articular
- Nodular formation in cutaneous/subcutaneous tissues but may also occur in deep body tissues
- Infarction and/or hemorrhage of the nails, folds of the feet, and hands
- Carpal tunnel syndrome
- Lymphadenopathy
- Anemia
- Pleuritis/pulmonary nodules
- Pericarditis
- Vasculitis

Small joints of the hands and feet are usually affected first. The proximal interphalangeal and metacarpophalangeal joints of the fingers along with the wrists, knees, ankles, and toes are commonly involved. Larger joints may become affected as the disease progresses. Although there may be asymmetric findings initially, joint involvement tends to be symmetric. Deformities can occur after months to years. The most common joint deformities are ulnar deviation of the fingers, hyperextension of the distal interphalangeal joint with flexion of the proximal interphalangeal joint (boutonnière deformity), flexion of the distal interphalangeal joint with extension of the proximal interphalangeal joint (swan-neck), and knee deformities. An example of finger deformities is shown in Figure 20–1. Physical impairment results from progressive joint disease and can have a major impact on the quality of life for most patients.

Although RA primarily affects the musculoskeletal system, other systemic involvement includes cardiac, pulmonary, central nervous system, cutaneous, gastrointestinal, and hematopoietic systems. Twenty to 35% of patients have subcutaneous nodules (Harris, 1997a; Tierney et al, 1999). These rheumatoid nodules

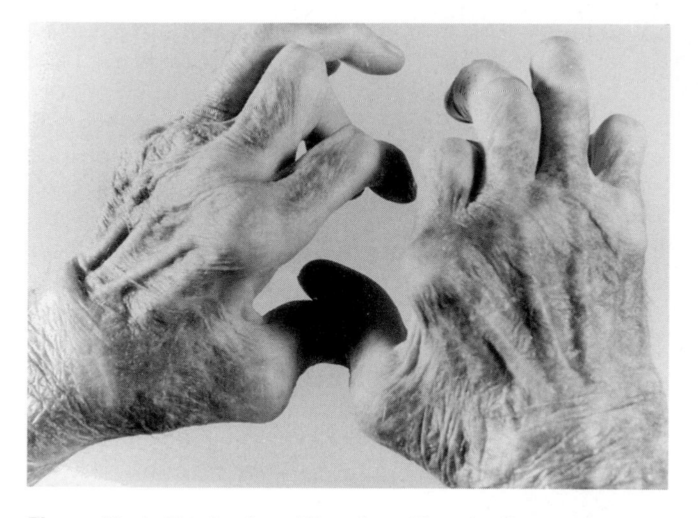

Figure 20–1. Hands of an RA patient. Note the finger deformities bilaterally. The metacarpal and proximal interphalangeal joints are affected most severely. Significant impairment results from this level of deformity. (*Reprinted with permission from Mahoney BP. Rheumatologic disease and associated ocular manifestations.* J Am Optom Assoc. *1993;64:403–415.*)

are the most common extra-articular finding of seropositive patients, and are characterized as firm, round, subcutaneous masses most commonly found on the extensor surfaces of the forearms (Kanski & Thomas, 1990). Clinical manifestations also include vasculitis and atrophy of the skin and muscle. A common neurologic complication in RA is entrapment neuropathy resulting from proliferative synovitis. Carpal tunnel syndrome results from compression of the median nerve and can often cause symptoms in RA patients. Pulmonary findings include pleuritis, interstitial lung fibrosis, and nodules. Other extra-articular findings include lymphadenopathy, splenomegaly, leukopenia, thrombocytopenia, and acute pericarditis.

Ocular

The ocular manifestations of RA are summarized in Table 20–2. Ocular conditions associated with RA include keratoconjunctivitis sicca, episcleritis, scleritis,

TABLE 20–2. OCULAR MANIFESTATIONS OF RHEUMATOID ARTHRITIS

- Dry eye
    - Keratoconjunctivitis sicca
    - Filamentary keratitis
    - Secondary bacterial keratitis
- Paracentral or peripheral corneal ulceration
- Episcleritis
- Anterior scleritis:
    - Nonnecrotizing
    - Necrotizing
- Posterior scleritis

and corneal ulceration. Although anterior uveitis occurs in other rheumatic diseases, it is not more common in RA patients than in the general population (Bacon & Moots, 1997).

Keratoconjunctivitis Sicca

The most common ocular manifestation of RA is keratoconjunctivitis sicca. Patients usually present with symptoms of dryness, sandy or gritty sensation, foreign-body sensation, burning, tearing, or photophobia. Symptoms may be worse at the end of the day or in windy, dry environments. The diagnosis of dry eye can be made by examining the corneal pretear film meniscus and evaluating the cornea with the use of fluorescein and rose bengal staining. Keratoconjunctivitis sicca can progress to a filamentary keratitis.

Episcleritis and Scleritis

The incidence of episcleritis and scleritis is higher in RA patients as compared to the general population. Most studies have found an incidence of <1% for either episcleritis or scleritis in patients with RA. Episcleritis and scleritis can be classified by their anatomical location and their clinical appearance (Watson & Hayreh, 1976). Episcleritis is classified as simple or nodular. An example of episcleritis in an RA patient is shown in Figure 20–2.

Scleritis is differentiated into anterior and posterior forms. Anterior scleritis is described as diffuse, nodular, or necrotizing. Necrotizing scleritis is subdivided into forms with inflammation or without inflammation (scleromalacia perforans).

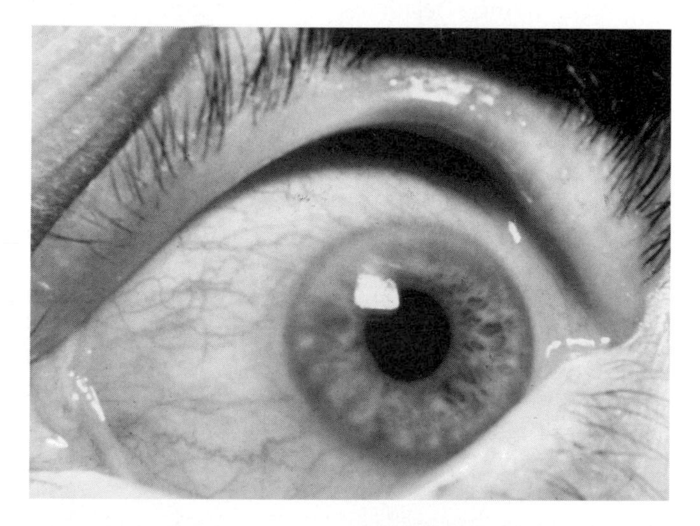

Figure 20–2. Episcleritis in an RA patient. This patient had recurrent episodes of episcleritis that responded well to topical steroid use. No corneal involvement manifested during any of the active episodes. (*Courtesy of Dr. Brian Mahoney.*)

Patients with episcleritis or scleritis usually present with complaints of redness and pain. Slit-lamp examination reveals injection of the fine plexus of the superficial episcleral vessels or of the larger vessels of the deep sclera. In differentiating an episcleritis from a scleritis, the episcleral vessels are finer in caliber and lie more superficially. In scleritis, the deeper scleral vessels are involved along with the more superficial episcleral vessels. In both episcleritis and scleritis, there should be no other conjunctival inflammatory changes besides mild dilation of the overlying conjunctival vessels. Conjunctival discharge should not be present. Patients with episcleritis generally complain of discomfort rather than pain, whereas patients with scleritis often complain of severe pain (Watson & Hayreh, 1976). The condition may be bilateral and affect any quadrant. A nodule may result from localized edema of the episclera or sclera. Photophobia and lacrimation are not routinely associated with episcleritis or scleritis, but when these symptoms are severe they often are indicative of a necrotizing process (Watson & Hayreh, 1976).

Scleritis tends to be more severe in patients with RA as compared to patients with idiopathic scleritis (de la Maza et al, 1994a). Classification of the scleritis helps to determine the prognosis as well as the treatment and management of the patient. Diffuse anterior scleritis is the most common form of scleritis in RA patients (Harper & Foster, 1998). It is also the most benign form of scleritis. Patients may present with diffuse redness and swelling of the episclera and sclera. In nodular anterior scleritis, the nodule is deep red, immobile, and separate from the overlying episcleral tissue. There may be multiple nodules.

Necrotizing scleritis may present with or without inflammation. The inflammatory form of necrotizing scleritis is the most serious. Presenting complaints include severe pain, redness, and vision loss. The presence of an avascular patch of episcleral tissue associated with an area of scleral edema is an important presenting sign (Cobo, 1983). The adjacent cornea may also be affected. Treatment is more difficult and may require systemic steroids or cytotoxic agents. Complications include keratitis, glaucoma, cataract, uveitis, scleral thinning, global perforation, and vision loss. Inflammatory necrotizing scleritis may correlate with systemic vasculitis (Foster et al, 1984). Without appropriate treatment, these patients may die within 5 years as a result of systemic vasculitis (Foster, 1980). Therefore, scleritis can be an important indicator of more serious systemic disease.

Necrotizing scleritis without inflammation is also known as scleromalacia perforans. In this condition, painless thinning of the sclera exposes the underlying uveal tissue. Scleromalacia perforans is more common in patients with long-standing RA and does not have the complications that are seen in the inflammatory form of scleritis (Harper & Foster, 1998; Narsing et al, 1985). Global perforation is very rare. Patients are asymptomatic, and treatment is not necessary. Posterior scleritis may be associated with anterior scleritis. The presenting symptoms of posterior scleritis are pain, decreased vision, and redness. In severe cases, there may be proptosis or diplopia. Funduscopic signs include a circumscribed area of scleral inflammation, choroidal folds, retinal striae, choroidal detachment, exudative macular detachment, cystoid macular edema, peripheral retinal detachment, and disc edema. Uveitis and glaucoma are other ocular findings.

Keratopathy

The most common keratopathy seen in RA is that secondary to keratoconjunctivitis sicca (Harper & Foster, 1998). Severe dry eye may lead to a filamentary keratitis or a secondary bacterial infection. The cornea may also be involved in anterior scleritis. The incidence of corneal involvement in scleritis ranges from 36 to 50% in patients with RA (de la Maza et al, 1994a; McGavin et al, 1976). Corneal involvement usually results from an extension of the scleral inflammatory process. Patterns of peripheral corneal involvement in scleritis include sclerosing keratitis, acute stromal keratitis, furrowing (limbal guttering), and corneal ulceration (Robin et al, 1986).

Sclerosing keratitis is the most common keratopathy associated with scleritis (Robin et al, 1986). It may present as a peripheral thickening and grayish opacification of the stroma adjacent to the area of scleritis. Progression of the keratitis may result in scarring, vascularization, and lipid deposition. In acute stromal keratitis, there are superficial or midstromal peripheral infiltrates associated with nonnecrotizing scleritis. Eventually this may result in vascularization and scarring (Robin et al, 1986).

Peripheral corneal furrowing is also associated with rheumatoid scleritis (Figure 20–3). It may start as an area of sclerosing keratitis, but it progresses circumferentially to involve the entire periphery. In necrotizing scleritis, there may be severe thinning associated with the peripheral corneal furrowing. Peripheral ulcerative keratitis (PUK) is the most severe form of keratitis associated with scleritis. The peripheral ulceration is sterile and appears to be autoimmune-mediated. The incidence is 31% in patients with rheumatoid-associated scleritis (Harper & Foster, 1998). PUK is usually located adjacent to the area of scleral inflammation and more often is associated with necrotizing disease. Severe PUK may result in perforation and

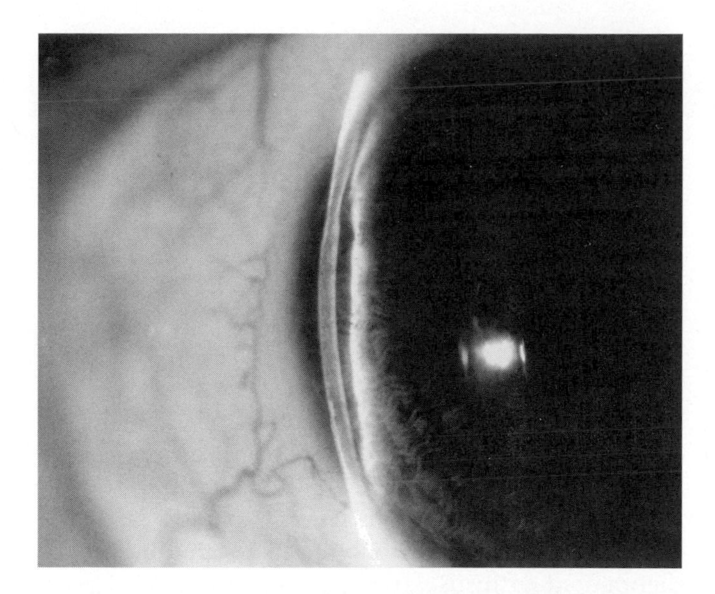

Figure 20–3. Peripheral corneal thinning in an RA patient. Note the stromal loss in a circumferential pattern near the limbus of the cornea. This was present bilaterally and was not accompanied by corneal perforation. No dry eye was present and no ocular treatment was necessary. (*Reprinted with permission from Mahoney BP. Rheumatologic disease and associated ocular manifestations.* J Am Optom Assoc. *1993;64:403–415.*)

destruction of the globe (Messmer & Foster, 1995). Both necrotizing scleritis and PUK are associated with systemic vasculitis (Foster et al, 1984; McGavin et al, 1976; Watson & Hayreh, 1976). Because visceral vasculitis is associated with a higher mortality rate, these patients need aggressive systemic therapy in order to preserve the globe as well as to prolong life (Messmer & Foster, 1995; Vollertsen et al, 1986).

A keratopathy can also occur without scleritis. Paracentral corneal ulceration is a sterile keratitis that affects the central area of the cornea. It is less common than PUK (Harper & Foster, 1998). Both forms of ulceration can result in corneal thinning and perforation even without any obvious signs of inflammation (Adachi et al, 1998; Harper & Foster, 1998). Studies have shown through conjunctival biopsy that the underlying etiology may be an active vasculitis (Kervick et al, 1992). Another contributing factor in sterile ulceration is the production of conjunctival collagenase (Eiferman et al, 1979).

Corneal involvement can also be associated with episcleritis in patients with RA. A keratopathy may occur in up to 15% of cases of rheumatoid episcleritis, and it is usually milder than that seen with scleritis (Robin et al, 1986). Peripheral stromal edema and infiltration may occur adjacent to the episcleral inflammation, eventually causing opacification and vascularization. These changes do not develop into ulceration (de la Maza et al, 1994b).

> Necrotizing scleritis or peripheral ulcerative keratitis can be an important indicator of more serious underlying systemic disease.

Other Ocular Manifestations

Rheumatoid nodules have been reported on the upper eyelid of an RA patient with severe disease (Carter et al, 1976). Bilateral episcleral nodules were observed in another RA patient (Harper & Foster, 1998). A patient with seropositive rheumatoid disease developed a bilateral superior oblique tendon sheath syndrome. Most fundus lesions are caused by posterior scleritis, but cotton-wool spots have been reported in an RA patient (Meyer et al, 1978). Another case report describes an RA patient who presented with a retinitis consistent with progressive outer retinal necrosis (PORN), possibly resulting from immunosuppression therapy (Bryan et al, 1998). Treatment regimens for RA also may have ocular side effects. Ocular manifestations include corneal deposits, lens opacification, chrysiasis (gold deposition), retinopathy, and optic neuropathy. Ocular side effects of systemic medications are discussed later in this chapter.

DIAGNOSIS

Systemic

The criteria used in diagnosing RA are listed in Table 20–3. Patients are diagnosed with RA if they have at least four of the seven criteria. Laboratory findings and radiographic studies help to make the initial diagnosis and help to monitor the progression of the disease.

Diagnostic Findings

The most important serologic finding is the presence of rheumatoid factors (RFs). RFs are autoantibodies directed against an abnormal IgG, and are found in

TABLE 20–3. DIAGNOSTIC CRITERIA FOR RHEUMATOID ARTHRITIS

1. Morning stiffness (≥1 hour)
2. Swelling of three or more joints
3. Swelling of hand joints (proximal interphalangeal, metacarpophalangeal, or wrist)
4. Symmetric swelling
5. Subcutaneous nodules
6. Serum rheumatoid factor
7. Radiographic changes

Four criteria must be met for diagnosis.

over 75% of RA patients. RFs are seen in 1 to 5% of healthy persons (Lipsky, 1998). High titers of rheumatoid factors commonly correlate with severe rheumatoid disease. Rheumatoid factors also may be present in patients with systemic lupus erythematosus, Sjögren syndrome, and less frequently in scleroderma or polymyositis. Elevated titers may also be seen in conditions such as syphilis, sarcoidosis, infective endocarditis, tuberculosis, leprosy, and parasitic infections; in the elderly; and in asymptomatic relatives of patients with autoimmune disease. Conversely, a negative rheumatoid factor by routine lab testing does not exclude the diagnosis of RA.

Antinuclear antibodies (ANAs) may be present in 20% of patients (Tierney et al, 1999). The erythrocyte sedimentation rate (ESR) is often elevated, and the degree of elevation may correlate with disease activity (Blackburn & Chatham, 1997; Stites et al, 1994). A normochromic, normocytic anemia is common in patients with active disease (Arnett, 1996). The white cell count may be normal or slightly elevated, but leukopenia (low white cell count) can occur with splenomegaly. The platelet count is commonly elevated and can correlate with the severity of joint inflammation. Synovial fluid analysis may help to determine the degree of inflammation.

X-ray Findings

Soft tissue swelling and juxta-articular demineralization are the initial x-ray findings. The earliest changes are seen in the wrists or feet. Later, joint-space narrowing results from destruction of the articular cartilage. Bony erosions develop at the junction of the synovial membrane and bone. Loss of cartilage and laxity of ligaments result in maladjustment and subluxation of the joints.

Differential Diagnosis

Diagnosis of RA can be difficult, especially early in the disease and in acute presentations. The clinical findings of subcutaneous nodules and the presence of RFs are helpful, but are not specific differential features. A complete medical evaluation, usually including synovial fluid analysis, is indicated for definitive diagnosis.

Differential diagnosis of RA includes other rheumatic disease such as systemic lupus erythematosus (SLE), Reiter syndrome, gout, psoriatic arthritis, degenerative osteoarthritis, and chronic inflammatory bowel disease. Additional conditions such as rubella vaccination, parvovirus infection, sarcoidosis, Lyme disease, and infectious mononucleosis can mimic early rheumatoid arthritis. The more common conditions considered in the differential diagnosis of RA are listed in Table 20–4. A suggested workup for the differential diagnosis of RA is listed in Table 20–5. Which tests are ordered would depend upon clinical presentation and suspicion.

Ocular

Ocular manifestations of RA can be detected by a thorough anterior and posterior segment evaluation. Gross inspection in natural light helps to identify the characteristic bluish hue of scleritis that may be missed with biomicroscopy. Slit-lamp examination with a red-free filter may help to identify any avascular areas of the sclera (Watson & Hayreh, 1976). If posterior scleritis is suspected, B-scan ultrasonography is a helpful ancillary test (Benson, 1988).

TABLE 20–4. DIFFERENTIAL DIAGNOSIS OF RHEUMATOID ARTHRITIS (RA)

	RA	Osteoarthritis	SLE	Gout	Reiter
Sex predilection	Female	Male/Female	Female	Male	Male
Rheumatoid factor	+	–	+	–	–
Subcutaneous nodules	+	–	+	+ (tophi)	–
Joint involvement	Polyarticular, symmetric, PIP/MCP joints	Monoarticular, asymmetric, DIP joints	Polyarticular, symmetric, PIP/MCP joints	Monoarticular (early), asymmetric	Polyarticular, asymmetric
Associated findings	Low-grade fever, malaise, weight loss, morning stiffness	Increase with age; pain increases through the day and with use	Butterfly rash (+) ANA	Sodium urate crystals in synovial fluid	Urethritis, conjunctivitis

PIP: proximal interphalangeal joints; MCP: metacarpophalangeal joints; DIP: distal interphalangeal joints; SLE: systemic lupus erythematosus; ANA: antinuclear antibodies; tophi: subcutaneous deposits of crystalline uric acid.

TABLE 20–5. DIAGNOSTIC TESTS FOR RHEUMATOID ARTHRITIS

- CBC (complete blood count)
- ESR (erythrocyte sedimentation rate)
- RF (serum rheumatoid factor)
- ANA (antinuclear body)
- Serum uric acid estimation
- Serological tests for syphilis
  - RPR (rapid plasma reagin) or VDRL (venereal disease research laboratory)
  - FTA abs (fluorescent treponemal antibody absorption test)
- Urinalysis
- X-rays
  - Involved joints
  - Chest
  - Sacroiliac
- Synovial fluid analysis

TREATMENT AND MANAGEMENT

Systemic

There is no known cure for RA nor any means of preventing it. Early diagnosis of RA optimizes the management of the disease. The goals of treatment include (1) relieving pain and stiffness, (2) reducing inflammation, (3) protecting joint function and muscle strength, (4) controlling systemic involvement, and (5) minimizing undesirable drug side effects. More recent studies have advocated early, more aggressive therapy to prevent irreversible joint damage that occurs within 1 to 2 years of disease onset (American College of Rheumatology, 1996; Hochberg, 1999). Table 20–6 summarizes the systemic treatment of RA.

> Early, more aggressive therapy may prevent irreversible joint damage that can occur within 1 to 2 years of disease onset.

An interdisciplinary approach optimizes management of RA patients. Physical therapy is effective in decreasing the symptoms of RA. A balanced program of rest and exercise along with heat or cold therapy helps to alleviate symptoms as well as maintain strength and mobility. Bed rest may be needed on a regular basis to relieve inflammation and fatigue. Specific joints may need to be immobilized through the use of braces, splints, or crutches (Borigini & Paulus, 1995).

Medical management of RA usually involves use of (1) nonsteroidal anti-inflammatory drugs (NSAIDs) and simple analgesics; (2) oral or intra-articular glucocorticoids; and (3) disease-modifying antirheumatic drugs (DMARDs) which include antimalarials, D-penicillamine, sulfasalazine, gold compounds, methotrexate, and immunosuppressive or cytotoxic drugs.

TABLE 20–6. SYSTEMIC TREATMENT AND MANAGEMENT OF RHEUMATOID ARTHRITIS

- Rest
- Physical therapy
- Aspirin
- NSAIDs
- Corticosteroids
- Antimalarial medications (hydroxychloroquine)
- Gold salts
- Sulfasalazine
- Methotrexate
- D-penicillamine
- Other cytotoxic or immunosuppressive agents
- Orthopedic and surgical intervention

Aspirin and NSAIDs have analgesic and anti-inflammatory effects, but do not alter the progression of the disease. These drugs have toxic side effects which include gastric irritation, platelet dysfunction, rash, liver dysfunction, and bone marrow depression. The gastrointestinal side effects are the most common and can result in gastric ulceration and bleeding. NSAIDs inhibit prostaglandins by inhibiting cyclooxygenase enzymes. There are two separate enzymes, cyclooxygenase 1 and 2. Cyclooxygenase 1 is present in many cells and tissues including the stomach and the platelet and produces prostaglandins that may be beneficial to renal and gastric function, whereas cyclooxygenase 2 is involved in the inflammatory response (Smith, 1998). Celecoxib (Celebrex) is a selective cyclooxygenase 2 inhibitor that has been recently approved to relieve signs and symptoms of RA. Because of its specificity for the COX-2 pathway, it has promising therapeutic benefit because of less gastrointestinal toxicity. However, adverse gastrointestinal effects have been reported. Long-term studies are needed to compare the adverse effects of COX-2 inhibitors and nonselective NSAIDs.

Although corticosteroids have a powerful anti-inflammatory effect, they do not alter the progression of the disease. In addition, symptoms often reccur when the drugs are discontinued. Intra-articular injection of corticosteroids may help relieve symptoms for a period of months. However, degenerative arthritis may result from multiple intra-articular corticosteroid injections. Low-dose systemic corticosteroids, eg, 5 to 10 mg prednisone daily, may be indicated in patients who have not responded well with other therapies. Side effects of corticosteroid therapy include hyperadrenocorticism, weight gain, diabetes mellitus, hypertension, osteoporosis, myopathy, mental disturbances, infections, glaucoma, and cataracts.

Disease-modifying antirheumatic drugs are also called slow-acting antirheumatic drugs and remission-inducing drugs. These agents, which include antimalarials, D-penicillamine, sulfasalazine, gold compounds, and immunosuppressive agents, have diverse mechanisms of action. Although NSAIDs and glucocorticoids help alleviate symptoms, joint damage may progress. DMARDs reduce or prevent joint damage, thus preserving joint integrity and function. As many as two thirds of patients clinically improve over the course of weeks to months with these drugs (American College of Rheumatology, 1996). Each of these drugs has significant toxic effects, and patients need to be monitored carefully.

Hydroxychloroquine (Plaquenil) is the most common antimalarial drug used to treat RA. Its mechanism of action is unknown, but it appears to affect monocyte function. It may take 1 to 6 months for maximum therapeutic benefit. Dosages range from 200 to 600 mg per day. Side effects include skin rashes, nausea and vomiting, myopathy, and retinal toxicity.

Gold salt therapy is used less frequently because of its toxic side effects. Gold can be administered intramuscularly, which is most common, or orally. Clinical improvement may take 3 to 6 months. Toxic reactions include dermatitis, photosensitivity, stomatitis, neutropenia, proteinuria, aplastic anemia, peripheral neuropathy, nephritis, pneumonitis, and keratitis.

Penicillamine can also be used in the treatment of RA. Similar to gold, it is a slow-acting nonsteroidal anti-inflammatory agent which may take up to 6 months to take effect. Side effects include rash, loss of sense of taste, nausea and vomiting, anorexia, proteinuria, aplastic anemia, and thrombocytopenia. Sulfasalazine has an efficacy similar to that of gold and penicillamine. Side effects include neutropenia (low white count) and thrombocytopenia (low platelet count). Improvement may be observed within 2 months of treatment with sulfasalazine.

Methotrexate is often the initial DMARD prescribed because it is effective and is well tolerated over the long term (Kremer, 1998). Methotrexate has immunosuppressive, cytotoxic, and anti-inflammatory effects (Wigley, 1995). It may produce maximum benefit in 2 to 6 weeks. The most common side effects are gastric irritation and stomatitis (inflammation of the mouth). Less common side effects include bone marrow suppression and liver toxicity. Other immunosuppressive agents used in the treatment of RA include azathioprine, cyclophosphamide, and chlorambucil.

The DMARD leflunomide (Arava) was recently approved for decreasing the structural damage of RA (Elliott & Chan, 1998). Leflunomide causes the cell arrest of lymphocytes involved in the autoimmune process (Fox, 1998). The reduction of lymphocyte activity decreases the damage mediated by the cytokines and antibodies. Side effects include diarrhea and rash, with less severe toxicities such as pulmonary toxicity and bone marrow suppression, which is seen with methotrexate. Another recently approved DMARD is etanercept (Enbrel), which inhibits tumor necrosis factor or TNF (Clinical Pharmacology, 1999). TNF plays a role in RA by mediating cytokines that cause inflammation and joint destruction. These newer drugs provide promising treatment options for patients who have an inadequate response to traditional therapies.

Surgical intervention may help correct or compensate for joint damage. Arthroplasty may help maintain or improve joint motion. Arthrodesis (fusion of bones across a joint space) can correct deformity and alleviate pain, but results in loss of motion. A synovectomy may decrease inflammation and prevent joint damage, but the synovium often grows back and symptoms reoccur.

Management of patients with RA may require a combination of therapies to adequately control the disease. Newer therapies hope to minimize adverse side effects. Early more aggressive treatment helps to prevent irreversible joint damage and disability. In the future, genetic markers may help to identify patients at risk for developing severe disease.

Ocular

An overview of the treatment of the ocular sequelae of RA is listed in Table 20–7. Ocular lubricants are the main treatment modality for keratoconjunctivitis sicca. Lubricant treatment may not eliminate all epithelial staining. An improvement in symptoms as well as decreased staining may be considered a therapeutic success. Temporary or permanent punctal plugs and punctal ablative procedures are other treatment options. When secondary infection occurs, antibiotic treatment is indicated. If keratoconjunctivitis sicca progresses to a filamentary keratitis, treatment includes debridement of the filaments and lubrication with artificial tears and ointment. In severe cases a bandage contact lens may be helpful.

The treatment of rheumatoid episcleritis depends on the severity and chronicity. If mild inflammation is present, the episcleritis may resolve on its own. More severe or chronic forms may require topical vasoconstrictors or steroids. Short-term use of a topical steroid is optimal, but longer-term use may be needed if there is corneal involvement. Oral NSAIDs can be used as an adjunctive therapy in recurrent cases of episcleritis.

Treatment of scleritis depends on the type and severity of the scleritis. Topical steroids alone are not effective. Oral NSAIDs can be effective with some pa-

TABLE 20–7. OCULAR TREATMENT AND MANAGEMENT OF RHEUMATOID ARTHRITIS

Dry Eye
- Ocular lubricants
- Punctal occlusion

Filamentary Keratitis
- Filament removal
- Heavy lubrication
- Bandage contact lens

Corneal Ulceration (Sterile)
- Systemic steroids
- Immunosuppressive or cytotoxic agents

Episcleritis
- Artificial tears
- Topical vasoconstrictor/antihistamine
- Topical steroids
- Oral NSAIDs

Anterior Scleritis
- Nonnecrotizing
  - NSAIDs (indomethacin)
  - Systemic steroids
- Necrotizing
  - Immunosuppressive or cytotoxic agents

Posterior Scleritis
- Systemic or retrobulbar injections of steroids
- Antiprostaglandins (aspirin)
- Immunosuppressive or cytotoxic agents

tients. Oral corticosteroids may be needed to sufficiently control the inflammation. Treatment for posterior scleritis includes systemic or retrobulbar injections of corticosteroids.

Antiprostaglandins such as oxyphenbutazone, indocin, and aspirin also can be effective therapy (Benson, 1988; Wakefield & McCluskey, 1989). Periocular steroid injections are contraindicated in anterior scleritis, because they may cause global perforation (Cobo, 1983). In severe cases of necrotizing or posterior scleritis, a referral to a rheumatologist is indicated for more aggressive therapy. These patients need immunosuppressive or cytotoxic agents to prevent perforation and destruction of the globe. Surgical procedures may be required to adequately manage necrotizing scleritis and peripheral ulcerative keratitis.

Treatment of corneal involvement in rheumatoid scleritis is directed at controlling the scleral inflammation with systemic steroids and/or immunosuppressive agents. Topical corticosteroids may be used to treat sclerosing keratitis, but they are contraindicated in corneal furrowing and ulceration because of the possibility of perforation. Topical collagenase inhibitors, bandage soft contact lenses, or cyanoacrylate glue may be more effective therapy in these patients (Robin et al, 1986). Surgical conjunctival resection may stop the progression of corneal furrowing. Lamellar or penetrating keratoplasty may prevent perforation or may restore vision after the control of the scleritis (Robin et al, 1986).

Comanagement with a rheumatologist is important in treating ocular disease in RA patients. Increasing the strength or dosage of systemic medications can be effective in controlling ocular inflammation. In addition, systemic medications may need to be modified or discontinued to prevent ocular side effects.

Detecting or monitoring ocular side effects of systemic medications is important for the eyecare practitioner. Table 20–8 lists some of the ocular side effects of medications commonly used in the treatment of RA.

Ocular side effects of NSAIDs include transient blurred vision, diplopia, whorl keratopathy, and photosensitivity. Indomethacin may have additional side effects of subconjunctival and retinal hemorrhages. There have been some reports of a rare idiosyncratic optic nerve response from certain NSAIDs. The optic neuropathy may cause a unilateral or bilateral decrease in visual acuity. If the medication is discontinued, visual acuity usually returns to normal within a few months, although color vision may take longer to return. If the medication is not discontinued, permanent vision loss may result. Ibuprofen, as well as other NSAIDs, can also cause pseudotumor cerebri (Katzman et al, 1981). Therefore, if patients complain of vision loss, it is important to rule out any optic nerve abnormalities.

There are a number of ocular side effects of corticosteroids, but two of the most important are posterior subcapsular cataract (PSC) and glaucoma. It has

TABLE 20–8. OCULAR SIDE EFFECTS OF RHEUMATOID ARTHRITIS MEDICATIONS

Medication	Side Effect
NSAIDs	Transient blurred vision
	Diplopia
	Photosensitivity
	Whorl keratopathy (eg, indomethacin)
	Optic neuropathy
	Retinal or subconjunctival hemorrhages
Corticosteroids	Posterior subcapsular cataract
	Glaucoma
Gold salts	Corneal and conjunctival deposits
	Lens deposits
Chloroquine/Plaquenil	Whorl keratopathy
	Pigmentary retinopathy
	Toxic maculopathy
Methotrexate	Punctate keratitis
	Periorbital edema
	Blepharitis
	Conjunctival hyperemia
	Photophobia

been well established that both topical and oral corticosteroid use can cause PSC or a secondary glaucoma.

Patients receiving gold therapy may develop ocular chrysiasis (gold deposition). Gold deposition is more common in the conjunctiva and cornea, and less common in the lens and retina. Visual acuity is not affected. Ocular chrysiasis is reversible after discontinuing gold therapy. Deposition of gold in the cornea or lens does not necessitate stopping therapy unless corneal ulceration occurs.

Ocular side effects of methotrexate include periorbital edema, blepharitis, conjunctival hyperemia, increased lacrimation, and photophobia. The drug has been found in the tears and may cause ocular irritation, requiring lubricant therapy but not discontinuation of the drug.

Corneal deposits of presumed antimalarial salts can occur with use of chloroquine and hydroxychloroquine. According to Easterbrook (1993), these deposits may occur in up to 90% of patients taking chloroquine, but in less than 5% in those taking hydroxychloroquine. These corneal changes are usually asymptomatic and are reversible when treatment is discontinued.

The retinopathy associated with chloroquine or hydroxychloroquine can range from fine macular mottling with loss of the foveal reflex to a bull's-eye maculopathy with concentric rings of hyper- and hypopigmentation. In advanced cases, attenuated retinal arterioles and optic nerve pallor may be observed. The retinopathy may be irreversible, have a delayed onset, or progress after discontinuing the medication. There is a much higher incidence of retinopathy associated with chloroquine as compared to hydroxychloroquine (Weiner et al, 1991).

According to Levy et al, 1997 and Bernstein, 1991, there is an extremely low risk of hydroxychloroquine retinopathy when these criteria are met: (1) the maintenance dosage is less than 6.5 mg/kg/day, (2) duration of treatment is less than 10 years, and (3) there is no history of renal insufficiency because hydroxychloroquine is excreted by the kidney. As an example, a person weighing 70 kg (or 154 pounds) should not be taking more than 455 mg of hydroxychloroquine per day. In a study of 1207 patients, Levy and colleagues (1997) found an incidence of hydroxychloroquine retinopathy of 0.4%. In Easterbrook's prospective study (1993) of 2000 patients treated with antimalarials, he found only three patients with definite hydroxychloroquine retinopathy. All three were taking dosages greater than 6.5 mg/kg/day. Patients should have an initial evaluation within 4 weeks of onset of treatment. Methods to detect retinopathy include visual acuity, color vision, automated visual field of central 10°, Amsler grid, ophthalmoscopy, and serial color photographs. Amsler grid testing at home may help to detect an early paracentral scotoma. Fluorescein angiography, electroretinography, and electrooculography may give variable results (Cruess et al, 1985; Easterbrook, 1993). The drug manufacturer recommends examinations every 6 months, but others believe patients may be followed at 9- to 12-month intervals (Bernstein, 1991; Bird & Morgan, 1998; Easterbrook, 1993; Levy et al, 1997; Morsman et al, 1990; Ruiz & Saatci, 1991).

> There is an extremely low risk of hydroxychloroquine retinopathy when these criteria are met: (1) the maintenance dosage is less than 6.5 mg/kg/day, (2) duration of treatment is less than 10 years, and (3) there is no history of renal insufficiency.

DISEASE COURSE AND PROGNOSIS

RA can result in significant disability and a higher than expected mortality rate. A minority of patients will improve spontaneously or achieve remission, usually within 2 years of diagnosis of the disease (Tierney et al, 1999). However, most patients have chronic disease progression and functional disability. RA patients have six times the probability of severe activity limitations and 10 times the work disability rate as the general population. Approximately 50% of RA patients are unable to work within 10 years of diagnosis (Arnett, 1996). Life expectancy may be shortened by 7 years in males and 3 years in females (Harris, 1997a). The higher mortality rate correlates with the degree of disability and results from infection, heart disease, respiratory failure, renal failure, and gastrointestinal disease. Complications of therapy contribute to the increased mortality rate (Stites et al, 1994). Positive RF, poor functional status, more than 30 inflamed joints, and extra-articular manifestations are possible risk factors for early death (Tierney et al, 1999). Patients with these risk factors need early and aggressive treatment to help prevent the complications of severe disease.

CONCLUSION

Rheumatoid arthritis is a chronic polyarticular inflammatory disease that primarily affects women. The progressive joint disease can result in significant functional impairment and disability. The most common ocular manifestation is keratoconjunctivitis sicca. Less common ocular findings include anterior and posterior segment inflammation. Necrotizing scleritis and peripheral ulcerative keratitis may correlate with serious underlying systemic disease requiring aggressive systemic treatment. The eyecare practitioner plays a major role in managing ocular manifestations of RA as well as detecting any ocular side effects from medications used in treating RA. Comanagement with a rheumatologist or internist helps to provide optimal patient care.

REFERENCES

Adachi W, Nishida K, Quantock AJ, et al. Ultrastructural alterations in the stroma adjacent to non-inflammatory corneal perforations associated with long standing RA. *Br J Ophthalmol.* 1998;82:1445–1446.

American College of Rheumatology. Guidelines for the management of RA. *Arthritis Rheum.* 1996;39:713–722.

Arnett FC. Rheumatoid arthritis. In: Bennett JC, Plum F, eds. *Cecil Textbook of Medicine.* Philadelphia: WB Saunders; 1996:1459–1466.

Bacon PA, Moots RJ. Extra-articular rheumatoid arthritis. In: Koopman WJ, ed. *Arthritis and Allied Conditions: A Textbook of Rheumatology.* 13th ed. Baltimore: Williams & Wilkins; 1997:1071–1088.

Baker DG, Rabinowitz JL. Current concepts in the treatment of rheumatoid arthritis. *J Clin Pharmacol.* 1986;26:2–21.

Beasley RP, Willkens RF, Bennett PH. High prevalence of rheumatoid arthritis in Yakima Indians. *Arthritis Rheum.* 1973;16:743.

Beers MH, Berkow R. Diffuse connective tissue disease. In: *The Merck Manual of Diagnosis and Therapy.* Whitehouse Station: Merck; 1999:416–423.

Benson WE. Posterior scleritis. *Surv Ophthalmol.* 1988;32: 297–316.

Bernstein HN. Ocular safety of hydroxychloroquine. *Ann Ophthalmol.* 1991;23:292–296.

Bird H, Morgan AW. Hydroxychloroquine. In: Van de Putte LB, Furst DE, Williams HJ, Van Riel PL, eds. *Therapy of Systemic Rheumatic Disorders.* New York: Marcel Dekker; 1998:113–129.

Blackburn Jr WD, Chatham WW. Laboratory findings in rheumatoid arthritis. In: Koopman WJ, ed. *Arthritis and Allied Conditions: A Textbook of Rheumatology.* 13th ed. Baltimore: Williams & Wilkins; 1997:1092.

Borigini MJ, Paulus HE. Rheumatoid arthritis. In: Weisman MH, Weinblatt ME, eds. *Treatment of the Rheumatic Diseases.* Philadelphia: WB Saunders; 1995;31–51.

Bryan RG, Myers FL, Madison W. Progressive outer retinal necrosis in a patient with rheumatoid arthritis. *Arch Ophthalmol.* 1998;116:1249.

Calabro JJ. Rheumatoid arthritis. A potentially crippling disease that may attack at any age. *Clin Symp.* 1971;23:2–10.

Carter BT, Sanborn GE, Humphries MK. Rheumatoid nodules of the upper lid. *Arch Ophthalmol.* 1976;94:2127–2128.

Clinical Pharmacology. 1999 [Online]. Available: http://www.cponline.gsm.com (May 1999).

Cobo M. Inflammation of the sclera. *Int Ophthalmol Clinics.* 1983;23:159–171.

Cruess AF, Schachat AP, Nicholl J, Augsburger JJ. Chloroquine retinopathy. Is fluorescein angiography necessary? *Ophthalmology.* 1985;92:1127–1129.

Cullom RD, Chang B. *The Wills Eye Manual.* Philadelphia: JB Lippincott; 1994:123–126.

de la Maza MS, Foster CS, Jabbur NS. Scleritis associated with rheumatoid arthritis and with other systemic immune-mediated diseases. *Ophthalmology.* 1994a;101:1281–1288.

de la Maza MS, Jabbur NS, Foster CS. Severity of scleritis and episcleritis. *Ophthalmology.* 1994b;101:389–396.

Easterbrook M. Ocular safety of hydroxychloroquine. *Semin Arthritis Rheum.* 1993;23(suppl 1):62–67.

Eiferman RA, Carothers DJ, Yankeelov JA. Peripheral rheumatoid ulceration and evidence for conjunctival collagenase production. *Am J Ophthalmol.* 1979;87:703–709.

Elliott WT, Chan J. Leflunomide (Arava). *Therapeutics & Drug Alert.* 1998;3:35–37.

Firestone GS. Etiology and pathogenesis of rheumatoid arthritis. In: Kelley WN, Ruddy S, Harris Jr ED, Sledge CB, eds. *Textbook of Rheumatology.* 5th ed. Philadelphia: WB Saunders; 1997:851.

Foster CS. Immunosuppressive therapy for external ocular inflammatory disease. *Ophthalmology.* 1980;87:140–150.

Foster CS, Forstot SL, Wilsone LA. Mortality rate in rheumatoid arthritis patients developing necrotizing scleritis or peripheral ulcerative keratitis. Effects of systemic immunosuppression. *Ophthalmology.* 1984;91:1253–1263.

Fox RI. Mechanism of action of leflunomide in rheumatoid arthritis. *J Rheumatol Suppl.* 1998;53:20–26.

Fraunfelder FT, Grove JA. *Drug-Induced Ocular Side Effects* 4th ed. Baltimore: Williams & Wilkins; 1996:58–63, 145–162, 288–293, 366–368.

Harper SL, Foster CS. The ocular manifestations of rheumatoid disease. *Int Ophthalmol Clin.* 1998;38:1–19.

Harris Jr ED. Clinical features of rheumatoid arthritis. In: Kelley WN, Ruddy S, Harris Jr ED, Sledge CB, eds. *Textbook of Rheumatology.* 5th ed. Philadelphia: WB Saunders; 1997a:898–900.

Harris Jr ED. *Rheumatoid Arthritis.* Philadelphia: WB Saunders; 1997b:241.

Hochberg MC. Adult and juvenile rheumatoid arthritis: Current epidemiologic concepts. *Epidemiol Rev.* 1981;3:27–44.

Hochberg MC. Early aggressive DMARD therapy: The key to slowing disease progression in rheumatoid arthritis. *Scand J Rheumatol Suppl.* 1999;112:3–7.

Kanski JJ, Thomas DJ. *The Eye in Systemic Disease.* 2nd ed. London: Butterworth-Heinemann; 1990:39–41.

Katzman B, Lu LW, Tiwari RP, Bansal R. Pseudotumor cerebri: An observation and review. *Ann Ophthalmol.* 1981; 13:887–892.

Kervick GN, Pflugfelder SC, Haimovici R, et al. Paracentral rheumatoid corneal ulceration. Clinical features and cyclosporine therapy. *Ophthalmology.* 1992;99:80–88.

Kremer JM. Methotrexate and emerging therapies. *Rheum Dis Clin North Am.* 1998;24:651–658.

Lamberts DW. Dry eye and tear deficiency. *Int Ophthalmol Clin.* 1983;23:123–130.

Larsen BA, Alderdice CA, Hawkins D, et al. Protective HLA-DR phenotypes in rheumatoid arthritis. *J Rheumatol.* 1989; 16:455–458.

Levy GD, Munz SJ, Paschal J, et al. Incidence of hydroxychloroquine retinopathy in 1,207 patients in a large multicenter outpatient practice. *Arthritis Rheum.* 1997;40:1482–1486.

Lipsky PE. Rheumatoid arthritis. In: Fauci AS, Braunwald E, Isselbacher KJ, Wilson JD, et al, eds. *Harrison's Principles of Internal Medicine.* New York: McGraw-Hill; 1998:1880–1888.

MacGregor A, Ollier W, Thomson W, et al. HLA-DRB1* 0401/0404 genotype and rheumatoid arthritis: Increased association in men, young age at onset, and disease severity. *J Rheumatol.* 1995;22:1032–1036.

Mahoney BP. Rheumatologic disease and associated ocular manifestations. *J Am Optom Assoc.* 1993;64:403–415.

McGavin DD, Williamson J, Forrester JV, et al. Episcleritis and scleritis. A study of their clinical manifestations and association with rheumatoid arthritis. *Brit J Ophthalmol.* 1976;60:192–226.

Messmer EM, Foster CS. Destructive corneal and scleral disease associated with rheumatoid arthritis. Medical and surgical management. *Cornea.* 1995;14:408–417.

Meyer E, Scharf J, Miler B, et al. Fundus lesions in rheumatoid arthritis. *Ann Ophthalmol.* 1978;10:1583–1584.

Mody GM, Hill JC, Meyers OL. Keratoconjunctivitis sicca in rheumatoid arthritis. *Clin Rheumatol.* 1988;7:237–241.

Morsman CD, Livesey SJ, Richards IM, et al. Screening for hydroxychloroquine retinal toxicity: Is it necessary? *Eye.* 1990;4:572–576.

Narsing AR, Marak GE, Hidayat AA. Necrotizing scleritis. A clinicopathologic study of 41 cases. *Ophthalmology.* 1985; 92:1542–1549.

Physicians' Desk Reference. 53rd ed. Montvale, NJ: Medical Economics; 1999:2799.

Robin JB, Schanzlin DJ, Verity SM, et al. Peripheral corneal disorders. *Surv Ophthalmol.* 1986;31:1–36.

Ruiz RS, Saatci OA. Chloroquine and hydroxychloroquine retinopathy: How to follow affected patients. *Ann Ophthalmol.* 1991;23:290–291.

Smith TJ. Cyclooxygenases as the principal targets for the actions of NSAIDs. *Rheum Dis Clin North Am.* 1998;24: 501–523.

Stastny P. Association of the B cell alloantigen DRW4 with rheumatoid arthritis. *N Engl J Med.* 1978;298:869–871.

Stites DP, Terr AI, Parslow TG. *Basic & Clinical Immunology.* 8th ed. Norwalk, CT: Appleton & Lange; 1994:392–397.

Tierney DW. Ocular chrysiasis. *J Am Optom Assoc.* 1988; 59:960–962.

Tierney LM, McPhee SJ, Papadakis MA. *Current Medical Diagnosis & Treatment.* 38th ed. Stamford, CT: Appleton & Lange; 1999:804–811.

Vollertsen RS, Conn DL, Ballard DJ, et al. Rheumatoid vasculitis: Survival and associated risk factors. *Medicine.* 1986;65:365–375.

Wakefield D, McCluskey P. Cyclosporin therapy for severe scleritis. *Brit J Ophthalmol.* 1989;73:743–746.

Watson PG, Hayreh SS. Scleritis and episcleritis. *Brit J Ophthalmol.* 1976;60:163–191.

Weinblatt ME. Treatment of rheumatoid arthritis. In: Koopman WJ, ed. *Arthritis and Allied Conditions: A Textbook of Rheumatology.* 13th ed. Baltimore: Williams & Wilkins; 1997:1131.

Weiner A, Sandberg MA, Gaudio AR, et al. Hydroxychloroquine retinopathy. *Am J Ophthalmol.* 1991;112:528–534.

Whitson WE, Krachmer JH. Adult rheumatoid arthritis. In: Gold DH, Weingeist TA, eds. *The Eye in Systemic Disease.* Philadelphia: JB Lippincott; 1990:61–64.

Wigley FM. Rheumatoid arthritis. In: Barker LR, Burton JR, Zieve PD, eds. *Principles of Ambulatory Medicine.* 4th ed. Baltimore: Williams & Wilkins; 1995:943–964.

Wollheim FA. Rheumatoid arthritis—The clinical picture. In: Madison PJ, Isenberg DA, Woo P, Glass DN, eds. *Oxford Textbook of Rheumatology.* 2nd ed. Oxford: Oxford University Press; 1998:1004–1005.

Chapter 21

JUVENILE RHEUMATOID ARTHRITIS

Gina A. Dell'Arciprete, Catherine Pace Watson

Juvenile rheumatoid arthritis (JRA) is a group of arthritides whose systemic and ocular manifestations can be severely disabling. These disorders can be classified by clinical characteristics into pauciarticular JRA, polyarthritic JRA, and systemic onset JRA (SoJRA). The ocular sequelae vary for each category of JRA, as do the systemic features. The major ocular manifestations of JRA—anterior uveitis, cataracts, and band keratopathy—cause more severe vision loss than other types of rheumatic diseases. The systemic and ocular prognosis for most JRA patients is good with early detection and treatment.

EPIDEMIOLOGY

Systemic

The annual incidence of JRA in the United States ranges from 7.8 to 13.9 per 100,000 children (Gäre, 1998; Pachman & Poznanski, 1992) under 16 years old. JRA affects females more than males in at least a 2:1 ratio (Gäre, 1998; Harper & Foster, 1998). Polyarticular JRA represents 30 to 40% and pauciarticular JRA accounts for 40 to 50% of all cases in the United States. Pauciarticular and polyarticular JRA predominate in females. SoJRA, only 10 to 20% of all cases, occurs with equal frequency in males and females. It generally occurs in children under 5 years of age. Fifty percent of SoJRA cases develop polyarticular JRA within a year of onset of the disease (Pachman & Poznanski, 1998). SoJRA has the highest morbidity and mortality rates of all forms of JRA.

Ocular

Chronic nongranulomatous anterior uveitis is the major ocular complication of JRA. It occurs in 14 to 21% of children with JRA (Dollfus, 1998; Harper & Foster, 1998). Ocular involvement occurs in 78 to 91% of pauciarticular JRA, in 7 to 14% of polyarticular JRA, and in 1 to 6% of SoJRA (Dollfus, 1998). Uveitis is seen more commonly in females than in males.

PATHOPHYSIOLOGY/DISEASE PROCESS

Systemic

The systemic onset of JRA is insidious in most cases. Upper respiratory infections, trauma, and heredity have been implicated as precipitating factors for the development of JRA; however, their roles still remain unclear. In all forms of JRA, even severe cases, young children often do not complain of pain; rather, they limit the use of the affected extremity. The differentiation is based upon the number of affected joints and other accompanying signs and symptoms (Table 21–1).

TABLE 21–1. SYSTEMIC MANIFESTATIONS OF JUVENILE RHEUMATOID ARTHRITIS

	Pauciarticular	Polyarticular	Systemic Onset
Articular Features			
Characteristics	1–4 joints	5 or more joints	1 or more joints
Joints involved	Knees	Small joints of hands, cervical and temporomandibular joints; knees, hips, ankles	Knees, wrists, ankles
Serology	(+/−) ANA (−) RF	Usually (−) ANA (+/−) RF	(−) ANA (−) RF
Associated HLA alleles	A2, DR5, w6, w52, w8, DR6, DR8	DRw8.1, DQw4, DP3, Dw4, Dw14, DR4	DR4, DR5, DR8
Extra-Articular Features of Systemic Onset JRA			
• Fever[a]	• Macular rash	• Anemia	
• Koebner phenomenon	• Serosal inflammation	• Anorexia	
• Hepatosplenomegaly	• Lymphadenopathy	• Myopathy	
• Growth retardation	• Pericarditis		

[a]Fever may occur in all types of JRA.

- *Pauciarticular*—arthritis affecting one to four joints
- *Polyarticular*—arthritis affecting five or more joints
- *Systemic*—arthritis affecting one or more joints, preceded by at least two weeks of daily spiking fever (Harper & Foster, 1998)

Pauciarticular or oligoarticular JRA, is the most prevalent type of JRA. This form of the disease affects one to four joints in children under 5 years old, and is more common in females than males. Monoarthritis may occur in one third to one half of the cases. The large joints, especially the knee, are most often affected. Although the child may not complain of pain, the affected joint is generally warm and swollen. Disease onset is insidious, with a limp often the first sign. The arthritis associated with pauciarticular JRA is rarely destructive and often transient (Pelkonen, 1998).

Systemically, low-grade fever, mild anemia, and fatigue sometimes occur. Rheumatoid factor (RF) is negative and antinuclear antibody (ANA) testing is positive in 50% of cases. ANA testing is positive in 90% of those with uveitis. Although these children test HLA-B27 negative, there is an association with HLA-A2, HLA-DR5, -w6, -w8, and -w52 (Cassidy, 1997).

Polyarticular JRA affects five or more joints. This form of JRA affects females more commonly than males. ANA testing is generally negative but can be positive in a small percentage of cases. Polyarticular JRA is broken down further by positive or negative rheumatoid factor.

In the more common rheumatoid factor–negative polyarticular JRA, onset can be insidious or precipitated by trauma, infection, or an immunologic stimulus such as an immunization. Usually small joints of the fingers and hands are affected, although cervical joints and the temporomandibular joint may also be affected. Weight-bearing joints, especially knees, hips, and ankles, can be involved. Joint involvement occurs bilaterally. The affected joints will be warm and swollen, though not necessarily painful unless the hip is involved. Joint stiffness occurs especially after rest. In children under 5 years of age, fusiform swelling (spindle-shaped swelling) between joints may occur rather than swelling at the joint. A low-grade fever may be noted, and in some cases, tachycardia out of proportion to the fever can be detected. An increase in frequency of HLA alleles DRw8.1, DQw4, and DP3 may be found (Cassidy, 1997).

A small percentage of cases of polyarticular JRA are rheumatoid factor positive. In these children, clinical features are indistinguishable from the adult form of rheumatoid arthritis (RA), and the arthritis can be severe. A majority of these children are DR-4, Dw4, and -w14 positive (Cassidy, 1997), but HLA-B27 negative.

Systemic onset JRA (SoJRA) was initially described in 1897 by George Frederick Still. This form of JRA, often called Still disease, mimics infectious disease more than any of the others.

SoJRA is characterized by arthritis that may not be present initially, but develops within the first few months of onset. In this form, arthritis can affect various joints, especially knees, wrists, and ankles, and in severe cases can persist into adulthood.

Daily spiking fevers are present. These fevers last at least 2 weeks but can continue for months. In many cases these children are admitted into hospitals with fevers of unknown origin.

An evanescent macular rash commonly appears over the trunk and proximal extremities. Koebner phenomenon (linear streaks in areas that are subjected to pressure) may be present. Blood testing is negative both for RF and ANA.

Serosal inflammation is often present, with pericarditis being the most common and potentially fatal form. Myocarditis is a rare but also potentially fatal complication (Schneider & Laxer, 1998). Hepatosplenomegaly is common, as is generalized lymphadenopathy. Anorexia, anemia, and growth retardation have also been reported.

Ocular

Ocular manifestations (Table 21–2) are most common in the pauciarticular form of JRA. Chronic anterior uveitis usually appears before the onset of arthritis but may occur after the onset in 6 to 24% of cases. In 67 to 89% of patients the uveitis is bilateral. The uveitis is often asymptomatic and therefore often remains undiagnosed until vision loss is substantial.

There is no relationship between joint inflammation and the presence or exacerbation of the uveitis (Dollfus, 1998). Most patients will present with uveitis within 7 years of the onset of the arthritis. The majority of ocular complications are related to chronic uveitis. Cataract formation occurs in 50% of eyes with chronic anterior uveitis secondary to JRA. The cataracts are a result of prolonged topical and systemic corticosteroid treatment, as well as the chronic ocular inflammation. Band keratopathy, which occurs in up to 77% of patients with chronic anterior uveitis, results from aggressive ocular inflammation rather than abnormal calcium deposition. Loss of visual acuity occurs when the visual axis is affected (Harper & Foster, 1998).

TABLE 21–2. OCULAR MANIFESTATIONS OF JUVENILE RHEUMATOID ARTHRITIS

- Chronic nongranulomatous anterior uveitis—usually bilateral
- Complications secondary to chronic anterior uveitis and its treatment:
  - Cataract
  - Band keratopathy
  - Glaucoma
  - Hypotony
  - Macular edema
  - Epiretinal membranes
- Rare:
  - Posterior uveitis
  - Tractional retinal detachment
  - Disc neovascularization
  - Inflammatory optic neuropathy
  - Acquired Brown syndrome

Glaucoma is estimated to occur in 15 to 45% of JRA patients with uveitis (Harper & Foster, 1998). Glaucoma in JRA patients, like cataracts, is due to corticosteroid treatment and chronic ocular inflammation. Hypotony can also occur from long-term inflammation and repeated ocular surgical procedures. Posterior uveitis is rare (Dollfus, 1998). Macular edema, inflammatory optic neuropathy, and epiretinal membranes may also occur as the result of incompletely treated inflammation. In extremely rare cases, tractional retinal detachment, disc neovascularization, or acquired Brown syndrome may occur. Acquired Brown syndrome is believed to be caused by an inflammatory mass that restricts the passage of the superior oblique tendon through the trochlea (Wang, 1984).

DIAGNOSIS

Systemic

There is no single clinical finding or laboratory test that will make the diagnosis of JRA, but rather multiple tests (Table 21–3) are selected to rule out other likely causes. JRA can be further classified into subgroups

TABLE 21–3. DIAGNOSTIC TESTS FOR JUVENILE RHEUMATOID ARTHRITIS

Systemic
- ANA
- RF
- X-ray of involved joints
- ESR
- CBC w/differential
- Serum complement
- C-reactive protein
- Lyme titer
- HLA-B27

Ocular

Tests typical for uveitis workup:
- CBC w/differential
- Serum chemistry
- ESR
- ANA
- RF
- Fluorescent treponemal antibody absorption/rapid plasma reagin
- Serum angiotensin-converting enzyme
- Purified protein derivative
- Chest x-ray

Consider tests for:
- HLA-B27
- Toxoplasmosis
- Toxocariasis
- Herpes simplex
- Herpes zoster
- Cytomegalovirus
- Epstein–Barr virus

based on disease characteristics noted during the first 6 months of symptoms.

In children under 16 years of age, arthritic symptoms must persist for at least 6 weeks to justify a diagnosis of JRA. The most clinically significant diagnostic tests for JRA include erythrocyte sedimentation rate (ESR), complete blood count (CBC) with differential, ANA, RF, serum complement, C-reactive protein, and radiologic evaluation.

In many cases, a diagnosis of JRA is based on exclusion of other disease entities (Table 21–4). Some of the more common disorders that need to be excluded are rheumatic fever, systemic lupus erythematosus, and the spondyloarthropathies. In endemic geographic areas, Lyme disease should be considered as well. Hematologic diseases such as the leukemias, hemophilia, and sickle cell anemia can also mimic JRA.

Immunogenetic studies in JRA can be considered, but associations are generally weak. Diagnosis should be made based upon the clinical presentation and evaluation.

TABLE 21–4. DIFFERENTIAL DIAGNOSIS OF JUVENILE RHEUMATOID ARTHRITIS

Systemic
- Infection
  - Tuberculosis
  - Lyme arthritis
  - Reactive arthritis
  - Septic arthritis
  - Rheumatic fever
  - Osteomyelitis
- Oncologic disorders
  - Neuroblastoma
  - Bone tumors
- Hematologic disorders
  - Leukemias
  - Hemophilia
- Rheumatologic and inflammatory disorders
  - Spondyloarthropathies
  - Systemic lupus erythematosus
  - Polyarteritis nodosa
  - Inflammatory bowel-related arthritis
  - Psoriatic arthritis
  - Scleroderma
  - Sarcoidosis
  - Villonodular synovitis
- Other
  - Endocrinopathies (eg, juvenile diabetes mellitus)
  - Mucopolysaccharidoses
  - Chondrocalcinosis
  - Castleman disease
  - Familial Mediterranean fever
  - Kawasaki disease

Ocular—Anterior Uveitis
- Ankylosing spondylitis
- Trauma
- Sarcoidosis
- Syphilis
- Inflammatory bowel disease
- Lyme disease
- Fuchs heterochromic iridocyclitis
- Reiter syndrome
- Tuberculosis
- Herpes simplex
- Herpes zoster

Ocular

Laboratory testing should attempt to rule out common causes of uveitis in children (Tables 21–3 and 21–4). Ocular complications of JRA are diagnosed most accurately by biomicroscopic examination. Females with a positive ANA are at the highest risk for developing chronic uveitis. The chronic anterior uveitis in JRA is nongranulomatous and characteristically asymptomatic by virtue of its insidious nature. Adding to the difficulty involved in diagnosing uveitis in JRA patients is the fact that those affected are often very young and may not be aware of any ocular changes or capable of communicating them. As a result, many patients present with advanced ocular involvement (e.g., posterior synechiae, band keratopathy, cataracts).

> Uveitis occurs most commonly in young females with pauciarticular ANA positive JRA with disease onset before the age of 2.

> Children with chronic anterior uveitis are often asymptomatic. They commonly do not have visual complaints until significant vision loss has occurred. Early detection and treatment can decrease the incidence of serious complications.

TREATMENT AND MANAGEMENT

Systemic

The treatment goals for JRA include control of pain, prevention of loss or restoration of range of motion, and promotion of normal growth and development. To this end, a treatment program should be multifaceted. Physical and occupational therapy are generally combined with a pharmacologic regimen (Tables 21–5).

First-line therapy for JRA patients are nonsteroidal anti-inflammatory drugs (NSAIDs) and analgesics such as acetylsalicylic acid, naproxen, and tolmetin. Drawbacks include limited efficacy and hepatotoxicity. A second or third NSAID may be added before advancing to second-line agents.

Slow-acting antirheumatic drugs (SAARDs) constitute the second line of therapy in JRA. Common SAARDs are hydroxychloroquine and sulfasalazine. These drugs seldom exert any clinically demonstrable effect before 4 to 12 weeks of treatment.

Gold compounds or penicillamine can be used in children with progressing polyarticular arthritis who are not responsive to NSAIDs alone or NSAIDs and SAARDs in combination.

Methotrexate is a disease-modifying antirheumatic drug (DMARD) that has been used in children with polyarticular JRA previously unresponsive to NSAIDs. Although the mechanism of action is unknown, it is thought that methotrexate affects immune function. At low dosages, it ameliorates symptoms of inflammation but has not been shown to have any beneficial effect on bone erosions or other radiologic changes that result in impaired joint use and function. Effects have been seen as early as 3 to 6 weeks after initiation of therapy.

The third line of pharmacologic treatment involves the use of glucocorticoids. Glucocorticoids may be useful in cases that are resistant to more conservative forms of treatment. These drugs can be used in combination with NSAIDs and other antirheumatic drugs. Oral prednisone is used in severe cases. Prednisolone and triamcinolone can be used intraarticularly if there are one or two joints that continue to show disease activity in a child who has responded well to other therapies. Glucocorticoids are most effective against systemic manifestations such as fever and rash. They have little effect against the process of arthritic joint damage. The most significant adverse affect of this type of therapy in children is growth retardation. In the most severe cases, methylprednisolone can be used in intravenous pulse therapy. However, these children need to be monitored constantly for electrolyte and fluid imbalance as well as cardiac arrhythmia.

Immunosuppressive agents and cytotoxic agents such as azathioprine, cyclophosphamide, and chlorambucil are used only in approved experimental protocols. These drugs should be reserved for cases of life-threatening disease or unremitting progression.

Intravenous immunoglobulin (IVIG) is an experimental therapy that has been considered as a means to wean young patients off corticosteroids. It has been shown to be effective when used in parallel with other courses of therapy such as NSAIDs and methotrexate. Its mechanism of action is unknown, but IVIG may reduce the immune response. Its antirheumatic effect, if any, is unclear.

Other experimental therapies include cyclosporine, immune modulators (e.g., anti-CD5-ricin) and antibiotic therapy (minocycline).

Orthopedic surgery in some children can decrease the mechanical impairment of joint motion. Arthroscopy is the surgical method of choice. Total joint replacement is usually only considered after bone growth has ceased.

Ocular

Serious visual loss can be prevented with early detection and aggressive treatment of anterior uveitis in JRA patients. Significant visual loss (less than 20/200) can occur in up to 75% of patients with advanced eye disease (Dollfus, 1998). Glaucoma, cataract, and band keratopathy are complications of chronic anterior uveitis that was either undiagnosed or not treated appropriately.

Visual outcome often can be predicted by the severity of the initial ocular findings (e.g., advanced uveitis with posterior synechiae) and visual acuity. Young female pauciarticular JRA patients with a positive ANA have the highest risk of developing chronic anterior uveitis and should be examined every 3 months for at least 7 years after the onset of JRA. Table 21–5 lists recommended ocular follow-up schedules for all forms of JRA.

Concurrent systemic therapy may adequately control the articular inflammation but have minimal effect on ocular inflammation. Topical corticosteroid therapy and short-acting cycloplegic agents are the primary treatment for anterior uveitis in JRA patients. Long-acting cycloplegic agents, such as atropine, have been used but should be avoided due to the risk of induced amblyopia and synechiae in the dilated position, in addition to potential systemic side effects. In mild cases, a short-acting cycloplegic can be instilled at bedtime to minimize the cycloplegic effects during the day. Topical steroid therapy should be tailored to the severity of the uveitis as well as the response to treatment. Steroid dosage should be tapered slowly until there are no inflammatory cells in the anterior chamber. The presence of mild flare is not as significant as the presence inflammatory cells. The persistent, chronic nature of anterior uveitis in JRA patients usually requires that treatment continue over months or possibly years.

Uveitis unresponsive to topical steroid treatment will most likely not respond significantly to systemic steroid treatment. Anterior sub-Tenon's steroid injections may result in a better response, but may require general anesthesia in very young patients. Intraocular pressure must be monitored regularly during steroid therapy.

TABLE 21–5. TREATMENT AND MANAGEMENT OF JUVENILE RHEUMATOID ARTHRITIS

Systemic
Articular
- Exercise:
  - Physical and occupational therapy
- NSAIDs/analgesics:
  - ASA, naproxen, tolmetin
- SAARDs:
  - Hydroxychloroquine, sulfasalazine
- If unresponsive to NSAIDs +/− SAARDs:
  - Gold salts, penicillamine, methotrexate
- Glucocorticoids:
  - Prednisone, triamcinolone, methylprednisolone
- Experimental:
  - IV immunoglobulin, cyclosporine, immune modulators, antibiotics
- Orthopedic surgery

Extra-Articular
- Fever: analgesics/monitor
- Macular rash, lymphadenopathy, hepatosplenomegaly: monitor
- Growth retardation: growth hormone
- Pericarditis: hospitalization

NOTE: Extra-articular manifestations may influence overall treatment of JRA (e.g., systemic medication changes, hospitalization)

Ocular
- Anterior uveitis
  - Topical cycloplegics: cyclopentolate 1%, homatropine 5%
    - Dose dependent upon severity of inflammation
  - Topical steroids: prednisolone acetate 1%
    - Dose dependent upon severity of inflammation
  - Recommended monitoring/follow-up schedules:
    - Pauci-JRA (+) ANA
      - Every 2–3 months for 7 years, biannually thereafter
    - Pauci-JRA (−) ANA
      - Every 4–6 months for 7 years, biannually thereafter
    - Poly-JRA (+) ANA
      - Every 3 months for 7 years, biannually thereafter
    - Poly-JRA (−) ANA
      - Every 6 months for 7 years, biannually thereafter
    - SoJRA
      - Annually
- Glaucoma
  - Topical treatment
    - Surgery—trabeculodialysis
  - Band keratopathy
    - Ocular lubricants
    - Chelation
  - Cataract
    - Surgery
    - Aphakic corrective lenses—spectacle and contact

Systemic NSAIDS may help decrease the amount of steroid needed to control the anterior uveitis. If the uveitis still does not respond, or in those patients in whom the side effects of chronic steroid treatment need to be minimized, cytotoxic and immunosuppressive agents may be considered. Due to the long-term toxicity of these agents, careful monitoring of serum levels and co-management with a rheumatologist are crucial.

Secondary glaucoma in JRA is difficult to manage and the visual prognosis is poor. Topical treatment only provides temporary control. Topical carbonic anhydrase inhibitors may be beneficial. Trabeculodialysis has a higher success rate than filtration surgery in children.

If band keratopathy develops, chelation and debridement should be undertaken to restore corneal integrity and improve visual acuity. Lubricant therapy with unpreserved ophthalmic ointments and artificial tears is necessary when epithelial disruption is present in symptomatic patients.

Cataract management in JRA is also difficult. Anterior uveitis should be inactive or at least well controlled before surgery; however, delaying surgery can lead to amblyopia in some cases. A lensectomy–vitrectomy procedure (removal of lens, posterior lens capsule, and anterior vitreous) without intraocular lens implantation has been advocated for JRA children in an attempt to avoid cyclic membrane formation. Intraocular lens implantation is contraindicated in children with JRA. In some instances, the intraocular lens may be a stimulus for intraocular inflammation and provide structural support for inflammatory membranes. Therefore, these patients will need visual rehabilitation through aphakic spectacle and contact lens correction. Amblyopia also requires appropriate therapy. Complications include hypotony, glaucoma, macular edema, uveitis, hyphema, choroidal detachments, and phthisis.

CONCLUSION

JRA is a group of arthritides that develop in childhood. The overall prognosis is good, especially with early detection and multidisciplinary management. However, the subtle nature of the early clinical findings can make early detection of JRA difficult. Recognition and proper treatment can significantly reduce systemic and ocular morbidity.

REFERENCES

American Academy of Pediatrics Section on Rheumatology and Section on Ophthalmology. Guidelines for ophthalmologic examinations in children with juvenile rheumatoid arthritis. *Pediatrics.* 1993;92:295.

Boone MI, Moore TL, Cruz OA. Screening for uveitis in juvenile rheumatoid arthritis. *J Pediatr Ophthalmol Strabismus.* 1998;34:41–43.

Cassidy JT. Juvenile rheumatoid arthritis. In: Kelley WN, Harris Ed, Ruddy S, Sledge CB, eds. *Textbook of Rheumatology.* Philadelphia: Saunders; 1997:1207.

Dana MR, Merayo-Lloves J, Schaumberg DA, Foster CS. Visual outcomes prognosticators in juvenile rheumatoid arthritis associated uveitis. *Ophthalmology.* 1997;104:236.

Dollfus H. Eye involvement in children's rheumatic diseases. *Baillieres Clin Rheumatol.* 1998;12:309.

Foster CS, Barrett F. Cataract development and cataract surgery in patients with juvenile rheumatoid arthritis-associated iridocyclitis. *Ophthalmology.* 1993;100:809–817.

Gäre BA. Epidemiology. *Baillieres Clin Rheumatol.* 1998; 12:191.

Giles CL. Uveitis in childhood—Part I. Anterior. *Ann Ophthalmol.* 1989;21:13–28.

Harper SL, Foster CS. The ocular manifestations of rheumatoid disease. In: Jakobiec FA, Colby K, eds. *Int Ophthalmol Clin.* 1998;38.

Kanski JJ. Juvenile arthritis and uveitis. *Surv Ophthalmol.* 1990;34:253–267.

Kanski JJ, Shun-Shin A. Systemic uveitis syndromes in childhood: An analysis of 340 cases. *Ophthalmology.* 1984; 91:1247–1252.

Pachman LM, Poznanski AK. Juvenile rheumatoid arthritis. In: McCarty DJ, Koopman WJ, eds. *Arthritis and Allied Conditions.* Philadelphia: Lea & Febiger; 1992:1021.

Pachman LM, Poznanski AK. Recent advances in the diagnosis and care of the child with arthritis. *The Child's Doctor. Journal of the Children's Memorial Hospital.* 1998; Spring.

Pelkonen PM. Juvenile arthritis with oligoarticular onset. *Baillieres Clin Rheumatol.* 1998;12:273.

Probst LE, Holland EJ. Intraocular lens implantation in patients with juvenile rheumatoid arthritis. *Am J Ophthalmol.* 1996;122:161.

Schneider R, Laxer RM. Systemic onset juvenile rheumatoid arthritis. *Baillieres Clin Rheumatol.* 1998;12:245.

Tugal-Tutkun I, Havrlikova K, Powers WJ, Foster CS. Changing patterns in uveitis of childhood. *Ophthalmology.* 1996;103.

Uziel Y, et al. Intravenous immunoglobulin therapy in systemic onset juvenile rheumatoid arthritis: A follow-up study. *J Rheumatol.* 1996;23:910.

Wang FM, Wertenbaker C, Behrens MM, Jacobs JJ. Acquired Brown's syndrome in children with juvenile rheumatoid arthritis. *Ophthalmology.* 1984: 91:23–26.

Wolf MD, Litchter PR, Ragsdale CG. Prognostic factors in the uveitis of juvenile rheumatoid arthritis. *Ophthalmology.* 1987;94:1242.

Chapter 22

ANKYLOSING SPONDYLITIS

Miriam Rolf

Ankylosing spondylitis (AS), also known as Marie-Strümpell or Bechterew's disease, is an inflammatory arthropathy that was first described in the late nineteenth century. It is most prevalent in young men. It characteristically involves the sacroiliac joint and occasionally the spinal cord, giving rise to symptoms of back pain, stiffness, and discomfort. AS is the prototype for the spondyloarthropathies, a group of rheumatoid-negative inflammatory disorders that share a variety of clinical, radiological, genetic, and pathologic features. Diseases included in this classification are ankylosing spondylitis, Reiter syndrome, and psoriatic arthritis. AS was one of the first spondyloarthropathies to be associated with ocular inflammatory disease. Acute nongranulomatous iridocyclitis is the primary ocular sequela evident in AS. It frequently manifests prior to any other symptoms, often leading to the diagnosis of AS.

EPIDEMIOLOGY

Systemic

AS is mainly observed in young males. The adult form of AS usually presents between puberty and 35 years of age, with a peak age of onset in the middle to late 20s. Onset after the fourth decade is very uncommon (Osial et al, 1993). Juvenile AS develops before the age of 16, usually beginning at 8 to 10 years of age (Wong et al, 1996). Men were once thought to be affected with AS ten times more frequently than women. These statistics are probably not accurate since AS appears to be underdiagnosed in women, given its milder course (Smith & Nozik, 1989; Wong et al, 1996). Recent estimates of a male-to-female ratio ranging between 5:1 and 1:1 are thought to be more accurate (Osial et al, 1993).

In the early 1970s two independent research groups, led by Brewerton and Schlosstein, found a remarkable association between the major histocompatability antigen, HLA-B27, and AS (Brewerton et al, 1973; Schlosstein et al, 1971). HLA-B27 is a class I major histocompatability complex marker that is present in 6 to 8% of the normal Caucasian population in the United States and 3% of normal African-Americans. However, HLA-B27 is present in 90% of patients with AS (Osial et al, 1993; Rosenbaum, 1999; Toussirot & Wending, 1998). This predisposing factor is more common in certain ethnic groups than others, resulting in a strikingly uneven distribution of AS. The highest frequency of AS is found in Native American Indians and Alaskan Eskimos, whereas the disease is almost nonexistent in African-Americans and Japanese (Oliveri et al, 1998). Although the genetic linkage to HLA-B27 has been established, the exact mode of inheritance is not fully understood. AS occurs in approximately 1 to 2% of the Caucasian population, but the frequency among first-degree relatives who are HLA-B27 positive is 20 times that of the normal population (Osial et al, 1993; Schlosstein et al, 1971).

Ocular

AS is the most frequently identified systemic disease associated with recurrent iridocyclitis, or acute anterior uveitis. In fact, it is estimated that 50% of patients with acute anterior uveitis who are HLA-B27 positive suffer from some form of rheumatic disease, especially a spondyloarthropathy (Rothova et al, 1987). Kimura and associates (1966) identified approximately 35% of uveitis patients as having probable or definite AS. Acute iridocyclitis occurs in approximately 25% of all AS patients during the course of their disease (Rosenbaum, 1999). The uveitis is not related to the severity of the primary rheumatic disease. Oftentimes the uveitis can present years prior to the joint and skeletal signs and may aid in the diagnosis of the condition.

PATHOPHYSIOLOGY/DISEASE PROCESS

Systemic

The seronegative spondyloarthropathies (SPAs) constitute a large group of rheumatic disorders with common genetic, clinical, and radiologic characteristics. The presence of central or axial involvement is their most characteristic clinical feature. Diseases included in this classification include ankylosing spondylitis, Reiter syndrome, and psoriatic arthritis. AS is the prototype for the SPAs and is a progressive inflammatory arthropathy with a predilection for the axial skeleton (Table 22–1). The sacroiliac joint is affected most severely, and the vertebral column is affected less extensively. Peripheral joint involvement is also relatively common, and several organ systems including the heart, lungs, and kidneys may be affected. Fortunately, the overall course of the disease is usually benign and fewer than 20% of patients develop significant disability (Kettering, 1996).

TABLE 22–1. CHARACTERISTIC FEATURES OF ANKYLOSING SPONDYLITIS

Systemic
Common in young adult males
Sacroiliitis of the spinal cord and sacroiiliac joint
Extra-articular manifestations—heart, lung, kidney
Peripheral joint complications
Strong association with HLA-B27
Chronic lower back pain or stiffness

Ocular (Uveitis)
Unilateral presentation
Sudden onset
Nongranulomatous with fine keratic precipitates
Propensity for posterior synechiae to develop
High rate of recurrence, with alternation between eyes common
Complete resolution of inflammation between attacks

The etiology of AS is unknown. Its pathogenesis is believed to be multifactorial in nature, with viral and bacterial infections implicated as triggering mechanisms. Current research is focused on its genetic component, specifically the HLA-B27 molecule. In 1997, Ren and colleagues reported on the existence of AS "protective" B27 alleles. The B*2706 allele present in Singaporeans and Thais and the B*2709 allele found in Sardinians appear to prevent the development of AS. Hence, researchers have suggested that a causative agent generates arthritogenic peptides capable of binding effectively to susceptible AS B27 subtypes, but not to other protected subtypes (ie, alleles B*2706 and B*2709).

> AS typically presents in young adult males with lower back pain that is alleviated by exercise.

Symptoms of inflammatory back disease secondary to AS are clinically manifested as progressive stiffening of the spine with pain. The typical clinical presentation is a young adult male with lower back pain or morning stiffness that is alleviated with physical activity. The pain is insidious in onset, lasts several months in duration, is exacerbated by rest, and can radiate into the buttocks and thighs. Involvement of the dorsal spine and rib cage can cause ill-defined dorsal spinal pain and pleuritic-type chest pain. A flexed or bent-over posture often relieves the back pain, but if left untreated can lead to joint fusion and subsequent kyphosis.

Enthesopathy is a distinct pathologic feature of AS, and it explains many of the ill-defined symptoms of this condition. It is an inflammatory reaction at the entheses, the cartilaginous sites of attachment of tendons and ligaments to bone. This inflammatory reaction leads to localized pain or stiffness, as well as deposition of new bone. An ankylosed joint occurs when the bones comprising that joint fuse and become immobile.

Spondylitis occurs in approximately 50% of patients with AS (El-Khoury et al, 1996). It begins at the thoracolumbar and lumbosacral junctions and then moves cephalad. Enthesitis of the sacroiliac joint starts with subchondral bony erosions and cartilage destruction. It is followed by a reactive formation of bone growth from the ilium that spans the width of the joint. The cartilage that separates the joint ossifies and the

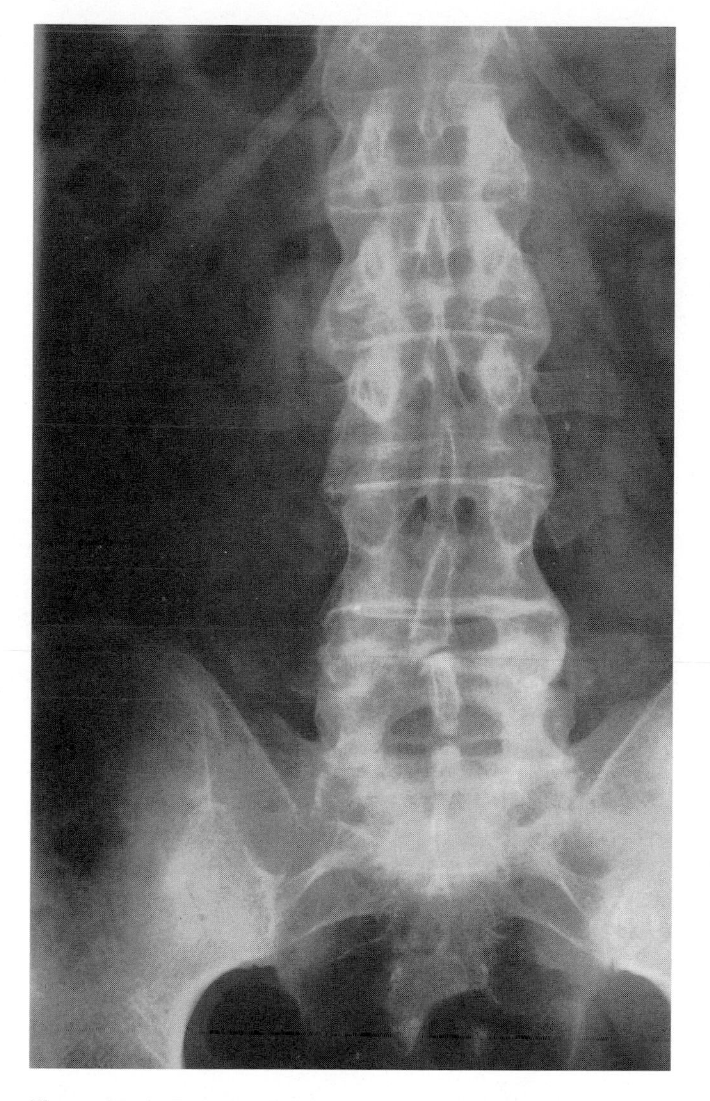

Figure 22–1. Frontal radiograph of a 48-year-old-male with AS illustrating complete fusion of the sacroiliac joints and complete spinal fusion (bamboo spine) consistent with the disease.

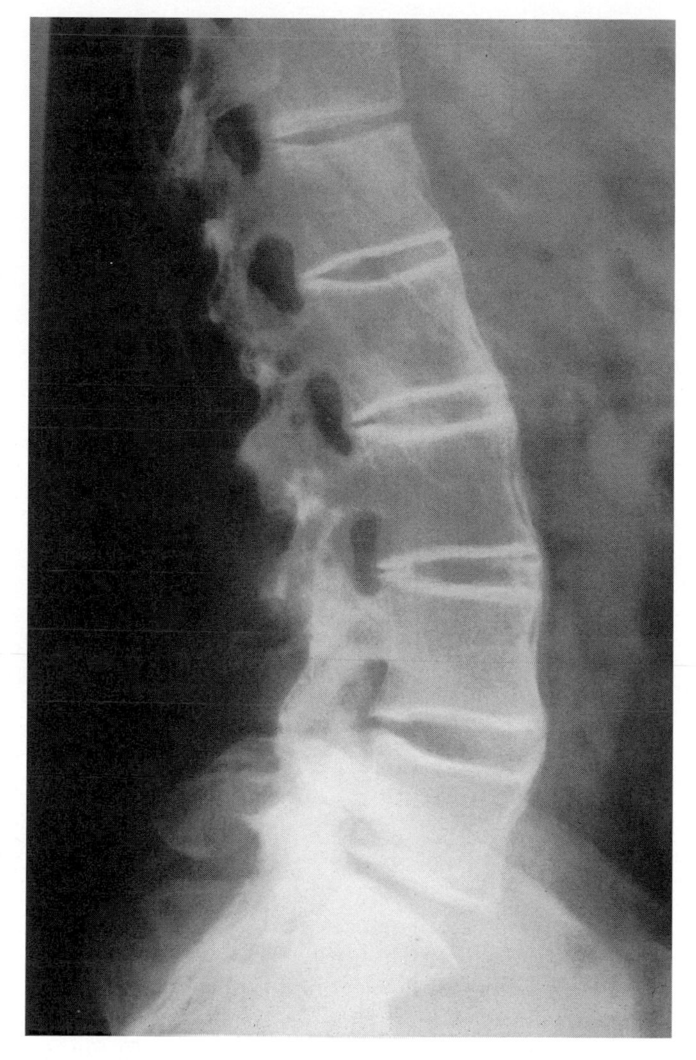

Figure 22–2. Lateral radiograph of the same patient shown in Figure 22–1 illustrating complete fusion of the axial skeleton and kyphosis of the spine.

joint eventually fuses. Sacroiliitis tends to be a symmetric process as viewed in the pelvic radiograph (Figure 22–1).

Enthesopathy of the vertebral column is associated with the development of syndesmophytes. Syndesmophytes are vertical bony spurs that represent ossification of the outer fibers of the annulus fibrosus. The annulus fibrosus is the ring of fibrocartilage and fibrous tissue forming the circumference of the intervertebral disc. The spurs ascend the spinal cord in a sequential and symmetric fashion, resulting in complete fusion of the vertebral bodies. At times the spurs can bulge beyond the margins of the vertebral bodies and give rise to the radiographic bamboo appearance of the spine (Figure 22–2). Although this feature is most characteristic of AS, few individuals progress to the classic ankylosed spine. After the ossification process is completed, the pain subsides and osteoporosis develops, making the spine vulnerable to pathologic fractures.

Variations in the typical clinical presentation exist for females and juvenile-onset patients. Both groups tend to develop peripheral joint disease before back pain. In addition, females generally have a later onset and a milder course than males with less involvement of the ascending spine.

Cardiovascular involvement in AS patients is typically associated with long-standing and severe disease. However, it also has been documented in mild or even subclinical presentations of AS. Its estimated frequency is 3 to 10% and it may be the only clinical sign of the disease (Oliveri et al, 1998). Inflammatory changes at the aortic valve result in dense fibrosis of the valves, as well as fibrotic changes of the adjacent atrioventricular nodal tissue, the aortic wall, and myocardial septum. These fibrotic changes result in aortic regurgitation, which can cause aortic insufficiency and complete heart block. Additional cardiovascular abnormalities include conduction disturbances and less frequently, angina and pericarditis.

Pulmonary fibrosis is a rare manifestation of AS which is characterized by slow, progressive fibrosis and cystic changes within the lung apices. Secondary fungal infection (eg, *Aspergillus*) may develop and can be fatal. Clinically it is associated with cough, dyspnea, sputum production, and occasionally hemoptysis. Respiratory failure secondary to severe thoracic spine involvement can also occur. These pulmonary changes manifest after the fifth decade, typically many years after presentation of the joint disease.

Although once thought to be a relatively rare complication of AS, subclinical renal abnormalities were detected in 35% of AS patients evaluated in a Brazilian study (Nabokov et al, 1996). Possible mechanisms of kidney damage include the long-term adverse effects of NSAIDs, an increased incidence of glomerulonephritis, and renal deposition of amyloid. Additional prospective studies are necessary to elucidate the long-term significance of renal involvement in this disease.

Extraspinal involvement occurs in 30 to 40% of AS patients and presents concurrently with the onset of back disease (Oliveri et al, 1998). The large peripheral joints of the hips, shoulders, and knees are primarily affected, whereas the smaller distal joints are generally spared. Arthritis progression to joints of the upper extremities can also involve the rib cage. This may lead to chest pain, decreased chest expansion, and associated breathing difficulties.

Ocular

Ocular involvement occurs in approximately 25% of patients during the course of AS (Rosenbaum, 1999). There is no temporal relationship between the onset of eye disease and the onset of back disease. In addition, the activity of the spondylitis does not necessarily parallel the activity of the eye disease.

> The propensity for keratic precipitates in AS uveitis mandates prompt and aggressive treatment.

The hallmark of AS iridocyclitis is its acute onset. The inflammation typically follows a very reproducible pattern with unilateral presentation. Oftentimes a prodrome of vague discomfort or foreign-body sensation precedes observable inflammation by 24 to 48 hours. Ocular inflammation is usually confined to the anterior segment. Patients typically present with symptoms of pain, photophobia, and decreased vision along with accompanying signs of intense conjunctival injection, fine nongranulomatous keratic precipitates, and an anterior chamber reaction. Posterior synechiae develop rapidly and occur more frequently in AS iridocyclitis than in other form of anterior uveitis (Rosenbaum, 1999). Generally, the structures of the posterior segment are spared, but macular edema may occur after multiple recurrences. Severe case presentations may involve hypopyon formation, vitreal opacification, or hypotony. Cataracts and secondary glaucoma are more likely to result from therapy than from the inflammation itself.

> Acute onset of ocular inflammation is the hallmark of ankylosing uveitis and it may aid in its systemic diagnosis.

Uveitis associated with AS has a strong tendency to recur and may present in the alternate eye. The inflammation typically responds well to topical corticosteroids and cycloplegics. With appropriate treatment the uveitis should resolve completely within 2 to 3 months of onset without complication. This complete resolution of inflammation between attacks is highly suggestive of uveitis associated with HLA-B27 and helps to distinguish it from other forms of recurrent uveitis (eg, Behçet disease) (Rosenbaum, 1999). In general, the visual prognosis for patients with AS is excellent unless complications, such as macular edema and vitreal opacification, supervene.

DIAGNOSIS

Systemic

There is no specific diagnostic test for AS. Diagnosis relies upon patient and family history, clinical presentation, and radiographic and serologic test results that are consistent with the disease. This information will help support a clinician's physical examination and assist in ruling out mimicking disorders (Tables 22–2, 22–3, and 22–4). The most useful tests are x-rays of the pelvis and lumbosacral spine, followed by HLA-B27 typing.

Similar to other spondyloarthropathies, AS can be difficult to diagnose in its early stages. This is particularly true in physically active patients because exer-

TABLE 22–2. DIAGNOSIS OF ANKYLOSING SPONDYLITIS

Imaging studies:
1. X-rays to detect fusion of the axial skeleton (bamboo spine) and the sacroiliac joints
2. CT scans and technetium bone scans may also be helpful initially
3. Echocardiogram and chest x-ray may detect extra-articular manifestations

Patient history: chronic morning lower back pain and stiffness that improves with exercise

Physical exam: Schober test illustrates degree of spinal flexion (see text)

Laboratory testing: does not give a definitive diagnosis

cise delays the osteoblastic process that ankyloses the joints (Krongard & De Vos, 1996; Beckingsgal et al, 1984). Several classification criteria have been established to aid in the diagnosis of AS and other spondyloarthropathies. (Tables 22–5 and 22–6 are two examples). Some authorities view criteria classifications as too restrictive, delaying the diagnosis of insidious cases. They recommend that classification criteria be used as general guidelines only.

Patient history and physical examination are essential to the clinical diagnosis of the disease. Approximately 75% of AS patients present with chronic lower back pain and stiffness, especially upon awakening. The Schober test may be included as part of the physical examination to measure lumbar spine mobility. This diagnostic maneuver also provides a useful gauge of disease progression and clinical severity. In this test a line is drawn over the spinous process of the fifth lumbar vertebra while the patient is standing upright. At the midpoint, a span is measured 10 cm above and 5 cm below this line. The distance between these two points is then remeasured while the patient is in full flexion. An increase of more than 5 cm is considered indicative of normal lumbar mobility. An increase of less than 5 cm suggests spinal rigidity.

Radiographic studies are instrumental in the diagnosis of AS. X-rays provide an objective finding to detect joint fusion or calcification of the cartilaginous spaces, even in asymptomatic patients. Rosenbaum and Wernick (1990) reported that approximately 50% of patients with anterior uveitis without an obvious cause had an undiagnosed systemic illness. A spondyloarthropathy often was determined to be the underlying disease mechanism (Wong et al, 1996). Although sacroiliitis is considered to be the hallmark of AS, it may present before unequivocal radiographic changes appear. In the first few months of the disease the sacroiliac changes may be detectable only by computed tomography (CT) or technetium bone scanning. CT scanning is also more sensitive in identifying active sacroiliac joint inflammation. Despite these advantages, standard x-rays are considered to be more cost-effective for routine patient evaluations. As the inflammatory nature of the disease progresses, erosion and sclerosis of the sacroiliac and peripheral joints are evident on standard radiographic film. X-rays of the vertebral column reveal intervertebral joint calcification, giving the characteristic bamboo appearance associated with advanced AS.

Although typically ordered in conjunction with radiographic testing, routine lab assays also are nonspecific for AS and may provide minimal assistance in its diagnosis. The value of HLA-B27 typing is especially controversial. Despite its high sensitivity and specificity, HLA-B27 testing cannot be used to diagnose AS in randomly selected persons. HLA-B27 is present in 8 to 10% of the normal American population and the test is

TABLE 22–3. LABORATORY REFERENCE VALUES IN ANKYLOSING SPONDYLITIS (AS)

Test	Normal Values	Values in AS
HLA-B27	Requires clinical correlation	90% positive
CRP	<0.8 mg/dL	Elevated
ANA	Negative	Negative
ESR	Values depend on the method used Male age/2; (Female age +10)/2	Elevated
RF factor	0–69 IU/mL (nonreactive)	Negative test

TABLE 22–4. SYSTEMIC DIFFERENTIAL DIAGNOSIS OF ANKYLOSING SPONDYLITIS

Rheumatoid arthritis

Other spondyloarthropathies—Reiter syndrome, psoriatic arthritis, inflammatory bowel disease

Diffuse idiopathic skeletal osteoarthropathy

TABLE 22–5. CLINICAL CRITERIA LIST FOR THE DIAGNOSIS OF ANKYLOSING SPONDYLITIS

1. Low back pain greater than 3 months' duration, unrelieved by rest
2. Pain and stiffness in the thoracic cage
3. Limited chest expansion
4. Limited motion in the lumbar spine
5. Past or present evidence of iridocyclitis
6. Bilateral radiographic sacroiliitis
7. Radiographic syndesmophytosis

Diagnosis requires four of the first five criteria, or criteria 6 and 7.
Modified from: Bluestone R. Ankylosing spondylitis. In McCarty DJ, ed. Arthritis and Allied Conditions. *Philadelphia: Lea & Febiger; 1985.*

TABLE 22–6. DIAGNOSTIC CRITERIA FOR ANKYLOSING SPONDYLITIS (AS) (MODIFIED NEW YORK CRITERIA)

1. Lower back pain not relieved by rest of at least 3 months' duration
2. Lumbar restriction in the frontal and sagittal planes
3. Decreased chest expansion compared to normal age-matched values
4. Unilateral sacroiliitis (grades 3 or 4)
5. Bilateral sacroiliitis (grades 2 or 3)

Definite AS if criterion 4 or 5 above, along with any other criterion, is observed.

positive in many nonspecific forms of iridocyclitis. The presence of the HLA-B27 haplotype may be viewed simply as a predisposing factor for AS, but does not imply eventual development of the disease. Other lab results consistent with AS include an elevated C-reactive protein (CRP) and erythrocyte sedimentation rate (ESR), seronegative values for the antinuclear antibody (ANA) test and rheumatoid factor (RF factor), and findings consistent with mild anemia.

Additional specialty tests such as echocardiogram and chest radiography may be utilized as needed to identify patients with less common pulmonary and cardiac complications of AS.

Ocular

The diagnosis of anterior uveitis is generally straightforward, but determining its exact cause can be challenging even to an astute clinician. Ocular assessment of these patients includes a comprehensive history, a thorough physical exam, and a complete eye evaluation paying particular attention to the characteristics (Table 22–7) and possible sequelae of the inflammation. Iridocyclitis secondary to AS has its own unique qualities that differentiate it from other forms of anterior uveitis. Symmetry, suddenness of onset, distribution and type of keratic precipitates, duration, and tendency to recur are some of the features that must be evaluated when constructing a differential diagnosis (Table 22–8). Appropriate laboratory and radiographic testing should be ordered if the history and ocular presentation supports its diagnostic value.

TABLE 22–7. OCULAR DIAGNOSIS OF UVEITIS IN ANKYLOSING SPONDYLITIS (AS)

Hallmarks of AS Uveitis	
Symmetry	Unilateral
Onset	Acute
Duration	Self-limited; complete resolution in 6–8 weeks with treatment
Continuity	Recurrent; may alternate to opposite eye
KPs	Fine, nongranulomatous
Complications	Posterior synechiae, cataracts, glaucoma, macular edema
Location	Anterior

Ocular Presentation

Symptoms
- Prodromal discomfort
- Pain
- Photophobia
- Decreased vision
- Redness

Signs
- Ciliary injection
- Fine granulomatous KPs
- Anterior chamber reaction
- Increased/decreased IOP
- Posterior synechiae

TREATMENT AND MANAGEMENT

Systemic

Aggressive medical treatment is not necessary for most patients with AS. The goal of treatment is to relieve pain and stiffness, preserve joint and spine function, and prevent disability. This objective is achieved by vigorous exercise and physical therapy in conjunction with the judicious use of nonsteroidal anti-inflammatory drugs (NSAIDs) (Table 22–9). Daily exercise that is directed toward the preservation of functional posture, joint mobility, muscle strength, and deep breathing is most beneficial.

Since the course of the disease cannot be altered, NSAIDs play a supportive role in the treatment of AS. However, they are still considered the mainstay of treatment by reducing pain and stiffness in most patients. Several NSAIDs are available that offer similar beneficial results, but none has demonstrated superiority over phenylbutazone. Unfortunately, the routine use of phenylbutazone is precluded due to the severe hematological side effects associated with long-term use. Indomethacin is now considered the NSAID of choice, and it is typically prescribed for morning and bedtime use during periods of acute flare-up. All NSAIDs share common side effects, most notably gas-

TABLE 22–8. OCULAR DIFFERENTIAL DIAGNOSIS OF ANKYLOSING SPONDYLITIS

Fuch's heterochromic iridocyclitis
Reiter syndrome
Behçet disease
Lyme disease
Psoriatic arthritis

TABLE 22–9. SYSTEMIC TREATMENT/MANAGEMENT OF ANKYLOSING SPONDYLITIS

Anti-inflammatories
- NSAIDs (ie, indomethacin)
- Local injection of corticosteroids to treat enthesopathy and peripheral arthritis

Physical therapy/exercise
Orthopedic surgical intervention, if necessary
Pulmonary, renal, and cardiac complications are managed by their respective specialists

TABLE 22–10. OCULAR TREATMENT/MANAGEMENT OF ANKYLOSING SPONDYLITIS

Topical cycloplegic and steroid preparations:
- i gtt homatropine 5% or cyclopentolate 2% ophth soln bid–tid
- i gtt prednisolone acetate 1% ophth susp q 1h–qid (depending on severity)

Oral steroid tablets or periocular steroid injection may be required for severe presentations
Vitrectomy, cataract surgery, glaucoma medication when warranted

trointestinal upset. The administration of H_2 receptor antagonists, prostaglandin analogs, or Prilosec in conjunction with the NSAID usually alleviates the unwanted gastrointestinal side effects (Toussirot & Wending, 1998). The development of specific isoforms of NSAIDs that could eliminate toxicity while still providing analgesia is still being researched (Toussirot & Wending, 1998).

Other forms of medications have been utilized to treat AS when NSAIDs are poorly tolerated or ineffective, or symptoms are severe. Sulfasalazine has proven to be effective in such cases and has shown good tolerability in clinical trials. Beneficial results are mainly evident in patients with peripheral joint involvement. The long-term effects on spinal mobility are not known.

Immunosuppressive agents appear to have little to offer in the management of AS. Other second-line treatments such as methotrexate and gold salts require properly designed, controlled studies to evaluate their effectiveness.

Some specific manifestations of AS such as enthesopathy and peripheral arthritis can be best managed by local injections of corticosteroids. Extra-articular manifestations of AS, such as kidney, cardiac, and lung complications, require parallel management with their respective specialists. Orthopedic surgical intervention is necessary if significant joint disease affects the hips or knees.

Ocular

Iridocyclitis associated with AS can frequently be managed by conventional therapy using topical steroids and cycloplegics (Table 22–10). The goals of therapy include preservation of vision, reduction of ocular pain, elimination of the inflammation, and prevention of postinflammatory sequelae. Management requires vigilance and a flexible approach to treatment. 1% prednisolone acetate ophthalmic suspension and 5% homatropine ophthalmic solution are considered the standard therapeutic agents, but the exact dosage must be determined on an individual case basis. Due to the propensity for keratic precipitate development in severe cases, hourly administration of corticosteroids as well as a stronger, longer-lasting cycloplegic agent may be necessary. In severe or chronic presentations, a periocular injection or a loading dose of systemic steroids may be required.

The topical steroids are tapered gradually as the inflammation resolves, as evidenced by the decrease of cells and flare detected in the anterior chamber. Most episodes of anterior uveitis resolve within 2 to 6 weeks, but frequent recurrences will warrant a very slow taper over several weeks.

The use of systemic NSAIDs may also be effective in controlling ocular inflammation. Unfortunately, most patients have recurrences despite their use. Dougados and colleagues (1993) demonstrated that the use of sulfasalazine reduced the occurrence of acute anterior uveitis. Its application in AS management still warrants further investigation.

Vitrectomy, cataract surgery, and glaucoma therapy are implemented on an individual basis when needed. In conjunction with routine rheumatic evaluations, eye doctors should monitor patients with AS on a regular basis, typically every 6 to 12 months, or when they experience prodromal symptoms consistent with iridocyclitis.

CONCLUSION

AS is a chronic inflammatory disorder of the cartilaginous joints of the axial skeleton that typically presents during the second or third decade of life. It affects males more severely than females. It is characterized by the inflammatory reaction it elicits in the axial skeleton and peripheral joints. Physical impairment is usually minor despite its long course. AS rarely is associated with mortality and does not require aggressive treatment and management. NSAIDs remain the mainstay of treatment in conjunction with physical exercise.

Clinical trials are underway to investigate alternate treatment modalities. Recurrent, nongranulomatous iridocyclitis is commonly associated with AS. Although the inflammation associated with this disease is often intense, complete resolution of the inflammation can usually be obtained with conventional ocular therapy. Early diagnosis is imperative to minimize the complications associated with chronic anterior uveitis and to prevent vision loss. Continued research is necessary to fully define the manifestations of this rheumatic disease and more importantly to determine its etiology.

REFERENCES

Abel GS, Terry JE. Ankylosing spondylitis and recurrent anterior uveitis. *J Am Optom Assoc.* 1991;62: 844–848.

Azouz EM, Duffy CM. Juvenile spondyloarthropathies: Clinical manifestations and medical imaging. *Skeletal Radiol.* 1995;24:399–408.

Barozzi L, Olivieri I, De Matteis M, et al. Seronegative spondyloarthropathies: Imaging of spondylitis, enthesitis and dactylitis. *Euro J Radiol.* 1998;27:512–517.

Beckingsgal AB, Williams D, Gibson JM, et al. *Klebsiella* and acute anterior uveitis. *Br J Ophthalmol.* 1984;68:866–868.

Bluestone R. Ankylosing spondylitis. In: McCarty DJ, ed. *Arthritis and Allied Conditions.* Philadelphia: Lea & Febiger; 1985.

Brandt J, Rudwaleit M, Eggens L, et al. Increased frequency of Sjögren's syndrome in patients with spondyloarthropathy. *J Rheumatol.* 1998;25:718–724.

Brewerton DA, Caffrey M, Nicholls A, et al. Acute anterior uveitis and HL-A27. *Lancet.* 1973;2:994–996.

Burgos-Vargas R, Pacheco-Teno C, Vazquez-Mellado J. Juvenile-onset spondyloarthropathies. *Pediatr Rheumatol.* 1997; 23:569–598.

Calin A. The Individual with ankylosing spondylitis: Defining disease status and the impact of the illness. *Br J Rheumatol.* 1995;34:663–672.

Calin A, Fries JF. Striking prevalence of ankylosing spondylosis in "healthy" W27 positive males and females: A controlled study. *N Eng J Med.* 1975;293:835–839.

Careless DJ, Inman RD. Acute anterior uveitis: Clinical and experimental aspects. *Semin Arthritis Rheum.* 1995; 24:432–441.

Catterall RD, Perkins ES. Uveitis and urogenital disease in the male. *Br. J Ophthalmol.* 1961;45:109–116.

Dougados M. Diagnostic features of ankylosing spondylitis. *Br. J Rheumatol.* 1995;34:301–303. Editorial.

Dougados M, Berenbaum F, Maetzel A, et al. The use of sulfasalazine for the prevention of attacks of acute anterior uveitis associated with spondyloarthropathy. *Rev Rheum.* 1993;60:80–82.

El-Khoury GY, Kathol MH, Brandses EA. Seronegative spondyloarthropathies. *Radiol Clin North Am.* 1996;34:343–356.

Espinoza LR. Spondyloarthropathies. In: *Lippincott's Primary Care Practice.* Philadelphia: Lippincott; 1998;2:81–86.

Fischbach F. *A Manual of Laboratory and Diagnostic Tables.* 4th ed. Philadelphia: Lippincott; 1992.

Gran JT, Husby G. Clinical, epidemiologic, and the therapeutic aspects of ankylosing spondylitis. *Curr Opin Rheumatol.* 1998;10:292–298.

Harley JB, Scoffield RH. The spectrum of ankylosing spondylitis. *Hosp Pract.* 1995; July 15;37–46.

Keat A. Why the joint, why the eye? *Clin Rheumatol.* 1996; 15(suppl 1):19–21.

Kettering JM, Towers JD, Rubin DA. The seronegative spondyloarthropathies. *Semin Roentgenol.* 1996;31:220–228.

Kimura SJ, Hogan MJ, O'Connor GR, et al. Uveitis and joint disease: A review of 191 cases. *Trans Am Ophthalmol Soc.* 1966;64:301.

Krongard DFA, De Vos D. Diagnosis of ankylosing spondylitis. *Radiol Technol.* 1996;68:163–165.

Kuipers JG, Raybourne RB, Williams KM, et al. Specificities of human TAP alleles for HLA-B27 binding peptides. *Arthritis Rheum.* 1996;39:1892–1895.

Lyons JL, Rosenbaum JT. Uveitis associated with inflammatory bowel disease compared with uveitis associated with spondyloarthropathy. *Arch Ophthalmol.* 1997;115:61–64.

Nabokov AV, Shabunin MA, Smirnon AV. Renal involvement in ankylosing spondylitis (Bechterew's disease). *Nephrol Dial Transplant.* 1996;11:1172–1175.

Nuki G. Ankylosing spondylitis, HLA-B27, and beyond. *Lancet.* 1998;351:767–768.

O'Connor RG. Endogenous uveitis. In: Krauss-Makiw E, O'Connor RG, eds. *Uveitis: Pathophysiology and Therapy.* 2nd ed. New York: Thieme; 1986.

Oliveri I, Barozzi L, Padula A, et al. Clinical manifestations of seronegative spondyloarthropathies. *Euro J Radiol.* 1998; 27:53–56.

Osial TA Jr, Cash JM, Eisenbeis CH Jr. Arthritis-associated syndromes. *Prim Care.* 1993;20:857–882.

Petty RE. Is ankylosing spondylitis in childhood a distinct entity? *J Rheumatol.* 1996;23:2013–2014. Editorial.

Ren EC, Koh WH, Sim D, et al. Possible protective role of HLA-B*2706 for ankylosing spondylitis. *Tissue Antigens.* 1997;49:67–69.

Rosenbaum JT. Anterior uveitis and systemic disease. In: Yanoff M, Duker JS, eds. *Ophthalmology.* St. Louis: Mosby; 1999.

Rosenbaum JT, Wernick R. Selection and interpretation of laboratory tests for patients with uveitis. *Int Ophthalmol Clin.* 1990;30:238–242.

Rothova A, Van Veenendaae WG, Linssen A, et al. Clinical features of acute anterior uveitis. *Am J Ophthalmol.* 1987; 103:137–145.

Scharf Y, Zonis S. Histocompatability antigens (HLA) and uveitis. In: Cottier E, ed. *Current Research. Surv Ophthalmol.* 1980;24:220–228.

Schlosstein L, Terasaki PI, Bluestone R. High association of an Hl-A antigen, W27, with ankylosing spondylitis. *N Engl J Med.* 1971;288:704–706.

Smith RE, Nozik RA. Iridocyclitis associated with arthritis syndromes (ankylosing spondylitis, Reiter's syndrome,

juvenile rheumatoid arthritis). *In:* Smith RE, Nozik RA, eds. *Uveitis: A Clinical Approach to Diagnosis and Management.* 2nd ed. Baltimore: Williams & Wilkins; 1989.
Strobel ES, Fritschka E. Case report and review of the literature: Fatal pulmonary complication in ankylosing spondylitis. *Clin Rheumatol.* 1997;16:617–622.
Toussirot E, Wending D. Current guidelines for the drug treatment of ankylosing spondylitis. *Drugs.* 1998;56:225–240.
Vilar MJP, Cury SE, Ferry MB, et al. Renal abnormalities in ankylosing spondylitis. *Scand J Rheumatol.* 1997;26:19–23.
Wakefield D, Montanaro A, McClusky P. Acute anterior uveitis and HLA-B27. In: Cotlier E, Weinreb R, eds. *Current Research. Surv Ophthalmol.* 1991;36(3):223–232.
Wong SG, Durdin JC, Thompson LR. Anterior uveitis associated with ankylosing spondylitis, Reiter's syndrome, and sarcoidosis. *South J Optom.* 1996;14:4–9, 21–26.

Chapter 23

PSORIATIC ARTHRITIS

John E. Conto

Psoriatic arthritis (PsA) is an uncommon seronegative spondyloarthropathy (arthritis of the spine) that is distinguished from other inflammatory arthropathies by the presence of characteristic psoriatic skin and nail disease. The arthritis may be mild to severe, with single or multiple peripheral joints becoming affected. The degree of joint involvement is quite variable, and often several different patterns concurrently exist. Sacroiliitis and spondylitis may be seen in patients with PsA, but are less commonly present than in patients with ankylosing spondylitis(AS) or Reiter syndrome (RS). A genetic predisposition for psoriasis and seronegative arthritis has been supported by family and HLA studies. The inheritance pattern is thought to be a dominant inherited multifactorial trait with variable penetrance. Environmental factors are thought to play a role in the development of PsA, including bacterial antigen induction, retrovirus antigen reaction, trauma, and immunologic agents.

Ocular involvement in PsA ranges from a mild purulent conjunctivitis to a nongranulomatous uveitis similar to that seen in RS or AS. Episcleritis may develop rarely. Unlike many other inflammatory arthropathies, keratoconjunctivitis sicca does not often occur in conjunction with PsA.

EPIDEMIOLOGY

Systemic

- The frequency of PsA in patients with psoriasis has been reported to be between 5 and 42%.
- The estimated incidence of PsA in the general population of the United States is thought to be 0.1 to 1%.
- Males and females are affected equally.
- The peak age of onset appears to be in the fourth or fifth decades.

Ocular

- Generalized ocular inflammation occurs in about 30% of patients.
- Conjunctivitis has been reported in approximately 20% of cases.
- Anterior uveitis appears in an estimated 7 to 16% of patients.

PATHOPHYSIOLOGY/DISEASE PROCESS

Systemic (Table 23–1)

- Usually has a slow onset, but can develop acutely in one third of patients.

TABLE 23–1. SYSTEMIC MANIFESTATIONS OF PSORIATIC ARTHRITIS

Psoriasis
Symptoms
- Mild to moderate itching

Signs
- Discrete erythematous lesions
- Scaling and flaking of the skin

Psoriatic Nail Disease
Signs
- Discoloration
- Ungual bed separation
- Cracking and ridging
- Nail pitting

Psoriatic Arthritis
Symptoms
- Joint pain
- Joint stiffness

Signs
- Joint swelling of fingers and toes
- Sacroiliitis
- Asymmetric changes of the DIP joints
- Bony ankylosis
- "Pencil-in-cup" or "fishtail" deformities of phalanges

- The disease course includes periods of exacerbation and remission.
- The psoriasis often precedes the arthritis by several years, although in 15 to 20% of cases the arthritis occurs before the development of the skin lesions.
- Discrete erythematous lesions with scaling and flaking of the surrounding skin produce mild to moderate itching.
- Nail involvement is seen in about 80% of patients, and the severity of the arthritis appears to be related to the degree of nail changes.
- Nail manifestations include discoloration, thickening of the distal nail, separation at the ungal bed, ridging, cracking, and nail pitting (Figure 23–1).
- Joint involvement is typified by a synovitis, which is indistinguishable from that seen in rheumatoid arthritis (RA).
- Early arthritic changes usually involve the small finger joints, but the knee, hip, ankle, and wrist can also be involved.
- Several arthritic patterns can present in isolation or in combination:
  - The asymmetric oligoarticular form is the most common, with a pattern similar to the peripheral arthropathy seen in AS or RS.

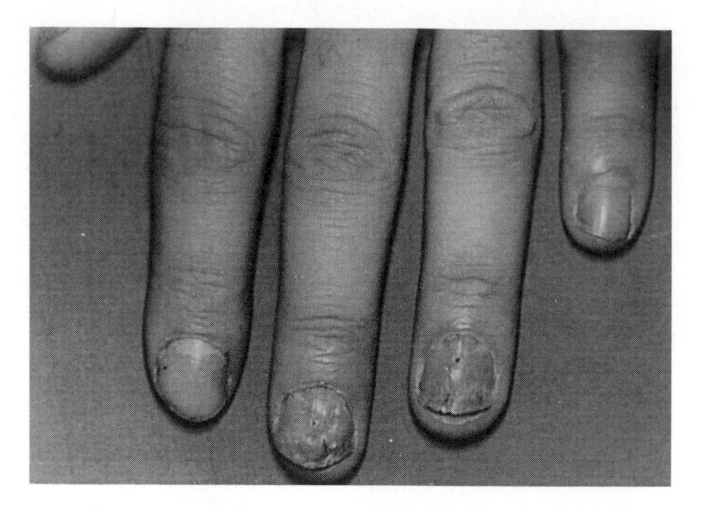

Figure 23–1. Psoriatic nail manifestations: discoloration, distal nail thickening, ridging, cracking, and nail pitting. (*Reprinted with permission from Gawkrodger DJ.* An Illustrated Colour Text of Dermatology. *New York: Churchill Livingstone; 1992.*)

  - Symmetrical polyarthritis is the next most common with a similar clinical presentation to RA.
  - Predominant distal interphalangeal (DIP) joint arthritis is characterized by isolated involvement of the fingers, and is most often associated with the nail disease.
  - The least common forms are predominant axial arthritis, which closely resembles AS, and deforming erosive arthritis or arthritis mutilans, which causes progressive osteolysis and severe distortion of involved digits (Figure 23–2).
- Patients with PsA tend to have less functional loss, and they do not lose as much time from work, as patients with RA.

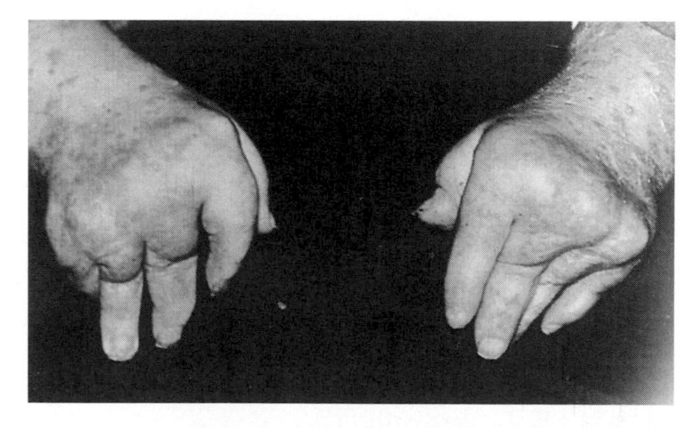

Figure 23–2. Deforming arthritis mutilans with severe distortion of the digits and hands. (*Reprinted with permission from Gawkrodger DJ.* An Illustrated Colour Text of Dermatology. *New York: Churchill Livingstone; 1992.*)

- Mortality due to PsA is rare, and when death occurs, it is usually from complications related to medical therapy.
- The exact cause is unknown, but genetic, immunological, and environmental factors are thought to be involved:
  - Psoriasis-related genes have been found on the short arm of chromosome 6, and the long arm of chromosome 4 and chromosome 17.
  - The HLA antigens B13, B17, B27, B37, B38, B39, Cw6, DR4, and DR7 have been implicated as susceptibility markers.
  - Increasing evidence suggest that psoriasis is a primary T-cell-mediated autoimmune disease with secondary keratinocyte activation and proliferation.
  - Environmental factors such as viral and bacterial agents have been implicated in the development of PsA.

Ocular (Table 23–2)

- Ocular symptoms of minor irritation, injection, foreign-body sensation, or photophobia may occur.
- The conjunctivitis is superficial, occasionally accompanied by a mucopurulent discharge, and is generally short in duration, but may follow a chronic course.
- The acute nongranulomatous anterior uveitis is unilateral, most often seen in patients with sacroiliitis, and may be recurrent and alternate between the eyes.
- Posterior segment involvement is rare, and complications, such as cystoid macular edema or cataract, are uncommon if initial treatment of the anterior uveitis is adequate.
- Keratoconjunctivitis sicca is uncommon.
- Episcleritis occurs infrequently and is usually self-limiting.

TABLE 23–2. OCULAR MANIFESTATIONS OF PSORIATIC ARTHRITIS

Symptoms
- Irritation
- Injection
- Photophobia
- Foreign-body sensation
- Decreased vision

Signs
- Mucopurulent conjunctivitis
- Anterior uveitis
- Episcleritis
- Keratoconjunctivitis sicca

DIAGNOSIS

Systemic

- Currently there are no valid classification criteria for PsA.
- The diagnosis is made in the presence of psoriasis or psoriatic nail disease, along with the characteristic signs of the spondyloarthritis (Table 23–3).
- There are no characteristic laboratory abnormalities:
  - Rheumatoid factor (RF) is negative in the vast majority.
  - Erythrocyte sedimentation rate (ESR) may be elevated, but is nonspecific.
  - Anemia may be present, but is also nonspecific.
  - Analysis of the synovial fluid may show inflammatory components.
- There has been an increased linkage of psoriasis and PsA with several HLA antigens, including HLA-B13, B17, B27, B37, B38, B39, Cw6, and DR7.
- Radiographic findings may demonstrate the following:
  - Asymmetric changes of the DIP joints, terminal phalanges, and sacroiliac joint.
  - Other radiographic features, not characteristic of PsA alone, are bony ankylosis or destruction of the joints of the hands and feet, and bony proliferation of the distal joints.
  - Progressive erosion of the phalanges may appear as "pencil-in-cup" or "fishtail" deformities.
- In general, PsA is differentiated from the other arthropathies (Table 23–4) based upon the presence of the characteristic skin disease:
  - Joint tenderness in PsA is less than in RA.
  - PsA joints often have a purplish discoloration not commonly seen in other forms of arthritis.
  - Distal joint inflammation distinguishes PsA from osteoarthritis.
  - DIP joint involvement is uncommon in RA.

TABLE 23–3. DIAGNOSTIC TESTS FOR PSORIATIC ARTHRITIS

Complete blood count (CBC)—demonstrates anemia
ESR—elevated
RF—negative
HLA typing—HLA-B27 most common
Synovial fluid analysis—inflammatory components
X-ray/CT of involved joints—sacroiliac, spine, wrist, phalanges

TABLE 23–4. SYSTEMIC AND OCULAR DIFFERENTIAL DIAGNOSIS OF PSORIATIC ARTHRITIS

- Osteoarthritis
- Rheumatoid arthritis
- Ankylosing spondylitis
- Reiter syndrome

- The arthritic digits often have characteristic psoriatic nail changes.
- Dactylitis (whole digit inflammation) is typical for PsA although it may occur in RS.
- In patients with peripheral arthritis and psoriasis, the presence of enthesitis (inflammation at the site of the tendon insertion of the bone) supports a diagnosis of PsA versus RA with psoriasis.
- Psoriatic spondyloarthropathy results in less pain and less restriction of spinal movement than that seen in AS.

Ocular

- The conjunctivitis and anterior uveitis are similar in clinical appearance to those seen in RS or AS.
- The anterior uveitis is typically nongranulomatous, acute in onset, unilateral, and recurrent, with frequent development of synechiae.
- The anterior uveitis may be accompanied by dry eye or keratitis and may be indistinguishable from that seen in AS.
- Differentiation of PsA as the cause from other similar etiologies is based on the systemic findings.

> PsA should be considered as the etiology of a nongranulomatous anterior uveitis if characteristic skin and nail signs are present in conjunction with a spondyloarthropathy.

TREATMENT AND MANAGEMENT

Systemic (Table 23–5)

- The psoriasis is usually mild, requiring no treatment, but when necessary, it is treated with topical medications including tar, corticosteroid creams, and UVB light or systemic medications, including methotrexate, psoralens with UVA light (PUVA), retinoic acid derivatives, or cyclosporine.

TABLE 23–5. TREATMENT AND MANAGEMENT OF PSORIATIC ARTHRITIS

Systemic

Psoriasis

- White petrolatum or crude coal tar ointment (bid to involved areas)
- Anthralin ointment or cream (0.1 to 1%)
- Topical corticosteroid creams (e.g., triamcinolone acedtonide 0.1% bid)
- UVB light therapy (280 to 320 nm)
- Methotrexate (5–15 mg/week)
- Psoralen with UVA light (PUVA) (e.g., methoxsalen PO followed by exposure to UVA [330 to 360 nm])
- Retinoic acid derivatives (e.g., 0.5–1 mg/kg/day isotretinoin PO)

Psoriatic arthritis

- NSAIDs (e.g., ibuprofen 400–800 mg qid, aspirin 3–6.5 g/day)
- Intra-articular glucocorticosteroid injections (e.g., triamcinolone hexacetonide)
- Antimalarials (e.g., hydroxychloroquine 200–600 mg daily)
- Penicillamine (250–750 mg/day PO)
- Sulfasalazine (500 mg–3 g/day PO)
- Methotrexate (2.5–20 mg in single dose/week)
- Azathioprine (1–2.5 mg/kg/day)
- Cyclosporine (up to 5 mg/kg/day)
- Parenteral gold compounds (e.g., gold thioglucose IM)
- Exercise and physical therapy
- Surgical joint reconstruction

Ocular

Conjunctivitis/episcleritis

- Vasoconstrictors (e.g., naphazoline hydrochloride 0.025% bid)
- Cold compresses
- Artificial lubricants (e.g., 2% methylcellulose q4h to qid)

Anterior uveitis

- Topical corticosteroids (e.g., 1% prednisolone acetate q1h-qid)
- Cycloplegics (e.g., 2% homatropine bid)

Keratoconjunctivitis sicca

- Artificial lubricants (e.g., 2% methylcellulose q4h to qid)
- Punctal plugs
- Local environmental humidity

Abbreviations: bid, twice a day; g, gram; h, hour; IM, intramuscularly; kg, kilogram; mg, milligram; nm, nanometer; PO, orally; q, each, every; qid, four times daily.

- Mildly active arthritis is treated with nonsteroidal anti-inflammatory drugs (NSAIDs) with indomethacin more effective than aspirin or ibuprofen.
- Synovitis may be managed with local glucocorticoid injections. Oral steroids are rarely necessary.
- Slow-acting antirheumatic drugs (SAARDs) that are effective include antimalarials, penicillamine, sulfasalazine, methotrexate, azathioprine, and cyclosporine A.
  - Mild cases of PsA—sulfasalazine.
  - More severe cases of PsA—methotrexate and cyclosporine.

- Many of these drugs have toxic side effects that limit their broad use.
- Parenteral or oral gold has been used with various degrees of success in severe erosive cases, although about one third of patients will have a severe skin reaction.
- Physical therapy and exercise are helpful in preserving the range of motion of the involved joints.
- Hand and ankle splints may prevent contracture from developing.
- Surgical reconstruction of damaged joints can be considered when extreme functional loss occurs, but has a less favorable result than in RA.

Ocular (Table 23–5)

- The conjunctivitis follows a benign course, usually resolving over a period of 7 to 10 days; however, supportive therapy with cold compresses, vasoconstrictors, and ocular lubricants may be helpful for subjective relief.
- Acute anterior uveitis can be managed with varying dosages of topical corticosteroids, depending on the severity of anterior chamber reaction, and cycloplegic agents.

CONCLUSION

PsA is an arthropathy that is seen with psoriatic skin or nail disease. The clinical course is often benign, but can be quite variable in the overall effect on physical function. Many joints are affected, from the small distal joints of the digits to the larger joints of the spine or hip. Like the other seronegative arthropathies, PsA can have associated ocular findings, most commonly conjunctivitis or anterior uveitis. The ocular complications are usually mild, without long-standing sequelae.

REFERENCES

Al-Khonizy W, Reveille JD. The immunogenetics of the seronegative spondyloarthropathies. *Baillieves Clin Rheumatol.* 1998;12:567–588.

Alonso JCT, Perez AR, Castrillo JMA, et al. Psoriatic arthritis (PsA): A clinical immunological and radiological study of 180 patients. *Br J Rheumatol.* 1991;30:245–250.

Banares A, Hernandez-Garcia C, Fernandez-Gutierrez B, Jover JA. Eye involvement in the spondyloarthropathies. *Rheum Dis Clin N Am.* 1998;24:771–784.

Dieppe PA, Doherty M, Macfarlene D, Maddison P. Psoriatic arthropathy. In: Dieppe PA, Doherty M, Macfarlene D, Maddison P, eds. *Rheumatology Medicine.* Edinburgh: Churchill Livingstone; 1985:86–90.

Dougados M, Revel M, Khan MA. Spondyloarthropathy treatment: Progress in medical treatment, physical therapy and rehabilitation. *Baillieves Clin Rheumatol.* 1998;12: 717–736.

Espinoza LR, van Solingen R, Cuellar ML, Angulo J. Insights into the pathogenesis of psoriasis and psoriatic arthritis. *Am J Med Sci.* 1998;316:272–276.

FitzGerald O, Kane D. Clinical, immunopathogenic, and therapeutic aspects of psoriatic arthritis. *Curr Opin Rheumatol.* 1997;9:295–301.

Furst DE. Update on clinical trials in the rheumatic diseases. *Curr Opin Rheumatol.* 1998; 10:123–128

Gladman DD. Clinical aspects of the spondyloarthropathies. *Am J Med Sci.* 1998;316:234–238.

Gladman DD. Psoriatic arthritis. *Rheum Dis Clin N Am.* 1998;24:829–844.

Gladman DD. Psoriatic arthritis: Review of current concepts. *Isr J Med Sci.* 1991;27:228–232.

Lambert JR, Wright V. Eye inflammation in psoriatic arthritis. *Ann Rheum Dis.* 1976;35:354–356.

Leczinsky CG. The incidence of arthropathy in a ten-year series of psoriasis cases. *Acta Derm Venereol.* 1948;28:483–485.

Marcussion J. Psoriasis and arthritic lesions in relation to the inheritance of HLA genotypes. *Acta Derm Venereol.* 1979; 59(suppl 82):1–48.

Melvin JL. Rheumatic disease in the adult and child. In: Melvin JL. *Occupational Therapy and Rehabilitation.* 3rd ed. Philadelphia: Davis; 1989:88–92.

Michet CJ, Conn DL. Psoriatic arthritis. In: Kelley WN, Harris ED, Ruddy S, Sledge CB, eds. *Textbook of Rheumatology.* 3rd ed. Philadelphia: Saunders; 1989:1053–1063.

Moll JMH, Wright V. Psoriatic arthritis. *Semin Arthritis Rheum.* 1973;3:55–78.

Olivieri I, Cantini F, Salvarani C. Diagnostic and classification criteria, clinical and functional assessment, and therapeutic advances for spondyloarthropathies. *Curr Opin Rheumatol.* 1997;9:284–290.

Wright V. Psoriatic arthritis. In: Kelley WN, Harris ED, Ruddy S, Sledge CB, eds. *Textbook of Rheumatology.* 2nd ed. Philadelphia: Saunders; 1985:1021–1031.

Chapter 24

REITER SYNDROME

Chung Yong Song

Reiter syndrome (RS) belongs to the class of disorders known as the seronegative spondyloarthropathies. Seronegativity implies that RS is rheumatoid factor negative. Reiter syndrome is characterized by the classic triad of arthritis, urethritis, and conjunctivitis. Some feel the high occurrence of mucocutaneous lesions warrants changing the clinical triad to a tetrad. Keratoderma blennorrhagicum, circinate balanitis, and painless oral ulcers are examples of the mucocutaneous lesions encountered in RS patients. RS shares the spondyloarthropathy class with ankylosing spondylitis (AS), psoriasis, ulcerative colitis, and Crohn disease. These conditions present with radiologic sacroiliitis with or without spondylitis (inflammation of the spine) and peripheral inflammatory arthritis. In 1981, the American College of Rheumatology defined RS as "an episode of peripheral arthritis of more than one month duration occurring in association with urethritis and/or cervicitis." The pathogenesis of RS is thought to involve the interaction between bacterial antigens, bacterial phlogistic (inflammatory) components, and the immune system combined with a genetic predisposition (HLA-B27). There is no curative treatment for RS, but various forms of management from antibiotics and immunosuppressive agents to physical therapy and pain management have been used with success. The major ocular manifestations are conjunctivitis and uveitis. The conjunctivitis is noninfectious and self-limiting. However, the uveitis must be treated promptly because it can be recurrent and difficult to manage.

EPIDEMIOLOGY

Systemic

RS is thought to be the most common cause of peripheral arthritis in young men 15 to 35 years of age. It affects males five times more frequently than females. When RS occurs following enteric infection, the male-to-female ratio is 1:1, but reaches as high as 9:1 when occurring after sexually acquired infections. RS is much more common among Caucasians than African-Americans. HLA-B27 is present in 8% of normal Caucasians and 3% of normal African-Americans. In RS patients, the prevalence of HLA-B27 increases to 80% of Caucasians and 50 to 60% of African-Americans. Overall, HLA-B27 is found in 60 to 90% of RS patients. RS is rare in children, particularly young girls. Almost all cases in children and the elderly follow an enteric infection.

The estimated incidence of RS is 3 to 4 per 100,000 males in the United States. The risk of developing RS in the general population is approximately 0.2%. The risk increases to 2% in a population positive for HLA-B27, and increases further to 20 to 25% in an HLA-B27 population following an enteric infection. Two percent of patients with nonspecific urethritis also develop RS.

Approximately half of RS patients will develop some kind of disability that is considered to be permanent and show active disease about 20 years after diagnosis. The incidence of RS in HIV patients is between 2 and 11%, but recently is found to be increasing in Africa (Cuellar, 1998). The indigenous population of the eastern tip of Chukotka Peninsula of Siberia has a higher frequency of HLA-B27 (40%) and spondyloarthropathies (2%) than the Caucasian population (Krylov et al, 1995). HIV infection more than triples the risk of developing RS in HLA-B27 patients (Winchester et al, 1988). There have also been rare reports of RS after bacillus Calmette-Guérin (BCG) therapy for bladder carcinomas and after hepatitis B vaccination (Saporta et al, 1997).

Ocular

Ocular findings occur in approximately 50% of RS patients following a sexually acquired infection and 75% of RS patients following an enteric infection. The most common ocular manifestation is bilateral conjunctivitis, which occurs in 33 to 100% of RS patients. Anterior uveitis will develop in 20 to 40% of RS patients during the course of their disease and occurs in 5 to 10% at initial presentation. Conversely, 50% of all acute anterior uveitis patients are positive for HLA-B27.

PATHOPHYSIOLOGY/DISEASE PROCESS

Systemic

Stoll first recorded a patient exhibiting the classic triad of RS in 1776. Sir Benjamin Brodie also described a similar syndrome in a patient in 1818. In 1916, Hans Reiter described a case of arthritis, nongonococcal urethritis, and conjunctivitis in a World War I cavalry officer after a bout of dysentery from an enteric infection. RS can also develop after a venereal infection as the other major "trigger" cause. Ahvonen and coworkers used the term "reactive arthritis" to describe an aseptic arthritis after failing to isolate pathogens from knee aspirate in 1969. Reactive arthritis is defined as an acute, sterile synovitis associated with a localized infection elsewhere in the body. The terms RS and reactive arthritis are used interchangeably in the literature. Other terms such as sexually acquired reactive arthritis (SARA) and enteric reactive arthritis (ERA) have been proposed to distinguish the trigger infection. Undifferentiated seronegative arthritis (USNA) has been used to describe a reactive arthritis without an identified initiating infection. Brewerton and colleagues first described the association between RS and the major histocompatibility complex (MHC) class I specificity of the human leukocyte antigen (HLA) B27 in 1973. RS shares this association of HLA-B27 with the other spondyloarthropathies.

The etiology of RS is as yet unknown. However, theories of pathogenesis have evolved over the last few decades. An enteric or venereal trigger infection may be involved in initiating the disease. There is crucial evidence supporting the interplay of bacterial antigens or components and an abnormal host "autoimmune" response in the development of this disease. The presence of HLA-B27 may serve as a predisposing factor. The presence of TAP (transporters associated with antigen processing) alleles may also contribute to the susceptibility to RS (Barron et al, 1995). It seems likely that transport of bacterial antigens from the site of the initial infection to the affected joint occurs. There has been controversy surrounding "asepticity" or "sterility" of aspirate from the inflamed joint in the past. Researchers have rarely been able to isolate microorganisms from the joints of RS patients (Hughes & Keat, 1994). Newer immunohistochemical methods have identified chlamydial bacterial antigens and enteric bacteria such as *Yersinia* and *Salmonella* in the joints. In addition, high titers of specific antibody to both *Chlamydia* and *Salmonella* have been found in synovial fluid, supporting the presence of bacterial antigens in the joint. Moreover, other studies have implied that bacterial antigens can persist in the joint itself or other reservoir sites, disseminating to the joint for many years and perhaps accounting for the recurrence of RS symptoms (Hughes & Keat, 1994). Intact chlamydial RNA was found in synovial tissue using reverse transcription polymerase chain reaction (PCR) indicating viable and metabolically active *Chlamydia* (Gerard et al, 1998). The detection of bacterial RNA/DNA by PCR in joint tissue has also yielded mixed results and awaits further research. Furthermore, bacterial components have been shown to induce inflammation (phlogistic) in experimental models.

In males RS usually follows a venereal infection, whereas in females it usually follows dysentery. The major venereal pathogen is *Chlamydia trachomatis*. The major enteric pathogens are *Shigella flexneri* and *Salmonella enteritidis* (Table 24–1). Unlike septic arthritis, it is not the pathogens that directly cause the arthritis. The patient's immune response, mediated by peptides (CD4+ and/or CD8+ T lymphocytes) derived from microbes, leads to the arthropathy. Lavery and Lisse (1994) found that elevated tryptase levels in synovial fluid support the theory that mast cell activation is involved in the pathogenesis of RS. Segal (1996) proposed an alternative theory, which stated that peptidergic nerves can transmit signals from abdominal and pelvic areas to lumbosacral joints via the spinal cord, predisposing them to arthritis.

TABLE 24–1 PATHOGENS ASSOCIATED WITH REITER SYNDROME

Enteric Organisms
- *Shigella flexneri*
- *Salmonella enteritidis*
- *Salmonella typhimurium*
- *Yersinia enterocolitica*
- *Yersinia pseudotuberculosis*
- *Campylobacter jejuni*
- *Salmonella heidelberg*
- *Salmonella paratyphi*
- *Salmonella choleraesuis*
- *Escherichia coli*
- *Cryptosporidia*
- *Entamoeba histolytica*
- *Giardia lamblia*
- *Clostridium difficile*
- *Shigella sonnei*
- *Strongyloides stercoralis*
- *Taenia saginata*
- *Leptospira icterohaemorrhagica*

Urogenital Organisms
- *Chlamydia trachomatis*
- *Chlamydia psittaci*
- *Neisseria gonorrhoeae*
- *Ureaplasma urealyticum*

RS usually occurs in young white males (15 to 35 years old) with a recent history of dysentery or urethritis. Symptoms of oligoarthritis (two to four joints) present within 1 month of the dysentery or urethritis/cervicitis along with painful enthesopathy (especially the Achilles tendon). Clinical signs include mucocutaneous lesions such as keratoderma blennorrhagicum, circinate balanitis, and painless oral ulcers. Conjunctivitis usually occurs within a few days of the dysentery or urethritis.

The leading cause of enteric infection in children includes *Salmonella, Shigella, Yersinia,* and *Campylobacter.* Diarrhea with or without vomiting is the initial symptom in 65% of these cases. Typically, a fever and diarrhea first presents followed by conjunctivitis and then genitourinary, joint, and skin findings.

The systemic manifestations of RS are numerous (Table 24–2). The clinical course and prognosis for RS is varied. Less than one third of RS patients show the classic triad. The term "incomplete RS" is given to patients who do not exhibit all three of the classic symptoms but follow a clinical course similar to classic RS. This may be due in part to the nonsimultaneous presentation of the symptoms and the intentional/unintentional under-reporting of genitourinary and ocular symptoms. Patients who develop the classic triad seem to run an intermittent, milder course than those who develop incomplete RS. The disease also tends to affect females less severely than males. At the onset of the disease, fever, malaise, and weight loss are common symptoms. For patients with SARA, the symptoms usually resolve in the majority of cases within 6 months. Half of these patients will have recurrence of symptoms in the future.

In the early 1960s, aseptic arthritis after *Salmonella* gastroenteritis (ERA) was differentiated from *Salmonella* septic arthritis. Salmonellosis aseptic arthritis typically presents 3 weeks or less following the onset of gastroenteritis. There is no sex predilection and only a small percentage of patients develop arthritis after salmonellosis. Samuel and co-workers (1995) confirmed that a disproportionately large number of patients who develop post-*Salmonella* reactive arthritis are HLA-B27 positive. A minority of these patients had extra-articular manifestations of RS. The most common symptoms were joint pain (67%), joint stiffness(52%), conjunctivitis (41%), and mouth ulcers (25%). C-reactive protein testing and CD8 levels tended to be higher in cases with higher levels of arthritic activity. Sixty percent of the men and 66% of the women were HLA-B27 positive. In this study, the classic RS triad was present in only 22% of patients and incomplete RS was present in 44%.

TABLE 24–2. SYSTEMIC MANIFESTATIONS OF REITER SYNDROME

Articular
- Polyarthritis
- Sacroiliitis
- Enthesitis

Extra-Articular
- Urethritis/cervicitis
- Conjunctivitis/uveitis
- Painless oral ulcers
- Keratoderma blennorrhagicum
- Circinate balanitis
- Amyloidosis
- Aortitis
- Pulmonary fibrosis
- Prostatitis

Uncommon
- Protrusio acetabuli (sinking of the acetabulum with protrusion of the femoral head through it causing limitation of the hip joint)
- Epileptic seizures
- Thrombophlebitis
- Hyperprolactinemia
- Systemic vasculitis
- Coronary artery stenosis

Urethritis is characterized by difficult and painful urination. There may be blood in the urine as well as a transient sterile purulent discharge. Prostatitis has been reported in up to 80% of RS men. For female patients, cervicitis, vaginitis, reactive salpingitis, and sterile pyuria may occur. These urogenital symptoms may develop even after enteric infections.

The venereal or enteric infection is followed days to weeks later by the arthropathy. The arthritis is usually asymmetric, polyarticular (although it can start as monoarticular), and involves the large weight-bearing joints such as the knee and ankle. As the disease progresses, it can involve the fingers and wrists. Sacroiliitis presents in half of RS patients.

Enthesitis (Figure 24–1) is the painful inflammation of a tendon or ligament attachment to a bone. The most commonly affected enthesitis sites are the heel insertions of the Achilles tendon and plantar fascia, insertions of the patella tendon, insertions of the ischial tuberosities, pubic symphysis, and iliac crest. Calcaneous changes may be evident on both the plantar and posterior aspects of the heel bone (Sartoris, 1994). Secundini and co-workers (1997) found that the lower aspect of the calcaneous was involved in 100% of patients studied with RS. Talalgia (heel pain) is an early symptom in RS affecting either the posterior aspect of the heel or the plantar surface of the heel. Dactylitis, a variation of enthesitis, has been associated with 28% of RS patients. Osteoporosis, joint space loss, and marginal erosions with adjacent proliferation of the joints can be found in these patients.

Mucocutaneous lesions occur in about half of RS patients. Painless ulcers can affect various mucous tissues such as the buccal mucosa, tongue, palate, pharynx, and lips. The keratoderma blenorrhagicum (Figure 24–2) of RS histologically resembles pustular psoriasis. It is the most common of the cutaneous lesions and usually presents on the palms and plantar surfaces as hyperkeratotic/crusted papules. When present on the penis, it is called circinate balanitis and its appearance differs depending upon circumcision. Nail abnormalities may range from small subungual pustules to onycholysis (loosening of nail from the nail bed) and subungual hyperkeratosis.

Pulmonary fibrosis mimicking tuberculosis has been observed in RS. Typical cardiovascular complications result from an inflammation resulting in fibrosis of the aortic wall and myocardial septum. This can lead to cardiac conduction deficits and aortic regurgitation. Warren and colleagues (1998) reported gout as a rare complication in an RS patient.

Ocular

Conjunctivitis is the initial symptom in up to two thirds of patients with RS. Recurrences of ocular manifestations can mirror the pattern of systemic articular involvement. Although the exact mechanism is unknown, it has been theorized that antibodies to bacterial pathogens cross-react with HLA lymphocytes and bind to ocular structures, causing the ocular reaction.

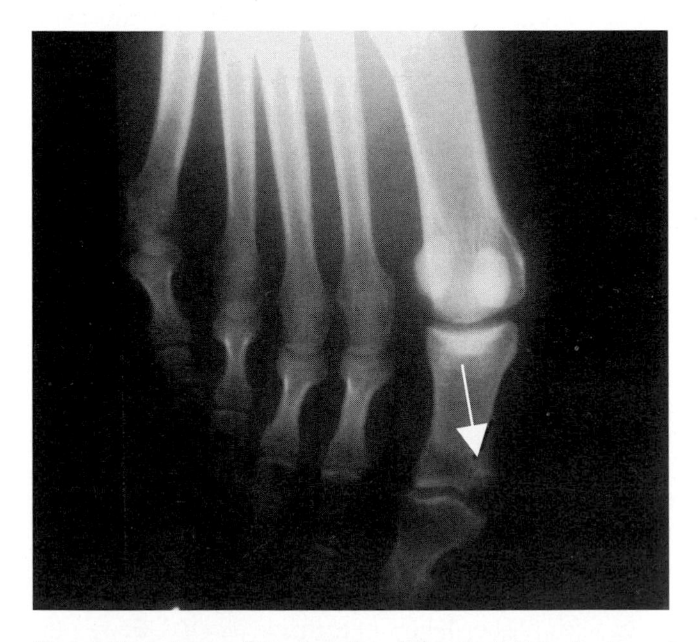

Figure 24–1. X-ray of the feet of an RS patient. Note the loss of bone at the lateral aspects of the joints of the toes (*arrow*). This patient had symptoms of tendinitis and had previously been treated for a chlamydial infection. He experienced nonspecific ocular irritation of both eyes on a recurrent basis following the chlamydial infection.

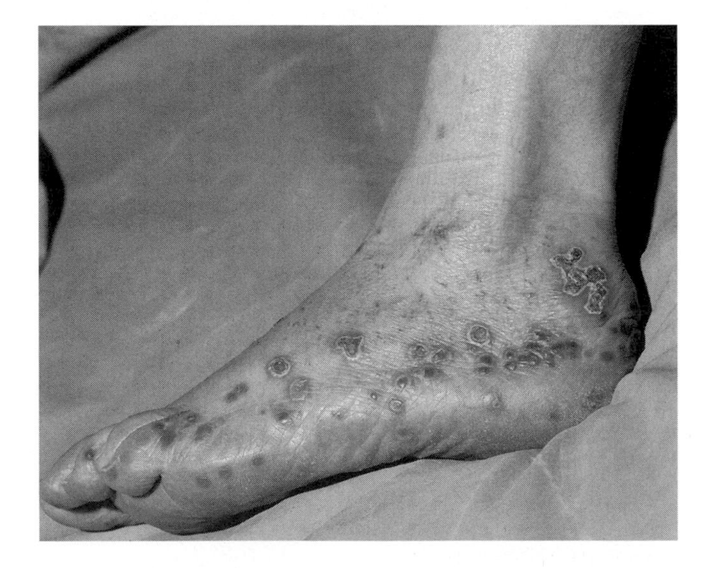

Figure 24–2. Reiter syndrome, Keratoderma blennorrhagicum. Multiple, annular, hyperkeratotic plaques with central clearing on the sole of the foot. (*With permission from Fitzpatrick TB et al.* Color Atlas and Synopsis of Clinical Dermatology. *3rd ed. New York: McGraw-Hill; 1997: 393.*)

TABLE 24–3. OCULAR DIFFERENTIAL DIAGNOSIS OF REITER SYNDROME CONJUNCTIVITIS AND/OR UVEITIS

- Viral conjunctivitis (recent upper respiratory infection with conjunctival follicles)
- Allergic conjunctivitis (itching and conjunctival chemosis with a history of hay fever or contact with an allergen)
- Bacterial conjunctivitis (profuse purulent discharge and matted shut eyelids upon awakening)
- Idiopathic uveitis

Many ocular findings are associated with RS (Table 24–3). The most common are conjunctivitis and anterior uveitis. The conjunctivitis is unilateral or bilateral and occurs in one third to one half of RS patients. It is typically noninfectious with little to no purulent discharge and self-limiting in less than 2 weeks. Conjunctival injection, episcleritis, and scleritis, along with a mild papillary reaction, may be observed. Superficial punctate keratitis can accompany these ocular findings and usually resolves without complication. However, subepithelial infiltrates and corneal ulcers with perforation have been reported as a rare but severe outcome.

Acute nongranulomatous anterior uveitis (usually unilateral) is the major ocular finding that must be treated. Photophobia, pain, blurred vision, and tearing are the typical presenting symptoms. Numerous cells and dense flare with small to medium-sized keratic precipitates tend to influence the formation of posterior synechiae. Spillover of cells from the anterior chamber may create the appearance of vitritis. Aggressive management of the inflammation is necessary to prevent synechiae. Chronic recurrent uveitis with RS needs to be appropriately managed to prevent cataract, recalcitrant secondary glaucoma, and persistent cystoid macular edema. The typical course of the anterior uveitis is 2 to 6 weeks. Hypopyon has been reported as a rare ocular complication in RS uveitis (D'Alessando et al, 1991).

DIAGNOSIS

Systemic

The diagnosis of RS can be made with a thorough history and physical exam. The incomplete form of RS (in which the classic triad is not present) is more common. Previous enteric or venereal infection with subsequent conjunctivitis, peripheral arthritis, urethritis/cervicitis, conjunctivitis/uveitis, and mucocutaneous lesions can help establish the diagnosis. However, less than one third of patients with RS present with all three of the classic findings. Laboratory testing (Table 24–4) may reveal the following: negative rheumatoid factor (RF), negative antinuclear antibody (ANA), positive HLA-B27, mild anemia and leukocytosis, elevated erythrocyte sedimentation rate (ESR), elevated C-reactive protein (CRP), elevated serum creatinine, and sacroiliitis with joint involvement on plain films. The lab tests are not specific, and the examiner must be wary of false-negatives and false-positives.

TABLE 24–4. DIAGNOSTIC TESTS USED IN THE DIAGNOSIS OF REITER SYNDROME

Major
- HLA-B27 serologic typing
- Rheumatoid factor (RF)
- Antinuclear antibody (ANA)
- Complete blood count with differential (CBC with differential)
- Erythrocyte sedimentation rate (ESR)
- C-reactive protein (CRP)
- Serum creatinine
- Plain films

Additional
- Magnetic resonance imaging with or without contrast
- Ultrasound
- Bone scintigraphy
- Arthrocentesis

The differential diagnoses (Table 24–5) of RS are gonococcal arthritis, rheumatoid arthritis, AS, and pso-

TABLE 24–5. SYSTEMIC DIFFERENTIAL DIAGNOSIS OF REITER SYNDROME

	Differentiating Characteristics (versus RS)
Major	
• Septic arthritis (gonococcal)	Resolves rapidly with antibiotics
• Psoriasis	Equal male to female ratio, predominant dermatologic changes
• Ankylosing spondylitis	Lacks a trigger infection and usually presents with complete spinal fusion
• Rheumatoid arthritis	Typically will have a positive rheumatoid factor and rheumatoid nodules
• Inflammatory bowel disease Ulcerative colitis Crohn disease	Presence of abdominal pain, diarrhea, and fever with weight loss
Minor	
• Calcium pyrophosphate deposition disease	
• Osteoarthritis	
• Lyme arthritis	
• Systemic lupus erythematosus	
• Sjögren disease	
• Sarcoidosis	
• Kawasaki disease	
• Gout	
• Whipple disease	

riasis. Other conditions such as inflammatory bowel disease, Lyme arthritis, systemic lupus erythematosus, and gout must also be considered.

PCR is found to be superior to serological typing to determine HLA-B27 positivity (Kirveskari et al, 1997). PCR may also be helpful in differentiating gonococcal arthritis from RS (Liebling et al, 1994). Psoriasis and RS have been theorized as belonging to a disease continuum. The dermatologic lesions of psoriasis are frequently indistinguishable from the skin lesions of RS (Romani et al, 1996). Magnetic resonance imaging (MRI) of the finger or toe revealing flexor tenosynovitis is considered to be the gold standard for dactylitis, although physical examination can be adequate. Bone scintigraphy is more sensitive than radiography for evaluation of talalgia (Lin et al, 1995). MRI with contrast of the involved joints may be useful in differentiating rheumatoid arthritis from RS (Jevtic et al, 1995).

Approximately half of RS patients have sacroiliitis and axial joint disease. Anteroposterior and oblique tunnel view radiography of the sacroiliac region is an important diagnostic tool in RS. X-rays of the lower body joints may also show inflammation causing erosion with adjacent areas of bony proliferation.

The differential diagnosis of recurrent aphthous stomatitis is Behçet disease, Crohn disease, SLE, and other spondyloarthropathies (Livneh et al, 1996).

Ocular

The ocular finding of conjunctivitis as part of the clinical triad is critical in making the diagnosis of RS. The biomicroscope should allow the examiner to assess the hyperemia and mixed papillary reaction of the conjunctiva. Differential diagnoses (Table 24–6) include viral conjunctivitis (recent upper respiratory infection, follicles), bacterial conjunctivitis (profuse purulent discharge and matted shut lids), and allergic conjunctivitis (itch, chemosis, and history of hay fever or contact with allergen). The presentation of systemic complaints (eg, arthritis, urethritis, mucocutaneous lesions, and heel pain) may prompt the examiner to consider the diagnosis of noninfectious conjunctivitis associated with RS.

Anterior uveitis is diagnosed based upon the biomicroscopic findings of cells, flare, and keratic precipitates. A dilated fundus examination must be performed to rule out a posterior uveitis or any retinal involvement. Chronic uveitis may lead to posterior synechiae, cataract, cystoid macular edema, and secondary glaucoma. The systemic history must be carefully reviewed. The presence of keratitis and episcleritis, both rare in RS, must be investigated to rule out other possible causes.

TABLE 24–6. OCULAR MANIFESTATIONS OF REITER SYNDROME

Common
- Conjunctivitis
- Anterior uveitis
- Posterior synechiae
- Secondary glaucoma
- Cystoid macular edema
- Cataract

Uncommon
- Corneal ulcer
- Episcleritis
- Scleritis
- Keratitis
- Subepithelial infiltrates
- Hypopyon
- Multifocal choroiditis

TREATMENT

Systemic

There is no curative treatment for RS. However, there are many forms of palliative therapy (Table 24–7). Hans Reiter treated his RS patients with arsenicals without apparent benefit. Short-term antibiotic therapy with sulphonamides and penicillin was also ineffective in early RS patients.

When urethritis is present, tetracycline for 2 weeks may be prescribed. Lymecycline, a form of tetracycline,

TABLE 24–7. SYSTEMIC TREATMENT OF REITER SYNDROME

Arthralgia
- NSAID (eg, naproxen 500 mg bid)
- Corticosteroid (eg, prednisone 20 mg bid)
- Physical therapy
- Mesalamine (eg, 250 mg qd to qid)
- Olsalazine, sulfasalazine (eg, 500 mg qid)
- Tetracycline (eg, 250–500 mg qid for 3–4 weeks), doxycycline, minocycline, and lymecycline
- Erythromycin (eg, 250 mg qid)
- Cytotoxic and immunosuppressive agents (eg, cyclosporin 4 mg/kg qd)

Dermatologic
- Topical calcipotriene (eg, 15 gm bid for hyperkeratosis)
- Corticosteroids (eg, 40 mg qd)
- Phototherapy and PUVA
- Methotrexate (eg, 7.5 mg per week) and etretinate (eg, 50 mg qd)

Reiter Syndrome with HIV Disease
- All of the above in conjunction with infectious disease (ID) specialist
- Zidovudine (eg, 250 mg qid for AIDS also with ID specialist)

has been utilized to treat both postchlamydial RS and postdysenteric RS for 3 months with dimunition of the arthritis. Toussirot and co-workers (1997) found that it significantly reduced the arthritis in postchlamydial RS while having no effect on postdysenteric RS. The incidence of RS after a new episode of sexually transmitted diseases was significantly lower in patients given erythromycin or tetracycline as compared to patients who were prescribed penicillin or placebo. In another study, bromocriptine mesylate brought on an acute remission in four male RS patients (Bravo et al, 1992).

Oral nonsteroidal anti-inflammatory drugs (NSAIDs) are the mainstay of treatment for the arthralgia in RS. Indomethacin, once the NSAID of choice, has been supplanted by other NSAIDs such as etodolac, ketoprofen, and tolmetin. Patients with reactive arthritis who are not treated successfully with NSAIDs can be given sulfasalazine 2000 mg/day. Clegg and colleagues (1996) found this treatment to be well tolerated and effective in alleviating symptoms. Solomon and associates (1991) reported a 33% beneficial response rate with sulfasalazine in patients with severe RS. They also reported cyclosporine to be effective for RS.

Controversy surrounds the use of immunosuppressive agents, especially in HIV patients. Etretinate is also reported to be effective for the treatment of the joint manifestations in HIV-associated RS (Weitzul & Duvic, 1997). Sulfasalazine possibly shows improvement of CD4 counts in RS patients with HIV (Disla et al, 1994). Zwillich and co-workers (1994) reported positive results after treatment with mesalamine and olsalazine.

Keratoderma blennorrhagicum has been treated successfully in some RS patients with chlortetracycline or streptomycin. Oral doxycycline and topical calcipotriene may also be prescribed for the dermatologic lesions resembling psoriasis (Thiers, 1997).

Dactylitis associated with spondyloarthropathies may be treated with immunosuppressive agents (eg, gold, methotrexate, and sulfasalazine) (Rothschild et al, 1998). A spondylitis functional index (SFI) can be used to monitor RS. SFI is a self-reported measure of patient performance when receiving treatment for a spondyloarthropathy (Moncur et al, 1996). Physical therapy in the form of an extension exercise program is also beneficial in the treatment of axial skeleton manifestations.

TABLE 24–8. OCULAR TREATMENT OF REITER SYNDROME

Conjunctivitis
- Vasoconstrictors (eg, naphazoline qid)
- Ocular lubricants (eg, carboxymethylcellulose qid)

Uveitis
- Topical steroids (eg, prednisolone acetate 1% q1h–qid)
- Topical cycloplegics (eg, homatropine 2–5% tid)
- Sub-Tenon steroid injections (eg, triamcinolone 40 mg q3 weeks)
- Systemic corticosteroids (eg, prednisone 60–100 mg PO qd)
- Systemic immunosuppressants (eg, methotrexate, azathioprine, cyclosporin)

Secondary Glaucoma
- Topical IOP-lowering agents (eg, timolol qd or bid, brimonidine bid)
- Iridectomy/iridotomy

Keratitis and/or Corneal Ulcer
- Topical antibiotics (eg, ciprofloxacin q1/2h-qid, tobramycin q2h-qid, bacitracin ointment qhs)

Cystoid Macular Edema
- Systemic NSAID (eg, indomethacin 25 mg po tid)
- Topical NSAID (eg, ketorolac qid)

Ocular

The treatment of the ocular manifestations of RS is summarized in Table 24–8. The conjunctivitis of RS can be unilateral or bilateral, mucopurulent or nonpurulent. It is always self-limiting in 2 weeks or less, is noninfectious, and precedes the onset of arthritis. Supportive therapy with vasoconstrictors and ocular lubricants are sufficient for this condition. Antibiotic use is not necessary because of the lack of an infectious microorganism. Anterior uveitis in RS is usually acute, unilateral, and nongranulomatous. This can be contrasted to uveitis from inflammatory bowel disease (ulcerative colitis and Crohn disease), in which it is usually bilateral, posterior, and chronic (Lyons & Rosenbaum, 1997). Anterior uveitis in RS is treated aggressively with topical corticosteroids and cycloplegics. For more recalcitrant cases, sub-Tenon steroid injections and/or systemic use of corticosteroids or immunosuppressants may be necessary. Special care must be taken not to withdraw the topical steroids too early because this can cause the condition to recur. Treatment should be continued for several weeks after the uveitis has resolved. Recurrent bouts of uveitis may necessitate a low-dose maintenance regimen of a topical corticosteroid. The use of an oral NSAID may be helpful in controlling the ocular inflammation severity and recurrence. Topical or systemic corticosteroid usage may lead to steroid response glaucoma, and these patients should be treated with intraocular pressure (IOP)–lowering medications and discontinuation or modulation of steroid usage. Secondary glaucoma from posterior synechiae or impaired trabecular outflow also may need to be controlled with peripheral iridectomy or iridotomy and IOP-lowering medications. Cataract formation from chronic uveitis can be managed by cataract extraction. Cystoid macular edema can be difficult to manage, but topical NSAID usage can ameliorate the condition. Keratitis and episcleritis may occur with or without conjunctivitis. Topical antibiotic usage may be indicated for prophylaxis as well as for the treatment of corneal ulcers; however, this is a rare occurrence.

CONCLUSION

RS is a multisystem disease that can follow a relatively benign or chronic debilitating course. The potential for vision loss from chronic recalcitrant uveitis can be devastating. As such, one must be aggressive when treating this condition. In recent decades, a considerable amount of work has been done to link the presence of HLA-B27 and enteric or genitourinary infection to the course of RS. The treatment for RS has been changing throughout the years and newer medicines seem promising. Through genetic science, the future may even hold a curative therapy. Treatment of the RS patient includes physical therapy and potentially harmful medicines. Therefore, appropriate management must consist of a multidisciplinary approach in which the eyecare practitioner can serve a pivotal role in treating ocular complications and communicating with other healthcare providers. Proper diagnosis and management will allow improvement in the RS patient's quality of life.

REFERENCES

Ahvonen P, Sievers K, Aho K. Arthritis associated with *Yersinia enterocolitica* infection. *Acta Rheumatol Scand.* 1969;15:232–253.

Altman EM, Centeno LV, Mahal M. AIDS-associated Reiter's syndrome. *Ann Allergy.* 1994;72:307–316.

Azouz EM, Duffy CM. Juvenile spondyloarthropathies: Clinical manifestations and medical imaging. *Skeletal Radiol.* 1995;24:399–408.

Baggia S, Lyons JL, Angell E, et al. A novel model of bacterially-induced acute anterior uveitis in rats and the lack of effect from HLA-B27 expression. *J Invest Med.* 1997; 45:295–301.

Banares A, Jover JA, Fernandez-Gutierrez B, et al. Patterns of uveitis as a guide in making rheumatologic and immunologic diagnoses. *Arthritis Rheum.* 1997;40:358–370.

Barozzi L, Olivieri I, De Matteis M, et al. Seronegative spondylarthropathies: Imaging of spondylitis, enthesitis and dactylitis. *Eur J Radiol.* 1998;27:S12–17.

Barron KS, Reveille JD, Carrington M, et al. Susceptibility to Reiter's syndrome is associated with alleles of TAP genes. *Arthritis Rheum.* 1995;38:684–689.

Barth WF. Office evaluation of the patient with musculoskeletal complaints. *Am J Med.* 1997;102:3S–10S.

Bauman C, Cron RQ, Sherry DD. Reiter syndrome initially misdiagnosed as Kawasaki disease. *J Pediatr.* 1996;128:366–369.

Beutler AM, Schumacher HR Jr, Whittum-Hudson JA, et al. Case report: In situ hybridization for detection of inapparent infection with *Chlamydia trachomatis* in synovial tissue of a patient with Reiter's syndrome. *Am J Med Sci.* 1995;310:206–213.

Beutler AM, Whittum-Hudson JA, Nanagara R, et al. Intracellular location of inapparently infecting *Chlamydia* in synovial tissue from patients with Reiter's syndrome. *Immunol Res.* 1994;13:163–171.

Boehni U, Christen B, Greminger P, et al. Systemic vasculitis associated with seronegative spondyloarthropathy (Reiter's syndrome). *Clin Rheumatol.* 1997;16:610–613.

Branigan PJ, Gerard HC, Hudson AP, et al. Comparison of synovial tissue and synovial fluid as the source of nucleic acids for detection of *Chlamydia trachomatis* by polymerase chain reaction. *Arthritis Rheum.* 1996;39: 1740–1746.

Braun J, Bollow M, Remlinger G, et al. Prevalence of spondylarthropathies in HLA-B27 positive and negative blood donors. *Arthritis Rheum.* 1998;41:58–67.

Braverman PK, Srasburger VC. Sexually transmitted diseases. *Clin Pediatr.* 1994;33:26–37.

Bravo G, Zazueta B, Lavalle C. An acute remission of Reiter's syndrome in male patients treated with bromocriptine. *J Rheumatol.* 1992;19:747–750.

Bryant GA. Reiter's syndrome. *Orthop Nurs.* 1998;17:57–62.

Burgos-Vargas R, Pacheco-Tena C, Vazquez-Mellado J. Juvenile-onset spondyloarthropathies. *Rheum Dis Clin North Am.* 1997;23:569–598.

Careless DJ, Inman RD. Acute anterior uveitis: Clinical and experimental aspects. *Semin Arthritis Rheum.* 1995;24: 432–441.

Clegg DO, Reda DJ, Weisman MH, et al. Comparison of sulfasalazine and placebo in the treatment of reactive arthritis (Reiter's syndrome). *Arthritis Rheum.* 1996;39: 2021–2027.

Cron RQ, Sherry DD. Reiter's syndrome associated with cryptosporidial gastroenteritis. *J Rheumatol.* 1995;22: 1962–1963.

Cuellar ML. HIV infection-associated inflammatory musculoskeletal disorder. *Rheum Dis Clin North Am.* 1998;24: 403–421.

D'Alessandro LP, Forster DJ, Rao NA. Anterior uveitis and hypopyon. *Am J Ophthalmol.* 1991;112:317–321.

Disla E, Rhim HR, Reddy A, et al. Improvement in CD4 lymphocyte count in HIV-Reiter's syndrome after treatment with sulfasalazine. *J Rheumatol.* 1994;21:662–664.

El-Khoury GY, Kathol MH, Brandser EA. Seronegative spondyloarthropathies. *Radiol Clin North Am.* 1996;34: 343–357.

Erdesz S, Shubin SV, Shoch BP, et al. Spondyloarthropathies in circumpolar populations of Chukotka (Eskimos and Chukchi): Epidemiology and clinical characteristics. *J Rheumatol.* 1995;21:1101–1104.

Fischel JD, Lipton J. Acute anterior uveitis in juvenile Reiter's syndrome. *Clin Rheumatol.* 1996;15:83–85.

Geppert MJ, Mizel MS. Management of heel pain in the inflammatory arthritides. *Clin Orthop.* 1998;349:93–99.

Gerard HC, Branigan PJ, Schumacher HR, et al. Synovial *Chlamydia trachomatis* in patients with reactive arthritis/Reiter's syndrome are viable but show aberrant gene expression. *J Rheumatol.* 1998;25:734–742.

Gusis SE, Riopedre AM, Penise O, et al. Protrusio acetabuli in seronegative spondyloarthropathy. *Semin Arthritis Rheum.* 1993;23:155–160.

Hansen CP, Mortenson S. Epididymo-orchitis and Reiter's disease. Two infrequent complications after intravesical bacillus Calmette-Guérin therapy. *Scand J Urol Nephrol.* 1997;31:317–318.

Hoogland YT, Alexander EP, Patterson RH, et al. Coronary artery stenosis in Reiter's syndrome: A complication of aortitis. *J Rheumatol.* 1994;21:757–759.

Horowitz S, Horowitz J, Taylor-Robinson D, et al. *Ureaplasma urealyticum* in Reiter's syndrome. *J Rheumatol.* 1994;21: 877–882.

Hughes RA, Keat AC. Reiter's syndrome and reactive arthritis: A current view. *Semin Arthritis Rheum.* 1994;24:190–210.

Jara LJ, Silveira LH, Cuellar ML, et al. Hyperprolactinemia in Reiter's syndrome. *J Rheumatol.* 1994;21:1292–1297.

Jevtic V, Watt I, Rozman B, et al. Distinctive radiological features of small hand joints in rheumatoid arthritis and seronegative spondyloarthritis demonstrated by contrast-enhanced (Gd-DTPA) magnetic resonance imaging. *Skeletal Radiol.* 1995;24:351–355.

Kellner H, Fuessi HS, Herzer P. Seronegative spondyloarthropathies in HIV-infected patients: Further evidence of uncommon clinical features. *Rheumatol Int.* 1994;13: 211–213.

Kellner H, Wen J, Wang J, et al. Serum antibodies from patients with ankylosing spondylitis and Reiter's syndrome are reactive with HLA-B27 cells transfected with the *Mycobacterium tuberculosis* hsp60 gene. *Infect Immun.* 1994;62:484–491.

Kettering JM, Towers JD, Rubin DA. The seronegative spondyloarthropathies. *Semin Roentgenol.* 1996;31:220–228.

Kirchner JT. Reiter's syndrome. A possibility in patients with reactive arthritis. *Postgrad Med.* 1995;97:111–112,115–117, 121–122.

Kirveskari J, Kellner H, Wuorela M, et al. False-negative serological HLA-B27 typing results may be due to altered antigenic epitopes and can be detected by polymerase chain reaction. *Br J Rheumatol.* 1997;36:185–189.

Krylov M, Erdesz S, Alexeeva L, et al. HLA class II and HLA-B27 oligotyping in two Siberian native population groups. *Tissue Antigens.* 1995;46:382–386.

Krylov MY, Reveille JD, Alexeeva LI, et al. HLA-B27 subtypes among the Chukotka native groups. *Arch Immunol Ther Exp (Warsz).* 1995;43:135–138.

Kuipers JG, Raybourne RB, Williams KM, et al. Specificities of human TAP alleles for HLA-B27 binding peptides. *Arthritis Rheum.* 1996;39:1892–1895.

Lauhio A, Leirisako-Repo M, Landevirta J, et al. Double-blind placebo-controlled study of three month treatment with lymecycline in reactive arthritis with special reference to chlamydial arthritis. *Arthritis Rheum.* 1991;34:6–14.

Lavery JP, Lisse JR. Preliminary study of the tryptase levels in the synovial fluid of patients with inflammatory arthritis. *Ann Allergy.* 1994;72:425–427.

Liebling MR, Arkfeld DG, Michelini GA, et al. Identification of *Neisseria gonorrhoeae* in synovial fluid using the polymerase chain reaction. *Arthritis Rheum.* 1994;37:702–709.

Lin WY, Wang SJ, Lang JL, et al. Bone scintigraphy in evaluation of heel pain in Reiter's disease: Compared with radiography and clinical examination. *Scand J Rheumatol.* 1995;24:18–21.

Livneh A, Zaks N, Katz J, et al. Increased prevalence of joint manifestations in patients with recurrent aphthous stomatitis. *Clin Exp Rheumatol.* 1996;14:407–412.

Lyons JL, Rosenbaum JT. Uveitis associated with inflammatory bowel disease compared with uveitis associated with spondyloarthropathy. *Arch Ophthalmol.* 1997;115:61–64.

Magro CM, Crowson AN, Peeling R. Vasculitis as the basis of cutaneous lesions in Reiter's disease. *Hum Pathol.* 1995;26:633–638.

Martin DH, Mroczkowski TF. Dermatologic manifestations of sexually transmitted diseases other than HIV. *Infect Dis Clin North Am.* 1994;8:533–582.

Miller-Blair DJ, Tsuchiya N, Yamaguchi A. Immunologic mechanisms in common rheumatologic diseases. *Clin Orthop.* 1996;326:43–54.

Moncur C, Cannon G, Shaw M, et al. Inter-observer reliability of the spondylitis functional index instrument for assessing spondyloarthropathies. *Arthritis Care Res.* 1996; 9:182–188.

Nanagara R, Li F, Beutler A, et al. Alteration of *Chlamydia trachomatis* biologic behavior in synovial membranes. Suppression of surface antigen production in reactive arthritis and Reiter's syndrome. *Arthritis Rheum.* 1995;38: 1410–1417.

Olivieri I, Barozzi L, Padula A, et al. Clinical manifestations of seronegative spondyloarthropathies. *Eur J Radiol.* 1998; 27:S3–S6.

Pancaldi P, Van Linthoudt D, Alborino D, et al. Reiter's syndrome after intravesical bacillus Calmette-Guérin treatment for bladder carcinoma. *Br J Rheumatol.* 1993;32: 1096–1098.

Peterson MC. Clinical aspects of *Campylobacter jejuni* infections in adults. *West J Med.* 1994;161:148–152.

Peterson MC. Rheumatic manifestations of *Campylobacter jejuni* and *C. fetus* infections in adults. *Scand J Rheumatol.* 1994;23:167–170.

Reveille JD. HLA-B27 and the seronegative spondyloarthropathies. *Am J Med Sci.* 1998;316:239–249.

Rodriguez J, Diaz F, Collazos J. Thrombophlebitis and Reiter's syndrome. *Postgrad Med.* 1994;70:145–146.

Romani J, Puig L, Baselga E, et al. Reiter's syndrome-like pattern in AIDS-associated psoriasiform dermatitis. *Int J Dermatol.* 1996;35:484–488.

Rothschild B. Reactive arthritis and Reiter's syndrome. *Compr Ther.* 1994;20:441–444.

Rothschild BM, Pingitore C, Eaton M. Dactylitis: Implications for clinical practice. *Semin Arthritis Rheum.* 1998;28:41–47.

Samuel MP, Zwillich SH, Thomson GT, et al. Fast food arthritis—A clinico-pathologic study of post-*Salmonella* reactive arthritis. *J Rheumatol.* 1995;22:1947–1952.

Saporta L, Gumus E, Karadag H, et al. Reiter syndrome following intracavitary BCG administration. *Scand J Urol Nephrol.* 1997;31:211–212.

Sartoris DJ. Radiography of articular disorders in the foot. *J Foot Ankle Surg.* 1994;33:518–525.

Secundini R, Scheines EJ, Gusis SE, et al. Clinicoradiological correlation of enthesitis in seronegative spondyloarthropathies (SNSA). *Clin Rheumatol.* 1997;16:129–132.

Segal AH. Anatomic predilection of the spondyloarthropathies—A case of the nerves? *J Rheumatol.* 1996;23:491–494.

Solomon G, Brancato L, Winchester R. An approach to the HIV positive patient with a spondyloarthropathic disease. *Rheum Dis Clin North Am.* 1991;17:43–59.

Taylor-Robinson D, Gilroy CB, Horowitz S, et al. *Mycoplasma genitalium* in the joints of two patients with arthritis. *Eur J Clin Microbiol Infect Dis.* 1994;13:1066–1069.

Thiers BH. The use of topical calcipotriene/calcipotriol in conditions other than plaque-type psoriasis. *J Am Acad Dermatol.* 1997;37:S69–S71.

Thomas DG, Roberton DM. Reiter's syndrome in an adolescent girl. *Acta Paediatr.* 1994;83:339–340.

Thomson GT, McKibbon C, Inman RD. Mesalamine therapy in Reiter's syndrome. *J Rheumatol.* 1994;21:570–572.

Toussirot E, Despaux J, Wendling D. Do minocycline and other tetracyclines have a place in rheumatology? *Rev Rhum Engl Ed.* 1997;64:474–480.

Warren KJ, Kazi S, Nassar NN. Gout in a patient with Reiter's syndrome. *Cutis.* 1998;61:85–86.

Weitzul S, Duvic M. HIV-related psoriasis and Reiter's syndrome. *Semin Cutan Med Surg.* 1997;16:213–218.

Winchester R, Brancato L, Itescu S, et al. Implications from the occurrence of Reiter's syndrome and related disorders associated with advanced HIV infection. *Scand J Rheumatol suppl.* 1988;74:89–93.

Yamaguchi A, Ogawa A, Tsuchiya N, et al. HLA-B27 subtypes in Japanese with seronegative spondyloarthropathies and healthy controls. *J Rheumatol.* 1996;23:1189–1193.

Zwillich SH, Ritchlin CT. Olsalazine in Reiter's syndrome. *J Rheumatol.* 1994;21:2169–2170.

Chapter 25

SYSTEMIC LUPUS ERYTHEMATOSUS

Nancy N. Wong

Systemic lupus erythematosus (SLE) is a chronic multisystem disease process of unknown etiology. The pathophysiology is characterized by autoantibody production resulting in immune complex deposition and tissue damage. Lupus manifestations involving the renal, cardiac, and nervous systems may result in morbidity. Additionally, ocular manifestations commonly encountered include keratoconjunctivitis sicca and lupus retinopathy. Moreover, ocular complications may represent a marker of systemic disease activity. Hence, early recognition of ocular findings associated with systemic lupus prompts both ocular and systemic treatment.

EPIDEMIOLOGY

Systemic

The estimated prevalence of SLE in the United States ranges from 15 to 50 per 100,000 population (Hahn, 1998). The incidence of SLE in the United States is estimated to be 25.5 per million among white females. However, incidence levels increase two to three times among African-American and Hispanic females. Elevated incidence levels are also observed among persons of Polynesian and Native American descent (Von Feldt, 1995). In addition to the racial predilection, SLE also demonstrates gender differences. Females represent 90% of SLE cases (Hahn, 1998). Onset typically occurs between the first and fourth decades of life (Von Feldt, 1995). The disease course demonstrates periods of increased activity punctuated with intervals of relative quiescence.

Systemic lupus erythematosus may represent a continuum of disease processes with varying levels of manifestations and severity. Discoid lupus erythematosus is a chronic dermatological condition characterized by localized circumscribed cutaneous lesions. Such lesions resemble those observed in SLE patients. However, discoid lupus patients fail to demonstrate antinuclear antibodies (ANA) commonly observed in SLE patients (Nguyen & Foster, 1998). Similarly, antinuclear antibodies are also observed in drug-induced lupus. Medications such as procainamide, hydralazine hydrochloride, phenytoin, isoniazid, chlorpromazine hydrochloride, methyldopa, and quinidine have been associated with the development of drug-induced lupus (Rich, 1996).

Ocular

Approximately 30% of SLE patients demonstrate ocular manifestations. Keratoconjunctivitis sicca (KCS) is the most common ophthalmic manifestation occurring in approximately 25% of SLE patients. Retinal vasculitis is observed in approximately 5% of SLE patients (Reddy and Foster, 1994).

Systemic lupus erythematosus is an immune-mediated disease with multisystemic manifestations.

PATHOPHYSIOLOGY/DISEASE PROCESS

The etiology of SLE remains elusive. The disease is the result of autoantibody production and abnormal immunoregulation (Davies, 1996). The immune system fails to recognize "self" antigens and mounts an immune response against the antigens. The resultant autoantibody production has been observed against multiple antigens. Ninety-five percent of SLE patients demonstrate autoantibodies to nuclear antigens or antinuclear antibodies. Other prominent antigens to which autoantibodies are produced include native double-stranded DNA (anti-dsDNA), proteins complexed to RNA (anti-Sm and anti-Ro), phosphoprotein (anti-La), and phospholipids (anticardiolipin and lupus anticoagulant) (Reddy & Foster, 1994). Table 25–1 lists autoantibodies observed in systemic lupus erythematosus. Antigen–autoantibody recognition results in the formation of immune complexes in the circulation. Complex formation activates the complement system. Chemotactic factors and leukocytes infiltrate the complex site, resulting in inflammation. Progressive inflammation results in tissue damage.

Diagnosis is dependent on satisfaction of 4 out of 11 criteria determined by the American Rheumatological Association.

Systemic

Symptoms associated with SLE patients include myalgia, arthralgia, fatigue, fever, headaches, and weight loss. The disease is chronic with periods of remission and exacerbation.

Systemic lupus erythematosus demonstrates multisystemic findings (Table 25–2). Musculoskeletal manifestations, which include arthralgia, arthritis, and myalgia, are observed in 95% of SLE patients. Arthral-

TABLE 25–1. AUTOANTIBODIES IN SYSTEMIC LUPUS ERYTHEMATOSUS

Specificity (Antigen)	Clinical Importance/Comments
Nuclear	Multiple antigens detected; sensitive when HEp-2 or WIL-2 cells used; quite nonspecific
Native (double-stranded) DNA	Highly specific for SLE; seen in about 70% of lupus patients; associated with nephritis and disease activity
Denatured (single-stranded) DNA	High titers in SLE; lower titers in other diseases
Sm (protein complexed to small RNA)	Highly specific for SLE; seen in 50% of SLE patients
Histones	More common in drug-induced SLE (95%)
Nuclear ribonucleoprotein (RNP)	Seen in SLE and other diseases; highest titers in MCTD
Ro (SSa; RNA polymerase)	Seen in primary Sjögren syndrome and SLE
La (SSb; protein complexed to small RNA)	Seen in primary Sjögren syndrome and SLE
Nucleolar	Seen in scleroderma, primary Sjögren syndrome, and SLE
Phospholipid	
Cardiolipin	Seen in SLE and other diseases; gives false-positive VDRL
Clotting factors	Called lupus anticoagulants; cause prolonged PTT; associated with venous and arterial thrombosis
Endothelial surface antigens	May contribute to thrombosis
Platelet surface antigens	Associated with thrombocytopenia and abnormally small platelets
Erythrocyte surface antigens	Occasionally associated with hemolysis
Lymphocyte surface antigens	May be associated with leukopenia and abnormal T-cell function
Neuronal antigens	High titers are correlated with diffuse CNS lupus

CNS, central nervous system; DNA, deoxyribonucleic acid; MCTD, mixed connective tissue disease; PTT, partial thromboplastin time; RNA, ribonucleic acid; SLE, systemic lupus erythematosus; VDRL, Venereal Disease Research Laboratory.

Reprinted with permission from: Reddy CV, Foster CF. Systemic lupus erythematosus. In: Albert DM, Jakobiec FA, eds. Principles and Practice of Ophthalmology. *Philadelphia: W.B. Saunders; 1994:286.*

gia and arthritis are characterized by joint stiffness, especially in the morning. Many patients develop joint deformities. Jaccoud arthropathy, a nonerosive deformity of the hand, is observed in 10% of lupus patients (Figure 25–1). The skeletal involvement of SLE often resembles that observed in rheumatoid arthritis. Hence, many SLE patients may be misdiagnosed with rheumatoid arthritis (Boumpas et al, 1995b). A severe skeletal complication in lupus patients is osteonecrosis in which avascular necrosis of the bone occurs. Chronic corticosteroidal therapy may be a risk factor for osteonecrosis development (Petri, 1998).

Hematological manifestations are encountered in 85% of SLE patients. The most common hematological condition encountered is chronic anemia. The anemia

TABLE 25–2. SYSTEMIC MANIFESTATIONS OF SYSTEMIC LUPUS ERYTHEMATOSUS

- Systemic symptoms (95%)
  - Myalgia
  - Fatigue
  - Fever
  - Headache
  - Weight loss
  - Rash
- Musculoskeletal (95%)
  - Arthralgia
  - Arthritis
  - Myalgia
  - Myopathy
  - Joint deformities
- Hematological (85%)
  - Anemia
  - Leukopenia
  - Thrombocytopenia
  - Lymphopenia
- Dermatological/mucocutaneous (80%)
  - Malar rash
  - Discoid rash
  - Alopecia
  - Raynaud phenomena
- Renal (50%)
  - Proteinuria
  - Nephropathy
- Cardiac (50%)
  - Pericarditis
  - Myocarditis
  - Valvulopathy
  - Accelerated atherosclerosis
- Pulmonary (50%)
  - Pleurisy
  - Pleural effusions
  - Lupus pneumonitis
  - Pulmonary hypertension
- Neurological (50%)
  - CNS vasculitis
  - Cranial and peripheral neuropathies
  - Functional dysfunction
  - Organic brain syndromes

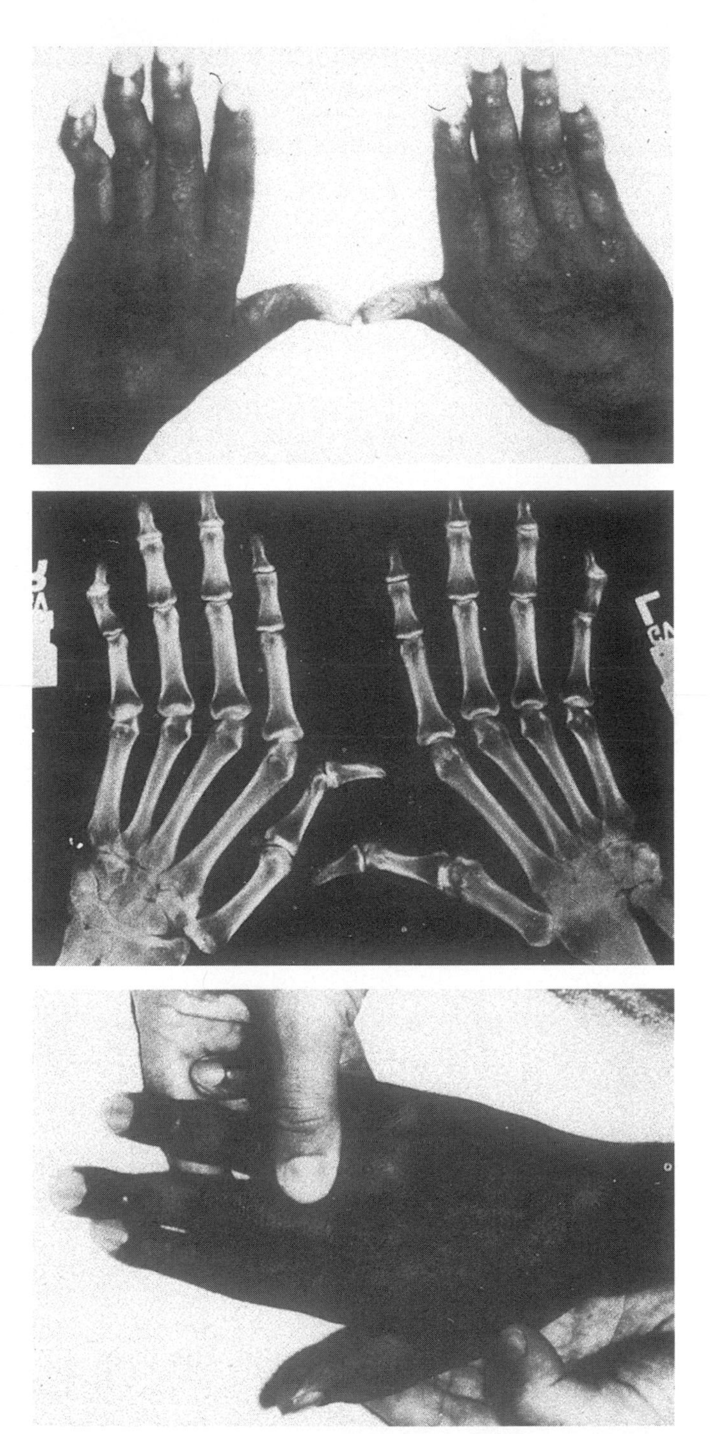

Figure 25–1. Jaccoud arthropathy. (*Reprinted with permission from: Boumpas DT, Fessler BJ, Austin HA, et al. Systemic lupus erythematosus: Emerging concepts (Part 2: Dermatologic and joint disease, the antiphospholipid antibody syndrome, pregnancy and hormonal therapy, morbidity and mortality, and pathogenesis*). Ann Int Med. *1995;123:42–53.*)

may be an iatrogenic effect from chronic medications employed in the treatment of the disease process. Chronic nonsteroidal anti-inflammatory and immunosuppressive medical therapy have been associated with anemia. Leukopenia (depressed white blood cell count) may result from the production of antineutrophil autoantibodies. Thrombocytopenia (reduced platelet levels) has been associated with antiplatelet autoantibodies. Antiplatelet autoantibodies bind to platelet surface glycoproteins. The platelets are subsequently ingested by macrophages.

Dermatological and mucocutaneous lesions are encountered in approximately 80% of SLE cases. The classical malar rash is exhibited in approximately 50% of lupus patients (Figure 25–2). The erythematosus lesion extends from both cheeks and crosses the nose in a butterfly pattern. Many SLE patients demonstrate photosensitivity to ultraviolet light. Exposure to solar radiation may precipitate dermatological rashes and aggravate systemic disease activity (Boumpas et al, 1995b). The lesions often present following exposure to sunlight and resolve within several days to weeks (Hay & Smith, 1995). Twenty-five percent of SLE patients demonstrate discoid cutaneous manifestations characterized by discrete round erythematosus lesions. Discoid lesions localized to the scalp often result in alopecia (Schur, 1996).

Renal manifestations have been reported in approximately 50% of systemic lupus cases. Lupus nephropathy is initiated by the production of autoantibodies, especially autoantibodies to DNA. Antigen–autoantibody complexes deposit in the subendothelial region of the glomerular capillary wall. Complement activation results in capillary wall injury necrosis and fibrosis (Boumpas et al, 1995a).

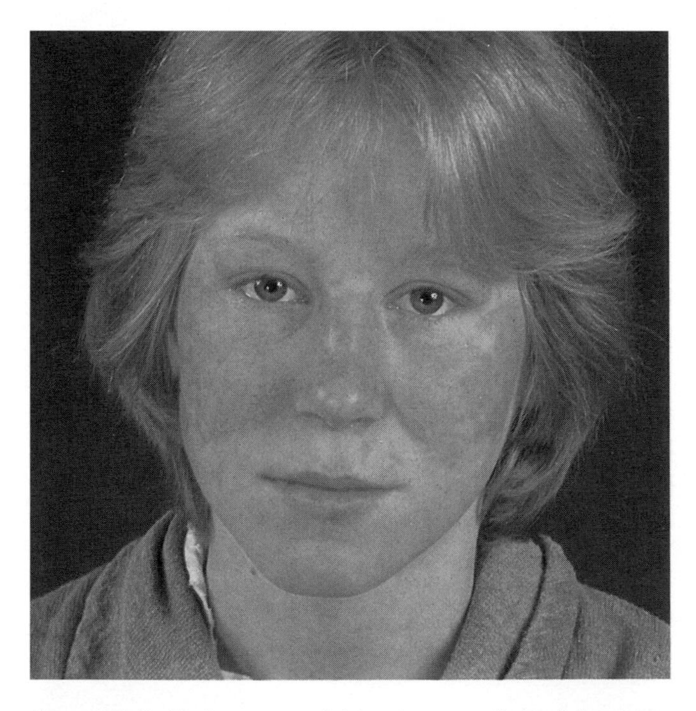

Figure 25–2. Erythematous, slightly edematous, "butterfly" rash typical of SLE. (*Photo courtesy of Machiel Polano, MD, Clinic of Dermatology, University Hospital, Leiden, Netherlands*).

Cardiac manifestations occur in about 50% of SLE patients. Noninfectious cardiac valvular disease has received increased attention in SLE with the development of advanced imaging procedures such as transthoracic and transesophageal echocardiography. Echocardiographic studies have suggested valve disease in 18 to 40% of SLE patients. The disease is characterized by verrucae vegetations composed of fibrin, fibrous tissue, hematoxylin bodies, and minimal inflammatory cells adherent to the cardiac valves, in particular the mitral valve. Such noninfectious valve abnormalities in SLE patients have been termed Libman—Sacks endocarditis (Joffe et al, 1996). Progressive valvulopathy may result in altered cardiac hemodynamics, valve stenosis, or blood regurgitation. The production of autoantibodies to phospholipids (anticardiolipin and lupus anticoagulant) also have been associated with valvular disease (Joffe et al, 1996). Accelerated atherosclerosis often is observed in lupus patients. The pathogenesis may be secondary to elevated serum cholesterol levels following chronic corticosteroid administration. Circulating immune complexes may promote intracellular accumulation of the serum cholesterol. Additional cardiac manifestations include pericardial effusion and myocarditis.

Pulmonary complications are observed in about 50% of the SLE population. Pulmonary involvement may be subdivided into acute and chronic disease processes. Acute conditions include rare complications such as alveolar hemorrhage and lupus pneumonitis. Chronic manifestations include interstitial lung disease and pulmonary hypertension. Pulmonary hypertension has been associated with elevated levels of antiribonucleoprotein antibodies (Schur, 1996).

Neurological manifestations (50%) present with symptoms of headache, anxiety, depression, and mood swings. Lupus vasculitis and vasculopathy may result in cranial and peripheral neuropathies. Thrombosis may result in strokes (Schur, 1996). Additional neurological manifestations include seizures, Bell palsy, organic brain syndrome, and psychosis (Jabs et al, 1986).

Ocular

The most common ocular manifestation (Table 25–3) of SLE is keratoconjunctivitis sicca with or without xerostomia. KCS is observed in approximately 25% of SLE patients. Additional ocular manifestations include

TABLE 25–3. OCULAR MANIFESTATIONS OF SYSTEMIC LUPUS ERYTHEMATOSUS

- Anterior segment manifestations
  - Keratoconjunctivitis sicca
  - Superficial punctate keratitis
  - Conjunctivitis
  - Episcleritis
  - Scleritis
- Posterior segment manifestations
  - Lupus retinopathy
  - Proliferative retinopathy
  - Vaso-occlusive disease
  - Choroidopathy
- Neuro-ophthalmic manifestations
  - Anterior ischemic optic neuropathy
  - Posterior ischemic optic neuropathy
  - Pupillary abnormalities
  - Retrochiasmal disease
  - Internuclear ophthalmoplegia
- Iatrogenic manifestations
  - Bull's eye maculopathy
  - Keratopathy
  - Glaucoma
  - Cataracts

superficial punctate keratitis with or without recurrent corneal erosions, conjunctivitis, episcleritis, and diffuse and nodular scleritis. Peripheral corneal furrowing (Figure 25–3) has been reported in lupus patients. The peripheral cornea often is affected by systemic vasculitic conditions due to the presence of vascularized collagen tissue adjacent to the limbus. The presence of blood vessels and lymphatics adjacent to the peripheral cornea leaves the tissue susceptible to ocular involvement of systemic vasculitic and autoimmune disorders (Robin et al, 1986). In rare cases, interstitial keratitis and marginal corneal melts have been documented (Arffa, 1997). Other uncommon ocular manifestations include periorbital edema, necrotizing scleritis (Nguyen & Foster, 1998), uveitis (Gold et al, 1972), and extraocular myositis (Grimson & Simons, 1983).

Retinal lesions are the second most common ocular manifestation. Classical lupus retinopathy (Figure 25–4) is characterized by cotton-wool spots (CWS) in isolation or surrounded with hemorrhages. The CWS corresponds to avascular zones on fundus fluorescein angiography. Lupus retinopathy may result from immune complex infiltration of vasculature walls, vascular constriction, and hyaline thrombosis. Histopathological studies have failed to demonstrate the presence of inflammatory cells suggestive of a true vasculitis (Nguyen & Foster, 1998). Lupus retinopathy may parallel systemic disease activity (Klinkhoff et al, 1986). Rarely, lupus retinopathy progresses to a severe vasculitis characterized by diffuse arteriolar occlusion and

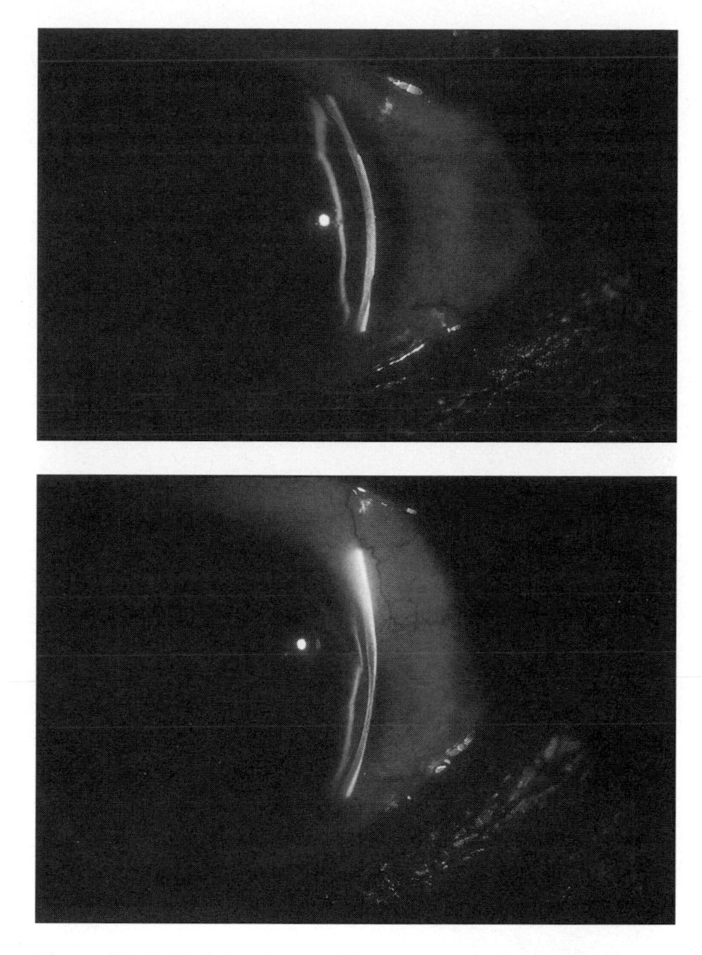

Figure 25–3. Peripheral corneal furrowing in SLE. (*Photo courtesy of Monica Everett, OD.*)

extensive capillary nonperfusion. Nonperfusion may result in neovascularization and proliferative retinopathy. Proliferative disease includes retinal and disc neovascularization.

Large-caliber vaso-occlusions such as central retinal artery occlusion (CRAO), branch retinal artery occlusion (BRAO), central retinal vein occlusion (CRVO), and branch retinal vein occlusion (BRVO) have been observed in SLE patients. An association has been demonstrated between large vessel occlusion and antiphospholipid antibodies, in particular, lupus anticoagulant (Hall et al, 1984). Autoantiphospholipids interact with negatively charged phospholipids located on vascular endothelial cell membranes and give rise to venous and/or arterial thrombosis (Levine et al, 1988). The vessel walls demonstrate fibrinoid degeneration and hyaline thrombosis (Reddy & Foster, 1994). Vasculature occlusion results in retinal nonperfusion and neovascularization.

A rare complication of SLE is choroidopathy. Immune complex infiltration of the choroidal vasculature

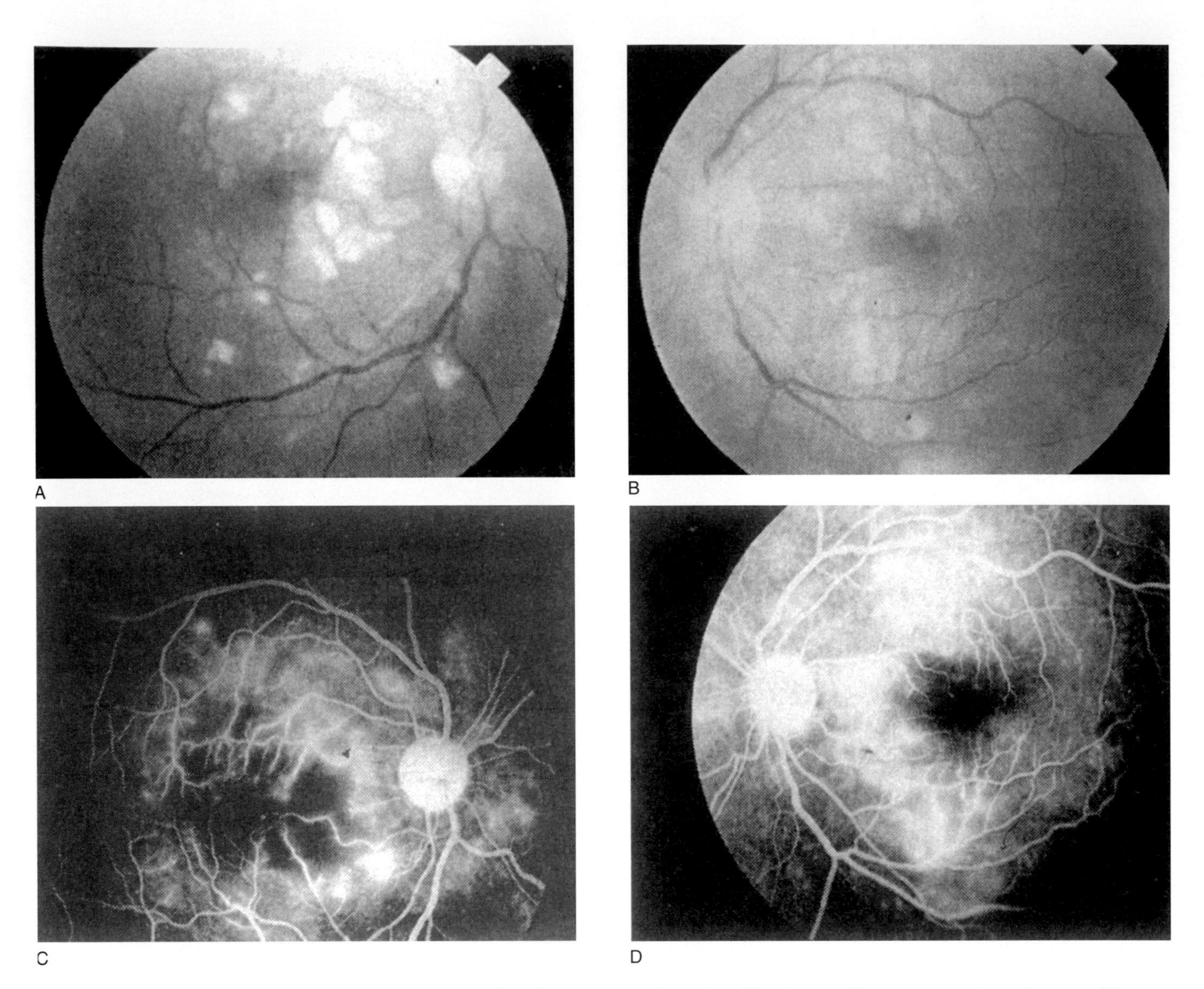

Figure 25–4. Lupus retinopathy with corresponding fluorescein angiography. (*Reprinted with permission from: Nguyen QD, Foster CS. Systemic lupus erythematosus and the eye.* Int Ophthalmol Clin. *1998;38:33–60.*)

has been observed in histological studies. Complement activation in response to the complex depositions results in vasculitis and inflammation (Graham et al., 1985). The choroidopathy damages the overlying retinal pigment epithelium (RPE). Subretinal transudation ensues causing serous RPE and/or neurosensory retinal detachments (Jabs et al, 1988).

Neuro-ophthalmological complications may manifest throughout the neural pathway. Optic nerve diseases include anterior and posterior ischemic neuropathies. The neuropathy may result from occlusion of small vessels supplying the neuronal tissue. Mild ischemia produces demyelination, whereas advanced disease gives rise to axonal damage (Jabs et al, 1986). Additional rare neuro-ophthalmological manifestations include cranial nerve palsies, transient ptosis, orbital pseudotumor (Mahoney, 1993), retrochiasmal defects, pupillary abnormalities, and internuclear ophthalmoplegia (Reddy & Foster, 1994).

DIAGNOSIS

Systemic

In 1982, the American Rheumatological Association established a revised criteria for the diagnosis of SLE (Table 25–4). The diagnosis of SLE is achieved when patients demonstrate 4 of the 11 criteria serially or

TABLE 25–4. THE 1982 REVISED CRITERIA FOR CLASSIFICATION OF SYSTEMIC LUPUS ERYTHEMATOSUS

Criterion	Definition
1. Malar rash	Fixed erythema, flat or raised, over the malar eminences, tending to spare the nasolabial folds
2. Discoid rash	Erythematous raised patches with adherent keratotic scaling and follicular plugging; atrophic scarring may occur in older lesions
3. Photosensitivity	Skin rash as a result of unusual reaction to sunlight by patient history or physician observation
4. Oral ulcers	Oral or nasopharyngeal ulceration, usually painless, observed by a physician
5. Arthritis	Nonerosive arthritis involving two or more peripheral joints, characterized by tenderness, swelling, or effusion
6. Serositis	(a) Pleuritis—convincing history of pleuritic pain or rub heard by a physician or evidence of pleural effusion OR (b) Pericarditis—documented by ECG or rub or evidence of pericardial effusion
7. Renal disorder	(a) Persistent proteinuria greater than 0.5 g/day or greater than 3+ if quantitation not performed OR (b) Cellular casts—may be red cell, hemoglobin, granular, tubular, or mixed
8. Neurologic disorder	(a) Seizures—in the absence of offending drugs or known metabolic derangements, eg, uremia, ketoacidosis, or electrolyte imbalance OR (b) Psychosis—in the absence of offending drugs or known metabolic derangements, eg, uremia, ketoacidosis, or electrolyte imbalance
9. Hematologic disorder	(a) Hemolytic anemia—with reticulocytosis OR (b) Leukopenia—less than 4000/mm^3 total on two or more occasions OR (c) Lymphopenia—less than 1500/mm^3 on two or more occasions OR (d) Thrombocytopenia—less than 100,000/mm^3 in the absence of offending drugs
10. Immunologic disorder	(a) Positive LE cell preparation OR (b) Anti-DNA (antibody to native DNA in abnormal titer) OR (c) Anti-Sm (presence of antibody to Sm nuclear antigen) OR (d) False-positive serologic test for syphilis known to be positive for at least 6 months and confirmed by *Treponema pallidum* immobilization or fluorescent treponemal antibody absorption test
11. Antinuclear antibody	An abnormal titer of antinuclear antibody by immunofluorescence or an equivalent assay at any point in time and in the absence of drugs known to be associated with "drug-induced lupus" syndrome

The classification is based on 11 criteria. For the purpose of identifying patients in clinical studies, a person shall be said to have systemic lupus erythematosus if any 4 or more of the 11 criteria are present, serially or simultaneously, during any interval of observation.

Reprinted with permission from: Tan EM, Cohen AS, Fries JF, et al. The 1982 revised criteria for the classification of systemic lupus erythematosus. Arthritis Rheum. *1982;25:1271–1277.*

simultaneously during any interval of observation (Tan et al, 1982).

Laboratory investigations (Table 25–5) play an important role in the diagnosis of SLE. Moreover, laboratory studies also may provide an index of systemic disease activity. More than 95% of SLE patients demonstrate positive antibody findings for components of the cell nucleus in the fluorescent antinuclear antibody test (FANA). Positive ANA findings are highly suggestive of lupus. However, ANA findings are not specific for SLE because antinuclear antibodies are also produced in multiple collagen vascular diseases (Table 25–6). FANA has replaced the use of the lupus erythematosus (LE) cell preparation test for assessing ANA. The

TABLE 25–5. DIAGNOSTIC TESTS IN SYSTEMIC LUPUS ERYTHEMATOSUS

Laboratory Test	Normal Values	SLE Values
Antinuclear antibody[a]	ANA titer <1:20	ANA titer ≥1:80[a]
Complete blood count (CBC) with differential	Negative Coombs test White blood cells 4400–11,300/mm³ Lymphocytes	Positive Coombs test (anemia) Leukopenia <4000/mm³ Lymphopenia <1500/mm³
Platelet count	150,000–450,000/mm³	Thrombocytopenia <100,000/mm³
Urinalysis	1–2 RBC/WBC per 400 × power field	Hematuria, pyuria, cylindruria, active urine sediment
Chemistry panel	Serum creatinine Protein excretion rate Proteinuria	>265μmol/L (>3 mg/dL) >150 mg/day >0.5 g/day
FTA-ABS	Nonreactive	False-positive[b]
VDRL	Nonreactive	False-positive[b]
RPR	Nonreactive	False-positive[b]
Westergren ESR	♂ = Age/2 ♀ = (Age + 10)/2	>25 mm/hour correlates with disease activity

[a]If ANA titer ≥ 1:80, assay for additional autoantibodies (eg, anti-DNA, anti-Ro, anti-La).
[b]Autoantibodies to phospholipids (anticardiolipin) may result in false-positive syphilis results.

LE cell preparation demonstrates low sensitivity and variable specificity (Pisetsky et al, 1997). Elevated levels of ANA, low complement levels, high levels of cryoglobulins, and increased levels of circulating immune complexes as measured by the Raji cell assay are suggestive of increased disease activity (Nguyen & Foster, 1998). During episodes of disease activity, the heightened presence of immune complexes results in activation of the complement system. Activation results in decreased serum complement levels that can be measured by assessing total hemolytic complement activity, C3 and C4 protein levels, or the presence of complement split products (Pisetsky et al, 1997).

Additional laboratory testing that should be obtained if a patient demonstrates positive FANA findings includes evaluation of sera antibodies to native double-stranded DNA (anti-dsDNA) and antibodies to the small nuclear ribonucleoprotein complex (anti-Sm). Autoantibodies to DNA represent an index marker of systemic disease activity. In particular, increased renal disease activity is associated with increased levels of anti-DNA. Other laboratory findings supportive of lupus renal dysfunction include proteinuria, elevated creatinine levels, and elevated blood urea nitrogen (BUN) levels. Additionally, renal biopsies may reveal lupus nephritis (Pisetsky et al, 1997).

TABLE 25–6. DIFFERENTIAL DIAGNOSIS OF SYSTEMIC LUPUS ERYTHEMATOSUS

- Rheumatoid arthritis
- Sjögren syndrome
- Dermatological conditions
- Hematological disorders
- Polymyositis
- Scleroderma

SLE patients also may exhibit autoantibodies to a protein complexed to RNA [anti-Ro (SS-A)] and a phosphoprotein [anti-La (SS-B)]. Elevated levels of both autoantibodies also have been demonstrated in patients with Sjögren syndrome. Moreover, anti-Ro is associated with the HLA-DR2 and HLA-DR3 alleles. These two alleles appear to exert an effect on certain autoantibodies, which in turn results in lupus-related clinical findings (Nguyen & Foster, 1998).

A complete blood count with differential may reveal anemia, leukopenia, and/or thrombocytopenia. Anemia may arise from autoantibody production (anti-Rh) against red blood cells, resulting in hemolysis. Immune-mediated hemolytic anemia results in a positive Coombs test. Leukopenia with white blood cell counts of less than 4000/μL may result from antineutrophil antibody production. Thrombocytopenia with platelet counts of <100,000/μL may arise from antiplatelet antibody production. A prolonged partial thromboplastin time (PTT) often is observed in patients with antiphospholipid antibodies (anticardiolipin and lupus anticoagulant) that interfere with coagulation (Levine et al, 1988). Antiphospholipids can result in false-positive findings on the fluorescent treponema antibody absorption (FTA-ABS) test (Schur, 1996) and the Venereal Disease Research Laboratory (VDRL) and rapid plasma reagin (RPR) tests for syphilis (Pisetsky et al, 1997).

Ocular

Ocular findings are not included in the diagnostic criteria for SLE. However, early recognition of ocular lupus manifestations may point toward early treatment of patients who have not been formally diagnosed with SLE. Moreover, proper diagnosis of lupus eye disease may prevent subsequent vision loss.

Examination should include a thorough patient and familial history. High concordance of lupus in monozygotic twins suggests a genetic predisposition (Nguyen & Foster, 1998). Important initial testing includes visual acuity assessment and pupillary testing. Both provide information regarding the integrity of the neuro-ophthalmic pathway, which may be affected in central nervous system (CNS) lupus. Anterior segment examination should evaluate for discoid lesions, blepharitis, and KCS. Posterior segment examination should include observation of the optic nerve and retinal fundus grounds. Retinal manifestations present indications for further study via fundus fluorescein angiography. Angiography may reveal hypofluorescence (nonperfusion and arteriolar occlusion) or hyperfluorescence (neovascularization). Additionally, iatrogenic ocular sequelae also results from chronic use of medications to treat systemic lupus (Table 25–3). Intraocular pressures should be monitored in patients undergoing steroidal therapy. Ocular fundi of patients receiving antimalarial agents should be evaluated for maculopathy.

TREATMENT AND MANAGEMENT

Systemic

To date, no known cure for SLE exists. Treatment is aimed toward alleviating symptomology (Table 25–7). Lupus patients should be counseled on the use of protective sunscreen and avoidance of exposure to ultraviolet radiation in order to prevent exacerbation of dermatological lesions. Advanced skin lesions are responsive to hydroxychloroquine therapy (~200 to 800 mg/day) (Nguyen & Foster, 1998). Patients with severe mucocutaneous disease who are intolerant of antimalarial agents may benefit from dapsone or retinoids. Moreover, thalidomide has been demonstrated to be effective against cutaneous lesions. However, thalidomide use has been limited due to the teratogenic effects (Petri, 1998).

TABLE 25–7. SYSTEMIC TREATMENT OF SYSTEMIC LUPUS ERYTHEMATOSUS

- Sunscreen and avoidance of solar radiation
- Nonsteroidal anti-inflammatory agents
- Antimalarial agents
  - Hydroxychloroquine (200–800 mg/day)
  - Chloroquine (250 mg/day)
- Corticosteroids
  - Methylprednisolone (1–2 g/day)
  - Prednisone (mild 5–10 mg/day; severe 100–300 mg/day)
- Immunosuppressive agents
  - Cyclophosphamide (~2 mg/kg/day)
  - Azathioprine (~0.5 mg/kg/day)
  - Methotrexate (~7.5–15 mg/week)
  - Cyclosporine (~2.5 mg/kg/day)
- Plasmapheresis

Nonsteroidal anti-inflammatory agents (NSAIDs) represent the initial therapeutic agent employed for the treatment of arthralgia and arthritis. However, chronic NSAID therapy may precipitate renal complications. If successful treatment fails to be achieved with NSAID therapy, antimalarial agents represent the second-line medication. Antimalarial agents such as hydroxychloroquine (200 to 400 mg/day) or chloroquine (250 mg/day) may act by altering lysosomal function. This results in interference of antigen processing and autoimmunity activation. Alternatively, advanced arthritic disease may be treated with low-dose corticosteroids (prednisone 5 to 10 mg/day) (Pisetsky et al, 1997).

Combination therapy of corticosteroid and immunosuppressive agents is employed in the treatment of renal disease. Patients with proliferative glomerulonephritis receive intravenous steroid (1 to 2 gm methylprednisolone/day) and high-dose oral prednisone (100 to 300 mg/day) in conjunction with pulse cyclophosphamide. Major side effects of cytotoxic cyclophosphamide therapy include bone marrow suppression, malignancy, infection, and ovarian failure. Alternative immunosuppressive agents include azathioprine, methotrexate, and cyclosporine. In refractory renal disease, plasmapheresis may be attempted with or without combined immunosuppressive therapy (Pisetsky et al, 1997).

Similarly, patients in CNS crisis are managed with intravenous and/or oral corticosteroids in conjunction with cytotoxic agents. Plasmapheresis may be indicated if CNS complications fail to resolve with high-dose corticosteroid therapy. Additionally, lupus patients with elevated levels of antiphospholipids are at increased risk for strokes. Antiplatelet and anticoagulation therapy may be indicated to prevent such thrombotic events (Pisetsky et al, 1997).

Ocular

Eye care of SLE patients requires treatment of lupus eye disease and management of ocular sequelae secondary to systemic medical therapy (Table 25–8). Keratoconjunctivitis sicca may be managed with ocular lubricants, lid hygiene, and punctal occlusion. Avoidance of ultraviolet radiation may prevent the exacerbation

TABLE 25–8. OCULAR TREATMENT OF SYSTEMIC LUPUS ERYTHEMATOSUS

- Dry eye management (eg, ocular lubricants and punctal occlusion)
- Laser photocoagulation
- Vitrectomy
- Retinal repair procedures
- Management of iatrogenic ocular conditions
  - Glaucoma
  - Cataracts
  - Bull's eye maculopathy

of lid discoid lesions (Nguyen & Foster, 1998). Retinal vasculitis, which parallels systemic disease activity, demonstrates therapeutic benefits from isolated corticosteroid and cytotoxic therapy or combination therapy (Neumann & Foster, 1995). Neovascularization resulting from proliferative retinopathy or vasoocclusive disease requires treatment with laser photocoagulation. Advanced retinal diseases may require vitrectomy and retinal repair procedures.

SLE patients undergoing hydroxychloroquine or chloroquine therapy should be monitored at 6-month intervals for adverse side effects. The medications may result in RPE pigmentary changes that progress to the formation of a bull's eye maculopathy (Figure 25–5). Early detection of RPE mottling changes and prompt reduction or discontinuation of antimalarial agents may result in reversal of the retinopathy. In contrast, retinopathy progression may result in impaired color vision, visual field disturbances, and metamorphopsia. Additionally, hydroxychloroquine and chloroquine also result in keratopathy. Early keratopathy is characterized by punctate deposition on the corneal epithelium. Progressive changes result in the formation of a whorl-like pattern. Keratopathy is associated with symptoms of reduced vision, glare, halos, and photophobia (Bartlett & Jaanus, 1989).

Finally, patients on corticosteroid therapy should be evaluated for increased intraocular pressure. Steroidal responders should be managed with antiglaucoma therapy. Lupus patients receiving chronic steroid therapy may also demonstrate early development of posterior subcapsular cataracts.

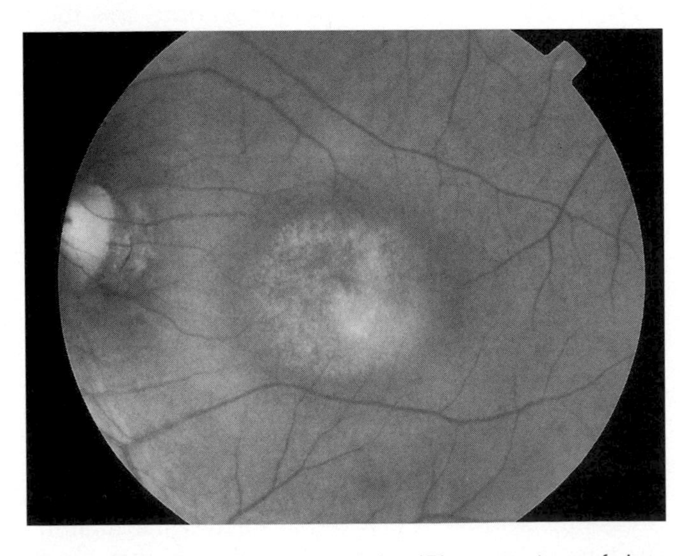

Figure 25–5. Bull's eye maculopathy. (*Photo courtesy of Joan Portello, OD.*)

CONCLUSION

Systemic lupus erythematosus is an autoimmune disease of unknown etiology. The pathogenesis involves the production of autoantibodies against multiple antigens. Autoantibody–antigen complex formation results in complement activation and multisystemic tissue damage.

Lupus presents with multiple ophthalmic manifestations. Common ocular complications include discoid skin lesions and keratoconjunctivitis sicca. However, ocular morbidity may be associated with lupus retinopathy and neuropathy. Early recognition of lupus eye symptomology and findings in an undiagnosed SLE case may be indicative of further evaluation via a rheumatology consult. Prompt diagnosis and treatment can facilitate partial or complete disease remission. Additionally, routine evaluations should be performed to monitor for the development of adverse sequelae secondary to medications employed in the treatment of systemic lupus disease.

REFERENCES

Arffa RC. *Grayson's Diseases of the Cornea,* 4th ed. St. Louis: Mosby–Year Book; 1997:485–493.

Bartlett JD, Jaanus SD. Ocular effects of systemic drugs. In: Bartlett JD, Jaanus SD, eds. *Clinical Ocular Pharmacology,* 2nd ed. Boston: Butterworth-Heinemann; 1989:801–842.

Boumpas DT, Austin HA, Fessler BJ, et al. Systemic lupus erythematosus: Emerging concepts (Part 1: Renal, neuropsychiatric, cardiovascular, pulmonary, and hematologic disease). *Ann Intern Med.* 1995a;122:940–950.

Boumpas DT, Fessler BJ, Austin HA, et al. Systemic lupus erythematosus: Emerging concepts (Part 2: Dermatologic and joint disease, the antiphospholipid antibody syndrome, pregnancy and hormonal therapy, morbidity and mortality, and pathogenesis). *Ann Intern Med.* 1995b; 123:42–53.

Davies KA. Complement, immune complexes and systemic lupus erythematosus. *Br J Rheumatol.* 1996;35:5–23.

Gold D, Feiner L, Henkind P. Retinal arterial occlusive disease in systemic lupus erythematosus. *Arch Ophthalmol.* 1977;95:1580–1585.

Gold DH, Morris DA, Henkind P. Ocular findings in systemic lupus erythematosus. *Br J Ophthalmol.* 1972;56: 800–804.

Graham EM, Spalton DJ, Barnard RO, et al. Cerebral and retinal vascular changes in systemic lupus erythematosus. *Ophthalmology.* 1985;92:444–448.

Grimson BS, Simons KB. Orbital inflammation, myositis and systemic lupus erythematosus. *Arch Ophthalmol.* 1983;101: 736–738.

Hahn BH. Systemic lupus erythematosus. In: Fauci AS, Braunwald E, Isselbacher KJ, et al, eds. *Harrison's Principles of Internal Medicine,* 14th ed. New York: McGraw-Hill; 1998:1874–1880.

Hall S, Buettner H, Luthra HS. Occlusive retinal vascular disease in systemic lupus erythematosus. *J Rheumatol.* 1984; 11:846–850.

Hay EM, Smith ML. Systemic lupus erythematosus and lupus-like syndromes. *Br Med J.* 1995;310:1257–1261.

Jabs DA, Hanneken AM, Schachat AP, Fine SL. Choroidopathy in systemic lupus erythematosus. *Arch Ophthalmol.* 1988;106:230–234.

Jabs DA, Miller NR, Newman SA, et al. Optic neuropathy in systemic lupus erythematosus. *Arch Ophthalmol.* 1986; 104:564–568.

Joffe II, Jacobs LE, Owen AN, et al. Noninfective valvular masses: Review of the literature with emphasis on imaging techniques and management. *Am Heart J.* 1996;131: 1175–1183.

Klinkhoff AV, Beattie CW, Chalmers A. Retinopathy in systemic lupus erythematosus: Relationship to disease activity. *Arthritis Rheum.* 1986;29:1152–1156.

Levine SR, Crofts JW, Lesser R, et al. Visual symptoms associated with the presence of a lupus anticoagulant. *Ophthalmology.* 1988;95:686–692.

Mahoney BP. Rheumatologic disease and associated ocular manifestations. *J Am Optom Assoc.* 1993;64(6):403–415.

Neumann R, Foster CS. Corticosteroid-sparing strategies in the treatment of retinal vasculitis in systemic lupus erythematosus. *Retina.* 1995;15:206–212.

Nguyen QD, Foster CS. Systemic lupus erythematosus and the eye. *Int Ophthalmol Clin.* 1998;38:33–60.

Petri M. Treatment of systemic lupus erythematosus: An update. *Am Fam Physician.* 1998;57:2753–2760.

Pisetsky DS, Gilkeson G, St. Clair EW. Systemic lupus erythematosus (diagnosis and treatment). *Med Clin N Am.* 1997;81:113–128.

Reddy CV, Foster CF. Systemic lupus erythematosus. In: Albert DM, Jakobiec FA, eds. *Principles and Practice of Ophthalmology.* Philadelphia: W.B. Saunders; 1994:2894–2901.

Rich MW. Drug-induced lupus. *Postgrad Med.* 1996;100: 299–307.

Robin JB, Schanzlin DJ, Verity SM, et al. Peripheral corneal disorders. *Surv Ophthalmol.* 1986;31:1–36.

Schur PH. Systemic lupus erythematosus. In: Bennett JC, Plum F, eds. *Cecil Textbook of Medicine,* 20th ed. Philadelphia: W.B. Saunders; 1996:1475–1483.

Tan EM, Cohen AS, Fries JF, et al. The 1982 revised criteria for the classification of systemic lupus erythematosus. *Arthritis Rheum.* 1982;25:1271–1277.

Von Feldt JM. Systemic lupus erythematosus. *Postgrad Med.* 1995;97:79–94.

Chapter 26

GIANT CELL ARTERITIS/ POLYMYALGIA RHEUMATICA

Richard J. Madonna

Giant cell arteritis (GCA) is a systemic vasculitis with a predilection for the cranial arteries that almost always affects the elderly. Vision loss, in the form of an anterior ischemic optic neuropathy, is due to involvement of the ophthalmic artery, and is usually severe and permanent. Unilateral ocular involvement will proceed to bilateral involvement, usually in 1 to 10 days, if there is no therapeutic intervention. Importantly, transient monocular blindness, photopsia, or transient binocular visual loss may precede permanent vision loss in a number of cases.

Polymyalgia rheumatica (PMR) is a poorly understood syndrome marked by aching and stiffness in the torso and proximal limbs. It too almost always occurs in elderly patients. It is clear that these two conditions are linked. They occur in the same population and often in the same individual. Symptoms of PMR may precede, occur simultaneously with, or follow clinical GCA. In fact, PMR may be a milder form of GCA. In a genetically predisposed individual over the age of 50 years, some unknown factor may precipitate one of the syndromes; some other factor then may be able to shift the process to the other one at a later time (Hunder, 1997).

EPIDEMIOLOGY

Systemic

GCA rarely occurs in persons under age 50 and has an average age of onset of approximately 70 years. The incidence of biopsy-proven GCA in persons 50 years of age and older varies between 0.5 and 25.4 per 100,000 (Ghanchi & Dutton, 1997). An autopsy study detected histological evidence of arteritic lesions in the temporal artery and aorta in 16 of 1097 autopsies. This discrepancy probably represents those with subclinical arteritis (Ostberg, 1971). The disease is found predominantly in Caucasians, and is more common in women than men.

Annual incidence of PMR is reported to be close to 1 in 2000 but it may be present in as many as 1 in 200 persons (Salvarani et al, 1995). Like GCA it occurs predominantly in Caucasians, and is more common in women than men.

Ocular

Visual symptoms have been reported in 14 to 70% of cases of GCA (Ghanchi & Dutton, 1997). Unilateral or bilateral, partial or complete vision loss is the most common ocular complication. The visual loss usually is due to anterior ischemic optic neuropathy but may be due to posterior ischemic optic neuropathy, retinal artery occlusion, choroidal ischemia, orbital ischemia, or cortical ischemia. Fifty to seventy-five percent of cases with unilateral ocular involvement will proceed to bilateral involvement without therapeutic intervention. Vision loss is not associated with PMR unless the condition evolves into GCA or is found concurrently with GCA.

Vision loss is not associated with PMR unless the condition evolves into GCA or is found concurrently with GCA.

PATHOPHYSIOLOGY/DISEASE PROCESS

Systemic

GCA is an obliterative vasculitis of unknown etiology affecting medium and large-sized arteries. Inflammation leads to structural changes within the artery, reduction of blood flow, and finally, ischemia. Electron microscopy shows early damage to the smooth muscle cells. Persistent inflammation causes segmental fragmentation of the elastic lamina, swollen endothelium, smooth muscle necrosis, and cellular infiltration with lymphocytes, plasma cells, macrophages, histiocytes, eosinophils, fibroblasts, and giant cells. The cellular infiltrate is affected by steroid treatment, but the characteristic histological features are present for weeks after the initiation of steroid use. The presence of giant cells on biopsy is not essential for the diagnosis of GCA if other histologic features are present. Histologic changes may be segmental or focal, called segmental "skip lesions," and may lead to false-negative results on biopsy.

Superficial temporal, occipital, vertebral, ophthalmic, and posterior ciliary arteries are the most frequently affected vessels, but the coronary arteries and aorta also have been shown to be involved (Freddo et al, 1999). Inflammatory involvement may be correlated to the amount of elastic tissue in the artery. Intracranial vessels, having minimal internal elastic lamina, are involved minimally. The same may hold true for smaller vessels.

The role of the immune system in GCA has been investigated. Cellular immunity appears to play a greater role than humoral immunity in the disease. Lymphocytic infiltration is marked by a greater number of CD4 cells as compared to CD8 cells.

It has always been thought that arteritis is not present in patients with PMR. However, new studies showed that cytokine mRNA from lymphocytes and macrophages was found in temporal artery biopsies of patients with PMR as well as GCA. This was the first time that vascular involvement in PMR was demonstrated. Additionally, tissue from patients with PMR lacked evidence of interferon-gamma, a cytokine that is elevated in GCA. This substance may be critical in the progression to overt arteritis (Weyand et al, 1994).

Clinically, GCA is marked by nonspecific symptoms such as fever, malaise, weight loss, anorexia, night sweats, and depression. Severe proximal muscle pain is common. Headache, which may be frontal, temporal, or occipital, appears insidiously and becomes severe. Neck pain occurs frequently. Partial temporal artery occlusion leads to jaw claudication. Neck pain and jaw claudication may be the symptoms most closely associated with GCA (Hayreh et al, 1997). The temporal artery is often tortuous, nodular, red, and tender (Figure 26–1). The temporal artery and scalp may be so tender that patients are unable to comb their hair, wear a hat, or sleep on a pillow. Conversely, occult GCA, without systemic manifestations, is not uncommon and the clinician should be alert to its existence (Table 26–1).

PMR is characterized by pain and morning stiffness in the neck, shoulders, lumbar area, and thighs. The stiffness often subsides over the course of the day.

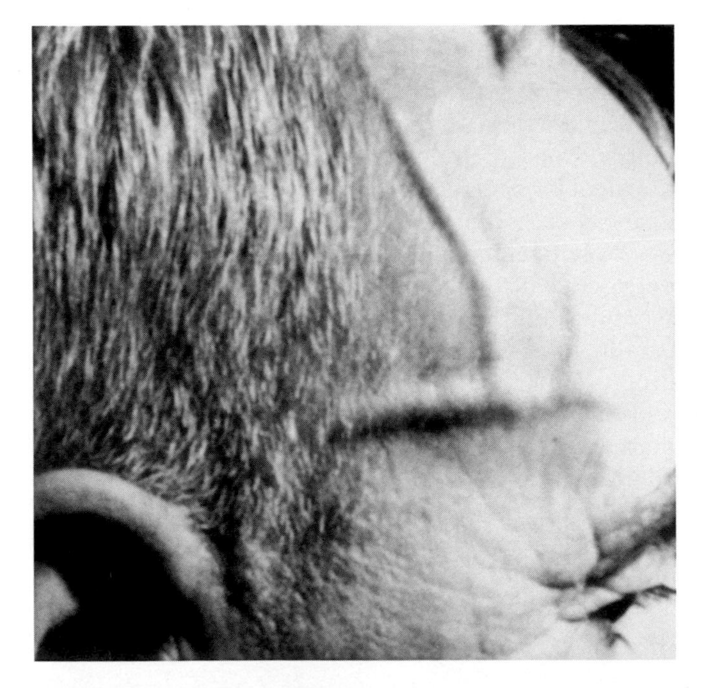

Figure 26–1. Temporal arteritis with typical appearance of the swollen, tender, inflamed temporal artery with involvement of both the anterior and posterior branches. (*Reprinted with permission from Healey LA, Wilske KR.* The Systemic Manifestations of Temporal Arteritis. *New York: Grune & Stratton; 1978.*)

TABLE 26–1. SYSTEMIC MANIFESTATIONS OF GIANT CELL ARTERITIS/POLYMYALGIA RHEUMATICA

GCA
Headache
Neck pain
Jaw claudication
Proximal muscle pain
Prominent, tender temporal artery
Fever
Malaise
Night sweats
Weight loss
Anorexia
No symptoms
PMR
Pain
Morning stiffness: neck and proximal joints
Mild synovitis: knees, wrists, other
Many of the symptoms of GCA

Mild synovitis of the knees, wrists, or other joints may be present. Pain is often disproportionate to the degree of observable swelling (Table 26–1).

> "Occult" GCA, without systemic manifestations, may occur in about 1 in 5 patients with GCA.

Ocular

Most ocular manifestations are due to partial or total vascular occlusion in the territory of the ophthalmic artery. Patients may present with transient visual loss (amaurosis fugax) consistent with partial arterial occlusion. Total vascular occlusion usually manifests as an anterior ischemic optic neuropathy but can occur anywhere along the visual pathway (Table 26–2).

Arteritic anterior ischemic optic neuropathy (AAION), the most common cause of visual loss in GCA, usually manifests as sudden, painless, relatively permanent vision loss in one eye. Vision loss varies from minimal to profound but is typically worse than in nonarteritic anterior ischemic optic neuropathy (NAION). The disc is edematous and often pale because of occlusion of the posterior ciliary arteries (Figure 26–2). Splinter hemorrhages and cotton-wool spots may be present. There is usually a significant afferent pupillary defect. The classic visual field defect is an

TABLE 26–2. OCULAR MANIFESTATIONS OF GIANT CELL ARTERITIS/POLYMYALGIA RHEUMATICA

GCA
Transient visual loss
Anterior ischemic optic neuropathy
Posterior ischemic optic neuropathy
Central retinal artery occlusion
Ocular motor nerve palsies
Anterior segment ischemia
Posterior segment ischemia with resultant neovascular glaucoma
Cerebral ischemia with visual pathway infarction
PMR
None unless concurrent GCA

A

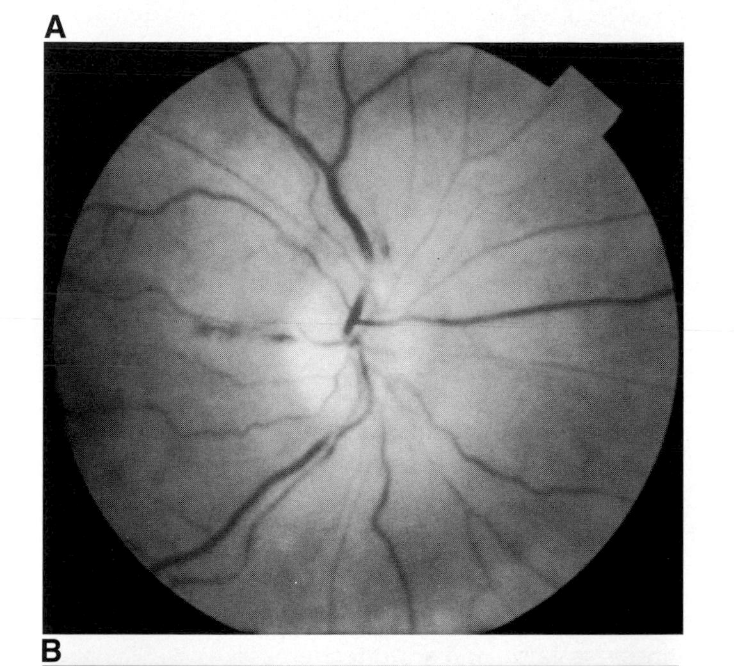

B

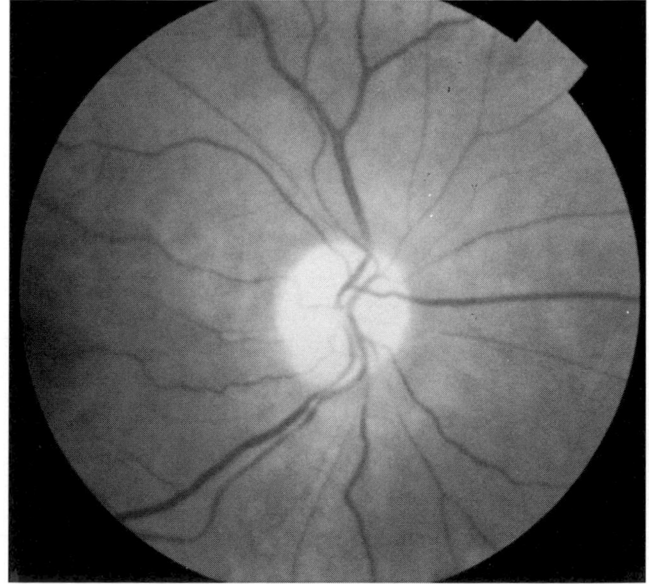

Figure 26–2. A. Acute anterior ischemic optic neuropathy secondary to GCA. Note the elevation of the nerve head with blurred disc margins and adjacent flame hemorrhages. **B.** Atrophic appearance of the same nerve head several months later. (*Courtesy of Dr. Jerome Sherman.*)

altitudinal defect but sectoral, central, and a variety of other defects have been described. Disc swelling resolves over the course of 2 to 3 months, leaving sectoral or general disc pallor often with cupping. As stated previously, AAION will involve the second eye rapidly if steroid treatment is not instituted.

Visual system vascular occlusion may cause other less common manifestations of GCA. These include posterior ischemic optic neuropathy (PION); central retinal artery occlusion; ocular motor nerve palsies; anterior segment ischemia leading to corneal edema, iritis, hypotony, and cataract; posterior segment ischemia with resultant iris and angle neovascularization and neovascular glaucoma; and cerebral ischemia leading to visual pathway infarction, including occipital lobe stroke and cortical blindness.

DIAGNOSIS

Systemic

PMR and GCA probably represent two forms of the same disease with the major difference being the risk of blindness in patients with GCA. Laboratory findings typical of patients with GCA are often similar in those with PMR.

The diagnosis of GCA should be considered in all patients 50 years of age and older with classic symptoms of the disease: headache, neck pain, jaw claudication, muscle ache, fever of unknown origin, flu-like illness, malaise, and scalp tenderness, as well as sudden or unexplained loss of vision. In the presence of a plethora of these symptoms, a clinical diagnosis can be made. PMR is a clinical diagnosis that should be considered in older patients with pain and stiffness in the shoulder and pelvic girdle often associated with fever, malaise, and weight loss.

The Westergren erythrocyte sedimentation rate (ESR) usually is elevated in GCA although normal ESRs have been reported in up to 22.5% of cases of GCA (Hayreh et al, 1997). The normal ESR is higher in females than in males, and increases with age. A general rule of thumb for normal ESR determination by the Westergren method is as follows: Normal male ESR $\leq$ (age in years)/2; and normal females ESR $\leq$ (age in years + 10)/2. The ESR in GCA often is elevated markedly to 50 mm/hour and higher. The ESR is similarly elevated in PMR.

The ESR should not be used as the sole criterion for diagnosing GCA. Age and a number of hematological factors including anemia, malignancy, and hypercholesterolemia influence the ESR. A normal ESR should not dissuade the clinician from further evaluation or treatment when the clinical picture strongly suggests GCA. Patient complaints consistent with GCA despite normal laboratory and biopsy findings may still warrant treatment to prevent catastrophic visual or systemic results. Additionally, patients with GCA already may be on corticosteroid therapy for symptoms of PMR, thereby lowering the ESR.

> GCA must still be considered in the patient with normal ESR if there is strong systemic evidence of the disease.

The level of C-reactive protein (CRP) produced by the liver increases in infection and inflammation and is correlated with disease activity in GCA. A CRP > 2.45 mg/dL was found to be 100% sensitive in the diagnosis of GCA as compared to 92% sensitivity for an ESR above 47 mm/hour. CRP levels change more quickly than the ESR in measuring both disease activation and response to treatment. The combination of an ESR > 47 mm/hour and C-reactive protein > 2.5 mg/dL was 97% specific for the diagnosis of GCA in one study (Hayreh et al, 1997).

> The use of ESR and CRP together is becoming standard in the laboratory investigation of GCA.

Protein synthesis increases in GCA, causing an increase in plasma viscosity. Plasma viscosity has been shown to correlate with disease activity in GCA. Combined results of ESR and plasma viscosity may increase diagnostic reliability greater than either of the two tests alone (Ghanchi & Dutton, 1997).

Laboratory testing should also include a complete blood count (CBC) with differential to rule out any other systemic disease involvement. Patients with GCA and PMR often have a normochromic normocytic anemia. The clinician should remember that anemia can artificially elevate the ESR although usually not to the levels seen in GCA. A markedly increased platelet count has been reported in a patient with GCA, and this may have diagnostic and prognostic value. The platelet count was reduced after steroid treatment. Reduction of CD8+ lymphocytes has been used to discriminate between patients with GCA and PMR and those with other diseases. Anticardiolipin antibodies were present in almost 50% of patients with GCA and PMR in one study population. These antibodies disappeared in 56% of these patients after treatment. The levels of $alpha_2$ globulin and fibrinogen are also commonly elevated, and there is an increased incidence of human leukocyte antigen (HLA) B8 and B10 in GCA.

Temporal artery biopsy (TAB) remains the gold standard for diagnosis of GCA. A positive TAB confirms the presence of the disease, but a negative one does not rule out the condition. New headache, jaw claudication, temporal artery abnormality on examination, and absence of synovitis are most highly associated with a positive TAB; negative biopsies are more typically found in those without jaw claudication and normal temporal artery in the presence of synovitis (Hunder, 1997). The biopsied artery should be at least 25 mm in length to ensure that diseased artery is biopsied. So-called "skip lesions" can be avoided if an appropriate arterial length is analyzed. In cases where there is a high suspicion of GCA and normal biopsy, a second biopsy of the suspected artery or biopsy of the contralateral temporal artery may provide diagnostic information.

> A second biopsy of the suspected temporal artery or a biopsy of the contralateral artery should be performed if the initial biopsy is normal but the index of suspicion for the disease is high.

Color Doppler ultrasonography has been utilized in patients with GCA. A dark halo around the temporal artery (which disappeared after steroid treatment) was observed in 73% of patients with symptomatic GCA, but was not present in controls (Schmidt et al, 1997). Information is lacking on whether ultrasonography can detect those without symptoms of GCA who would have positive TABs (occult GCA). Color Doppler ultrasonography may be useful in distinguishing those patients with GCA from those with PMR or from normals. Peak systolic velocity in the superficial temporal artery was considerably reduced in patients with GCA when compared to those with PMR or normals (Table 26–3).

The differential diagnosis of GCA and PMR includes any condition that causes the symptom complex seen in these conditions and an elevated sedimentation rate (Table 26–4). This includes but is not limited to malignant disorders, infections, and other arthritides.

TABLE 26–3. DIAGNOSTIC TESTS FOR GIANT CELL ARTERITIS/POLYMYALGIA RHEUMATICA

GCA
Systemic
Westergren erythrocyte sedimentation rate (ESR)[a]
C-reactive protein (CRP)[a]
Temporal artery biopsy (TAB)[a]
Plasma viscosity
CBC with differential
Levels of CD4 and CD8 lymphocytes
Anticardiolipin antibodies
$Alpha_2$ globulin and fibrinogen
HLA B8 and B10
Color Doppler ultrasonography
Ocular
Fluorescein angiogram
PMR
Westergren erythrocyte sedimentation rate
CBC with differential
Laboratory findings often overlap with those seen in GCA
Color Doppler ultrasonography

[a]Primary tests.

Ocular

Vision loss due to AION is the most common ocular finding in GCA. Patients usually have profound vision loss in one eye, afferent pupillary defect, and dense altitudinal or sectoral visual field loss. The optic nerve is usually markedly edematous and may either be hyperemic or whitish ("pale edema") with equal likelihood. Disc edema resolves over the course of 2 to 3 months leaving a pale, cupped nerve. Retinal hemorrhages and cotton-wool spots may be present.

Clinical signs may be useful in helping distinguish arteritic AION from NAION. Patients with NAION typically have less severe vision loss, do not have pale edema, and go on to develop vision loss in the opposite eye much less often. Fluorescein angiographic

TABLE 26–4. DIFFERENTIAL DIAGNOSIS OF GIANT CELL ARTERITIS/POLYMYALGIA RHEUMATICA (GCA/PMR)

Systemic
Malignancies
Infections
Arthritides
Ocular
Arteritic anterior ischemic optic neuropathy (AION)
nonarteritic ischemic optic neuropathy (NAION)
Diabetic papillopathy
Compressive optic neuropathy
Inflammatory optic neuropathy
Infectious optic neuropathy
Other causes of optic neuropathy
Central retinal artery occlusion (CRAO)
Embolic etiology
Infectious etiology
Inflammatory etiology
Oculomotor nerve palsies
Microvascular disease
Compressive disease

findings in patients with arteritic AION are consistent with complete occlusion of the posterior ciliary artery circulation to the eye; patients with NAION most commonly have transient or incomplete perfusion deficits. The clinician should never differentiate arteritic AION from NAION on clinical findings alone. All patients over age 50 with AION should have appropriate laboratory studies performed at presentation. TAB is indicated in those patients in whom there is a high level of suspicion for the disease.

> In the older patient, NAION should never be differentiated from AAION on clinical impressions alone.

PION is a much less common complication of GCA in which visual loss is found in the setting of a normal fundus exam but with an afferent pupillary defect. Ischemia of the retrolaminar optic nerve from nutrient vessel occlusion is felt to be responsible.

Central retinal artery occlusion (CRAO), oculomotor nerve palsies, and transient visual loss are less common presenting signs of GCA. Older patients presenting with these conditions should be evaluated for GCA.

In addition to NAION, the differential diagnosis of arteritic AION includes any condition that can cause optic nerve swelling, including diabetic papillopathy and compressive, inflammatory, or infectious lesions. CRAO from GCA must be contrasted with CRAO from embolic, inflammatory, or infectious processes. Oculomotor nerve palsy from microvascular disease, such as diabetes, is the major differential for diplopia in GCA, although compressive etiologies must be considered, particularly with third-nerve palsy. If transient monocular vision loss is noted, carotid occlusive disease must be considered.

TREATMENT AND MANAGEMENT

Systemic

Corticosteroids are the mainstay of treatment (Table 26–5) of GCA because they decrease arterial inflammation, thereby increasing blood flow to affected organs. Traditionally, the disease has been treated with oral prednisone but intravenous methylprednisolone has been used recently. The goal of steroid therapy is the preservation of vision in the fellow eye in patients who have lost vision or prevention of vision loss in both eyes of those whose vision has not been affected.

TABLE 26–5. TREATMENT AND MANAGEMENT OF GIANT CELL ARTERITIS/POLYMYALGIA RHEUMATICA

GCA
With vision loss
Immediate erythrocyte sedimentation rate (ESR) and Creative protein (CRP)
IV methylprednisolone 1–2 g/day for 3 days
Temporal artery biopsy (TAB)
Oral prednisone 1 g/day
Steroid taper guided by disease activity until maintenance dose reached
Without vision loss
Immediate ESR and CRP
Oral prednisone 1–2 mg/kg/day
TAB
Steroid taper guided by disease activity until maintenance dose reached
PMR
Oral prednisone 10–15 mg daily
Gradual taper to maintenance dose of 2.5–7.5 mg (may continue for years)

Note: complications of steroid therapy should be anticipated and carefully monitored.

There have been reports of significant visual improvement in eyes with AAION following steroid therapy, but this should not be expected.

There is no single accepted treatment for the patient with GCA. A reasonable approach to the patient presenting with visual loss and suspected GCA starts with ordering of immediate ESR and CRP. If the laboratory results are conclusive or clinical symptomatology is overwhelming, corticosteroid treatment should begin. Intravenous (IV) methylprednisolone 1 to 2 g/day is recommended for patients with vision loss or amaurosis. IV treatment should continue for at least 3 days, whereupon the patient is switched to oral prednisone of at least 1 mg/kg/day. Oral prednisone should be used for those without vision loss with a starting dose of 1 to 2 mg/kg/day. TAB should be performed at the onset of treatment to confirm the diagnosis.

Steroid dosage is reduced slowly based on disease activity as measured by improvement in systemic symptoms and a decrease in the ESR and CRP. Patients should be followed at 1- to 2-week intervals to monitor the response to treatment and identify a minimum suppressive steroid dose. A maintenance dose of 7.5 mg often is adequate after 6 to 9 months, with most patients able to discontinue treatment after 2 years (Ghanchi & Dutton, 1997).

Complications of high-dose, long-term corticosteroid treatment always must be kept in mind. Calcium and vitamin D supplements should be provided to reduce the risk of bone fracture due to osteoporosis in this high-risk group. Other complications such as impaired glucose metabolism, risk of infection, peptic ulcer, and fluid retention, must also be carefully monitored.

Immunosuppressive and cytotoxic agents have been investigated as alternatives to steroid treatment for GCA, particularly in those cases of steroid-resistant or relapsing disease. Reports of success with cyclosporine or cyclophosphamide have not been substantiated through clinical trials. Presently, methotrexate probably is considered the most useful of these secondary agents.

PMR is managed with relatively low-dose oral corticosteroid treatment. Initial dosages of 10 to 15 mg daily with gradual taper to maintenance therapy of 2.5 to 7.5 mg are usually adequate to alleviate symptoms. Therapy may need to be continued for years (Table 26–5).

Ocular

Ocular therapy is simply systemic therapy whose primary goal is to prevent visual loss in the fellow eye. There are reports of significant visual improvement if treatment begins within 24 to 36 hours of visual loss, particularly with systemic steroids. Unfortunately, some cases progress to bilateral vision loss despite aggressive steroid therapy. Ocular side effects of steroid therapy include glaucoma and posterior subcapsular cataracts.

CONCLUSION

GCA is an inflammatory obliterative arteritis leading to ischemia from occlusion of medium and large-sized arteries. Older patients presenting with unilateral severe vision loss, diplopia, or transient vision loss associated with systemic complaints such as headache, jaw claudication, and neck pain should be suspected of having the disease. An ESR and CRP should be ordered immediately; definitive diagnosis is made by temporal artery biopsy. Treatment with high-dose steroids should not be delayed if clinical signs point to the diagnosis. Delay in treatment could lead to irreversible vision loss.

PMR is a clinical syndrome marked by aching and stiffness in the proximal limbs and torso, and is closely related to GCA. It requires low-dose corticosteroid treatment to alleviate symptoms. PMR is not usually associated with vision loss unless GCA occurs simultaneously or subsequently.

REFERENCES

Freddo TAB, Price M, Kase C, Goldstein MP. Myocardial infarction and coronary artery involvement in giant cell arteritis. *Optom Vis Sci.* 1999;76:14–18.

Galetta SL. Vasculitis. In: Miller NR, Newman NJ, eds. *Walsh & Hoyt's Clinical Neuro-Ophthalmology.* Baltimore: Williams & Wilkins; 1998:3725–3886.

Ghanchi FD, Dutton GN. Current concepts in giant cell (temporal) arteritis. *Surv Ophthalmol.* 1997;42:99–123.

Hayreh SS, Podhajsky PA, Raman R, et al. Giant cell arteritis: Validity and reliability of various diagnostic criteria. *Am J Ophthalmol.* 1997;123:285–296.

Hayreh SS, Podhajsky PA, Zimmerman B. Ocular manifestations of giant cell arteritis. *Am J Ophthalmol.* 1998; 125:509–520.

Hunder GG. Giant cell arteritis in polymyalgia rheumatica. *Am J Med.* 1997;102:514–516.

Ostberg G. Temporal arteritis in a large necropsy series. *Ann Rheum Dis.* 1971;30:224–235.

Salvarani C, Gabriel SE, O'Fallon WM, Hunder GG. The incidence of giant cell arteritis in Olmstead County, Minnesota: Apparent fluctuations in a cyclic pattern. *Ann Intern Med.* 1995;123:192–194.

Schmidt WA, Kraft HE, Vorpahl K, et al. Color duplex ultrasonography in the diagnosis of temporal arteritis. *N Engl J Med.* 1997; 337:1336–1342.

Weyand CM, Hicok KC, Hunder GG, Goronzy JJ. Tissue cytokine patterns in patients with polymyalgia rheumatica and giant cell arteritis. *Ann Intern Med.* 1994;121:484–491.

Chapter 27

SJÖGREN'S SYNDROME

Harriette Moutopoulos Canellos

Sjögren's syndrome (SS) is an autoimmune disorder characterized by decreased lacrimal and salivary gland secretion resulting in keratoconjunctivitis sicca and xerostomia, respectively. These conditions together are known as the sicca complex. The pathophysiology of this condition is thought to be due to lymphocytic and plasma cell infiltration leading to the destruction of the lacrimal and salivary glands. In close to 60% of patients with SS, this infiltration may extend to extraglandular organs such as skin, upper and lower respiratory tracts, vagina, kidneys, and central and peripheral nervous systems (Anaya & Talal, 1997). SS may exist as either a primary condition or in association with other autoimmune diseases (secondary Sjögren's syndrome) such as rheumatoid arthritis or systemic lupus erythematosus.

EPIDEMIOLOGY

The absolute incidence of SS is unknown, but its estimated prevalence is 1 to 3% of the world population. Many people go undiagnosed. Nine out of ten persons afflicted with SS are women, with a mean age of 50 years. However, SS also can occur in younger persons. SS does not have any race or ethnic predilection. Twelve percent of patients have one or more relatives with SS (Carsons & Harris, 1998). Approximately 50% of people with SS are described as having secondary SS (SS Foundation, 1998).

PATHOPHYSIOLOGY/DISEASE PROCESS

The exact etiology of SS is unknown. It may be due to the interaction of genetic, hormonal, neuroendocrine, viral, and other environmental factors. Viruses, including those of the herpes virus and retrovirus families, have been linked to SS. In particular, the Epstein–Barr virus has shown a close association with the development of this condition. SS is characterized by a mixed cellular infiltration of exocrine glands, which consists predominantly of lymphocytes. This lymphoproliferation in the lacrimal and salivary gland usually starts in the central perivascular region of the lobule. As the infiltration progresses, it expands in a centrifugal fashion toward the periphery of the lobule, encompassing epithelial ducts and ultimately replacing secretory acini. The proliferation leads to the characteristic epimyoepithelial islet formation in SS patients. Perivascular lymphocytic infiltrates may also interrupt the normal neural innervation of the gland. This results in dysfunction and eventual destruction of the salivary and lacrimal glands (Pflugfelder et al, 1994).

The clinical presentation of SS can be quite variable. Those patients afflicted with primary SS usually present with a more aggressive development of severe ocular and oral manifestations. In contrast, secondary SS tends to have a more slowly developing insidious presentation. The connective tissue disease associated with SS usually precedes or is synchronous with the

TABLE 27–1. SYSTEMIC AND OCULAR MANIFESTATIONS OF SJÖGREN'S SYNDROME

Oral • Xerostomia • Fissures of mouth and tongue • Oral yeast infections • Dental caries	• Splenomegaly • Lymphoma
Salivary Glands • Enlarged parotid glands	**Gastrointestinal** • Gastritis
Nasopharyngeal • Dry nose • Decreased smell • Epistaxis • Difficulty speaking • Dry pharynx • Dysphagia	**Dermatologic** • Dry, rough skin • Purpuric rash • Skin ulceration • Urticaria
Tracheobronchial • Chronic cough • Bronchitis • Interstitial pneumonitis	**Gynecological** • Vaginal dryness • Vulvar discomfort • Yeast infections
Renal • Tubular acidosis • Interstitial nephritis • Renal calculi • Hypokalemia • Glomerulonephritis	**Musculoskeletal** • Arthralgias • Arthritis • Myalgias
Hepatic • Biliary cirrhosis • Hepatomegaly	**Neurologic** • Multiple sclerosis-like syndrome • Cranial nerve palsies • Peripheral neuropathies
Immunologic/Hematologic • Elevated ESR • (+) ANA • (+) RF • Anemia • Hypergammaglobulinemia	**Endocrine** • Thyroiditis **Other** • Vasculitis • Raynaud's phenomenon **Ocular** • Keratoconjunctivitis sicca • Filamentary keratitis • Corneal erosions • Blepharitis • Bacterial keratitis

sicca complex. Table 27–1 summarizes the systemic and ocular manifestations of SS.

Ocular

Tears and saliva have both lubricating and immunologic properties. With a decrease in these substances, discomfort, mucous membrane drying, and a potential for secondary infection may result. The aqueous layer of the tear film is affected in SS. The tear meniscus becomes diminished or absent. This decrease in moisture results in an ocular surface devoid of its previous luster. Tear lysozymes, produced by the acinar and tubular epithelial cells of the lacrimal gland, are significantly reduced. Patients typically complain of a scratchy, foreign-body sensation. The symptoms are due to contact between the palpebral conjunctiva and the finely pitted and irregular corneal and bulbar conjunctival surfaces. Symptoms generally worsen toward the end of the day. With chronic insult, corneal opacification and pannus can occur.

Although SS causes a defect in the aqueous aspect of the tear film, mucin and oil are produced in their normal quantities. Because of the decrease in the aqueous component, the mucin and oil are not solubilized, but are deposited in the conjunctival cul de sac. This results in the production of long strings of mucin. Patients will often complain of the blurred vision caused by these disruptions of the corneal surface. Environmental factors such as wind may also cause increased patient discomfort.

Because of compromise of the tear film, large areas of epithelium can slough off. Epithelial filaments formed by the loose epithelium and the blinking process can adhere to the cornea. Mucin filaments can form as a result of mucous particles adhering to small defects in the corneal epithelium (Figure 27–1). In addition, the conjunctival blood vessels become injected due to the process of vasodilation. Blepharitis may develop in many of these patients, as well as a secondary bacterial keratitis caused by the compromised ocular surfaces.

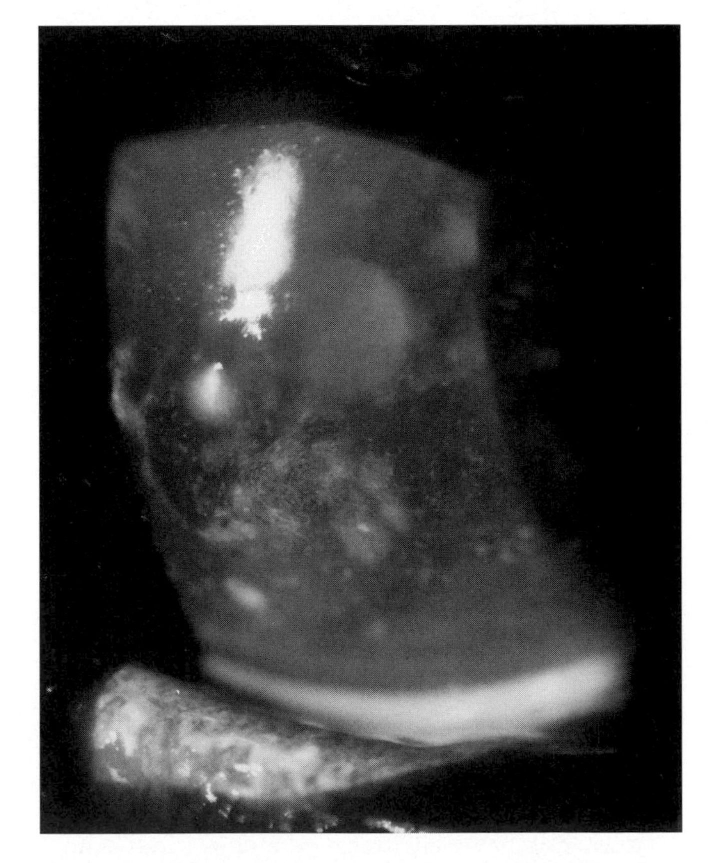

Figure 27–1. Filamentary keratitis in a Sjögren's syndrome patient. This 61-year-old patient has rheumatoid arthritis. Note the diffuse epithelial staining with fluorescein. Heavy dye uptake by the filament is observed. Filament stripping and heavy lubrication were sufficient to control this episode of keratitis.

Scar formation and ulceration may result. These ocular manifestations present with varying degrees but can be severe and debilitating.

Oral

Both the major (parotid, submandibular) and minor (gingival, palantine) salivary glands are affected in SS. Oral manifestations include painful fissures at the corners of the mouth, tongue, and mucous membranes. The diminished salivary flow predisposes the patient to periodontal disease and oral yeast infections such as *Candida.* Infiltration of lymphocytes into the parotid or submandibular glands can cause pain and swelling. Fifty percent of these patients have enlarged parotid glands, which can be symmetrical, recurrent, and accompanied by fever, tenderness, or erythema (Carsons & Harris, 1998). This swelling can result in the classic "chipmunk" appearance of the face.

Systemic

Mucous membrane drying of the nasopharynx can result in epistaxis (nosebleeds), alterations in smell and taste, and difficulty speaking. This dysphasia is secondary to pharyngeal dryness or esophageal dysmotility. Chronic atrophic gastritis is another common digestive tract complication. Involvement of the tracheobronchial mucosa can lead to chronic cough, bronchitis, or lymphocytic interstitial pneumonitis.

Xerosis of the skin occurs in about 50% of SS patients (Carsons & Harris, 1998). Sweat and sebaceous gland dysfunction can lead to roughness, cracking, and fissures. These fissures can become red, itchy, and infected. Occasionally, red, annular, or scaly lesions resembling psoriasis develop.

Gynecological complications in women with SS include vaginal dryness, vulvar discomfort, and yeast infections. Many women complain of painful intercourse. There is a slightly higher incidence of recurrent fetal death and congenital heart block in mothers with SS.

Raynaud's phenomenon occurs in approximately 20% of SS patients (Talal, 1992). Vasculitis affecting small vessels and medium-sized arteries can develop and cause purpuric rash, skin ulceration, and urticaria, especially involving the legs. When vasculitis involves the viscera, it can lead to hepatomegaly, splenomegaly, and glomerulonephritis. Other kidney involvement includes interstitial nephritis and renal tubular acidosis. Renal calculi and hypokalemic muscle weakness are other possible clinical presentations of renal involvement. Primary biliary cirrhosis is the most common form of liver involvement.

Peripheral and central nervous system dysfunction may occur in SS. Peripheral nervous system involvement includes sensorimotor and autonomic neuropathy. Symptoms may include paresthesia or dysesthesia. Carpal tunnel syndrome is not uncommon. Dysfunction of the trigeminal nerve is the most common cranial neuropathy, resulting in facial pain and numbness, as well as loss of taste and smell. Central nervous system lesions are multifocal, and may mimic CNS involvement in multiple sclerosis. Perivascular inflammatory infiltrates have been found in patients with neuropathy, suggesting an underlying necrotizing vasculitis (St. Clair, 1993).

Joint pain, myalgias, and fatigue are common symptoms in SS. Arthralgia and arthritis are common joint manifestations. Rheumatoid arthritis, systemic lupus erythematosus, scleroderma, and polymyositis are connective tissue diseases most commonly associated with SS. Approximately 25% of SS patients have rheumatoid arthritis (Talal, 1992). If the arthritis does not develop within the first year of the sicca complex, then the probability drops to only 10% (Anaya & Talal, 1997).

Other diseases associated with SS include hypothyroidism and lymphoma. Hypothyroidism can develop in up to 20% of SS patients (Dry.Org, 1998). Lymphoma occurs in less than 5% of SS patients (Carsons & Harris, 1998). However, patients with SS are reported to have a relative risk 44 times greater than that of the general population for the development of lymphoma (Horsfall & Isenberg, 1994). Undifferentiated B-cell lymphoma or a well-differentiated immunocytoma are the more common presentations. Lymphoma may arise in exocrine glands, but also may include other organs such as the reticuloendothelial system, lungs, gastrointestinal tract, and kidneys.

> The eyecare provider should be aware that there is an associated autoimmune disorder in 50% of Sjögren's syndrome patients and a risk of lymphoma in 5%. Therefore, successful management requires a multidisciplinary approach.

DIAGNOSIS

A diagnosis of SS is made when two out of three of the following criteria are met:

1. Keratoconjunctivitis sicca
2. Positive lip biopsy confirming the presence of immune cells or lymphocytes identified as causing the dry mouth

3. Associated extraglandular connective tissue disease, or other autoimmune disorders such as rheumatoid arthritis or lupus

Table 27–2 summarizes the appropriate tests for the diagnosis of SS.

> Sjögren's syndrome is an autoimmune disorder that occurs primarily in females with a mean age of 50 and is characterized by keratoconjunctivitis sicca and xerostomia.

Ocular

Ocular symptoms usually assist in the diagnosis of keratoconjunctivitis sicca. Burning, foreign-body sensation, grittiness, and dry eye complaints are common throughout the course of the day. Photophobia, blurred vision, general ocular irritability, and complaints of redness also are common. These patients can sometimes remove thick, ropy strands of mucin from their eyes. The Schirmer test evaluates aqueous tear production and is primarily used to diagnose keratoconjunctivitis sicca. In the Schirmer I test, a folded strip of filter paper is placed over the lower lid between the bulbar and palpebral conjunctiva. The amount of wetting is measured after 5 minutes. The test is considered positive if there is less than 5 mm of wetting. The phenol red thread test, which is similar to the Schirmer test, can also be used to aid in the diagnosis. Also, a low tear breakup time and a diminished or absent tear meniscus are evident in these patients. The tear film will also contain increased amounts of particulate material.

Superficial punctate keratopathy is noted on biomicroscopic examination, most prominently in the inferior cornea and adjacent conjunctiva, because of insufficient lubrication. The integrity of the cornea and conjunctiva can be assessed with fluorescein and rose bengal dyes. Fluorescein dye detects areas devoid of epithelium as well as areas of drying. Rose bengal staining detects devitalized cells. Fluorescein also stains the corneal filaments present in filamentary keratitis (see Figure 27–1). With long-standing insult, corneal erosions may develop, as well as corneal opacification and neovasculariation. Enlargement of the lacrimal gland is not common.

Antimicrobial enzymes such as lysozyme and lactoferrin are usually diminished or absent in SS. β_2 microglobulin levels in tears are elevated (St. Clair, 1993). These tests are useful in research settings but have limited importance clinically. Conjunctival and lacrimal gland biopsies reveal lymphocytic infiltration and aid in the diagnosis, but lacrimal gland biopsy rarely is done because of the risk of hemorrhage and damage to the secretory ducts.

In order to correctly diagnose SS, it is important to understand that other ocular conditions are associated with dry eye signs and symptoms not caused by SS (Table 27–3). For example, keratitis could be a result of lagophthalmos caused by seventh cranial nerve palsy, proptosis, eyelid retraction from thyroid eye disease, or senile ectropion. Blepharitis, trichiasis, contact lens–related disorders, conjunctivitis, and ocular infections can all cause dryness and corneal irritation. In addition, ocular toxicity from topical eye medications (e.g., neomycin, gentamicin, topical beta-blockers) can result in keratitis. Any topical ophthalmic drop containing preservatives may also result in keratitis. Some systemic medications (e.g., antihistamines, antidepressants, antipsychotics, antiseizure medications, muscle relaxants, diuretics, and beta-blockers) may produce ocular dryness, as well as dryness of the mouth and other mucous membranes.

TABLE 27–2. DIAGNOSIS OF SJÖGREN'S SYNDROME

Primary SS

Requires two of the following three criteria to be present:

1. Ocular—dry eye (keratoconjunctivitis sicca)
   Schirmer I test: less than 5 mm wetting in 5 minutes
   AND
   Positive rose bengal and/or fluorescein staining of cornea and conjunctiva
2. Oral—dry mouth
   Abnormal biopsy of labial salivary gland: focus score of 1 or greater
3. Systemic—serologic evidence of extraglandular connective tissue disease or autoimmune disorder
   (+) rheumatoid factor
   OR
   (+) antinuclear antibody
   OR
   (+) Ro (SS-A) or La (SS-B) antibodies

Secondary SS

Requires presence of signs and symptoms of SS described above plus diagnosis of an autoimmune disorder such as:

1. Rheumatoid arthritis
   OR
2. Systemic lupus erythematosus
   OR
3. Scleroderma
   OR
4. Polymyositis

Oral

Oral and nasopharyngeal evaluation will reveal dryness, macular erythema, inflammation, ulceration of the mucous membranes, and increased dental caries.

TABLE 27–3. DIFFERENTIAL DIAGNOSIS OF SJÖGREN'S SYNDROME

Systemic
- Hepatitis C
- Hepatic cirrhosis
- Diabetes
- Hyperlipoproteinemia
- Sarcoidosis
- Hemochromatosis
- Tuberculosis
- Amyloidosis
- Chronic pancreatitis
- HIV
- Multiple sclerosis
- Viral infections
- Anxiety
- Depression
- Pre-existing lymphoma
- Chronic fatigue syndrome
- Systemic medications with anticholinergic effects

Ocular
- Blepharitis
- Conjunctivitis
- Ocular infections
- Contact lens–related problems
- Keratitis due to lagophthalmos/ectropion
- Toxicity from topical medications and preservatives in medications
- Environmental factors

The labial salivary gland biopsy is widely used to assess the salivary component in SS (Table 27–2). A positive biopsy reveals the presence of focal lymphocytic infiltrates and damage to acinar and ductal epithelium. The focus scoring method is used to measure lymphocytic infiltration. A focus is defined as 50 or more mononuclear cells per 4 mm^2 of examined tissue. The presence of one or more foci is considered diagnostic for the oral component of SS (Fox & Saito, 1994). Salivary glands can also be evaluated by measuring flow rate (sialometry). This test is not very specific or sensitive. Sialography images the anatomical structure of the parotid gland. It is uncomfortable for the patient and usually is not necessary to diagnose SS. Salivary gland scintigraphy provides a functional evaluation of all salivary glands and correlates with minor salivary gland biopsy.

Systemic

Seventy percent of SS patients have significant titers of antinuclear antibodies (ANA), and 80% have significant titers of rheumatoid factor (RF) (Anaya & Talal, 1997). Patients frequently have autoantibodies to intracellular ribonucleoproteins Ro (SS-A) and or La (SS-B). SS-A antibodies occur in 65% of SS patients, but are also found in patients with other connective tissue disorders. SS-B antibodies are found in 40% of SS patients, and more often in those with primary SS (Carsons & Harris, 1998). Both autoantibodies also are found in systemic lupus erythematosis. The erythrocyte sedimentation rate (ESR) may be elevated in SS or an associated connective tissue disorder. In 50% of SS patients, gamma globulins are elevated. They can be used to monitor the progression of the disease. Patients with elevated gamma globulins tend to have polymyopathy, renal tubular acidosis, or vasculitis as part of the disease process. β_2 microglobulin levels may be increased, especially in patients with renal disorders and lymphoproliferative disease. Increased levels of cryoglobulins occur in up to one third of SS patients. Approximately 25% of SS patients are anemic (Anaya & Talal, 1997).

SS, along with other autoimmune diseases, is associated with the presence of certain histocompatibility antigens. Patients with primary SS may test positively for the HLA-B8 DR3 gene. Patients with secondary SS and those with rheumatoid arthritis test positively for the HLA-DR4 gene (Carsons & Harris, 1998). It has been found that autoimmune diseases run in families, but the inheritance pattern is not predictable in SS. Therefore, the likelihood of passing SS to one's children is not high, and a relative may develop an autoimmune disease other than SS.

The diagnosis of SS often is not straightforward since other disease processes can mascarade as SS (see Table 27–3). For example, glandular swelling and dryness may occur in hepatitis C, hemochromatosis, diabetes, sarcoidosis, tuberculosis, amyloidosis, hepatic cirrhosis, hyperlipoproteinemia, and chronic pancreatitis (Fox, 1994). Additionally, salivary gland infiltrates and parotid swelling can develop in patients with HIV. The increased anticholinergic activity seen in some patients with multiple sclerosis results in clinical sicca symptoms. Viral infections, anxiety, depression, and lymphoproliferative diseases also are associated with sicca symptoms. Finally, symptoms of fatigue, fibromyalgia, and high titers of ANA are also found in chronic fatigue syndrome, which therefore, also must be included in the differential diagnosis. Under these circumstances, it is important to utilize lab tests and medical examination findings to obtain a correct diagnosis of SS (Table 27–2).

TREATMENT AND MANAGEMENT

Ocular

Although there is no cure, management of patients with SS is directed at reducing symptoms and preventing complications and disease progression by recognition and early treatment of the glandular and extraglandular manifestations. Treatment of the ocular manifestations of SS (Table 27–4) involves the frequent application of unpreserved artificial tears. Higher-viscosity agents, such as carboxymethylcellulose, can be used to extend tear film retention time and some may also provide mechanical protection of epithelial cells. In addition, lubricating ointments should be prescribed at night. Punctal occlusion, with collagen or silicone plugs, can be used to retain the precorneal tear film. Punctal plugs can be used as adjunctive therapy and are effective for chronic dry eye complaints. Other punctal procedures such as laser occlusion and electrocautery are not used very often.

Treatment for filamentary keratitis includes lubrication, sodium chloride drops and ointment, and acetylcysteine 10% drops, which break up mucous strands and filaments. Debridement of corneal filaments can be achieved with fine forceps or a sterile cotton-tipped applicator. If the symptoms are significant, a bandage soft contact lens may be considered. However, contact lenses should be used with caution because of the potential for exacerbation of dryness, keratitis, and secondary infection. A lateral tarsorrhaphy decreases the exposure area of the ocular surface and is only considered if other treatment methods fail. Moisture chambers and side shields attached to glasses are used in order to help prevent tear evaporation. Bacterial keratitis must be treated appropriately with antibiotics. Patients with blepharitis must be educated on lid hygiene and may require treatment with an antibiotic.

Patients with SS should receive regular examinations from their primary eyecare provider every 3 to 6 months depending upon their symptoms and ocular complications. In severe cases, even the best efforts of the eyecare provider cannot overcome the ocular surface damage and the symptoms that are associated with it. The patient's quality of life can be compromised.

TABLE 27–4. TREATMENT AND MANAGEMENT OF SJÖGREN'S SYNDROME

Systemic
- Creams/ointments for xerosis of the skin
- Sterile lubricants/moisturizers for vaginal dryness
- Antifungal creams for vaginal yeast infections
- Nonsteroidal anti-inflammatory agents (oral)
- Corticosteroids (oral)
- Immunomodulating agents: hydroxychloroquine, methotrexate, cyclophosphamide

Oral
- Dental hygiene
- Saliva substitutes
- Sugar-free gum and lozenges
- Increased water intake
- Mucolytic agents
- Saline nasal sprays
- Humidifiers
- Antifungal tablets/creams for yeast infections

Ocular
- Frequent application of artificial tears
- Lubricating ointments at night
- Punctal occlusion
- Debridement of filaments in filamentary keratitis
- Lid hygiene/antibiotic for blepharitis
- Antibiotic for bacterial keratitis
- Moisture chambers/glasses with side shields
- Lateral tarsorrhaphy if condition severe

Oral

Management of oral complications (Table 27–4) involves dental prophylaxis, such as the use of dental floss, toothpastes, and mouth rinses especially made for dry mouth; topical application of fluoride; and routine dental care. Saliva substitutes in the form of sprays can increase parotid flow rates for a short period of time. Oral yeast infections can be treated with antifungal tablets. Cheilitis (cracking at the angles of the cheek), usually due to *Candida* infection, can be treated with topical antifungal creams. These patients need to consume liquids regularly, especially during meals and often during sleep hours. The use of sugar-free gum and lozenges may help stimulate salivary flow.

Saline sprays help restore moisture to the nose. Humidifiers help to loosen up secretions and are especially helpful in dry climates and at high altitudes. Lavaging the sinuses with a saline irrigation system will help to remove dry, crusted secretions in patients with recurrent sinus blockage. Mucolytic agents can be used to break up thick, sticky secretions.

Systemic

Dermatologic and gynecologic symptoms must be addressed in patients with SS. Skin dryness is treated with creams and ointments. Vaginal mucosal problems can be treated with sterile lubricants, moisturizers, and antifungal creams for yeast infections. Because of the slightly increased risk of fetal death and congenital heart block, it is important that patients planning pregnancy be under the care of both an obstetrician experienced in handling patients with autoimmune diseases and a rheumatologist in order to provide the best care for both mother and fetus.

The major systemic medications used in SS patients consist of nonsteroidal anti-inflammatory drugs (NSAIDs), corticosteroids, and immunomodulating drugs. These medications have little effect on glandular disease and generally do not relieve symptoms of keratoconjunctivitis sicca or xerostomia. NSAIDs are commonly used in the treatment of arthralgias and myalgias. Systemic corticosteroids, because of adverse side effects, generally are reserved for persons with internal organ involvement, such as the lung, kidney, or nervous system, or those who develop vasculitis. Corticosteroids may also be used in patients with secondary SS for their underlying connective tissue disease.

Immunomodulating agents include hydroxychloroquine, methotrexate, and cyclophosphamide. Hydroxychloroquine is also useful in patients with rheumatoid arthritis and systemic lupus erythematosus. Hydroxychloroquine, depending on the dose, can cause corneal edema and a whorl-like pattern of pigment deposition in the corneal epithelium. These changes tend to be reversible upon discontinuation of the drug. Irreversible pigmentary disturbances can occur in the retina and form the classic bull's eye maculopathy. Other findings include arteriolar narrowing, optic disc pallor, visual field changes, decrease in visual acuity, and possible color vision changes and night blindness. These patients require careful monitoring for ocular side effects (generally every 6 months).

Methotrexate is commonly used in secondary SS when rheumatoid arthritis is the primary condition. It is sometimes used in patients with primary SS who have internal organ involvement. Cyclophosphamide has substantial side effects, and its use is limited to seriously ill patients with internal organ involvement or vasculitis. It can also be used as part of a chemotherapy regimen in those patients who develop lymphoma. Malignant lymphoma should be treated appropriately with chemotherapy, radiotherapy, or surgery. See Table 27–4 for a summary of the treatment and management of SS.

CONCLUSION

Sjögren's syndrome is a complex condition, not only causing keratoconjunctivitis sicca and xerostomia, but also involving extraglandular organs and systems. Although SS is a chronic illness, nearly all patients can lead productive lives. It is important that eyecare providers keep in mind that there are other common conditions that mimic the ocular manifestations in SS. A thorough case history probing ocular, oral, and other organ systems can help the practitioner make or rule out the diagnosis of Sjögren's syndrome.

Once the diagnosis of SS has been made, the optimal management of the SS patient involves a multidisciplinary approach. Medical care is rendered from the patient's rheumatologist, eyecare provider, dermatologist, dentist, otolaryngologist, and gynecologist. Although SS is usually a relatively benign disease, early detection and immediate initiation of appropriate and aggressive treatment of extraglandular lymphoproliferation is extremely important. SS, like many chronic conditions, requires stringent patient compliance. Therefore, proper patient education can be regarded as the most important component of the management of the SS patient.

REFERENCES

Anaya JM, Talal N. Sjögrens syndrome and connective tissue diseases associated with other immunologic disorders. In: Koopman WJ, ed. *Arthritis and Allied Conditions.* Baltimore: Williams & Wilkins; 1997:1561–1575.

Carsons S, Harris E, eds. *The New Sjögren's Syndrome Handbook.* New York: Oxford University Press; 1998.

Dry.Org. Internet Resources for Sjögren's Syndrome [Online]. Available: http://www.dry.org/ss95gui.html [1998, December 30].

Fox RI. Epidemiology, pathogenesis, animal models, and treatment of Sjögren's syndrome. *Curr Opin Rheumatol.* 1994a;6:501–508.

Fox RI. Vth International Symposium on Sjögren's Syndrome Clinical Aspects and Therapy. *Clin Rheumatol.* 1995;14 (suppl 1):17–19.

Fox RI, Kang Ho II. Pathogenesis of Sjögren's syndrome. *Rheum Dis Clin North Am.* 1992;18:517–538.

Fox RI, Saito I. Criteria for the diagnosis of Sjögren's syndrome. *Rheum Dis Clin North Am.* 1994b;20:391–407.

Friedlaender MH. Ocular manifestations of Sjögren's syndrome: Keratoconjunctivitis sicca. *Rheum Dis Clin North Am.* 1992;18:591–608.

Horsfall A, Isenberg D, eds. *Autoimmune Diseases Focus on Sjögren's Syndrome.* United Kingdom: Bios Scientific Publishers; 1994.

Pflugfelder SC, Crouse CA, Atherton SS. Epstein–Barr virus and the lacrimal gland pathology of Sjögren's syndrome. *Adv Exp Med Biol.* 1994;350:641–646.

St. Clair WE. New developments in Sjögren's syndrome. *Curr Opin Rheumatol.* 1993;5:604–612.

Sjögren's Syndrome Foundation. What is Sjögren's Syndrome [Online]. Available: http://www.sjogrns.com/whatis.htm[1998, December 30].

Sullivan DA, Sato EH. Potential therapeutic approach for the hormonal treatment of lacrimal gland dysfunction in Sjögren's syndrome. *Clin Immunol Immunopathol.* 1992; 64:9–16.

Talal N. Immunologic and viral factors in Sjögren's syndrome. *Clin Exp Rheumatol.* 1990;5(suppl 8):23–26.

Talal N. Sjögren's syndrome: Historical overview and clinical spectrum of disease. *Rheum Dis Clin North Am.* 1992; 18:507–515.

Toda I, Shinozaki N, Tsubota K. Hydroxypropyl methylcellulose for the treatment of severe dry eye associated with Sjögren's syndrome. *Cornea.* 1996;15:120–128.

Vitali C, Bombardieri S. Diagnostic criteria for Sjögren's syndrome: The state of the art. *Clin Exp Rheumatol.* 1990; 8:13–16.

Chapter 28

SARCOIDOSIS

Esther S. Marks

Sarcoidosis is a multisystemic granulomatous disease of unknown etiology. It was first described by the British physician Jonathon Hutchinson in 1898 as a dermatologic disorder termed Mortimer's malady (named for one of his patients). The current name sarcoidosis was derived from the term "sarkoid" coined by the Norwegian dermatologist Caesar Boeck in 1899, who felt the granulomatous skin lesion resembled a sarcoma. In 1909, Schumacher, a German physician, was the first to describe ocular involvement in sarcoidosis, in the form of an anterior uveitis.

Sarcoidosis is characterized most commonly by bilateral hilar lymphadenopathy, pulmonary infiltration, and dermatologic and ocular manifestations. In the nearly 100 years since it was first described, advances in diagnostic technology have significantly furthered the understanding of the pathogenesis of sarcoidosis, although medical researchers still remain puzzled as to the inciting agent.

EPIDEMIOLOGY

Systemic

The epidemiology of sarcoidosis varies around the world. In the United States, sarcoidosis has an age-adjusted annual incident rate of 10.9 per 100,000 Caucasians, and 35.5 per 100,000 African-Americans (Joint Statement, 1999). Several studies report the disease to be more virulent in African-Americans. There appears to be a slight female predilection. Peak incidence occurs in the third and fourth decades of life, although there appears to be another peak in the fifth to seventh decades, particularly in females. Reports of seasonal outbreaks and spatial clusters have lent credence to an infectious or environmental etiologic agent. Analyses of familial clusters suggest a polygenic mode of inheritance for sarcoidosis susceptibility.

Sarcoidosis involves many systems. Close to 95% of patients have pulmonary involvement. Muscle involvement is present in at least 50% of patients with little symptomatology. Although renal granulomas are common (demonstrated in up to 40% of patients), kidney dysfunction is unusual. Other manifestations include bone and joint involvement (up to 35%), dermatologic manifestations (25%), splenomegaly (up to 15%), hepatomegaly (up to 20%), bone marrow involvement (17%), neurologic manifestations (10%), endocrine involvement (up to 10%), clinically significant cardiac involvement (5%), clinically evident salivary gland involvement (5%), and mucous membrane manifestations (5%). The gastrointestinal system and the pancreas are rarely affected.

The course of the disease is highly variable, characterized by exacerbations and spontaneous or therapy-induced remissions. Chronic or progressive disease occurs in up to 30% of patients, whereas spontaneous regressions occur in approximately 65% of patients. In the United States, most sarcoidosis-related deaths (up to 5% of patients) are due to pulmonary complications, although cardiac and central nervous system complications are also responsible (Joint Statement, 1999).

Ocular

Ocular manifestations may occur in 17 to 64% of patients, although a frequency of 20 to 25% is most often cited. The reported frequencies of specific types of ocular manifestations are quite variable; however, the most common finding is anterior granulomatous uveitis, occurring in 50 to 85% of patients with ocular involvement. Posterior segment lesions of the choroid and retina may occur in 25%, and optic nerve involvement in as few as 5%. Sarcoidosis of the skin of the eyelid has been variably reported as occurring in 12 to 27%, and conjunctival granulomas in 44 to 56%. Keratoconjunctivitis sicca, secondary to lacrimal gland involvement, has been reported in as few as 4% and as many as 66%.

PATHOPHYSIOLOGY/DISEASE PROCESS

The etiology of sarcoidosis has been variably ascribed to infectious agents (viruses, mycobacteria, spirochetes, fungi), environmental factors (pine pollens, peanut dust, clay eating, hairsprays), drugs, chemicals, or an autoimmune dysfunction. Despite continuing controversy regarding its etiology, the pathogenesis of sarcoidosis has become clearer.

Sarcoidosis is characterized by noncaseating granuloma formation in multiple systems. These granulomas are composed mainly of epithelioid cells, as well as some giant cells. Activated T lymphocytes interact with monocytes, macrophages, and other inflammatory cells, encouraging the formation of granulomas and eventual fibrosis and hyalinization. Heightened cell-mediated immune processes (in particular elevated T-lymphocyte helper/suppressor ratios) occur at disease sites, and are depressed in the blood and at unaffected sites. Humoral immunity is elevated, with increases in many serum immunoglobulins.

Systemic

Sarcoidosis falls into two general groups: subacute/acute and chronic. The subacute/acute patient tends to have an abrupt onset of asymptomatic bilateral hilar lymphadenopathy, sometimes with parenchymal infiltration, and occasional erythema nodosum. The majority of these patients experience spontaneous resolution of the disorder without treatment within 2 years. The chronic sarcoidosis patient has usually had 2 or more years of symptoms. Onset is more insidious, consisting of pulmonary infiltrates, progressive dermatologic lesions, hepatosplenomegaly, and chronic ocular and other system involvement. The prognosis is generally poorer in chronic sarcoidosis. Treatment usually is required to relieve symptoms and signs.

Clinical presentation depends on the organ system or tissues affected and the degree of resulting dysfunction (Table 28–1). The vast majority of patients demonstrate pulmonary involvement (Figure 28–1). This usually begins as an alveolitis and proceeds to granuloma and fibrosis formation. The most common pulmonary symptoms are cough (mild to severe), dyspnea (mild to severe), wheezing, frequent chest pain, and occasional hemoptysis. Pleural effusion occasionally may occur, although pneumothorax is rare. Constitutional symptoms—malaise, weight loss, fever, fatigue—occur in approximately 30% of patients and may be quite disabling. Hilar, cervical, axillary, epitrochlear, inguinal, and supraclavicular lymphadenopathy are exceedingly common. The nodes are firm and nontender.

> Pulmonary involvement is overwhelmingly the most common systemic manifestation of sarcoidosis.

Dermatologic lesions, representing granulomatous infiltration, occur in about one quarter of patients. Erythema nodosum, common in European, Puerto Rican, and Mexican patients, is rare in African-American patients. It may erupt quite suddenly and severely in acute sarcoidosis, with tender red nodules often on the legs, accompanied by joint pain. Despite the severity of symptoms, this manifestation confers a favorable prognosis for spontaneous resolution of both the skin lesions and other concurrent sarcoid symptoms. Löfgren syndrome is a symptom complex characterized by erythema nodosum and bilateral hilar lymphadenopathy, with or without arthritis. It too, has a very favorable prognosis.

Other cutaneous manifestations may occur, often associated with chronic disease, requiring treatment or sometimes regressing on their own. The lesions may be plaque-like, papular, nodular, or infiltrative. The most common sites of involvement are the face (especially around the mouth, nose, and eyes), neck, and extensor surfaces of the extremities. These lesions may cause serious disfigurement such as in lupus pernio (more common in African-American females) involving the face and nose. Even scars may become infiltrated by granulomas. Dermatologic lesions usually

TABLE 28–1. SYSTEMIC MANIFESTATIONS OF SARCOIDOSIS

Pulmonary Involvement[a]
Alveolitis, followed by granulomatous infiltration, and fibrosis
Occasional pleural effusion, rare pneumothorax
Symptoms include cough, dyspnea, wheezing, chest pain, hemoptysis
Lymph Node Involvement
Firm and nontender enlargement of various nodes, especially hilar and mediastinal
Others include cervical, axillary, epitrochlear, inguinal, and supraclavicular
Constitutional Symptoms
Weight loss, anorexia
Fatigue, general malaise
Dermatologic Involvement
Erythema nodosum (Löfgren syndrome: erythema nodosum, bilateral hilar lymphadenopathy, with(out) arthritis)
Plaque-like, nodular, papular, or infiltrative lesions of the face (especially around the nose, mouth, and eyes), neck, and extensor surfaces of the extremities
Lupus pernio—disfiguring lesions of the face and nose
Scar infiltration
Mucous Membrane and Salivary Gland Involvement
Nasal cavity, sinuses, and larynx; enlarged parotid glands
Symptoms include nasal congestion, sinus headache, and hoarseness
Nasal septum perforation results in saddle nose deformity
Bone and Joint Involvement
Most commonly affects hands and feet with painful sausage swelling
Nasal bones, skull, axial skeleton, and long bones may also be affected
Bone cysts, lattice-like lesions, or punched-out lesions may occur
Acute migratory polyarthritis (ankles, knees, wrists, elbows, proximal interphalanges)
Chronic mono- or oligoarticular arthritis (knees or ankles)
Arthritic symptoms: painful, red, inflamed joints with limitation of motion
Neurologic and Muscular Involvement
Cranial nerve palsies, most commonly the VII, followed by the IX and X, VIII, and others
All types of peripheral neuropathies with paresthesias, neuralgias, muscle weakness, and atrophy
Tendon reflexes may be decreased or absent
Asymptomatic muscle infiltration more common than myopathy
Aseptic meningitis with headache, fever, and neck rigidity
Space-occupying granulomatous lesions throughout CNS (predilection for the base of the brain) with headaches, papilledema, lethargy, visual acuity and field loss, and seizures
Reticuloendothelial Involvement
Hepatosplenomegaly
Occasional serious liver dysfunction: hepatitis, cirrhosis, portal hypertension
Hypercalcemia and hypercalciuria may lead to nephrolithiasis and/or nephrocalcinosis
Cardiac Involvement
Cardiomyopathy, congestive heart failure, angina, valvular incompetence, and arrhythmias
Cor pulmonale and sudden death
Other Involvement
Gastrointestinal, pancreatic, and reproductive system involvement
Endocrine involvement may lead to diabetes insipidus and panhypopituitarism

[a]Most common manifestations.

are accompanied by mucous membrane, joint, and bone lesions.

Bone lesions in sarcoidosis may include cysts, punched-out lesions, or lattice-like lesions. Most commonly the hands and feet are involved, followed by the nasal bones, skull, axial skeleton, and ends of long bones. They may be asymptomatic, or present as painful, sausage swelling, with resulting bone deformity. Acute arthritis, particularly a migratory polyarthritis, involving the joints of the ankles, knees, wrists, elbows, and proximal interphalanges, is more common in females with sarcoidosis. Joints are red, inflamed, and tender. Pain and limitation of motion are characteristic. The arthritis may last a couple of weeks

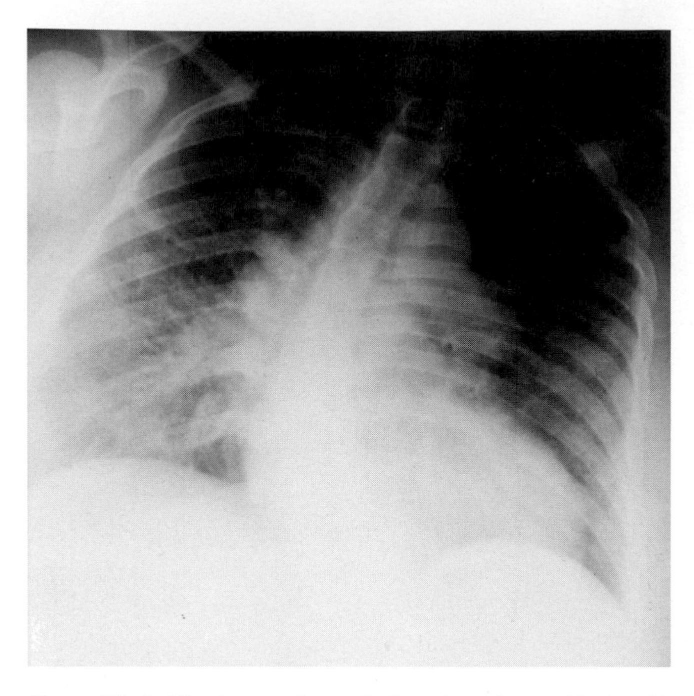

Figure 28–1. Chest x-ray demonstrating stage 2 sarcoidosis with bilateral hilar lymphadenopathy and pulmonary infiltrates.

to several months without permanent joint changes. Chronic arthritis is usually mono- or oligoarticular, involving the knees or ankles.

Mucous membrane involvement includes the nasal cavity, sinuses, and larynx. Patients may complain of sinus headaches, nasal congestion, and hoarseness. If nasal septum perforation from granulomatous infiltration occurs, the patient develops a saddle nose deformity. Salivary gland involvement also may occur with nontender bilateral parotid gland enlargement. This usually indicates chronic sarcoidosis. Parotid gland involvement often is accompanied by lacrimal gland infiltration resulting in a sicca complex of dry mouth and eyes.

Neurologic manifestations commonly involve the cranial nerves and meninges. Facial nerve palsy is the most common sign of neurosarcoidosis, occurring in greater than 50% of patients, and usually is caused by lower motor neuron dysfunction. It may be unilateral or bilateral, and may appear alone or along with other cranial nerve palsies. Most often it is transient. Various theories have been suggested to explain the pathogenesis of this palsy including compression by a swollen parotid gland and demyelinization. None have been substantiated. Other commonly involved cranial nerves are the optic nerves, the glossopharyngeal and vagus nerves (resulting in hoarseness), and the auditory nerves (resulting in deafness). These manifestations carry a poorer prognosis. The remaining cranial nerves are less commonly involved. Peripheral neuropathy may occur with paresthesias, neuralgias, and weakness or atrophy of muscles. Tendon reflexes may be depressed or absent. Several types of neuropathy have been described with sarcoidosis including Guillain–Barré syndrome. Muscular involvement is most commonly asymptomatic although myopathy has been observed.

Aseptic meningitis due to granulomatous infiltration of the meninges has been reported in up to one quarter of neurosarcoidosis patients. Fever, headache, and neck rigidity are common symptoms in both the acute and chronic forms. Seizures have also been reported in up to one quarter of patients with neurologic involvement, and generally indicate a poor prognosis. Although uncommon, space-occupying granulomatous lesions have been reported throughout the central nervous system, with a predilection for the base of the brain. Symptoms, common to most space-occupying masses, include headaches, seizures, decreased visual acuity, papilledema, and lethargy.

Both the liver and spleen may be enlarged asymptomatically. Occasionally, serious liver dysfunction may result in hepatitis, cirrhosis, or portal hypertension. Bone marrow and kidney involvement are also usually asymptomatic. However, hypercalcemia and the associated hypercalciuria may lead to nephrolithiasis (kidney stones) or nephrocalcinosis (diffuse kidney calcification). Hypercalcemia results from the production of 1,25-dihydroxy vitamin D by sarcoid granulomas. This increases the resorption of calcium from the gastrointestinal tract.

Although cardiac granulomatous infiltration may occur in up to one third of sarcoidosis patients, it is clinically significant in only 5%. It may lead to cardiomyopathy, congestive heart failure, angina, valvular incompetence, arrhythmias, or sudden death. The most common cardiac manifestation of sarcoidosis is cor pulmonale. This results from pulmonary hypertension due to extensive pulmonary disease. Prognosis is quite poor.

Although granulomatous involvement of the gastrointestinal tract, pancreas, reproductive system, and the endocrine system is rare, two disorders deserve mention. Diabetes insipidus should be suspected in a sarcoidosis patient presenting with polydipsia and polyuria. It is the result of involvement of the hypothalamic–pituitary axis. Panhypopituitarism is also reported secondary to sarcoidosis.

The mortality rate in sarcoidosis is primarily due to the complications of pulmonary insufficiency and cardiac involvement. Overall, the rate as reported is up to 5%.

Ocular

Manifestations of sarcoidosis may involve almost any ocular structure or tissue, and may be the presenting sign of the disease (Table 28–2). Uveitis, particularly anterior, is the most common ocular manifestation. It may present as subacute or chronic (as an incidental discovery on routine examination). If symptomatic, the patient may complain of a red, watery, photophobic, and blurry eye. The uveitis may be unilateral or bilateral, and is characterized by cells and flare, mutton fat keratic precipitates, and occasionally, iris nodules, although a nongranulomatous presentation may occur. Patients may not develop symptoms until complications occur, such as anterior and posterior synechiae (Figure 28–2), secondary glaucoma, secondary cataract, band keratopathy, or cystoid macular edema. Recurrent or chronic uveitis is usually associated with chronic sarcoidosis.

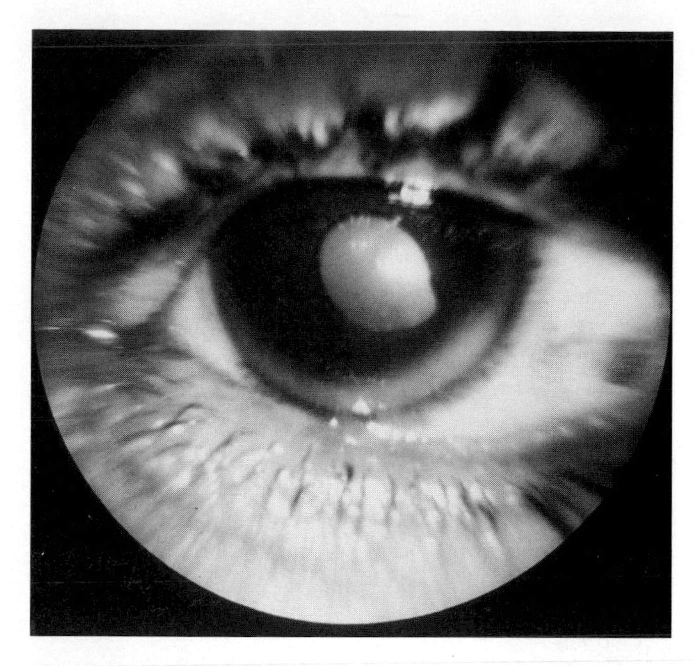

Figure 28–2. Chronic granulomatous uveitis resulting in posterior synechiae.

TABLE 28–2. OCULAR MANIFESTATIONS OF SARCOIDOSIS

Lid/Adnexal Involvement
Granulomatous lid lesions—papular, nodular, ulcerative, or plaque-like
Lacrimal gland enlargement with displacement of globe and distension of lid
Anterior Segment Involvement
Conjunctival (palpebral and fornix) granulomatous nodules—symptoms of irritation
Keratoconjunctivitis sicca—symptoms of sore, gritty, burning eyes
Anterior uveitis[a]
May be asymptomatic
Symptoms include red, watery, photophobic, blurred vision
Signs include cells, flare mutton fat KPs, vitreal spillover
If long-standing, may have posterior and/or anterior synechiae, secondary glaucoma, secondary cataracts, cystoid macular edema, and band keratopathy
Uveoparotid fever (Heerfordt syndrome): fever, parotid enlargement, and uveitis
Posterior Segment Involvement
Vitreal opacities—snowballs, string-of-pearls
Posterior uveitis or periphlebitis with retinal perivenous sheathing and yellow white exudates (candle wax drippings)
Rare occlusion of retinal veins
Neovascularization of disc or retina
Yellow-gray choroidal granulomas with or without overlying vitritis and vasculitis
Neuro-ocular Involvement
Cranial nerve palsy (restricted motilities, diplopia, ectropion, and lagophthalmos possible)
Papilledema secondary to intracranial lesions (headache, visual field defects, and visual acuity loss possible)
Direct optic nerve infiltration (disc edema, visual acuity loss, dyschromatopsia, visual field defects)
Optic atrophy (visual acuity loss, relative afferent pupillary defect)
Toxic Drug Effects
Steroids—cataract formation, glaucoma
Chloroquine—corneal deposits, bull's eye retinopathy

[a]Most common manifestations.

Posterior segment involvement most commonly presents as a periphlebitis or posterior uveitis (chorioretinitis). The vitreous may demonstrate spillover of inflammatory cells from an anterior uveitis, or present with fluffy snowballs or "string-of-pearls" opacities. Retinal veins may demonstrate yellow-white perivascular exudates ("candle wax drippings"). Sheathing of the vessels may occur anywhere in the fundus. Retinal and optic nerve neovascularization, believed to be due to capillary nonperfusion, may lead to vitreous hemorrhage and tractional retinal detachment. Initially, patients may be asymptomatic or present with blurry vision. Frank occlusion of the central retinal vein or one of its branches is rare. Choroidal granulomas may occur, appearing as yellow-grey lesions with or without an overlying vitreitis, or accompanying vasculitis.

Keratoconjunctivitis sicca may develop secondary to lacrimal gland infiltration. Patients may present with dry, gritty, burning eyes. Conjunctival involvement in sarcoidosis results in the formation of granulomas described as yellow nodules. These are most often found in the fornices and on the palpebral conjunctiva. Large nodules may produce irritation. Progressive cicatricial conjunctivitis has also been reported, with symptoms of chronic conjunctivitis—sore, red, itchy eyes. Granulomas of the skin of the eyelid also may occur. These may be nodular, papular, ulcerative, or plaque-like.

Neuro-ocular manifestations include extraocular muscle dysfunction secondary to cranial nerve palsies, papilledema secondary to intracranial sarcoid mass lesions, disc edema secondary to intraocular inflammation, and granulomatous involvement of the optic nerve at its head, intraorbital, or intracranial locations. Patients may report diplopia in the case of cranial nerve palsies and visual field defects from optic nerve involvement due to an intracranial mass lesion, along with painless loss of visual acuity and color vision, particularly with direct optic nerve infiltration. Optic atrophy may result when the optic nerve is compromised.

Ocular manifestations may occur in isolation or precede or occur concurrently with other manifestations. Certain symptom complexes may occur. Heerfordt syndrome, also known as uveoparotid fever, is characterized by fever, parotid gland enlargement, facial nerve palsy, and uveitis.

DIAGNOSIS

Systemic

Diagnosis (Table 28–3) requires a clinical and radiographic picture compatible with sarcoidosis, histologic confirmation of noncaseating granulomas via biopsy, and the elimination of other diseases, eg, tuberculosis (Table 28–4), that produce similar clinical pictures. Initial examination must include a thorough history and physical examination to reveal past or current signs and symptoms consistent with sarcoidosis. This should be followed by routine nonspecific hematologic tests (including erythrocyte sedimentation rate (ESR) or C-reactive protein (CRP), serum chemistries (including calcium and liver function tests), urinalysis, and chest x-rays. Tissue biopsy is the best diagnostic tool. Transbronchial lung biopsy (TLB) is the recommended procedure, although the patient should be carefully examined for a potentially less invasive site for biopsy—skin, lip, or superficial lymph node (Joint Statement, 1999).

Further tests used to determine the presence of sarcoidosis include serum angiotensin-converting enzyme (ACE), serum lysozyme, gallium scan, tuberculin skin testing (PPD) and anergy panel, Kveim–Siltzbach skin test, and when indicated, pulmonary function tests (PFTs) and bronchoalveolar lavage (BAL). Central nervous system involvement may require cerebrospinal fluid (CSF) examination, computerized tomography (CT), and magnetic resonance imaging (MRI). Electrocardiograms (ECGs), Holter monitoring, thallium scans, and echocardiography may be needed to reveal possible cardiac involvement. Many of these laboratory and imaging tests are nonspecific, and therefore must be interpreted in the context of the clinical picture.

TABLE 28–3. DIAGNOSTIC TESTS FOR SARCOIDOSIS

Systemic
Complete blood count (CBC)
Serum chemistries (including calcium, liver enzymes, creatinine, BUN)
Erythrocyte sedimentation rate (ESR) or C-reactive protein (CRP)
Serum angiotensin-converting enzyme (ACE)
Serum lysozyme
Urinalysis
Purified protein derivative (PPD) and anergy panel
Chest x-ray (CXR)
Pulmonary function tests (PFTs)
Tissue biopsy[a]
  Easily accessible site, eg, skin, lip, superficial lymph node
  Transbronchial lung biopsy (TLB)
If available:
  Kveim–Siltzbach skin test
When indicated:
  Bronchoalveolar lavage (BAL)
  Computerized tomography (CT)
  Magnetic resonance imaging (MRI)
  Cerebrospinal fluid (CSF) examination
  Electrocardiogram (ECG)
  Holter monitoring
  Thallium scan
  Echocardiography

Ocular
CBC
Serum chemistries
Serum ACE
CXR
PPD with anergy panel
Syphilis serology
Toxoplasmosis titers
ANA
Fluorescein and/or indocyanine green angiography
Tissue biopsy of conjunctival or lacrimal granuloma[a]
If inconclusive, consider:
  Serum lysozyme
  CT, MRI, or gallium scans
  PFTs
  Tissue biopsy eg, skin, lymph node, lung[a]
If available:
  Kveim–Siltzbach skin test

[a]Provides definitive diagnosis.

Routine laboratory tests may reveal a leukopenia (specifically lymphopenia and decreased T-lymphocyte helper/suppressor ratios) or thrombocytopenia, with occasional anemia, eosinophilia, monocytosis, and elevated ESR. Hypercalcemia, hypercalciuria, proteinuria, and abnormal liver function tests also may occur.

Elevated ACE levels have been observed in 34 to 90% of patients with active sarcoidosis. The sarcoid granulomas produce ACE, an enzyme that catalyzes the conversion of angiotensin I to the vasoconstrictor angiotensin II. However, ACE levels are elevated in a

TABLE 28–4. DIFFERENTIAL DIAGNOSIS OF SARCOIDOSIS (ABBREVIATED)

Systemic—Pulmonary Involvement
Mycobacteria, especially—*tuberculosis*
Histoplasmosis
Coccidioidomycosis
Cryptococcosis
Aspergillosis
Blastomycosis
Leprosy
Tumor-related granulomas
Wegener granulomatosis
Hypersensitivity pneumonitis
Beryllium disease
Interstitial pneumonia
Drug reactions
Aspiration of foreign matter

Ocular–Anterior Uveitis (Usually Granulomatous)
Granulomatous:
- Syphilis
- Tuberculosis
- Lyme disease
- Leprosy

Nongranulomatous:
- Anklyosing spondylitis
- Reiter syndrome
- Psoriatic arthritis
- Inflammatory bowel disease
- Juvenile rheumatoid arthritis
- Systemic lupus erythematosus
- Behçet disease

number of other diseases (eg, lymphoma, tuberculosis, cirrhosis, diabetes mellitus, Gaucher disease, and leprosy to name a few). The same is true of serum lysozyme levels. This enzyme is produced by the sarcoid granulomas, and therefore is usually elevated in active disease. However, it also may be elevated in other disease processes.

Chest radiography in sarcoidosis, although nonspecific, has been widely studied. Many diseases may present similarly, eg, tuberculosis, lymphoma, and carcinoma. Therefore, diagnostic tests to exclude other diseases must also be considered, such as the culturing of sputum, blood, and CSF to eliminate the possibility of an infectious etiology, e.g., tuberculosis.

A widely used staging (or typing) method has been devised for interpreting chest x-ray results, despite controversy concerning whether or not patients pass through the stages in a sequential fashion. Stage 0 denotes a clear chest x-ray, even though the patient may have abnormal pulmonary function. This stage may occur either early or late in the disease. Stage 1 is characterized by bilateral hilar lymphadenopathy, usually a manifestation of early disease that resolves within 1 to 2 years. Stage 2 represents bilateral hilar lymphadenopathy plus parenchymal infiltration, which does not carry as good a prognosis although symptoms usually resolve. Stage 3 presents as pulmonary infiltration only, whereas stage 4 is characterized by fulminant infiltration and fibrosis. Patients with stage 4 sarcoidosis have the least favorable prognosis, as they may develop respiratory failure, pneumothorax, and cor pulmonale. In addition to chest x-rays, radiography of suspected bone and/or joint involvement may be performed looking for punched-out lesions, cysts, and lattice-like lesions.

Patients suspected of having restrictive pulmonary disease should undergo PFTs. Although nonspecific in nature, these tests may provide information concerning the presence of infiltrative lung disease, even prior to being visible on radiography. Forced vital capacity and forced expiratory volume are often reduced.

Tissue biopsy provides histologic confirmation of noncaseating granulomas. Tissue samples should first be obtained from easily accessible sites (e.g., skin, mucous membranes, conjunctiva, or lacrimal gland) if available. If not, transbronchial lung biopsy or biopsies of lymph nodes, liver, or skeletal muscle may be considered.

Characteristic immune changes in sarcoidosis include increased humoral immunity, ie, elevations in serum complement, circulating immune complexes, and autoantibodies; depressed peripheral cell-mediated immunity, ie, lymphopenia and cutaneous anergy (on tuberculin skin testing [PPD], and anergy panels); and increased cell-mediated immunity at disease sites as seen with bronchoalveolar lavage (BAL). BAL uses a fiberoptic bronchoscope in the distal airway. Saline is instilled and then removed by suction. Elevated levels of T lymphocytes are recovered in active pulmonary sarcoidosis.

The Kveim–Siltzbach skin test, another immunological test for sarcoidosis, is believed to be a delayed hypersensitivity reaction to some unknown antigen. A saline suspension of human sarcoidal tissue is injected intradermally in the flexor surface of the forearm. Approximately 4 to 6 weeks later, a positive result will demonstrate the appearance of a nodule that may be biopsied to reveal noncaseating granuloma formation. Positive results are found in 59 to 94% (75% being the most commonly stated figure) of sarcoidosis patients, with a very low false-positive rate. Although less invasive than lung biopsy or bronchoalveolar lavage, the skin test has several disadvantages. It is limited by the excessive length of time necessary to obtain positive results; it requires the avoidance of systemic steroids for the duration of the test; and most importantly, the Kveim antigen is not commercially available.

Examination of CSF is usually reserved for aiding in the diagnosis of meningitis. Meningeal involvement in neurosarcoidosis may reveal elevated protein levels, normal or decreased glucose levels, and pleocytosis. The CSF may also be cultured to rule out an infectious etiology.

Imaging techniques other than chest radiography may be utilized for diagnosis of intra- or extrathoracic sarcoidosis. The routine use of chest CT scans for the diagnosis of pulmonary sarcoid is often advocated because of reported higher sensitivity (Hansell & Kerr, 1991). CT and MRI scans are especially useful in the diagnosis of neurosarcoidosis. Gallium scans are also useful because gallium 67 has been found to accumulate in active sarcoidal tissue. It is particularly helpful in delineating lacrimal gland, parotid gland, and intrathoracic involvement. However, its use is limited in abdominal and skeletal evaluation, because normal bone and abdominal viscera will absorb gallium. Studies are ongoing into other imaging techniques that may aid in the diagnosis of sarcoidosis such as positron emission tomography (PET) (Mañá, 1997)

Ocular

Ocular manifestations may be readily diagnosed (see Tables 28–3 and Table 28–4) with a comprehensive eye examination. Evaluation may reveal decreased visual acuity, dyschromatopsia, pupil abnormalities, or restricted motilities secondary to neuro-ocular involvement or intraocular inflammation. Slit-lamp biomicroscopy may reveal an apparently prolapsed lacrimal gland, lid swelling and erythema, a displaced globe, a dry eye, superficial punctate keratitis, symblepharon formation, or conjunctival or lid nodules. Intraocular inflammation will manifest characteristically with cells, flare, and keratic precipitates (usually mutton fat), along with potential complications such as posterior or anterior synechiae, increased intraocular pressure (secondary glaucoma), secondary cataract, band keratopathy, and cystoid macular edema in long-standing cases.

Posterior segment involvement may be visualized with dilated fundus examination. Vitreal opacities, perivenous retinal yellow exudates and sheathing, choroidal granulomas, neovascularization of the optic nerve or retina, papilledema, or optic nerve pallor may be revealed. Fluorescein, and more recently, indocyanine green angiography may assist in the evaluation of chorioretinal involvement and neovascularization.

> Sarcoidosis should always be considered in a patient presenting with a granulomatous uveitis.

Intraocular inflammation suspected to be secondary to sarcoidosis should be investigated with routine diagnostic tests including an ESR or CRP, serum ACE level, chest x-ray, PPD with anergy panel, syphilis serology, toxoplasmosis titers (for posterior uveitis), and antinuclear antibody testing to rule out an autoimmune etiology. A lacrimal gland mass, optic nerve involvement, or cranial nerve palsy requires imaging techniques—CT, MRI, or gallium scans of the head and orbits to rule out tumors, demyelinating diseases, vascular lesions, etc. Conjunctival or lacrimal gland biopsy should be considered to demonstrate noncaseating granulomas. Patients suspected to have sarcoidosis should be evaluated by an internist for medical management, and further evaluation by a dermatologist, neurologist, or pulmonary specialist may be indicated.

TREATMENT AND MANAGEMENT

Systemic

Patients with asymptomatic hilar lymphadenopathy do not require treatment. Routine chest x-rays every 6 months should be performed until the adenopathy disappears (usually within 1 to 2 years). However, patients with symptomatic or progressive intrathoracic disease, persistent constitutional symptoms, or sarcoidosis involving other organ systems require systemic medical therapy (Table 28–5).

Corticosteroids are the mainstay of sarcoidosis treatment, although optimal dose and duration have never been clinically studied in randomized, prospective trials. A 2-week loading dose, followed by a taper to a 6- to 12-month maintenance dose, followed by another taper (as long as a relapse does not occur) are usually recommended. Medication may be given daily or its equivalent on alternate days. Local administration of corticosteroids may be useful. Steroid inhalers or nasal sprays may alleviate local symptoms. Intralesional injections of steroids may resolve certain cutaneous lesions. Complications due to steroid therapy may result, e.g., weight gain, diabetes mellitus, hypertension, cataracts, and glaucoma. Therefore, the patient on systemic corticosteroid therapy must be closely monitored. Despite immune suppression from steroid therapy, there have been reports of sarcoidosis patients concurrently infected with the human immunodeficiency virus (HIV) that have been effectively treated with corticosteroids (Lee & Chronister, 1999; Lowery et al, 1990).

Cytotoxic drugs are used in chronic or refractory disease. Methotrexate also has been found to be effective in refractory cases, and in the treatment of disfiguring cutaneous sarcoidosis. Azathioprine has been

TABLE 28–5. TREATMENT AND MANAGEMENT OF SARCOIDOSIS

SYSTEMIC

- Asymptomatic bilateral hilar lymphadenopathy monitored every 6 months with chest x-ray without treatment
- Symptomatic or progressive pulmonary disease, cardiac disease, neurologic disease, and hypercalcemia require medical therapy

Corticosteroids

- Oral corticosteroids
  - Therapy may be daily or its equivalent on alternate days
  - Oral prednisone 30–40mg qd × 2 weeks
  - Taper to maintenance dose × 6–12 months, then slow taper
- Local corticosteroids
  - Steroid inhalers or nasal sprays may be used for airway involvement
  - Intralesional injections for cutaneous lesions

Cytotoxic agents

- Methotrexate
  - Used in patients with chronic disease and cutaneous sarcoidosis
  - 10–25mg/weekly, repeated if relapse occurs
- Azathioprine
  - Used in patients with chronic disease
  - 50–200 mg/day
- Others
  - Cyclophosphamide 50–150 mg/day orally; 500–2000 mg every 2–4 weeks intravenously

Noncytotoxic agents

- (Hydroxy)chloroquine
  - Used to treat hypercalcemia and cutaneous sarcoidosis; 200–400 mg qd
- Cyclosporine
  - Used in chronic disease and refractory neurosarcoidosis, 5–10 mg/kg/day
- Ketoconazole
  - Used to treat hypercalcemia
- NSAIDs
  - Used for musculoskeletal symptoms and erythema nodosum

Anticytokines

- Thalidomide
  - Possible use in severe cutaneous sarcoidosis
- Pentoxifylline
  - May be beneficial at 400 mg tid

Radiation therapy

- Used in selected cases of neurologic disease

Surgical treatment

- Cardiac pacemakers or defibrillators
- Intervention for expanding intracranial masses or increased intracranial pressure
- Lung and other organ transplantation in end-stage disease

OCULAR

- Comanagement with the healthcare team
- Recalcitrant anterior uveitis, posterior segment and orbital involvement; require standard systemic treatment with oral prednisone, although additional local ocular therapy may be necessary
- Anterior uveitis
  - Topical prednisolone acetate 1% q 1–6 hours
  - Topical cycloplegia e.g., scopolamine 0.25% bid to tid
  - Periocular steroid injections if recalcitrant
  - Antiglaucoma medications if necessary
- Eyelid lesions
  - Intralesional injection of steroids
- Cicatricial conjunctivitis
  - Subconjunctival or sub-Tenon steroid injection
- Keratoconjunctivitis sicca
  - Artificial tears solution prn
  - Artificial tears ung qhs if indicated
  - Punctal occlusion if necessary
- Chorioretinal involvement
  - Systemic steroids required but in higher doses, e.g., 60–100 mg prednisone qd with taper
  - If cystoid macular edema exists, consider acetazolamide 250 mg qd or an NSAID, e.g., indomethacin 25 mg tid × 6 weeks
  - Retinal capillary nonperfusion and neovascularization may require panretinal photocoagulation
  - Vitrectomy and retinal detachment repair if necessary
- Toxic drug effects
  - Monitor patients on prednisone for cataract formation and glaucoma development
  - Monitor patients on chloroquine for corneal deposits, decreased visual acuity, and bull's eye retinopathy

Abbreviations: bid, twice a day; q, each, every; qd, every day; tid, three times a day.

found to be useful in severe refractory cases. Although effective, chlorambucil has been replaced with other drugs beacause of its high toxicity/malignancy rate. Cyclophosphamide is also limited by high toxicity.

Noncytotoxic drugs, including antimalarials, cyclosporine, ketoconazole, and anticytokines, have been used effectively in sarcoidosis. The antimalarial chloroquine is used to treat cutaneous sarcoidosis. A daily loading dose for 2 weeks followed by a 6-month maintenance dose has been particularly efficacious in disfiguring skin involvement. Hydroxychloroquine (Plaquenil) is also used. Should chloroquine treatment be instituted, a preliminary ocular examination and follow-up examinations every 6 months must be performed to rule out the development of toxic ocular side effects. Cyclosporine has been limited to refractory neurosarcoidosis and chronic disease due to its toxicity levels. Nonsteroidal anti-inflammatory drugs (NSAIDs) are particularly useful in the treatment of musculoskeletal symptoms and erythema nodosum. The antifungal ketoconazole is effective in treating hypercalcemia in sarcoidosis patients by lowering circulating 1,25-dihydroxyvitamin D and serum calcium levels. Tumor necrosis factor (TNF) is a cytokine that mediates part of the inflammatory response in sarcoidosis. Both thalidomide and pentoxyfylline, drugs with anti-TNF activity, have been reported to be beneficial, although further studies are needed (Baughman & Lower, 1997).

Radiation therapy has been used in a limited number of cases of neurosarcoidosis, although surgical intervention may be required in cases of expanding intracranial masses or increased intracranial pressure. Cardiac involvement may necessitate the placement of pacemakers or defibrillators. In end-stage cases, successful lung and other organ transplantation have been reported.

Ocular

The treatment of ocular sarcoidosis varies according to the ocular tissue(s) involved (see Table 28–5). The presence of other organ involvement also determines treatment protocol. Many ocular manifestations may be managed with topical, local, and/or systemic steroids.

Anterior uveitis is treated with the standard protocol of topical steroids and cycloplegic agents. Antiglaucoma medications may be required in cases of secondary glaucoma. Recalcitrant anterior uveitis, as well as cicatricial conjunctivitis, may be relieved with subconjunctival or sub-Tenon steroid injections. Lid lesions may respond to intralesional injections of steroids. Systemic steroids are required with anterior uveitis unresponsive to topical and injected steroids, posterior segment manifestations, and orbital involvement (e.g., lacrimal gland enlargement).

Patients on topical or systemic steroids, as well as patients on antimalarials, must be monitored for potential toxic effects. Although steroids may cause the development of cataracts or glaucoma, both these complications may be treated successfully (cataract extraction or medical glaucoma therapy) without necessarily discontinuing the medication. However, should a patient develop toxic ocular complications from (hydroxy) chloroquine, a prompt decrease in dose or total withdrawal may be required to avoid irreversible vision loss from a dose-related pigmentary retinopathy (bull's eye retinopathy). Patients on antimalarials should be examined every 6 months for changes in visual acuity, color vision, Amsler grid, retinal changes, and corneal deposits. Amsler grid monitoring at home should be encouraged.

Prophylactic panretinal photocoagulation may be considered for retinal capillary nonperfusion. The goal is to prevent proliferative retinopathy. However, retinal and/or optic nerve neovascularization often occurs despite prophylaxis, requiring further photocoagulation. Vitrectomy and retinal detachment surgery may be required.

Keratoconjunctivitis sicca symptoms should be relieved with topical lubricants. The severity will determine the appropriate treatment regimen. Occasionally, punctal occlusion may be required.

CONCLUSION

Sarcoidosis is a granulomatous disease characterized by pulmonary, cutaneous, ocular, and other organ system involvement. Although the pathogenesis of the disease has been elucidated, the etiology still remains unknown despite intensive research. Frequent ocular involvement, often presenting as the initial manifestation of the disease, may lead to the correct systemic diagnosis. Therefore, the eyecare provider is an integral member of the healthcare team managing the sarcoidosis patient.

REFERENCES

Alexander LJ. Ocular manifestations of sarcoidosis. In: *Primary Care of the Posterior Segment.* Norwalk, CT: Appleton & Lange; 1989: 194–196.

Arnold WJ. Sarcoidosis. In: Kelley WN, Harris ED, et al, eds. *Textbook of Rheumatology.* Philadelphia: WB Saunders; 1993: ch 83.

Austin JHM. Pulmonary sarcoidosis: What are we learning from CT? *Radiology.* 1989;171:603–604.

Badrinas F, et al. Seasonal clustering of sarcoidosis. *Lancet* 1989;ii:455–456.

Bascom R, Johns CJ: The natural history and management of sarcoidosis. *Adv Intern Med.* 1986;31:213–241.

Baughman RP, Lower EE. Steroid-sparing alternative treatments for sarcoidosis. *Clinics Chest Med.* 1997;18:853–864.

Bell NH. Endocrine complications of sarcoidosis. *Endocrinol Metab Clin North Am.* 1991;20:645–654.

Brownstein S, et al. Sarcoidosis of the eyelid skin. *Can J Ophthalmol.* 1990;25:256–259.

Chapelon C, et al. Neurosarcoidosis: Signs, course and treatment in 35 confirmed cases. *Medicine.* 1990;69:261–276.

Collison JMT, Miller NR, Green WR. Involvement of orbital tissues by sarcoid. *Am J Ophthalmol.* 1986;102:302–307.

Drosos AA, et al. The forgotten cause of sicca complex: Sarcoidosis. *J Rheumatol.* 1989;16:1548–1551.

Duker JS, Brown GC, McNamara JA. Proliferative sarcoid retinopathy. *Ophthalmology.* 1988;95:1680–1686.

Ferry AP. The eye and rheumatic diseases. In: Kelley WN, Harris ED, et al, eds. *Textbook of Rheumatology.* Philadelphia: WB Saunders; 1993:516–517.

Geggel HS, Mensher JH. Cicatricial conjunctivitis in sarcoidosis: Recognition and treatment. *Ann Ophthalmol.* 1989; 21:92–94.

Hansell DM, Kerr IH. The role of high resolution computed tomography in the diagnosis of interstitial lung disease. *Thorax.* 1991;46:77–84.

Hosoda Y, Yamaguchi M, Hiraga Y. Global epidemiology of sarcoidosis: What story do prevalence and incidence tell us? *Clin Chest Med.* 1997;18:681–694.

Jabs DA, Johns CJ. Ocular involvement in chronic sarcoidosis. *Am J Ophthalmol.* 1986;102:297–301.

James DG, Williams WJ. Kveim-Siltzbach test revisited. *Sarcoidosis.* 1991;8:6–9.

Johns CJ, Scott PP, Schonfeld SA. Sarcoidosis. *Ann Rev Med.* 1989;40:353–371.

Joint Statement of the American Thoracic Society (ATS), the European Respiratory Society (ERS) and the World Association of Sarcoidosis and Other Granulomatous Disorders (WASOG): Statement on sarcoidosis. *Am J Respir Crit Care Med.* 1999;160:736–755.

Jordan DR, et al. Optic nerve involvement as the initial manifestation of sarcoidosis. *Can J Ophthalmol.* 1988; 23:232–237.

Jordan DR, et al. The diagnosis of sarcoidosis. *Can J Ophthalmol.* 1988;23:203–207.

Karma A, Huhti E, Poukkula A. Course and outcome of ocular sarcoidosis. *Am J Ophthalmol.* 1988;106:467–472.

Kimmel AS, et al: Branch retinal vein occlusion in sarcoidosis. *Am J Ophthalmol.* 1989;107:561–562.

Lee AK, Chronister CL. Sarcoidosis-related anterior uveitis in a patient with human immunodeficiency virus. *J Am Optom Assoc.* 1999;70:384–390.

Lieberman J. Enzymes in sarcoidosis: Angiotensin-converting-enzyme (ACE). *Clin Lab Med.* 1989;9:745–755.

Lightman S, Chan CC. Immune mechanisms in chorioretinal inflammation in man. *Eye.* 1990;4:345–353.

Lowery WS, et al. Sarcoidosis complicated by HIV infection: Three case reports and a review of the literature. *Am Rev Respir Dis.* 1990;142:887–889.

Mañá J. Nuclear imaging: ^{67}Gallium, ^{201}Thallium, ^{18}F-labeled fluoro-2-deoxy-D-glucose positron emission tomography. *Clin Chest Med.* 1997;18:799–812.

Mayers M. Ocular sarcoidosis. *Int Ophthalmol Clin.* 1990; 30:257–263.

Moller DR. Etiology of sarcoidosis. *Clin Chest Med.* 1997; 18:695–706.

Newman LS, Rose CS, Maier LA. Sarcoidosis. *N Engl J Med.* 1997;337:1224–1234.

Rothova A, et al. Risk factors for ocular sarcoidosis. *Doc Ophthalmol.* 1989;72:287–296.

Sharma OP. *Sarcoidosis: Clinical Management.* London: Butterworths; 1984.

Sharma OP, Sharma AM. Sarcoidosis of the nervous system: A clinical approach. *Arch Intern Med.* 1991;151:1317–1321.

Siltzbach LE, et al. Course and prognosis of sarcoidosis around the world. *Am J Med.* 1974;57:847–852.

Silver MR, Messner LV. Sarcoidosis and its ocular manifestations. *J Am Optom Assoc.* 1994;65:321–327.

Spaide RF, Ward DL. Conjunctival biopsy in the diagnosis of sarcoidosis. *Br J Ophthalmol.* 1990;74:469–471.

Stampfl DA, et al. Sarcoidosis causing duodenal obstruction: Case report and review of gastrointestinal manifestations. *Dig Dis Sci.* 1990;35:526–532.

Stanford MR, Graham EM. Systemic associations of retinal vasculitis. *Int Ophthalmol Clin.* 1991;31:23–33.

Thomas PD, Hunninghake GW. Current concepts of the pathogenesis of sarcoidosis. *Am Rev Respir Dis.* 1987; 135:747–760.

Tingey DP, Gonder JR. Ocular sarcoidosis presenting as a solitary choroidal mass. *Can J Ophthalmol.* 1992;27:25–29.

Toews GB, Lynch JP. Editorial commentary: Methotrexate in sarcoidosis. *Am J Med Sci.* 1990;300:33–36.

Toner GC, Bosl GJ. Sarcoidosis, "sarcoid-like lymphadenopathy," and testicular germ cell tumors. *Am J Med.* 1990;89:651–656.

Weinreb RN, Tessler H. Laboratory diagnosis of ophthalmic sarcoidosis. *Surv Ophthalmol.* 1984;28:653–664.

Winterbauer RH, Kirtland SH, Corley DE. Treatment with corticosteroids. *Clin Chest Med.* 1997;18:843–851.

Wolfensberger TJ, Herbort CP. Indocyanine green angiographic features in ocular sarcoidosis. *Ophthalmology.* 1999; 106:285–289.

Zic JA, et al. Treatment of cutaneous sarcoidosis with chloroquine: Review of the literature. *Arch Dermatol.* 1991; 127:1034–1040.

Chapter 29

INFLAMMATORY BOWEL DISEASE

Susan P. Schuettenberg

Inflammatory bowel disease (IBD) is a term used to describe a variety of chronic bowel afflictions ranging from mild to severe. Although ocular complications are not frequent, they may occur. Inflammatory bowel disease is usually divided into two categories: ulcerative colitis (UC) and Crohn's disease (CD). UC is an inflammatory disease of the colon characterized by diffuse inflammation of the colon's mucosal layer. CD is found throughout the gastrointestinal tract and involves full-thickness inflammation of the gut wall.

EPIDEMIOLOGY

Systemic

IBD is found to be more common among Caucasians than African-Americans. It affects an equal number of men and women. Although IBD is a disease of the young adult (peak occurrences between age 15 and 35), it can occur at any age. The incidence of IBD is higher in the Jewish population, especially those of Ashkenazi heritage. Two to five percent of IBD patients will have at least one affected relative.

Worldwide, the incidence of UC has been found to be 6 to 8 cases per 100,000, and its prevalence is numbered at 50 to 70 cases per 100,000. Although the incidence of CD is set at 2 cases per 100,000, with a prevalence of 20 to 40 cases per 100,000, many feel that this disease is on the rise.

Ocular

The overall frequency of extraintestinal manifestations of IBD is approximately 35%. On average, 10% of all patients with CD have ocular complications. With UC, ocular manifestations occur much less frequently and are much less severe. Posterior segment involvement has also been reported, but the incidence is less than 1% of patients with IBD.

PATHOPHYSIOLOGY/DISEASE PROCESS

Systemic

The cause of IBD remains unknown. Although there is a strong genetic predisposition for the disease, environmental influences probably play a role. Research is currently underway to identify the genes responsible for IBD. In addition, a higher than normal prevalence of haplotype HLA-B27 has been found among IBD patients. An autoimmune etiology is theorized since immune complexes have been found circulating in patients' blood. These are thought to be the cause of the many extraintestinal manifestations. Alteration of the mucosal barrier of the intestine allows for microorganisms to act as antigens. This in turn elicits an immune response from the lymph tissue of the intestines. The resultant antigen–antibody complexes circulate systemically, and once deposited in distant tissue provoke an inflammatory response, causing tissue damage.

UC and CD are chronic conditions characterized in most patients by exacerbations and remissions that range from mild to severe and even life-threatening (Table 29–1).

UC is restricted to the mucosal lining of the colon, and usually involves the rectum. The major symptoms are abdominal pain and bloody diarrhea. Fever, weight loss, anorexia, dehydration, and anemia can occur in those patients with severe colitis. Patients may present in a number of ways, ranging from proctitis alone (inflammation of the anus and rectum) to pancolitis (inflammation of the entire colon). The prognosis is good for those patients with proctitis as the sole manifestation, but for those presenting with pancolitis, hospitalization is required. For cases of mild colitis, remission can be achieved through medical or surgical treatment (colectomy).

An extreme case of UC can result in a condition termed toxic megacolon. This complication is marked by dilation of the colon (more than 6 cm in diameter) with extreme thinning of the bowel wall. The patient becomes critically ill and is at risk for perforation of the colon with resulting peritonitis. This is a life-threatening situation with a high rate of mortality.

TABLE 29–1. SYSTEMIC MANIFESTATIONS OF INFLAMMATORY BOWEL DISEASE

Ulcerative Colitis
- Crampy lower abdominal pain, relieved with bowel movement
- Bloody diarrhea
- Fever, weight loss, anorexia
- Proctitis
- Pyoderma gangrenosum
- Kidney stones
- Bowel carcinoma
- Erythema nodosum

Endoscopy reveals:
- Only *mucosal* involvement
- Bowel foreshortening
- Blurred vascular pattern
- Deep ulcerations
- Pseudopolyps

Crohn's Disease
- Constant abdominal pain, usually in the lower right quadrant, relieved with bowel movement
- Formed or diarrheal stool, usually *not* bloody
- Fever, weight loss >5% body weight, malnutrition
- Intermittent bowel obstruction
- Aphthous ulcers
- Perianal/perirectal abscesses
- Bowel carcinoma
- Liver and kidney involvement
- Arthritis

Endoscopy reveals:
- Involvement of *all* layers of bowel wall
- Strictures
- Fistulas
- Skip lesions
- String signs

Prolonged periods of spontaneous remission can occur in cases of UC, with a patient enduring only minimal symptoms. Clinically, the course of the disease may vary, with more than half of all UC patients suffering a relapse within 1 year of diagnosis. Most patients suffering from UC have a normal lifespan, with death occurring only as a result of a severe complication such as bowel perforation or the development of carcinoma of the colon.

The inflammatory lesions of CD may be found throughout the gastrointestinal tract, from the mouth to the anus and rectum. Unlike UC, bowel involvement in CD tends to be irregular and discontinuous.

Crohn's disease can be subdivided by bowel distribution. In approximately 30% of patients, the inflammation involves the small intestine only (especially the terminal ileum). This is called regional enteritis. Another 30% suffer from inflammation of the colon alone, and this is termed Crohn's colitis, granulomatous colitis, or Crohn's disease of the colon. The final 40% have ileocolitis, with involvement of the ileum and parts of the large intestine (usually the ascending colon).

Unpredictable flare-ups and spontaneous remissions mark the clinical course of this disease. Diarrhea, abdominal pain (especially in the lower right quadrant), weight loss exceeding 5% of total body weight, vomiting, dehydration, and a low-grade fever signal the onset of a flare-up. If the small intestine is extensively involved, intermittent bowel obstruction is likely to occur. Perianal or perirectal abscesses may also be present. The mortality rate is found to increase with the duration of CD, with as many as 10% dying due to complications such as sepsis and peritonitis.

Extraintestinal manifestations of IBD are quite common. For example, UC is characterized by nephrolithiasis (kidney stones), erythema nodosum (an inflammatory reaction of subcutaneous fat resulting in tender red nodules of the skin), and an indolent necrotic skin lesion termed pyoderma gangrenosum. Patients with UC also have a high incidence of colonic cancer.

CD is marked by arthritis (both ankylosing and migratory), renal disorders, liver function abnormalities, and bowel carcinoma. In addition, stomatitis (inflammation of the mouth) and aphthous ulcers of the buccal mucosa (superficial ulcers of the mouth) are frequent findings.

One serious complication that occurs in up to 30% of children and adolescents with IBD is delayed growth and development. Decreased nutritional intake due to malabsorption from the affected bowel is partially responsible for this problem. Therefore, an aggressive nutritional program is extremely important in preventing or reversing growth retardation and delayed sexual maturation.

The extraintestinal manifestations found in IBD may on occasion precede a bowel flare-up, and are often the most disabling part of the disease. Not only do these complications occur after the diagnosis of IBD has been made, but they can also be a presenting symptom. Most will be relieved by an improvement in the colitis or following treatment or surgery.

Ocular

The ocular manifestations found in both UC and CD may (1) precede the onset of the disease or an acute attack of either form of IBD; (2) follow the same pattern of exacerbation and remission as the systemic disease; or (3) present as a chronic condition with exacerbations and remissions of its own. The ocular complications may range from benign to blinding.

Ocular manifestations of UC are relatively rare, but when present, the most common is uveitis (Figure 29–1). For those patients suffering from CD, uveitis and episcleritis are among the most common findings. In addition, conjunctivitis and keratopathy as well as other ocular manifestations have been reported (Table 29–2).

In the IBD literature, keratopathy is the general term used to describe any corneal involvement ranging from stromal infiltrates to corneal ulcers. Conjunctival changes associated with CD have been divided into three patterns: granuloma formation, fibrovascular membrane proliferation, and blepharoconjunctivitis. Scleritis, although a less common ocular complication, is important because it is one of the most sight-threatening ocular manifestations of IBD (Figure 29–2).

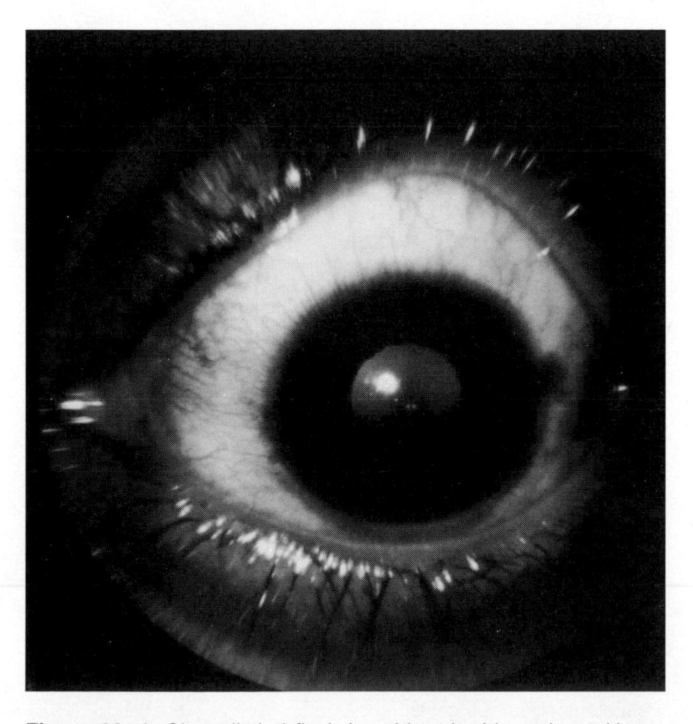

Figure 29–1. Circumlimbal flush is evident in this patient with anterior uveitis.

TABLE 29–2. OCULAR MANIFESTATIONS OF INFLAMMATORY BOWEL DISEASE

Crohn's Disease	
• Episcleritis	Common
• Uveitis	Common
• Blepharitis	Rare
• Conjunctivitis	Rare
• Keratitis	Rare
• Scleritis	Rare
• Scleromalacia perforans	Rare
• Xerophthalmia	Rare
• Cataracts	Rare
• Orbital myositis	Rare
• Proptosis	Rare
• Optic disc edema	Rare
• Central serous retinopathy	Rare
• Macular hemorrhage	Rare
• Macular edema	Rare
• Neuroretinitis	Rare
• Exudative retinal detachment	Rare
• Choroidal folds	Rare
• Retrobulbar neuritis	Rare
• Endophthalmitis	Rare
• Orbital cellulitis	Rare
Ulcerative Colitis	
Uveitis	Rare
Optic neuritis	Rare

DIAGNOSIS

Systemic

The diagnosis of IBD (Table 29–3) is based on the presenting signs and symptoms (Table 29–1). Laboratory studies are *not* considered to be beneficial in the diagnosis of IBD, except to rule out other etiologies.

The diagnosis of UC requires a view of the sigmoid colon via endoscopy, revealing a red mucosa that bleeds easily, the absence of a normal mucosal blood vessel pattern, and possible pseudopolyps. Radiographic findings may include a foreshortened colon with a narrowed lumen, strictures, deep ulcerations, and pseudopolyps (Figure 29–3). A biopsy of the rectal mucosa is necessary to rule out carcinoma or amebiasis (colitis caused by the *Entamoeba histolytica* parasite), and a stool sample is needed to exclude bacterial diarrhea (Table 29–4).

The diagnosis of CD also is one of exclusion, and is based on endoscopy and radiologic studies, including

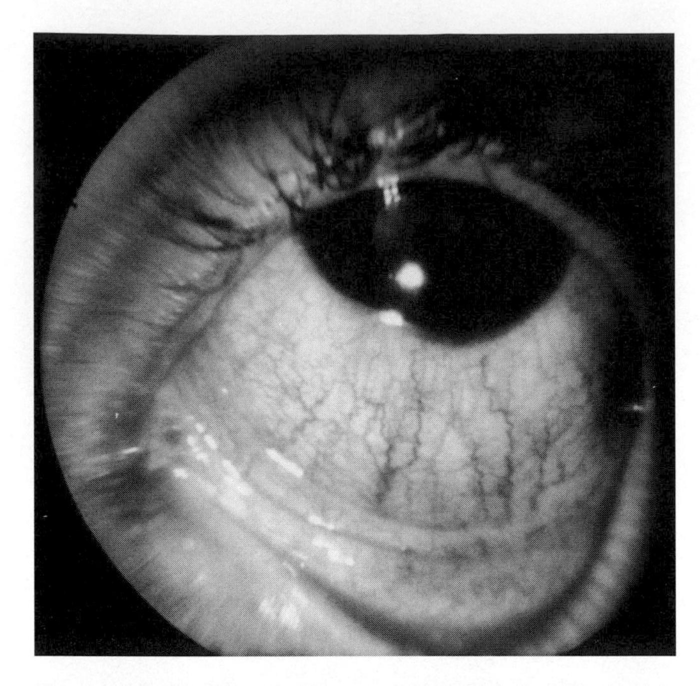

Figure 29–2. Nodular scleritis secondary to Crohn's colitis. Nodule appears at the 7 o'clock position at the limbus. (*Reprinted with permission from Schuettenberg SP. Nodular scleritis, episcleritis, and anterior uveitis as ocular complications of Crohn's Disease.* J Am Optom Assoc. *1991;62:377–381.*)

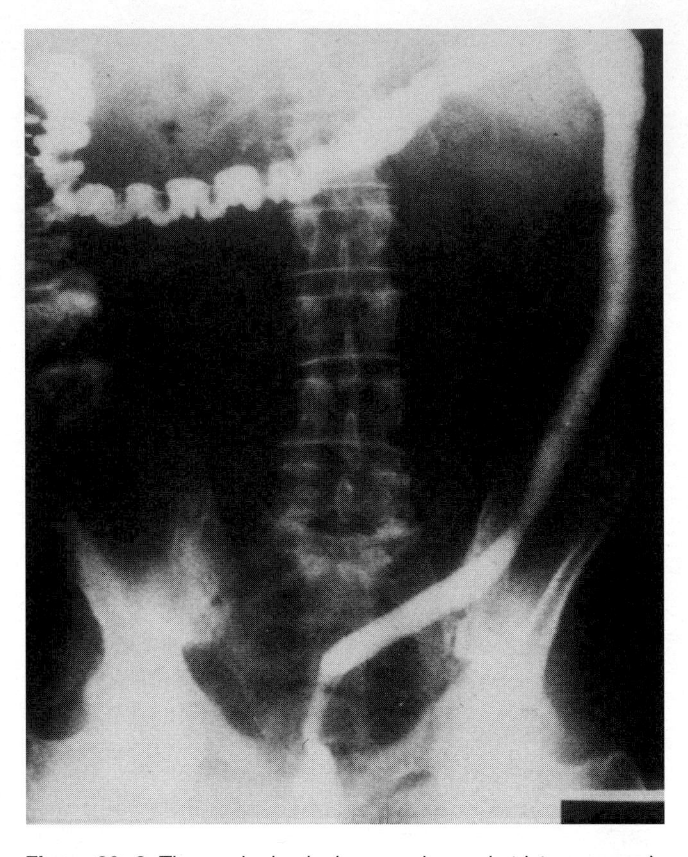

Figure 29–3. The marked colonic narrowing and strictures seen in this x-ray can be characteristic of chronic ulcerative colitis. (*Reproduced from* Hospital Medicine, *September 1990, with the permission of Cahner's Publishing Co.*)

a barium enema. Biopsy of the bowel will reveal full-thickness inflammation of the bowel wall, with granulomas found in the serosa. This results in adhesions between adjacent loops of the intestine and to other abdominal organs. Major radiographic findings include intestinal strictures, longitudinal ulcers, and internal bowel fistulas (bowel to bowel, bladder, vagina, abdominal wall, or skin), which can contribute to nutritional problems. In addition, "skip" areas—sections of normal intestine intervening between diseased bowel—can occur. A reduction in the size of the intestinal lumen of the small bowel is termed the "string sign," and also is characteristic of CD. Again, there is no truly reliable lab test to indicate the activity of the disease.

Ocular

The eyecare professional must be aware that ocular manifestations can occur prior to, during, or after a bout of IBD. Therefore, IBD should be considered in the systemic differential diagnosis of a patient who presents with recurrent episcleritis, recurrent uveitis, or scleritis.

> The ocular manifestations of IBD (as well as the other extraintestinal manifestations) may occur before, during, or after a bowel flare-up. They can sometimes be the presenting symptom of IBD.

TABLE 29–3. DIAGNOSTIC TESTS FOR INFLAMMATORY BOWEL DISEASE

Systemic
- Stool sample
- Endoscopy with biopsy
- Radiographic studies

Ocular
- HLA-B27
- X-ray of sacroiliac joint

TABLE 29–4. DIFFERENTIAL DIAGNOSIS OF INFLAMMATORY BOWEL DISEASE

Systemic
Carcinoma of colon
Amebiasis
Bacterial diarrhea
Ischemic colitis
Pseudomembranous colitis

Ocular
Reiter's syndrome

Reiter syndrome can occasionally be marked by arthritis, uveitis, and diarrhea, and therefore should enter into the differential diagnosis (see Table 29–4).

TREATMENT AND MANAGEMENT

Systemic

The goal of therapy in the treatment of IBD is to control the disease activity by decreasing the bowel inflammation, reducing the abdominal pain, controlling the episodes of diarrhea, and optimizing nutrition, thereby improving the quality of life. The medical treatment of CD and UC requires the use of many of the same agents, and will be discussed together (Table 29–5).

TABLE 29–5. TREATMENT AND MANAGEMENT OF INFLAMMATORY BOWEL DISEASE

Systemic

Ulcerative colitis
- Supportive measures (bed rest, change in eating habits)
- Aminosalicylates (sulfasalazine, mesalamine, olsalazine)
- Corticosteroids (orally or topically)
- Surgical intervention (colectomy) if unresponsive to treatment

Crohn's disease
- Supportive measures
- Aminosalicylates
- Antibiotics (Flagyl, Cipro, Biaxin)
- Corticosteroids (orally or topically)
- Immunosuppressants (azathioprine, 6-mercaptopurine, cyclosporine, methotrexate)
- Surgical intervention (colectomy) if unresponsive to treatment

Ocular

Conjunctivitis
- Topical steroid therapy

Episcleritis
- Warm/cold compresses prn
- Artificial tears qid
- Moderate cases: add topical decongestant qid
- Severe cases: topical NSAID or mild steroid

Keratopathy (depending on type of corneal involvement)
- Topical antibiotic (Polytrim)
- Topical steroid

Uveitis
- Topical steroid qid to q4h depending on severity
- Mydriatic/cycloplegic bid

Scleritis
- Topical steroid q4h or more for patient comfort
- Indomethacin (75–100 mg PO daily) or flubiprofen (300 mg PO daily)
- If unresponsive or severe, add prednisone (60–80 mg PO daily, taper once the pain has subsided, then discontinue after 2 weeks)
- Combined therapy using lower dosages of NSAID and corticosteroid if treatment fails or patient cannot tolerate required doses
- If unremitting, penicillamine or cyclophosphamide
- Scleral inlay grafts if scleral perforation occurs (rare)

Abbreviations: bid, twice a day; NSAID, nonsteroidal anti-inflammatory drug; PO, orally; prn, as required; q, each, every; qid, four times daily.

Mild to moderate acute IBD is treated with supportive measures such as bed rest and a change in eating habits, including removing roughage from the diet. Conventional medical management utilizes oral or topical steroids, antibiotics, and aminosalicylates. Those agents containing 5-aminosalicylic acid (5-ASA) include sulfasalazine, mesalamine, and olsalazine sodium. An anti-inflammatory agent, 5-ASA is the active ingredient that locally inhibits the synthesis of prostaglandins and leukotrienes (compounds that are mediators of the inflammatory reaction). If the 5-ASA therapy is not sufficient, corticosteroid therapy may be helpful either alone or in conjunction with the 5-ASA. Oral prednisone or a topical enema therapy (of hydrocortisone, prednisolone, or budesonide) can be administered. When the acute attack of IBD has subsided, 5-ASA should be continued because it decreases the incidence of future flare-ups. Chronic steroid therapy is sometimes required for those patients who cannot achieve a remission without it, or in those whose disease flares up whenever steroids are tapered.

The use of antibiotics is somewhat controversial in the management of IBD. The mechanism of action is unknown, but those studies that have been undertaken show a definite benefit for patients with CD. Treatment includes the use of metronidazole (Flagyl), ciprofloxacin (Cipro), clarithromycin (Biaxin), and tetracycline.

Immunosuppressant agents have become the accepted therapy for those patients with intractable IBD, despite their significant side effects. The potent immunosuppressants involved are azathioprine, 6-mercaptopurine (6-MP), cyclosporine, and methotrexate. Moreover, recent trials of immunomodulatory treatments using cytokines (interleukins) and anticytokines are promising. The majority of patients utilizing these treatments suffer from CD, since refractory cases of UC are referred for surgery (colectomy and ileoanal pouch anastomosis).

Treatment of toxic megacolon (an extreme case of acute UC) consists of immediate hospitalization and initiation of high doses of corticosteroids and broad-spectrum antibiotics. If the dilation of the colon continues, emergency colectomy is the treatment.

Twenty to twenty-five percent of all UC patients will require surgical treatment. This consists of a total colectomy and is considered a "cure," since UC is confined to the colon. A colectomy is necessary when the colitis is either unremitting or unresponsive to therapy.

Surgical treatment for CD is helpful in controlling the disease, but it will not cure the patient. Bowel resection is reserved for the complicated cases of CD—those with fistula formation, bowel narrowing, abscesses, toxic megacolon (much less common in CD), and bowel perforation. However, many are reluctant to advise surgery since there is a 50 to 75% recurrence rate over a 5-year period. Often, those patients who have suffered from CD for a number of years will have had much of their small intestine removed, since new lesions are always developing.

Ocular

In cases of both UC and CD, steroid therapy is particularly indicated in the treatment of extraintestinal manifestations, including ocular complications (see Table 29–5). The steroid therapy will help keep the bowel inflammation in check, thereby reducing the likelihood of other complications. Most ocular problems occur after a flare-up has begun, but they have been found to precede the bowel inflammation as well.

The most common ocular complications found in patients with IBD are anterior uveitis, episcleritis, keratopathy, and conjunctivitis.

Uveitis is treated with a course of topical steroids and mydriatic or cycloplegic agents. The frequency and duration of the medication depends on the presentation and severity of each case. Typically, the steroid is tapered to prevent a rebound of the inflammation.

Episcleritis is usually treated with supportive measures: warm/cold compresses several times a day, artificial tears, topical decongestants, or topical nonsteroidal anti-inflammatory drugs (NSAIDs). In severe cases, some have been known to use a mild steroid.

The treatment of the keratopathy varies from the use of topical antibiotics to topical steroid therapy, depending on the type of corneal involvement.

The conjunctival changes associated with CD have been successfully treated with topical steroid therapy (Wright, 1980).

The treatment of scleritis can begin with topical steroid therapy for patient comfort, but this is rarely sufficient to control the condition. Systemic NSAIDs such as indomethacin or flurbiprofen are then added to suppress the destructive process until remission occurs naturally. For unresponsive scleritis or severe inflammation such as necrotizing scleritis, systemic steroids are needed. Patients with IBD may already be on a course of steroids for the bowel inflammation, but if they are not, then daily doses of prednisone are initiated, tapered once the pain has subsided, and then discontinued after 2 weeks. If either of these treatments fails to control the inflammation, or if the patient cannot tolerate the dosage required, then combination therapy using lower dosages of both the corticosteroid and the NSAID can be initiated.

In unremitting cases of scleritis, cytotoxic immunosuppressive agents such as penicillamine or cyclophosphamide may be used, but with extreme caution due to their severe systemic side effects. Subconjunctival injections of steroids are to be avoided, because this action may accelerate the deterioration of the sclera. Surgical treatment (scleral inlay grafts) is useful only in the rare case of perforation.

Since ocular involvement may occur during a bout of IBD, treatment of the bowel inflammation with steroids and anti-inflammatory agents will have a beneficial effect on any ocular complication.

CONCLUSION

Inflammatory bowel disease primarily affects younger patients, and may range from mild to severely debilitating. Existing treatment protocols may be beneficial, although the side effects of long-term corticosteroid use may be problematic. Removal of the diseased colon will ultimately cure UC, but no known cure exists for CD. Ocular complications can occur at any point in the disease process (even prior to diagnosis); therefore, IBD should be considered in the systemic differential diagnosis of a patient with recurrent uveitis, recurrent episcleritis, or scleritis. Appropriate intervention early in the course of the disease is particularly beneficial.

REFERENCES

Bonner GF. Current medical therapy for inflammatory bowel disease. *South Med J.* 1996;89:556–566.

Botoman VA, Bonner GF, Botoman DA. Management of inflammatory bowel disease. *Am Fam Physician.* 1998; 57:57–68.

Crohn BB. Ocular lesions complicating ulcerative colitis. *Am J Med Sci.* 1925;169:261–267.

Ernst BB, Lowder CY, Meisler DM, et al. Posterior segment manifestations of inflammatory bowel disease. *Ophthalmology.* 1991;98:1272–1280.

Evans JP, Eustace P. Scleromalacia perforans associated with Crohn's disease. *Br J Ophthalmol.* 1973;57:330–335.

Greenstein AJ, Janowitz HD, Sachar DB. The extraintestinal complications of Crohn's disease and ulcerative colitis: A study of 700 patients. *Medicine.* 1976;55:401–412.

Hopkins DJ, Horan E, Burton IL, et al. Ocular disorders in a series of 332 patients with Crohn's disease. *Br J Ophthalmol.* 1974;58:732–737.

Knox DL, Schachat AD, Mustonen E. Primary, secondary and coincidental ocular complications of Crohn's disease. *Ophthalmology.* 1984;91:163–173.

Korelitz BI, Coles RS. Uveitis (iritis) associated with ulcerative and granulomatous colitis. *Gastroenterology.* 1967; 52:78–82.

Lyons JL, Rosenbaum JT. Uveitis associated with inflammatory bowel disease compared with uveitis associated with spondylarthropathy. *Arch Ophthalmol.* 1997;115:61–64.

Macoul KL. Ocular changes in granulomatous ileocolitis. *Arch Ophthalmol.* 1970;84:95–97.

Mondino BJ, Phinney RB. Treatment of scleritis with combined oral prednisone and indomethacin therapy. *Am J Ophthalmol.* 1988;106:473–479.

O'Morain C. *Crohn's Disease: Treatment and Pathogenesis.* Boca Raton, FL: CRC; 1987.

Petrelli EA, McKinley M, Troncale FJ. Ocular manifestations of inflammatory bowel disease. *Ann Ophthalmol.* 1982; 14:356–360.

Present DH. Inflammatory bowel disease: Extraintestinal manifestations. *Mt Sinai J Med.* 1983;50:126–132.

Rankin GB, Watts HD, Melnyk CS, Kelley ML. National cooperative Crohn's disease study: Extraintestinal manifestations and perianal complications. *Gastroenterology.* 1979; 77:914–920.

Robinson M. Optimizing therapy for inflammatory bowel disease. *Am J Gastroenterol.* 1997;92:12S–17S.

Rosenthal S, Snyder J, Hendricks K, et al. Growth failure and inflammatory bowel disease: Approach to treatment of a complicated adolescent problem. *Pediatrics.* 1983; 72:481–490.

Rutgeerts P, Lofberg R, Malchow H, et al. A comparison of budesonide with prednisolone for active Crohn's disease. *N Engl J Med.* 1994;331:842–845.

Schachter H, Kirsner J. *Crohn's Disease of the Gastrointestinal Tract.* New York: Wiley; 1980:12–124.

Sedwick LA, Klingele TG, Burde RM, et al. Optic neuritis in inflammatory bowel disease. *J Clin Neuro-ophthalmol.* 1984; 4:3–6.

Sleisenger MH, Fordtran JS. *Gastrointestinal Disease: Pathophysiology, Diagnosis and Management.* Philadelphia: Saunders; 1989:1327–1358.

Strauss RE. Ocular manifestations of Crohn's disease: Literature review. *Mt Sinai J Med.* 1988;55:353–356.

Watson P. Diseases of the sclera and episclera. In: Duane TD, ed. *Clinical Ophthalmology.* Philadelphia: Harper & Row; 1989;1–30.

Watson PG. The diagnosis and management of scleritis. *Ophthalmology.* 1980;87:716–720.

Wright P. Conjunctival changes associated with inflammatory disease of the bowel. *Trans Ophthal Soc UK.* 1980; 100:96–97.

Section VII

SKELETAL AND CONNECTIVE TISSUE DISORDERS

Chapter 30

PAGET DISEASE

Margaret McNelis

Paget disease, also known as osteitis deformans, is a chronic, progressive disorder of bone characterized by abnormal osteoclastic activity. Abnormal and accelerated bone formation and resorption can cause prominent skeletal deformities as well as vascular and nervous systems manifestations. Ocular involvement can occur as a result of local bone deformity causing compression of the optic nerve, globe, or lacrimal duct. Angioid streaks are also found in patients with Paget disease.

EPIDEMIOLOGY

Systemic

Paget disease affects between 0.1 and 3.0% of the population by the fifth decade, and 11% in their ninth decade. It is most prevalent in persons from the United Kingdom and their descendants. More recently, however, the incidence and severity appears to be falling. One study showed men with polyostotic disease had low-activity forms, compared to women, who tended toward moderate- or high-activity disease.

Ocular

Angioid streaks are found in 8 to 15% of patients with Paget disease. In addition, there is a clear association of optic neuropathy; however, the incidence is not known.

PATHOPHYSIOLOGY/DISEASE PROCESS

Systemic

The etiology of Paget disease is unknown, but there appears to be a hereditary predisposition. A viral etiology has also been proposed, with possible links to measles, respiratory syncytial virus, and canine distemper virus. The pathophysiologic mechanism is one of excessive bone resorption followed by the production of abnormal new bone, leading to structural and functional alterations of the skeleton and adjacent tissues.

The disease takes place in three phases, and each may occur simultaneously in one or more bones. The osteolytic phase is characterized by excessive osteoclastic bone resorption and increased vascularity of the affected bone. The osteoclasts in Paget disease are especially large, sometimes containing up to 100 nuclei. This stage is followed by the mixed phase, in which simultaneous osteolytic and osteoblastic activity occurs, with the deposition of lamellar (also called pagetic) bone. Lastly, in the osteosclerotic phase, dense, less vascular bone is laid down in a mosaic pattern. The most commonly affected bones are the cranium (osteoporosis circumscripta), clavicles, pelvis, and long bones, especially in the lower extremities. When there is vertebral involvement, it usually occurs in the thoracic and lumbar region.

Skeletal findings include deformity and pathologic "chalkstick" (the bone breaks cleanly) fractures, which can occur as a result of the abnormal bone activity. Symptoms may include deep bone pain and warmth over the affected areas. Other systems can be affected, depending upon the site(s) of bone malformation (Table 30–1). Loss of lumbar lordosis and paraparesis may result from pagetic dorsal or cervical vertebra in spinal artery steal syndrome. When the cranium is involved, the superficial temporal artery may become more prominent. Basilar invagination may develop as the skull base softens and weight of the cranium increases (Figure 30–1). As this occurs, the basilar arteries may become compressed, leading to severe brainstem and cerebellar dysfunction. Neurological symptoms may suggest compression of the brain, spinal cord, and peripheral and cranial nerves. These symptoms include headaches with Valsalva maneuver or straining, trigeminal neuralgia, hemifacial spasm, and numbness or weakness of the extremities. Later, flexor spasms and sphincter difficulties may develop. Similar complications arise from hydrocephalus, when communication between the ventricular–aqueductal system is impaired.

> Sudden pain, despite treatment, may indicate a fracture or neoplasm at the pagetic bone site.

TABLE 30–1. SYSTEMIC MANIFESTATIONS OF PAGET DISEASE

Skeletal System
- Skeletal deformities of cranium, clavicles, long bones (especially lower extremities), vertebrae (thoracic and lumbar region) (C)
- Chalkstick fractures (C)
- Basilar invagination of the skull, compressing basilar artery and leading to severe brainstem and cerebellar dysfunction, hydrocephalus (M)
- Dental complications (C)
- Bone tumors: osteogenic sarcoma; fibrosarcoma; multiple myeloma; lymphatic leukemia (R)

Hearing Loss
- Secondary to (1) bone changes and vascular ischememic damage to 8th cranial nerve and (2) conduction loss from ossicle sclerosis and otitis media from chronic eustachian tube obstruction (M)

Vascular Abnormalities Secondary to Pagetic Bone Changes
- Arterial calcification (C)
- Congestive heart failure (M)
- Vascular ischemia of neural structures secondary to shunting of blood through hypervascular pagetic bone (pagetic steal) (M)
- Temporal artery prominence (M)
- Heart block from intracardiac calcification (R)

C, common; M, more frequently than rarely; R, rare.

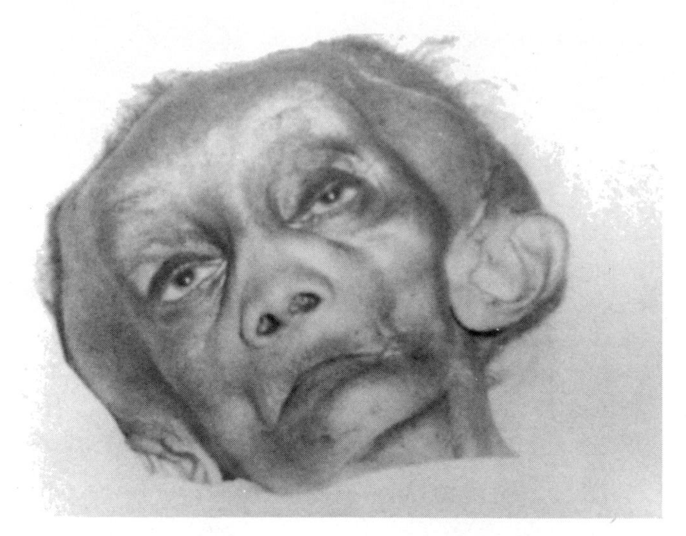

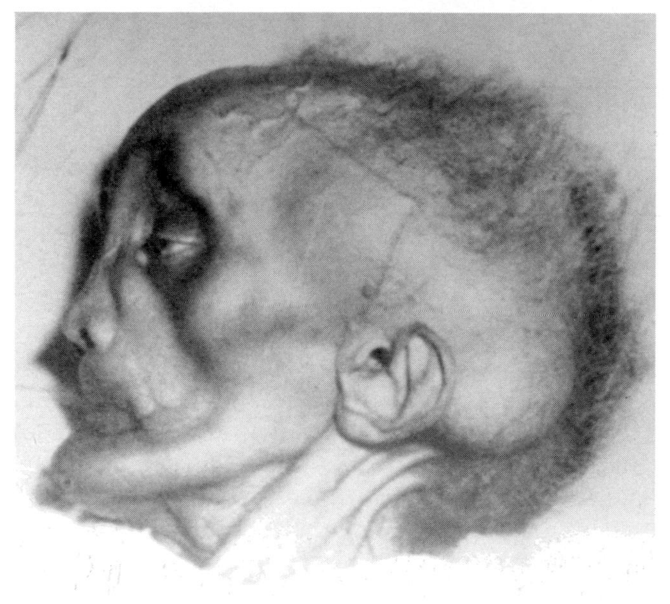

Figure 30–1. Increased cranium size due to bony malformation. (*Reprinted with permission from Renie WA.* Goldberg's Genetic and Metabolic Eye Disease. *2nd ed. Boston: Little, Brown; 1986:484.*)

Dental complications include loosening and loss of teeth from osteolytic disease, and malocclusion from overgrowth of bone. Infections may follow dental surgery.

Several serious vascular abnormalities may develop secondary to the pagetic bone changes. These include congestive heart failure, heart block from intracardiac calcification, and arterial calcification. Shunting of blood through hypervascular pagetic bone also leads to vascular ischemia of neural structures. This phenomenon is known as "pagetic steal."

Hearing loss is extremely variable and occurs in 30 to 50% of patients with skull involvement. Sensory neural loss is due primarily to temporal bone and petrous ridge changes with resultant vascular ischemic damage to the eighth cranial nerve. These patients may also report tinnitus and vertigo. Conductive hearing loss can also occur as a result of ossicle sclerosis and chronic otitis media from constriction of the eustachian tube.

The most serious complication of Paget disease is the development of primary bone tumors. These tumors almost always arise in pagetic bone. The most frequent tumor is the osteogenic sarcoma. Less than 1% of Paget patients develop this tumor; however, in patients who have multiple pagetic sites (or polyostotic disease), it may occur in as many as 10% of patients. The second most common tumor is the fibrosarcoma. Occasional occurrence of hematopoietic tumors, such as multiple myeloma and lymphatic leukemia, have also been reported. All of these tumors are aggressive and lethal.

Ocular

Ocular compromise in Paget patients may occur due to local bone deformity, angioid streaks, and metabolic and/or vascular disturbances (Table 30–2). Angioid streaks are the most common ocular manifestation. Clarkson and Altman (1982) reviewed active cases of Paget disease. They found that those patients with angioid streaks had been diagnosed for a longer period of time and had more sites of the disease than those with normal eye findings. This implies a correlation between disease duration and amount of ocular involvement. This study also indicated that approximately 20% of patients with active skull involvement developed angioid streaks. These may become complicated by subretinal neovascularization and disciform macular scars. Ocular symptoms may include metamorphopsia or scotomas if subretinal neovascularization occurs.

TABLE 30–2. OCULAR MANIFESTATIONS OF PAGET DISEASE

Angioid Streaks in Retina
- Can cause subretinal neovascularization and disciform macular scar

Local Bone Deformity
- Optic neuropathy
- Extraocular muscle palsy
- Exophthalmos
- Epiphora secondary to lacrimal duct obstruction

Vascular Disturbances
- Optic neuropathy

Other
- Increased intraocular pressure and glaucoma
- Chondrosarcoma

Optic neuropathy may be caused by local bone compression to the optic nerve. Interestingly, Eretto and colleagues (1984) found that only 2 of 9 patients with Paget disease exhibiting visual field defects associated with optic neuropathy had optic canal encroachment, indicating another cause for the neuropathy, possibly a result of pagetic "steal." Elevation of intraocular pressure, glaucoma, and orbital chondrosarcoma have also been reported.

Local bone compression of the globe or cranial nerves can cause exophthalmos or extraocular muscle involvement with subsequent diplopia. Patients may complain of epiphora if the lacrimal duct is compressed.

DIAGNOSIS

Systemic

Paget disease is rarely diagnosed before the age of 35, and is often a spurious finding when x-ray or blood examinations are performed for another disorder. Diagnosis is based on clinical signs and symptoms, as well as laboratory testing (Table 30–3). Elevation of the serum alkaline phosphatase (an index of osteoblastic activity) is more than twice the upper normal limit in Paget disease. Elevation of urinary pyrodinoline excretion is a sensitive marker of bone resorption, found in 73% of Paget patients. Characteristic radiographic findings will confirm the diagnosis. Technetium-99 diphosphonate bone scans are used to determine the extent of bony involvement, and are the most sensitive means to detect active lesions of Paget disease, although this is not a specific test for the disease (Figure 30–2). In this test, the scanning agent is adsorbed (attached) onto "hot" areas, indicating regions of increased bone vascularity and mineralization. Confirmational x-rays are then taken of the positive regions of the scans. Bone biopsy is rarely necessary, but may occasionally be used when differentiating "burned

TABLE 30–3. DIAGNOSTIC TESTS UTILIZED IN PAGET DISEASE

Systemic
- Bone scan
- X-ray
- CT/MRI
- Serum alkaline phosphatase
- Urinary hydroxyproline and pyridinoline

Ocular
- Fundus photography
- Fluorescein angiography
- Amsler grid
- Westergren ESR, if sudden loss from neuropathy

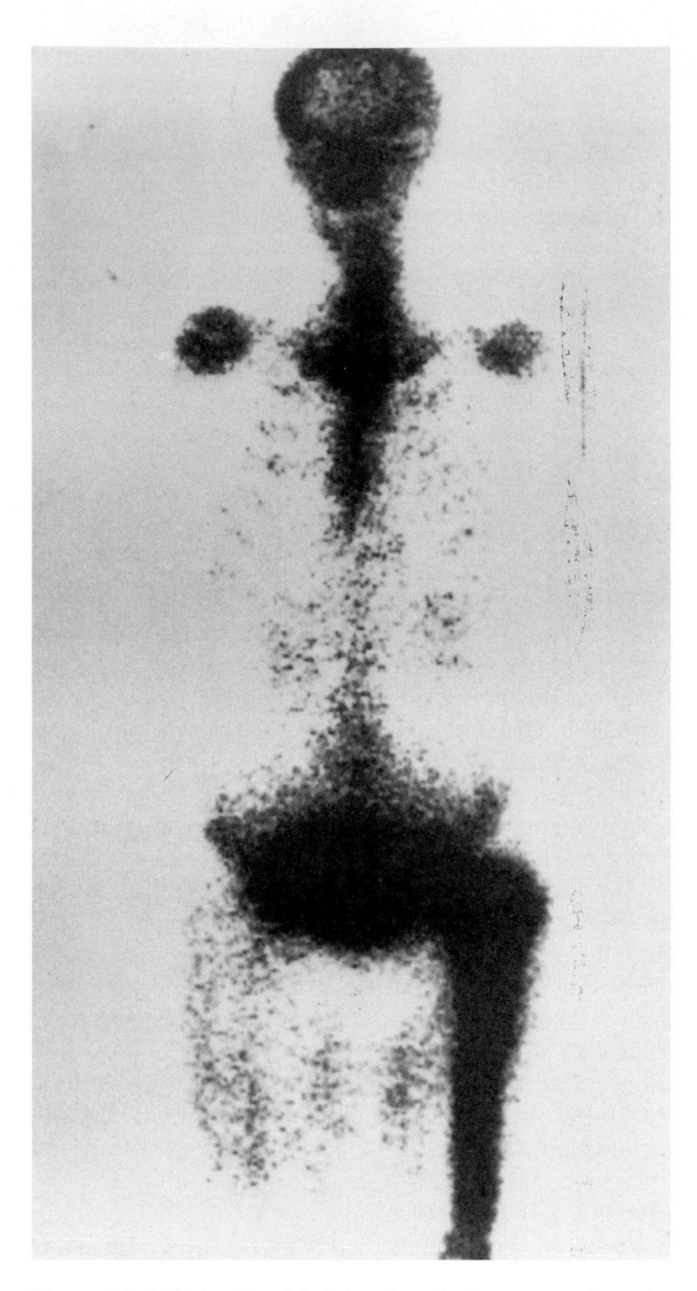

Figure 30–2. Technetium-99 diphosphonate bone scan shows increased areas of vascularity and mineralization, particularly in the left femur. (*Reprinted with permission from Singer FR.* Paget's Disease of Bone. *New York: Plenum; 1977:108.*)

out" Paget sites from primary hyperparathyroidism, osteomyelitis, and osteomalacia (Table 30–4).

Some patients have elevated serum metabolites of vitamin D. Serum concentration of calcium and inorganic phosphorous is normal, but urinary calcium may be elevated and may lead to renal calculi. If serum calcium or inorganic phosphorous are abnormal, other disease entities must be ruled out, such as malignancy or primary hyperparathyroidism.

TABLE 30–4. DIFFERENTIAL DIAGNOSIS OF PAGET DISEASE

Systemic
- Ankylosing spondylitis
- Rheumatoid arthritis
- Gout
- Primary hyperparathyroidism
- Renal osteodystrophy
- Osteoporosis
- Osteomalacia

Ocular
Angioid streaks:
- High myopia
- Pseudoxanthoma elasticum
- Sickle-cell disease
- Acromegaly
- Ehlers–Danlos syndrome
- Pituitary tumor
- Lead poisoning
- Senile elastosis

Optic neuropathy—must rule out:
- Ischemic syndromes
- Nutritional deficiency
- Toxic etiologies
- Anemia

Ocular

Diagnosis of angioid streaks is made by fundoscopy and fluorescein angiography. They appear in the peripapillary area and radiate outward, roughly in the directions of the extraocular muscles. They may appear reddish to gray, depending on the amount of fundus pigmentation present.

Clinical signs of optic neuropathy will be evident on fundus and visual field examinations as well as through patient history. Forced ductions can be used to differentiate muscle entrapment versus cranial nerve palsy in cases of extraocular muscle paralysis. Exophthalmos secondary to bone deformity can be measured through exophthalmometry. If the lacrimal duct is obstructed, symptoms of epiphora along with clinical signs of blockage (Jones dye test) will help make the diagnosis. X-ray and CT scan of the involved areas can be used to confirm the diagnosis.

TREATMENT AND MANAGEMENT

Systemic

Most patients with Paget disease require no therapy or only mild analgesic agents such as aspirin or indomethacin for pain in affected areas. Patients with pain and asymptomatic patients with at-risk pagetic lesions should receive antiresorptive therapy. Table 30–5 includes a summary of treatment and manage-

TABLE 30–5. TREATMENT AND MANAGEMENT OF PAGET DISEASE

Skeletal Involvement
- No treatment if bone involvement is minor
- Analgesics for pain in affected areas
- Salmon calcitonin injections in courses, or human calcitonin, as alternative therapy
- Orthopedic surgery
- Antiresorptive therapy
- Occipital craniotomy in cases with basilar compression
- Chemotherapy or radical resection with bone tumors

Hearing Loss
- Calcitonin and disodium etidronate

Ocular Involvement
- **Angioid streaks**
  Routine fundus examination and visual field examination
  Home Amsler grid monitor
  Fluorescein angiography
  Laser surgery, when indicated for SRNVM
- **Bone deformity causing muscle paralysis, exophthalmos**
  No specific treatment, follow only with supportive measures
  Debulking of bones
- **Optic neuropathy caused by pagetic "steal"**
  Surgical debulking
  Systemic salmon calcitonin, bisphosphonates, or mithramycin
- **Lacrimal obstruction**
  Monitor, supportive measures
  Local debulking of bones

ment of Paget disease. Orthopedic surgery, including total hip replacement, can aid in ambulation when needed. These patients also respond well to salmon calcitonin injections of 40 μg daily or on alternate days. Salmon calcitonin causes an inhibition of the ongoing bone resorptive process by decreasing the number of osteoclasts. It has been shown to relieve bone pain and help heal osteolytic lesions. It also reduces increased cardiac output and may cause the reversal of some neurological damage. Due to the formation of antibodies to salmon calcitonin, its long-term efficacy tends to diminish with time. Some of these patients do well when switched to human calcitonin. Patients tend to respond best when they receive intermittent courses of therapy, rather than remaining on it chronically. Recent advances have been made in the administration of calcitonin in the form of a nasal spray for patients with milder disease. This has good acceptance in geriatric cases where subcutaneous injection is less convenient.

Both sensorineural and conductive hearing loss have been reported to stabilize and occasionally reverse with combination therapy of calcitonin and disodium etidronate, a bisphosphonate. It can be taken orally at 5 mg/kg of body weight with similar results to calcitonin. Several new bisphosphonates include risedronate, alendronate, pamidronate, and tiludronate. These are used in 3-day to 6-month courses and can provide prolonged remission up to 30 months from the end of the course. Side effects can include bilateral anterior uveitis, episcleritis, and ototoxicity.

Cytotoxic agents such as mithramycin have been used to suppress several manifestations of the disease by inhibiting bone resorption and reducing hypercalcemia. They offer dramatic relief from bone pain but they are also highly toxic to hepatic, renal, and platelet tissue and are reserved for patients unresponsive to other therapy.

Patients with basilar compression may require occipital craniotomy for decompression of neurologic structures. In cases of sarcoma, chemotherapy has been largely ineffective, and radical resection of the affected limb has the best outcome for survival.

Ocular

Complete dilated fundus ophthalmoscopic examination and visual fields are indicated in Paget patients. Ocular management consists of laser therapy to subretinal neovascularization when serous detachment of the macula is a possible threat. Prophylactic photocoagulation of angioid streaks is contraindicated, as it may stimulate new vessel growth. Angioid streaks without neovascularization should be followed at least every 6 months by stereo fundus photography and fluorescein angiography, when indicated. The patient should also self-monitor for any changes with a home Amsler grid. If optic neuropathy or lacrimal duct obstruction results from a compressive lesion, surgical debulking is an option. However, this is of limited aid due to excessive bleeding and regrowth of the surgical site. Optic neuropathy is thought to be caused by bony compression and pagetic "steal" of vascular supply secondary to hypervascular bone lesions. Although it is difficult to restore neural function, treatment is the systemic administration of salmon calcitonin, sodium etidronate, or mithramycin.

CONCLUSION

Paget disease is a common disorder of bone, which can lead to many systemic manifestations. In addition to skeletal deformities, advanced disease affects the vascular and nervous system, including the eyes. Its manifestations can occur in various forms and degrees in the affected sites. Although a specific etiology remains elusive, recent developments in medicine have proven helpful in reducing its severity. The eyecare practitioner can play an important role in management of the patient with Paget disease through education, follow-up, and timely referral when indicated.

REFERENCES

Altman RD. Paget's disease of bone: Rheumatologic complications. *Bone.* 1999;24(suppl):47S–48S.

Ankrom MA, Shapiro JR. Paget's disease of bone (osteitis deformans). *J Am Geriatr Soc.* 1998;46:1025–1033.

Ballin M. Parathyroidism in reference to orthopedic surgery. *J Bone Jt Surg.* 1933;15:120.

Berman L. The endocrine treatment of Paget's disease. *Endocrinology.* 1932;16:109.

Clarkson JG, Altman RD. Angioid streaks. *Surv Ophthalmol.* 1982;26:235.

Cooper C, Dennison E, Schafheutle K, et al. Epidemiology of Paget's disease of bone. *Bone.* 1999;24 (suppl):3S–5S.

Cundy T, Wattie D, Busch S, et al. Paget's disease in New Zealand: Is it changing? *Bone.* 1999;24 (suppl):7S–9S.

D'Agostino HR, Barnett CA, Zielinski XJ, Gordan GS. Intranasal salmon calcitonin treatment of Paget's disease of bone. Results in nine patients. *Clin Orthop.* 1988;230: 223–228.

Davis AE Jr. Simultaneous occurrence of osteitis deformans and Hodgkin's disease. *JAMA.* 1960;173:153.

Delmas PD, Meuniere PJ. The management of Paget's disease of bone. *N Engl J Med.* 1997;336:558–566.

Eretto P, Krohel GB, Shihab ZM, et al. Optic neuropathy in Paget's disease. *Am J Ophthalmol.* 1984;97:505.

Federman JL, Shields JA, Tomer TL. Angioid streaks. Fluorescein angiographic features. *Arch Ophthalmol.* 1975;93:951.

Foldes J, Shamir S, Brautbar C, et al. HLA-D antigens and Paget's disease of bone. *Clin Orthop.* 1991;266:301–303.

Foldes J, Shamir S, Kidroni G, Menczel J. Vitamin D in Paget disease of bone. *Clin Orthop.* 1989;243:275–279.

Fraser WD. Paget's disease of bone. *Curr Opin Rheumatol.* 1997;9:347–354.

Gagel RF, Logan C, Mallette LE. Treatment of Paget's disease of bone with salmon calcitonin nasal spray. *J Am Geriatr Soc.* 1988;36:1010–1014.

Gass JDM, Clarkson JG. Angioid streaks and disciform macular detachment in Paget's disease (osteitis deformans). *Am J Ophthalmol.* 1973;75:576.

Haddad JG. Paget's disease of bone. In: Stein J, ed. *Internal Medicine.* 3rd ed. Boston: Little, Brown; 1990:2361–2364.

Healey JH, Buss D. Radiation and pagetic osteogenic sarcomas. *Clin Orthop Sep.* 1991;270:128–134.

Krane SM. Paget's disease of bone. *Clin Orthop.* 1977;127:24.

Kukita A, Chenu C, McManus LM, et al. Atypical multinucleated cells form in long-term marrow cultures from patients with Paget's disease. *J Clin Invest.* 1990;85:1280–1286.

Lando M, Hoover LA, Finerman G. Stabilization of hearing loss in Paget's disease with calcitonin and etidronate. *Arch Otolaryngol Head Neck Surg.* 1988;114:891–894.

Lewis T, Tesh AS, Lyles KW. Caring for the patient with Paget's disease of bone. *Nurse Pract.* 1999;24:50–58.

McKusick VA. *Heritable Disorders of Connective Tissue.* 4th ed. St. Louis: Mosby; 1960:718–723.

McMurtry CT. Paget's disease: A review. *Veterans Health System J.* 1999;11:23–27.

Mills BG, Singer FR. Nuclear inclusions in Paget's disease of bone. *Science.* 1976;194:201.

Monfort J, Rotes Sala D, Romero AB, et al. Epidemiological, clinical, biochemical and imaging characteristics of monostotic and polyostotic Paget's disease. Bone. 1999; 24(suppl):13S–14S.

Mooy CM, De Klein A, van den Bosch W, et al. Orbital chondrosarcoma developing in a patient with Paget disease. *Am J Ophthalmol.* 1999;127:619–621.

Muff R, Dambach MA, Perrenaud A, et al. Efficacy of human calcitonin in patients with Paget's disease refractory to salmon calcitonin. *Am J Med.* 1990;89:181–184.

O'Doherty DP, Dickerstaff DR, McCloskey EZ, et al. A comparison of the acute effects of subcutaneous and intranasal calcitonin. *Clin Sci.* 1990;78:215–219.

Paton D. *The Relation of Angioid Streaks to Systemic Disease.* Springfield: Thomas; 1972:38–46.

Potter HG, Schneider R, Ghelman B, et al. Multiple giant cell tumors and Paget's disease of bone: Radiographic and clinical correlations. *Radiology.* 1991;180:261–264.

Proops D, Bayley D, Hawke M. Paget's disease and the temporal bone—A clinical and histopathological review of six temporal bones. *J Otolaryngol.* 1985;14:20–29.

Rassmussen H, Bordier P. *The Physiologic and Cellular Basis of Metabolic Bone Disease.* Baltimore: Williams & Wilkins; 1974:272–304.

Rebel A, Malkani K, Basle M, Bregeon C. Osteoclast ultrastructure in Paget's disease. *Clin Orthop.* 1987;217:4.

Rosenkrantz JA, Gluckman EC. Co-existence of Paget's disease of bone and multiple myeloma: Case reports of two patients. *Am J Roentgenol Rad Ther Nuc Med.* 1957;78:30.

Shields JA, Federman JL, Tomer TL, et al. Angioid streaks. Ophthalmoscopic variations and diagnostic problems. *Br J Ophthalmol.* 1975;59:257.

Singer FR. Paget's disease of bone. In: Wyngaarden JB, Smith LH, eds. *Cecil's Textbook of Medicine.* 17th ed. Philadelphia: Saunders; 1985:1461–1463.

Singer FR. *Paget's Disease of Bone.* New York: Plenum; 1977: 93–102, 121–158.

Siris ES. A potent new bisphosphonate for Paget's disease of bone. *Am J Med.* 1996;101:339–340.

Tiegs RD. Paget's disease of bone: Indications for treatment and goals of therapy. *Clin Ther.* 1997;19:1309–1329.

Verhoeff FH. Histological findings in a case of angioid streaks. *Br J Ophthalmol.* 1948;32:531.

Chapter 31

MARFAN SYNDROME

Margaret McNelis

Marfan syndrome is composed of a group of connective tissue disorders that exhibit characteristic skeletal, cardiovascular, and ocular abnormalities with a wide range of expressivity. The typical presentation of a Marfan syndrome patient is that of a tall individual with long, thin arms and legs, hypermobile joints, and a long face. It has been suggested that Abraham Lincoln may have had Marfan syndrome, as well as the composer Rachmaninov, who wrote piano music that is best played by very long, hyperextensible hands. Subluxation of the crystalline lens is the most common ocular manifestation of this disease.

EPIDEMIOLOGY

Systemic

Marfan syndrome occurs in 4 to 6 per 10,000 births. Between 5 and 35% of these cases are new mutations and are associated with an increased paternal age. Sporadic cases tend to be more severely affected than familial ones. The disease shows no racial or sexual predilection. Skeletal involvement is found in every patient with Marfan syndrome. Aortic involvement occurs in 80% of patients with the disease.

Ocular

Subluxation of the crystalline lens occurs in 50 to 58% of patients with Marfan syndrome, with little effect on acuity in most patients. Visual acuity is 20/40 or better in 60% of patients with lens subluxation. Glaucoma occurs in 8% of patients, secondary to lens dislocation or a congenital angle anomaly. Retinal detachment is found in 9% of patients with dislocated lenses. Iris transillumination is present in about 10% of patients, and approximately 20% of patients with Marfan syndrome are strabismic.

PATHOPHYSIOLOGY/DISEASE PROCESS

Systemic

While once considered to be exclusively autosomal dominantly transmitted with variable penetrance, Marfan syndrome is now thought to be comprised of several molecular defects that cause a group of phenotypically similar disorders. It has been linked to a defect in the fibrillin gene on chromosome 15. A phenotypically similar but distinct disorder, congenital contractural arachnodactyly, has been linked to a defect in the fibrillin gene on chromosome 5, and it is probably this disorder that Antoine Marfan described in 1896.

Fibrillin is a major component of the microfibrils found in the connective tissue space of blood vessel walls and the suspensory ligaments of the crystalline lens. Fibrillin is probably a family of connective tissue proteins, rather than a single protein in itself, and

Marfan-like changes may arise when mutations occur on other fibrillin genes. This may account for the variability in phenotypes of different Marfan patients.

Skeletal abnormalities of Marfan syndrome manifest as long, spiderlike fingers (arachnodactyly; Figure 31–1) and armspan equal to or greater than height. The Marfan patient is tall within his or her family, with the upper segment of the body (head to pubic bone) much shorter than the lower segment (pubic bone to floor). Scoliosis is frequent and is the most debilitating of the skeletal complications. Overgrowth of the ribs can cause sternal displacement inward (pectus excavatum) or outward (pectus carinatum or pigeon chest). The number and severity of skeletal abnormalities in Marfan syndrome increase during puberty.

The joints will be hyperextensible, and repeated dislocations of the hips, clavicles, patellas, and mandibles may occur. Patients usually have a high arched palate and an abnormal smallness of the jaw. Other variable physical signs include a broad nasal bridge, large floppy low-set ears, partially cleft palate, inguinal hernia, femoral fracture, overlapping toes, foot deformities, decreased muscle tone, diminished reflexes, and peripheral muscle wasting.

Mitral valve prolapse is common, characterized by midsystolic click and late systolic murmur on auscultation. An association has been made between mitral valve prolapse and cerebrovascular events such as transient ischemic attacks, retinal vascular emboli, and stroke. See Chapter 4 for a more complete discussion of valve disorders. Aortic involvement is the most common cause of death. Histologic examination of Marfan aortas exhibit cystic medial necrosis with focal fragmentation of the elastic fibers in the media. Structurally altered cardiac valves may give rise to bacterial endocarditis, arrhythmias, rupture of the chordae tendineae, sudden mitral insufficiency, and sudden death.

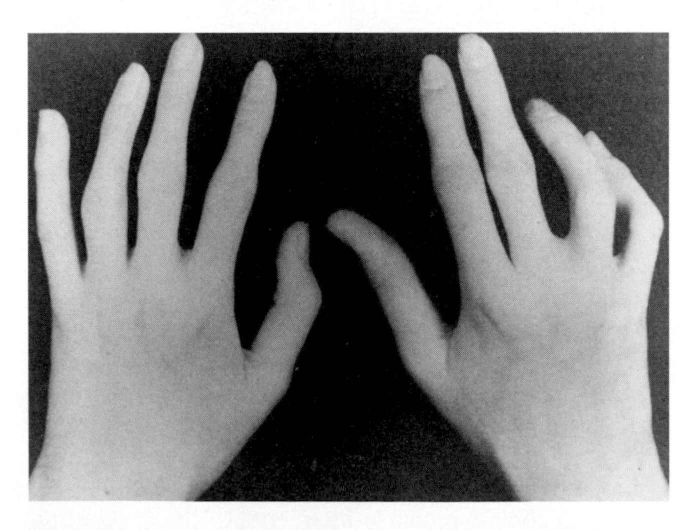

Figure 31–1. Long, spiderlike fingers in a patient with Marfan syndrome (*Reprinted with permission from McKusick VA.* Heritable Disorders of Connective Tissue. *4th ed. St. Louis: Mosby; 1960:172.*)

Marfan patients may also exhibit skin folds and stretch marks in places where body fat has been neither gained nor lost. These patients are also more prone to inguinal hernias, as well as other hernia types. Spontaneous pneumothorax and bullous emphysema have been reported, but the incidence is unknown. A high frequency of sleep apnea in these patients has also been noted, perhaps due to a floppy, easily collapsible pharynx.

Various central nervous system manifestations have been documented (Table 31–1), as well as an association with schizophrenia.

Ocular

The major ocular sign in Marfan syndrome is ectopia lentis, or bilateral displacement of the crystalline lenses (Figure 31–2). The lenses will almost always be displaced upward in a superotemporal direction, usually occurring in utero. This type of dislocation is incomplete, and nonprogressive, and accommodation is possible because the zonules remain attached to the lens. This is to be differentiated from the ectopia lentis found in homocystinuria, in which the zonules rupture and the lenses dislocate down and in. In these cases, accommodative function is impaired. Lenticular astigmatism may be induced with lens subluxation, depending on the degree of dislocation. Phakic eyes are more commonly myopic in the Marfan patient.

> Marfan syndrome may be present in a patient with iridodonesis, ectopia lentis, and transillumination defects of the iris.

Increased axial length can cause moderate to severe myopia and the risk of spontaneous retinal detachment increases with increased axial length. The choroid in these patients may be thin, displaying various degrees of scleral crescents, but staphylomas are uncommon. Peripheral retinal degenerations may also occur, leading to retinal detachment. Other peripheral retinal manifestations include prominent areas of white without pressure, lattice degeneration, retinal holes, and less commonly, retinoschisis. Colobomas of the iris, lens, and optic nerve have been associated with Marfan syndrome.

TABLE 31–1. SYSTEMIC MANIFESTATIONS OF MARFAN SYNDROME

Skeletal
- Arachnodactyly (C)
- Armspan that exceeds height (C)
- Hyperextensible joints (C)
- High, arched palate (C)
- Small jaw bones (C)
- Hernias (C)
- Flat feet and foot deformities (C)
- Scoliosis (C)
- Pectus excavatum/carinatum (C)
- Broad nasal bridge (M)
- Large, floppy, low-set ears (M)
- Partially cleft palate (M)
- Femoral fracture (M)
- Overlapping toes (M)

Cardiovascular
- Mitral valve prolapse (C)
- Arrhythmias (C)
- Dilated ascending aorta; rupture or aneurysm of aorta (C)
- Cerebrovascular accidents such as transient ischemic attacks, strokes (C)
- Structurally altered cardiac valves with resultant bacterial endocarditis, arrhythmia, rupture of chordae tendineae, sudden mitral insufficiency (C)

Cutaneous
- Skin folds and stretch marks (C)

Muscular System
- Decreased muscle tone (C)
- Diminished reflexes (C)
- Peripheral muscle wasting (M)

Pulmonary System
- Spontaneous pneumothorax (R)
- Bullous emphysema (R)
- Sleep apnea (R)

Central Nervous System
- Dural ectasia such as lumbosacral meningocele (a congenital hernia in which the meninges protrude through an opening in the skull or spinal column) (M)
- Dilated cisterna magna (M)
- Learning disability (M)
- Hyperactivity with or without attention deficit disorder (M)
- An association with schizophrenia has been suggested (R)

C, common; M, more frequently than rarely; R, rare.

Horner syndrome has been reported in cases of carotid artery dissection. Intracranial vessel dissection may also cause other cranial nerve palsies and ophthalmoplegia, as well as tinnitis, amaurosis, scintillating scotomata, and artery occlusions of the eye.

Relatively flat corneas are typical in Marfan syndrome, but a few cases of keratoconus have also been reported. Corneal diameter may be increased up to 14 mm without an increase in intraocular pressure.

As is common in many other connective tissue disorders, the anterior chamber angle in Marfan syndrome is deep with structural abnormalities. Glaucoma may occur due to pupil block, congenital angle anomalies, or anterior lens subluxation. If glaucoma occurs, further stretching of the globe, which already may have an increased axial length, may cause retinal detachment.

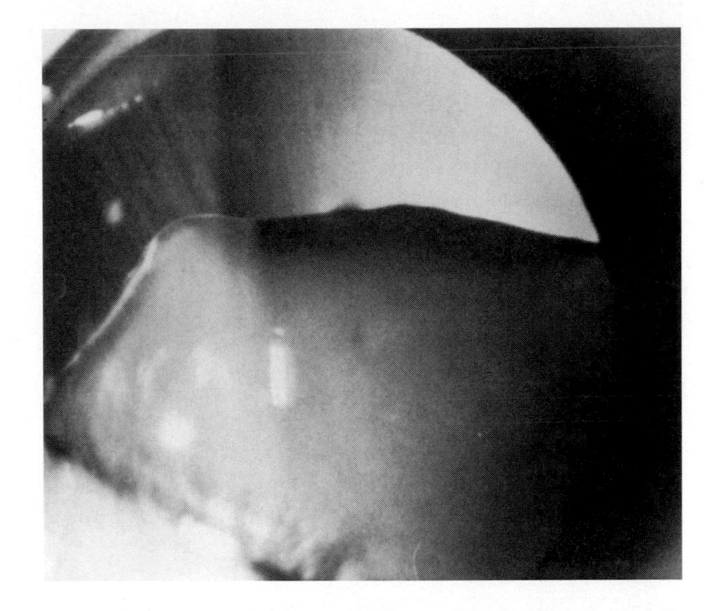

Figure 31–2. Ectopia lentis in a Marfan patient in which the lens is displaced in an upward direction (*Reprinted with permission from Renie WA, ed.* Goldberg's Genetic and Metabolic Eye Disease. *2nd ed. Boston: Little, Brown; 1986:395.*)

Retinal arterial occlusions associated with emboli from inflamed mitral valve leaflets have been reported.

Due to the thinness of the sclera in Marfan syndrome, as well as other connective tissue disorders, it often appears blue. Upon careful observation, iridodonesis may be seen, as may heterochromic irides. The iris dilator muscle is often hypoplastic, causing miotic pupils that dilate poorly, and the pupils are occasionally eccentric. Iris topography is also reduced, giving it a smooth appearance. The iris transilluminates in about 10% of patients, more prominently at the iris base.

Cases of microspherophakia and cataracts have been reported in conjunction with Marfan syndrome. Coloboma of the fundus and macula have also been reported.

Reiger anomaly, characterized by a prominent anteriorly displaced Schwalbe line, iris strands to Schwalbe line, and anterior iris–stromal hypoplasia, has been reported in three cases of Marfan syndrome. This is an autosomal dominant disorder, and presently there does not appear to be a common embryologic or metabolic factor associating the two disorders.

Acquired Brown syndrome, which is defined as an inflammation of the microfibrillar fibers of the superior oblique tendon, is accompanied by diplopia and pain in upgaze, and has also been associated with Marfan syndrome. Other binocular complications associated with Marfan syndrome include amblyopia, strabismus, anisometropia, and rarely, nystagmus. Table 31–2 gives a complete list of the ocular manifestations of Marfan syndrome.

DIAGNOSIS

Systemic

Diagnosis of Marfan syndrome (Table 31–3) is made based primarily upon skeletal, ocular, and cardiovascular manifestations. Patients with arachnodactyly and armspan equal to or greater than height may be suspected to have the disease. Most of these patients' height is in the 95th percentile or greater for their age. Signs of hyperextensible joints, such as a history of repeated dislocations of the hips, clavicles, patellas, and mandible, or other systemic features, may lend further evidence to the diagnosis. On physical examination, a murmur or click on auscultation may be detected.

In the absence of a family history of Marfan syndrome, diagnosis is based upon skeletal involvement as well as manifestations in at least two other systems. If one (or more) first-degree relatives are affected, diagnosis requires the involvement of two systems, of which one manifestation should be major.

Diagnostic echocardiographic findings (Table 31–4) include a dilated ascending aorta, and late in the disease, left ventricular failure. Echocardiography also provides a more definitive diagnosis of mitral valve prolapse.

Tissue biopsies will indicate a disruption in the elastic fibers in the blood vessel walls. There will be increased collagen deposition overall, and proliferation of smooth muscle cells. Several Marfan cases have shown decreased synthesis of type I collagen. In some patients, urinary hydroxyproline levels are elevated, indicating increased collagen turnover.

Ocular

Marfan syndrome may be diagnosed after the discovery of bilateral lens subluxation on routine eye examination. Other causes of lens subluxation (eg, homocystinuria), (Table 31–5) must be ruled out. Very rarely, the less com-

TABLE 31–2. OCULAR MANIFESTATIONS OF MARFAN SYNDROME

Sclera/Conjunctiva
- Blue sclera (M)
- Flat or increased corneal diameter (R)
- Keratoconus (R)
- Increased axial length (M)

Iris, Pupil, and Angle Anomalies
- Iridodonesis (C)
- Reiger anomaly (C)
- Deep anterior chamber angle (C)
- Heterochromic irides (C)
- Miotic pupils that dilate poorly secondary to hypoplastic iris dilator (C)
- Reduced iris topography (giving a smooth appearance) or iris transillumination defects (more prominent at iris base) (C)

Lens
- Ectopia lentis (C)

Glaucoma
- Secondary glaucoma from pupil block, congenital angle anomalies, or anterior lens subluxation (M)

Retina
- Retinal detachment (C)
- Peripheral retinal degenerations such as white without pressure, lattice degeneration, retinoschisis, and retinal holes (M)
- Retinal arterial occlusions (R)

Binocular
- Strabismus (C)
- Amblyopia (C)
- Anisometropia (M)
- Nystagmus (R)

Other
- Enophthalmos (C)
- Down-slanting palpebral fissures (M)
- Colobomas (M)
- Brown tendon sheath syndrome (R)

C, common; M, more frequently than rarely; R, rare.

TABLE 31–3. MARFAN SYNDROME: CRITERIA FOR DIAGNOSIS[a]

Criteria	Hard Manifestations	Soft Manifestations
Ocular features	Subluxated lenses	Myopia
Cardiovascular features	Aortic dilatations	Mitral valve prolapse
Skeletal features	Severe scoliosis Deformity of anterior chest	Tall stature Joint laxity Arachnodactyly

[a]In the presence of a family history of the disease, a minimum of two criteria must be present to make a diagnosis of Marfan syndrome. In the absence of family history, three criteria must be present.

Adapted with permission from Cohen PR, Schneiderman P: Clinical manifestations of Marfan syndrome. Int J Dermatol. *1989;23:292.*

TABLE 31–4. DIAGNOSTIC TESTS UTILIZED IN MARFAN SYNDROME

- MRI to determine extent of aortic dilation
- Echocardiogram
- X-ray
- In ectopia lentis, negative cyanide–nitroprusside test for disulfides in the urine (to rule out homocystinuria)

TABLE 31–5. DIFFERENTIAL DIAGNOSIS OF MARFAN SYNDROME

Systemic

Marfan syndrome resembles congenital contractural arachnodactyly (CCA).

- They may be distinguished molecularly by defects of fibrillin on chromosomes 15 and 5, respectively.
- Management is the same for both disorders.
- Ocular and aortic manifestations are absent in CCA.

Ocular

Differentials between ectopia lentis in Marfan syndrome:

- The lens is generally subluxed up and out in Marfan syndrome.
- The lens is generally subluxed down and in from homocystinuria.
- Diagnosis of homocystinuria is confirmed by excess homocystine in the urine.

mon manifestations discussed in the ocular natural history section earlier in the chapter will be found on routine examination.

TREATMENT AND MANAGEMENT

Systemic

Life expectancy has dramatically improved in the last 20 years, largely due to advances in cardiovascular surgery and medical therapy. Currently there is no treatment for the fundamental defect that produces Marfan syndrome (Table 31–6). Severe scoliosis may warrant the use of a brace, or spinal fusion. There has been an attempt to prevent the severity of scoliosis in young girls by administering estrogen, thereby speeding up puberty and shortening the amount of time for scoliosis to progress. The effect of this therapy is unknown, but these young women have not grown to as great a height as would be expected with the disease. Orthotics are used in the treatment of foot deformities.

Annual echocardiograms should be performed in order to monitor the progression of aortic dilatation. When the diameter is greater than 50% normal size, echocardiograms are done every 6 months. Surgery is warranted when the diameter of the aortic root reaches 5.5 centimeters. The procedure of choice now is total aortic root replacement with a composite valve and coronary implantation. A β-blocker is typically prescribed to prevent further aortic enlargement. Low-impact aerobic sports such as swimming and cycling are encouraged for patients to maintain good cardiovascular fitness, but contact sports and isometric exercises should be discouraged. Particularly thorough physical examinations are recommended before participation in sports activities, since many of these people are of superior athletic build, and not yet diagnosed. In the cases of aortic aneurysm or rupture, surgical intervention is necessary. Smoking is associated with aortic graft failure, and is strictly avoided. This includes secondhand smoke as well.

TABLE 31–6. TREATMENT AND MANAGEMENT OF MARFAN SYNDROME

Cardiovascular Complications

- Echocardiogram every 6 months or annually
- Surgical intervention for aortic dilatation, aneurysm, or rupture, when indicated
- Systemic β-blockers
- Low-impact aerobic sports

Skeletal Complications

- Braces or spinal fusion for severe scoliosis
- Estrogen therapy in young females (efficacy has not yet been determined)
- Orthotics for foot deformities

Ocular Complications

- Appropriate phakic/aphakic prescriptions as early as possible to prevent amblyopia
- Annual fundus evaluation to detect retinal complications; retinal consultation and repair of retinal detachment, as indicated
- Mydriatics and miotics to reposition subluxated lenses
- Treatment of secondary glaucoma with standard regimen
- Sub-Tenon steroid injections in Brown syndrome

Ocular

Reduced visual acuity may result from delayed or inadequate correction of refractive error. Therefore, it is important to fit children early with appropriate phakic/aphakic prescriptions to prevent amblyopia from developing. Because the lens maintains normal accommodative function, it is not removed unless it induces a secondary glaucoma or prevents adequate visualization of the retina. In cases where subluxation occurs into the anterior chamber and causes a secondary glaucoma, mydriatics are used to reposition the lens, sometimes followed by chronic miotic ophthalmic drops to maintain its position. Standard medical glaucoma therapy is indicated in chronic open-angle glaucoma. Retinal detachments are treated with surgical repair. In the case of Brown syndrome, sub-Tenon steroid injections near the trochlea have relieved both symptoms and diplopia.

CONCLUSION

Marfan syndrome manifests as abnormalities in several tissue systems leading to skeletal, ocular, cardiovascular, and cutaneous manifestations. It is not uncommon for an eyecare provider to be the first to discover this disorder in a patient with bilaterally subluxated lenses. Management of these patients is interdisciplinary, and prompt referral to the appropriate healthcare provider is indicated.

REFERENCES

Adams JN, Trent RJ. Aortic complications of Marfan's syndrome. *Lancet.* 1998;352:1722–1723.

Allen RA, Straatsma BR, Apt L, Hall MO. Ocular manifestations of the Marfan syndrome. *Trans Am Acad Ophthalmol Otolaryngol.* 1967;71:18.

Barnett HJM, Boughner DR, Taylor DW, et al. Further evidence relating mitral valve prolapse to cerebral ischemic events. *N Engl J Med.* 1980;302:139.

Bergen RL, Cangemi FE, Glassman R. Bilateral arterial occlusion secondary to Barlow's syndrome. *Ann Ophthalmol.* 1982;14:673–675.

Braverman AC. Exercise and the Marfan syndrome. *Jo Am Coll Sports Med.* 1998:S387–395.

Cheitlin M. Thromboembolic studies in the patient with a prolapsed mitral valve. *Circulation.* 1979;60:46.

Cistulli PA, Sullivan CE. Sleep disorders in Marfan's syndrome. *Lancet.* 1991;337:1359–1360.

Collins M, Swann PG, See ML. Case report: Marfan's syndrome. *Clin Exp Optom.* 1988;71:58–59.

Cullom RD, Cullom ME. Two neuro-ophthalmic episodes separated in time and space. *Surv Ophthalmol.* 1995;40:217–224.

Eaton L, Meiner S. Marfan syndrome: Identification and management. *Med Surg Nurs.* 1999:113.

Good WV, Corbett TD. Acquired Brown's syndrome in association with Marfan's syndrome. *Binoc Visn Q.* 1991;6:101–102.

Gott VL, Pyeritz RE, MacGovern GJ, et al. Surgical treatment of aneurysms of the ascending aorta in the Marfan syndrome. *N Engl J Med.* 1986;314:1070–1074.

Grin TR, Nelson LB. Rieger's anomaly associated with Marfan's syndrome. *Ann Ophthalmol.* 1987;19:380–384.

Halme T, Savunen T, Aho H, et al. Elastin and collagen in the aortic wall: Changes in the Marfan syndrome and annuloaortic ectasia. *Exp Mol Pathol.* 1985;43:1–12.

Joseph KN, Kane HA, Milner RS, et al. Orthopedic aspects of the Marfan phenotype. *Clin Orth Rel Res.* 1992;277:251–261.

Kainulainen K, Pulkkinen L, Savolainen A, et al. Location on chromosome 15 of the gene defect causing the Marfan syndrome. *N Engl J Med.* 1990;323:935–939.

Kanski J. *Clinical Ophthalmology.* London: Butterworths; 1984:8.17–8.18.

Krupin T. Marfan syndrome, lens subluxation, and open-angle glaucoma. *J Glaucoma.* 1999:8;393–399.

Lee B, Godfrey M, Vittale E, et al. Linkage of Marfan syndrome and a phenotypically related disorder to two different fibrillin genes. *Nature.* 1991;330–333.

Maddox BK, Sakai LY, Keene BR, Glanville RW. Connective tissue microfibrils. *J Biol Chem.* 1989;264:21381–21385.

Maslen CL, Corsen GM, Maddox BK, et al. Partial sequence of a candidate gene for the Marfan syndrome. *Nature.* 1991;352:334–337.

Maumenee IH. The eye in the Marfan syndrome. *Trans Am Ophthalmol Soc.* 1981;79:684.

McKusick VA. The defect in Marfan syndrome. *Nature.* 1991;352:279–281.

Morse RP, Rockenmacher S, Pyeritz RE, et al. Diagnosis and management of infantile Marfan syndrome. *Pediatrics.* 1990;86:888–894.

Nelson LB, Maumenee IH. Ectopia lentis. In: Renie WA, ed. *Goldberg's Genetic and Metabolic Eye Disease.* 2nd ed. Boston: Little, Brown; 1986:389–395.

Pyeritz RE. The Marfan syndrome. *Am Fam Physician.* 1986;34:83–94.

Pyeritz RE. Marfan syndrome. In: Emery AEH, Rimoin DL, eds. *Principles and Practice of Medical Genetics.* New York: Churchill Livingstone; 1983;2:820–835.

Pyeritz RE, McKusick VA. The Marfan syndrome: Diagnosis and management. *N Engl J Med.* 1979;300:772–777.

Robert L. Inborn metabolic disorders of the eye. In: Peyman GA, Sanders DR, Goldberg MF, eds. *Principles and Practice of Ophthalmology.* Philadelphia: Saunders; 1980:1746–1749.

Sirota P, Frydman M, Sirota L. Schizophrenia and the Marfan syndrome. *Br J Psychiatry.* 1990;157:433–436.

Skovby F, McKusick VA. Estrogen treatment for tall stature in girls with the Marfan syndrome. *Birth Defects.* 1977;13:155.

Traboulsi EI, Aswas MI, Jalkh AE, Malouf JE. Ocular findings in mitral valve prolapse syndrome. *Ann Ophthalmol.* 1987;19:354–359.

Tsipouras P, Del Mastro R, Sarfarazi M, et al. Genetic linkage of the Marfan syndrome, ectopia lentis, and congenital contractural arachnodactyly to the fibrillin genes on chromosomes 15 and 5. *N Engl J Med.* 1992;326:905–909.

Woerner EM, Royalty K. Marfan syndrome: What you need to know. *Postgrad Med.* 1990;87:229–236.

Worobec-Victor SM, Bain MAB. Oculocutaneous genetic diseases. In: Renie WA, ed. *Goldberg's Genetic and Metabolic Eye Disease.* 2nd ed. Boston: Little, Brown; 1986:510–511.

Zito G. Neurological complications of mitral leaflet prolapse. *Lancet.* 1979;1:784.

Chapter 32

EHLERS–DANLOS SYNDROME

Margaret McNelis

Ehlers–Danlos (ED) syndrome is an inherited disorder of collagen synthesis whose manifestations may include skin abnormalities, joint hyperextensibility, and the increased tendency to bruise. The majority of subtypes were previously divided into 11 groups, most of which were autosomal dominant in inheritance. The classification of Ehlers–Danlos syndrome has recently been revised into six subtypes, based upon the molecular cause of each type. The Ehlers–Danlos subtypes include classical, hypermobility, vascular, kyphoscoliotic (ocular scoliotic), arthrochalasia, and dermatosparaxis. The other forms that were previously described as types V through XI are rare, and their relationship to ED syndrome is uncertain. The ocular–scoliotic type (previously known as type IV) is much less frequently encountered than previously thought (Beighton et al, 1997). The various subtypes of the disease result from different mutations of the gene that produces type III procollagen. These mutations appear to affect the synthesis, organization, and degradation of collagen fibrils. Ocular findings in Ehlers–Danlos syndrome include keratoconus, prominent epicanthal folds, angioid streaks, microcornea, and blue sclera.

EPIDEMIOLOGY

Systemic

Ehlers–Danlos syndrome occurs in approximately 1 per 200,000 persons. About 80% exhibit the classical form (types I or II), 10% the hypermobility type, 4% the vascular type, and 6% the remaining types.

Ocular

Prominent epicanthal folds are found in 25% of classical Ehlers–Danlos syndrome. Blue scleras are found in less than 10%, most commonly ocular–scoliotic. Eight percent exhibit moderate myopia, while 7% are strabismic. Loose, easily everted upper eyelids and widely spaced eyes are common in these patients, but epidemiologic data are not available.

PATHOPHYSIOLOGY/DISEASE PROCESS

Systemic

The type of Ehlers–Danlos syndrome determines the natural history of the disease (Table 32–1). This can be predicted from familial and biochemical studies and can also be used to determine potential pregnancy and surgical risks. Classical-type Ehlers–Danlos is comprised of two groups, previously known as types I and II. Type I Ehlers–Danlos syndrome is inherited in an autosomal dominant manner and clinical features include very soft, hyperextensible skin (Figure 32–1), extreme joint hypermobility, easy bruising, and poor wound healing and scarring. Hernias occur in 10 to 20% of patients, as well as premature birth in 50% due to weakness of fetal membranes. Mitral valve prolapse is common, usually manifesting by adolescence, and

TABLE 32–1. SYSTEMIC MANIFESTATIONS OF EHLERS–DANLOS SYNDROME

- Soft, hyperextensible skin
- Thin, atrophic "cigarette-paper" scarring
- Joint hypermobility
- Easy bruising
- Poor wound healing
- Hernias secondary to weak tissues
- Premature birth secondary to weak fetal membranes
- Mitral valve prolapse, "floppy" mitral valve syndrome
- Recurrent joint dislocations
- Degenerative arthritic changes
- Scoliosis
- Arterial rupture
- Traumatic or spontaneous carotid cavernous sinus fistula
- Cardiovascular and GI complications secondary to fragile vessels rupturing, and/or intestinal rupture or perforation

often in early childhood. Life expectancy of this type is normal.

Type II (Mitis) Ehlers–Danlos syndrome is also inherited in an autosomal dominant pattern. It presents with milder features than type I. Joint hypermobility is usually limited to the hands and feet. Skin changes are mild to absent, displaying the characteristic thin, atrophic "cigarette paper" scars at trauma prone sites. Life expectancy is also normal in this type.

The hypermobility subtype also has an autosomal dominant inheritance pattern and exhibits marked joint laxity and soft skin with minimal extensibility and bruisability. Recurrent dislocations and early degenerative arthritic changes due to unstable joints may require surgery. These patients also demonstrate signs of prolapsed mitral valve (also referred to as "floppy mitral valve" syndrome).

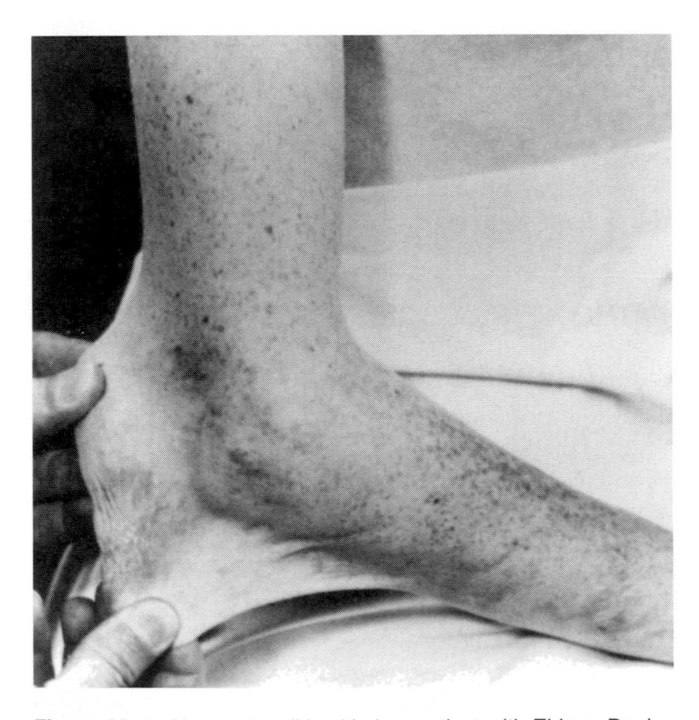

Figure 32–1. Hyperextensible skin in a patient with Ehlers–Danlos syndrome. (*Reprinted with permission from Perry HO, Bietti G. Ocular involvement in dermatologic disease. In: Mousoff F, ed.* The Eye in Systemic Disease. *St. Louis: Mosby, 1980:413.*)

Autosomal dominant and autosomal recessive forms of the vascular subtype (type IV) exist. This type has the worst prognosis for life because of such effects on the cardiovascular system as ruptured aorta or intracranial vessels. Gastrointestinal system afflictions such as intestinal perforation are often life threatening. One half of patients die before the age of 40.

Ocular

Myopia and strabismus are common findings in patients with Ehlers–Danlos syndrome (Table 32–2). Epicanthal folds and blue sclera are other less commonly encountered manifestations. Microcornea, retinal detachment, keratoconus, and angioid streaks have also been associated with this syndrome. Due to hyperextensibility of the skin, easy eversion of the upper eyelid is possible (Méténier sign).

Ocular signs of Ehlers–Danlos, unique to the ocular–scoliotic type (type VI, previously) include keratoglobus and corneal haze at the level of Bowman layer. Glaucoma is often present by the third decade, and retinal detachment by the fourth. Vitreoretinal degeneration and angioid streaks with associated neovascularization and disciform scarring occur with minimal trauma. Corneas or globes may rupture upon minimal trauma. Rare cases of ectopia lentis have also been reported.

TABLE 32–2. OCULAR MANIFESTATIONS OF EHLERS–DANLOS SYNDROME

- Myopia
- Strabismus
- Prominent epicanthal folds
- Blue sclera
- Microcornea
- Retinal detachment
- Keratoconus
- Angioid streaks
  - Neovascularization and disciform scarring with minimal trauma
- Keratoglobus
- Corneal haze at Bowman membrane
- Secondary glaucoma
- Vitreoretinal degeneration
- Rupture of cornea or globe with minimal trauma
- Ectopia lentis
- Lid laxity (Méténier sign)
- Staphyloma

DIAGNOSIS

Systemic

Diagnosis and differentiation (Table 32–3) is primarily made through physical examination following signs of skin, joint, and bruising abnormalities, along with detailed family history to determine the mode of inheritance, as well as tissue biopsy (Table 32–4). Prenatal diagnosis of the vascular subtype (previously type IV) is possible via type III collagen analysis.

> Suspect vascular Ehlers–Danlos syndrome in a young to middle-aged patient with a spontaneous carotid cavernous fistula.

Ocular

Routine ocular examination may reveal any ocular manifestation of Ehlers–Danlos syndrome. External and anterior segment evaluation may reveal epicanthus, strabismus, myopia, blue sclera, microcornea, corneal haze, keratoconus, or keratoglobus. Angioid streaks, subsequent macular scarring and retinal detachment may be found on dilated fundus examination.

TREATMENT AND MANAGEMENT

Systemic

Management of Ehlers–Danlos syndrome is mostly through supportive measures (Table 32–5). Some forms of Ehlers–Danlos syndrome have had beneficial results from 2 to 4 g of ascorbic acid per day. These patients should avoid trauma, but if it occurs, it is important to provide lacerations and wounds with good support, because it takes a longer period of time for these patients to heal. Physical therapy is important to maintain strength and stability of hypermobile joints.

These patients are challenging surgical candidates because of tissue weakness in suturing, excessive bleeding, and very slow wound healing. Surgery is generally avoided in the more severe cases except in emergency. When possible, genetic counseling may be helpful.

TABLE 32–3. DIFFERENTIAL DIAGNOSIS OF EHLERS–DANLOS SYNDROME

Systemic
- Severe neonatal form of Marfan syndrome

Ocular
- Brittle cornea syndrome (ocular–scoliotic type)

TABLE 32–4. DIAGNOSTIC TESTS UTILIZED IN EHLERS–DANLOS SYNDROME

- Urinary hydroxylysyl pyridinoline and lysyl pyridinoline levels
- Collagen analysis via skin biopsy

Ocular

Ocular treatment poses many risks to patients with Ehlers–Danlos syndrome (Table 32–5). In the case of strabismus, surgery may or may not be advised, depending on the degree of ocular tissue compromise. Contact lenses may be used to correct the corneal irregularities of keratoconus. This may be accomplished with rigid gas-permeable lenses, soft lenses, or a piggyback combination.

Special consideration needs to be given to those patients who develop retinal detachments, due to the fragility of the globe and the possibility of rupture under stress. This characteristic makes scleral buckling risky, and detachments are usually repaired with laser photocoagulation or cryotherapy. In certain cases of macular degeneration, laser therapy may be indicated.

CONCLUSION

Ehlers–Danlos syndrome is a group of generalized collagen disorders. The organs most dramatically affected include the skin, joints, and skeletal system, gastrointestinal tract, and the cardiovascular system. Ocular manifestations are variable, and although they may not appear to be sight threatening, the fragility of the globe may make these patients risky candidates for ocular surgery.

TABLE 32–5. TREATMENT AND MANAGEMENT OF EHLERS–DANLOS SYNDROME

Systemic
- 2–4 g ascorbic acid daily to stimulate collagen synthesis, promote wound healing, and reduce vessel fragility
- Avoidance of trauma
- Appropriate supportive measures to promote healing of wounds
- Physical therapy
- Genetic counseling

Ocular
- Contact lenses for corneal irregularities
- Extreme care during or avoidance of unnecessary surgery

REFERENCES

Arkin W. Blue scleras with keratoglobus. *Am J Opthalmol.* 1964;58:678–672.

Bahn CF, Falls HF, Varley GA, et al. Classification of corneal endothelial disorders based on neural crest origin. *Ophthalmology.* 1984;91:558–563.

Beighton P. *The Ehlers–Danlos Syndrome.* London: Heinemann; 1970.

Beighton P. Serious ophthalmological complications in the Ehlers–Danlos syndrome. *Br J Ophthalmol.* 1970;54:263–268.

Beighton P, DePaepe A, Steinmann B, et al. Ehlers–Danlos syndromes: Revised nosology, Villefranche 1997. *Am J Med Genet.* 1998;77:31–37.

Biglan AW, Brown SI, Johnson BL. Keratoglobus and blue sclera. *Am J Ophthalmol.* 1979;83:225–233.

Burrows N. The molecular genetics of the Ehlers–Danlos syndrome. *Clin Exp Dermatol.* 1999;24:99–106.

Byers P. Ehlers–Danlos syndrome: Recent advances and current understanding of the clinical and genetic heterogeneity. *J Invest Ophthalmol.* 1994;103(suppl):47S–57S.

Byers PH. Type IV Ehlers–Danlos syndrome. In: Akeson W, Bornstein P, Glimcher MJ, eds. *Proceedings of the Workshop on Heritable Disorders of Connective Tissue.* St. Louis: Mosby; 1982:61–101.

Cole WG, Evans R, Sillence DO. The clinical features of Ehlers–Danlos type VII due to a deletion of 24 amino acids from the pro-alpha 1(I) chain of type I procollagen. *J Med Genet.* 1987;24:698–701.

Eyre DR, Shapiro FD, Aldridge JF. A heterozygous collagen defect in a variant of the Ehlers–Danlos syndrome type VII. *J Biol Chem.* 1985;260:11322–11329.

Fox R, Pope FM, Narcisi P, et al. Spontaneous carotid cavernous fistula in Ehlers–Danlos syndrome. *J Neurol Neurosurg Psychiatr.* 1988;51:984–986.

Gorlin RJ, Cohen MM. Craniofacial manifestations of Ehlers–Danlos syndromes, Cutis Laxa syndromes, and Cutis Laxa-like syndromes. In: Frias JL, Paul NW, eds. *Craniofacial Structures in Connective Tissue Disorders.* New York: Wiley-Liss; 1988:47–61.

Greenfield G, Romano A, Stein R, Goodman RM. Blue sclera and keratoconus: Key features of a distinct disorder of connective tissue. *Clin Genet.* 1973;4:8–16.

Gregoratos N, Bartsocas CS, Papas K. Blue sclera with keratoglobus and brittle cornea. *Br J Ophthalmol.* 1971; 55:424–426.

Gurwood A, Mastrangelo D. Understanding angioid streaks. *J Am Optom Assoc.* 1997;68:309–314.

Hollister DW. Ehlers–Danlos type VIII. *Clin Res.* 1980;28:99A.

Hood OJ, Horton WA, Duvic M. Ehlers–Danlos syndrome caused by an apparent structural mutation in the carboxy portion of pro-alpha 2(I). *Am J Hum Genet.* 1987; 41:A100.

Hyams SW, Dar H, Neumann E. Blue sclera and keratoglobus. Ocular signs of a systemic connective tissue disorder. *Br J Ophthalmol.* 1969;53:53–58.

Kaplan JA, LaFranco FP, Garoon I. Hereditary retinal detachment and vitreoretinal dysplasias. In: Renie WA, ed. *Goldberg's Genetic and Metabolic Eye Disease.* 2nd ed. Boston: Little, Brown; 1986:411–422.

May MA, Beauchamp GR. Collagen maturation defects in Ehlers–Danlos keratopathy. *J Ped Ophthalmol Strab.* 1987; 24:78–82.

McDermott M, Holladay J, Liu D. Corneal topography in Ehlers–Danlos syndrome. *J Cataract Refract Surg.* 1998; 24:1212–1215.

McKusick VA. The Ehlers–Danlos syndrome. In: McKusick VA: *Heritable Disorders of Connective Tissue.* 4th ed. St. Louis: Mosby; 1972:292–360.

Meyer E, Ludatscher RM, Zonis S. Collagen fibril abnormalities in the extraocular muscles in Ehlers–Danlos syndrome. *J Ped Ophthalmol Strab.* 1988;25:67–72.

Miura S, Shirakama A, Ohara A, et al. Fibronectin receptor on polymorphonuclear leukocytes in families of Ehlers–Danlos syndrome and other hereditary connective tissue diseases. *J Lab Clin Med.* 1990;116:363–368.

Nelson LB, Maumenee IH. Ectopia Lentis. *Surv Ophthalmol.* 1982;27:143–160.

Paton D. *The Relation of Angioid Streaks to Systemic Disease.* Springfield, IL: Thomas; 1972:62–63.

Perry HO, Bietti G. Ocular involvement in dermatologic disease. In: Mausolf FA, ed. *The Eye in Systemic Disease.* 2nd ed. St. Louis: Mosby; 1980:413–415.

Pinnell SR, Krane SM, Kenzora JE, Glimachen MJ. A heritable disorder of connective tissue, hydroxylysine-deficient collagen disease. *N Engl J Med.* 1972;286:1013–1020.

Pollack J, Custer P, Hart W. Ocular complications in Ehlers–Danlos syndrome type IV. *Arch Ophthalmol.* 1997;115: 416–419.

Pope F, Burrows N. Ehlers–Danlos syndrome has varied molecular mechanisms. *J Med Genet.* 1997;34:400–410.

Pope FM, Narcisi P. Nicholls AC, Lieberman M. Clinical presentation of Ehlers–Danlos syndrome type IV. *Arch Dis Child.* 1988;63:1016–1025.

Robertson I. Keratoconus and the Ehlers–Danlos syndrome. A new aspect of keratoconus. *Med J Aust.* 1975;1:571–573.

Sato K, Ikeda T. Fluorescein angiographic features of neovascular maculopathy in angioid streaks. *Jpn J Ophthalmol.* 1994;38:417–422.

Schievink WI, Piepgras DG, Earnest F, Gordon H. Spontaneous carotid cavernous fistula in Ehlers–Danlos syndrome type IV. Case report. *J Neurosurg.* 1991;74:991–998.

Siegel RC, Black CM, Baily AJ. Cross-linking of collagen in the X-linked Ehlers–Danlos type V. *Biochem Biophys Res Commun.* 1979;88:281–287.

Steinmann B, Tuderman L, Peltonen L, et al. Evidence for a structural mutation of procollagen type I in the Ehlers–Danlos syndrome VII. *J Biol Chem.* 1980;255:8887–8893.

Stewart RE, Hollister DW, Rimoin DL. A new variant of the Ehlers–Danlos syndrome: An autosomal disorder of fragile skin, abnormal scarring, and generalized periodontitis. *Birth Defects.* 1977;13:85–93.

Thomas IT, Frias JL. The cardiovascular manifestations of genetic disorders of collagen metabolism. *Ann Clin Lab Sci.* 1987;17:377–382.

Vissing H, D'Alessio M, Lee B, et al. Multiexon deletion in the procollagen III gene is associated with mild Ehlers–Danlos syndrome Type IV. *J Biol Chem.* 1991;266:5244–5248.

Wenstrup RJ, Murad S, Pinnell SR. Ehlers–Danlos syndrome type VI: Clinical manifestations of collagen lysyl hydroxylase deficiency. *J Pediatr.* 1989;115:405–409.

Wirtz MK, Keene DR, Hori H, et al. In vivo and in vitro noncovalent association of excised alpha 1 (I) amino-terminal propeptides with mutant pN alpha 2(I) collagen chains in native mutant collagen in a case of Ehlers–Danlos syndrome, type VII. *J Biol Chem.* 1990;265:6312–6317.

Chapter 33

OSTEOGENESIS IMPERFECTA

Margaret McNelis

Osteogenesis imperfecta (OI), also known as fragilitas ossium and maladie de Lobstein, is an inherited disorder of connective tissue. It affects bone, joints and ligaments, skin, eyes, and ears. The classic clinical triad of OI includes blue sclera, deafness, and bone fracture.

EPIDEMIOLOGY

Systemic

OI has a frequency of greater than 1 in every 20,000 births. There is no sex or racial predilection.

Ocular

Blue scleras are most frequent in type I OI. No further epidemiological data are available regarding the ocular manifestations of OI.

PATHOPHYSIOLOGY/DISEASE PROCESS

Systemic

There are four varieties of OI. All four types exhibit a disorder of type I collagen synthesis in all affected tissues. Type I collagen is the major structural protein of bone, skin, and vessels. It also provides tensile strength and sites for anchoring cells and platelet aggregation. Unaffected family members may be carriers of an abnormal gene of connective tissue. Table 33–1 contains a summary of the systemic manifestations of OI. Dentin protein analysis shows that although OI teeth may appear clinically normal, the majority of collagen in all types of OI dentin is abnormal.

OI type I is the mildest and most common form. It is inherited as autosomal dominant in two varieties, with and without dental abnormalities. When dental abnormalities are present, decreased production of pulp and dentin produce irregular yellowish-blue teeth. Brittleness of bone and multiple fractures may be present at birth. Nonunion of fractures occurs in all forms of OI much more frequently than normals. This can lead to repeated fractures at a progressively deformed site. This improves after puberty, but returns with pregnancy and menopause. Easy bruising results from poor coagulability and capillary fragility. Mitral valve prolapse and aortic dilatation may also be seen. Deafness occurs in about one third of patients due to otosclerosis beginning in the second to third decades, along with a progressive sensorineural hearing loss that develops independently. Loose joints and tendons result in flat feet, kyphosis (hunchback), and frequent dislocations.

OI type II, the most severe type of the disease, is the perinatal lethal form. It is a result of a sporadic dominant mutation, or can be inherited recessively. Almost all bones break in utero, leading to marked deformity

TABLE 33–1. SYSTEMIC MANIFESTATIONS OF OSTEOGENESIS IMPERFECTA

Bone
- Bony fragility and brittleness causing multiple fractures (type I,II,III)
- Bone deformity secondary to repeated fractures (types I,II,III)
- Compressive fractures (types I,II,III)
  Leading to an increased susceptibility to large hematomas or intracranial hemorrhages
- Short stature (types I,III)

Joints and Ligaments
- Loose joints and tendons may cause flat feet, kyphosis, frequent joint dislocations (types I,III)
- Severe kyphoscoliosis can lead to respiratory failure

Skin
- Thin and translucent skin (type IV)
- Tears at the corners of the mouth and groin (type IV)
- Easy bruising and hemorrhaging (type IV)
- Hyperplastic scars
- Excessive sweating
- Abnormal temperature regulation
- Malignant hyperthermia

Ears
- Otosclerosis leading to hearing loss (types I,III)
- Sensorineural hearing loss (types I,III)

Teeth
- Abnormal dentin and pulp leading to irregular teeth (types I,III,IV)

Cardiovascular
- Aortic regurgitation, floppy mitral valve, fragile vessels (type IV), premature vascular calcifications

Gastrointestinal
- Constipation

of limbs. Dismemberment can also occur during birth. If the infant survives delivery, he or she rarely lives longer than a few days.

OI type III, less severe than type II, is inherited in a heterogeneous autosomal recessive manner. There are numerous fractures at birth; however, bones are better developed than type II, with the infant's condition nearly normal. These children develop short stature and severe bone deformities, which are often independent of fracture. Kyphoscoliosis is dramatic, and can ultimately lead to respiratory failure. There is moderate looseness of joints, and variable dental and hearing changes. Chronic abdominal pain and constipation are associated with severe acetabular protrusion.

OI type IV has the most variable presentation of the four, and is transmitted both recessively and in a dominant form. Joint and hearing involvement are less frequent than in other types. The skin appears thin and translucent. Skin tears at the corners of the mouth and groin areas may occur. This type can be almost indistinguishable from Ehlers-Danlos syndrome when joints are involved. Some patients show significant cardiovascular alterations such as aortic regurgitation, floppy mitral valves, fragile blood vessels, and hypocoagulability. These may all lead to an increased susceptibility to large hematomas, compressive skull fractures, and intracranial hemorrhages.

Ocular

Electron microscopy of the scleral tissue of all OI patients reveals fibrils that resemble immature collagen. These fibrils are more translucent and uniformly arranged than normal, allowing uveal blood and pigment to become clinically visible as a blue cast. Blue sclera (Figure 33–1) are most frequent in type I. The degree of blueness is dependent upon the severity of collagen defect, and there is significant variability in color, due to the high heterogeneity of the disease. OI is associated with reduced ocular rigidity, although there does not seem to be a correlation between the degree of blueness of the sclera and amount of reduction in rigidity.

Corneal fibril arrangements are similar to those found in the sclera. This may manifest as reduced cen-

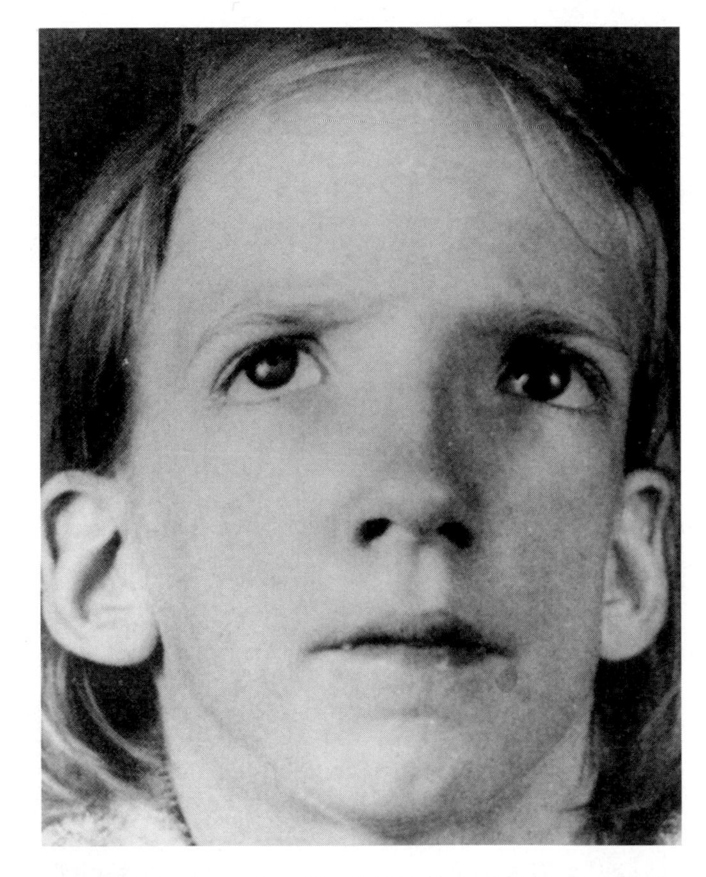

Figure 33–1. Blue sclera. (*Reprinted with permission from McKusick VA.* Heritable Disorders of Connective Tissue. *4th ed. St. Louis: Mosby, 1972:417.*)

TABLE 33–2. OCULAR MANIFESTATIONS OF OSTEOGENESIS IMPERFECTA

Blue Sclera
- Associated with reduced ocular rigidity

Corneal Collagen Irregularities
- Can lead to decreased central corneal thickness, keratoconus, megalocornea, anterior embryotoxin

Other
- Congenital glaucoma
- Crystalline lens dislocation
- Zonular cataract formation
- Partial color blindness
- Choroidal sclerosis
- Subhyaloid hemorrhage
- Optic neuropathy/atrophy secondary to skull fractures causing optic nerve compression

tral corneal thickness, keratoconus, megalocornea, or anterior embryotoxin.

Congenital glaucoma, crystalline lens dislocation, zonular cataract formation, partial color blindness, and choroidal sclerosis have been described in association with OI, as well as a report of subhyaloid hemorrhage (Table 33–2). Optic neuropathy and atrophy may occur in the more severe forms in which skull fractures cause optic nerve compression.

DIAGNOSIS

Systemic

Diagnosis of OI types I and II can be made in utero by ultrasound early in the second trimester, or by chorionic villus sampling in the first trimester in families with a previously affected fetus. At birth, multiple fractures in an infant without a history of abuse may lead to diagnosis of any type; however, it may be more difficult to distinguish until later in life, when the diagnosis is aided by family history, pedigree, and x-rays (Table 33–3). Hypercalciuria occurs in OI children and can be detected through blood testing. Its magnitude reflects the severity of the skeletal disease. This may predict the stature of the child when he or she is older. Bone biopsy is of limited use in OI. Differential diagnosis includes juvenile osteoporosis, osteomalacia, and rickets, and is distinguished through biochemical measures of calcium, phosphorous, parathyroid hormone, and vitamin D (Table 33–4).

TABLE 33–3. DIAGNOSTIC TESTS UTILIZED IN OSTEOGENESIS IMPERFECTA

- X-rays
- Bone mineral density
- Skin biopsy
- Collagen analysis

TABLE 33–4. DIFFERENTIAL DIAGNOSIS OF OSTEOGENESIS IMPERFECTA (OI)

Systemic
- OI must be distinguished from abuse (intracranial injury, lacerations, burns are unlikely in OI).

Ocular
- Retinal hemorrhage should raise suspicion of child abuse.

Ocular

Blue sclera is the most obvious ocular finding in OI and may be helpful in the diagnosis of this disease. In addition, lens subluxation, choroidal sclerosis, and retinal and subhyaloid hemorrhages may be found following birth trauma.

> Retinal hemorrhages are unlikely in OI and should be reported to the patient's pediatrician and radiologist when abuse is suspected.

TREATMENT AND MANAGEMENT

Systemic

Systemic therapy for all types of OI (Table 33–5) is primarily through orthopedic measures such as using lightweight external bracing, molded seating, and surgical

TABLE 33–5. TREATMENT AND MANAGEMENT OF OSTEOGENESIS IMPERFECTA

Orthopedic Measures
- Braces
- Molded seating
- Surgical straightening with long-bone rodding

Physical Therapy
- Swimming and exercise to maintain muscle tone and range of motion

Hearing
- Hearing aids
- Surgical management

Genetic Counseling

Ocular
- Standard management (contact lenses) for keratoconus
- Standard glaucoma management
- Low-vision devices if visual impairment present

straightening with long-bone rodding. Physical therapy and swimming to maintain muscle tone and range of motion are crucial. Surgical intervention is indicated if neurologic symptoms arise, related to brainstem compression. Long-bone rodding is used in cases of recurrent fracture or nonunion. Progressive hearing loss has been treated surgically with stapes operations, but results have been disappointing. Cyclic administration of pamidronate appears to increase bone mineral density and decrease pain in children with severe osteopenia. Genetic counseling is recommended in families of patients with OI.

Ocular

Management of the ocular manifestations of OI is limited (Table 33–5). No treatment exists or is necessary for blue sclera, and it does not appear that these eyes are more prone to rupture than normal eyes. Keratoconus is managed in a standard manner, with appropriate contact lenses. Glaucoma is also managed with standard medical treatment. If vision becomes severely impaired, low-vision devices may become necessary; however, it is important to keep in mind limitations in mobility due to bone deformities (eg, kyphoscoliosis). Yoked base-up prisms may be helpful for reading in a case of severe kyphoscoliosis or impaired head and neck movement.

CONCLUSION

OI is a generalized disorder of connective tissue that manifests itself specifically in the bones and eyes, as well as other tissues and systems. It can occur sporadically, or can be inherited either dominantly or recessively, displaying a wide variety of penetrance. There is limited therapy available; however, many advances have been made in understanding its mechanism and genetics. The eyecare practitioner may play an important role in the diagnosis and management of this disorder.

REFERENCES

Ablin DS. Osteogenesis imperfecta: A review. *Can Assoc Radiol J.* 1998;49:110–123.

Beighton P, Winship I, Behari D. The ocular form of osteogenesis imperfecta: A new autosomal recessive syndrome. *Clin Genet.* 1985;28:69–75.

Brons JT, van der Harten HJ, Wladmiroff JW, et al. Prenatal ultrasonographic diagnosis of osteogenesis imperfecta. *Am J Obstet Gynecol.* 1988;159:176–181.

Byers PH, Bonadio JF. Osteogenesis imperfecta: Clinical heterogeneity. In: Brown KS, Salinas CS, Paul NW, eds. *Craniofacial Mesenchyme in Morphogenesis and Malformation.* New York: Liss; 1983:65–75.

Chan CC, Green WR, de la Cruz ZC, et al. Ocular findings in osteogenesis imperfecta congenita. *Arch Ophthalmol.* 1982;100:1459–1463.

Chines A, Petersen DJ, Schranck FW, Whyte MP. Hypercalcuria in children severely affected with osteogenesis imperfecta. *J Pediatr.* 1991;119:51–57.

Engelbert RH, Pruijs HE, Beemer FA. Osteogenesis imperfecta in childhood: Treatment strategies. *Arch Phys Med Rehabil.* 1998;79:1590–1594.

Gage JP, Francis MJ, Smith R. Abnormal amino acid analyses obtained from osteogenesis imperfecta dentin. *J Dent Res.* 1988;67:1097–1102.

Gamble JG, Rinsky LA, Strudwick J, Bleck EE. Non-union of fractures in children who have osteogenesis imperfecta. *J Bone Joint Surg.* 1988;70:439–443.

Garretsen TJ, Cremers CW. Stapes surgery in osteogenesis imperfecta: analysis of postoperative hearing loss. *Ann Otol Rhinol Laryngol.* 1991;100:120–130.

Gerber LH, Binder H, Weintrob J, et al. Rehabilitation of children and infants with osteogenesis imperfecta. A program for ambulation. *Clin Orthop.* 1990;251:254–262.

Glorieux FH, Bishop NJ, Plotkin H, et al. Cyclic administration of pamidronate in children with severe osteogenesis imperfecta. *N Engl J Med.* 1998;339:947–952.

Kaiser-Kupfer MI, McCain L, Shapiro JR, et al. Low ocular rigidity in patients with osteogenesis imperfecta. *Invest Ophthalmol Vis Sci.* 1981;20:807–809.

Khalil M. Subhyaloid hemorrhage in osteogenesis imperfecta tarda. *Can J Ophthalmol.* 1983;18:251–252.

Krane SM. Heritable and developmental disorders of connective tissue. In: Stein IJ. *Internal Medicine.* 3rd ed. Boston: Little, Brown; 1990:1818–1820.

Marini JC. Osteogenesis imperfecta—Managing brittle bones. *N Engl J Med.* 1998;339:986–987.

McKusick VA. *Heritable Disorders of Connective Tissue.* 4th ed. St. Louis: Mosby; 1972:390–454.

Minch CM, Kruse RW. Osteogenesis imperfecta: A review of basic science and diagnosis. *Orthopedics.* 1998;21:558–567.

Miura S, Shirakami A, Ohara A, et al. Fibronectin receptor on polymorphonuclear leukocytes in families of Ehlers–Danlos syndrome and other hereditary connective tissue diseases. *J Lab Clin Med.* 1990;116:363–368.

Moriwake T, Seino Y. Recent progress in diagnosis and treatment of osteogenesis imperfecta. *Acta Paediatr Jpn.* 1997;39:521–527.

Nager GT. Osteogenesis imperfecta of the temporal bone and its relation to otosclerosis. *Ann Otol Rhinol Laryngol.* 1988;97:585–593.

Nogami H, Oohira A. Defective association between collagen fibrils and proteoglycans in fragile bone of osteogenesis imperfecta. *Clin Orthop.* 1988;232:284–291.

Opheim O. Loss of hearing following the syndrome of van der Hoeve–de Kleyn. *Acta Otolaryngol.* 1968;65:337.

Pedersen U, Bramsen T. Central corneal thickness in osteogenesis imperfecta and otosclerosis. *J Otorhinolaryngol Relat Spec.* 1984;46:38–41.

Rowe DW. Osteogenesis imperfecta. In: Wyngaarden JB, Smith LH, eds. *Cecil Textbook of Medicine.* 17th ed. Philadelphia: Saunders; 1985:1151–1152.

Smith R, Francis MJO, Sykes B. The eye and collagen in osteogenesis imperfecta. In: *The Eye and Inborn Errors of Metabolism.* Oxford: National Foundation–March of Dimes at the Radcliff Infirmary; 1975:563–568.

Starman BJ, Eyre D, Charbonneau H, et al. Osteogenesis imperfecta. The position for substitution for glycine by cysteine in the triple helical domain of the pro alpha 1(I) chains of type I collagen determines the clinical phenotype. *J Clin Invest.* 1989;84:1206–1214.

Tosi LL. Osteogenesis imperfecta. *Curr Opin Pediatr.* 1997; 9:94–99.

Verstreken M, Claes J, Van de Hening PH. Osteogenesis imperfecta and hearing loss. *Acta Otorhinolaryingol Belg.* 1996; 50:91–98.

Section VIII

PHAKOMATOSES

Chapter 34

NEUROFIBROMATOSIS

Joan K. Portello

Neurofibromatosis (NF) is a member of the group of diseases called the phakomatoses. These hereditary disorders are characterized by the appearance of multiple benign tumors called hamartomas involving various body tissues. Hamartomas are not true neoplasia, but consist of disorganized overgrowth of cells appropriate for that organ. NF is characterized by small pigmented skin lesions (café-au-lait spots), followed by the development of multiple peripheral nerve tumors (neurofibromas and schwannomas). Several different forms of NF have been identified. The most common are referred to as NF type 1 (NF-1) and NF type 2 (NF-2).

The systemic and ocular manifestations of NF can be extremely variable in severity because of the incomplete penetrance of this autosomal dominant condition, as well as its variable age-dependent expression. Familial expressivity does not contribute to the severity of the disease in future generations.

NF may have been first recognized as early as the mid-1600s. In 1882, the German pathologist Frederick Daniel von Recklinghausen described in his classic treatise a disorder comprised of multiple fibromas of the skin and their relationship to multiple neuromas. He is credited for giving the disease the eponym von Recklinghausen disease.

Possibly the most famous victim of NF was Joseph Carey Merrick, born August 5, 1862. He was known as the Elephant Man because his forehead was distinctly grooved toward the middle, with enlarged swellings on either side resembling those of an Indian elephant. Although Merrick died at the age of 27, photographs, casts of his head and limbs, and reconstruction of his skeletal bones have provided information about his disorder. Although it is believed (Seward, 1990) that Merrick probably suffered from NF, the possibility exists that he may have suffered from other diseases involving bone and skin malformations (Tibbles & Cohen, 1986).

EPIDEMIOLOGY

Systemic

NF-1, an autosomal dominant disorder, affects approximately 1 out of every 4000 live births worldwide. There is a prevalence of 30 cases of NF-1 per 10,000 of the total population in a given year. In the United States alone over 100,000 patients have been diagnosed with NF-1. Spontaneous mutations are accountable for about 50% of all new cases reported. Riccardi (1989a) provided substantiating data that sporadic mutations may be correlated with advanced paternal age. NF-2, also autosomal dominant, has a frequency of 1 in 50,000 individuals worldwide, with just under 1000 cases reported in the United States. There is no race or sex predilection for NF-1 or NF-2.

Approximately 94% of NF-1 patients have one or more dermal café-au-lait spots and approximately 75%

have six or more. One or more café-au-lait spots are present in approximately 42% of patients with NF-2 and virtually no cases have six or more spots. Plexiform neurofibromas (involving a proliferation of Schwann cells from the inner aspect of nerve sheaths that follow the nerve pathway to possibly involve the spinal roots and spinal cord) occur in over 50% of patients diagnosed with NF. Riccardi (1989a), observed that at least 85% of women with neurofibromatosis developed areolar neurofibromas after puberty. Bilateral acoustic neuromas are present in 95% of NF-2 patients and approximately 5% of NF-1 patients.

Ocular

Over 50% of the patients with NF-1 have ocular features. Iris melanocytic hamartomas, known as Lisch nodules, are the most common ocular finding, occurring in approximately 90% of NF-1 and 3% of NF-2 patients. Choroidal hamartomas, the second most common ocular finding, are present in 35% of patients. Approximately 70% of optic nerve gliomas or pilocytic astrocytomas of the optic pathways (2 to 5% of all childhood brain tumors) occur in NF-1 (Listernick et al, 1997). A significant number of NF-2 patients have cataracts as the sole ocular manifestation. In a study by Ragge and colleagues (1995) it was reported that posterior subcapsular or capsular, cortical or mixed lens opacities occurred in 67% of patients with NF-2. Similarly, a study by Mautner and co-workers (1996) found posterior subcapsular cataracts in 63% of NF-2 patients. Retinal hamartomas have been found in as few as 8% and as many as 22% of NF-2 patients (Parry et al, 1994; Ragge et al, 1995). Epiretinal membranes have been reported in NF-2 (Kaye et al, 1992; Landau & Yasargil, 1993). Some studies suggest epiretinal membranes may be associated with retinal hamartomas in NF-2 (Bouzas et al, 1992; Parry et al, 1994).

PATHOPHYSIOLOGY/DISEASE PROCESS

Systemic

In order to clarify any pre-existing inconsistencies in the terminology of different types of NF, the Panel for the National Institute of Health Consensus Development on Neurofibromatosis in 1987 devised a classification for this disease. The panel acknowledged that two distinctive forms of NF exist, but that variability of these forms also may be found. These other forms with variability are quite difficult to classify at this time due to insufficient clinical and/or genetic criteria.

NF type 1, or NF-1, is most common, involving peripheral nervous system manifestations, specifically neurofibromas, as described by von Recklinghausen. NF type 2, or NF-2, primarily has central nervous system manifestations, specifically bilateral acoustic neuromas. Frequently, patients with bilateral acoustic neuromas suffer from progressive hearing loss. A specific allele has been identified on different chromosomes for these two distinct categories. In some cases the clinical and pathological criteria for NF-1 and NF-2 overlap. When this occurs, the syndrome is referred to as NF-3. Other variants of neurofibromatosis (NF-4 through NF-8) have also been reported (Riccardi, 1989b). Segmental NF-5, which is a rare form of neurofibromatosis, is characterized by cutaneous and neural defects limited to only one body region or a single dermatomal segment. Patients diagnosed with NF-5 have a negative family history of neurofibromatosis (Hager et al, 1997). However, a case report noted NF-1 was diagnosed in a child of a parent with segmental NF (Boltshauser et al, 1989).

Genetic linkage studies have shown the NF-1 gene to be linked to the nerve growth factor receptor on the long distal arm of chromosome 17 at 17q11.2 (Fountain et al, 1989). The mapping of the NF-2 allele has been localized to chromosome 22 at 22q11 (Karnes, 1998). The genes identified in both NF-1 and NF-2 act as tumor suppressor genes. Research has shown that this information can be used in DNA analysis to permit molecular prenatal or presymptomatic diagnosis. It has not been determined whether distinct genetic loci or variable expression of the NF gene is responsible for the variant forms.

It is very difficult to describe a singular natural history of NF given its tremendous diversity (Figure 34–1). Café-au-lait spots are often present at birth or within the first 5 years of life. These dermal spots usually increase in number and size by adulthood but do not cause any adverse effects. Multiple freckling within skin folds, usually in the axillary region and/or the groin area, is another attribute found in NF-1 patients. Hamartomas involving neural tissue are termed neurofibromas. It is not known what causes neurofibromas to be present initially, to progress, or to recur. The higher levels of sex hormones present during puberty and during pregnancy may stimulate growth of the tumors. Circulating nerve growth factor, which stimulates growth of the peripheral nervous system, has been implicated in systemic and orbital tumors.

> A single café-au-lait macule, noted in a young child, may be the presenting sign of neurofibromatosis; therefore, these patients should be monitored for subsequent development of any other systemic and/or ocular manifestations.

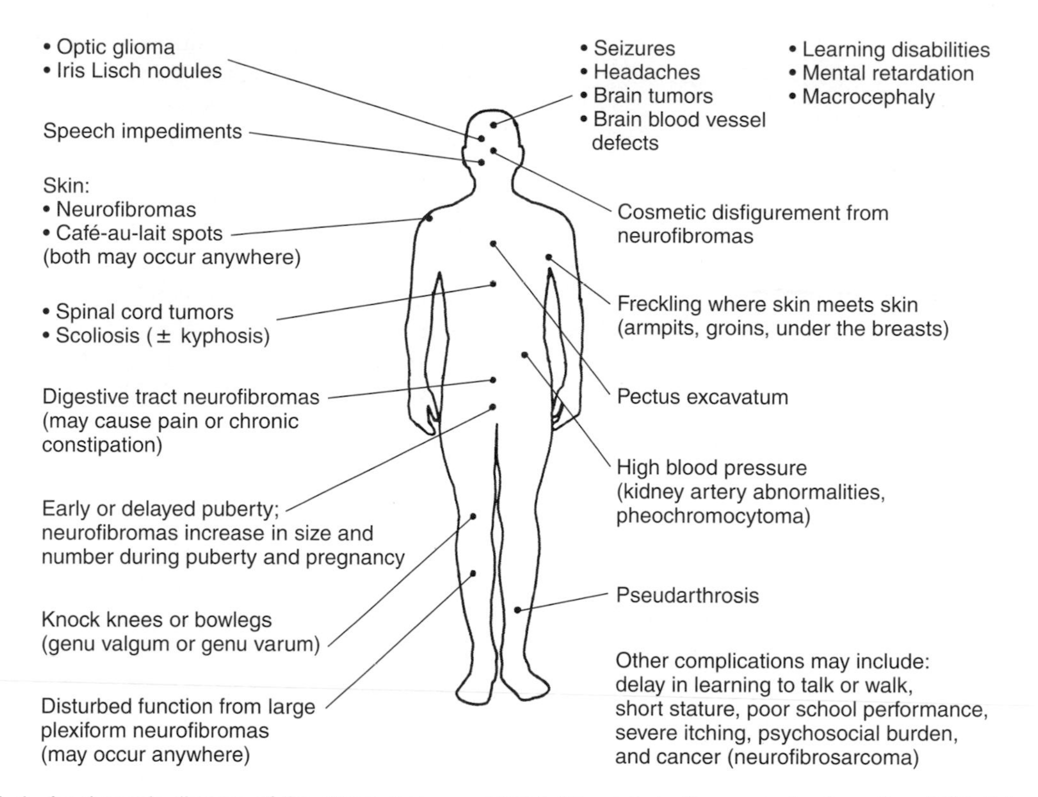

Figure 34–1. A schematic diagram of the clinical features of NF-1. (*Reprinted with permission from Powell PP. Schematic representation of von Recklinghausen neurofibromatosis (NF-1): An aid for patient and family education.* Neurofibromatosis. *1988;1:164–165.*)

Neurofibromas that arise from Schwann cells and perineural cells, fibroblasts, endothelial cells, pericytes, and mast cells occur in the central and peripheral nervous systems. At least three types of neurofibromas have been reported to occur in either NF-1 or NF-2, namely, cutaneous, subcutaneous, and plexiform. Cutaneous and subcutaneous neurofibromas are usually first noticeable at the time of puberty and increase in number throughout adulthood. Cutaneous neurofibromas are present in the integument and can be found on the face, trunk, and proximal limbs, usually sparing the shins. These flesh-colored, soft, vascular lesions vary in size from several millimeters to approximately 65 cm in diameter (Figure 34–2). They can number one and between thousands and typically are not associated with pain or tenderness. The tumors are mobile and as the dermis is moved, the tumor moves simultaneously. Cutaneous neurofibromas are less prominent in both size and number in NF-2 or other forms of the disease, compared with NF-1.

Subcutaneous neurofibromas are very solid tumors ranging anywhere in size from a few millimeters to 4 cm (Figure 34–3). They are associated with pain and tenderness. These tumors are located under the dermis. Therefore, if the skin moves, the tumor does not move with it. Subcutaneous neurofibromas are primarily present in NF-1, although paraspinal subcutaneous neurofibromas are present in both NF-1 and in NF-2 (Mautner et al, 1996).

The onset of plexiform neurofibromas may occur pre- or postpuberty. Plexiform neurofibromas may be further categorized into two subtypes: diffuse and nodular (Riccardi, 1989a). The diffuse plexiform neurofibroma is a soft and rubbery tumor with occasional

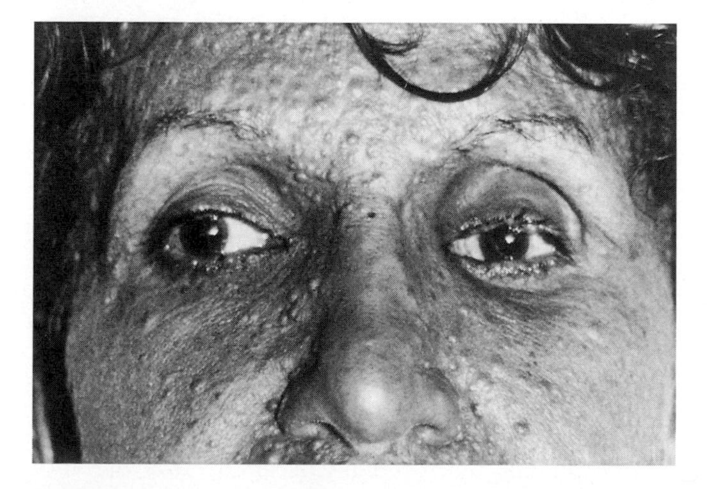

Figure 34–2. A 55-year-old white female with NF-1 and cutaneous neurofibromas of the face and left upper lid margin.

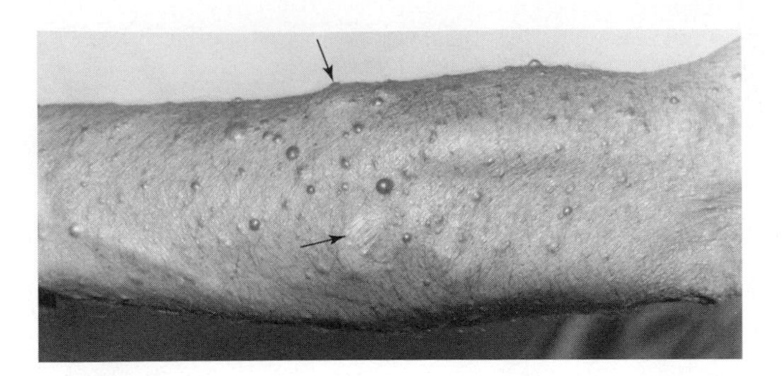

Figure 34–3. The same 55-year-old white female with NF-1 and subcutaneous neurofibromas of the arm.

overlying hyperpigmentation of the dermis. These tumors are usually localized and are caused by dysplasia of skin, muscles, and afferent blood vessels with subsequent overgrowth in that region. Nodular plexiform neurofibromas involve both the superficial and deep major and minor nerves. These painful and tender nodules tend to be dense and grow in an array of undulated strings along the nerves.

Other than being cosmetically unappealing and causing pruritus, cutaneous neurofibromas do not cause any serious threat to the patient's life. Involvement of either a paraspinal and/or nodular plexiform neurofibroma may lead to paraplegia or quadriplegia, and premature death has occurred due to these serious paralytic disorders (Poyhonen et al, 1997; Riccardi, 1989a). Diffuse plexiform neurofibromas not only have moderate to severe cosmetic abnormalities but, depending upon the location of the tumor, surgery may be necessary to prolong the patient's life. For instance, a diffuse plexiform neurofibroma found encompassing the trachea will require excision and occasionally tracheostomy.

Schwannomas rarely occur in NF-1, but will primarily affect the fifth and eighth cranial nerves in NF-2. Malignant schwannomas, although uncommon, decrease survival rate. Six percent or more of patients with NF-1 are likely to develop neurofibrosarcomas, usually from a pre-existing benign neurofibroma. This malignancy also contributes to premature death. Other invasive tumors associated with neurofibromatosis are meningiomas, ependymomas, and pheochromocytoma (tumor of the adrenal glands that leads to secondary hypertension). Neurofibromas of the gastrointestinal tract are found in approximately 10% of patients and can cause constipation.

Nontumorous characteristic features common to NF-1 are learning disabilities (diagnosed in 60% of NF-1 patients), speech impediments, seizures, headache, hydrocephalus, macrocephaly (seen in 16% of NF-1 patients), and premature or delayed puberty. Skeletal abnormalities include short stature, kyphoscoliosis (curvature of the lower and upper thoracic spine accompanying acute anteroposterior angulation), pseudarthrosis (a condition that mimics arthritis), sphenoid wing dysplasia, pectus excavatum (the sternum is abnormally concave), genu valgum/varum (knock-knee/bowleggedness), and pes planus (flat-footedness). Furthermore, Gabriel (1997) reported that the most common associated orthopedic manifestation of NF-1 is scoliosis. Vascular disorders (involvement of the afferent blood vessels) can affect the cerebral, gastrointestinal, and renal systems. Spinal and cerebral arachnoid cysts have also been reported (Table 34–1).

Ocular

Ocular involvement, especially in NF-1, may affect any part of the eye (Table 34–2). It can present during infancy before any systemic signs appear. One of the earliest signs and most common ophthalmic findings is the presence of iris Lisch nodules. These are found almost exclusively in NF-1 and may aid in the early diagnosis of NF (Figure 34–4). These melanocytic hamartomas are usually bilateral, small, well-defined elevated masses arising from the iris surface. They can appear as clear to yellow or brown in color. Lisch nod-

TABLE 34–1. SYSTEMIC MANIFESTATIONS OF NEUROFIBROMATOSIS

Skin Lesions
- Café-au-lait spots
- Freckling on skin folds

Peripheral Nerve Hamartomas
- Neurofibromas: cutaneous, subcutaneous, plexiform (diffuse and nodular)
- Schwannomas primarily affecting cranial nerves V and VIII
- Neurofibrosarcomas
- Meningiomas
- Ependymomas
- Pheochromocytomas

Central Nerve Tumors
- Bilateral/unilateral acoustic neuromas (vestibular schwannomas)
- Schwann cell tumors of the lining of the brain
- Meningiomas
- Ependymomas

Nontumorous Features
- Learning disabilities
- Speech impediments
- Seizures
- Headaches
- Hydrocephalus
- Macrocephaly
- Premature/delayed puberty
- Skeletal abnormalities: short stature, kyphoscoliosis, pseudoarthritis, sphenoid wing dysplasia, pectus excavatum, genu vulgum/varum, pes planus
- Vascular disorders affecting cerebral, gastrointestinal, and renal systems

TABLE 34–2. OCULAR MANIFESTATIONS OF NEUROFIBROMATOSIS

Anterior Segment and Adnexa
- Iris Lisch nodules
- Nodular plexiform neurofibromas of upper or lower lids
- Café-au-lait spots on eyelids
- Neurofibromas or schwannomas of conjunctiva, cornea, and/or orbit
- Corneal nerve thickening
- Decreased corneal sensitivity
- Exposure keratitis secondary to fifth- or seventh-nerve paralysis
- Hamartomas of anterior chamber

Glaucoma
- Congenital glaucoma
- Neovascular glaucoma

Cataracts
- Posterior subcapsular/anterior cortical/nuclear sclerotic

Retina and Choroid
- Choroidal hamartomas
- Retinal astrocytic hamartomas

Optic Nerve Tumors
- Optic nerve gliomas
- Chiasmal gliomas

Orbital Tumors
- Intraorbital/intracranial meningiomas
- Diffuse neurofibromas
- Orbital plexiform neurofibromas
- Orbital schwannomas (neurilemmomas)

ules become increasingly prevalent with age. The severity of the disease is independent of the number as well as the age of onset of these nodules.

> Lisch nodules are one of the earliest, most common ocular manifestations of neurofibromatosis.

During the progression of the disease, nodular plexiform neurofibromas may be found on the upper or lower lids. When they occur on the upper lid, they can create pseudoptosis, or if they occur on the lower lid, lagophthalmos may result. When palpated, they feel like a "bag of worms." If the lesions are large, they can be surgically removed, or if smaller, they can be debulked for cosmetic purposes. Café-au-lait spots may also exist on the eyelids. Neurofibromas and neurilemmomas (schwannomas) may be found on the conjunctiva, cornea, and/or orbit. However, conjunctival hamartomas are rare, and these lesions consist of small tumors found on the bulbar and/or palpebral conjunctiva.

Corneal nerve thickening is seen with NF-1. In NF-2, reduced corneal sensitivity and exposure of the cornea resulting in superficial keratitis, ulceration, and in severe cases perforation due to fifth-nerve involvement have been reported (Parry, 1990).

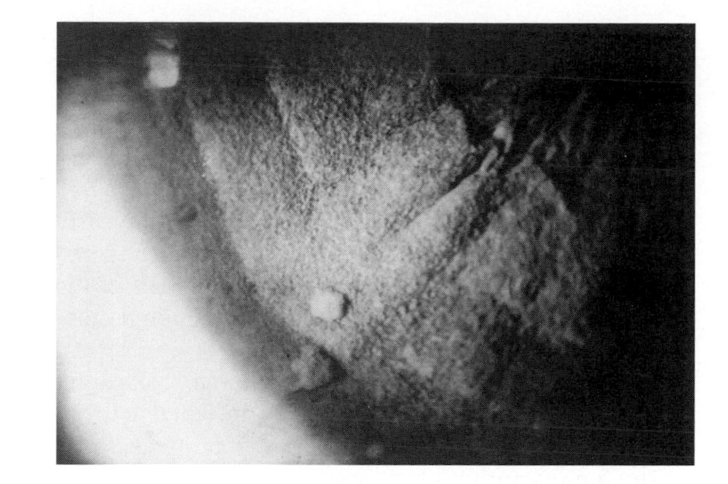

Figure 34–4. Iris Lisch nodules.

Other ophthalmic signs may include hamartomas in the anterior chamber angle, causing a decrease in aqueous outflow. Fifty percent of patients with lid neurofibromas also develop ipsilateral buphthalmos secondary to congenital glaucoma. Grant and Walton (1968) showed that congenital abnormal tissue growth, presumably a hamartoma, may cover most of the anterior chamber angle. This obstruction blocks aqueous outflow and results in glaucoma. Other studies suggest glaucoma could also be caused by a tumor thickening the choroid and ciliary body, thus closing the angle.

In adults with NF, neovascular glaucoma may be caused by the development of a fibrovascular membrane over the surface of the iris and trabecular meshwork. It is thought that the same mechanism that causes fibrovascular membrane formation in other systemic conditions is responsible for the neovascular membrane formation in NF. However, it is not known what precipitates this process.

Posterior subcapsular cataracts also may occur in NF-2 patients (at any age) and usually do not impede vision. Several reports have demonstrated that the disease also can be accompanied by anterior cortical and/or nuclear lens opacities (Bouzas et al, 1993; Mautner et al, 1996; Ragge et al, 1995).

Choroidal hamartomas are the second most common ocular finding in neurofibromatosis. They appear clinically as choroidal nevi, being flat or slightly elevated and yellow, light or dark brown, or black in color. Histologically they are a proliferation of Schwann cells rather than a proliferation of choroidal melanocytes. The lesions can be one to two optic disc diameters in size and as many as 2 to 20 in number.

Optic nerve gliomas (of astrocytic origin) and the less common chiasmal gliomas are the most common intraorbital tumors in NF. The highest incidence of optic nerve gliomas is within the first decade of life, with peak incidence between 2 to 6 years of age (Chutorian et al, 1964). Proptosis, an early ocular sign of an optic nerve glioma, may be followed by visual loss and motility restriction with severity depending upon the degree of the proptosis and the size of the tumor. In the early stages, the optic nerve becomes atrophic but has distinct borders. Disc elevation, swelling, or gliosis of the optic nerve will not be present. Optic nerve gliomas generally do not infiltrate the muscle cone or any orbital nerves. Evidence of an optic nerve glioma in a young child may become apparent before any other neurofibroma manifestations. Chiasmal pathway invasion by a growing intraorbital tumor is a rare occurrence. Chiasmal tumors often present with strabismus or nystagmus (especially in children) followed by hypothalamic disturbances and increased intracranial pressure.

> A child less than 6 years old who presents with an optic pathway glioma should be evaluated for neurofibromatosis.

Because of the variability of the natural history of optic nerve and chiasmal gliomas, it is difficult to predict visual prognosis in these patients. Optic nerve gliomas may recur after excision, never progress with or without radiation treatment, or may even improve with or without radiation treatment. Long-term survival with optic gliomas is more favorable than with chiasmal tumors. The initial presentation of increased intracranial pressure associated with chiasmal tumors usually leads to hydrocephalus. In these cases, cerebrospinal fluid bypass surgery has not been shown to increase the survival rate.

Intraorbital and intracranial meningiomas, typical of NF-2, occur less frequently than optic gliomas. Meningiomas that grow along the optic nerve or just behind the globe eventually result in a proptotic eye with vision loss. Meningiomas that infiltrate within the optic nerve will demonstrate signs of disc swelling and/or optic atrophy. Optic nerve optociliary shunt vessels, venous stasis retinopathy, and intraretinal hemorrhages tend to appear as the tumor progresses. Generally, intraorbital and intracranial meningiomas occur in the first decade of life, but they may present at any age. Early diagnosis and treatment is essential to preserve any functional vision. The survival rate is very good because meningiomas do not metastasize.

Retinal astrocytic hamartomas of the retinal nerve fiber layer or optic nerve (which are typical of tuberous sclerosis) are less common (Destro et al, 1991).

Orbital plexiform neurofibromas are usually accompanied by sphenooccipital bony deformities and defects in other parts of the skull. These bony defects may cause the patient's pulse to be transmitted to the cerebrospinal fluid, and result in pulsatile exophthalmos. Temporal lobe herniation through the bony deformities also may create a pulsatile exophthalmos (Jakobiec & Jones, 1991). Pulsating exophthalmos caused by neurofibromas occurs mostly in adulthood and should not be confused with carotid–cavernous sinus fistulas, arteriovenous malformations, large frontal mucoceles, or orbital varices. If left untreated, these benign slow-growing tumors can cause enormous craniofacial disfigurement.

DIAGNOSIS

Systemic

The National Institute of Health Consensus Development Conference on Neurofibromatosis in 1987 proposed diagnostic criteria for NF-1 and NF-2 (Tables 34–3 and 34–4). Although these guidelines greatly aid the healthcare practitioner in diagnosing this disease, *there can be overlap between the two categories.*

NF may be suspected on routine physical examination when dermal hamartomas are present. They may appear anywhere on the body. Another charac-

TABLE 34–3. DIAGNOSTIC CRITERIA FOR NF-1 AND NF-2

The clinical pathological entities to establish the diagnosis for NF-1 include two or more of the following:

1. Six or more café-au-lait macules of over 5 mm in greatest diameter in prepubertal persons and 15 mm or over in greatest diameter in postpubertal persons.
2. Two or more neurofibromas of any type or one plexiform neurofibroma (systemic and/or ocular).
3. Freckling in the axillary, inguinal, or other inguinal regions.
4. Optic glioma, unilateral or bilateral as best detected with magnetic resonance imaging techniques.
5. Two or more iris Lisch nodules as seen with a biomicroscope.
6. A distinctive osseous lesion such as sphenoid dysplasia or thinning of long bone cortices, with or without pseudarthrosis.
7. A first-degree relative (a parent, sibling, or offspring) with NF-1 by any of the above criteria.

The diagnostic criteria for NF-2 are met if a person has either of the following:

1. Bilateral eighth-nerve masses seen with appropriate imaging techniques such as magnetic resonance imaging or computerized tomographic scans.
2. A first-degree relative with NF-2 and either unilateral eighth-nerve mass or two of the following: neurofibroma(s), meningioma(s), glioma(s), schwannoma(s), or posterior subcapsular cataracts developing at any age.

From National Institutes of Health. Neurofibromatosis: National Institutes of Health Consensus Development Conference Statement. *Bethesda, MD: National Institutes of Health; July 1987.*

TABLE 34–4. DIFFERENTIAL DIAGNOSIS OF NEUROFIBROMATOSIS

Systemic
Proteus syndrome
Tuberous sclerosis
Von Hippel–Lindau disease
Sipple syndrome
Watson syndrome
McCune–Albright syndrome
Multiple mucosal neuroma syndrome
LEOPARD syndrome

Ocular
Iris Lisch nodules
Busacca nodules
Koeppe nodules
Retinal/choroidal hamartomas
Choroidal nevus
Malignant melanoma
Retinoblastoma
Hamartomas of the optic disc of retinitis pigmentosa
Optic nerve gliomas
Ischemic optic neuropathy
Pseudotumor
Optic neuritis or papillitis

teristic finding during routine physical examination is café-au-lait lesions, which may also occur anywhere on the body. Freckling in the skin folds, such as in the axillary and inguinal regions, is diagnosed on clinical examination, especially at puberty. A first-degree relative with NF-1 is helpful in establishing the diagnosis, although one should be aware that no set patterns differentiate hereditary from sporadic mutations.

Any individual who has a first-degree relative who tested positive for NF-2 and who presents with having hearing impairment should undergo a battery of diagnostic tests, including an audiogram, brainstem auditory-evoked responses, and a magnetic resonance imaging (MRI) procedure to aid in the potential diagnosis of NF-2 (Table 34–5).

Ocular

In an undiagnosed individual, Lisch nodules may be the most common initial sign of NF. Optic nerve gliomas or meningiomas are often the first evidence of NF in undiagnosed children. Optic nerve gliomas are best detected by contrast (gadolinium) MRI (magnetic resonance imaging), although computerized tomography (CT) is utilized in some cases. Furthermore, one study demonstrated the use of visual evoked potentials as a screening technique to aid in the detection of optic pathway gliomas in asymptomatic children with NF-1 (North et al, 1994). Indirect ophthalmoscopy may reveal astrocytic tumors of the retina or choroidal lesions in a patient with no previous visual symptoms.

TABLE 34–5. DIAGNOSTIC TESTS FOR NEUROFIBROMATOSIS

Systemic
Prenatal testing—chorionic villus sampling
Audiogram
Brainstem auditory-evoked responses and subsequent resection with preservation of hearing
MRI

Ocular
MRI with contrast
CT
Visual evoked potentials

If a young child has been diagnosed with a posterior subcapsular cataract and has no evidence of previous trauma, then a differential diagnosis should include NF, particularly NF-2 (see Tables 34–4 and 34–5).

TREATMENT AND MANAGEMENT

Systemic

The treatment of NF (Table 34–6) depends on the organs affected and the degree of severity. Although there is no cure for neurofibromatosis, early intervention in some cases may result in preservation of the organ. Modalities of treatment include surgical excision of tumors, radiation therapy, and chemotherapy. Surgical treatment is sometimes warranted for purely cosmetic reasons. Patients diagnosed with NF require physical examinations at least once a year. This is essential since the tumors can progress at any time.

Genetic counseling is imperative and should be suggested to patients as well as their families. Molecular prenatal diagnosis of NF-1 is now possible with chorionic villus sampling, and should be considered since a child born to an affected parent has a 50% chance of having NF-1. However, these tests do not predict clinical manifestations, severity, or complications of NF. Therefore, emphasis of the variability of the disorder should be stressed to each family member, as well as the understanding that although one child may have a mild case of NF, this does not always imply another child will manifest the same pattern. Psychosocial issues should be addressed such as cosmetic concerns and parental feelings of guilt. Patient/family educational information is available from the National Neurofibromatosis Foundation and the Acoustic Neuroma Association.

Ocular

Ocular treatment varies depending upon the extent and location of the ocular manifestations. Again, surgical intervention and/or radiotherapy may be indicated to

TABLE 34–6. TREATMENT AND MANAGEMENT OF NEUROFIBROMATOSIS

Systemic

Skin lesions

Cosmetic surgical removal of the lesions.

Peripheral nerve hamartomas

Monitor for any progression; if malignancy of the tumor ensues, then surgical intervention, radiation therapy, or chemotherapy is necessary.

Central nerve tumors

Monitor for any change in shape, size, or extension; if the tumor progresses, surgical treatment is necessary.

Ocular

Anterior segment and adnexa

Iris Lisch nodules: no treatment necessary.

Nodular plexiform neurofibromas of upper or lower lids: cosmetic surgical removal.

Exposure keratitis secondary to fifth- or seventh-nerve paralysis: standard dry eye treatment.

Hamartomas of anterior chamber: monitor for any progression; if severe, surgical intervention may be necessary.

Glaucoma

Congenital glaucoma: if intractable, enucleation is required.

Neovascular glaucoma: standard therapy.

Cataracts

Surgical intervention at any age when vision is compromised.

Retina and choroid

Surgical intervention with retinal detachment secondary to retinal or choroidal hamartomas.

Optic nerve tumors

Monitor utilizing MRI and CT imaging to document any progression of the tumor; if severe, surgical resection, radiotherapy, or chemotherapy may be warranted.

Orbital tumors

Monitor utilizing MRI and CT imaging to document any progression of the tumor or malignancy; if severe, surgical resection, radiation therapy, or chemotherapy is warranted.

preserve the functional components of the organ or to address cosmetic concerns.

Lid neurofibromas that cause secondary ptosis, entropion, or ectropion are surgically resected for both functional and cosmetic reasons. Optic nerve and chiasmal gliomas are either totally or partially excised, or radiotherapy is applied (Danoff et al,1980; Jenkin et al, 1993).

Surgical excision is the treatment of choice when dealing with orbital tumors since neurofibromas are radioinsensitive. Rarely is enucleation performed, and only if the orbital tumors are progressive or recurrent (Listernick et al, 1997).

Congenital glaucoma in infants is treated surgically by goniotomy. However, trabeculotomy is usually surgically performed if prominent iris adhesions exist. Otherwise, glaucoma secondary to neurofibromatosis is treated with standard therapy (Wong et al, 1995).

The majority of tumor findings in the eye are localized; however, all ocular findings such as Lisch nodules, choroidal hamartomas, retinal astrocytomas, and posterior lenticular changes should be carefully monitored over time for any change or growth (see Table 34–6).

CONCLUSION

Neurofibromatosis has a wide range of clinical expression. It can be so mild that it goes undiagnosed until adulthood or it can be evident at birth and include severe deformities with subsequent life-long complications. Once diagnosed, multidisciplinary management (i.e., neurologist, dermatologist, orthopedist, internist, eyecare provider) should provide follow-up care regularly. At present, research has permitted extensive genetic insight into this disease. Further genetic studies and investigation of the pathogenesis of NF are needed to perhaps prevent the complications of this disorder in the future.

REFERENCES

Binitie OP, Obikili AG. Pulsating orbital plexiform neurofibroma and optic nerve glioma. *East Afr Med J.* 1989; 66:362–364.

Boltshauser E, Stocker H, Mächler M. Neurofibromatosis type 1 in a child of a parent with segmental neurofibromatosis (NF-5). *Neurofibromatosis.* 1989;2:244–245.

Bouzas EA, Freidlin V, Parry DM, et al. Lens opacities in neurofibromatosis 2: Further significant correlations. *Br J Ophthalmol.* 1993;77:354–357.

Bouzas EA, Parry DM, Eldridge R, Kaiser-Kupfer MI. Familial occurrence of combined pigment epithelial and retina hamartomas associated with neurofibromatosis 2. *Retina.* 1992;12:103–107.

Burke JP, Bowell R, O'Doherty N. Proteus syndrome: Ocular complications. *J Pediatr Ophthalmol Strabismus.* 1988; 25:99–102.

Cawthon RM, Andersen LB, Buchberg AM, Xu GF. DNA sequence and genomic structure of EV12B, a gene lying within an intron of the neurofibromatosis type 1 gene. *Genomics.* 1991;9:446–460.

Chutorian AM, Schwartz SF, Evans RA, Carter S. Optic gliomas in children. *Neurology.* 1964;14:83–95.

Clementi M, Alessandra M, Franca A, et al. Linkage analysis of neurofibromatosis type 1. *Hum Genet.* 1991;87:91–94.

Danoff BF, Kramer S, Thompson N. The radiotherapeutic management of optic nerve gliomas in children. *Int J Radiat Oncol Biol Phys.* 1980;6:45–50.

Destro M, D'Amico DJ, Gragoudas ES, et al. Retinal manifestations of neurofibromatosis. *Arch Ophthalmol.* 1991; 109:662–666.

Eggers H, Jakobiec FA, Jones IA. Optic nerve gliomas. *Duane's Clin Ophthalmol.* 1991;2:1–17.

Fountain JW, Wallace MR, Bruce MA, et al. Physical mapping of a translocation breakpoint in neurofibromatosis. *Science.* 1989;244:1085–1087.

Gabriel KR. Neurofibromatosis. *Curr Opin Pediatr.* 1997; 9:89–93.

Good WV, Brodsky MC, Edwards MS, Hoyt WF. Bilateral retinal hamartomas in neurofibromatosis type 2. *Br J Ophthalmol.* 1991;75:190.

Grant WM, Walton DS. Distinctive gonioscopic findings in glaucoma due to neurofibromatosis. *Arch Ophthalmol.* 1968;79:127–134.

Grarretto NS, Ameriso S, Molina HA, et al. Type 2 neurofibromatosis with Lisch nodules. *Neurofibromatosis.* 1989; 2:315–321.

Hager CM, Cohen PR, Tschen JA. Segmental neurofibromatosis: Case reports and review. *J Am Acad Dermatol.* 1997;37:864–869.

Huson S, Dylan J, Beck L. Ophthalmic manifestations of neurofibromatosis. *Br J Ophthalmol.* 1987;71:235–238.

Jakobiec FA, Jones IS. Neurogenic tumors. *Duane's Clin Ophthalmol.* 1991;2:1–45.

Jenkin D, Angyalfi S, Becker L, et al. Optic glioma in children: Surveillance, resection, or irradiation? *Int J Radiat Oncol Biol Phys.* 1993;25:215–225.

Karnes PS. Neurofibromatosis: A common neurocutaneous disorder. *Mayo Clin Proc.* 1998;73:1071–1076.

Kaye LD, Rothner AD, Beauchamp GR, et al. Ocular findings associated with neurofibromatosis type 2. *Ophthalmology.* 1992;99:1424–1429.

Kobrin JL, Blodi FC, Weingeist TA. Ocular and orbital manifestations of neurofibromatosis. *Surv Ophthalmol.* 1979; 24:45–51.

Landau K, Yasargil G. Ocular fundus in neurofibromatosis type 2. *Br J Ophthalmol.* 1993;77:646–649.

Listernick R, Louis DN, Packer RJ, Gutmann DH. Optic pathway gliomas in children with neurofibromatosis 1: Consensus statement from the NF1 Optic Pathway Glioma Task Force. *Ann Neurol.* 1997;41:143–149.

Martyn LJ, Knox DL. Glial hamartoma of the retina in generalized neurofibromatosis. *Br J Ophthalmol.* 1972; 56:487–491.

Mautner V-F, Matthias L, Baser ME, et al. The neuroimaging and clinical spectrum of neurofibromatosis 2. *Neurosurgery.* 1996;38:880–885.

Michels VV, Whisnant JP, Garrity JA, Miller GM. Neurofibromatosis type 1 with bilateral acoustic neuromas. *Neurofibromatosis.* 1989;2:213–217.

Mulvihill JJ. Neurofibromatosis: History, nomenclature, and natural history. *Neurofibromatosis.* 1988;1:124–131.

National Institutes of Health. *Neurofibromatosis: National Institutes of Health Consensus Development Conference Statement.* Bethesda, MD: National Institutes of Health; July 1987.

National Institutes of Health Conference. Neurofibromatosis 1 (Recklinghausen disease) and neurofibromatosis 2 (bilateral acoustic neurofibromatosis). *Ann Intern Med.* 1990; 113:39–52.

National Institutes of Health Consensus Development Conference. Neurofibromatosis Conference Statement. *Arch Neurol.* 1988;45:575–578.

North K, Cochineas C, Tang E, Fagan E. Optic gliomas in neurofibromatosis type 1: Role of visual evoked potentials. *Pediatr Neurol.* 1994;10:426–429.

Obringer AC, Meadows AT, Elaine MD, Zackai MD. The diagnosis of neurofibromatosis-1 in the child under the age of 6 years. *AJDC.* 1989;143:717–719.

Parry DM. Gene mapping and tumor genetics. Neurofibromatosis 1 (Recklinghausen disease) and neurofibromatosis 2 (bilateral acoustic neurofibromatosis): An update. *Ann Intern Med.* 1990;113:39–52.

Parry DM, Eldridge R, Kaiser-Kupfer Ml, et al. Neurofibromatosis 2 (NF-2): Clinical characteristics of 63 affected individuals and clinical evidence for heterogeneity. *Am J Med Genet.* 1994;52:450–461.

Pou-Serradell A, Ugarte-Elola AC. Optic pathway gliomas in neurofibromatosis. *Neurofibromatosis.* 1989;2:227–232.

Powell PP. Schematic representation of von Recklinghausen neurofibromatosis (NF-1): An aid for patient and family education. *Neurofibromatosis.* 1988;1:164–165.

Poyhonen M, Niemela S, Herva R. Risk of malignancy and death in neurofibromatosis. *Arch Pathol Lab Med.* 1997; 121:139–143.

Pulst SM. Prenatal diagnosis of the neurofibromatoses. *Clin Perinatol.* 1990;17:829–843.

Ragge NK, Baser ME, Klein J, et al. Ocular abnormalities in neurofibromatosis 2. *Am J Ophthalmol.* 1995;120: 634–641.

Riccardi VM. Neurofibromatosis update. *Neurofibromatosis.* 1989a;2:284–291.

Riccardi VM. Is NF-1 always distinct from NF-2? *Neurofibromatosis.* 1989b;2:193–194. Editorial.

Rosner J. Clinical review of neurofibromatosis. *J Am Optom Assoc.* 1990;61:613–618.

Seiff SR, Brodsky MC, MacDonald G, et al. Orbital optic glioma in neurofibromatosis—magnetic resonance diagnosis of perineural arachnoidal gliomatosis. *Arch Ophthalmol.* 1987;105:1689–1692.

Seward GR. The Elephant Man. Part I. *Br Dent J.* 1990; 169:173–175.

Seward GR. The Elephant Man. Part II. *Br Dent J.* 1990; 169:210–216.

Seward GR. The Elephant Man. Part III. *Br Dent J.* 1990; 169:252–255.

Tibbles JA, Cohen MM. The Proteus syndrome: The Elephant Man diagnosed. *Br Med J.* 1986;293:683–685.

Wong PC, Dickens CJ, Hoskins Jr. HD. The developmental glaucomas. *Duane's Clin Ophthalmol.* 1995;3:1–17.

Chapter 35

TUBEROUS SCLEROSIS COMPLEX

Elizabeth B. Aksionoff

Tuberous sclerosis (TSC) complex was first described by Bourneville in 1880, and in 1908 Vogt associated the triad of epileptic seizures, mental retardation, and facial angiofibromas (adenoma sebaceum). Van der Hoeve was the first to associate retinal involvement with tuberous sclerosis in 1920. Tuberous sclerosis complex (Bourneville disease) is now recognized as a multisystem, hamartomatous disorder. It belongs to the class of neurocutaneous syndromes called the phakomatoses, which are characterized by disseminated hamartomas (tumor-like nodules) of the eye, skin, central nervous system, and viscera.

EPIDEMIOLOGY

Systemic

Population-based studies suggest a prevalence of 1 in 9000 for tuberous sclerosis. Other studies cite a prevalence of 1 in 6000 for newborns. The recent estimates of the frequency of tuberous sclerosis complex have increased because of new diagnostic studies to confirm the diagnosis. Now patients previously presumed to be asymptomatic or with milder manifestations can be diagnosed with the disease.

Signs of tuberous sclerosis may be present at birth; however, patients usually present during the third decade of life. Tuberous sclerosis is diagnosed in 25% of patients by age 2, 60% by age 10, and 80% by age 20. Because the gene for tuberous sclerosis is pleiotrophic and variable in expression, the estimates of incidence in the literature are quite variable.

Seizure disorders are found in 82 to 90% of the patient population and range from borderline to profound. The incidence of mental retardation is reported between 41 and 60%. Benign brain nodules may be detected in 14% of tuberous sclerosis patients by age 1 and in almost 60% by age 10. Giant-cell astrocytomas will develop in 2% of patients. An abnormal electroencephalograph (EEG) reading is found in 87% of those affected with tuberous sclerosis.

The incidence of skin lesions in tuberous sclerosis is 96%; by age 35, almost all patients will have the characteristic skin lesion, facial angiofibroma. There is an 86% incidence of hypomelanotic macules and 20% present with Shagreen patches. The skeletal system is affected in 40% of patients. Phalangeal cysts are found in the hands or feet of 66%.

Cardiac rhabdomyomas, as evidenced by echocardiogram, are found in 43% of patients with tuberous sclerosis. Renal angiolipomas occur in 50 to 80% of patients.

Ocular

Ocular involvement occurs in at least 50% of tuberous sclerosis patients. Benign astrocytic hamartomas of the retina or optic nerve occur in 50 to 87% of tuberous sclerosis patients.

PATHOPHYSIOLOGY/DISEASE PROCESS

Systemic

Tuberous sclerosis complex is a multisystem, hamartomatous disorder involving the brain, skin, viscera, and the eye (Table 35–1). It results from dysplasia of the neuroectodermal embryologic layer. Hamartomas are congenital anomalies of tissue formation arising from tissue normally present at the involved site. They typically contain large blood vessels and areas of calcification. Most hamartomas, although congenital, are usually inconspicuous at birth and become clinically apparent during the first two decades of life.

Inheritance of tuberous sclerosis is autosomal dominant, with low penetrance and variable expressivity. The disease has a high new mutation rate and may therefore appear as a sporadic condition in up to 80% of affected patients. Mutations in two genes, TSC1 and TSC2, cause TSC. Approximately half of the individuals and families have the TSC1 form of the gene and the other half have the TSC2 form. The TSC1 gene is located on chromosome 9 at loci 9q34. It codes for the tumor-suppressing protein hamartin. The TSC2 gene is found on chromosome 16 at loci 16p13 and codes for the protein tuberin. Sporadic mutations are more common in TSC2. These mutations often produce greater neurologic deficits.

TSC1 and TSC2 appear to function as tumor suppressor genes. The proteins hamartin and tuberin are involved in cellular pathways that modulate cellular differentiation, tumor suppression, and intracellular signaling. When the genes are damaged, tumor suppression is disrupted, allowing for a proliferation of tumors throughout the body. A "two hit" mechanism is proposed for the gene's action. A patient may inherit or acquire via mutation a deletion in one copy of the gene but will not develop TSC lesions unless there is a somatic mutation in the other copy.

It is difficult to predict the course of TSC in any patient. Depending on the manifestations, a patient may lead a normal life or show rapid systemic or neurological deterioration from the disease. The Tuberous Sclerosis Complex 2000 Cohort Study is underway to further elucidate TSC. It is a prospective study following the natural history of the physical and psychological problems associated with tuberous sclerosis in the first 250 children diagnosed with tuberous sclerosis in the United Kingdom after January 1, 2000.

TABLE 35–1. SYSTEMIC MANIFESTATIONS OF TUBEROUS SCLEROSIS

Central Nervous System
- Cerebral cortical malformations
- Astrocytic hamartomas
- Subependymal giant-cell astrocytomas
- The above can all lead to
  - Seizures
  - Mental retardation
  - Increased intracranial pressure
  - Hydrocephalus

Cutaneous
- Hypomelanotic macules (ash-leaf spots)
- Adenoma sebaceum
- Shagreen patches
- Subungual fibromas of fingers and toes
- Pitted hypoplasia of the teeth
- Café-au-lait spots
- Poliosis
- Vascular nevi

Visceral
- Renal angiomyolipomas may cause hematuria, uremia, hypertension
- Cardiac rhabdomyomas may cause cardiac arrhythmia
- Sclerotic areas of the calvarium and spine
- Phalangeal cysts
- Pleural cysts may cause emphysema, hemoptysis, recurrent pneumothorax

Other (Less Common) Hamartomas
- Liver
- Gastrointestinal tract
- Thymus
- Adrenal gland
- Pancreas

Central Nervous System

The neurological features of tuberous sclerosis are mental retardation and seizure disorder. "Tuber-shaped" cerebral cortical malformations are responsible for the effects of tuberous sclerosis on the central nervous system. Fibrillary gliosis is often associated with these cortical malformations.

Cortical tubers are large astrocytic hamartomas most commonly found in the cerebral cortex, but which occasionally may appear in the cerebellum, basal ganglia, and rarely in the brainstem and spinal cord. They may cause alterations in the normal convolutional pattern of the gyri.

Subependymal giant-cell astrocytomas are usually benign. These are most commonly found in the region of the basal ganglia and protrude into the lateral and third ventricles. They may grow to obstruct the foramen of Munro and cause hydrocephalus and increased intracranial pressure. The presenting symptoms of an expanding cranial mass may include headache, decreased vision, and/or vomiting.

The most common, and often first, manifestation of tuberous sclerosis is a seizure disorder. The seizures are a result of cerebral cortical malformations. Infantile spasms and tonic–clonic seizures are most common, but other types can occur. Older children and adults often develop complex partial or other focal seizures rather than the more generalized seizures of a younger age group. The seizures, or infantile spasms, usually begin in infancy or childhood, with repetitive myoclonic spasms of the head, neck, and limbs. These attacks are also known as "salaam attacks." They last for only a few seconds, but occur in groups of 10 to 50. These seizures may present as early as 4 months of age. With increasing age the infantile spasms become grand mal seizures. According to Pampliglione and Pugh (1975), 25% of children with seizures will develop other signs of tuberous sclerosis within 4 years. After the seizures present, the child may demonstrate a slowing in subsequent development. Although the seizures may arise from anywhere in the brain, they are usually concentrated in the periventricular distribution, where most of the tubers are found. There is a high correlation between seizures and irregularity on EEG.

Another manifestation of cerebral cortical malformations is mental retardation. Mental retardation is a common but not inevitable association with tuberous sclerosis.

There is a great deal of variability of the severity of seizures and mental retardation. Approximately one third of tuberous sclerosis patients will be of normal intelligence, with no significant health problems, while others may have severe mental retardation and/or seizures that are difficult to control. Developmental delays may also be evident from birth. Some degree of learning disability is found in 50% of tuberous sclerosis patients. Borberg (1951) found that 15% of mentally retarded patients develop normally until between the ages of 8 and 14, when they began to show signs of intellectual deterioration. This may be due to frequent uncontrolled seizures or increased intracranial pressure due to an obstruction of the foramen of Munro. The final level of neurological function most likely results from a combination of seizure severity and the size, location, and number of cerebral lesions.

Cutaneous

The earliest visible skin lesion associated with tuberous sclerosis is the hypomelanotic macule (Figure 35–1). This depigmented area, 1 to 2 cm in diameter, usually presents at birth. Hypomelanotic macules are a very common occurrence and are pathognomonic for tuberous sclerosis. They may be found on the trunk, limbs, or scalp and can range in number from 4 to 100. These lesions are called the "ash leaf" sign because they may resemble the shape of an ash tree leaf, oval at one end and tapered at the other, although they are quite variable in shape. These diagnostic lesions are often the first clinical sign of tuberous sclerosis.

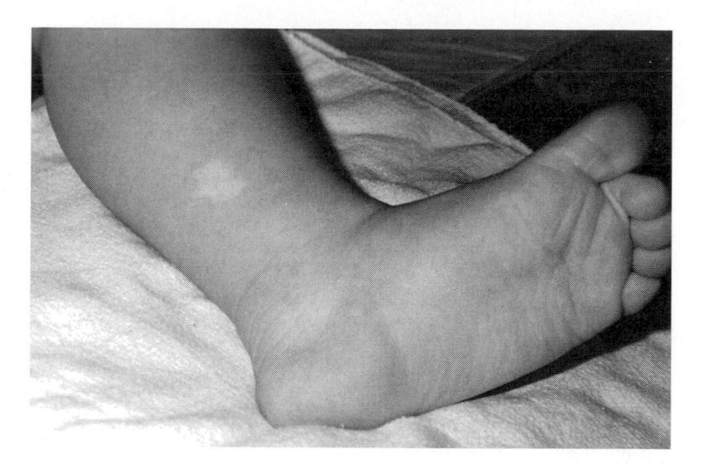

Figure 35–1. Hypomelanotic macule (ash-leaf spot) on the leg of a 1-year-old with tuberous sclerosis.

Facial angiofibromas or adenoma sebaceum are also common, and may be the only cutaneous sign of tuberous sclerosis. These are small, red-brown, raised nodules distributed in a butterfly pattern of the nasolabial fold, malar area, and on the chin. The angiofibromas are composed of hyperplastic vascular and connective tissue that displaces and alters the sebaceous glands. They are first visible at ages 2 to 5 and may be progressive to young adulthood. This condition is usually present in all affected individuals over age 35.

> A hallmark of tuberous sclerosis is the retinal astrocytic hamartoma. It may present as a flat, white semitransparent lesion of the superficial retina or an elevated, multinodular "mulberry lesion."

Shagreen patches, another cutaneous presentation, are fibrous plaques in the skin presenting with a waxy, yellow-brown, or flesh-colored appearance. These raised, irregular, rough areas of skin are most commonly found on the forehead, eyelids, back, or legs. Other less common cutaneous manifestations are listed in Table 35–1.

Visceral

The most commonly affected organ in tuberous sclerosis is the kidney. Polycystic renal disease is very common. Renal angiomyolipomas, usually benign multiple hamartomas of the kidneys, are common. They do not typically metastasize to other sites. They appear as nodules usually less than 2 cm in diameter. They may be solid or cystic, solitary or multiple, and unilateral or bilateral. The kidney tumors and cysts are usually asymptomatic. If symptoms do arise they may include pain, uremia, and other signs of renal failure as well as hypertension. Patients with tuberous sclerosis complex who have renal angiomyolipomas have a slightly greater risk of developing renal carcinoma than patients with renal angiomyolipomas without tuberous sclerosis.

Cardiac rhabdomyomas are usually benign, asymptomatic, whitish tumors less than a centimeter in size. They may appear as a solitary tumor, usually at the apex of the left ventricle, as multiple nodules throughout the heart, or as diffuse infiltration of the myocardium. Cardiac rhabdomyomas may be responsible for pulmonic or aortic stenosis. Possible presenting signs include cardiac arrhythmias, heart failure, or ECG changes.

Other less common visceral manifestations of tuberous sclerosis are listed in Table 35–1.

The lifespan is normal in those patients with tuberous sclerosis who show minimal manifestations of the disease. However, with severe epilepsy and mental retardation, the prognosis for life beyond the third decade is poor. The cause of death is usually due to seizures, associated tumors, or concurrent disease.

Ocular

The primary ocular manifestations of tuberous sclerosis are hamartomas of the retina and optic nerve. These benign lesions can develop as early as a few months of life. Solitary astrocytic hamartomas may be seen in normal individuals. However, in tuberous sclerosis, the astrocytomas may be bilateral and multifocal. The hamartomas have been classified into three different morphological types.

> Facial angiofibromas in a butterfly distribution on the face are characteristic for tuberous sclerosis.

Type 1 is the most common, usually appearing in the early stage of the disease, and located in the superficial retinal layers overlying the retinal blood vessels. They most commonly occur at or near the posterior pole, but may affect any part of the fundus. The hamartomas often arise in the retinal ganglion layer but may later involve all layers of the retina. The tumor is smooth and circular or oval in shape. It is relatively flat, although it might be slightly raised above the retina. It appears semitransparent and can range from grayish white to salmon in color, often with ill-defined margins. The lesion varies in size from one-half to three disc diameters in width. Its appearance may be very subtle and difficult to detect except for an abnormal light reflex or blurred underlying blood vessel. The lesion has little effect on the neighboring retina or choroid.

Type 2 is a well-circumscribed, calcified, white, opaque lesion that may be elevated and multinodular. This is considered the classic "mulberry"-type lesion (Figure 35–2). These astrocytic hamartomas are usually found at or around the optic disc and posterior pole. They range in size from one-half to three disc diameters in size. Some of these lesions have been known to dislodge and float freely in the vitreous and then possibly reattach and grow in other areas of the retina.

Type 3 is a combination of the first two varieties. The central core is calcified and nodular while the perimeter is smooth, semitranslucent, and salmon in color.

The hamartomas may be richly vascularized but present with varying degrees of vascularization. They usually do not grow over time; however, their appearance may change as they become calcified. The tumors are usually extramacular, arising in the inner retina, with little damage or vision loss. Hamartomas of the optic disc generally arise in the superficial layers of the papilla and interfere little with its structure or function. It is less common for the tumors to involve all layers of the retina or optic nerve, but the choroid and vitreous may be affected secondarily. Retinal detachments are rarely associated with the hamartomas.

Vascular malformations may occur at or adjacent to a large hamartoma. These malformations may lead to preretinal or vitreous hemorrhage. Papilledema

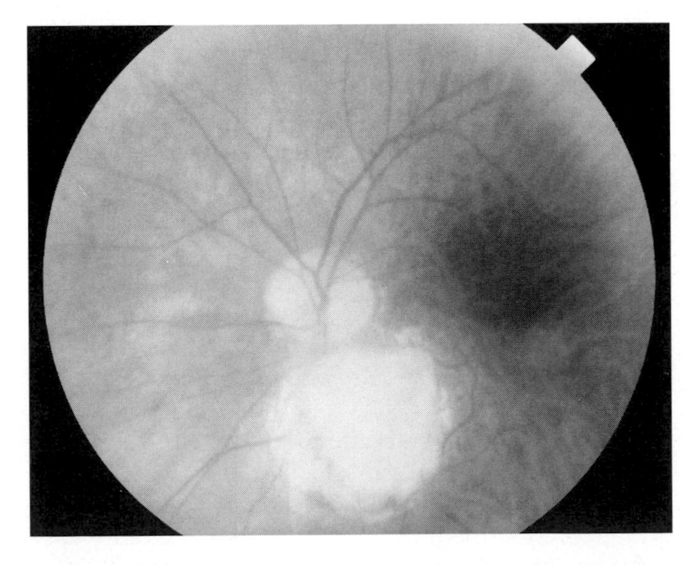

Figure 35–2. Solitary, multinodular retinal astrocytoma (type 2 or classic "mulberry" lesion).

and/or optic atrophy may occur and are signs of associated intracranial lesions.

Other retinal findings are less common, and include pigment epithelial defects such as peripheral retinal hypopigmentation and atypical colobomas. Although rare, localized areas of choroidal atrophy have been reported to occur at or adjacent to retinal astrocytomas.

Visual loss is more commonly due to intracranial lesions, especially paraventricular tumors resulting in raised intracranial pressure, papilledema, and subsequent optic atrophy. Intracranial tumors may also be responsible for diplopia and extraocular muscle paresis.

The main nonretinal manifestation of tuberous sclerosis is adenoma sebaceum of the eyelids. Other rare ocular manifestations are listed in Table 35–2.

TABLE 35–3. CRITERIA FOR DIAGNOSIS OF TUBEROUS SCLEROSIS[a]

Major Requirements
Facial angiofibromas (adenoma sebaceum)
Ungual fibromas
Cortical tubers
Subependymal hamartomas
Multiple retinal hamartomas
Fibrous plaque of the forehead

Minor Requirements
Infantile spasms
Hypopigmented macules
Shagreen patch
Single retinal hamartoma
Calcified subependymal or cortical lesion
Bilateral renal angiomyolipoma or cysts
Cardiac rhabdomyoma
First-degree relative with a primary diagnosis of tuberous sclerosis

[a]One major or two minor requirements are necessary for diagnosis.

DIAGNOSIS

Systemic

Although the original criteria for diagnosis of tuberous sclerosis included the triad of seizures, mental retardation, and adenoma sebaceum, this no longer holds true because of the variable presentation of this disease. A scheme for the diagnosis of tuberous sclerosis (Table 35–3) is based on the criteria set by Gomez (1979). To make the diagnosis, one of the major requirements, or two of the minor requirements, must be met.

The hypomelanotic macules are easily identified by reflecting ultraviolet light onto the skin from a Wood's lamp in a darkened room. This helps to identify lesions in an infant. The other cutaneous signs are easily identified by physical and dermatologic examination. A careful search for depigmented nevi is of particular diagnostic importance in early life. A skin biopsy of the hypopigmented macules will show melanocytes with decreased tyrosinase activity characteristic of tuberous sclerosis. This is in contrast to areas of vitiligo where there is an absence of melanocytes.

The diagnostic tests (Table 35–4) used for the central nervous system manifestations include the EEG, CT scan, or MRI. The EEG is abnormal in most patients and may show a grossly abnormal hypsarrhythmic pattern in one third of tuberous sclerosis patients. Hypsarrhythmia is characterized by high-voltage arrhythmic slow waves mixed with spike discharges showing a multifocal distribution.

MRI will show high signal lesions most commonly of the cerebral cortex, but also of the posterior fossa and brainstem (Figure 35–3). The MRI may also show hamartomas and gliotic areas of the brain. More severely affected patients tend to have a higher number of cerebral cortical lesions detected by MRI. In this manner, MRI is useful in predicting the clinical severity of tuberous sclerosis in younger children and those

TABLE 35–2. OCULAR MANIFESTATIONS OF TUBEROUS SCLEROSIS

- Adenoma sebaceum of the eyelids
- Retinal astrocytic hamartoma
- Optic nerve astrocytic hamartoma
- Papilledema secondary to increased intracranial pressure, which can lead to:
  - Optic atrophy secondary to chronic papilledema
  - Extracranial nerve paresis
- Pigment epithelial defects
- Atypical coloboma
- Poliosis
- Iris hypopigmentation

TABLE 35–4. CLINICAL EVALUATION AND TESTS UTILIZED TO DIAGNOSE TUBEROUS SCLEROSIS

- General physical examination with family history and examination of family members
- Wood's lamp skin testing
- Fundus examination
- Complete blood count
- Electrolyte testing
- CT or MRI of brain
- EEG
- Echocardiogram
- Abdominal CT
- Renal ultrasound
- Chest x-ray

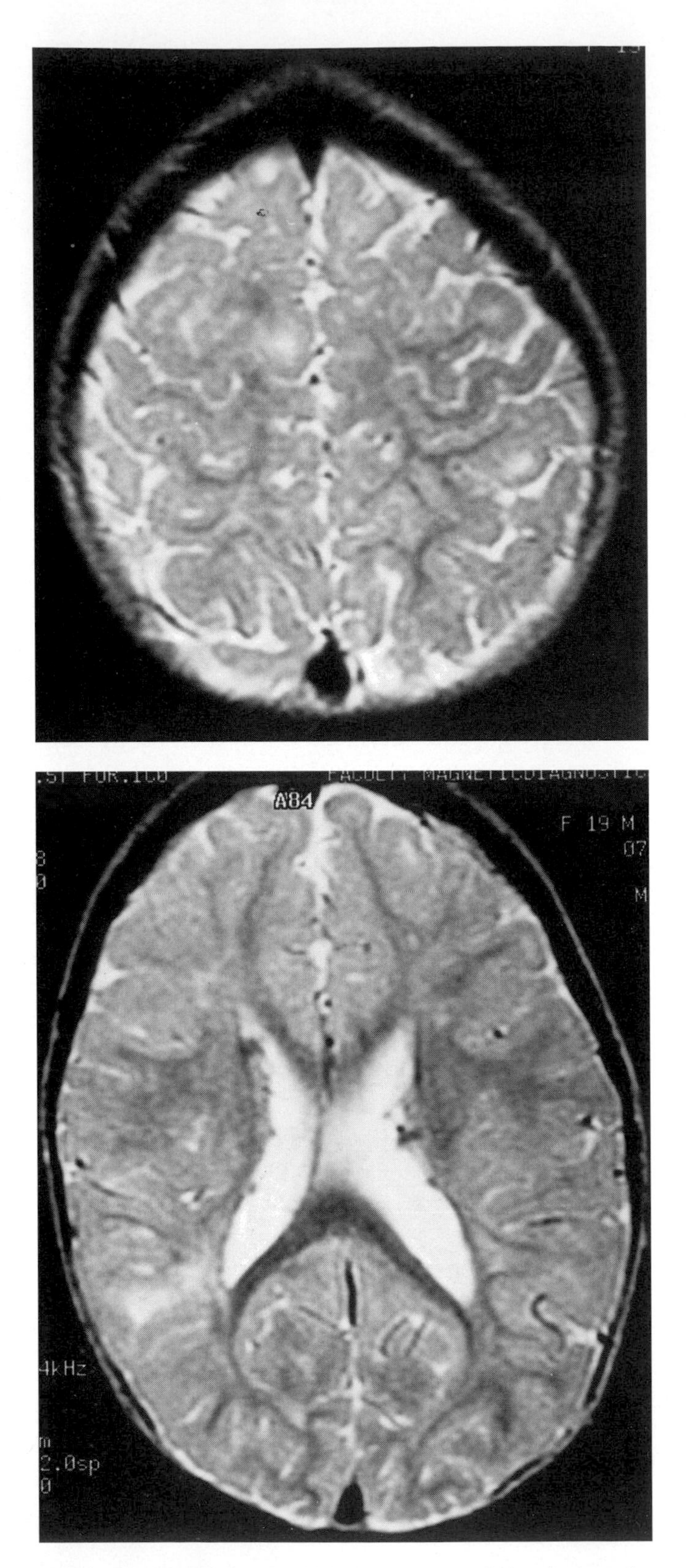

Figure 35–3. MRI showing high signal lesions (tubers) along the central sulcus and lateral ventricles.

newly diagnosed. MRI is recommended at 3-year intervals from time of diagnosis and every 6 months if a giant cell astrocytoma is detected.

Calcified lesions in the subependymal region or deeper can be identified by CT scan and will confirm the diagnosis of tuberous sclerosis. This imaging study will demonstrate multiple scattered calcium deposits located close to the wall of the lateral and third ventricle in the proximity of the foramen of Munro. A CT scan also best resolves periventricular calcific lesions. Fifty percent of patients with tuberous sclerosis will show evidence of intracranial calcified hamartomas. Cerebral cortical atrophy and mild to moderate ventricular dilatation may also be evident. Less commonly, lesions have been seen in the superficial brain parenchyma or the cerebellum.

Other useful diagnostic tests include positron emission tomography (PET) to study the seizure activity, and skull x-rays for intracranial calcifications. Nonimaging tests include blood work with a CBC and electrolyte analysis, urinalysis, blood pressure measurements, chest x-rays, abdominal CT scan, ultrasound of the kidney echocardiogram, ECG, and EEG.

Most of the visceral manifestations of tuberous sclerosis are asymptomatic and will be identified through diagnostic testing. At diagnosis of tuberous sclerosis complex, a renal ultrasound or CT scan should be performed to look for renal angiomyolipomas and/or cysts. Repeat ultrasound or CT is recommended every 3 years. Larger kidney tumors may present with hematuria and can be identified with intravenous pyelography. An echocardiogram is recommended to determine if cardiac rhabdomyomas are present. Cardiac rhabdomyomas are also usually asymptomatic; however, they may produce cardiac arrhythmias or obstruction of blood flow. There is no definitive test available yet for diagnosis of tuberous sclerosis in utero. Prenatal diagnosis of cardiac rhabdomyomas by fetal echocardiogram and ultrasound may be possible in certain instances.

Ocular

Comprehensive ocular evaluation may reveal retinal or optic disc astrocytic hamartomas. Visual fields and visual acuity are normal in the absence of a retinal hamartoma involving the macula or a central nervous system lesion affecting the visual pathways.

Fluorescein angiography can be used in the diagnosis of retinal hamartomas. The hamartomas will exhibit mild auto-fluorescence and late-phase staining. The mulberry lesions in particular are highly reflectile, and exhibit a marked autofluorescence that is obvious prior to injection of the dye or during the retinal arterial phase before the dye reaches the tumor circulation. During the venous phase, the tumors will appear hypofluorescent in comparison to the retinal and choroidal circulations. During the late venous stage, however, the phakomas fluoresce intensely. The type 1 lesions will also remain hypofluorescent up to the venous phase, and then a faint, diffuse hyperfluorescence occurs during the late venous phase. Small phakomas not noted ophthalmoscopically can be identified with angiography because of this hyperfluorescence. In this way, fluorescein angiography may be used as a screening tool to identify cases of suspected tuberous sclerosis.

Ultrasound B scan will show a strong echo with bright spots in the areas of calcified lesions.

An important differential diagnosis for the hamartomas of tuberous sclerosis is retinoblastoma of the optic nerve and retina. Other signs of tuberous sclerosis will help to make the diagnosis. Also, in tuberous sclerosis, the lesions will show little or no increase in size, while the retinoblastoma will increase dramatically.

The early-stage ocular lesions are characterized by opaque, white lesions that resemble myelinated nerve fibers. These are differentiated by bright fluorescence on angiography and are slightly raised above the surface of the retina in comparison to myelinated nerve fibers. These are also less discrete and lack the striate configuration of myelinated nerve fibers.

Inflammatory lesions such as early-stage toxocara or toxoplasmosis may cause a pale whitening of a focal region of retina and must be included in the differential diagnosis (Table 35–5).

Optic disc astrocytic hamartomas may be confused with optic disc drusen. The differentiating factor is that disc drusen lie within the disc while the hamartomas protrude above it and obscure the disc and retinal vasculature. Also to be considered in the differential diagnosis is optic disc glioma, which may present with disc swelling, or the disc may be obscured by a mass protruding above its surface.

TABLE 35–5. DIFFERENTIAL DIAGNOSIS OF ASTROCYTIC HAMARTOMA

- Retinoblastoma: Presents with a white retinal tumor but with a prominent feeder vessel, vitreous seeding, retinal detachment, and often no initial systemic signs. A retinoblastoma also frequently increases in size.
- *Toxocara:* Early lesions may be similar in appearance to flat, retinal hamartomas but TSC patients will test negative on an undiluted toxocara titer.
- Toxoplasmosis: Early lesions may appear similar to flat, retinal hamartomas but TSC patients will test negative on the anti-*Toxoplasma* antibody titer.
- Optic disc drusen: Disc drusen lie within the disc whereas optic disc hamartomas protrude above it to obscure the disc and the retinal vasculature.

TREATMENT AND MANAGEMENT

Systemic

Treatment of tuberous sclerosis is directed toward the alleviation of symptoms (Table 35–6). Tumors are not generally treated because growth and change of these lesions are rare. Anticonvulsant medication is used in the control of seizures. The seizures are often difficult to control with medication; however, long periods of remission may develop spontaneously. There is some controversy regarding the role of pertussis immunizations provoking the onset of infantile spasms in patients predisposed to seizures. In the past, pertussis immunization had been linked with seizure onset. Currently, many feel this not to be true; however, many physicians still may want to withhold this immunization in order to avoid any possible cause for seizure onset. The decision to administer this immunization may have to be made after discussion between the patient's neurologist, pediatrician, and parents.

Administration of ACTH or steroids may lead to an improvement in the EEG pattern and a cessation of the seizure attacks. The choice of antiepileptic drug is determined by the age of the patient and type of seizure. Surgery may benefit patients with focal areas causing intractable seizures. However, clinical relapse with a deterioration of the EEG is not infrequent. Occasionally surgical procedures are indicated in patients with severe seizures or expanding intracranial lesions. In some cases radiation therapy has been useful. Depending on the level of severity, patients with mental retardation may benefit from specialized schooling or vocational training. Children with milder developmental delays will benefit from early intervention for speech, occupational, or physical therapy as necessary.

TABLE 35–6. TREATMENT AND MANAGEMENT OF TUBEROUS SCLEROSIS

• Seizures	Anticonvulsant medication Adrenocorticotrophic hormone or steroids
• Mental retardation	Early intervention, specialized schooling, if necessary
• Visceral tumors	Careful monitoring and symptomatic treatment
• Cutaneous tumors	Cosmetic treatment
• Ocular tumors	Monitor Photodocumentation

Elimination of cutaneous and systemic lesions by dermabrasion and laser surgery is considered for cosmetic purposes. The adenoma sebaceum nodules can be treated but often result in regrowth and scarring. The tumors occurring in the visceral organs, kidney, and heart are usually benign and treated when complications arise. Hypertension resulting from the renal complications of tuberous sclerosis complex is treated with various antihypertensive medications. Most cardiac rhabdomyomas are asymptomatic but should be treated by a cardiologist if arrhythmias or other cardiac complications occur. However, careful monitoring of pulmonary, renal, and cardiac function is warranted.

Although cases do arise from spontaneous mutations, genetic counseling is important for the patient, his or her parents, and siblings. CT or MRI scans of asymptomatic relatives to detect a carrier is a component of genetic counseling and is essential to those directly at risk. The finding of intracranial calcification in a parent of an affected child is helpful to confirm that the disease was inherited in an autosomal dominant manner rather than through spontaneous mutation. Parents of affected individuals should undergo a thorough examination of the skin, ophthalmoscopic evaluation through a dilated pupil for phakomata, and cranial imaging such as x-ray, MRI, or CT scan. An echocardiogram, ultrasound, or CT study of the kidneys and a physical examination of skin and nails are indicated. With the major advances in isolating the location of the TSC genes, a prenatal test for tuberous sclerosis may be very close. The identification of the TSC1 and TSC2 genes and the proteins they code for allows us to learn more about their role in the disease process. This should lead to new therapies for seizures, developmental delays, and the tumors of tuberous sclerosis complex.

Ocular

Treatment of the ocular tumors is not indicated because the growth and change of these lesions are rare. Sequelae such as papilledema, vitreous hemorrhage, and retinal detachment are treated accordingly. Photodocumentation is indicated to ensure that a malignant lesion is not overlooked. For patients at risk for the disease or carrying the gene, yearly ophthalmoscopy is suggested.

CONCLUSION

Tuberous sclerosis is a disorder associated with a variable presentation of central nervous system, cutaneous, ocular, and visceral manifestations. Although the retinal hamartomas common in tuberous sclerosis are generally benign, the eyecare practitioner has a responsibility to refer patients presenting with ocular signs for neurological and systemic evaluations.

REFERENCES

Bansley D, Wolter JR. The retinal lesion in tuberous sclerosis. *J Pediatr Ophthalmol.* 1971;8:261–265.

Borberg A. Clinical and genetic investigations into tuberous sclerosis and Recklinghausen's neurofibromatosis. *Acta Psychiatr. Neurol.* 1951;71(suppl):2–239.

Brett EM. Neurocutaneous syndromes. In: Brett EM, ed. *Paediatric Neurology.* Edinburgh: Churchill Livingstone, 1991:571–576.

Cruess AF. Tuberous sclerosis and the eye. In: Ryan SJ, ed. *Retina.* St. Louis: Mosby; 1989;1:571–578.

Gomez MR. Neurocutaneous diseases. In: Bradley WG, Daroff RB, Fenichel GM, Marsden CD, eds. *Neurology in Clinical Practice.* Boston: Butterworth-Heinemann; 1991, 1323–1342.

Gomez MR. *Tuberous Sclerosis.* New York: Raven; 1979.

Green A, Johnson P, Yates J. The tuberous sclerosis gene on chromosome 9q34 acts as a growth suppressor. *Hum Mol Genet.* 1994;6:193–196.

Jones AC, Daniells CE, Snell RG, et al. Molecular genetics and phenotypic analysis reveals differences between TSC1 and TSC2 associated familial and sporadic tuberous sclerosis. *Hum Mol Genet.* 1997;6:2155–2161.

Krill AE. Tuberous sclerosis. In Krill AE, ed: *Krill's Hereditary Retinal and Choroidal Diseases.* Vol 2, *Clinical Characteristics.* Hagerstown, Md: Harper & Row; 1977:1219–1248.

Miller NR. Phakomatoses. In Miller NR, ed: *Walsh and Hoyt's Clinical Neuro-ophthalmology* Baltimore: Williams & Wilkins; 1988:1765–1788.

Pampiglione G, Moynahan EJ. The tuberous sclerosis syndrome, and clinical and EEG studies in 100 children. *J Neurol Neurosurg Psychiatr.* 1976;39:666–673.

Pampiglione G, Pugh E. Infantile spasms and subsequent appearance of tuberous sclerosis syndrome. *Lancet.* 1975; 2:1046.

Povey S, Burley MW, Attwood J, et al. Two loci for tuberous sclerosis: One on 9q34 and one on 16p13. *Ann Hum Genet.* 1994;58:107–127.

Roach ES, Williams DP, Laster DW. Magnetic resonance imaging in tuberous sclerosis. *Arch Neurol.* 1987;44:301–304.

Robertson DM. Ophthalmic manifestations of tuberous sclerosis. *Ann NY Acad Sci.* 1991;615:17–25.

Van Slegtenhorst M, de Hoogt R, Hermans C, et al. Identification of the tuberous sclerosis gene TSC1 on chromosome 9q34. *Science.* 1997;277:805–808.

Williams R, Taylor D. Tuberous sclerosis. *Surv Ophthalmol.* 1985;30:143.

Zion, V. M. Phakomatoses. In: Tasman W, Jaeger EA, eds. *Duane's Clinical Ophthalmology,* Philadelphia: Lippincott; 1992;5:6–7.

Chapter 36

STURGE–WEBER SYNDROME

Elizabeth B. Aksionoff

Sturge–Weber syndrome, also called encephalotrigeminal angiomatosis, is one of a group of congenital neurocutaneous syndromes called the phakomatoses. These syndromes are characterized by disseminated hamartomas (tumor-like nodules) of the eye, skin, and central nervous system.

Schirmer, in 1860, first associated buphthalmos with an ipsilateral facial nevus flammeus. In 1879, Sturge correlated unilateral buphthalmos, ipsilateral facial hemangioma, and contralateral epileptic seizures. It was not until 1922 that Weber established the triad of facial hemangioma, glaucoma, and cerebral dysfunction as the clinical entity, Sturge–Weber syndrome. Alexander and Norman (1960) believed that both facial and leptomeningeal angiomas must be present for the diagnosis of Sturge–Weber syndrome.

EPIDEMIOLOGY

Systemic

The incidence of Sturge–Weber syndrome is 1 in 50,000. Sturge–Weber syndrome shows no racial or sex predilection. Focal or generalized seizures are found in 80% of patients, with 50% occurring before the age of 1 year. Mental retardation occurs in 54 to 60%. Hemiplegia contralateral to the angiomas occurs in 31%.

Ocular

The most common ocular manifestations of Sturge–Weber syndrome are choroidal hemangiomas and glaucoma. Choroidal hemangiomas are found in 40% of patients, and of these, 88% will develop glaucoma. Exudative retinal detachments will occur in 50% of patients with choroidal hemangioma. There is a 30% incidence of glaucoma in Sturge–Weber syndrome, of which 60% of cases are congenital. The remaining 40% develop glaucoma before early adulthood. Iris heterochromia is found in 8% of these individuals.

PATHOPHYSIOLOGY/DISEASE PROCESS

Systemic

Sturge–Weber syndrome is believed to arise from a developmental error in a portion of the cephalic neural crest resulting in abnormal vasculature in the mesodermal derivatives of the supraocular dermis, choroid, and pia mater. Irregularity in the distribution and structure of small vessels results in abnormal proliferation of perivascular cells. Because these tumors are composed of cells normally present in this tissue, they are classified as hamartomas.

Sturge–Weber syndrome has no established genetic pattern. Its appearance is usually sporadic with variable expressivity.

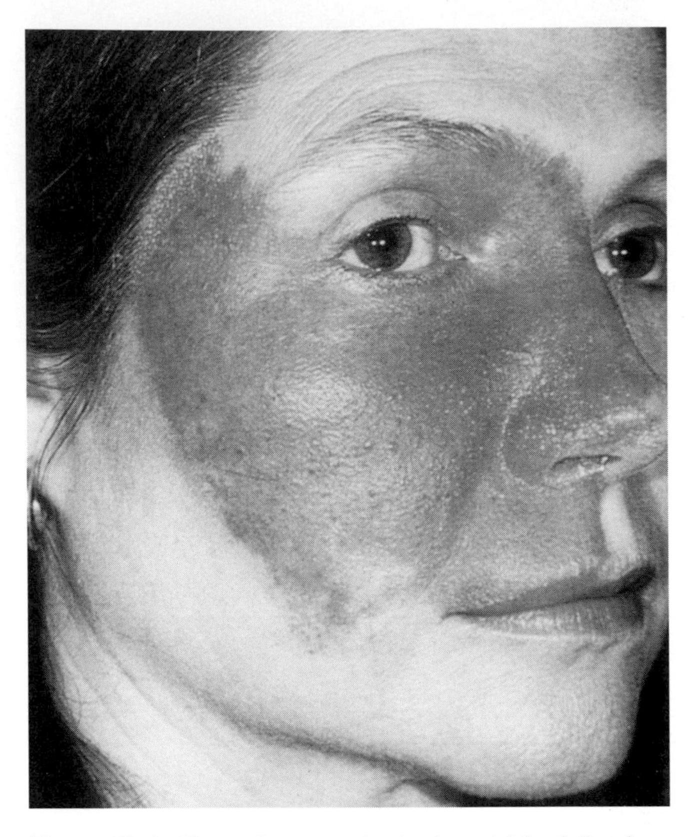

Figure 36–1. Nevus flammeus (port wine stain) of the face. (*Reprinted with permission from Habif TP.* Clinical Dermatology: A Color Guide to Diagnosis and Therapy. *2nd ed. St. Louis: Mosby, 1990:585.*)

Dermatologic

A common presenting feature of the disease is the nevus flammeus or port wine stain (Figure 36–1). This is a facial hemangioma within, but not always limited to, the distribution of the trigeminal nerve. The hemangioma primarily involves the ophthalmic and maxillary divisions, and rarely the mandibular division. The supraorbital region is almost always affected.

The hemangioma consists of large, dilated capillaries in the dermis and subcutaneous tissues, and is usually present at birth. It presents as irregular, flat, dull, red patches. The nevus may darken with age and become more nodular, but will not increase in size. The nevus flammeus is usually unilateral but may extend past the midline. Hypertrophy of the face may occur ipsilateral to the hemangioma. The globe on the affected side may become enlarged even in the absence of glaucoma. Hemangiomas of the oral or nasal cavity are also possible.

Central Nervous System

Angiomatosis of the cerebral leptomeninges, the layer overlying the cerebral cortex, occurs on the same side as the facial hemangioma and results in altered circulation of the underlying cerebral cortex. These areas show degenerative changes with subsequent calcification. Once the calcium is deposited, the lesions can be evaluated radiographically. Calcification is usually seen before the age of 1 year. These lesions increase in size up to the second decade of life and then stabilize. Usually the occipital or occipital–parietal regions of one of the cerebral hemispheres are affected, but the lesions may extend over an entire hemisphere. It is a rare exception if the brain lesions are not on the same side as the skin lesions.

Epileptic seizures are a frequent occurrence in Sturge–Weber syndrome. The seizures present early in life, with one half of patients developing them between the ages of 2 and 7 months. After seizure onset, development may be dramatically set back. When Sturge–Weber syndrome manifests with seizures in infancy, they may become intractable, with progressive hemiparesis, motor weakness, and mental retardation. The manifestations of seizure activity occur contralateral to the skin lesion. The type, frequency, and severity of seizures do not correlate with the extent of cutaneous involvement. They usually begin as partial seizures but become more generalized with time. Patients with seizures unresponsive to medical therapy may develop slowly progressive neurological deficits and ultimately become moderately or severely disabled.

Unilateral cerebral cortical angiomatoses and associated atrophy and calcification can lead to cerebral dysfunction. If present, mental retardation ranges from mild to profound deficiencies. Bilateral involvement of the brain is associated with earlier onset of seizures and a poorer prognosis for mental development.

Almost one third of patients will have some degree of transient hemiplegia or visual field defect contralateral to the facial angioma.

Visceral tumors have been associated with a wide range of organ systems. Visceral involvement is less common in Sturge–Weber syndrome than in the other phakomatoses (Table 36–1).

TABLE 36–1. SYSTEMIC MANIFESTATIONS OF STURGE–WEBER SYNDROME

- Nevus flammeus (port wine stain) along the distribution of the trigeminal nerve
- Seizure disorder
- Mental retardation
- Hemiparesis or hemiplegia contralateral to the nerves
- Angiomatosis of the cerebral leptomeninges ipsilateral to the nevus
- Visceral tumors of the lung, thymus, spleen, testes, ovaries, GI tract, pituitary, thyroid, pancreas

Many patients with Sturge–Weber syndrome die in their second or third decades from the progressive central nervous system manifestations.

Ocular

The first visible ocular manifestation of Sturge–Weber syndrome is usually the nevus flammeus of the eyelid. When the upper eyelid is involved, there is a greater correlation with glaucoma and intracranial angiomatosis. The nevus flammeus may cause the lid to become ptotic.

Choroidal hemangioma, the most common ocular manifestation, is a diffuse, flat, vascularized cavernous hemangioma usually located at the posterior pole, often temporal to the optic disc. It is usually unilateral, but may be bilateral if the facial angioma is bilateral. Histologically, the hemangioma is composed of dilated vascular channels lined by attenuated endothelial cells or fibrocytes. The tumor gives a diffuse red appearance to the retina, especially in contrast to the fellow eye. It is referred to as "tomato catsup" fundus.

Localized hemangiomas are less common but are associated with serous retinal detachments. These lesions are circular or oval, slightly elevated, and reddish-orange in color. The overlying retina may exhibit tortuosity and dilatation of the retinal vasculature. The retinal pigment epithelium above the choroidal hemangioma may exhibit drusen, areas of calcification, or atrophy. At this stage, visual function may not be affected. With time, cystoid degeneration of the overlying retina may occur, leading to exudation and retinal pigment alterations, as well as to exudative retinal detachments, subsequent iris neovascularization, and secondary glaucoma. Subretinal hemorrhage from the choroidal hemangioma may result in retinal detachment with forward displacement of the iris and angle closure secondary to peripheral anterior synechiae formation.

There are several theories on the pathogenesis of the glaucoma in Sturge–Weber syndrome. Some associate the disease with an angle anomaly in which there is an anterior insertion of the ciliary muscle and uveal tissue in the angle. The thick uveal meshwork, poorly developed scleral spur, and anteriorly inserted iris root lead to outflow obstruction. Another theory involves the presence of limbal and episcleral vascular malformations that increase the episcleral venous pressure and thus impede aqueous outflow, subsequently raising intraocular pressure.

Glaucoma may develop in infancy, childhood, or adulthood. Buphthalmos occurs if introcular pressure (IOP) is elevated in an infant less than 3 years of age, causing the cornea and sclera to enlarge. The glaucoma usually occurs on the same side as the facial hemangioma, especially if it involves the skin of the upper eyelid, tarsus, and conjunctiva. Patients with bilateral facial lesions may have glaucoma in either or both eyes. Visual acuity and field loss is variable depending on the severity of the glaucoma.

TABLE 36–2. OCULAR MANIFESTATIONS OF STURGE–WEBER SYNDROME

- Choroidal hemangioma
- Glaucoma
- Buphthalmos, if glaucoma occurs prior to 3 years of age
- Nevus flammeus of the eyelid; may also cause ptosis
- Iris heterochromia, caused by small iris hamartomas
- Serous or exudative retinal detachment
- Anomalous vessels of the episclera and conjunctiva
- Intracranial malformations may cause homonymous hemianopias and papilledema
- Retinal pigmentary atrophy/retinitis pigmentosa
- Choroidal coloboma
- Atrophic chorioretinitis
- Retinoblastoma

Large, anomalous blood vessels may be present in the conjunctiva, episcleral tissue, choroid, and retina. Episcleral hemangiomas are found in all Sturge–Weber patients with glaucoma (Phelps, 1978). An episcleral hemangioma may appear as a faint blue or purplish blush lying under the Tenon capsule and conjunctiva.

Iris heterochromia may occur, with the iris darker on the side of the facial nevus, because melanocytes are grouped into small hamartomas on the anterior surface of the iris.

Contralateral homonymous hemianopias with or without macular sparing may occur secondary to occipital intracranial lesions. The hemianopia probably occurs from a thrombosis of the vessels of the malformation that penetrate the cortex.

The retinal pigment epithelium (RPE) above the choroidal hemangioma may also exhibit changes. Drusen, areas of calcification, and RPE atrophy have been reported. Papilledema may result from increased intracranial pressure secondary to intracranial lesions. Other less commonly associated ocular manifestations of Sturge–Weber syndrome are included in Table 36–2.

DIAGNOSIS

Systemic

Nevus flammeus, present at birth, is the first presenting sign of Sturge–Weber syndrome, and is diagnosed by clinical appearance (Table 36–3). Occurrence of the nevus flammeus alone, without additional involvement of the eye or central nervous system, does not constitute a diagnosis of Sturge–Weber syndrome

TABLE 36–3. CLINICAL WORKUP AND DIAGNOSTIC TESTS UTILIZED IN THE DIAGNOSIS OF STURGE–WEBER SYNDROME

- General physical examination
- Ophthalmologic examination—including glaucoma workup
- CT scan or MRI
- EEG
- Ultrasound
- Fluorescein angiography

(Table 36–4). However, if glaucoma also exists, the diagnosis of Sturge–Weber syndrome can be made. Neurologic abnormalities are seldom evident at birth. Although seizures may not be initially present, neuroimaging and ocular evaluation is indicated if a nevus flammeus and/or glaucoma is diagnosed.

> The basic lesions of Sturge–Weber syndrome are ipsilateral vascular tumors of the skin, meninges, and choroid.

Computed tomography (CT) scans, especially axial and coronal views, are useful for the evaluation of the angiomatosis of the cerebral leptomeninges. They are more sensitive than x-rays to identify calcification and vascular lesions. The pathognomonic feature on radiographic studies is intracranial calcification arranged in parallel lines or "railroad tracks" showing a gyriform distribution. This is most commonly seen in the occipital or parietal lobes. Magnetic resonance imaging (MRI) is the method of choice to detect intracranial involvement, but abnormal calcifications are not appreciated as well as with CT scan. Enhancement with gadolinium-DTPA improves the diagnostic value of MRI, before neurological symptoms arise. Cerebral angiography may also serve to identify and determine the extent of the angiomatous malformation. It will show a lack of superficial veins, tortuosity, enlargement of the deep subependymal and medullary veins, and nonfilling of the superior sagittal sinus.

> On radiographic studies, intracranial calcifications arranged in parallel lines or "railroad tracks" are pathognomonic for Sturge–Weber syndrome.

TABLE 36–4. DIFFERENTIAL DIAGNOSIS OF STURGE–WEBER SYNDROME

Nevus flammeus (port wine stain): Glaucoma workup is negative; brain radiographic studies are negative

Seizures may be evaluated with electroencephalography. Patients with unilateral involvement will show ipsilateral signal attenuation on EEG. When seizures require surgical intervention, the presurgical workup can include MRI, positron emission tomography (PET), single-photon emission computed tomography (SPECT), and EEG to identify the area responsible for seizure activity.

> The hallmark of Sturge–Weber syndrome is the facial vascular lesion (port wine stain) affecting the area of the trigeminal nerve.

Ocular

External examination may reveal facial hemangioma, episcleral or conjunctival hemangioma, and iris heterochromia. Fundus examination may reveal hemangioma, glaucomatous optic nerve cupping, papilledema, retinal pigmentary atrophy, or retinal detachment.

> Choroidal hemangioma is the most common ocular manifestation of Sturge–Weber syndrome and is referred to as "tomato catsup" fundus.

Fluorescein angiography is a useful tool to diagnose choroidal hemangioma. A rapidly appearing, diffusely speckled background choroidal fluorescence beginning in the early transit phase with late staining is characteristic. In the absence of a retinal detachment, there is no leakage of the dye from the choroidal hemangioma into the retina. In isolated hemangiomas, the lesions fluoresce brightly during the early phases of angiography. An irregular lacy pattern may occur, probably due to the rapid filling of the cavernous channels of the hemangioma. Late hyperfluorescence of the tumor may result from the leakage of dye into the overlying subretinal space.

> If the nevus flammeus of Sturge–Weber syndrome is located on the upper eyelid, there is a greater correlation with glaucoma and intracranial angiomatosis.

A- and B-scan ultrasonography can be useful to assess choroidal thickening found with choroidal hemangioma. A-scan sonography will exhibit high internal reflectivity. The B scan will show a solid echogenic mass.

A complete glaucoma workup is mandatory for any patient with a nevus flammeus. Gonioscopy may reveal malformations of the anterior chamber and prominent iris processes adhering to the trabeculum, especially in those with the congenital form.

Visual fields are not only important to follow glaucoma patients but also to detect field defects associated with visual pathway lesions. Visual field defects may include contralateral homonymous hemianopsias associated with occipital leptomeningeal angiomas, or sectorial defects associated with hemangiomas of the choroid.

TREATMENT

Systemic

Epileptic seizures may be treated medically or surgically (Table 36–5). Anticonvulsant medications are effective in about one half of patients with seizures due to Sturge–Weber syndrome. Surgery, such as cerebral resections and hemispherectomy, is indicated only for patients with severe progressive disease unresponsive to medical management to avoid continued deterioration. Patients who develop intractable seizures in the first 6 months of life and unilateral hemispheric involvement should be considered for early resection of the involved hemisphere. There is evidence that with earlier intervention, less intellectual deterioration will occur.

Recent advances in neuroimaging techniques have made preclinical and early diagnosis of Sturge–Weber syndrome possible. This has allowed for early treatment with antiepileptic drugs to prevent or delay developmental anomalies or hemiplegias. Visceral tumors are rare and are only treated when symptoms arise from them. Cutaneous angiomas are usually asymptomatic and not treated. Facial cosmetics can be used to conceal the lesions. Laser therapy is an option for the cosmetic management of the facial nevus flammeus.

TABLE 36–5. TREATMENT AND MANAGEMENT OF STURGE–WEBER SYNDROME

- Seizures
  - Anticonvulsant medications
  - Surgical procedures: cerebral resection or hemispherectomy
- Mental retardation
  - Specialized schooling or vocational rehabilitation
- Facial nevus
  - Cosmetics
  - Laser surgery
- Glaucoma
  - Medical management
  - Surgical management: goniotomy, trabeculotomy, trabeculectomy, cyclocryotherapy
- Retinal detachment
  - Surgical management

Ocular

Follow-up eye care is important for Sturge–Weber patients, particularly if glaucoma or serous retinal detachment are present. Glaucoma in Sturge–Weber syndrome is variable in severity and subsequent treatment modalities (Table 36–5). It often responds poorly to medical management. If medical treatment fails or if the glaucoma is congenital, surgical intervention is necessary. Buphthalmos requires immediate treatment. Goniotomy is a common procedure in infants with congenital glaucoma. Trabeculotomy is performed if corneal clouding prevents visualization of the angle or previous goniotomy has failed. Another alternative used in the management of glaucoma in children with Sturge–Weber syndrome is cryocoagulation of the ciliary body in combination with topical medications. In adults, after medical management fails, argon laser trabeculoplasty may be attempted first. However, if the pressure reduction is insufficient, conventional surgery is the next alternative. Trabeculectomy bypasses any component of the glaucoma caused by elevated episcleral venous pressure, whereas goniotomy does not. If external filtration fails, cyclocryotherapy may be attempted as a last resort. Various other surgical techniques are employed including combined trabeculectomy and cyclocryotherapy, as well as combined trabeculotomy and trabeculectomy. Surgical glaucoma treatment may have complications such as intraoperative expulsive choroidal hemorrhage and choroidal effusion. It may be necessary to perform a posterior sclerotomy before opening the eye to prevent choroidal effusion.

Retinal detachment in Sturge–Weber patients is difficult to treat. When the retina is reattached, fibrous metaplasia of the RPE and cystoid degeneration of the retina overlying the choroidal hemangioma can cause poor visual prognosis.

CONCLUSION

Sturge–Weber syndrome is a congenital disorder involving hamartomas of the skin, central nervous system, and eye. It is characterized by facial hemangioma, glaucoma, and cerebral dysfunctions such as seizures and mental retardation. Although these entities may occur in isolation, Sturge–Weber syndrome is diagnosed when two or more systems are affected. Any patient presenting with a facial hemangioma in the trigeminal distribution or with idiopathic seizures must have comprehensive ocular and neurological evaluation to rule out other manifestations of this disease.

REFERENCES

Alexander GL, Norman RM. *The Sturge–Weber Syndrome.* Bristol, England: Wright: Stonebridge Press; 1960.

Awad AH, Mullaney PB, Al-Mesfer S, Zwaan JT. Glaucoma in Sturge–Weber syndrome. *JAAPOS.* 1999;3:40–45.

Brett EM. Neurocutaneous syndromes. In: Brett EM, ed. *Paediatric Neurology.* Edinburgh: Churchill Livingstone, 1991:580–583.

Garden JM, Bakus DA. Laser treatment of port wine stains and hemangiomas. *Dermatol Clin.* 1997;3:373–383.

Krill AE. *Sturge–Weber Syndrome Hereditary Retinal and Choroidal Diseases.* Vol 2, *Clinical Characteristics.* Hagerstown, Md: Harper & Row; 1977:1275–1290.

Mandal K. Primary combined trabeculotomy-trabeculectomy for early onset Sturge–Weber syndrome. *Ophthalmology.* 1999,106:1621–1627.

Miller NR. Phakomatoses. In: *Walsh and Hoyt's Clinical Neuro-ophthalmology.* Baltimore: Williams & Wilkins; 1988: 1800–1816.

Phelps CD. The pathogenesis of glaucoma in Sturge–Weber syndrome. *Ophthalmology.* 1978;85:276–286.

Susac JO, Smith JL, Scelfo RJ. The "tomato-catsup" fundus in Sturge–Weber syndrome. *Arch Ophthalmol.* 1974;92:69.

Tripatini B, Inpathi RC, Cibis GW. Sturge–Weber syndrome. In: Ryan SJ, ed. *Retina.* St. Louis: Mosby; 1991;1:443–447.

van Emelen C, et al. Treatment of glaucoma in children with Sturge–Weber syndrome. *J Pediatr Ophthalmol.* 2000; 37:29–34.

Weiss JS, Ritch R. Glaucoma in the phakomatoses. In: Ritch R, Shields MB, eds. *The Secondary Glaucomas.* St. Louis: Mosby; 1982, 28–50.

Zion VM. Phakomatoses. In: Tasman W, Jaeger EA, eds. *Duane's Clinical Ophthalmology.* Philadelphia: Lippincott; 1992;5:7–9.

Zupane ML. Update on epilepsy in pediatric patients. *Mayo Clini Proc.* 1996;71:899–916.

Chapter 37

VON HIPPEL–LINDAU DISEASE

Elizabeth B. Aksionoff

Von Hippel–Lindau (VHL) disease, also called retinocerebellar capillary hemangiomatosis, is one of a group of congenital syndromes called the phakomatoses. These syndromes are characterized by disseminated hamartomas (tumor-like nodules) of the eye, skin, and central nervous system. However, von Hippel–Lindau disease is the only phakomatosis without an associated skin lesion. It is a rare, hereditary disorder whose complete complex consists of angiomatosis of the retina, capillary hemangioblastomas of the central nervous system, and cysts or vascular tumors of the viscera. Retinal angiomatoses were first described by von Hippel in 1904. The correlation with hemangiomatous tumors of the cerebellum was made by Lindau in 1926.

EPIDEMIOLOGY

Von Hippel–Lindau disease shows no sexual or racial predilection. Its incidence is estimated at 1 in 32,000 births. It usually presents in the second to fourth decades of life, later than most of the other phakomatoses.

Headache is the presenting symptom in 90% of von Hippel–Lindau patients. Cerebellar hemangioblastomas may occur in 35 to 75% of patients. Retinal hemangioblastomas occur in 45 to 59% of patients with von Hippel–Lindau disease. Renal cell carcinoma has an incidence of 33% in those with von Hippel–Lindau disease and pheochromocytoma occurs in 17%. Half of the patients with cerebellar tumors also present with polycythemia. Cysts present in various visceral organs, with the pancreas (72%), kidney (59%), liver (17%), and epididymis (7%) the most common locations. The complete symptom complex is found in 20% of those with the cerebellar hemangioblastomas, and only 25% of patients with retinal angiomas develop neurological symptoms.

PATHOPHYSIOLOGY/DISEASE PROCESS

Systemic

Von Hippel–Lindau disease is characterized by angiomatosis of the retina, capillary hemangioblastomas of the central nervous system, and cysts or tumors of the viscera. The target organs in VHL are cerebellar and retinal cells producing hemangioblastomas; neural crest cells producing pheochromocytomas, paragliomas, and islet cell tumors; and glandular viscera producing renal, pancreatic, epididymal, and endolymphatic sac tumors.

VHL exhibits autosomal dominant inheritance with variable expression and incomplete penetrance. Incomplete penetrance of the gene allows the gene to be inherited but not expressed. Patients may be found to have VHL by diagnostic testing, yet be asymptomatic carriers. According to the "two hit" theory, when both copies of the gene are inactivated by mutation or loss, cell growth is uninhibited and tumors result.

Genetic linkage studies localized the gene to the short arm of chromosome 3 at loci 3p25-26. The VHL gene, discovered in 1993, is a tumor suppressor gene. It controls the VHL protein that regulates levels of growth factors promoting blood vessel growth. VHL protein produced by a healthy VHL gene suppresses tumor growth. When the VHL gene is mutated, the VHL protein is not produced to bind to elongins and regulate them. Elongins speed up the transcription process from DNA to RNA. With no regulation of elongins, cell growth goes out of control.

Generalized developmental dysgenesis of the neuroectoderm and mesoderm cause hemangioblastomas of the cerebellum (Figure 37–1), medulla, and spinal cord, which are the characteristic central nervous system lesions in von Hippel–Lindau disease. The hemangioblastomas are single or multiple cysts, fed and drained by large vessels. The cyst is fluid filled and contains a nodule of tumor cells in its wall. Hemangioblastomas are usually found in the posterior fossa, and they become symptomatic when they increase intracranial pressure or cause cerebellar dysfunction. Headache is the most common symptom occurring during the course of the disease, and may occur as a result of increased intracranial pressure or the direct affect of the hamartomas on the meninges. Signs of cerebellar dysfunction may include vomiting, ataxic gait, dysdiadochokinesia (the inability to perform rapidly alternating movements), vertigo, and dysmetria (movements overshooting their intended targets). Intracranial hemorrhage or compression of vital brainstem centers are the major causes of death in von Hippel–Lindau disease, secondary to cerebellar hemangioblastomas and less commonly to medullary hemangioblastomas.

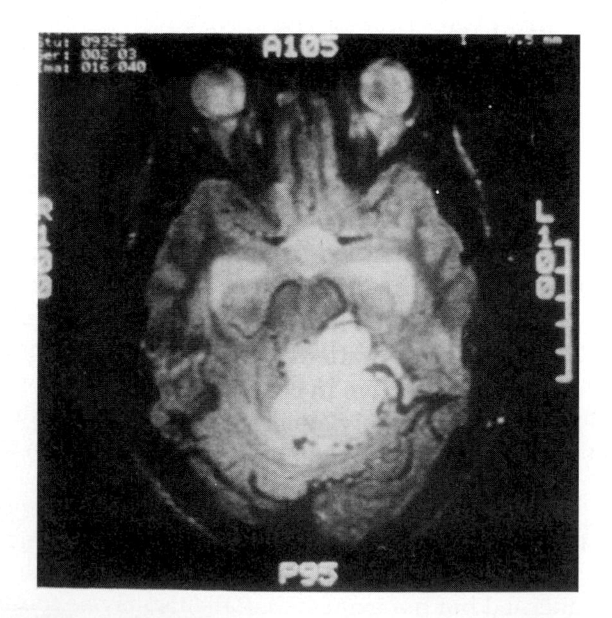

Figure 37–1. MRI with contrast shows cerebellar hemangioblastoma. (*Reprinted with permission from Burk RR: Von Hippel–Lindau disease (angiomatosis of the retina and cerebellum).* J Am Optom Assoc. *1991;62:384.*)

Less common systemic manifestations of von Hippel–Lindau disease are listed in Table 37–1. Spinal cord hemangioblastomas can cause pain, bilateral weakness of the extremities, and sensory disturbances. Renal cell carcinoma may present with hematuria, obstructive nephropathy, or an abdominal mass. This can be fatal secondary to metastasis or uremia. Pheochromocytoma, a tumor of the adrenal medulla, is often bilateral and can synthesize and release catecholamines into the blood, resulting in vasoconstrictive hypertension. Polycythemia, an increase in red cell count, may be found in patients with cerebellar tumors related to the erythropoietic activity of the CNS cyst fluid.

Ocular

Half the patients diagnosed with von Hippel–Lindau disease will eventually suffer visual loss. Angiomatosis retinae is often the first observed manifestation of von Hippel–Lindau disease, and usually is asymptomatic when it is discovered in the second or third decades. Although the angioma may occur anywhere in the retina, it is often found in the midperiphery (Figure 37–2). Angiomas often present bilaterally and may be multiple.

> Retinal hemangioblastoma is often the first observed manifestation of von Hippel–Lindau disease and is usually located in the mid-peripheral retina.

Welch (1970) divided the natural history of the retinal angioma into several stages (Table 37–2). Angiomas of the disc or peripapillary region usually do not have dilated feeder vessels and are the capillary type. There are two varieties, endophytic and exophytic. The endophytic type are circular, reddish, slightly elevated masses internal to the vasculature of

TABLE 37–1. SYSTEMIC MANIFESTATIONS OF VON HIPPEL–LINDAU DISEASE

- Hemangioblastomas of the cerebellum, medulla oblongata, spinal cord
- Hemangioblastomas of the pancreas
- Renal cell carcinomas
- Pheochromocytomas of the adrenal medulla
- Paragangliomas of the sympathetic chain
- Cysts and tumors of miscellaneous visceral organs: meninges, lung, liver, spleen, ovary, bladder, bones, skin, epididymis

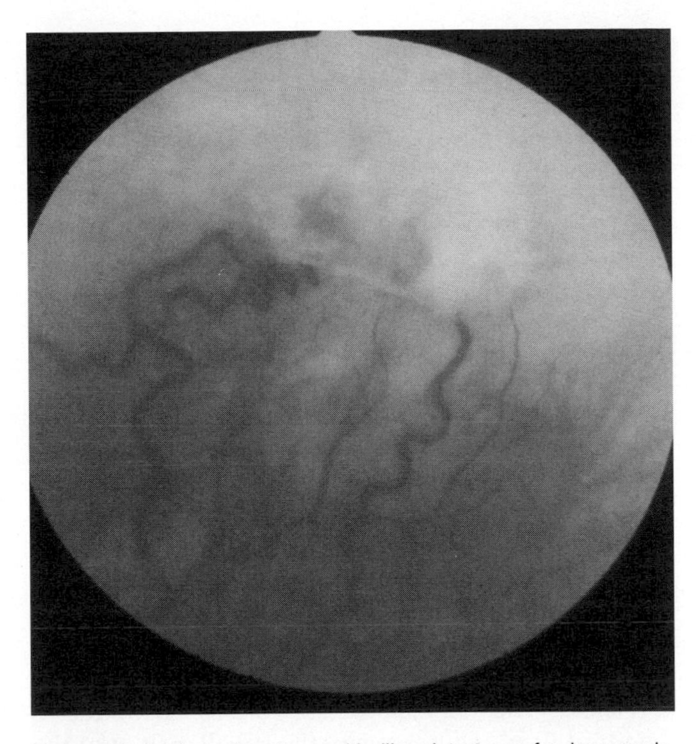

Figure 37–2. Retinal angioma with dilated, tortuous feeder vessels. *(Reprinted with permission from Burk RR: Von Hippel–Lindau disease (angiomatosis of the retina and cerebellum).* J Am Optom Assoc. *1991;62:385.*)

the optic disc. The earliest sign of the disc angioma is a small group of dilated capillaries usually on the temporal side. As it enlarges, this mass begins to resemble a nodule. These tumors give rise to surface neovascularization similar to the peripheral capillary hemangioma. The exophytic type is not seen as a distinct mass but as a blurring and elevation of the margin of the optic disc without prominent vascular channels.

TABLE 37–2. STAGES OF RETINAL ANGIOMA DEVELOPMENT

Stage 1: Preclassical
Microaneurysm-sized lesion consisting of a small capillary cluster
Endothelial cells of lesion are fenestrated, unlike a true capillary
Lack of tight junctions leads to leakage of plasma and blood components into the retina and subretinal space

Stage II: Classical
Larger lesion appearing as a small pink nodule or as a cluster of capillaries with associated dilated feeder vessels

Stage III: Exudation
Tumor enlarges, and secondary to incompetent capillary wall, lipid exudation into the retina and subretinal space occurs

Stage IV: Retinal Detachment
Internal limiting membrane is breached by a proliferation of fibrovascular tissue, causing vitreal traction and nonrhegmatogenous exudative retinal detachment

Stage V: End Stage
May include retinal hemorrhage, gliosis, neovascularization, rubeotic glaucoma, chronic uveitis, phthisis bulbi

TABLE 37–3. OCULAR MANIFESTATIONS OF VON HIPPEL–LINDAU DISEASE

- Angiomatosis retinae
- Optic disc or peripapillary angioma
- The above may cause
  - Exudation
  - Vitreous traction
  - Macular edema
  - Macular gliosis
  - Exudative retinal detachment
  - Neovascularization
  - Secondary glaucoma
  - Phthisis bulbi
- Cerebellar or central nervous system angiomas may cause
  - Papilledema
  - Cranial nerve dysfunctions
  - Nystagmus

Papillary, juxtapapillary, and peripheral angiomas may cause macular edema, the major cause of vision loss in von Hippel–Lindau disease. Even peripheral angiomas, especially those in the temporal fundus, may cause macular edema despite the presence of normal intervening retina. The maculopathy first presents as early edema or as discrete exudates in a star-shaped pattern. Further progression will result in a circular, elevated mass of subretinal exudate. This may lead to macular gliosis, extensive cystoid degeneration, and hole formation, resulting in a significant loss of central vision. These hemangiomas can lead to serous detachments of the peripapillary sensory retina and a ring of intraretinal lipid exudate. The angiomas may extend through a break in the internal limiting membrane and attach to the vitreous. If the vitreous produces traction on the tumor vessels, vitreous hemorrhage or retinal detachment may occur. This may lead to secondary glaucoma, chronic uveitis, and eventually a phthisical eye.

Increased intracranial pressure may lead to papilledema and subsequent optic atrophy as well as cranial nerve dysfunction, such as abducens nerve paresis. Nystagmus is a possible manifestation of cerebellar dysfunction resulting from cerebellar hemangioblastomas (Table 37–3).

DIAGNOSIS

Systemic

To make the diagnosis of von Hippel–Lindau disease, evidence of multisystem involvement must be present rather than isolated retinal, intracranial, or visceral lesions. Diagnosis is made when a patient has a hemangioblastoma of the central nervous system or retina and one or more of the following: first-degree relative with the disease; renal carcinoma; or renal, pancreatic, or epididymal cysts. Diagnosis is often difficult because of the variability in presentation. The first manifestation to become symptomatic is usually the retinal lesion, followed by CNS hemangioblastomas and visceral lesions.

Asymptomatic family members can be screened for VHL with a blood test. Patients with nonspecific findings such as renal cysts can be confirmed or ruled out as having VHL. Current methods of DNA testing can be utilized in patients with findings consistent with VHL but in the absence of family history. If a genetic test excludes VHL, only occasional screening of such patients is advised. If the genetic test is not definitive, diagnosis will be the result of imaging and ophthalmologic testing. Von Hippel–Lindau disease is usually diagnosed during routine physical or ocular examination (Table 37–4). Intracranial or visceral lesions may be discovered upon investigating the subjective symptoms or signs correlating with the involved areas. In these patients, complete blood chemistry (CBC) and urine analysis, which includes catecholamine, epinephrine, and norepinephrine levels, are recommended. Norepinephrine and epinephrine levels will help detect such manifestations as pheochromocytoma. Urine catecholamine levels should be checked every 1 to 2 years. If urine catecholamine levels are normal but blood pressure is elevated, plasma catecholamine levels should be taken. Any biochemical abnormalities warrant an abdominal computed tomography (CT) scan. A magnetic resonance imaging (MRI) of the abdomen will highlight renal carcinoma and other visceral lesions. For patients known to carry the VHL gene and for patients at risk of the disease, screening tests recommended by the NIH include enhanced MRI of the brain and spine and abdominal ultrasound every 2 years from age 11 and then abdominal CT from age 20 on.

Subjective complaint of headache is very common, and other symptoms indicating cerebellar or spinal cord involvement may occur, as described in the pathophysiology section. In the presence of these symptoms, CT of the head and upper cervical spinal cord are indicated, along with MRI of the brain.

Ocular

Von Hippel–Lindau disease may be diagnosed in an asymptomatic individual during routine ocular examination. These patients warrant a complete systemic workup as outlined in the systemic natural history section. Ocular diagnosis of von Hippel–Lindau disease is based upon the presence of retinal hemangioblastoma. Fluorescein angiography is a valuable tool in this diagnosis, and may be the only way to detect subclinical lesions. The enlarged capillaries act hemodynamically as shunts, with resultant enlargement of the afferent and efferent vessels. Because of the shunting mechanism, fluorescein travels through the tumor rapidly. The arterial phase shows a single, rapid-filling artery feeding each angioma, which also quickly fills with dye. The angioma will show varying amounts of dye leakage throughout the late phases. Also, due to the rapid flow of fluorescein, the lamellar flow of the vein may be disrupted. Without stereoscopic fluorescein angiography, retinal angiomas may be confused with papilledema, papillitis, choroiditis, choroidal neovascularization, or choroidal hemangioma.

If symptomatic, the ocular lesions may cause disturbances of vision, headache, papilledema, ocular motor dysfunction, or nystagmus. For the patient at risk for the disease, or carrying the gene, yearly ophthalmoscopy is advised.

Differential diagnosis (Table 37–5) includes Wyburn–Mason syndrome, Coats disease, and sickle-cell disease. In Wyburn–Mason syndrome and Coats disease, no tumor is present. Sea fans found in sickle-cell disease may simulate a capillary hemangioma; however, the sea fans do not have feeder vessel enlargement or produce the high-flow shunt seen in von Hippel–Lindau disease.

TABLE 37–4. CLINICAL EVALUATION AND TESTS UTILIZED TO DIAGNOSE VON HIPPEL–LINDAU DISEASE

- General physical examination
- Ophthalmologic examination
- CBC, electrolytes
- Urinalysis for catecholamine levels
- Abdominal and head CT
- Renal ultrasound
- MRI
- Fluorescein angiography

TABLE 37–5. DIFFERENTIAL DIAGNOSIS OF RETINAL HEMANGIOBLASTOMA

1. Wyburn–Mason syndrome: Presents with large dilated vessels from arteriovenous communications; however, no tumor is present. Lesions in Wyburn–Mason are commonly found in the superior temporal quadrant and posterior pole, whereas VHL hemangiomas are often in the peripheral retina.
2. Coat's disease: Aneurysmal dilation of blood vessels with subretinal exudate; however, no tumor is present.
3. Sickle-cell retinopathy: Sea fans do not have a feeder vessel enlargement or high-flow shunt activity seen with fluorescein angiography.

TREATMENT

Systemic

The systemic therapy of central nervous system (CNS) hemangioblastomas is often directed toward the alleviation of symptoms. However, asymptomatic cerebellar hemangioblastomas may be surgically removed to prevent complications of enlarging lesions. Hemangioblastomas of the spinal cord and brainstem are not treated if asymptomatic. Radiation therapy is warranted when symptoms arise (Table 37–6).

Cysts of the kidney, liver, and pancreas are usually asymptomatic and do not require treatment. However, early surgical removal of pheochromocytomas and renal cell carcinomas is indicated, because these are the most life-threatening lesions in von Hippel–Lindau disease.

Annual physical, kidney ultrasound, and neurological examinations are indicated in any patient at risk. This includes patients with a characteristic retina, CNS or visceral lesion, or a direct relative having the disease. The physical examination should include CBC and urine analysis. The neurological examination may include baseline CT scan of the head and upper cervical spinal cord. MRI of the brain, with particular attention to the posterior fossa, provides more information regarding the presence of cerebellar hemangioblastomas, and should be done when indicated.

Patients with any systemic manifestation of von Hippel–Lindau disease must have a comprehensive ocular examination to rule out the ocular manifestations of the disease.

TABLE 37–6. TREATMENT AND MANAGEMENT OF VON HIPPEL–LINDAU DISEASE

Systemic
- Cerebellar dysfunction
  Surgical removal
- Hemangioblastomas of the spinal cord and medulla
  Radiation therapy
- Pheochromocytomas
  Surgical removal
- Renal cell carcinomas
  Surgical removal
- Visceral lesions
  Symptomatic treatment

Ocular
- Preclassical angiomas
  Photodocumentation, 6-month follow-up
- Classical retinal angiomas
  Fluorescein angiography
  Argon photocoagulation, cryotherapy
- Retinal detachment
  Reattachment procedures
- Optic nerve angiomas
  Photocoagulation at first sign of exudation

By examining family members and/or through family history, an effort should be made to determine if the affected individual inherited the disease by autosomal dominant transmission or as a result of spontaneous mutation. This information is useful for genetic counseling. Knowledge of the VHL gene, and the proteins it encodes and what their functions are will aid in the development of medications and therapies for the various manifestations of VHL.

Ocular

The majority of tumors in von Hippel–Lindau disease progress and lead to serious visual loss. Therefore, indirect ophthalmoscopy is advised annually for family members of von Hippel–Lindau patients and every 6 months for those affected.

Retinal angiomas that are small, stable, and asymptomatic may be followed by photodocumentation (Table 37–4). Follow-up is important because of the great variability in tumor growth rate. When the tumors are small, photocoagulation may obliterate them with little complication. The tumor itself and not the abnormal vessels is treated in order to prevent tumor growth and its sequelae. Treatment destroys the angioma, leaving a pigmented scar and involuted feeder vessels. Treatment of the peripheral angioma will often resolve any macula edema produced by the angioma. Complications of photocoagulation include hemorrhage, exudative retinal detachment, and an increase in intraretinal lipid deposits.

For tumors larger than 0.8 disc diameter and those with subretinal fluid, cryotherapy is recommended. Several treatments may be necessary. Less posttreatment exudative detachment occurs after cryotherapy of large angiomas than after photocoagulation. For tumors greater than one disc diameter in size, a combination of cryotherapy followed by photocoagulation of the tumor itself is indicated. In instances of large tumors, multiple tumors, or vitreous membranes, vitrectomy should be considered. Penetrating diathermy and eye wall resection are other techniques used to treat large peripheral capillary hemangiomas. Proton beam irradiation is useful for large, advanced hemangioblastomas.

After treatment, patients should be followed with fluorescein angiography. Retreatment is indicated if the tumor persists in the pigmented scar or if fluorescein angiography shows the persistence of hyperfluorescence.

Intraretinal juxtapapillary capillary hemangiomas are difficult to treat because they are diffusely situated in the retina. Laser burns needed to destroy the abnormal vascular tissue must also penetrate the retinal tissue including the nerve fiber layer. When treated, there is a potential for full-thickness damage to the retina and disc, with resultant visual loss. If untreated, however, exudation, retinal detachment, and neovascular glaucoma may result from lesion growth. Treatment is usually indicated at the first sign of exudation.

For traction detachment or surface-wrinkling retinopathy, pars plana vitrectomy and membrane peeling may be used. Retinal detachments may require reattachment procedures such as scleral buckling.

Follow-up is recommended every 3 to 6 months depending on the extent of retinal findings. If a retinal or optic disc angioma is observed, a systemic workup with urinary catecholamine and CT or MRI of the head, upper cervical spinal cord, and abdomen are indicated.

CONCLUSION

Von Hippel–Lindau disease is a multisystem disease characterized by hemangioblastomas of the retina, hemangioblastomas of the central nervous system, and cysts or tumors of the viscera. This disease is of particular importance to the eyecare practitioner, because its first presenting signs are often ocular. Any retinal angioma should alert the practitioner to the need for a complete physical and neurological evaluation, because the associated renal cell carcinoma, pheochromocytoma, and cerebellar hemangioblastoma are potentially lethal lesions. Because the disease is autosomal dominant in nature, genetic counseling is advised.

There is growing optimism that the diagnosis of a potentially lethal lesion such as hemangioblastoma or renal cell carcinoma can be made earlier and more accurately with genetic testing.

REFERENCES

Annesley WH, Leonard BC, Shields JA, Tasman WS. Fifteen-year review of treated cases of retinal angiomatosis. *Ophthalmology.* 1977;83:446.

Choyke PL, Glenn GM, McClellan MW, et al. Von Hippel–Lindau disease: Genetic, clinical and imaging features. *Radiology.* 1995;146:629–642.

Couch V, Lindor NM, Kames PS, Michels VV. Von Hippel–Lindau disease. *Mayo Clin Proc.* 2000;75:265–272.

Duan L, Klausner R, et al. Inhibition of transcription elongation by the VHL tumor suppressor protein. *Science.* 1995; 269:1402–1406.

Duan L, Lineham WM, Klausner R, et al. Characterization of the VHL tumor suppressor gene product. *Proc Natl Acad Sci USA.* 1995;92:6459–6463.

Goldberg MF, Duke JR. Von Hippel–Lindau disease. *Am J Ophthalmol.* 1968;66:693–705.

Gomez MR. Neurocutaneous disease. In: Bradley WG, Daroff RB, Fenichel GM, Marsden CD, eds. *Neurology in Clinical Practice.* Boston: Butterworth-Heinemann; 1991.

Hardwig PW, Robertson DM. Von Hippel–Lindau disease: A familial, often lethal, multi-system phakomatosis. *Ophthalmology.* 1984;91:263–270.

Karsdorp N, Elderson A, Wittebol-Post D, et al. Von Hippel–Lindau disease: New strategies in early detection and treatment. *Am J Med.* 1994;97:158–168.

Krill AE. Von Hippel–Lindau disease. In: Krill AE, ed: *Krill's Hereditary Retinal and Choroidal Diseases.* Vol 2, *Clinical Characteristics.* Hagerstown, Md: Harper & Row; 1977: 1249–1274.

Latif F, Tory K, Gnarra J, et al. Identification of the von Hippel–Lindau disease tumor suppressor gene. *Science.* 1993; 260:1317–1320.

Maher ER, Iselius L, Yates JRW et al. Von Hippel–Lindau disease: A genetic study. *J Med Genet.* 1991;28:443–447.

Maher ER, Yates JRW, Harries R, et al. Clinical features and natural history of von Hippel–Lindau disease. *Quart J Med.* 1990;77:1151–1163.

Miller NR. Phakomatoses. In: Miller NR, ed: *Walsh and Hoyt's Clinical Neuro-ophthalmology.* Baltimore: Williams & Wilkins; 1988:1788–1800.

Nicholson DH. Capillary hemangioma of the retina and von Hippel–Lindau disease. In: Ryan SJ, ed. *Retina.* St. Louis: Mosby; 1989;1:563–570.

Ridley M, Green J, Johnson G. Retinal angiomatosis: The ocular manifestations of Von Hippel–Lindau disease. *Can J Ophthalmol.* 1986;21:276–283.

Welch RB. Von Hippel–Lindau disease: The recognition and treatment of early anastomosis retinae and the use of cryosurgery as an adjunct to therapy. *Trans Am Ophthalmol Soc.* 1970;68:367–424.

Zion, V.M. Phakomatoses. In: Tasman W, Jaeger EA, eds. *Duane's Clinical Ophthalmology.* Philadelphia: Lippincott; 1992;5:3–4.

Section IX

DERMATOLOGIC DISORDERS

Chapter 38

ATOPIC DERMATITIS

Michael Chaglasian

Atopic dermatitis (AD) is a chronic, relapsing skin disease of unknown etiology. It is characterized by eczematous inflammation in patients with a family history of atopy. Atopy is a term that identifies persons who have an IgE-mediated hypersensitivity to environmental allergens. In its most protracted course, the disease spans infancy, childhood, and adolescence, and may continue on into adulthood. It is also known as allergic eczema, infantile eczema, or allergic dermatitis. Ocular complications of AD were first noted in 1914 (Brunsting et al, 1955). Cataracts are very common and may appear at an early age. Other common ocular complications include keratoblepharoconjunctivitis, keratitis, and herpes simplex virus infection.

EPIDEMIOLOGY

Systemic

Surveys investigating the prevalence of AD vary as to the specific diagnostic criteria used. Most reports demonstrate that 2 to 5% of all children will exhibit some form of AD. In groups with a family history of atopy or asthma, the percentage may increase to 33%. The male-to-female ratio is about equal. Ninety percent of AD cases develop prior to age 5, most often within the first year of life. It rarely appears in adulthood (Leung et al, 1986). A strong genetic component is clearly present in AD, the inherited defect being within the immune system and as such it is considered an important component of the diagnostic criteria (Stevens et al, 1999). Uehara and Kimura (1993) found AD in 60% of children who had one parent with AD, and an 81% prevalence among those with two AD parents.

Ocular

Ocular complications are present in approximately 42% of patients (Garrity & Liesegang, 1984), with atopic keratoconjunctivitis the most common. Age and race characteristics of these patients are unknown. A slight male predominance may exist. Uehara (1981) studied 300 patients with AD and detected a prominent infraorbital fold of the lower eyelid in 25% of them, while finding it in only about 2% of the normal population. Anterior and posterior subcapsular cataracts are found in 13 to 25% of AD patients. The frequency of keratoconus in patients with AD is most likely between 0.5 and 1.5% (Brunsting et al, 1955; Garrity & Liesegang, 1984).

PATHOPHYSIOLOGY/DISEASE PROCESS

Systemic

The systemic complications of atopic dermatitis will generally begin in early childhood, and will primarily be limited to the skin. The hallmark symptom is an intense pruritis (itching) that may be generalized or local and is intermittent throughout the day. Pruritis may be aggravated by several factors, including exposure to soaps, wool, acrylic, lotions, low humidity, and sun.

The cutaneous manifestations of AD are continually changing in severity and appearance. Various morphologic skin lesions will present through periods of exacerbation and remission. Included among these dermatologic lesions are dermatitis, lichenification (a thickening and accentuation of skin markings), xerosis, and ichthyosis (keratinization of the skin). Often, an aggravating factor can be identified. Identification and removal of these factors may be the best therapy for the patient. Constant rubbing and scratching may cause or worsen some of these cutaneous findings.

Common areas that show patchy dermatitis in the infant include the cheeks (Figure 38–1), forearms, legs, and diaper area. The dermatitis is a scaly, rough, reddish area of skin. In days or weeks, further crusting and weeping of the area is frequent. As the child learns to crawl and walk, the affected areas shift to elbows, knees, wrists, and ankles. Lichenification replaces the erythematous dermatitis. The itching remains severe at this stage.

In later childhood, the disease may improve, or continued manifestations may appear including xerosis, lichenification, follicular eczema, fissuring and scaling of hands or feet, and skin hyper- or hypopigmentation. Many of these changes are self-induced from chronic scratching. Patients with atopic dermatitis have a tendency to develop generalized infections. The long-term weeping skin lesions are subject to secondary staphylococcal superinfections and thus require careful monitoring. Cutaneous, nonocular, viral infections from herpes simplex and vaccina are also common.

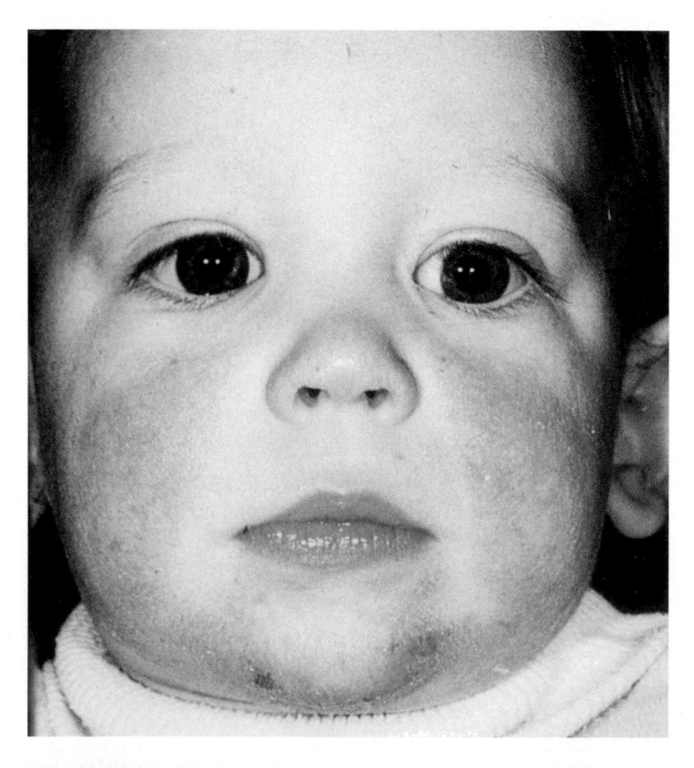

Figure 38–1. Atopic dermatitis of the cheeks. (*Reprinted with permission from Habif TP.* Clinical Dermatology: A Color Guide to Diagnosis and Therapy. *2nd ed. St. Louis: Mosby; 1990:77.*)

At around 2 years of age, half of the children with AD will demonstrate clear skin, whereas the other 50% will have continued recurrences up through ages 5 to 9. Those patients who have extended recurrences through adolescence are likely to have them continue into adulthood. The adult form of AD is usually more localized than the infantile or childhood forms. Areas of persistant eczematous irritation include the hands, face, neck, genitalia, or legs (Table 38–1).

Ocular

The ocular manifestations of atopic dermatitis are numerous (Table 38–2). Although an association of the disease with cataracts was first made in 1914, it was not until 1952 that Hogan described an "atopic keratoconjunctivitis" as a clinical entity. Other significant ocular manifestations include keratoconus, herpes simplex, anterior uveitis, and retinal detachment.

Ocular disease in patients with AD usually begins in the late teens and may persist for 20 years or more. Patients have a predictable history of dermatitis in early childhood, followed by occasional recurrences in adolescence. It has been noted that many of these patients will have a prominent fold of the lower eyelid, known as a Dennie–Morgan fold. The exact significance of this fold is uncertain, but it is likely to indicate past or present inflammation of the eyelid (Leung et al, 1986).

TABLE 38–1. SYSTEMIC MANIFESTATIONS OF ATOPIC DERMATITIS

Pruritis
Eczematous inflammation of hands, face, and neck
Dermatitis
Lichenification
Xerosis
Ichthyosis
Fissuring and scaling of hands and feet
Hypo- or hyperpigmentation of skin
Staphylococcal superinfections
Herpes simplex
Herpes zoster
Body Area Involved:
Infants: Cheeks, forearms, legs, diaper area
Mobile infants: Elbows, knees, wrists, ankles
Adults: Hands, face, neck, genitalia, legs

TABLE 38–2. OCULAR MANIFESTATIONS OF ATOPIC DERMATITIS

Prominent infraorbital fold of lower eyelid
Pruritis of the lids and periorbital skin
Foreign-body sensation
Decreased visual acuity (VA) secondary to cataract formation
Blepharitis
Thickening of lid margins
Superficial punctate keratitis
Keratoconjunctivitis
Symblepharon
Keratoconus
Herpes simplex
Cataracts
Less Frequently Reported:
Uveitis
Ocular hypertension
Branch retinal vein occlusion
Central serous choroidopathy
Retinal detachment

Atopic keratoconjunctivitis (Figure 38–2) is seen some time after localized cutaneous activity. It is bilateral and is characterized by pruritis, burning, and a slight mucous discharge. The eyelid will be mild to moderately erythematous and edematous. Blepharitis is a predominant finding (Tuft et al, 1990). Chronic eyelid inflammation and rubbing may lead to excoriation (loss of skin), lichenification, and lid eversion with secondary epiphora. The bulbar conjunctiva will be hyperemic and edematous during the acute phase. Further changes may include shrinkage of the fornix, symblepharon formation, Trantas dots, and inclusion cysts at the limbus (Hogan, 1953).

Hogan (1953) noted that early corneal signs begin with a superficial punctate keratitis at the superior limbal area. Over several years, areas of pannus may develop (Figure 38–3). A haziness to the anterior stroma is subsequently noted. If the ocular disease persists, marginal ulceration and vascularization can progress and lead to severe vision loss.

An impairment of the corneal epithelium has been noted by fluorophotometric evaluation. Yokoi and colleagues (1998) demonstrated that atopic dermatitis patients showed significantly higher fluorescein uptake, indicating that the "barrier" function of the corneal epithelium was impaired. Dogru and co-workers (1998) examined the tear function and the conjunctiva of 44 patients with AD. As compared to normals, 51% of the subjects had a tear film break time of less than 10 seconds, and Schirmer testing was abnormal in 62% of AD patients. The same group of patients also demonstrated goblet cell loss and squamous metaplasia by conjunctival impression cytology. This information highlights the importance of directing therapy toward the conjunctival epithelium in the early stages of the disease process.

The association between keratoconus and atopic disease has been noted and is well established. Keratoconus in AD patients follows the typical course of corneal thinning and ectasia with irregular astigmatism.

A high susceptibility to herpes simplex viral infection has been noted in several studies (Brunsting et al, 1955; Easty et al, 1975; Garrity & Liesegang, 1984). This corneal infection may be more difficult to manage in patients with AD.

The frequently occurring anterior subcapsular cataracts are often described as white, polygonal,

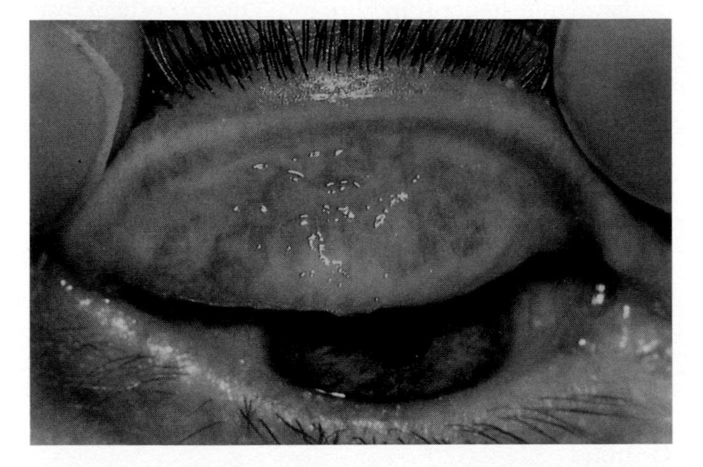

Figure 38–2. Prominent giant papillae with marked subepithelial sheets of fibrosis in a 42-year-old man with atopic keratoconjunctivitis. (*Reprinted with permission from Tuft SJ, Kemeny DM, Dart JKG, Buckley RJ. Clinical features of atopic keratoconjunctivitis.* Ophthalmology. *1991;98:150–158.*)

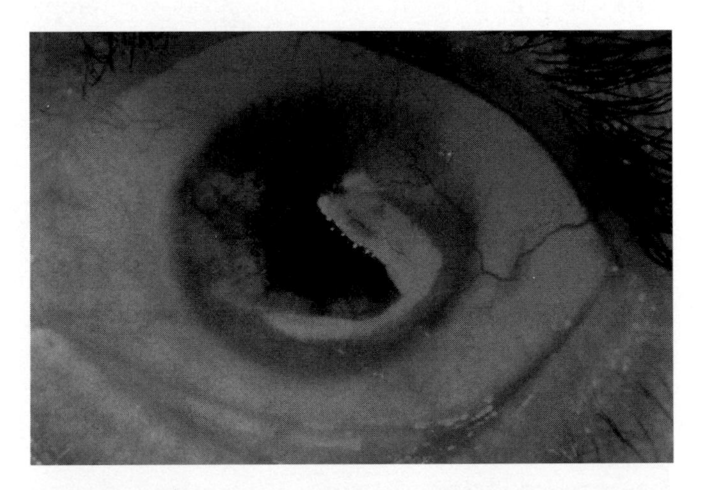

Figure 38–3. Peripheral corneal neovascularization and active pannus in a patient with recurrent atopic keratoconjunctivitis. (*Reprinted with permission from Foster CS, Calonge M. Atopic keratoconjunctivitis.* Ophthalmology. *1990;97:992–1000.*)

shield-like opacifications. Lens opacities usually first appear at age 20 and may either progress slowly or mature rapidly (Smolin & O'Connor, 1986). Since many AD patients may be treated with steroids, this etiology should be ruled out. Progression of cataracts has been associated with soft contact lens wear, facial skin lesions, and eye rubbing (Nagaki et al, 1999).

Other ocular manifestations have been less frequently reported. These include retinal detachment, uveitis, ocular hypertension, branch retinal vein occlusion, and central serous chorioretinopathy. In a 5-year review of young (less than 30 years old) patients who presented with retinal detachments, Nakatsu and colleagues (1995) found that 19% had a documented history of AD. Retinal dialysis and tears of the ciliary epithelium were often seen in these patients. The specific underlying pathogenesis of the detachments is unknown; however, self-inflicted ocular contusion by tapping the eyes has been suggested as one potential cause (Oka et al, 1994). The surgical repair of these tears typically has a good outcome.

DIAGNOSIS

Systemic

The multiple, varied, and ever-changing manifestations of atopic dermatitis have led to confusion in its diagnosis (Table 38–3). The diagnosis is primarily clinical and should be made based on criteria suggested by Hannifin and Rajka (1980) (Table 38–4). Thorough patient questioning usually reveals some prior family history of hayfever, asthma, allergic rhinitis, atopic dermatitis, or other atopic disease. A positive personal or family history of atopy and proper cutaneous features are principal criteria for diagnosis. The atopy patch test is used as a test for eczematous skin reactions to aeroallergens; the test is based on the presence of IgE molecules (Bruijnzeel-Koomen, 1998).

TABLE 38–3. DIFFERENTIAL DIAGNOSIS OF ATOPIC DERMATITIS

Systemic
Seborrheic dermatitis
Contact dermatitis
Nummular dermatitis
Wiskott–Aldrich syndrome
Hyper-IgE syndrome

Ocular
Seasonal allergic conjunctivitis
Vernal keratoconjunctivitis
Keratoconjunctivitis sicca
Keratoconus

TABLE 38–4. DIAGNOSTIC CRITERIA FOR ATOPIC DERMATITIS

Major Features
Personal/family history of atopy
Pruritis
Typical morphology and distribution
Tendency toward relapses or chronicity

Minor Features
Systemic
- Xerosis/ichthyosis/hyperlinear palms (prominent palm creases)
- Keratosis pilaris (horny or nutmeg-grater erosion on posterior arm or leg)
- Facial pallor
- Tendency toward nonspecific hand dermatitis
- Tendency toward repeated cutaneous infections
- White dermographism (skin swelling from scratching)

Ocular
- Infraorbital darkening
- Infraorbital lid fold
- Keratoconjunctivitis
- Keratoconus
- Anterior subcapsular cataracts

Laboratory diagnostic tests
- Immediate skin test reactivity
- Elevated serum IgE level
- Conjunctival histological studies

Adapted with permission from Hannifin JM, Rajka G. Diagnostic features of atopic dermatitis. Acta Derm Venereol. *1980;92(suppl 3):44–47.*

Laboratory findings may be significant for increased serum IgE levels (6000 ng/mL versus 780 ng/mL in normal patients). Although many patients with the disease will have elevated serum IgE levels, some studies show 50% of AD patients have normal levels. Thus, this feature should be considered nonspecific. Also, IgE values are not related to the degree of ocular manifestations. In vitro radioallergosorbent testing (RAST) can detect IgE antibodies. Approximately 85% of AD patients have positive RAST results for food and inhalant antigens (Beltrani, 1999). Unfortunately, the test has up to an 80% false-positive rate, and thus cannot be used as a stand-alone diagnostic test.

Additional lab testing may include looking for various inflammatory markers. Soluble interleukin-2, intercellular adhesion molecule-1, endothelial leukocyte adhesion molecule, and others have been studied as potential objective markers for AD (Kim & Honig, 1997). Further research will determine the clinical value of these new tests.

Ocular

Ocular diagnosis is made in patients with a history of atopic dermatitis and any of the ocular complications previously mentioned (Tables 38–2 and 38–4), most commonly atopic keratoconjunctivitis. See Table 38–3 for a list of differential diagnoses. Atopic keratoconjunctivitis can be diagnosed more definitively through conjunctival histopathologic studies that have demonstrated diagnostically specific changes (Foster et al, 1991). Some of these changes include epithelial invasion by mast cells and eosinophils, goblet cell proliferation and chronic mononuclear cell infiltration of the substantia propria (Hogan, 1962). Abnormal numbers of T cells, T helper/inducer cells, macrophages, and Langerhans' cells were found by Foster and co-workers (1991). These findings indicate that many cell types are involved in atopic keratoconjunctivitis and point out that successful long-term therapy cannot be solely aimed at mast cell stabilization. This is the rationale for systemic therapy in this topical disease.

In atopic dermatitis patients with ocular complications, serum IgE levels were significantly higher among those with cataracts as compared to those without cataracts (Uchio et al, 1998).

TREATMENT AND MANAGEMENT

Systemic

Treatment is directed toward any acute manifestations as well as the removal of all potentially inciting agents or antigens (Table 38–5). Most important is educating patients that they must avoid itching and scratching, since this will significantly hinder all treatment strategies. Damaged skin is treated aggressively, with an attempt to restore its normal condition and to control the pruritis. Treatment measures primarily include "tap-water" baths with water-trapping agents such as mineral oil and petrolatum USP (United States Pharmacopeia). Creams and lotions should be avoided because they often contain fragrances, solubilizers, and preservatives. Cold compresses and astringents are used to relieve itching. Secondary bacterial superinfections are best treated with systemic antibiotics. Systemic antihistamines and oral cromolyn sodium have been used with mixed results in helping control and reduce acute flare-ups. Topical steroids are very helpful in controlling the dermatitis and pruritis found in the follicular eczema and lichenification stages and remain the mainstay of therapy. The best agents are low- to mid-potency, in a cream or ointment base. Systemic steroids are reserved for refractory cases.

For severe, refractory AD, oral cyclosporin A (CSA) has been found to be effective. The immunosuppressive drug interferes with cytokine transcription in T cells. Unfortunately patients relapse upon discontinuation of the drug (Berth-Jones et al, 1997).

A new immunosuppressive agent, tacrolimus, has been utilized as a topical agent. While it is 10 to 100 times more potent than CSA at inhibiting T-cell activiation, it has minimal systemic absorption and toxicity. The initial results have been very promising, and multicenter trials have been initiated in Europe (Boguniewicz, 1997).

TABLE 38–5. TREATMENT AND MANAGEMENT OF ATOPIC DERMATITIS

Systemic
Avoidance of scratching
Removal of inciting agent (soaps, clothing)
"Tap-water" bath with bath oils for damaged skin
Cold compresses and astringents
Topical steroids (e.g., hydrocortisone acetate cream 0.5–1%; triamcinolone acetonide cream 0.025–0.5%)
Topical antipruritics
Bland emollient creams and lotions
Oral antihistamines
Ultraviolet phototherapy
Systemic steroids (rarely): prednisolone 5 mg qd; for short courses only
Systemic antibiotics (erythromycin) for staphylococcal control
Oral cyclosporine A (for recalcitrant cases) 5mg/kg/day

Ocular
Cold compresses
Artificial tear preparations
Decongestants
  Naphazoline 0.1% qid
  Phenylephrine 0.12% qid
Decongestant/antihistamine combinations
  Naphazoline/pheneramine (Vasoclear A, Naphcon A, Albalon A)
Cromolyn sodium 4% (Optichrom)
Topical steroids
  FML 0.1% qid
  Pred Mild 0.125%
  Inflammase Mild 0.125%
Topical steroids (ointments/creams)
  For periorbital skin hydrocortisone 1% cream
Oral antihistamines (for pruritis)
  Benadryl 25–50mg tid
  Allegra 60 mg bid
  Claritin 10 mg qd
Oral/topical cyclosporine A (currently under investigation)

Abbreviations: bid, twice a day; FML, fluorometholone; gd, every day; qid, four times daily; tid, three times a day.

In addition to avoidance, supportive, and pharmacologic treatment plans, patients with AD have other alternative therapies. Ultraviolet light (UV-A and UV-B) can cause significant improvement, though the exact mechanism is not understood. Caffeine (a phosphodiesterase inhibitor), oral evening primrose (for essential fatty acids), Chinese herbs (a combination of 10), hyposensitization, and behavior modification have all been described in the literature and as having a positive outcome on AD (Krafchik, 1999).

Ocular

Ocular management is also directed toward acute symptomatic relief (Table 38–5). For keratoconjunctivitis, cold compresses and topical decongestants or decongestant/antihistamines will relieve most patients. For more symptomatic presentations, topical steroids will provide a more rapid resolution. Low-potency, nonfluorinated corticosteroids (such as 1% hydrocortisone) should be the only preparations used on delicate facial skin (Woodmansee & Christiansen, 1998). Between the acute phases, artificial tear preparations are useful for corneal protection. Topical 4% cromolyn sodium has been used with some success for the relief of itching, inflammation, and lichenification. Its use can reduce the need for topical steroids.

In refractory cases of atopic keratoconjuctivitis the therapeutic benefits of systemic CSA have been noted (Hoang-Xuan et al, 1997). Over a mean treatment peroid of 37 months three of four patients demonstrated complete resolution of symptoms, while the fourth had significant improvement. Toxicity and side effects can develop, and further study is required to determine the appropriate maintenance dose. Topical CSA may show greater effectivity with less morbidity. Topical CSA has been investigated for a number of autoimmune ocular surface conditions. In atopic keratoconjunctivitis topical CSA was shown to decrease T-cell activation and reduce the number of conjunctival T cells, among other immunomodulatory effects (Hingorani et al, 1999). Further research needs to be done before topical CSA can have a greater clinical role.

> Early and aggressive topical therapy with lubricants, antihistamines, and mild steroids directed toward maintenance of the ocular surface epithelium may help to prevent future complications in atopic keratoconjunctivitis.

Patients who develop chronic keratoconjunctivitis may require systemic therapy in addition to their topical medications. Foster & Calonge (1990) recommend maximizing systemic antihistamine therapy.

Because of the increased corneal epithelial breakdown in keratoconic patients with AD, rigid gas-permeable contact lenses must be fit cautiously and patients followed closely, since corneal irritation is common in these patients. Frequent topical lubrication can improve patient success.

Cataract surgery is indicated for those patients with decreased acuity. Significant ocular complications are associated with cataract surgery in patients with atopic disease; thus, there is a higher risk for poor visual outcome (<20/100).

CONCLUSION

Atopic dermatitis is a relatively common, potentially chronic, superficial inflammation of the skin. Characterized by intense itching, it is commonly found in patients with a personal or family history of atopy. The skin is dry and pruritic; patchy lesions are distinguished by edema, erythema, excoriation, scaling, and hyperpigmentation. There are numerous ocular complications, most commonly keratoconjunctivitis and subcapsular cataracts. Decreased vision is most commonly a result of anterior or posterior subcapsular cataracts, although corneal disease (marginal inflammation and vascularization, stromal haziness, and HSV keratitis) can cause permanent visual loss. Although various topical treatment modalities offer patients some symptomatic relief, it is difficult to avoid permanent cutaneous or ocular damage in the chronic forms of the disease.

REFERENCES

Beltrani VS. Atopic dermatitis: The spectrum of disease. *J Cutan Med Surg.* 1999;3(suppl 2):8–15.

Berth-Jones J, Braham-Brown RA, Marks R, et al. Long-term efficacy and safety of cyclosporin in severe adult atopic dermatitis. *Br J Dermatol.* 1997;136:76–81.

Boguniewicz M. Advances in the understanding and treatment of atopic dermatitis. *Curr Opin Pediatr.* 1997; 9:577–581.

Bruijnzeel-Koomen C. The role of IgE in the pathogenesis of atopic dermatitis. *Allergy.* 1998;53(suppl 46):29–30.

Brunsting LA, Red WB, Bair HL. Occurrence of cataracts and keratoconus with atopic dermatitis. *Arch Dermatol.* 1955; 72:237–241.

Dogru M, Katakami C, Nakagawa N, et al. Impression cytology in atopic dermatitis. *Ophthalmology.* 1998;105:1478–1484.

Easty D, Enstwistle C, Funk A, Witcher J. Herpes simplex keratitis and keratoconus in the atopic patient: A clinical and immunologic study. *Trans Ophthalmol Soc UK.* 1975; 95:267–276.

Foster CS, Calonge M. Atopic keratoconjunctivitis. *Ophthalmology.* 1990;97:992–1000.

Foster CS, Rice BA, Dutt JE. Immunopathology of atopic keratoconjunctivitis. *Ophthalmology.* 1991;98:1190–1196.

Garrity JA, Liesegang TL. Ocular complications of atopic dermatitis. *Can J Ophthalmol.* 1984;19:21–24.

Hannifin JM, Lobitz WC Jr. Newer concepts of atopic dermatitis. *Arch Dermatol.* 1977;113:663–670.

Hannifin JM, Rajka G. Diagnostic features of atopic dermatitis. *Acta Derm Venereol.* 1980;92(suppl 3):44–47.

Hingorani M, Calder VL, Buckley RJ, et al. the immunomodulatory effect of topical cyclosporin A in atopic keratoconjunctivitis. *Invest Ophthalmol Vis Sci.* 1999;40:392–399.

Hoang-Xuan T, Prisant O, Hannouche D, Robin H. Systemic cyclosporine A in severe atopic keratoconjunctivitis. *Ophthalmology.* 1997;104:1300–1305.

Hogan MJ: Atopic keratoconjunctivitis. *Trans Am Ophthalmol Soc.* 1952;50:265–281.

Hogan MJ: Atopic keratoconjunctivitis. *Am J Ophthalmol.* 1953;36:937–947.

Katsura H, Hida T. Retinal detachment associated with atopic dermatitis. *Retina.* 1984;4:148–151.

Kim HJ, Honig PJ. Atopic dermatitis. *Curr Opin Pediatr.* 1997;10:367–392.

Krafchik BR. Treatment for atopic dermatitis. *J Cutan Med Surg.* 1999;3(suppl 2):16–23.

Leung DYM, Rhodes AR, Geha RS. Atopic dermatitis. In: Fitzpatrick TB, Eisen AZ, Wolf K, et al, eds. *Dermatology in General Medicine,* 3rd ed. New York: McGraw-Hill; 1986:1385–1411.

Nagaki Y, Hayasaka S, Kadoi C. Cataract progression in patients with atopic dermatitis. *J Cataract Refract Surg.* 1999; 25:96–99.

Nakatsu A, Wada Y, Kondo T. Retinal detachment in patients with atopic dermatitis. *Ophthamologica.* 1995;209:160–164.

Oka C, Ideta H, Nagasaki H, et al. Retinal detachment with atopic dermatitis similar to traumatic retinal detachment. *Ophthalmology.* 1994;101:1050–1054.

Smolin G, O'Connor GR. *Ocular Immunology.* Boston: Little, Brown; 1986:171–179.

Stevens SR, Kang K, Cooper KD. Atopic dermatitis: Introduction and overview. *J Cutan Med Surg.* 1999;3(suppl 2):2–7.

Tuft SJ, Kemeny DM, Dart JKG, Buckley RJ. Clinical features of atopic keratoconjunctivitis. *Ophthalmology.* 1991; 98:150–158.

Uchio E, Miyakawa K, Ikezawa Z, et al. Systemic and local immunological features of atopic dermatitis patients with ocular complications. *Br J Ophthalmol.* 1998;82:82–87.

Uehara M. Infraorbital fold in atopic dermatitis. *Arch Dermatol.* 1981;117:627–629.

Uehara M, Kimura C. Descendant family history of atopic dermatitis. *Acta Derm Venereol.* 1993;73:62–63.

Walker C, Craig TJ. Atopic dermatitis: A clinical review for the primary care physician. *JAOA.* 1999;99(suppl):5–10.

Woodmansee D, Christiansen S. Atopic dermatitis. *Pediatr Ann.* 1998;27:710–716.

Yokoi K, Yokoi N, Kinoshita S. Impairment of ocular surface epithelium barrier function in patients with atopic dermatitis. *Br J Ophthalmol.* 1998;82:797–800.

Chapter 39

ROSACEA

Michael Chaglasian

Rosacea dermatitis is a classic disorder affecting the cheeks, nose, forehead, chin, and eyes. Its characteristic rhinophyma (gross hypertrophy of the sebaceous glands of the nose) is a well-established hallmark, along with persistent erythema, telangiectasias, papules, and pustules. It is a syndrome of unknown etiology, although numerous associations and theories have been proposed.

The term rosacea is preferred over acne rosacea because the facial lesions are not similar to those found in acne vulgaris or cystic acne.

Ocular rosacea refers to patients with definitive ocular manifestations. Ocular involvement in rosacea is common and typically includes blepharitis, meibomianitis, chalazia, and a mild to severe keratitis. Left untreated, permanent visual loss is possible. Unfortunately, both conditions are widely underdiagnosed by eyecare practitioners. Treatment with oral tetracycline is very effective for both conditions.

EPIDEMIOLOGY

Systemic and Ocular

Rosacea affects adults 30 to 60 years of age. Women are twice as likely to have rosacea, without ocular signs, as men. However, ocular rosacea is equally divided between the sexes. Patients with ocular rosacea tend to be slightly older than those patients with facial manifestations alone. A positive family history may be elicited in up to 30% of rosacea patients. Despite being a relatively common condition, very little good epidemiologic data exist (Katz, 1998).

The specific distribution of rosacea among different races has not been well researched. The clinical impression is that it primarily affects fair-skinned Celtics and Northern Europeans. It was believed at one time that blacks were not affected, but it is now recognized that they also suffer from rosacea (Browning et al, 1986; Rosen & Stone, 1987).

Ocular involvement is present in upwards of 58% of patients. One third of all patients develop both ocular and facial manifestations simultaneously. Fifty percent develop skin lesions initially, whereas the remaining 20% will develop only ocular complications first (Borrie, 1953).

In a comprehensive review of 131 patients with ocular rosacea, Akpek and co-workers (1997) found an age range of 23 to 85 years (mean, 56 years); 10 patients were less than 30 years old. A majority (112) had cutaneous signs at presentation, whereas only 12 of them had been previously diagnosed. Surprisingly, 43% were women, much higher than had been noted in earlier reviews. None of the patients were black. Visual acuity was reduced at presentation in 13 patients, six of these required penetrating keratoplasty during the course of the disease. A total of seven patients were left with visual acuity of 20/400 or less.

PATHOPHYSIOLOGY/DISEASE PROCESS

Systemic

The cutaneous lesions of rosacea (Figure 39–1) have been well recognized for many centuries. Common patient complaints include facial flushing and warmth and painful pustules (small circumscribed elevations containing fluid, which are usually purulent) around the central one third of the face. They may first notice an erythematous blush over the cheeks and nose. The onset is slow and insidious and initially the lesions may be intermittent, though slow to resolve. Acneiform papules (small, solid, raised skin lesions) 2 to 3 mm in size begin to appear in the same area. Telangiectatic vessels also cover the cheeks, nose, and forehead. Rhinophyma can progress to prominent vascularity, swelling, and disfigurement. It usually occurs after other cutaneous lesions have been present for some time and may be more pronounced in males (Table 39–1).

The course of rosacea is prolonged with frequent recurrences. Transient skin papules and pustules resolve without scarring. After a few years the disease may spontaneously disappear (Fitzpatrick et al, 1992).

Numerous pathophysiological mechanisms have been suggested for rosacea. To date, none have been definitively established. Bacterial infection, specifically *Staphylococcus aureus,* has been linked to 60% of patients with rosacea; however, cultures of many patients are sterile. Climatic exposure to sun, wind, heat, or cold might exacerbate lesions, but evidence is not absolutely convincing.

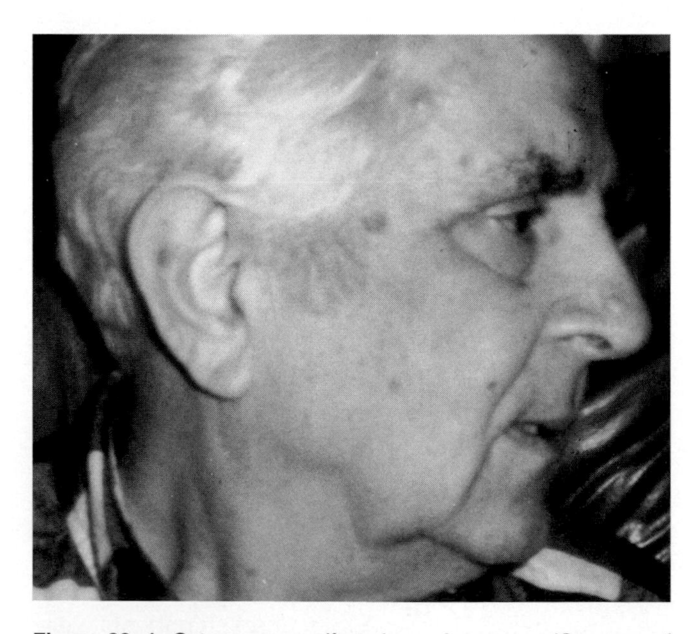

Figure 39–1. Cutaneous manifestations of rosacea. *(Courtesy of Dr. Diane T. Adamczyk.)*

TABLE 39–1. SYSTEMIC MANIFESTATIONS OF ROSACEA

Erythema
Flushing warmth
Pustules
Acneform papules
Telangiectatic vessels
Sebaceous gland hypertrophy
Rhinophyma

Extensive research has studied the hypertrophic sebaceous glands of patients with rosacea to determine an origin for the disease. No clear consensus has evolved; fatty acids in meibomian gland secretions are being studied as a possible route of irritation and tear disruption to the ocular surface (Browning & Proia, 1986).

The role of the follicle mite *Demodex folliculorum* in rosacea has also been investigated for many years. Initially, the mites were believed to be quite common in rosacea patients, but current literature proposes that the mites have a relatively insignificant role, if any, in the pathogenesis of rosacea.

In an editorial, Mindel and Rosenberg (1997) considered the gram-negative bacterium *Helicobacter pylori* as an underlying causative factor in both forms of rosacea. Residing in the stomach, *H. pylori* initiates a chain of reactions leading to an increase in the peptide hormone gastrin, which subsequently produces vasodilation of the skin and other ocular manifestations. Although there are several weaknesses in this theory, in the future antibiotic therapy directed towards *H. pylori* may be a component of the management plan.

In summary, multiple stimuli cause normal vessels to dilate and flush, leading to eythematous rosacea. The relase of inflammatory mediators like cytokines leads to telangiectasia and rhinophyma. Continued exacerbation of this cycle utimately leads to the classical clinical picture (Katz, 1998).

Ocular

The ocular manifestations in rosacea are numerous and nonspecific (Table 39–2). Except for a rare uveitis, they all appear on the ocular surface or eyelids. Commonly seen signs include blepharitis, meibomianitis, hordeola, chalazia, conjunctival hyperemia, punctate keratitis, epithelial erosions, and corneal vascularization leading to thinning or perforation.

Patients will typically present with complaints of foreign-body sensation, pain, or burning. The symptoms may be constant or intermittent, but are generally bilateral. They may be more marked than clinical findings would suggest. Other initial complaints include

TABLE 39–2. OCULAR MANIFESTATIONS OF ROSACEA

Symptoms
Foreign-body sensation
Pain, irritation
Burning
Photophobia
Redness
Epiphora
Decreased vision
Signs
Blepharitis
Meibomianitis
Disrupted tear film
Hordeola
Chalazia
Conjunctival hyperemia
Punctate keratitis
Epithelial erosions
Corneal vascularization
Corneal thinning, ulceration, perforation
Uveitis

red eyes, decreased vision, chalazia, and epiphora (Jenkins et al, 1979).

Blepharitis and meibomianitis are virtually universal findings in ocular rosacea patients. Inspissation of meibomian gland secretions will be noted during clinical examination. Zengin and colleagues (1995) reported on meibomian gland dysfunction in rosacea patients with and without ocular signs. They found abnormal meibomian gland secretions (plugging, volume, thickness) along with decreased production (Schirmer I) and decreased breakup time in patients with ocular rosacea.

Hordeola and chalazia are highly prevalent within the rosacea population. Lempert and co-workers (1979) found 64% of patients scheduled for chalazia excision to have clinically significant rosacea. Periorbital edema is a less common feature of rosacea, but may be seen as the initial presenting feature. Three patients with progressive, nonpruritic eyelid edema were found to have rosacea upon careful examination (Chen & Crosby, 1997). Unfortunately, these patients did not respond well to oral tetracycline therapy.

The tear film in rosacea patients has also been an area of study. Clinical examination reveals a significant disturbance to the ocular surface's protective layer. There is an excessive accumulation of debris, decreased tear breakup time (TBUT), and an oily, foamy consistency to the tears similar to that seen with seborrheic blepharitis (McCulley & Sciallis, 1977). Barton and colleagues (1997) investigated tear film composition in ocular rosacea patients in order to determine the underlying cause of ocular irritation. They found elevated concentrations of interleukin-1α in these patients. Interleukin-1α is known to be a fundamental proinflammatory cytokine, and thus could be a significant risk factor in the progression of ocular surface disease in ocular rosacea. This study also proposed that the elevated levels arise from reduced tear film turnover.

Controversy still exists as to whether or not there is an alteration in the tear film pH. Abelson and coworkers (1980) found an alkaline shift; Jaros and Coles (1983) found an acidic shift, whereas Browning (1985) did not find any diagnostically useful difference between rosacea patients and normal controls. Different methods of determining the tear film pH possibly may explain these conflicting results.

Many patients with ocular rosacea may also have a coexisting keratoconjunctivitis sicca. Lemp et al (1984) found almost 40% of rosacea patients with ocular manifestations to have a decreased Schirmer test. They concluded that this significantly contributed to patient symptomatology.

Corneal complications in ocular rosacea begin with a superficial punctate keratitis along the inferior two thirds of the cornea. The keratitis progresses with a dramatic peripheral vascularization, and subepithelial infiltrates central to the vessels may subsequently develop. Gross ulceration or infiltrate resolution causes further thinning of the cornea, which may ultimately lead to frank perforation of the cornea (Brown & Shahinian, 1978). Corneal erosions may develop at any time during active corneal disease. Other less common ocular findings include entropion, episcleritis, and iritis.

There are very few histologic or immunopathologic studies of ocular rosacea that help identify a pathophysiologic mechanism. Hoang-Xaun and associates (1990) studied the conjunctiva in patients with ocular rosacea. They found an overall increase of inflammatory cells, especially T helper/inducer cells, macrophages, and antigen-presenting cells. This finding suggests a type IV hypersensitivity reaction that accounts for conjunctival inflammation. An unidentified antigen may be reaching the globe through the meibomian gland secretions via the tear film. Therefore, ocular manifestations may be an exaggerated inflammatory response to this antigen and other toxic products.

DIAGNOSIS

Systemic and Ocular

No strict criteria have been established for the diagnosis of rosacea or ocular rosacea. Diagnosis is based on a clinical impression following identification of characteristic cutaneous lesions.

For rosacea, this would include erythema, telangiectasia, papules, pustules, and rhinophyma. The ocular findings in rosacea are too nonspecific to make a definitive diagnosis; thus, the facial features must be identified to confirm the diagnosis.

> The cutaneous signs of rosacea are often overlooked by eyecare practitioners when evaluating patients with chronic ocular irritation. Identifying these signs can cinch the diagnosis and thus allow the appropriate treatment to be initiated.

This presents a problem for the 20% of patients who develop ocular manifestations prior to facial. These patients often go undiagnosed, as specific testing for ocular rosacea has not been formulated. As previously discussed, tear pH results remain controversial. Browning and Proia (1986) have suggested a point-scale system for each clinical sign or symptom associated with ocular rosacea. Patients can be categorized as tentative, probable, or certain, depending on their total points.

Generally, if clinical suspicion is high, then initiation of proper therapy is warranted because the side effects are minimal. It is helpful to remember that symptoms are often more severe than the clinical appearance would suggest.

In conjunction with subjective assessments, practitioners may also employ a combination of objective tests that evaluate the tear film. Xeroscopy (a noninvasive measure of tear film stability), breakup time, fluorescein staining, rose bengal staining, fluorescein clearance testing, and Schirmer testing can all be used. In general the findings will point toward tear film irregularity and distortion, reduced TBUT, increased staining and fluorescein retention, and decreased aqueous production (Pflugfelder et al, 1998). Because these findings are seen in many other ocular surface disorders, they must be correlated with the appropriate signs and symptoms of ocular rosacea.

The differential diagnosis for rosacea (Table 39–3) includes seborrheic dermatitis, lupus erythematosus, cutaneous tuberous sclerosis, and acne vulgaris (teenage acne). It is differentiated from acne vulgaris by the lack of comedones (whiteheads), older age of the patient, and confinement of lesions to the face. In addition, the pustules of rosacea will resolve without scarring (Lempert et al, 1979).

TABLE 39–3. DIFFERENTIAL DIAGNOSIS OF ROSACEA

Systemic
Menopause
Essential telangiectasia
Contact dermatitis
Systemic lupus erythematosus
Seborrheic dermatosis
Acne vulgaris
Basal cell carcinomas (rhinophyma)
Ocular
Dry eye syndrome
Meibomian gland dysfunction
Seborrheic blepharitis
Chronic conjunctivitis
Cicatrizing conjunctivitis (pemphigoid)
Corneal ulcer
Recurrent epithelial erosion
Peripheral corneal neovascularization
Recurrent chalazia
Episcleritis

TREATMENT AND MANAGEMENT

Systemic

The treatment of choice for cutaneous lesions in rosacea is oral antibiotics (Table 39–4). Tetracycline 250 mg qid for 4 to 6 weeks and then tapered to a level that controls active flare-ups is the most widely prescribed medication. Within 3 to 6 weeks a dramatic improvement is noted in about 80% of patients. Some patients may be able to discontinue the drug, whereas others require a low maintenance dosage. Other prescribed antibiotics include ampicillin, erythromycin, and metronidazole. Tetracycline therapy does not improve the cutaneous erythema.

TABLE 39–4. TREATMENT AND MANAGEMENT OF ROSACEA

Systemic
Tetracycline 250 mg qid for 4–6 weeks
Doxycyline 100 mg qd for 4–6 weeks
Clarithromycin 250 mg bid for 2–4 weeks
Topical metronidazole gel 0.75%
Dietary restriction of alcohol and spicy foods
Isotretinoin
Dermabrasion
Carbon dioxide laser therapy
Ocular
The above plus:
Eyelid hygiene
Artificial tears
Topical antibiotics
Low-dose topical steroids
Keratoplasty

Abbreviations: bid, twice a day; qd, every day; qid, four times daily.

The long-acting tetracycline semisynthetic derivatives, doxycycline (Vibramycin) and minocycline (Minocin), also have proven effectiveness in the therapy of rosacea. They have the benefit of reduced administration and improved absorption with ingestion of dairy products. However, they are more costly for the patient. The contraindications and side effects of tetracycline therapy and its derivatives should be recognized by the practitioner.

An explanation for the therapeutic efficacy of tetracycline has been extensively researched. Current theories suggest a combination of bacterial eradication and decreased free fatty acid concentration in sebaceous gland secretions.

Clarithromycin has also been used in the treatment of rosacea. It offers significantly fewer side effects as compared to tetracycline and its derivatives. In a clinical trial patients demonstrated a positive response in 6 weeks (Torresani, 1997). Although it has not been clearly established, clarithromycin may work by reducing *H. pylori* levels, which can contribute to cutaneous/ocular rosacea.

Metronidazole has been utilized both as an oral and more recently as a topical agent in the therapy of rosacea. It is a synthetic derivative of nitroimidazole and has antibacterial, antiprotozoal, antihelminthic, and even some inhibitory influences on the immune system (anti-inflammatory). Oral dosages of 200 mg bid were found to be superior to placebo in the treatment of rosacea. In general, this medication is reserved for those patients who do not respond to the tetracyclines. Greater use of oral metronidazole is limited by concerns over toxicity with long-term use.

Topical metronidazole gel (MetroGel 0.75%) has become a very popular medication in rosacea management. Its usefulness has been well documented in several clinical trials (Aronson et al, 1987; Lowe et al, 1989; Nielsen, 1988). This safe and effective topical drug has no serious side effects or allergic reactions. Applied twice daily, its greatest actions are against the papules, pustules, and erythema of rosacea. It is not helpful for the telangiectasia. In a 6-month study of patients put on a maintenance dose of MetroGel (without concomitant oral antibiotics), only 23% experienced relapses of cutaneous signs, as compared to 42% of patients using placebo (Dahl et al, 1998). The mechanism of action for topical metronidazole gel is thought to be immunologic and anti-inflammatory and not antimicrobial (Schmadel & McEvoy, 1990).

The papules and pustules of rosacea patients with advanced cutaneous disease will respond well to a combination of topical and oral antibiotics. A common combination is 1000 mg/day of tetracycline with topical metronidazole, tapering the tetracycline as the condition improves.

In persistent and severe cases of ocular rosacea resistant to antibiotics, Kligman (1997) recommends low-dose isotretinoin (Accutane). Significant improvement is noted over 2 to 3 months, following which the dose is tapered.

Dietary restriction of alcohol, spicy foods, and hot beverages may help to improve skin lesions. These items are vasodilative, and clinical experience has shown that eliminating them can help improve cosmetic appearance. Stress reduction has also been advocated. Topical antibiotics or benzoyl peroxide are not beneficial to the rosacea patient.

Isotretinoin is used as adjunctive therapy with oral tetracyclines for patients with rhinophyma (Singer, 1998). For severe rhinophyma, more aggressive surgical treatment may be warranted. Dermabrasion, surgical reduction, and carbon dioxide laser therapy for hypertrophic sebaceous glands have been implemented for rosacea patients with persistent lesions. The CO_2 laser carbonizes superficial tissue, allowing it to be shaved off with a scalpel.

Ocular

Therapy for ocular manifestations of rosacea is not significantly different than treatment for its facial manifestations (Table 39–4). Tetracycline at similar dosages (250 mg qid for 4 to 6 weeks) has demonstrated its effectiveness throughout the literature. Frucht-Perry and associates (1989) investigated the use of doxycycline in ocular rosacea. Fourteen of their 16 patients did very well with a dosage of 100 mg qd for 4 to 6 weeks. One patient was switched to tetracycline because of ineffectiveness, and one patient failed to improve with either medication.

Concomitant lid hygiene therapy is recommended for all patients with ocular rosacea. Conventional combinations of dilute shampoo lid scrubs, warm compresses, and lid massage can help eliminate blepharitis, return meibomian gland secretions to normal, and decrease the incidence of hordeola and chalazia. Zengin and colleagues (1995) found that regular meibomian gland expression did not have a beneficial effect on the the tear film, whereas tetracycline therapy did improve tear breakup times. However, neither treatment improved aqueous tear production.

In a controlled study, the effects of topical metronidazole gel applied to the eyelid were compared to patients who just performed lid hygiene. Although both groups showed some improvement, 9 of 10 patients improved in the MetroGel group. Patients were instructed to apply the gel to a closed eyelid margin, being careful not to get gel on the ocular surface. There were no reports of ocular side effects during the 12-week treatment period. However, MetroGel has not been approved by the FDA for ophthalmic use (Barnhorst et al, 1996).

Patients with corneal involvement require careful monitoring because of the heightened risk for corneal ulceration and secondary infection. Systemic tetracycline is the primary therapeutic measure to thwart corneal complications. Patients should demonstrate improvement within 2 to 6 weeks of initiating therapy.

In treating 39 patients with cutaneous and ocular rosacea with 100 mg of doxycycline daily for 12 weeks, Quarterman and associates (1997) noted significant improvement in ocular signs and symptoms. This included erythema, telangiectasia, bulbar injection, papillary hypertrophy, and punctate epithelial erosions. In these patients the mean TBUT improved from 5.7 to 10.8 seconds. However, meibomian gland dysfunction showed only minimal improvement. Many of the cicatricial changes associated with chronic ocular rosacea will not be reversed with antibiotic therapy.

Topical antibiotics can be added prophylactically to patients with keratitis. Artificial tear preparations will provide symptomatic relief for patients as well as supplementing a deficient tear film in patients with coexisting dry eye. Topical steroids can be used for a short period of time (1 to 2 weeks) for iritis, peripheral keratitis, and episcleritis until the tetracycline takes affect. Low-dose steroids must be used because high concentrations may result in corneal melting.

For patients who proceed to develop corneal ulcerations and perforations, surgical management, either keratoplasty or conjunctival flaps, may be required.

CONCLUSION

Rosacea is a chronic, dermatologic disease of unknown etiology. It is characterized by recurrent episodes of inflammatory papules, facial erythema, and telangiectasias of the face. Potentially devastating visual complications may arise from the common ocular complications that are seen in this disease.

Oral antibiotics are the mainstay of treatment and work quite well for both the facial and ocular components of rosacea. Newer topical medications have also been proven to be beneficial. Patients with significant cutaneous involvement warrant a dermatology referral for more intensive therapy, including surgical treatment options. Patients should be educated that they may require long-term maintenance therapy to prevent bouts of reactivation.

Eyecare providers should remember that rosacea is often underdiagnosed because of overlooking the subtle facial features in patients who present with ocular signs and symptoms. Older patients who present with blepharitis, meibomianitis, and chalazia, especially if chronic or recurrent, should be carefully evaluated for rosacea.

REFERENCES

Abelson MB, Sadun AA, Udell IJ, Weston JH. Alkaline tear pH in ocular rosacea. *Am J Ophthalmol.* 1980;90:866–869.

Akpek EK, Merchant A, Pinar V, Foster CS. Ocular rosacea: Patient characteristics and follow-up. *Ophthalmology.* 1997;104:1863–1867.

Aronson IK, Rumsfield JA, West DP, et al. Evaluation of topical metronidazole gel in acne rosacea. *Drug Intell Clin Pharm.* 1987;21:346–351.

Barnhorst DA, Foster JA, Chern KC, et al. The efficacy of topical metronidazole in the treatment of ocular rosacea. *Ophthalmology.* 1996;103:1880–1883.

Barton K, Monroy DC, Nava A, et al. Inflammatory cytokines in the tears of patients with ocular rosacea. *Ophthalmology.* 1997;104:1868–1874.

Borrie P. Rosacea with special reference to its ocular manifestations. *Br J Dermatol.* 1953;55:458–463.

Brown SI, Shahinian L Jr. Diagnosis and management of ocular rosacea. *Ophthalmology.* 1978;85:779–786.

Browning DJ. Tear studies in ocular rosacea. *Am J Ophthalmol.* 1985;99:530–533.

Browning DJ, Proia AD. Ocular rosacea. *Surv Ophthalmol.* 1986;31:145–158.

Browning DJ, Rosenwasser G, Lugo M. Ocular rosacea in blacks. *Am J Ophthalmol.* 1986;101:441–444.

Chen DM, Crosby DL. Periorbital edema as an initial presentation of rosacea. *J Am Acad Dermatol.* 1997;37:346–348.

Dahl MV, Katz I, Krueger GG, et al. Topical metronidazole maintains remissions of rosacea. *Arch Dermatol.* 1998;134:679–683.

Fitzpatrick TB, Johnson RA, Polano MK, et al. *Color Atlas and Synopsis of Clinical Dermatology.* 2nd ed. New York: McGraw-Hill; 1992:10–11.

Frucht-Perry J, Chayet AS, Feldman ST, et al. The effect of doxycycline on ocular rosacea. *Am J Ophthalmol.* 1989;107:434–435.

Hoang-Xuan T, Rodrigyez A, Zalitas MM, et al. Ocular rosacea. *Ophthalmology.* 1990;97:1468–1475.

Jaros PA, Coles WH. Ocular surface pH in rosacea. *CLAO J.* 1983;9:333.

Jenkins MS, Bown SI, Lempert SL, Weinberg RJ. Ocular rosacea. *Am J Ophthalmol.* 1979;88:618–622.

Katz AM. Rosacea: Epidemiology and pathogenesis. *J Cutan Med Surg.* 1998;2(suppl 4):5–10.

Kligman AM. Ocular rosacea: Current concepts and therapy. *Arch Dermatol.* 1997;133:89–90.

Lemp MA, Mahmood MM, Weiler HH. Association of rosacea and keratoconjunctivitis sicca. *Arch Ophthalmol.* 1984;102:556–557.

Lempert SL, Jenkins MS, Brown SI. Chalazia and rosacea. *Arch Ophthalmol.* 1979;97:1652–1653.

Loss RJ Jr. Common dermatoses. In: Noble J, ed. *Textbook of General Medicine and Primary Care.* Boston: Little, Brown; 1987:638.

Lowe NJ, Henderson T, Millikan LE, et al. Topical metronidazole for severe and recalcitrant rosacea: A prospective open trial. *Cutis.* 1989;43:283–286.

McCulley JP, Sciallis GF. Meibomian keratoconjunctivitis. *Am J Ophthalmol.* 1977;84:788–793.

Mindel JS, Rosenberg EW. Is *Helicobacter pylori* of interest to ophthalmologists? *Ophthalmology.* 1997;104:1729–1730.

Nielsen PG. Metronidazole treatment in rosacea. *Int J Dermatol.* 1988;27:1–5.

Nielsen PG: Treatment of rosacea with 1% metronidazole cream. A double blind study. *Br J Dermatol.* 1983;108:327–332.

Pflugfelder SC, Tseng SCG, Sanabria O, et al. Evaluation of subjective assessments and objective diagnostic tests for diagnosing tear-film disorders known to cause ocular irritation. *Cornea.* 1998;17:38–56.

Quarterman MJ, Johnson DW, Abele DC, et al. Ocular rosacea: Signs, symptoms, and tear studies before and after treatment with doxycycline. *Arch Dermatol.* 1997;133:49–54.

Rosen T, Stone MS. Acne rosacea in blacks. *J Am Acad Dermatol.* 1987;17:70–73.

Salaman SSM. Tetracyclines in ophthalmology. *Surv Ophthalmol.* 1985;29:265–275.

Schmadel LK, McEvoy GK. Topical metronidazole: A new therapy for rosacea. *Clin Pharm.* 1990;9:94–101.

Singer MI. Drug therapy of rosacea: A problem-directed approach. *J Cutan Med Surg.* 1998;2(suppl 4):20–23.

Torresani C, Pavesi A, Manara GC. Clinical trial on clarithromycin versus cloxycycline in the treatment of rosacea. *Int J Dermatol.* 1997;36:938–946.

Zengin N, Tol H, Gunduz K, et al. Meibomian gland dysfunction and tear film abnormalities in rosacea. *Cornea.* 1995;14:144–146.

Chapter 40

CICATRICIAL PEMPHIGOID

Debra Bezan

Cicatricial pemphigoid is a progressive bullous (blister-forming) disease affecting the skin and mucous membranes. Cutaneous involvement occurs in only about 25% of cases, while ocular tissue involvement occurs in approximately 75 to 85% of cases and may be the initial sign of the disease.

EPIDEMIOLOGY

Cicatricial pemphigoid is a relatively rare disorder, with an estimated prevalence in the general population ranging from 1 in 10,000 to 1 in 60,000. It may occur in young adults, but is more common in older adults, with an average age of onset between 55 and 70 years. Cicatricial pemphigoid affects women about 1.7 times more often than men. Interestingly, 14 to 32% of cicatricial pemphigoid patients also have a history of ocular hypertension or glaucoma.

PATHOPHYSIOLOGY/DISEASE PROCESS

Systemic

The etiology of cicatricial pemphigoid is unknown, although it is generally thought to be a type II autoimmune disorder with the development of antibodies to components of the epithelial basement membrane. These antibodies then fix complement and ultimately lead to blister formation. Some cases appear to be related to use of topical drugs, including idoxuridine, timolol, epinephrine, dipivefrin, pilocarpine, demecarium, and echothiophate iodide. There have also been a few cases reported of cicatricial pemphigoid following an episode of erythema multiforme major (Stevens-Johnson syndrome).

There appears to be a genetic predisposition for developing cicatricial pemphigoid because there are some HLA subtypes that are associated with cicatricial pemphigoid, including B12, DR4, DR5, DQw3, DQB1, A2, B8, B35, and B49. It has been hypothesized that the drugs mentioned above may trigger cicatricial pemphigoid in genetically susceptible patients.

Subepidermal blister formation is the characteristic histologic finding in cicatricial pemphigoid. The histopathologic changes that occur are thought to be due to the binding of immunoglobulins (especially IgG) and complement to the basement membranes of skin and mucosa. The early or acute phases are characterized by subepithelial infiltration of T lymphocytes, macrophages, B cells, and plasma cells. Chronic phases produce some of the same inflammatory cells but also more neutrophils.

Bullous lesions of the oral mucosa are the most common systemic manifestation (Table 40–1). Other mucous membranes affected include those of the conjunctiva, nose, pharynx, larynx, esophagus, urethra, anus, and vagina. Complications associated with scar-

TABLE 40–1. SYSTEMIC MANIFESTATIONS OF CICATRICIAL PEMPHIGOID

- Triggered by certain drugs in some cases
- Bullous lesions of oral and other mucous membranes are common
- Occasional bullous skin lesions
- Progressive course

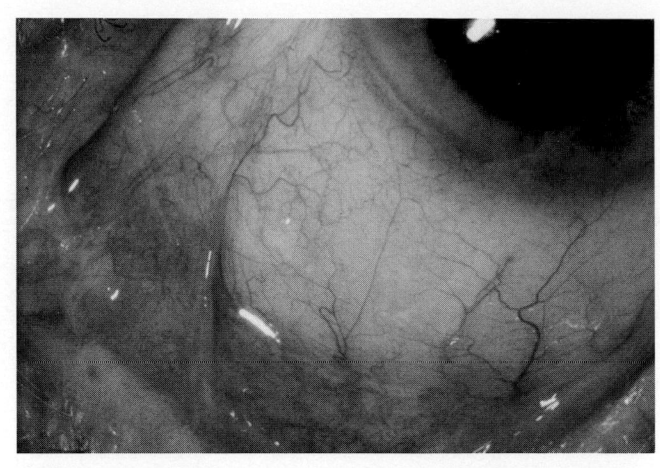

A

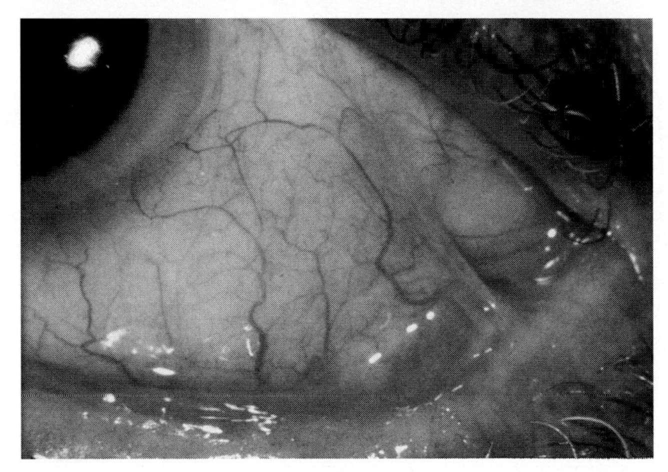

B

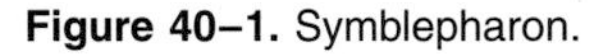

Figure 40–1. Symblepharon.

ring of the respiratory or gastrointestinal structures may result in death.

Skin lesions are less common than mucosal lesions. These fall into two categories: (1) nonscarring, recurrent vesiculobullous lesions, and (2) scarring localized plaques with overlying bullae.

> Cicatricial pemphigoid is a progressive autoimmune disorder that causes conjunctival scarring and severe dry eye.

Ocular

The ocular manifestations (Table 40–2) of cicatricial pemphigoid are bilateral though not necessarily symmetric. The conjunctiva is the most commonly affected ocular tissue and is involved in approximately two thirds of cases. Two systems have been developed to classify conjunctival changes that occur with cicatricial pemphigoid. The system developed by Foster and associates (1986) has the following four stages: (1) chronic conjunctivitis, rose bengal staining of the conjunctival epithelium, mucoid discharge, and subepithelial fibrosis; (2) conjunctival shrinkage and shortening of the inferior fornix; (3) development of symblepharon (Figure 40–1) along with other changes such as entropion, trichiasis, tear insufficiency, keratopathy, and corneal vascularization; and (4) severe dry eye, ocular surface keratinization, and ankyloblepharon (end stage). The system developed by Mondino and Brown (1981) grades cicatricial pemphigoid on a scale of 0 to 4 based on the percentage of visible conjunctival shrinkage: (0) no conjunctival shrinkage, (1) less than 25% shrinkage, (2) 25 to 50% shrinkage, (3) approximately 75% shrinkage, and (4) end stage with fornix obliteration.

TABLE 40–2. OCULAR MANIFESTATIONS OF CICATRICIAL PEMPHIGOID

- Chronic conjunctivitis
- Symblepharon
- Conjunctival shrinkage
- Entropion and trichiasis
- Corneal vascularization
- Severe dry eye
- Ocular surface keratinization
- Ankyloblepharon
- Restricted motility

The immunopathologic processes occurring in cicatricial pemphigoid result in hyperproliferation and poor differentiation of the conjunctival epithelial cells. There are also decreased numbers of mucin-producing goblet cells. These cellular changes cause squamous metaplasia of the epithelial cells resulting in abnormal keratinization.

These pathological changes also affect the tear film. The decreased numbers of conjunctival goblet cells result in less mucin in the tears. Conjunctival scarring blocks the ducts of the main and accessory lacrimal glands, which results in a decreased aqueous component of the tear film. In addition, entropion and trichiasis secondary to scarring cause faulty tear-spreading action.

Poor tear film quality, quantity, and spreading action result in corneal desiccation. Occasionally corneal bullae will form and erupt. These factors combined with mechanical trauma from cicatricial lid anomalies can cause significant epithelial defects and recurrent erosions. Changes in the tear film and mechanical trauma make the cornea more susceptible to secondary infection and ulceration. All of these factors may lead to corneal neovascularization, scarring, and loss of vision that can lead to legal blindness.

DIAGNOSIS

The diagnosis of cicatricial pemphigoid is based on history, clinical signs, and the progressive course of the disease (Table 40–3). Currently there are no laboratory tests available that are specific for cicatricial pemphigoid, although tissue biopsy and impression cytology may be used to confirm the diagnosis in many cases (Table 40–4). Immunoperoxidase techniques are more sensitive than immunofluorescent techniques for analyzing biopsy specimens.

Systemic

The cutaneous manifestations of cicatricial pemphigoid must be differentiated from other bullous skin diseases such as bullous pemphigoid or pemphigus vulgaris (Table 40–5).

Ocular

Ocular manifestations must be differentially diagnosed from other conditions that can demonstrate similar signs and symptoms. For example, symblepharon may be associated with Sjögren syndrome, sarcoidosis, atopic keratoconjunctivitis, or erythema multiforme as well as cicatricial pemphigoid. Conjunctival scarring can be a result of chemical (especially alkali) burns, trauma, or infection by *Chlamydia trachomatis,* adenovirus 8 and 19, herpes simplex, *Corynebacterium diphtheriae,* or β-hemolytic streptococcus. In addition to cicatricial pemphigoid, conjunctival shrinkage can be associated with erythema multiforme, scleroderma (progressive systemic sclerosis), or topical drug use.

TABLE 40–3. DIAGNOSTIC CRITERIA FOR CICATRICIAL PEMPHIGOID

- History
- Systemic signs including bullous lesions of skin and mucous membranes
- Ocular signs including conjunctivitis, conjunctival scarring (symblepharon), dry eyes, and corneal keratinization
- Progressive course
- Diagnostic tests are not specific but aid in confirming the diagnosis

TABLE 40–4. DIAGNOSTIC TESTING FOR CICATRICIAL PEMPHIGOID

- Tissue biopsy
- Impression cytology
- HLA testing

Note: Currently there are no diagnostic tests that are specific for cicatricial pemphigoid, but the above tests can add information useful in confirming the diagnosis.

TREATMENT AND MANAGEMENT

Systemic

The cutaneous lesions of cicatricial pemphigoid rarely need to be treated, as they tend to resolve spontaneously, often leaving atrophic scars (Table 40–6). Medical therapy for cicatricial pemphigoid centers around controlling the chronic inflammatory process involving the mucous membranes, and in particular trying to prevent sight-threatening changes in the ocular tissues. Corticosteroids and cytotoxic immunosuppressive drugs such as methotrexate, azathioprine, and cyclophosphamide have been used to control the inflammatory reaction in cicatricial pemphigoid with moderate success. Newer drugs that have shown promise in the treatment of cicatricial pemphigoid include oral dapsone and sulfapyridine and subconjunctival mitomycin-C.

TABLE 40–5. DIFFERENTIAL DIAGNOSIS OF CICATRICIAL PEMPHIGOID

Atopic keratoconjunctivitis
Chemical burn
Chronic use of topical ophthalmic pharmaceuticals
Erythema multiforme
Membranous or pseudomembranous conjunctivitis (bacterial or viral)
Sarcoidosis
Scleroderma
Sjögren syndrome
Trachoma

TABLE 40–6. TREATMENT AND MANAGEMENT OF CICATRICIAL PEMPHIGOID

- Systemic corticosteroids, immunosuppressives, dapsone and sulfapyridine to manage inflammation
- Lubricants, topical tretinoin, bandage lenses, and punctal occlusion to manage dry eye
- Surgical management of scarred tissues

Ocular

The signs and symptoms of dry eye are managed with ocular lubricants, moisture chambers, bandage contact lenses, and punctal occlusion. Topical tretinoin (vitamin A) therapy has been shown to be useful in reversing certain cases of squamous metaplasia. Tarsorrhaphy may be indicated for chronic corneal ulceration secondary to dry eye. Secondary infections may be managed with lid scrubs and topical and/or oral antibiotics. Topical and/or oral corticosteroids have been shown to be helpful in controlling the progression of cicatricial pemphigoid, but the ocular and systemic side effects from the dosages needed often render corticosteroids undesirable for long-term use.

When advanced cicatricial ocular changes have already occurred, surgical procedures may be performed to treat entropion, symblepharon, and ankyloblepharon. These procedures include tarsorrhaphy, allograft limbal transplantation, and amniotic membrane transplantation. Electrocautery or cryotherapy is useful in managing trichiasis. Penetrating keratoplasty has a low success rate in patients with cicatricial pemphigoid. If the cornea is severely scarred, a keratoprosthesis may be used to help the patient retain some usable vision.

CONCLUSION

Cicatricial pemphigoid is a progressive disease, presumably of autoimmune origin, that affects the skin and mucous membranes. The precise mechanism is not understood, but it is known that the use of certain topical glaucoma and antiviral medications is associated with the development of cicatricial pemphigoid in some cases.

Ocular manifestations include conjunctival inflammation, shrinkage, and scarring, entropion, trichiasis, dry eye, and corneal erosion, neovascularization, opacification, and restricted motilities. Management of this chronic, progressive disorder is often difficult. Strategies include using ocular lubricants, moisture chambers, and punctal occlusion for relief of dry eye symptoms, and using corticosteroids, cytotoxic immunosuppressive agents, or dapsone to control inflammation. In eyes with advanced scarring from cicatricial pemphigoid, surgical procedures may be needed to help the patient retain useful vision.

REFERENCES

Chan LS, Soong HK, Foster CS, et al. Ocular cicatricial pemphigoid occuring as a sequela of Stevens-Johnson syndrome. *JAMA.* 1991;266:1543–1546.

Donnenfeld ED, Perry HD, Wallerstein A, et al. Subconjunctival mitomycin C for the treatment of ocular cicatricial pemphigoid. *Ophthalmology.* 1999;106:72–79.

Elder MJ, Bernauer W. Cryotherapy for trichiasis in ocular cicatricial pemphigoid. *Br J Ophthalmol.* 1994;78:769–771.

Elder MJ, Leonard J, Dart JKG. Sulfapyridine—a new agent for the treatment of ocular cicatricial pemphigoid. *Br J Ophthalmol.* 1996;80:549–552.

Elder MJ, Lightman S. The immunological features and pathophysiology of ocular cicatricial pemphigoid. *Eye.* 1994;8:196–199.

Elder MJ, Lightman S, Dart JKG. Role of cyclophosphamide and high dose steroid in ocular cicatricial pemphigoid. *Br J Ophthalmol.* 1995;79:264–266.

Foster CS. Cicatricial pemphigoid. *Trans Am Ophthalmol Soc.* 1986;84:527–663.

Foster CS, Shaw CD, Wells PA. Scanning electron microscopy of conjunctival surfaces in patients with ocular cicatricial pemphigoid. *Am J Ophthalmol.* 1986;102:584–591.

Kristensen EB, Norn MS. Benign mucous membrane pemphigoid: Secretion of mucus and tears. *Acta Ophthalmol.* 1974;52:266–281.

Liesegang TJ. Conjunctival changes associated with glaucoma therapy: Implications for the external disease consultant and the treatment of glaucoma. Cornea. 1998; 17:574–583.

Louie TD. Ocular cicatricial pemphigoid: A case report. *J Am Optom Assoc.* 1998:69:153–160.

Mondino BJ. Cicatricial pemphigoid and erythema multiforme. *Ophthalmology.* 1990;97:939–952.

Mondino BJ, Brown SI. Ocular cicatricial pemphigoid. *Ophthalmology.* 1981;88:95–100.

Mondino BJ, Brown SI. Immunosuppressive therapy in ocular cicatricial pemphigoid. *Am J Ophthalmol.* 1983; 96:453–459.

Mondino BJ, Brown SI, Lempert S, Jenkins MS. The acute manifestations of ocular pemphigoid: Diagnosis and treatment. *Ophthalmology.* 1979;86:543–552.

Norn MS, Kristensen EB. Benign mucous membrane pemphigoid: Cytology. *Acta Ophthalmol.* 1974;52:282–290.

Ormerod LD, Fong LP, Foster CS. Corneal infection in mucosal scarring disorders and Sjögren's syndrome. *Am J Ophthalmol.* 1988;105:512–518.

Pouliquen Y, Patey A, Foster CS, et al. Drug induced cicatricial pemphigoid affecting the conjunctiva: Light and electron microscopic features. *Ophthalmology.* 1986;93:775–783.

Power WJ. Rodriguez A. Increasing the diagnostic yield of conjunctival biopsy in patients with suspected ocular cicatricial pemphigoid. *Ophthalmology.* 1995;102:1158–1163.
Sacks EH, Jakobiec FA Wieczorek R, et al. Immunophenotypical analysis of the inflammatory infiltrate in ocular cicatricial pemphigoid. Further evidence for a T-cell mediated disease. *Ophthalmology.* 1989;96:236–243.
Secchi AG, Tognon MS. Intraoperative mitomycin C in the treatment of cicatricial obliterations of conjunctival fornices. *Am J Ophthalmol.* 1996:122:728–730.
Smith RJ, Manche EE, Mondino BJ. Ocular cicatricial pemphigoid and ocular manifestations of pemphigus vulgaris. *Int Ophthalmol Clin.* 1997;37:63–75.
Tauber J, Melamed S, Foster CS. Glaucoma in patients with ocular cicatricial pemphigoid. *Ophthalmology.* 1989; 96:33–37.
Thoft RA, Friend J, Kinoshita S, et al. Ocular cicatricial pemphigoid associated with hyperproliferation of the conjunctival epithelium. *Am J Ophthalmol.* 1984;98:37–42.
Tsubota K, Satake Y, Ohyama M, et al. Surgical reconstruction of the ocular surface in advanced ocular cicatricial pemphigoid and Stevens-Johnson syndrome. *Am J Ophthalmol.* 1996;122:38–52.
Tugal-Tutkin I, Akova YA, Foster CS. Penetrating keratoplasty in cicatrizing conjunctival disease. *Ophthalmology.* 1995;102:576–585.

Chapter 41

ERYTHEMA MULTIFORME

Debra Bezan

Erythema multiforme (EM) is an acute, inflammatory condition of the skin and mucous membranes that is usually self-limiting. As the name multiforme implies, this condition takes on a number of forms. EM can be divided into two classifications: erythema multiforme minor (erythema multiforme of Hebra) and erythema multiforme major (Stevens–Johnson syndrome, ectodermosis erosiva pluriorificialis, dermatostomatitis, mucosal respiratory syndrome, or eruptive fever associated with stomatitis and ophthalmia).

EPIDEMIOLOGY

EM can occur at any age, but is most common in children and young adults. The peak occurrence is between the ages of 20 and 40. EM minor affects both sexes equally, while EM major affects males more often than females.

PATHOPHYSIOLOGY/DISEASE PROCESS

Systemic

The actual mechanism is unclear but there are a number of factors that can precipitate EM, including drugs, microbial infections, and other conditions including collagen vascular diseases, vaccinations, pregnancy, neoplasms, and radiation therapy. An estimated 58% of cases of EM appear to have a drug as the precipitating factor. There are over 40 different systemic drugs that have been implicated in triggering EM. These include sulfonamides, penicillins, salicylates, barbiturates, phenylbutazone, phenytoin, puroxicam, corticosteroids, allopurinol, arsenicals, and mercurials. Certain topical drugs of particular interest to eyecare practitioners have also been implicated, including sulfonamides, tropicamide, and proparacaine. In addition, cases of Stevens–Johnson syndrome have been reported secondary to oral acetazolamide and methazolamide.

Microbial infections have been determined to be the precipitating factor in approximately 15% of cases, with herpes simplex and *Mycoplasma pneumoniae* infections being the best documented. Some of the other triggering microbial infections and agents mentioned in the literature include infectious mononucleosis, psittacosis, influenza, adenovirus, coxsackievirus, *Yersinia,* tuberculosis, and histoplasmosis.

What causes such a diversity of agents to trigger EM is unknown; however, there appears to be a genetic predisposition for EM based on the association of certain HLA types such as HLA-Bw44 and HLA-DQB1*0601.

The pathophysiologic manifestations of EM are thought to be due to the deposition of immunoglobulins and complement at the dermal–epidermal junction and in the blood vessel walls of the dermis. EM is characterized by an infiltration of monocytes in the dermal layer. There is often a perivascular infiltration of lymphocytes and histiocytes around the dermal blood vessels. Subepithelial bullae form and the epidermal cells may become edematous or degenerate and become necrotic.

The systemic manifestations (Table 41–1) of EM may begin with prodromal flu-like symptoms including fever, headache, upper respiratory congestion, malaise, and prostration. These are more common with EM major than EM minor. The prodromal symptoms, if present, are followed by the characteristic dermal eruptions, which may be itchy or painful. The skin lesions are most commonly found on the extremities. Lesions occur more often on the trunk in EM major than EM minor. They begin as small red macules that usually develop into vesicles or bullae and may become necrotic (Figure 41–1). The lesions are termed "iris" or "target" lesions because they often have a characteristic "bull's-eye" appearance of a red center surrounded by a white zone surrounded by another red ring. Crops of skin lesions may continue to break out during the acute course of the disease.

EM minor primarily involves the skin with occasional limited involvement of the mucosa, while EM major (Stevens–Johnson syndrome) typically has both skin and mucous membrane involvement. It is more likely to affect the mouth, nose, conjunctiva, pharynx, larynx, trachea, esophagus, vagina, or urethra. Toxic epidermal necrolysis is a severe variation of EM major and characterized by widespread denuding of the epidermis.

The signs and symptoms of EM minor tend to last from 1 to 4 weeks, while EM major may last as long as 6 weeks. Both conditions usually resolve without extensive scarring of the skin, although focal areas of hyperpigmentation may remain. EM minor is more likely to recur than EM major.

Mortality is approximately 1% for EM minor but may range from 3 to 25% for EM major due to such complications as septicemia, pneumonitis, glomerulonephritis, myositis, and myocarditis.

TABLE 41–1. SYSTEMIC MANIFESTATIONS OF ERYTHEMA MULTIFORME

- Triggered by certain drugs and microbial infections
- Prodromal flu-like symptoms
- Bull's-eye skin lesions and mucous membrane involvement are common, especially in EM major (Stevens–Johnson syndrome)
- Self-limiting course

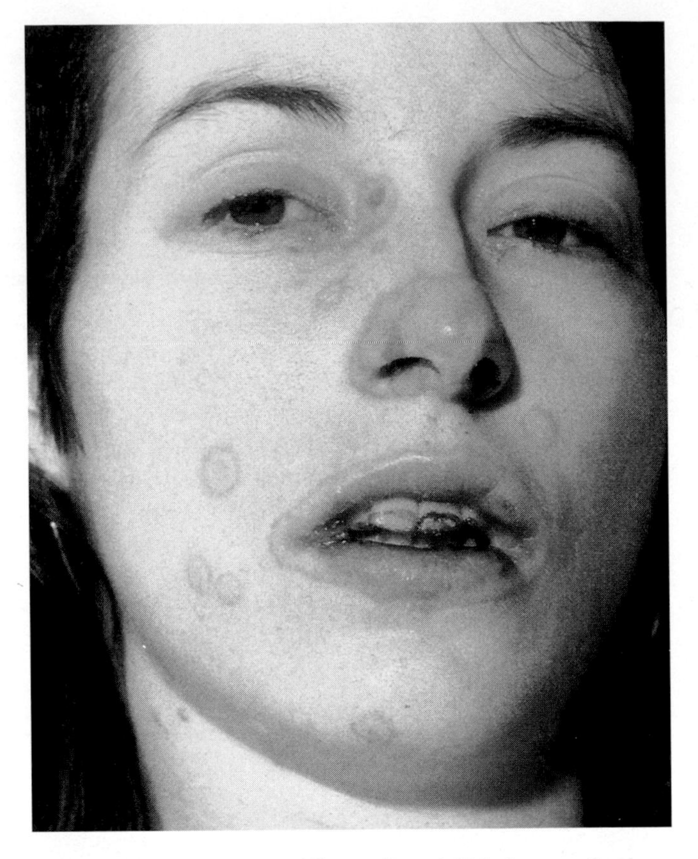

Figure 41–1. Erythema multiforme. Targetoid lesions on the face, with involvement of the oral mucous membranes and the eye (scleritis, periorbital edema, and bullae on the inner canthus). (*Reprinted with permission from Fitzpatrick TB, et al.* Color Atlas and Synopsis of Clinical Dermatology: Common and Serious Diseases. *2nd ed. New York: McGraw-Hill, 1992: 475.*)

Ocular

Ocular involvement is relatively common (Table 41–2) in EM major with a number of anterior segment tissues being affected (Figure 41–1). The lids are typically affected in the acute stage, which lasts 2 to 3 weeks. They may become edematous and hyperemic and show focal ulcerating or crusting lesions. In severe cases conjunctival scarring may result in late cicatricial entropion and trichiasis.

TABLE 41–2. OCULAR MANIFESTATIONS OF ERYTHEMA MULTIFORME

- Lid edema and focal ulcerations
- Conjunctival pseudomembranes or true membranes
- Occasional conjunctival and corneal scarring
- Occasional dry eye
- Occasional iritis or iridocyclitis

> Erythema multiforme, an acute inflammatory condition affecting mucous membranes, can be precipitated by ophthalmic pharmaceuticals including sulfonamides, tropicamide, proparacaine, acetazolamide, and methazolamide.

TABLE 41–4. DIAGNOSTIC TESTING FOR ERYTHEMA MULTIFORME

- Tissue biopsy
- HLA testing

Note: Currently there are no diagnostic tests that are specific for erythema multiforme but the above tests can add information useful in confirming the diagnosis.

The conjunctiva is one of the most common mucous membrane tissues to be affected by EM. Conjunctival involvement ranges from a mild transient injection to severe membrane formation and scarring. Pseudomembranes or true membranes are formed from an exudate composed of fibrin, neutrophils, other inflammatory cells, and necrotic epithelial cells. The development of later cicatricial complications of symblepharon and occasional ankyloblepharon depend on the severity of the inflammation. Episodes of conjunctival inflammation have been known to occur after EM major; however, recurrent bouts of EM major are less likely to involve the conjunctiva than the initial episode.

EM can cause a dry eye condition due to squamous metaplasia of the conjunctival epithelium and a decrease in the number of conjunctival goblet cells, resulting in poor mucin quantity and/or quality in the tear film. Scarring may also block the ducts of lacrimal glands, reducing tear production. If cicatricial entropion and trichiasis are present, the tears may not be spread properly across the ocular surface and further exacerbate a dry eye situation.

Poor tear-film quality, quantity, and spreading action can cause corneal and conjunctival desiccation. Mechanical trauma from lid abnormalities can also cause epithelial damage and make the cornea and conjunctiva more susceptible to secondary infection. Among the more serious infectious complications is corneal ulceration.

TABLE 41–3. DIAGNOSTIC CRITERIA FOR ERYTHEMA MULTIFORME

- History, especially for the previous use of pharmaceutical triggers
- Systemic signs including vesicular lesions of skin and/or mucous membranes
- Ocular signs including lid lesions, conjunctival inflammation and membrane formation, dry eyes, and occasional conjunctival scarring
- Self-limited course
- Diagnostic tests are not specific but aid in confirming the diagnosis

Although uncommon, iritis or iridocyclitis is another anterior segment manifestation of EM.

DIAGNOSIS

The diagnosis of EM is based on clinical signs and the natural history of the disease (Table 41–3). The presence of significant mucous membrane involvement is often used to differentiate EM major from EM minor. At present there are no specific laboratory tests that are useful in the diagnosis of EM (Table 41–4). However, a biopsy of the skin lesions has characteristic findings and helps confirm the diagnosis, although it will not identify the etiology.

Systemic

EM must be differentiated from other skin diseases (Table 41–5) with a similar appearance including urticarias, toxic erythemas, systemic lupus erythematosus, polyarteritis nodosa, bullous impetigo, pemphigus vulgaris, bullous pemphigoid, herpetic dermatitis, Behçet syndrome, and Reiter syndrome. A biopsy can help differentiate EM from these processes.

Ocular

EM must be differentially diagnosed from other conditions with similar ocular signs. Symblepharon, for example, may be associated with Sjögren syndrome, keratoconjunctivitis, sarcoidosis, or cicatricial pem-

TABLE 41–5. DIFFERENTIAL DIAGNOSIS OF ERYTHEMA MULTIFORME

- Behçet syndrome
- Bullous impetigo
- Bullous pemphigoid
- Herpetic dermatitis
- Pemphigus vulgaris
- Polyarteritis nodosa
- Reiter syndrome
- Systemic lupus erythematosus
- Toxic epidermal necrolysis (severe variant)
- Urticaria

phigoid in addition to EM. Conjunctival scarring similar to that seen in EM may be a result of chemical burns, trauma, trachoma, herpes simplex, diphtheria, or β-hemolytic streptococcus, and conjunctival shrinkage may be due to cicatricial pemphigoid, scleroderma, or topical drug use.

TREATMENT AND MANAGEMENT

Systemic

The treatment (Table 41–6) of EM involves identification and treatment of underlying factors such as *Mycoplasma pneumoniae* or *Mycobacterium tuberculosis,* if possible. If EM appears to be caused by drug use, the drug should be immediately discontinued.

Other therapies are primarily palliative or supportive. Skin lesions may be debrided, and topical and systemic antibiotics may be used to treat secondary infections. Topical and/or systemic corticosteroids may be used to control inflammation; however, there is evidence that they may prolong the course of the disease and increase the complication rate in some instances. In some severe cases (toxic epidermal necrolysis), fluid therapy may be needed to prevent systemic dehydration.

Ocular

Treatment of the ocular manifestations of EM includes the management of secondary dry eye with ocular lubricants, moisture chambers, bandage contact lenses, and punctal occlusion. Topical tretinoin may be helpful in reversing conjunctival squamous metaplasia by restoring normal cellular differentiation, and may also enhance goblet cell regeneration and mucin production. Stripping conjunctival membranes and frequent lysis of conjunctival adhesions with a glass rod may be of some benefit in preventing permanent scar formation. However, if cicatricial changes such as symblepharon and entropion do occur, surgical management may be indicated. Intraoperative injection of mitomycin-C may help prevent adhesion reformation. Electrocautery or cryotherapy may be used to treat secondary trichiasis. Tarsorrhaphy, allograft limbal transplantation, or amniotic membrane transplantation may be indicated for cases of chronic corneal ulceration due to dry eye.

TABLE 41–6. TREATMENT AND MANAGEMENT OF ERYTHEMA MULTIFORME

Systemic
- Treatment of underlying microbial infection if indicated
- Discontinue triggering drug if indicated
- Skin lesion debridement
- Topical and/or systemic antibiotics for secondary infection
- Topical and/or systemic corticosteroids to manage inflammation

Ocular
- Ocular lubrication, punctal occlusion
- Stripping of conjunctival membranes, lysis of conjunctival adhesions
- Topical tretinoin
- Surgical lid management

CONCLUSION

EM is a variable, self-limiting disorder that affects the skin and may also involve the mucous membranes. It can be divided into two subclassifications: EM minor and EM major (Stevens–Johnson syndrome). EM major is more likely to have ocular involvement than EM minor. Although the precise etiology is unclear, several factors are known to trigger EM, including certain systemic and topical pharmaceuticals and microbial infections. Management involves treatment of precipitating conditions, if possible, and palliative therapy for symptomatic relief. Treatment of ocular manifestations includes managing secondary dry eye and surgical repair of cicatricial conjunctival and lid anomalies.

REFERENCES

Anhalt GJ, Bahn CF, Diaz LA. Bullous diseases. *Int Ophthalmol Clin.* 1985;25:37–59.

Fitzpatrick TB, Johnson RA, Polano MK, et al. *Color Atlas and Synopsis of Clinical Dermatology: Common and Serious Diseases.* 2nd ed. New York: McGraw-Hill; 1992:474–477.

Flach AJ, Smith RS, Fraunfelder FT. Stevens–Johnson syndrome associated with methazolamide treatment reported in two Japanese women. *Ophthalmology.* 1995;102:1677–1680.

Foster CS, Fong LP, Azar D, Kenyon KR. Episodic conjunctival inflammation after Stevens–Johnson syndrome. *Ophthalmology.* 1988;95:453–462.

Genvert GI, Cohen EJ, Donnenfield ED, Blecher MH. Erythema multiforme after use of topical sulfacetamide. *Am J Ophthalmol.* 1985;99:465–468.

Hochman MA, Mayers M. Stevens–Johnson syndrome, epidermolysis bullosa, staphylococcal scalded skin syndrome, and dermatitis herpetiformis. *Int Ophthalmol Clin.* 1997;37:77–92.

Huff JC, Weston WL, Tonnesen MG. Erythema multiforme: A critical review of characteristics, diagnostic criteria and causes. *J Am Acad Dermatol.* 1983;8:763–775.

Mondino BJ. Cicatricial pemphigoid and erythema multiforme. *Ophthalmology.* 1990;97:939–952.

Nelson JD, Wright JC. Conjunctival goblet cell densities in ocular surface disease. *Arch Opthalmol.* 1984;102:1049–1051.

Ormerod LD, Fong LP, Foster CS. Corneal infection in mucosal scarring disorders and Sjögren's syndrome. *Am J Ophthalmol.* 1988;105:512–518.

Patz A. Ocular involvement in erythema multiforme. *Arch Ophthalmol.* 1950;43:244–256.

Power WJ, Ghoraishi M, Merayo–Lloves J, et al. Analysis of the acute ophthalmic manifestations of the erythema multiforme/Stevens–Johnson syndrome/toxic epidermal necrolysis disease spectrum. *Ophthalmology.* 1995;102:1669–1676.

Power WJ, Saidman SL, Zhang DS, et al. HLA typing in patients with ocular manifestations of Stevens–Johnson syndrome. *Ophthalmology.* 1996;103:1406–1409.

Rasmussen JE. Erythema multiforme in children: Response to treatment with systemic corticosteroids. *Br J Dermatol.* 1976;95:181–186.

Shelley WB. Herpes simplex virus as a cause of erythema multiforme. *JAMA.* 1967;201:153–156.

Soong HK, Martin NF, Wagoner MD, et al. Topical retinoid therapy for squamous metaplasia of various ocular surface disorders: A multicenter, placebo-controlled, double-masked study. *Ophthalmology.* 1988;95:1442–1446.

Tonnesen MG, Soter NA. Erythema multiforme. *J Am Acad Dermatol.* 1979;1:357–364.

Tsubota K, Satake Y, Ohyama M, et al. Surgical reconstruction of the ocular surface in advanced ocular cicatricial pemphigoid and Stevens–Johnson syndrome. *Am J Ophthalmol.* 1996;122:38–52.

Ward B, McCulley JP, Segal RJ. Dermatologic reaction in Stevens–Johnson syndrome after ophthalmic anesthesia with proparacaine hydrochloride. *Am J Ophthalmol.* 1978; 86:133–135.

Color Plates

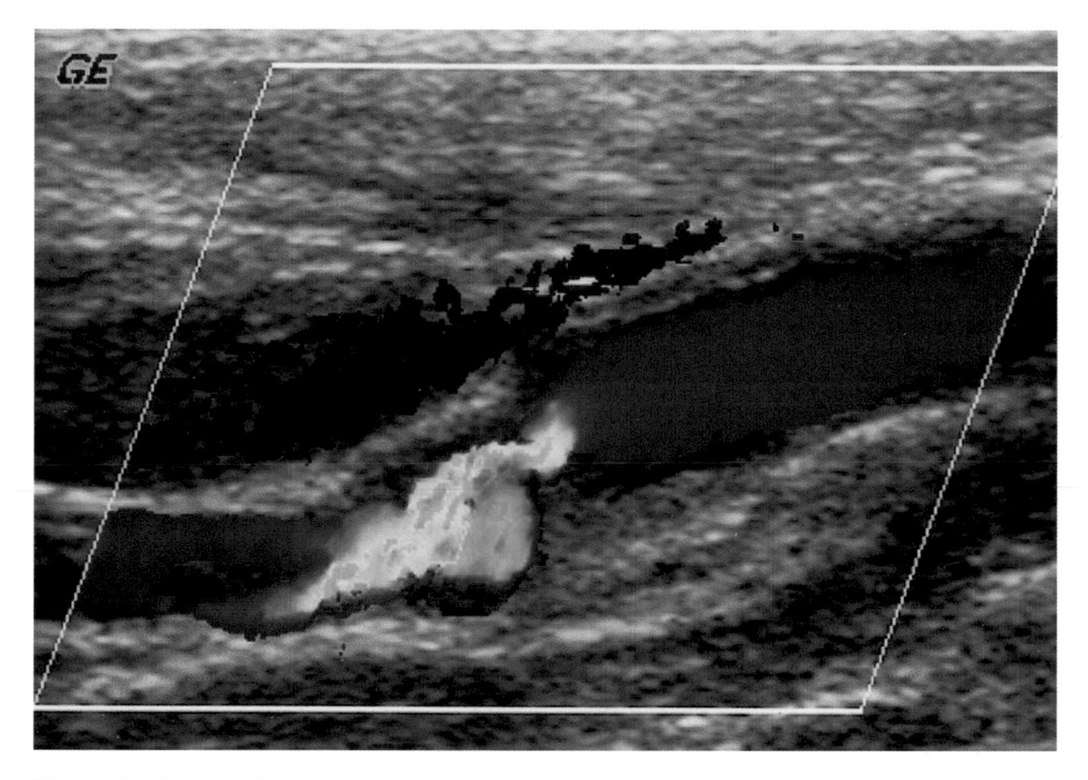

Plate 1. Duplex scan of an internal carotid artery plaque.

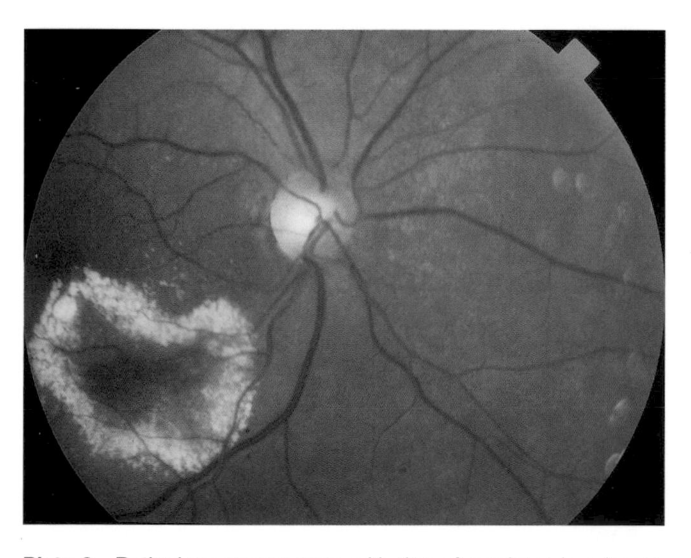

Plate 2. Retinal macroaneurysm with ring of exudates in a hypertensive patient.

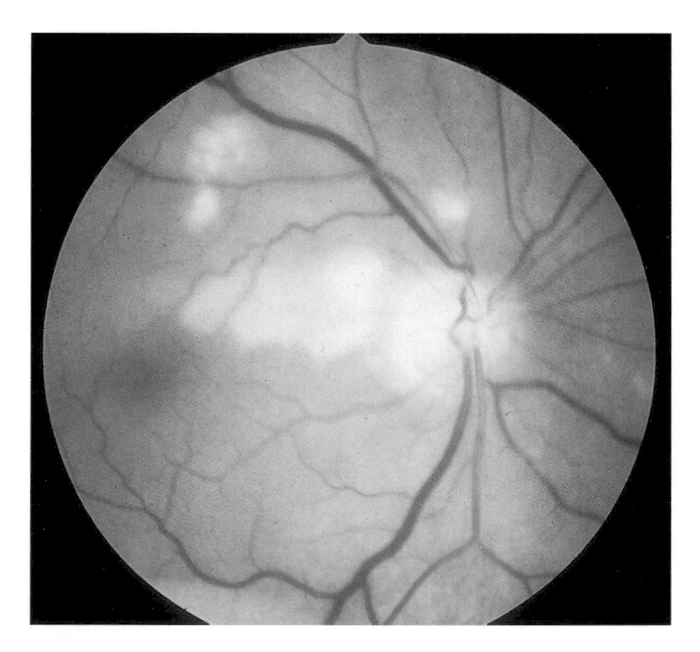

Plate 3. Cotton wool spots and ischemia due to a branch retinal artery occlusion secondary to cardiac valve disease.

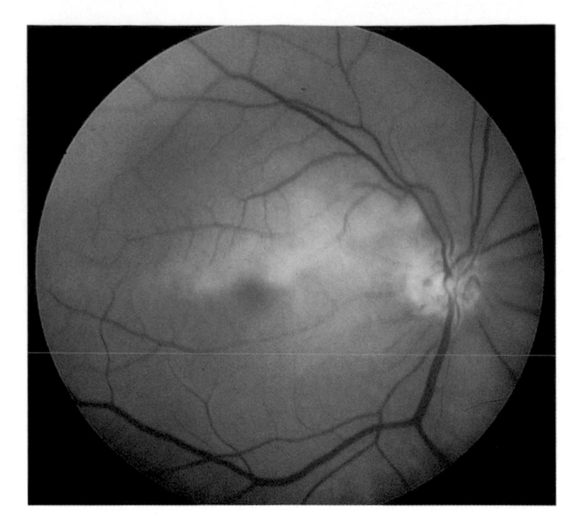

Plate 4. Combined disc edema and retinal ischemia secondary to nonarteritic anterior ischemic optic neuropathy and branch retinal artery occlusion in a patient with atrial fibrillation.

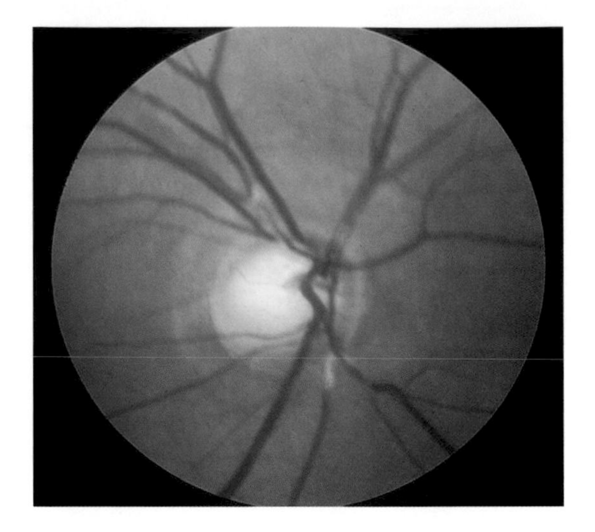

Plate 5. Multiple emboli adjacent to the optic nerve head in a patient with both calcific valvular disease and carotid artery disease.

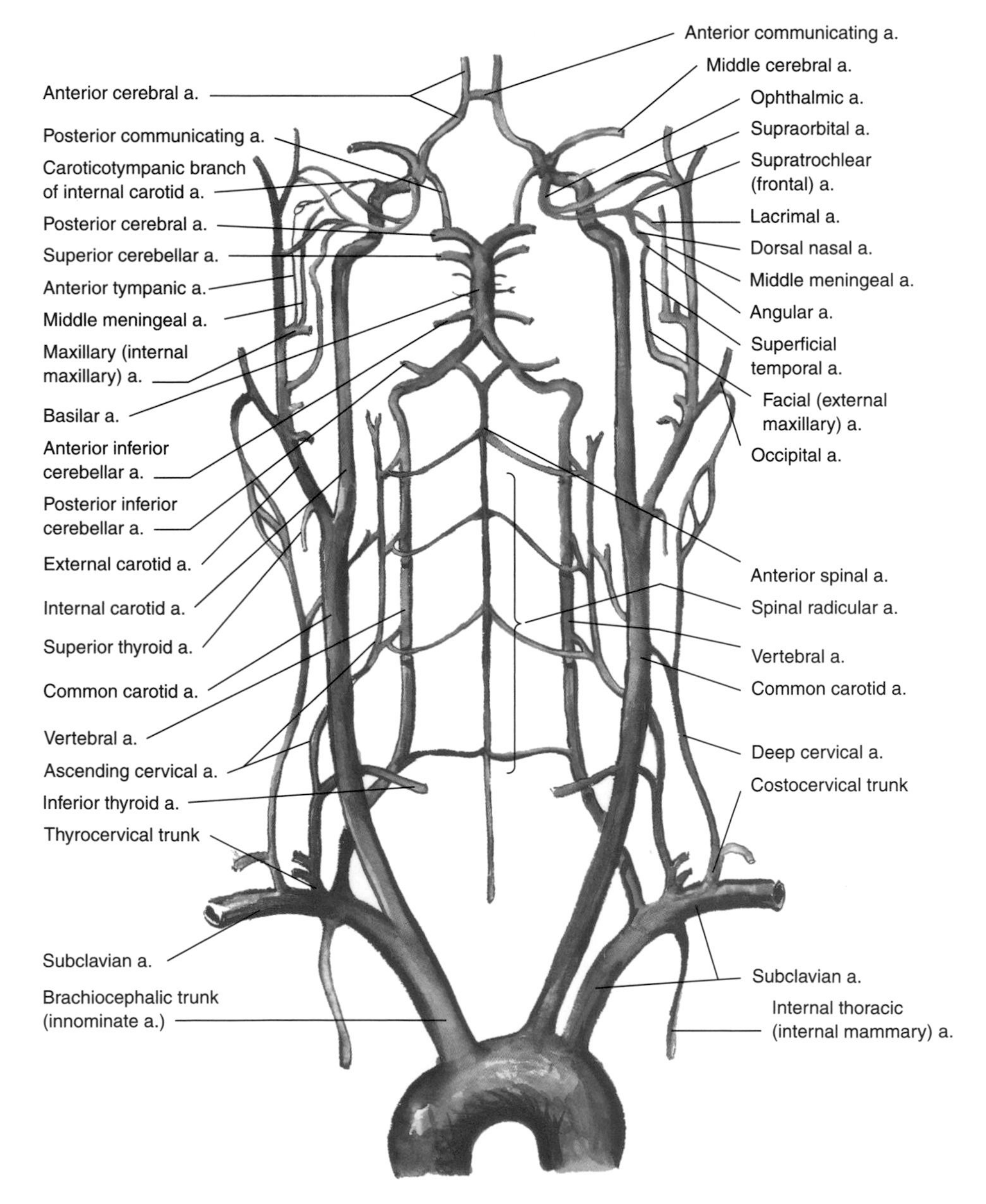

Plate 6. Cerebrovascular circulation.

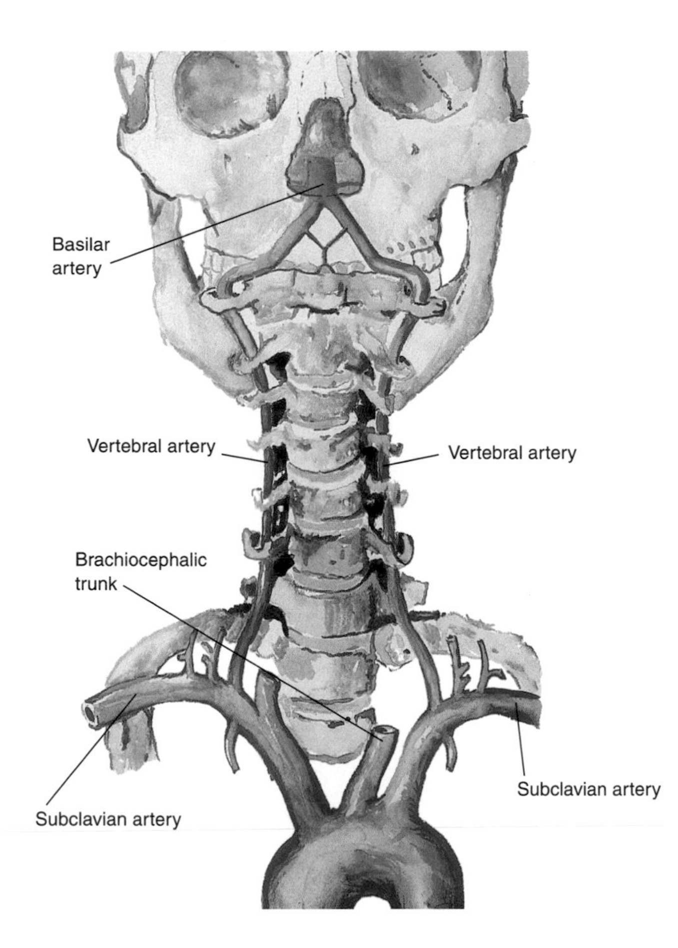

Plate 7. Course of the vertebral arteries.

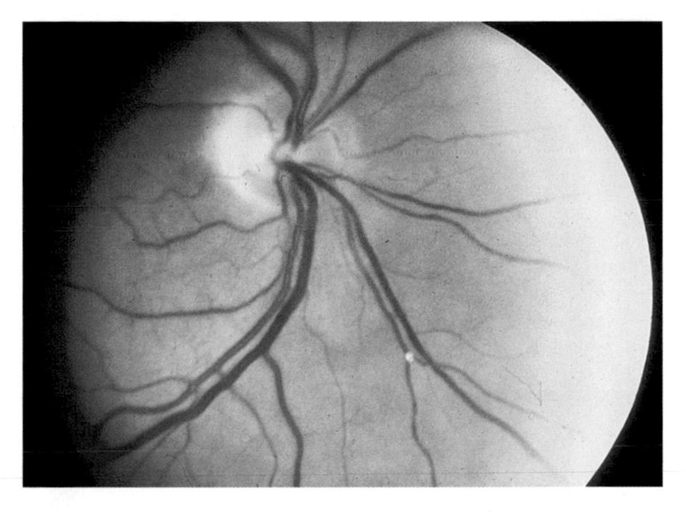

Plate 8. Hollenhorst plaque secondary to internal carotid artery disease.

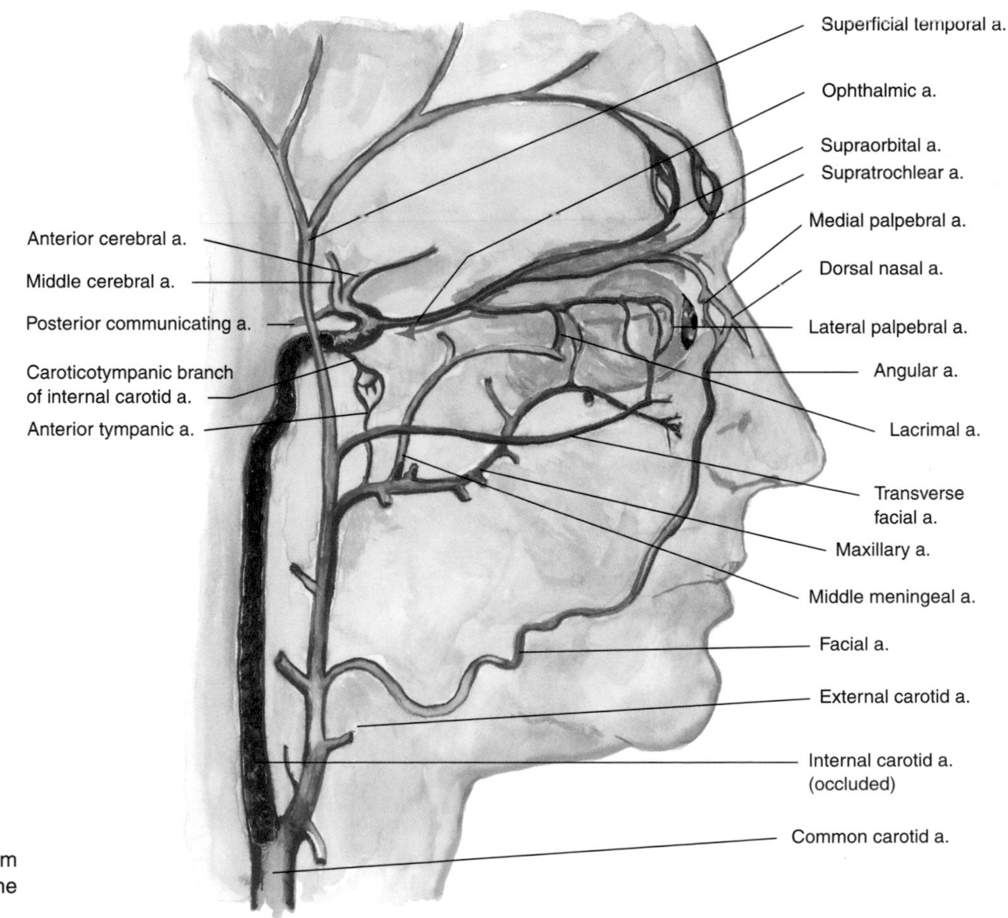

Plate 9. Retrograde blood flow from the superficial temporal artery to the ophthalmic artery.

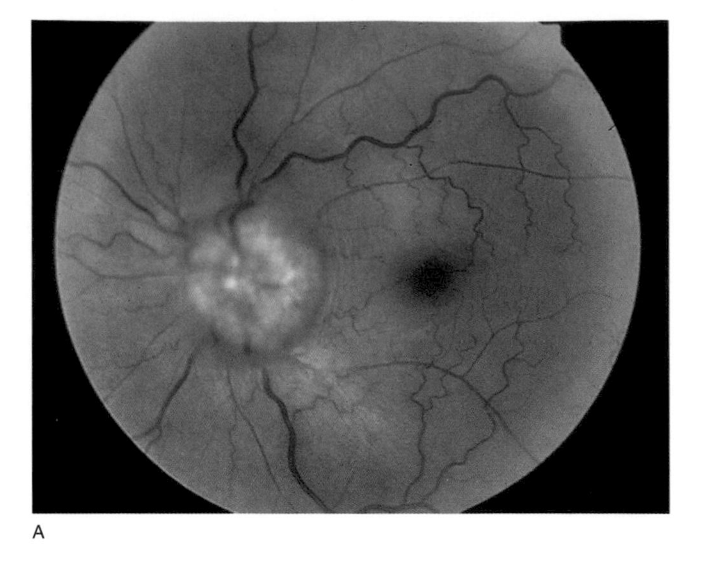

A

Plate 10 A, B. Chronic compensated papilledema. *(Reprinted with permission from L.J. Alexander, Primary Care of the Posterior Segment, 2nd ed., Norwalk, CT, Appleton & Lange, 1994).*

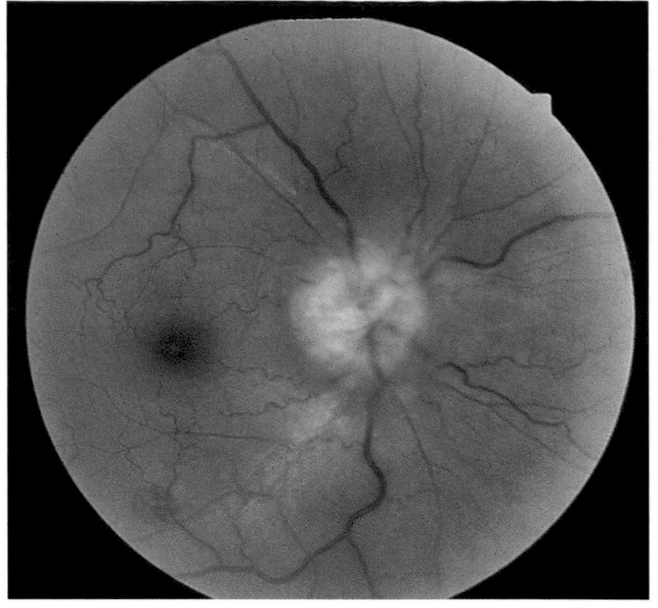

B

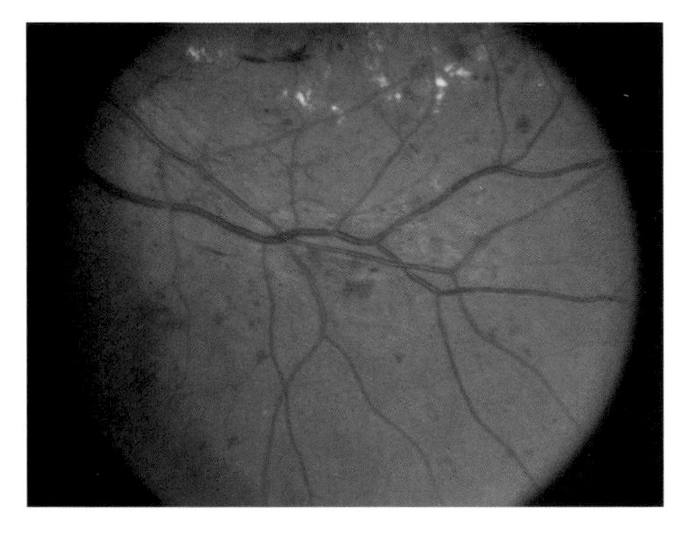

Plate 11. Severe nonproliferative diabetic retinopathy.

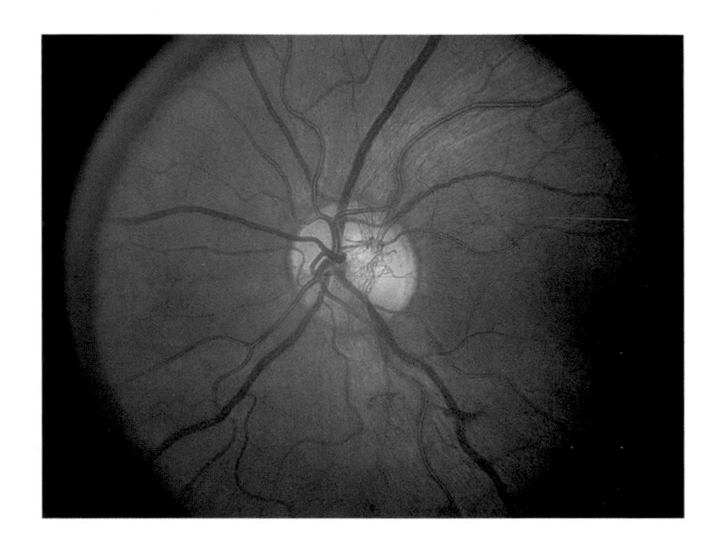

Plate 12. Proliferative diabetic retinopathy.

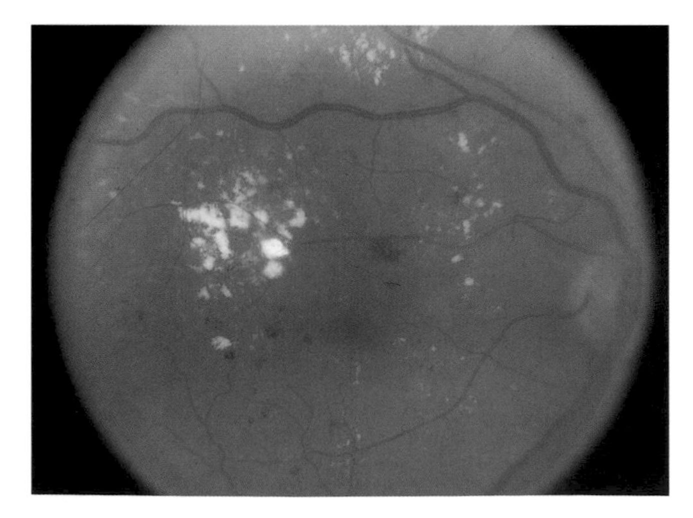

Plate 13. Diabetic macular edema.

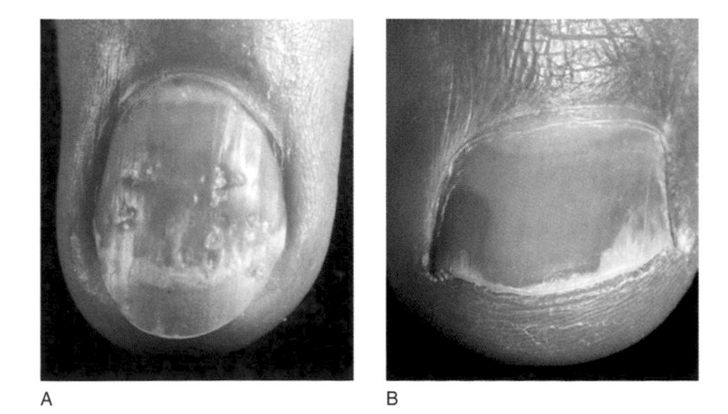

A B

Plate 14 A, B. Psoriatic nail manifestations. *(Reprinted with permission from T. B. Fitzpatrick et al., Color Atlas and Synopsis of Clinical Dermatology, 3rd ed., New York, McGraw-Hill, 1997).*

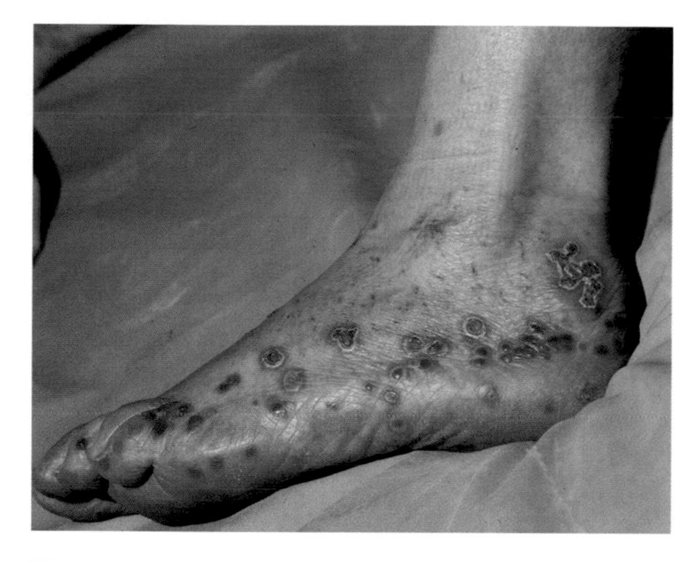

Plate 15. Keratoderma blennorrhagicum in a Reiter syndrome patient. *(Reprinted with permission from T. B. Fitzpatrick et al., Color Atlas and Synopsis of Clinical Dermatology, 3rd ed., New York, McGraw-Hill, 1997).*

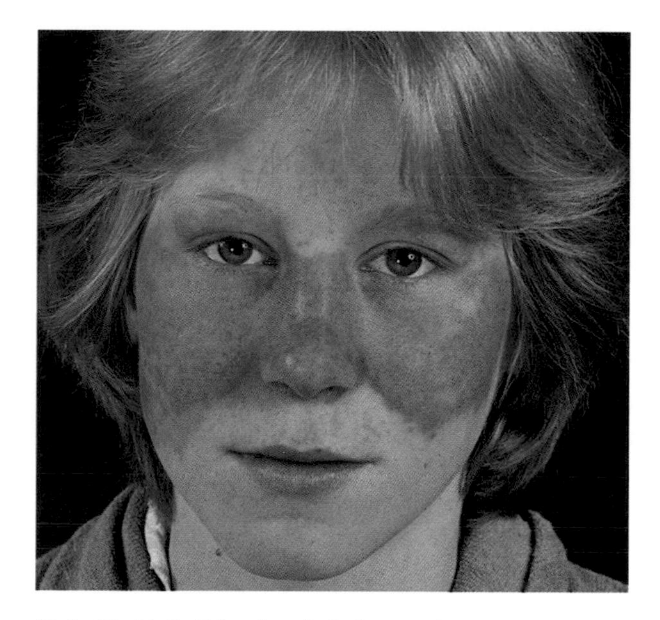

Plate 16. "Butterfly" rash typical of systemic lupus erythematosus. *(Reprinted with permission from T. B. Fitzpatrick et al., Color Atlas and Synopsis of Clinical Dermatology, 3rd ed., New York, McGraw-Hill, 1997).*

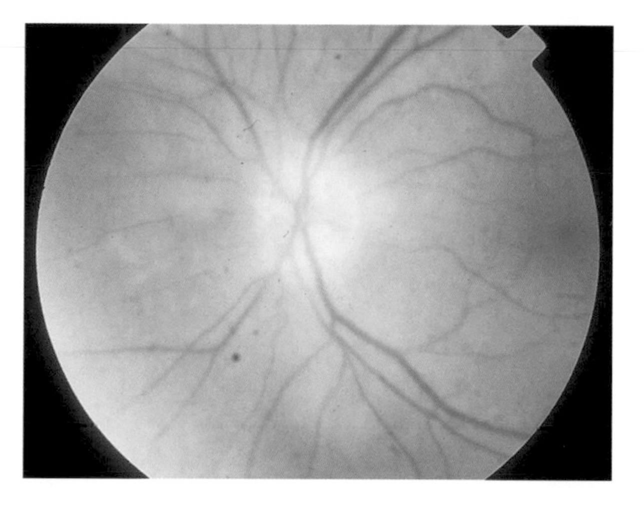

Plate 17. Arteritic AION in an 80-year-old man with giant cell arteritis. The disc is edematous, but not hyperemic (so-called "pale edema").

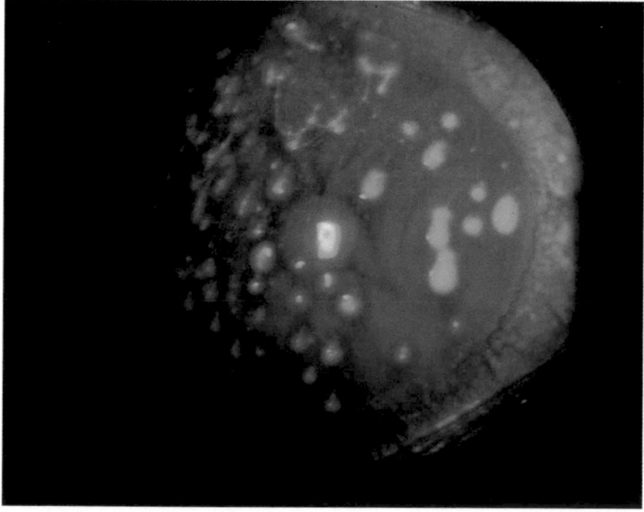

A

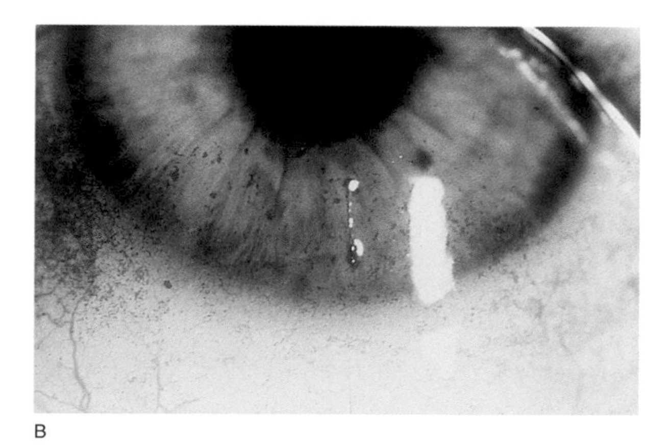

B

Plate 18 A, B. Filamentary keratitis in a patient with severe dry eye secondary to Sjogren's syndrome. (A) Filaments stained with fluorescein. (B) Filaments stained with rose bengal.

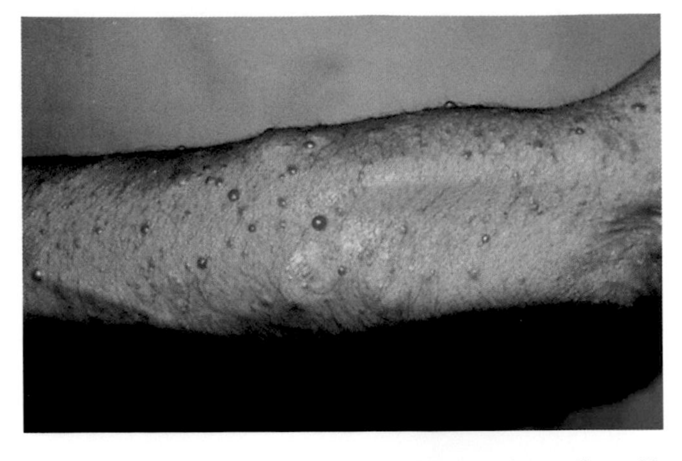

Plate 19. Subcutaneous neurofibromas of the arm in a patient with neurofibromatosis I.

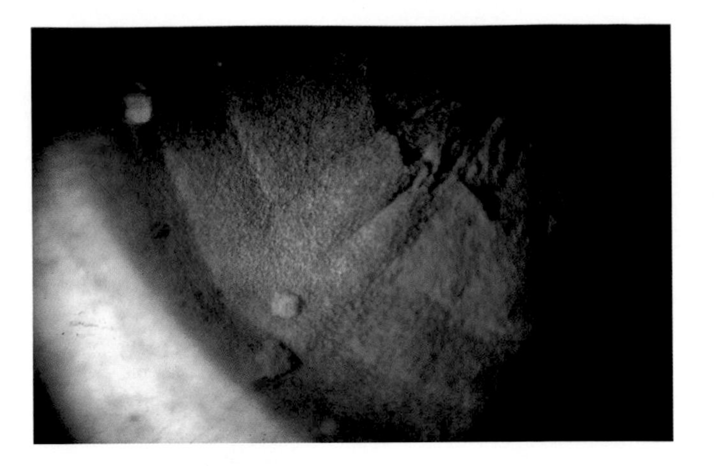

Plate 20. Iris Lisch nodules as seen in neurofibromatosis.

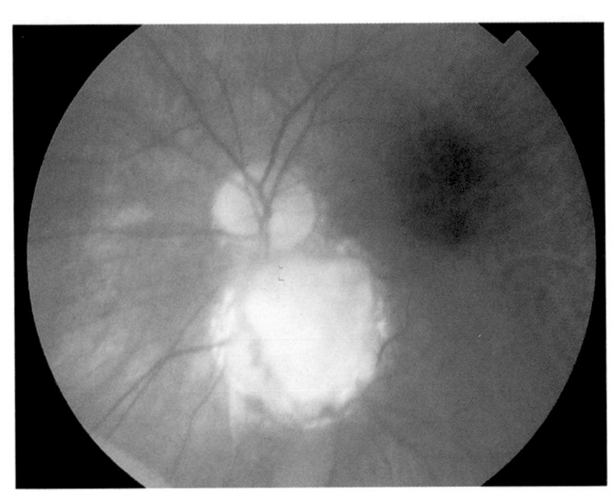

Plate 21. Astrocytoma in a patient with tuberous sclerosis.

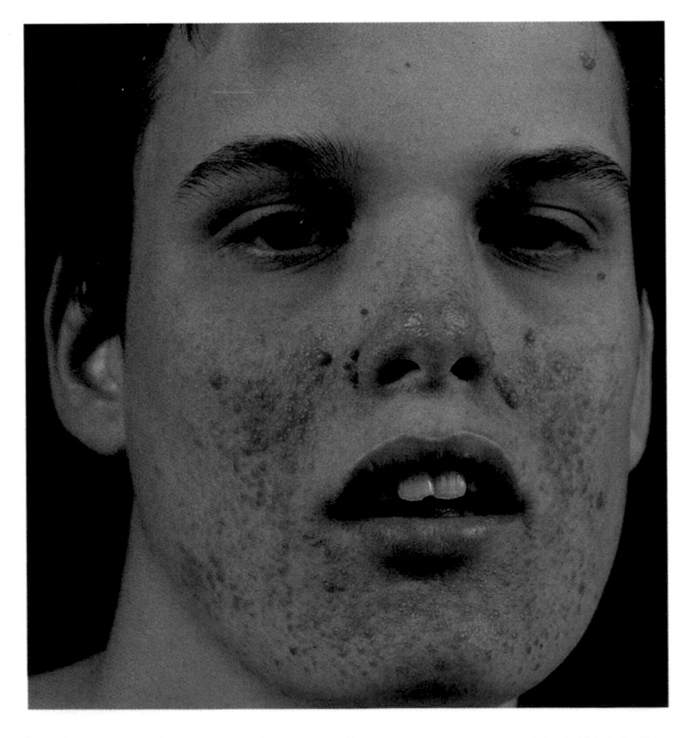

Plate 22. Adenoma sebaceum in tuberous sclerosis. *(Reprinted with permission from T. B. Fitzpatrick et al., Color Atlas and Synopsis of Clinical Dermatology, 3rd ed., New York, McGraw-Hill, 1997).*

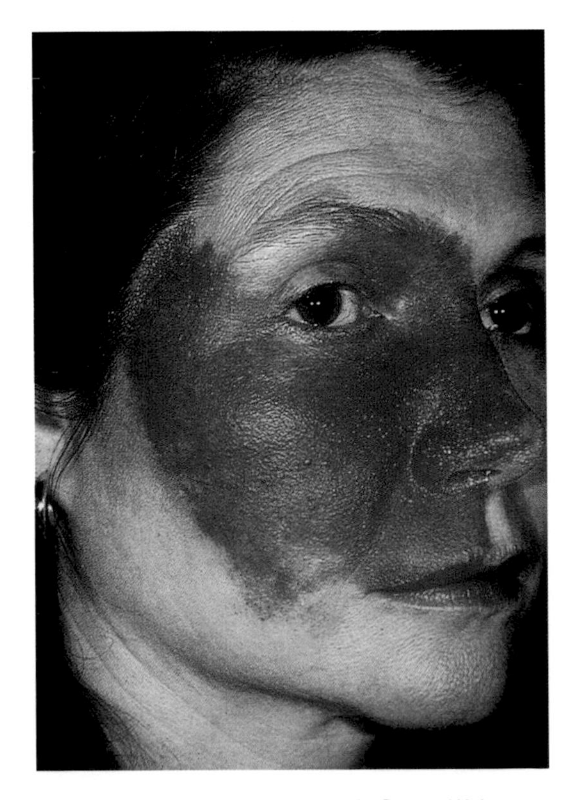

Plate 23. Nevus flammeus seen in Sturge-Weber.

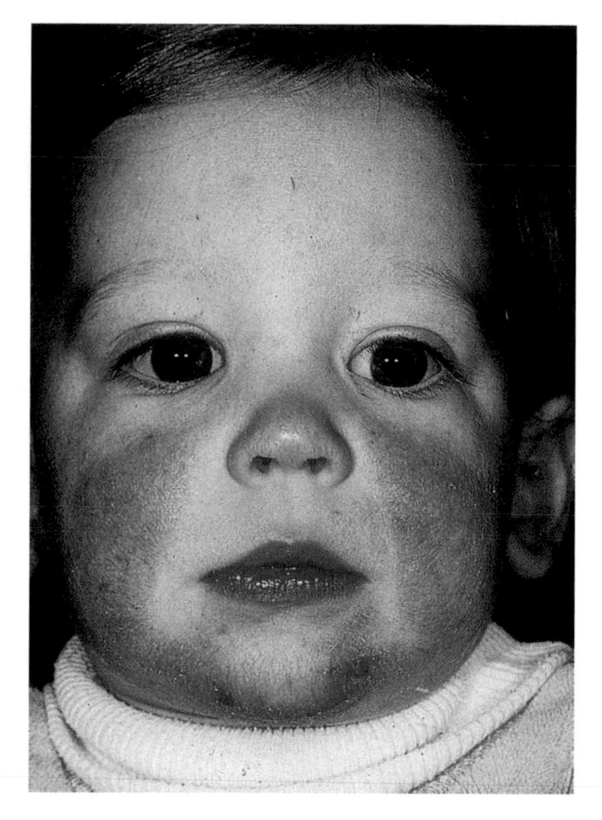

Plate 24. Atopic dermatitis of the cheeks. *(Reprinted with permission from Habif,TP, Clinical Dermatology: A Color Guide to Diagnosis and Therapy, 2nd ed., St Louis, Mosby, 1990, 77.)*

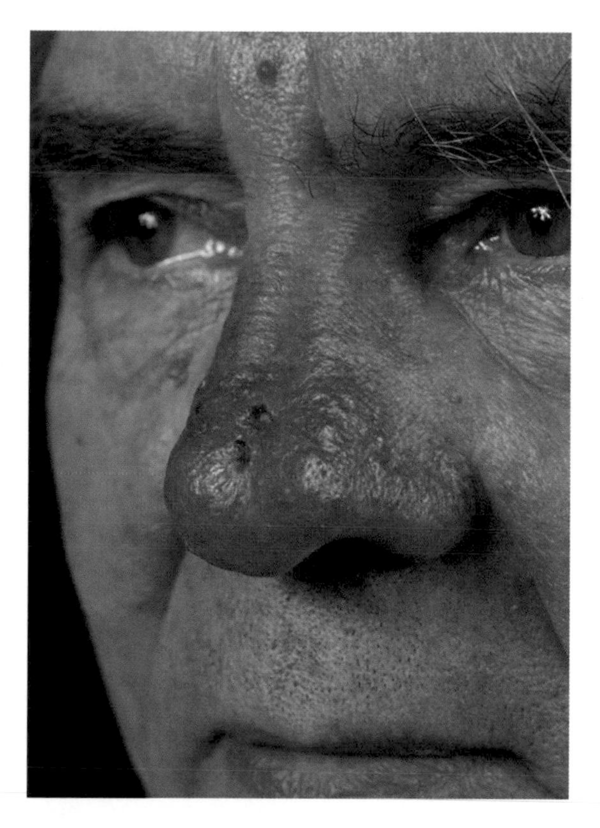

Plate 25. Rosacea. *(Reprinted with permission from T. B. Fitzpatrick et al., Color Atlas and Synopsis of Clinical Dermatology, 3rd ed., New York, McGraw-Hill, 1997).*

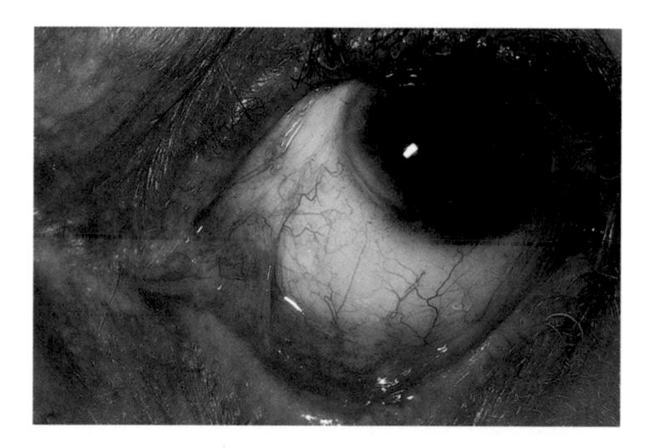

Plate 26. Symblepharon in cicatricial pemphigoid.

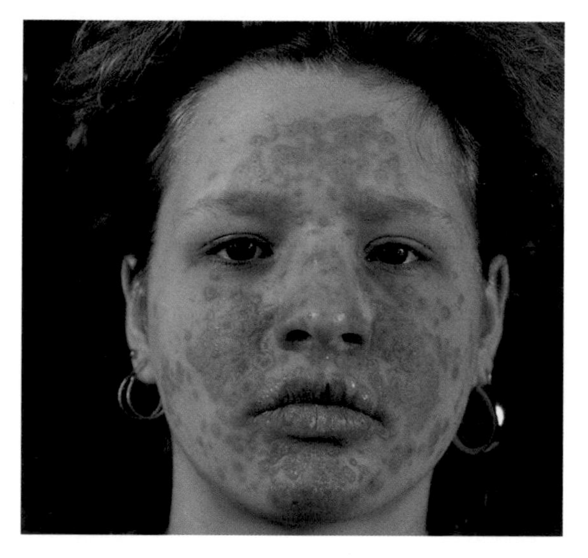

Plate 27. Erythema multiforme. *(Reprinted with permission from T. B. Fitzpatrick et al., Color Atlas and Synopsis of Clinical Dermatology, 3rd ed., New York, McGraw-Hill, 1997).*

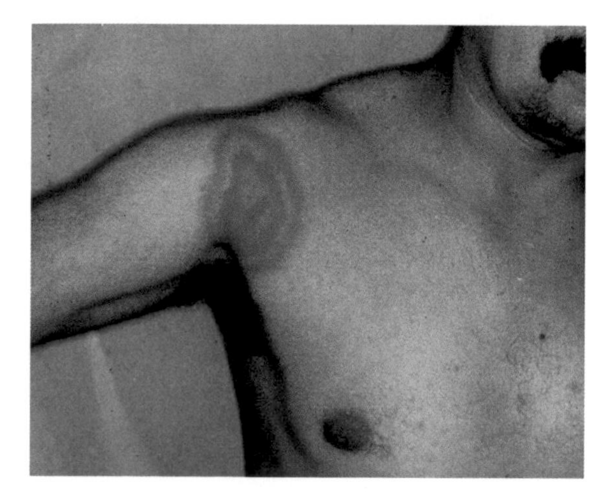

Plate 28. Typical erythema migrans in lyme disease.

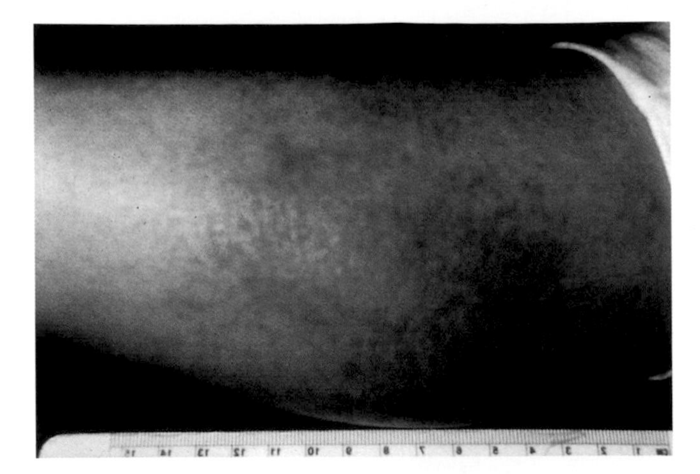

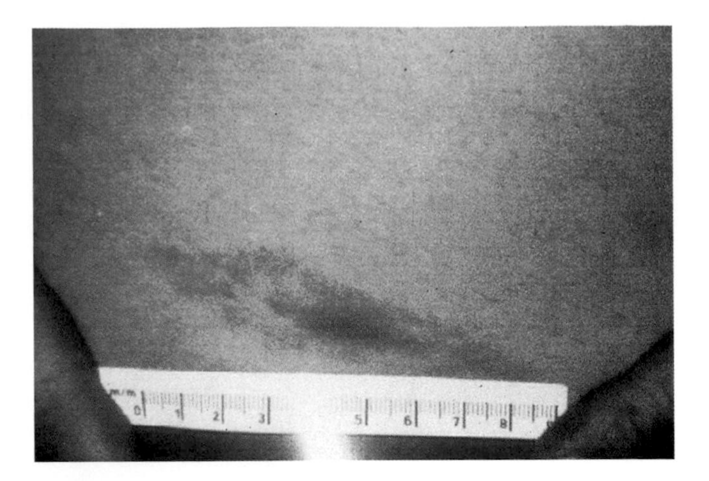

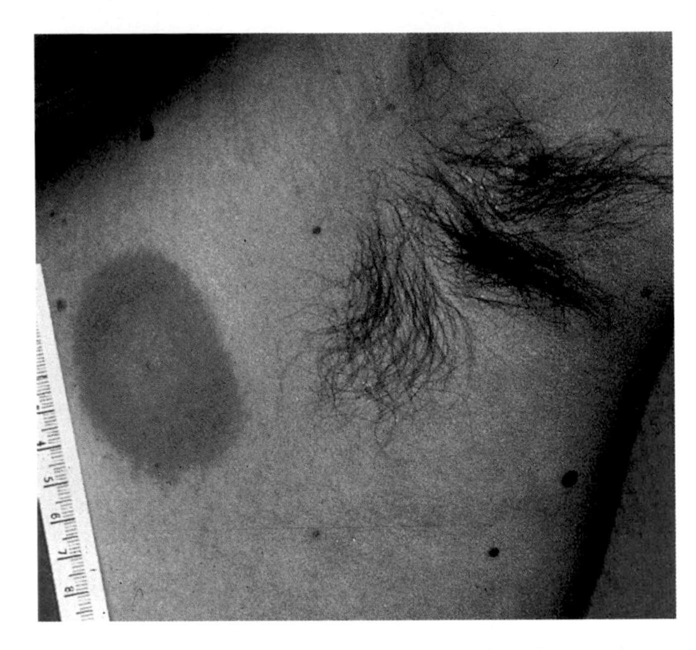

Plates 29, 30, 31. Varying appearances of erythema migrans lesions in Lyme disease.

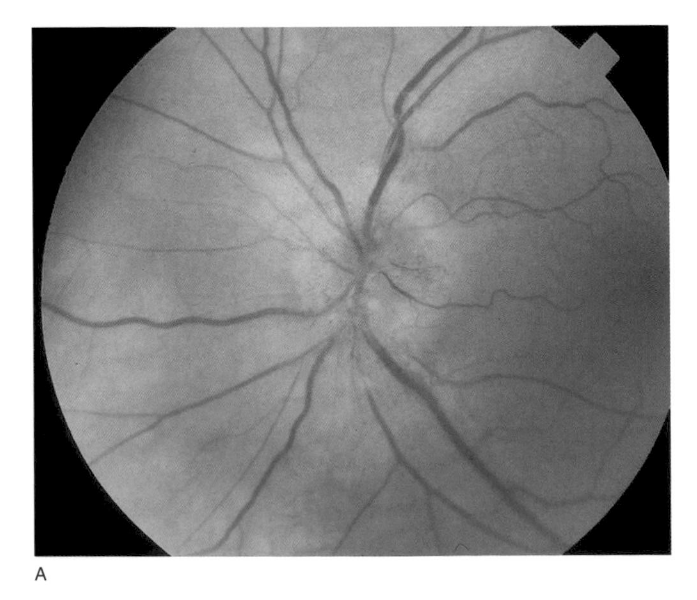

A

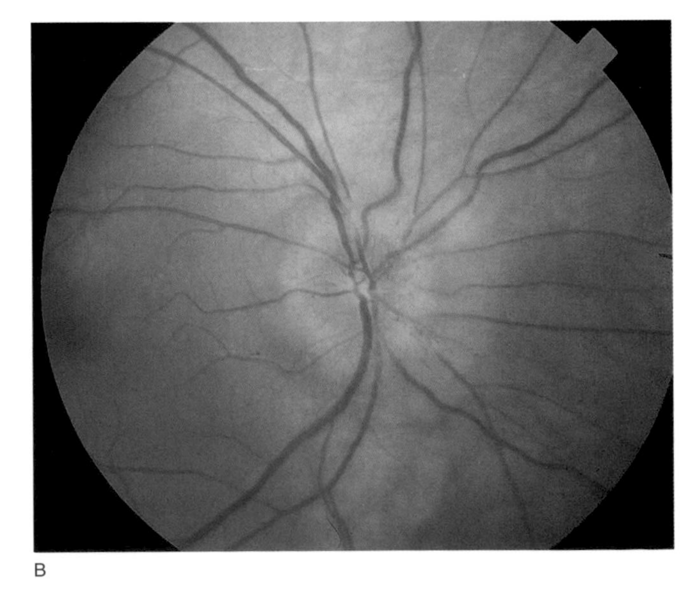

B

Plate 32 A, B. Bilateral disc edema in disseminated Lyme disease.

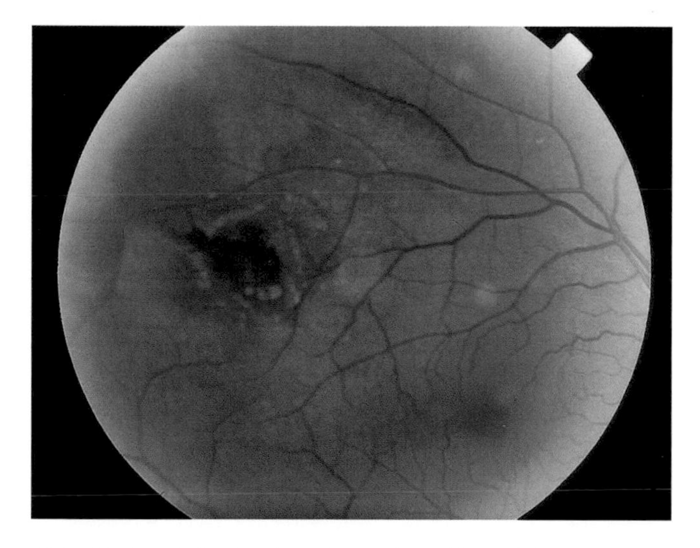

Plate 33. Focal chorioretinitis in a patient with syphilis.

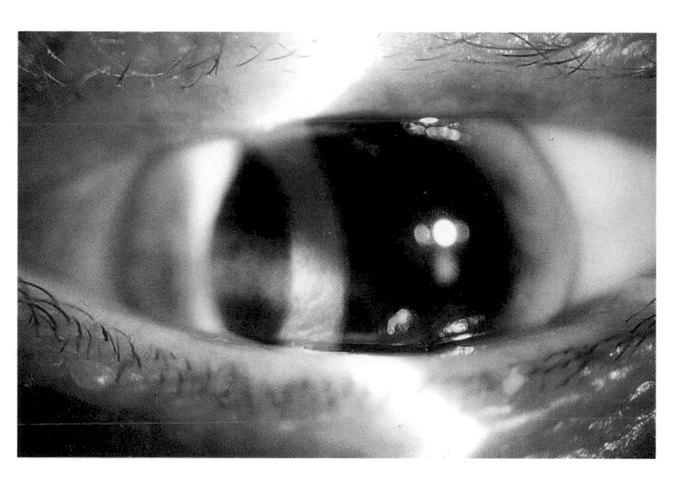

Plate 34. Interstitial keratitis in a syphilitic patient.

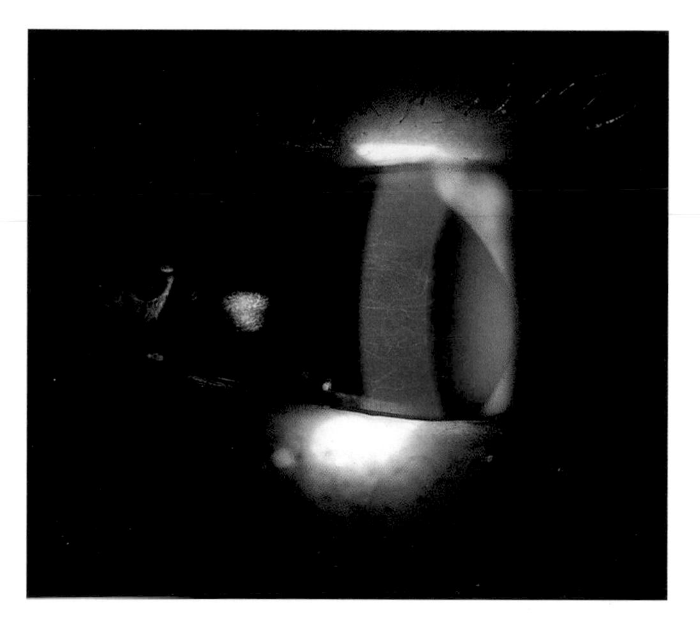

Plate 35. Ghost vessels secondary to interstitial keratitis in a syphilitic patient.

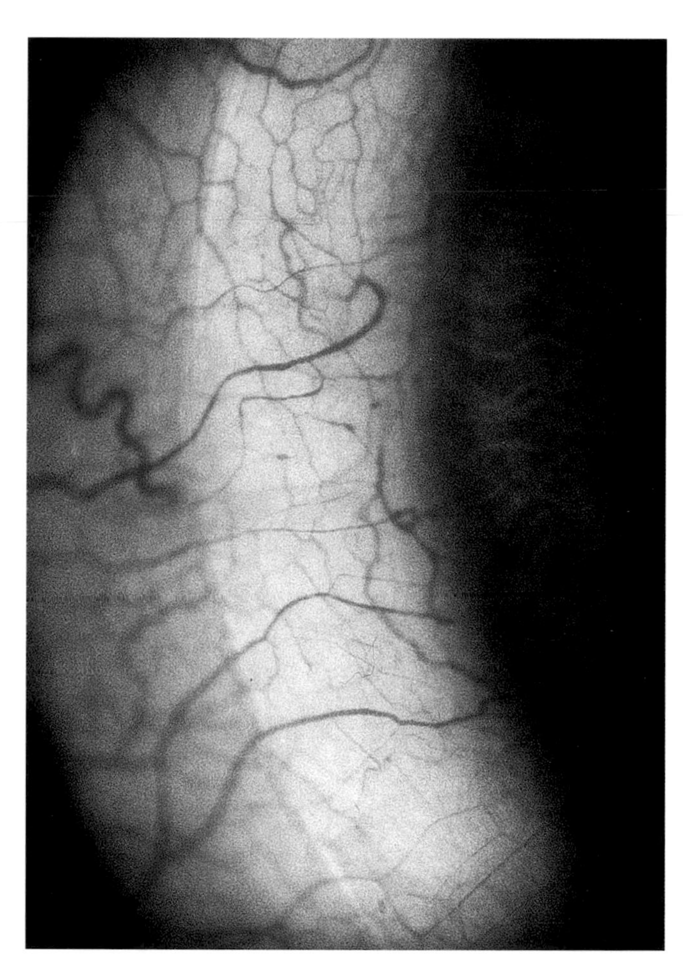

Plate 36. Conjunctival microvasculopathy as seen in HIV/AIDS patients.

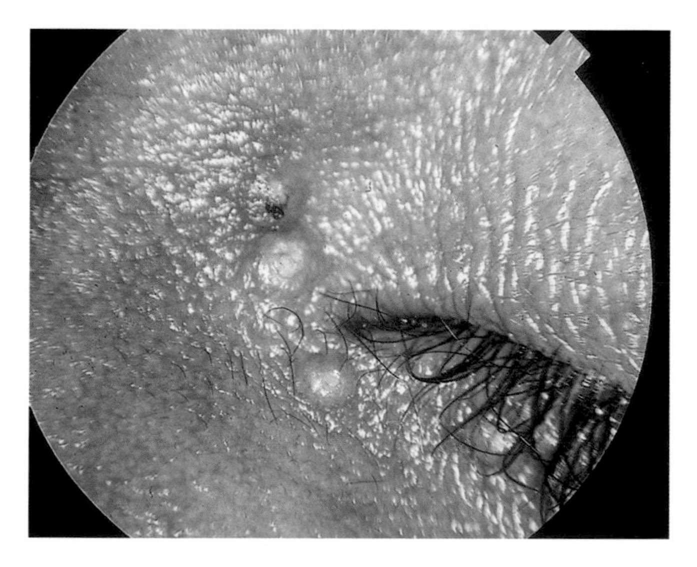

Plate 37. Molluscum contagiosum in an AIDS patient.

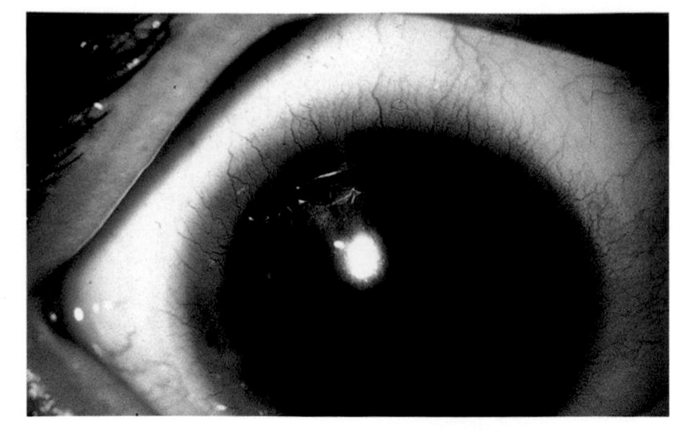

Plate 38. Microsporidial keratoconjunctivitis in an AIDS patient. *(Courtesy of Drs. J. Shovlin and G. Rossenwasser.)*

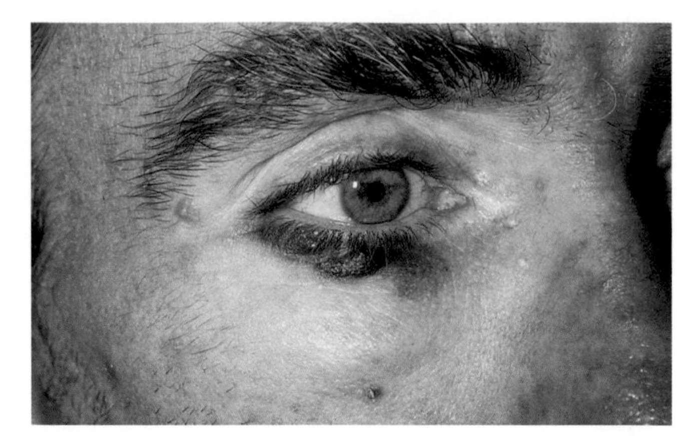

Plate 39. Kaposi's sarcoma of the conjunctiva and eyelid of an AIDS patient. *(Reprinted with permission from T. B. Fitzpatrick et al., Color Atlas and Synopsis of Clinical Dermatology, 3rd ed., New York, McGraw-Hill, 1997).*

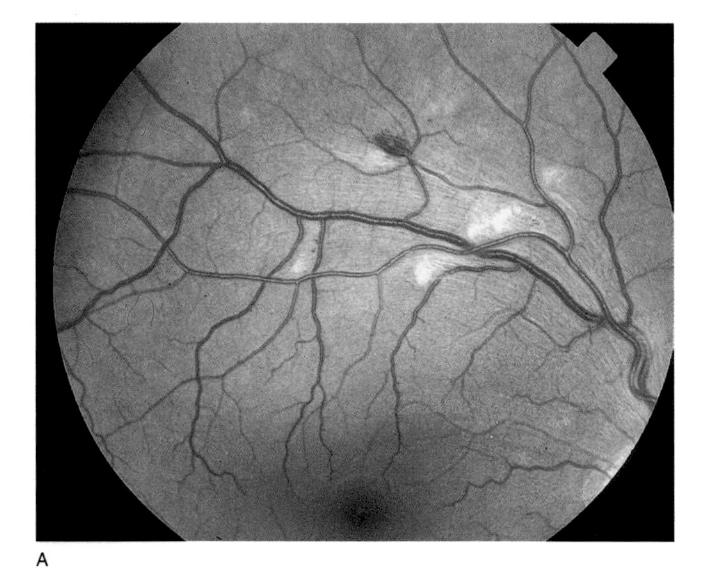

A

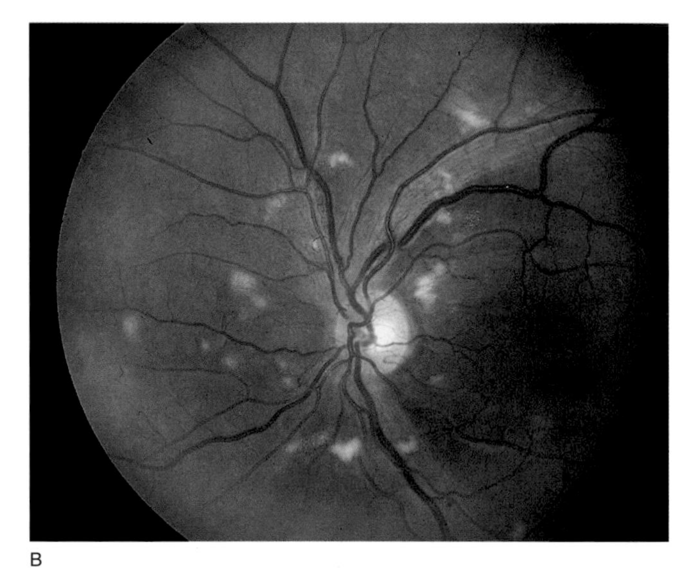

B

Plate 40 A, B. HIV retinopathy.

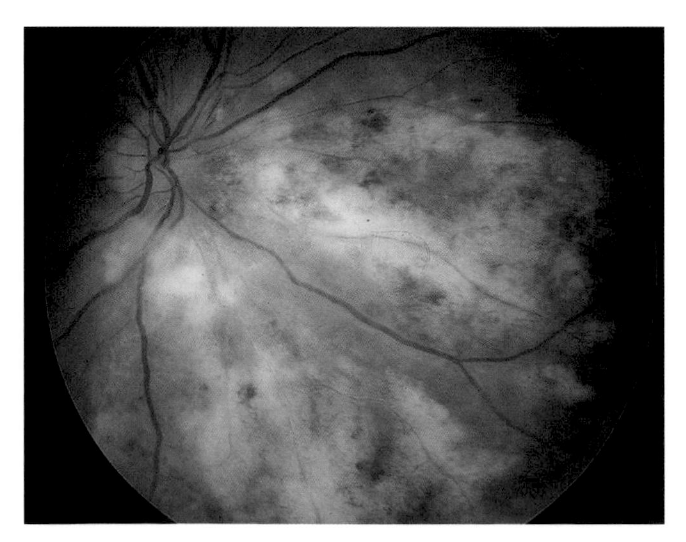

Plate 41. CMV retinitis in an AIDS patient.

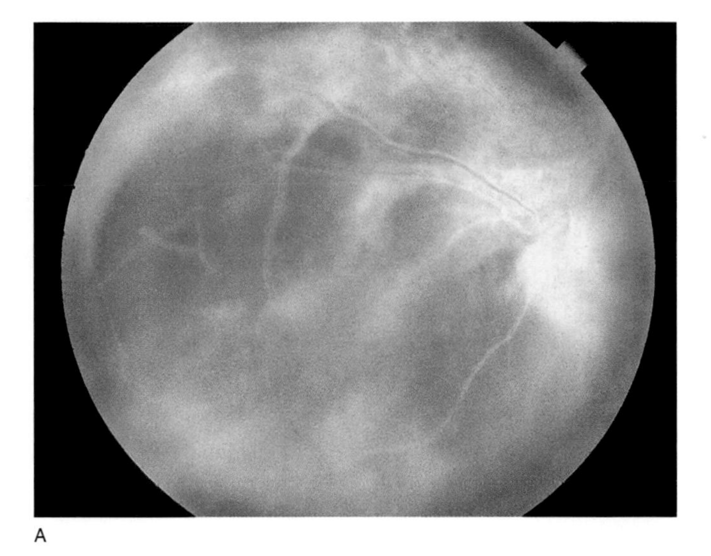

A

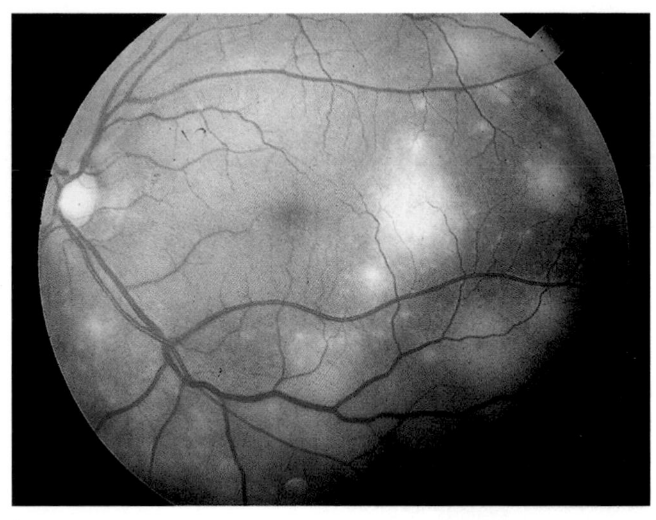

B

Plate 42 A, B. Progressive outer retinal necrosis in an AIDS patient.

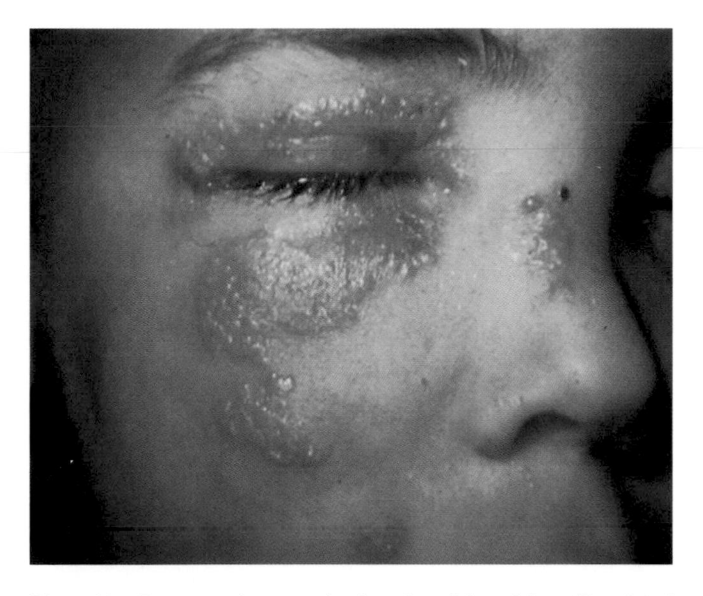

Plate 43. Recurrent herpes simplex virus lid vesicles. *(Reprinted with permission from S. Weinberg et al., Color Atlas of Pediatric Dermatology, 3rd ed., New York, McGraw-Hill, 1998).*

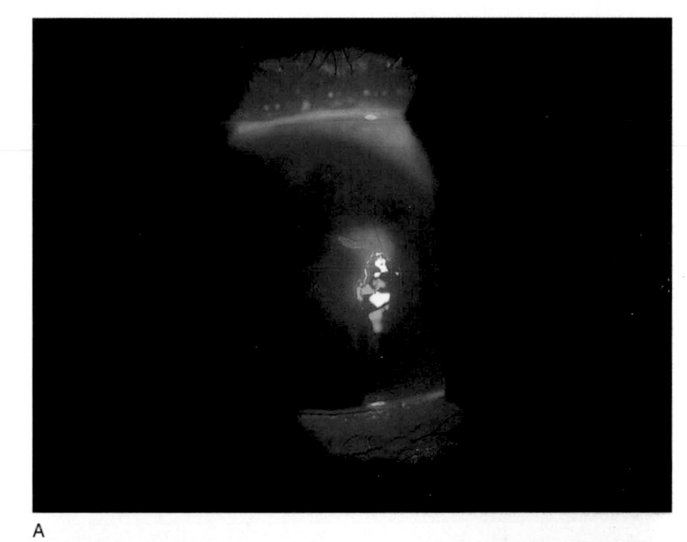

A

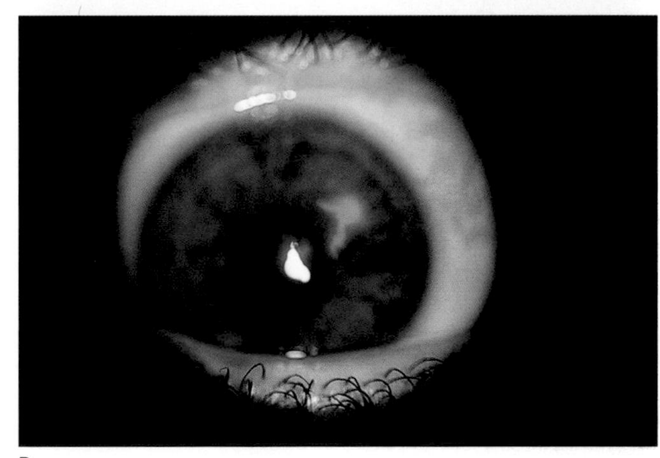

B

Plate 44 A, B. Classic herpes simplex dendritic keratitis.

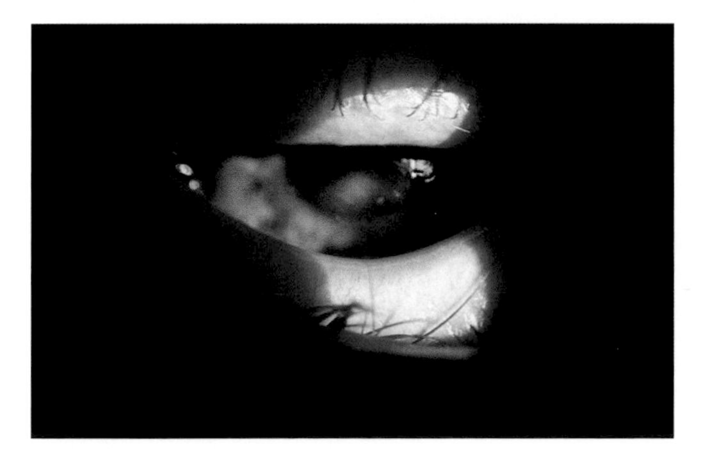

Plate 45. Stromal herpes simplex keratitis.

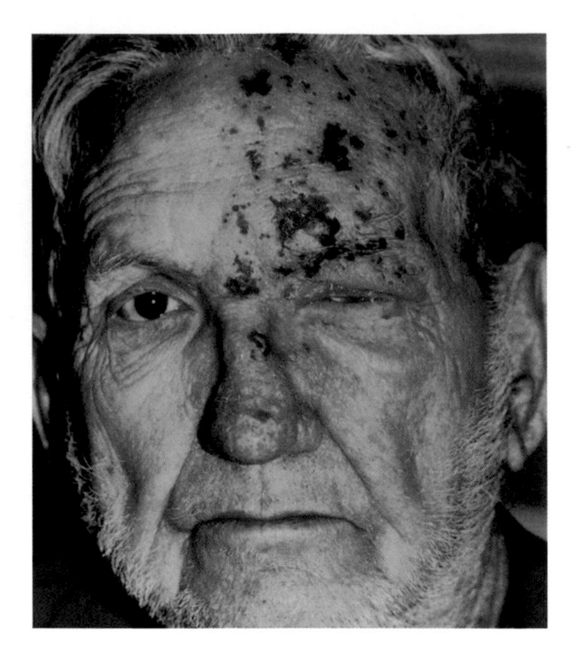

Plate 46. Herpes zoster ophthalmicus with cutaneous dissemination.

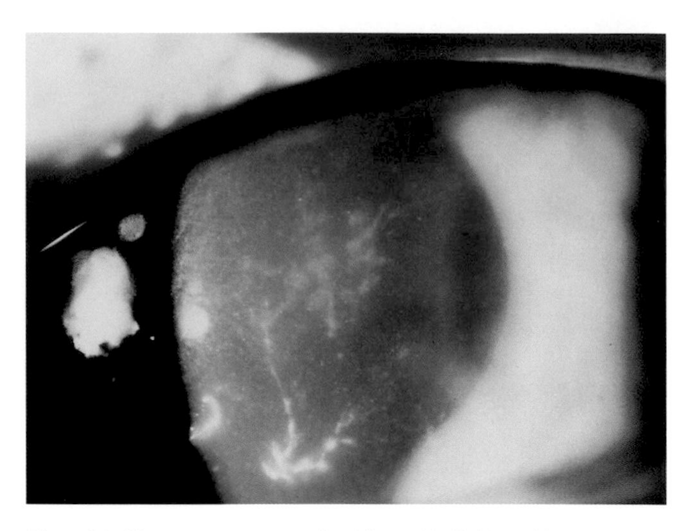

Plate 47. Herpes zoster pseudondrite epithelial keratitis.

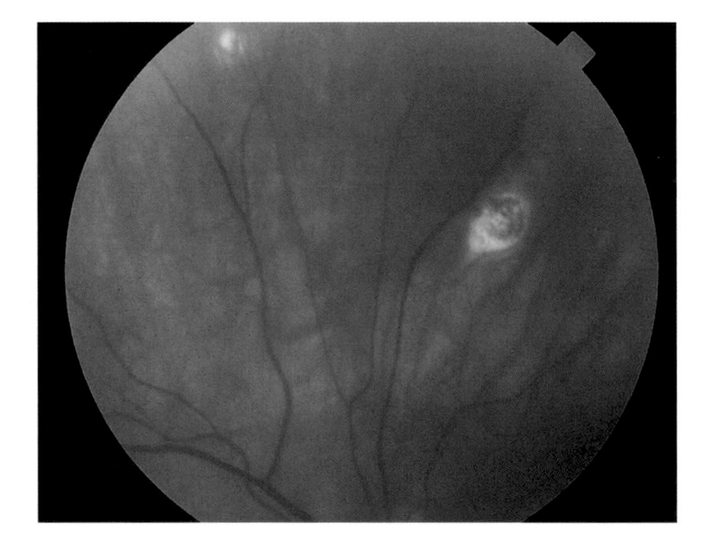

Plate 48. Peripheral atrophic histo spots.

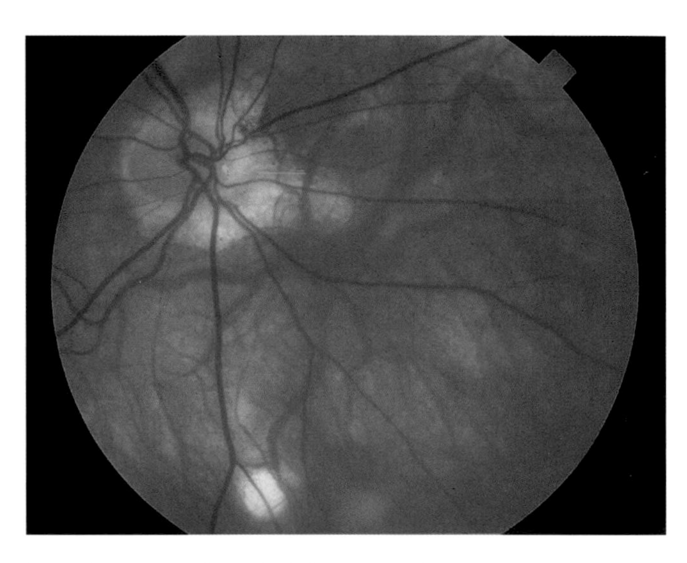

Plate 49. Peripapillary RPE changes in histoplasmosis.

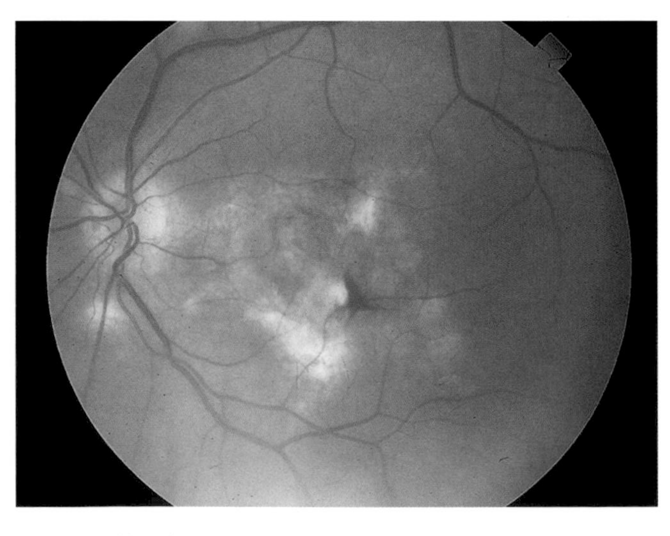

Plate 50. Macular scarring in histoplasmosis.

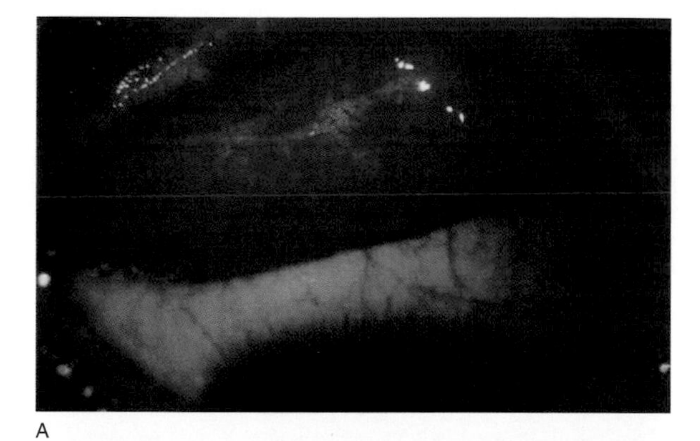

A

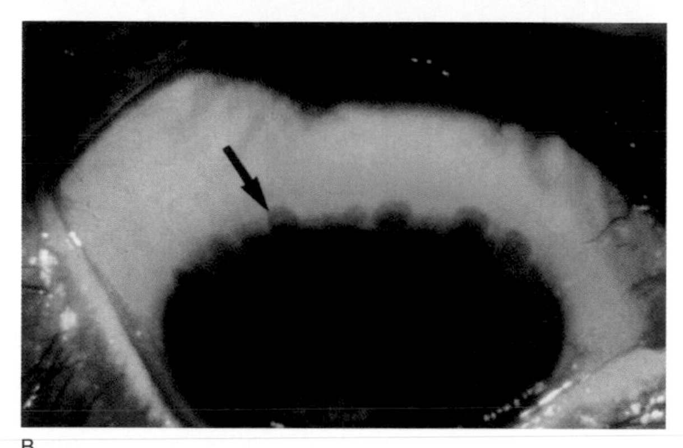

B

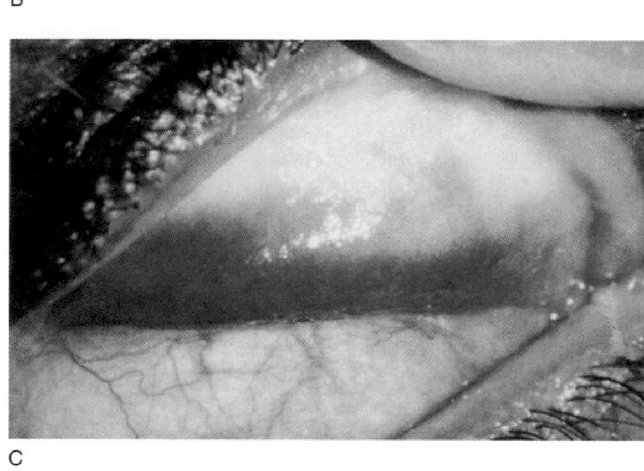

C

Plate 51 A, B, C. Severe pannus and scarring in endstage trachoma. *(Reprinted with permission from E.R. Mandel and M.D. Wagoner, Atlas of Corneal Disease, Philadelphia, WB Saunders, 1989. Used with permission.).*

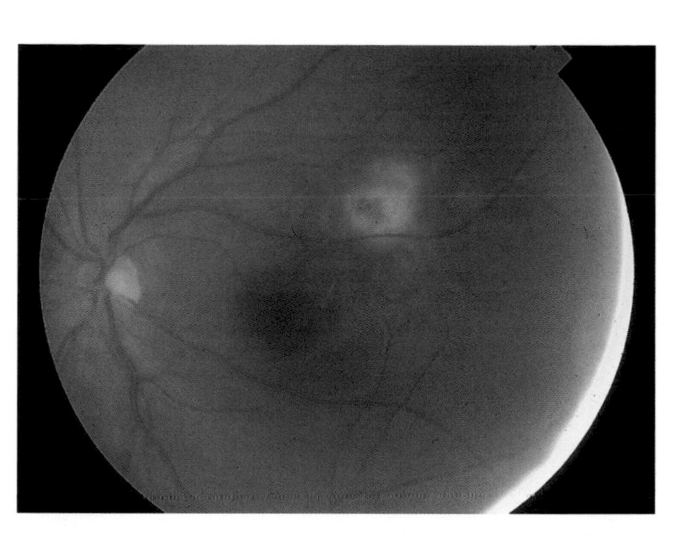

Plate 52. Active toxoplasmosis retinochoroiditis.

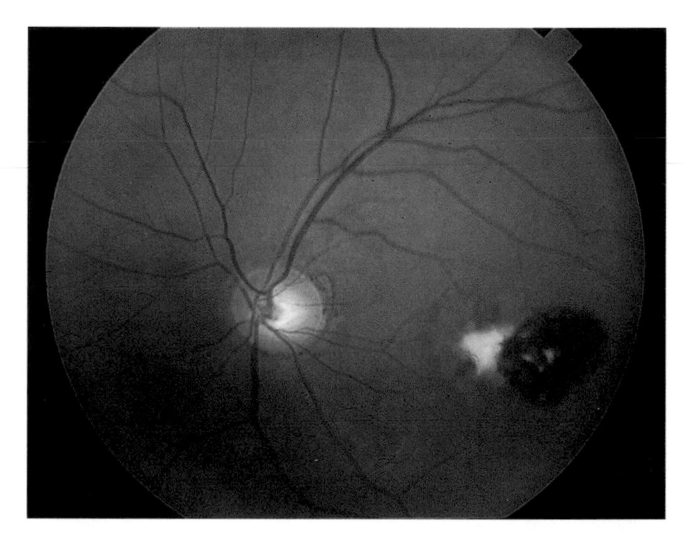

Plate 53. Healed toxoplasmosis retinochoroiditis lesion.

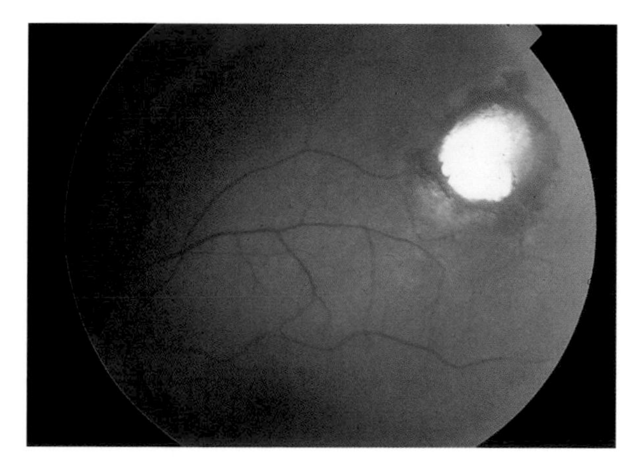

Plate 54. Macular toxoplasmosis retinochoroidal lesions.

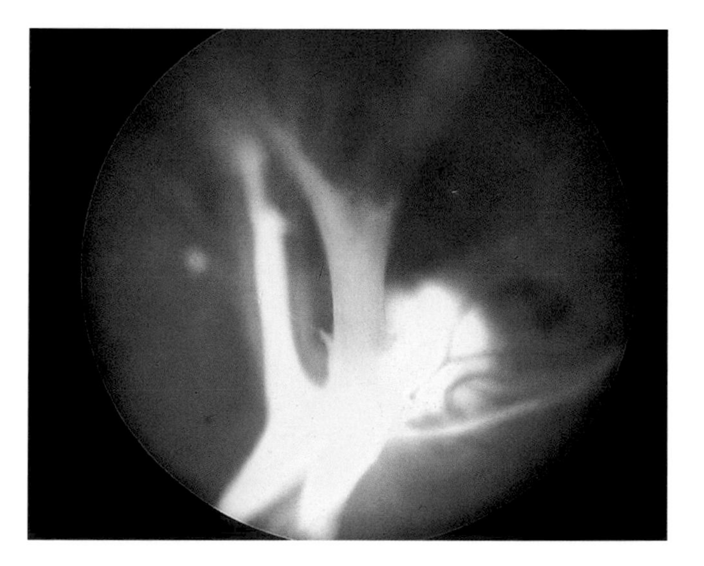

Plate 55. Toxocara canis vitreoretinitis.

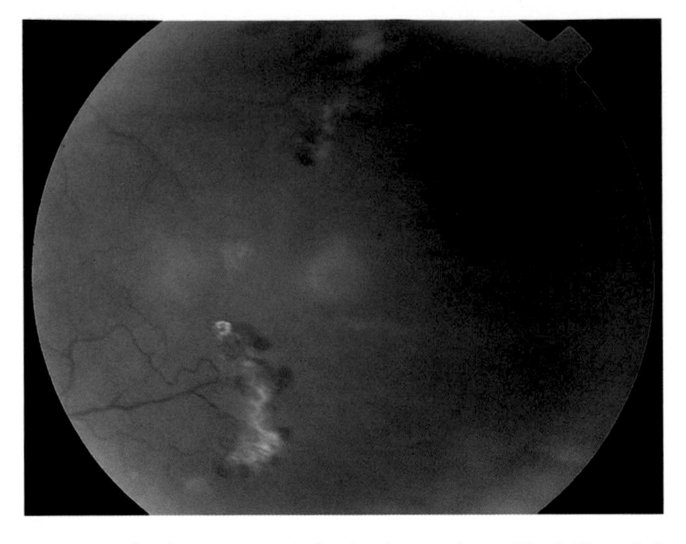

Plate 56. Seafan-neovascularization in a patient with sickle-cell C disease.

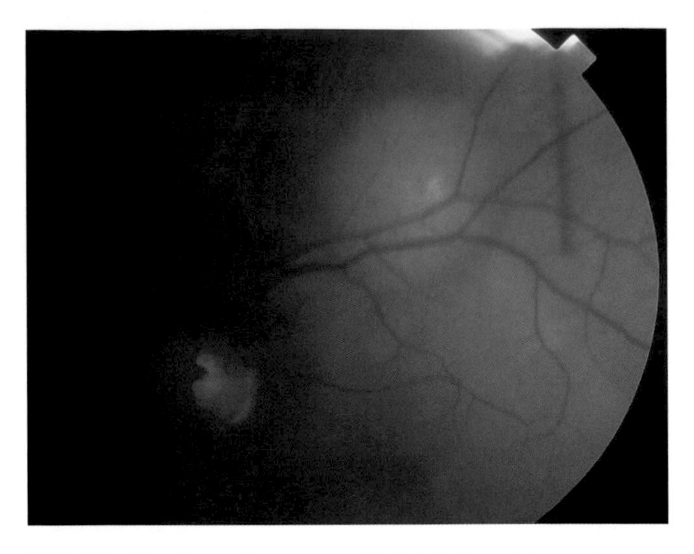

Plate 57. Nonrhegmatogenous retinal detachment from choroidal metastasis.

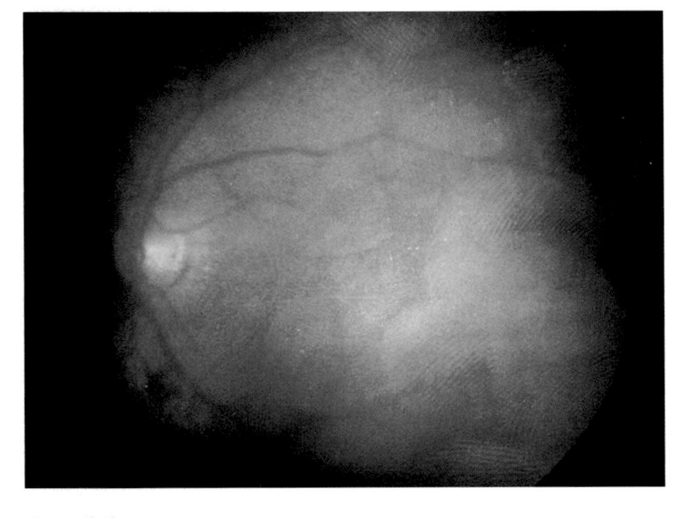

Plate 58A. Nonrhegmatogenous retinal detachment from choroidal metastasis in a patient with lung carcinoma.

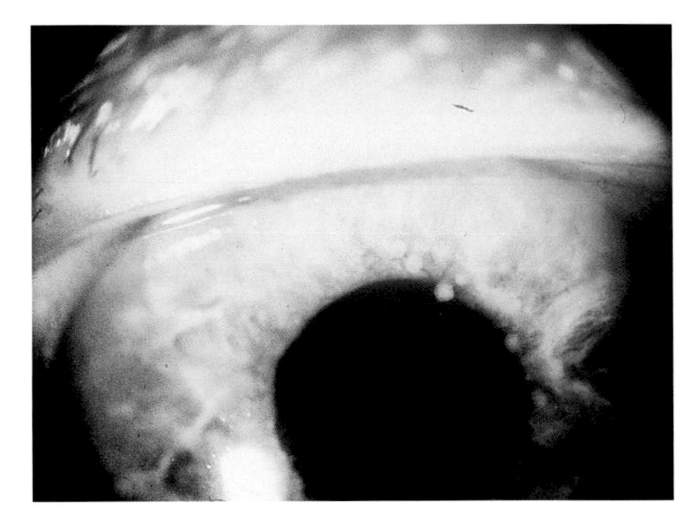

Plate 58B. Metastatic iris nodules in a patient with lung carcinoma.

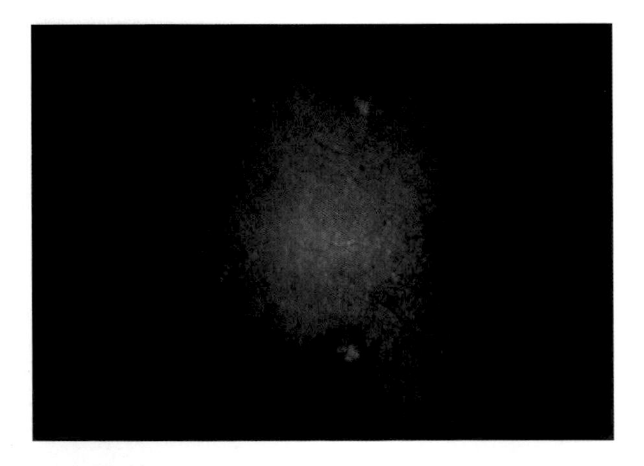

Plate 59. Eruptive xanthomas on the elbow of a diabetic patient with severe hypertriglyceridemia and hypercholesterolemia.

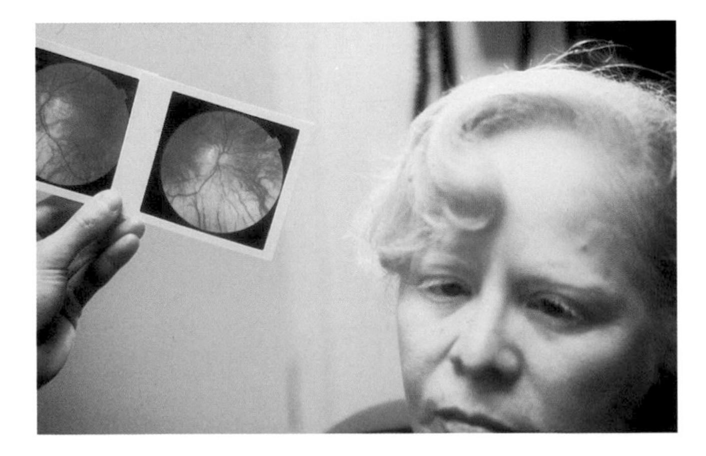

Plate 60. Classic tyrosinase-negative oculocutaneous albinism.

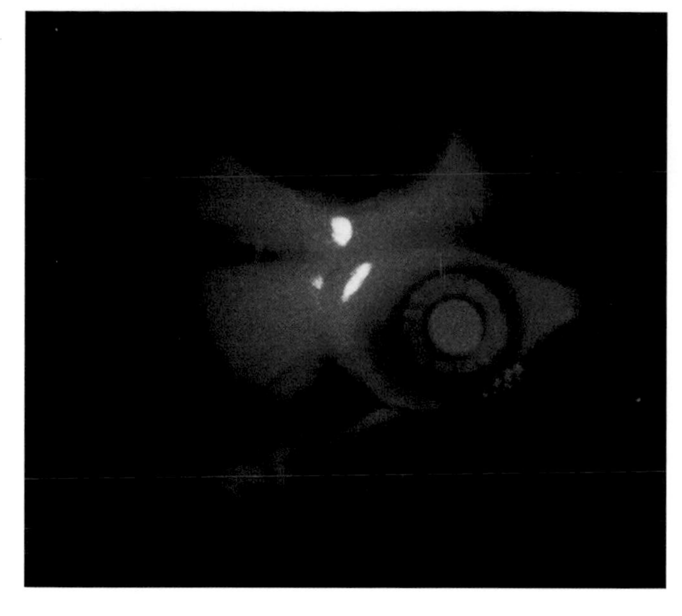

Plate 61. Iris transillumination in oculocutaneous albinism.

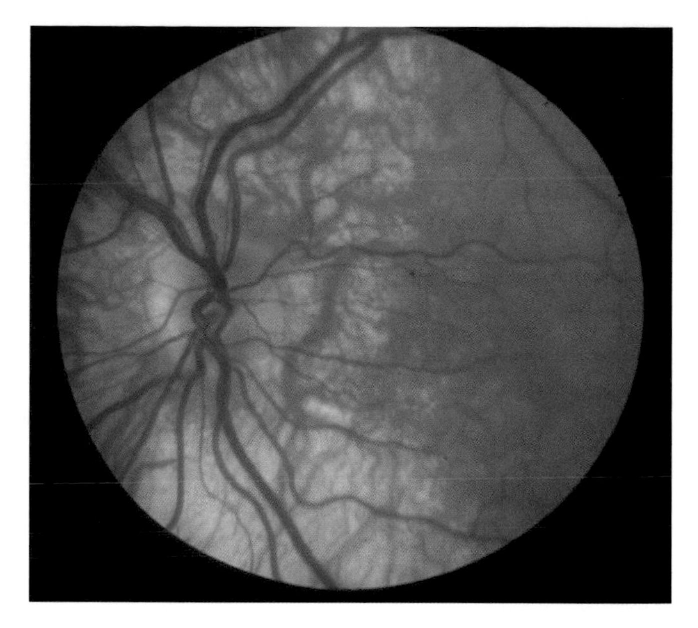

Plate 62. Macular-hypoplasia in an albinotic fundus.

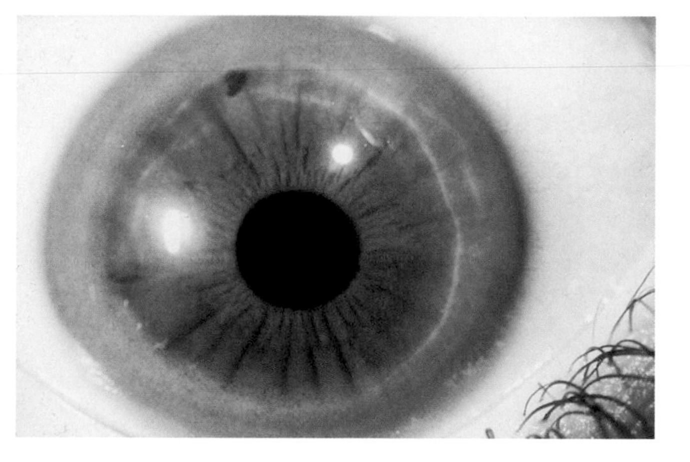

Plate 63. Kayser-Fleischer ring as seen in Wilson disease. *(Reprinted with permission from L.J. Catania, Primary Care of the Anterior Segment,* 2nd ed., *Norwalk CT, Appleton & Lange, 1995).*

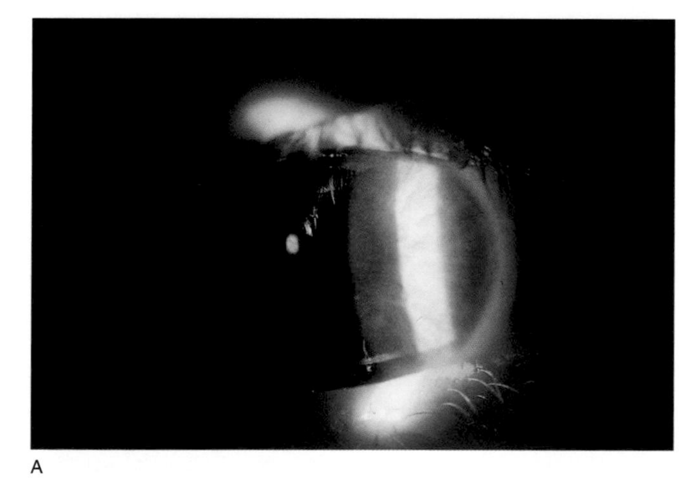

A

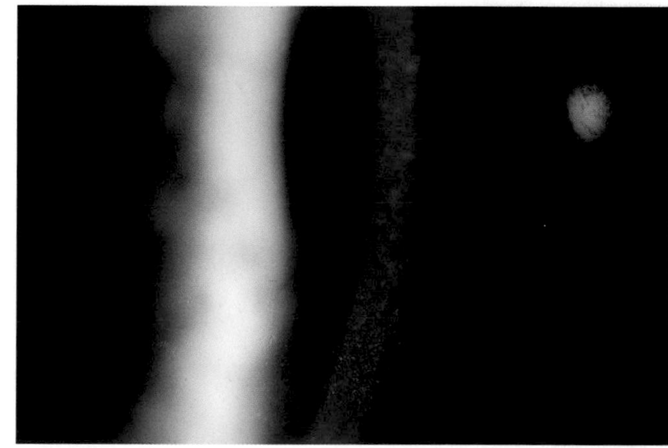

B

Plate 64 A, B. Corneal crystals seen in cystinosis.

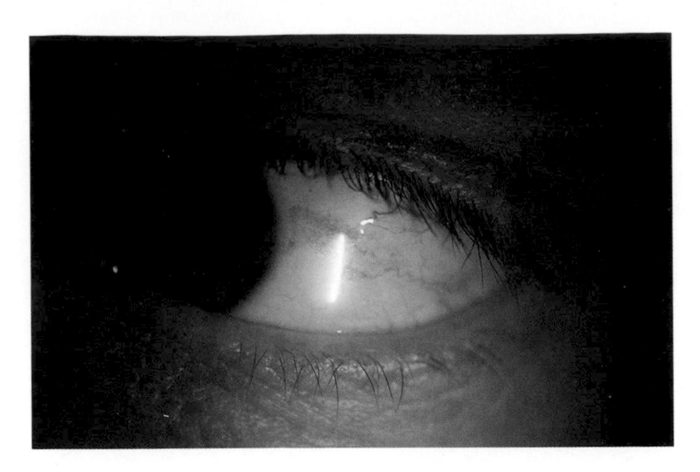

Plate 65. Bitot spot in vitamin A deficiency.

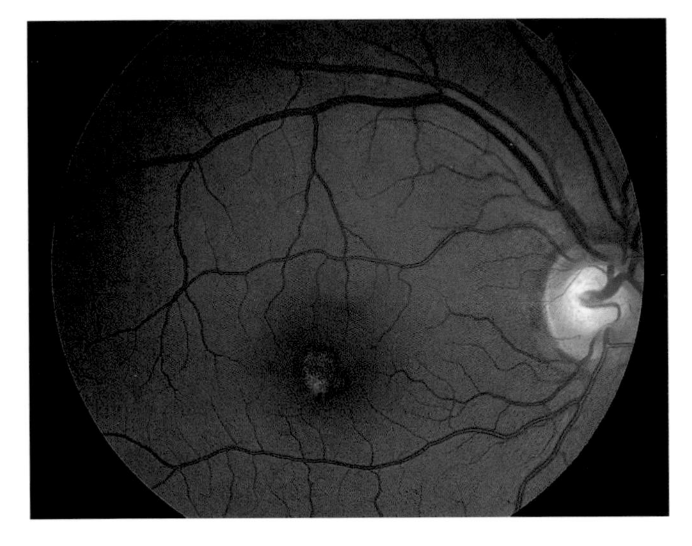

Plate 66. Solar maculopathy as seen in a sungazing drug abuser.

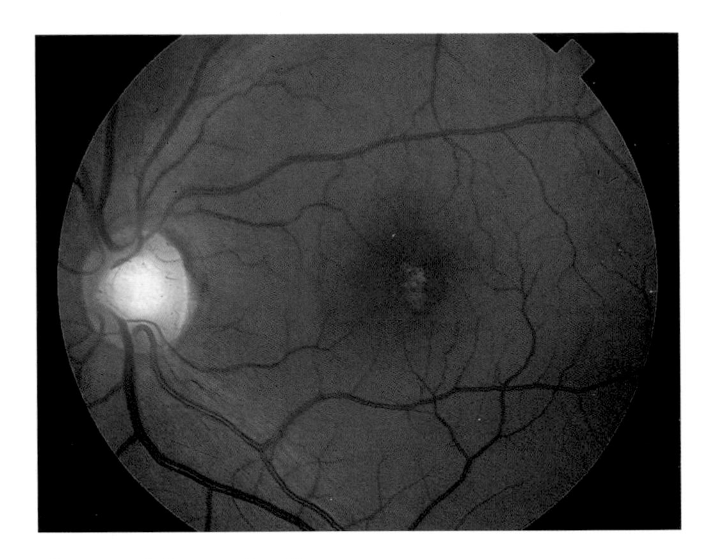

Plate 67. Solar maculopathy.

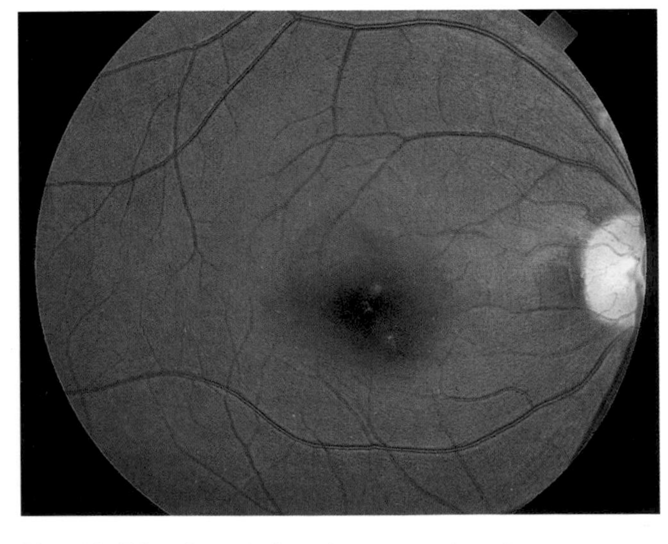

Plate 68. Talc retinopathy in an intravenous drug abuser.

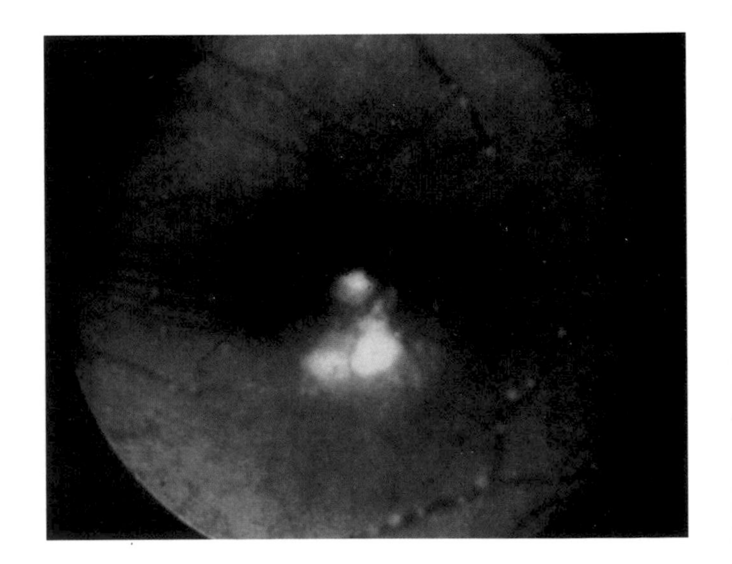

Plate 69. Candida retinitis.

Section X

INFECTIOUS DISORDERS

Chapter 42

TUBERCULOSIS

Esther S. Marks

Tuberculosis (TB) is an ancient granulomatous infection caused by *Mycobacterium tuberculosis*. Although it primarily affects the lungs, TB can attack many other tissues and organs, including most ocular structures, in particular the uvea. It has long been and continues to be a tremendous source of worldwide morbidity and mortality. In the past, a patient with consumption (TB) was relegated to a sanitorium until recovery or death occurred. Advances in medicine, both preventive and therapeutic, appeared to have set the stage for eradication of this disease. However, significant setbacks have occurred with the emergence of the HIV epidemic and new multidrug-resistant strains of TB (MDR-TB).

EPIDEMIOLOGY

Systemic

Tuberculosis continues to be a serious multinational health problem with a staggering 1.7 billion persons infected worldwide, approximately one third of the world's population (Sudre et al, 1992). Twenty million persons suffer from active disease. Approximately 8 million new cases and an estimated 3 million TB-related deaths occur each year (Kochi, 1991).

From 1953 (when national reporting of TB first began) to 1984, the United States experienced a steady annual decrease in the number of cases reported to the Centers for Disease Control and Prevention (CDC). However, in 1985 this downward trend halted, and from 1986 to 1992 the number of cases increased by 20% (McCray et al, 1997). This upward trend has been attributed to the HIV epidemic, increased immigration from TB-endemic countries, shrinking TB prevention and control programs, and the emergence of drug-resistant and MDR-TB. As a result of increased funding to state and local health departments for TB prevention and control programs, the number of reported cases fell by 5% in 1993, and has continued to fall on average 5 to 7% per year (Binkin et al, 1999; CDC, 1997).

In the United States almost 70% of all TB cases involve racial minorities, and approximately 86% of infected children (14 years and younger) are from ethnic minorities. The risk of TB is greatest among Asians and Pacific Islanders, followed by non-Hispanic African-Americans, Hispanics, Native Americans and Alaskan Natives, and lastly non-Hispanic whites (McCray et al, 1997). The presence of HIV infection appears to confer a 100 times greater risk of contracting TB, and homelessness a 150 to 300 times greater risk (Hamrick & Yeager, 1988). Although the case rate for the entire United States in 1996 was 8 per 100,000, a limited number of states and urban areas claim the majority of TB cases.

Many factors are known to carry an increased risk for TB. Certain genetic factors increase patient susceptibility. Diabetes mellitus, silicosis, gastrectomy, malnutrition, alcoholism, some hematologic disorders, certain malignancies, and disorders or medications resulting in immunosuppression (e.g., HIV infection or long-term corticosteroid use) confer poor resistance to TB infection or reactivation. Socioeconomic groups such as persons of low income and the medically underserved (e.g., the homeless and racial minorities) and demographic groups such as residents of poor housing, shelters, and correctional institutions, as well as residents of healthcare facilities such as mental institutions and nursing homes, also contribute to an increased risk. Persons new to the United States and born in high-TB-prevalence countries (e.g., the countries of Asia, Africa, and South America) have a higher risk of TB. TB continues to be a disease of the elderly (primarily due to reactivation of latent infection). Men are almost twice as likely as women to have active TB.

Only 5% of patients infected with TB will develop active disease within 1 year. Approximately 5% more will develop clinical disease later in life. Reactivation of latent TB accounts for about 90% of active TB cases in the United States. The remaining 10% are due to primary infection.

Active TB manifests overwhelmingly as pulmonary cases in males. Extrapulmonary TB accounts for less than 20% of all cases (Rieder et al, 1990). Lymphatic TB and pleural TB each account for approximately 25%, miliary TB (with or without meningeal TB) occurs in about 14%, genitourinary TB about 12.5%, bone and joint TB about 9%, and peritoneal, pericardial, renal, hepatic, and dermatologic TB account for the rest (Comstock & O'Brien, 1990). Overall, these extrapulmonary cases are more common in minorities, females, children (14 years and younger), and foreign-born persons.

Most alarming is the recent increase in drug-resistant TB cases, particularly MDR-TB. Most cases appear to occur in HIV clinics or wards involving HIV-infected patients or healthcare workers (Beck-Sagué et al, 1992). From 1982 to 1986, MDR-TB occurred in only 0.5% of new cases, and only 3% of recurrent cases. In 1991, MDR-TB occurred in 3.1% of new cases and 6.9% of recurrent cases (CDC, 1992a). In a study by Frieden and associates (1993), all New York City patients with available *Mycobacterium tuberculosis*–positive cultures in April 1991 were examined for TB drug susceptibility. A startling 33% were found to be resistant to one or more anti-TB medications. The main culprit appears to be prior inadequate treatment of TB, allowing reactivation and transmission of a now drug-resistant organism. However, the rates of drug-resistant TB in New York City have fallen to 6% of all TB cases (Lama & Frohman, 1998).

Ocular

The rate of ocular TB traditionally has been reported in the literature as extremely low (1 to 2%) (Biswas & Badrinath, 1996). However, Bouza and co-workers (1997), in a study of 100 cases of culture-proven TB, found the surprisingly high ocular TB rate of 18%. Further studies following strict diagnostic criteria are required to confirm the rate of ocular manifestations of TB.

PATHOPHYSIOLOGY/DISEASE PROCESS

The Organism

Thirty species are recognized in the genus *Mycobacterium.* Some, such as *M. avium* and *M. intracellulare,* are ubiquitous to the environment, posing a serious threat mainly in the immunocompromised (e.g., the *M. avium-intracellulare* [MAI] complex in AIDS patients). *Mycobacterium bovis* was a greater threat to humans prior to widespread dairy cattle tuberculin testing and the pasteurization of milk.

However, *M. tuberculosis* has remained a threat to humankind. An aerobic, acid-fast staining bacillus (AFB), *M. tuberculosis* does not contain or secrete toxins. It is slow-growing, requiring generation times of approximately 14 to 24 hours, and several weeks for isolation by culture.

Transmission

Mycobacterium tuberculosis most often is transmitted human to human via inhalation of aerosolized bacilli from sputum droplets. If an actively infectious patient talks, coughs, sneezes, or sings, a spray of sputum, infected with tubercle bacilli, is secreted. The larger particles expelled simply drop out of the air onto available surfaces. These particles rarely reaerosolize; therefore it is difficult to become infected by handling an infectious patient's belongings. Smaller particles evaporate. The now desiccated and quite light bacilli may float on air currents for some time before settling very slowly. The bacilli are rapidly killed by ultraviolet radiation, including daylight. Therefore, poorly ventilated, dark rooms may aid in the transmission of this infection.

Course of the Disease

Once inhaled, the bacilli travel via the bronchi to the alveoli of the lungs. The invading bacilli are engulfed by alveolar phagocytes. These phagocytes, usually unable to destroy the microorganisms, transport the bacilli to regional lymph nodes. Along the way, the pleural space may become infected. Dissemination from the lymph nodes may occur hematogenously. Approximately 3 to 8 weeks later, a hypersensitivity reaction to TB antigens occurs. At this point the host will respond positively to a tuberculin skin test. Granuloma formation occurs as host phagocytes are activated to better entrap and kill the bacilli. The result is foci of epithelioid cells, lymphocytes, and fibroblasts surrounding a central area of caseous necrosis. Some bacilli are capable of surviving within the phagocytes and foci for years.

Primary infection rarely leads to clinical disease. Only 10% of infected patients will develop active disease. Dissemination of TB may occur during the primary infection or may occur during a reactivation of a latent infection. Most infected sites heal, leaving scar tissue and calcification.

Systemic

Pulmonary TB

Active TB may present as either pulmonary or extrapulmonary (Table 42–1). Pulmonary TB is much more common, accounting for more than 80% of all cases, and is almost always symptomatic. Patients present with a chronic productive (mucoid or muco-purulent) cough, often of several weeks' duration. Hemoptysis (coughing up blood), although very common, is usually indicative of advanced disease. A low-grade fever, weight loss, anorexia, and fatigue may be present. A dull and aching chest pain may occur. Liquefaction of the caseous foci and microbial proliferation result in the formation of pulmonary cavities. Infrequently, pulmonary TB may present as an acute respiratory illness mimicking pneumonia or influenza. Pleurisy (inflammation of the pleura) with effusion (the leakage of fluid from lymphatics or blood vessels) may result.

> Pulmonary TB should always be suspected in a patient with chronic productive cough, hemoptysis, and chest pain.

Untreated pulmonary TB is a chronic, slowly progressive, and relapsing disease, although one third of patients may develop a stable nonprogressive course (Daniel & Tripathy, 1989). An untreated patient remains infectious for about 2 years, allowing the contagious patient to infect approximately 10 other persons per year depending on the housing conditions (Chaulet & Mulder, 1987).

TABLE 42–1. SYSTEMIC MANIFESTATIONS OF TUBERCULOSIS

General Constitutional Symptoms
- Low-grade fever
- Anorexia
- Weight loss
- Fatigue

Pulmonary TB
- Chronic productive (purulent or mucopurulent) cough
- Hemoptysis
- Dull aching chest pain
- Possible pleural effusion
- Rales on auscultation
- Classic x-ray: infiltrates, granulomas, with cavitation in apices of lungs
- Hilar and/or mediastinal lymphadenopathy
- (+) PPD and (+) AFB on sputum culture

Extrapulmonary TB

Miliary TB
- Multiple lesions on various organs
- Mild anemia and increased alkaline phosphatase
- Chest x-ray and PPD often (−)

TB meningitis
- Headache, abnormal behavior
- Altered consciousness, convulsions, coma
- (+) PPD
- CSF demonstrates increased protein, decreased glucose and chloride, pleocytosis, and (+) AFB culture

Pleural TB
- Pleural effusion
- Pleuritic pain
- (+) PPD and (+) AFB cultured from pleuritic fluid

Lymphatic TB
- Multiple granulomatous lymphadenitis
- Involves hilar, mediastinal, cervical, and supraclavicular
- (+) PPD, and (+) AFB culture of pus or lymph biopsy

Genitourinary TB
- Chronic recurrent urinary tract infections
- Nodular induration of prostate or vas deferens
- Pelvic inflammatory disease
- Amenorrhea
- Infertility
- (+) PPD, possible (+) AFB cultured from urine or biopsied from endometrium

Bone and joint TB
- Localized pain and swelling
- Possible abscesses
- Decreased joint spaces and joint damage
- (+) PPD

Other organ involvement
- Pericardium
- Liver
- Spleen
- Brain
- Skin

Abbreviations: AFB, acid-fast bacillus; CSF, colony-stimulating factor; PPD, purified protein derivative of tuberculin.

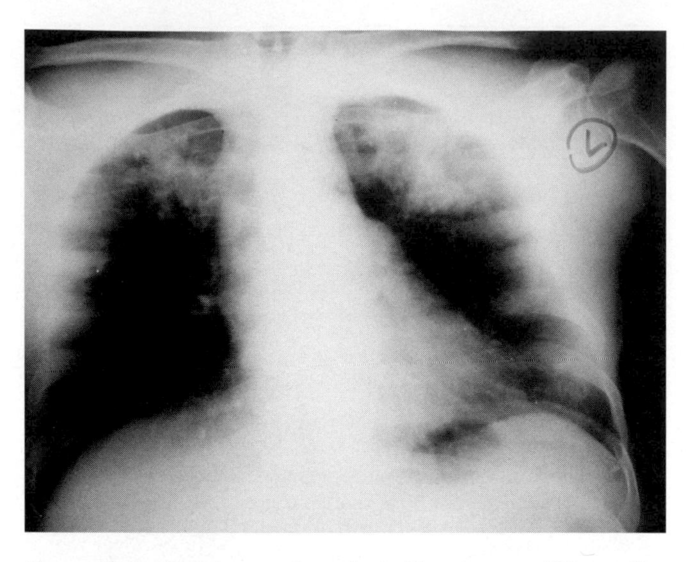

Figure 42–1. Chest x-ray of a patient with pulmonary TB revealing bilateral upper lung infiltrate, with lucencies in the infiltrate suggesting cavitation.

Extrapulmonary TB

Extrapulmonary TB, less than 20% of all TB cases, may take different forms. Hematogenous dissemination may result in miliary (millet seed size) TB. Multiple small lesions develop in the lungs, spleen, liver, and elsewhere. More common in the young and the elderly, the diagnosis may be missed because of the nonspecific symptoms, and often, negative chest x-ray and skin test. One exception is when TB meningitis occurs concurrently (usually in children). In this case (or when TB meningitis occurs in isolation), the symptoms are remarkable for headache, abnormal behavior, altered consciousness, and convulsions. Coma and death may occur without treatment.

Lymphatic TB is characterized by multiple granulomatous lymphadenitis. The hilar and mediastinal nodes are commonly involved, followed by the cervical and supraclavicular. Pleural TB (in the absence of pulmonary TB) is characterized by a pleural effusion, which progresses for 1 to 2 weeks, and pleuritic chest pain.

Genitourinary TB may present in a variety of ways, because any portion of the genitourinary tract may become involved. It may manifest as chronic recurrent urinary tract infections, nodular induration of the prostate or vas deferens, pelvic inflammatory disease, or amenorrhea. Infertility may result.

Bone and joint TB is believed to be caused by a reactivation of dormant foci. It most commonly involves the vertebrae of the spine (Pott disease), the large joints, and occasionally the long bones. Localized pain, swelling, and even abscess formation may occur, resulting in functional disability.

Peritoneal TB is thought to result from hematogenous dissemination, or extension from mesenteric lymph nodes or genitourinary involvement. Classically, it presents with painless ascites. However, it may also present as a fibroadhesive peritonitis, producing a tender abdomen, and abdominal masses.

Other organs may become involved in TB including the pericardium, liver, spleen, brain, and skin.

Ocular

Ocular disease secondary to systemic TB may manifest in a wide variety of ways (Table 42–2). Virtually all ocular structures (except the crystalline lens) may be affected. Most commonly, it affects the uvea, presenting as an anterior uveitis or disseminated choroiditis. Ocular manifestations may be due to hematogenous or contiguous spread of the organism (resulting in tubercle or granuloma formation in almost any ocular tissue), or due to a hypersensitivity reaction to TB proteins (resulting in phlyctenulosis, scleritis, retinal vasculitis, or most commonly uveitis). It may present during primary, latent, or reactivation infections. There also have been reports of ocular TB with no evidence of extraocular TB (Mansour & Haymond, 1990; Žorić et al, 1996).

Choroiditis may present with mild to severe vision loss, vitritis, disc swelling, choroidal or retinal yellow-white infiltrates, and anterior chamber reaction (usually granulomatous, although nongranulomatous also may occur). Periphlebitis with a macular exudative star and hemorrhages as well as neovascularization may occur. Anterior uveitis may present acutely, chronically, or recurrently. Acute episodes are marked by typical signs: circumlimbal injection, anterior chamber reaction with possible vitreal spillover, posterior synechiae, granulomatous keratic precipitates, and iris nodules. Signs and symptoms are greater in acute episodes.

> Tuberculosis should always be considered in the differential diagnosis of anterior or posterior uveitis, granulomatous or not, particularly in a patient at risk for TB.

Conjunctivitis may present as a unilateral red eye with a small nodule or painless ulcer on the palpebral conjunctiva. It may be surrounded by nodules or hypertrophic lesions. Regional lymphadenopathy can occur. Phlyctenular keratoconjunctivitis (Figure 42–2), once synonymous with TB, is now known to be due to a delayed hypersensitivity reaction to many different infectious organisms. The patient usually presents

TABLE 42–2. OCULAR MANIFESTATIONS OF TUBERCULOSIS[a]

Uveitis with or without Retinal Vasculitis
- May be acute, chronic, or recurrent
- Usually granulomatous
- Variable decrease in visual acuity
- Anterior: cells, flare, keratic precipitates, iris nodules
- Disseminated: vitreitis, vitreal hemorrhage, periphlebitis, macular exudative star, retinal hemorrhages, capillary closure, and neovascularization

Tubercles (Granulomas)
- May occur in lids, conjunctiva, sclera, cornea, uvea (especially the choroid), optic nerve, and orbit

Conjunctivitis
- Usually a small unilateral nodule or ulcer on the palpebral conjunctiva
- May be surrounded by nodules or hypertrophic lesions
- Local lymphadenopathy may occur
- Usually painless or foreign-body sensation
- (+) AFB in conjunctival scrappings

Phlyctenular Keratoconjunctivitis
- Unilateral or bilateral white nodule on bulbar conjunctiva or at limbus (may migrate toward corneal axis)
- Discomfort, photophobia
- Tearing, blepharospasm
- Secondary bacterial infection
- Corneal ulcer and scarring may occur
- Acuity may be affected if visual axis involved

Interstitial Keratitis
- Acute:
  - Tearing, photophobic painful red eye
  - Acuity variably affected depending on location of lesion
  - Unilateral corneal stromal patent blood vessels
  - Corneal edema and possible anterior chamber reaction
- Inactive:
  - Unilateral corneal stromal scarring with ghost vessels
  - Acuity variably affected depending on location of lesion

Scleritis
- Variably decreased acuity
- Varying pain, tearing, photophobia
- Conjunctival, episcleral, and scleral injection (diffuse or sectoral)
- Scleral nodules may be present
- Anterior chamber reaction may occur

Optic Neuropathy Secondary to EMB
- Decreased visual acuity
- Visual field defects (central or peripheral)
- Abnormal color perception (especially green)

[a]Almost all ocular structures (except the crystalline lens) may be affected by TB.

with a nodule on the bulbar conjunctiva, or at the limbus. The small white lesion is surrounded by an area of hyperemia. The lesion may migrate toward the central cornea, producing neovascularization and ulceration. The presentation may be unilateral or bilateral. Conjunctival injection is present, and a secondary bacterial infection may occur.

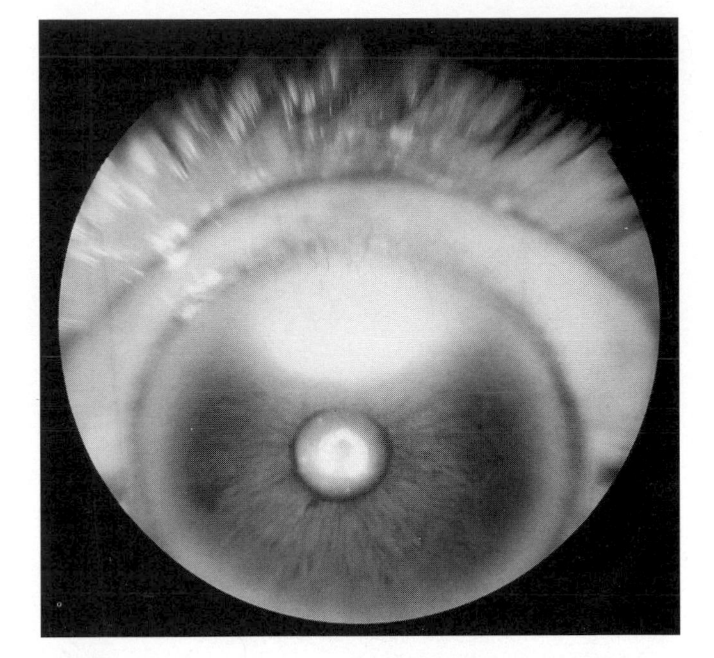

Figure 42–2. Corneal scarring secondary to old phlyctenular keratoconjunctivitis.

Unilateral interstitial keratitis may present acutely or as a sign of old disease. In the acute stage, the cornea will demonstrate patent stromal blood vessels, corneal edema, conjunctival injection, and possible anterior chamber reaction. In the inactive stage, the cornea will reveal stromal scarring with ghost vessels. In both stages, visual acuity may be decreased depending on the area of corneal involvement.

Scleritis may occur with usually moderate to severe pain. The conjunctival, episcleral, and scleral vessels will be inflamed diffusely or sectorally. Scleral nodules may be present, along with corneal involvement and anterior chamber reaction.

Toxic optic neuropathy (caused by the anti-TB medication ethambutol) may present with blurry vision. This may present as either decreased acuity or central visual field defects, or both. Patients may also complain of altered color vision.

DIAGNOSIS

The presumptive diagnosis of tuberculosis is obtained through careful history, physical examination, radiographic findings, and skin testing (Tables 42–3 and 42–4). Definitive diagnosis requires direct microscopy of a clinical specimen, usually a smear, laboratory identification and isolation of *M. tuberculosis* via culture, and drug sensitivity testing. Unfortunately, this organism is

TABLE 42–3. DIAGNOSTIC TESTS FOR TUBERCULOSIS

Systemic—Pulmonary TB
Presumptive diagnosis
- PPD with anergy panel
- Chest x-ray or CT scan

Definitive diagnosis
- Direct microscopy and culture of sputum or lung biopsy with drug sensitivity testing

Newer tests
- PCR assay
- Serum ELISA
- HPLC

Ocular—Uveal Involvement
CBC
Erythrocyte sedimentation rate (ESR) or C-reactive protein (CRP)
Serum chemistries
Serum ACE
Syphilis serology
ANA
Toxoplasmosis titer
Lyme titer
Fluorescein and/or indocyanine green angiography
PCR assay of ocular fluid or tissue

Abbreviations: ACE, angiotensin-converting enzyme; CBC, complete blood cell count; CT, computerized tomography; ELISA, enzyme-linked immunosorbent assay; HPLC, high-performance liquid chromatography; PCR, polymerase chain reaction; PPD, purified protein derivative.

very slow-growing; therefore, weeks may elapse prior to definitive diagnosis by culture.

The tuberculin skin test checks for a delayed hypersensitivity reaction of the skin to 0.1 mL (containing five test units) of intradermally injected purified protein derivative (PPD) of the *Mycobacterium.* The Mantoux technique of a single puncture is preferred over the Tine method of multiple punctures in which the amount of antigen delivered is difficult to control. The injection site should raise a wheal 6 to 10 mm in diameter. It must be evaluated 48 to 72 hours later to determine the presence and amount (in millimeters) of induration. Erythema need not be noted. Generally, a reaction of 10 mm or greater is considered positive; however, this varies with the health of the patient, as other conditions that alter cell-mediated immunity or delayed hypersensitivity reactions can alter reaction to the PPD. Patients with HIV/AIDS are usually considered positive with an induration of 5 mm or greater, as are patients who have had recent and close contact to TB, or those whose chest x-ray demonstrates presumptive TB. Approximately 15% of patients acutely ill with TB will have a negative PPD. These false-negative reactions may occur due to concurrent viral, bacterial, or fungal infections, lymphatic diseases, immunosuppressive medications or illnesses, age (in very young infants and in the elderly), surgery, stress, or live virus vaccinations.

TABLE 42–4. DIFFERENTIAL DIAGNOSIS OF TUBERCULOSIS

Systemic—Pulmonary TB
Sarcoidosis
Histoplasmosis
Atypical mycobacteria
Coccidioidomycosis
Cryptococcosis
Aspergillosis
Blastomycosis
Leprosy
Tumor-related granulomas
Wegener granulomatosis
Hypersensitivity pneumonitis
Interstitial pneumonia
Drug reactions
Aspiration of foreign matter

Ocular—Uveitis
Choroidal involvement
Infectious
- Syphilis
- Histoplasmosis
- Toxoplasmosis
- Toxocara
- Lyme disease
- Brucellosis

Yersinia
- Atypical mycobacteria
- *Pneumocystis carinii*
- Coccidioidomycosis
- Cryptococcosis
- Aspergillosis

Inflammatory/autoimmune
- Sarcoidosis
- Polyarteritis nodosa
- Rheumatoid arthritis
- Behçet disease
- Wegener granulomatosis
- Birdshot choroidopathy
- Acute posterior multifocal placoid pigment epitheliopathy
- Recurrent multifocal choroiditis
- Serpiginous choroidopathy

Other
- Neoplasm

Anterior uveitis
Granulomatous
- Syphilis
- Sarcoidosis
- Lyme disease
- Leprosy

Nongranulomatous
- Ankylosing spondylitis
- Reiter syndrome
- Psoriatic arthritis
- Inflammatory bowel disease
- Juvenile rheumatoid arthritis
- Systemic lupus erythematosus
- Behçet disease

Radiographic examination is required in a suspected case of TB regardless of the results of skin testing. Chest x-ray patterns may be quite varied. The appearance of infiltrates and cavitation, especially in the apices of the lungs, is characteristic of pulmonary TB. Hilar lymphadenopathy may or may not be present. Patients with concurrent HIV/AIDS may not demonstrate cavities, fibrosis, or granuloma formation because of their poor immune response. TB may also present in the middle or lower lobes, along with mediastinal lymphadenopathy and pleural effusion. Unfortunately, because characteristic patterns are not always seen, a misdiagnosis of pneumonia, malignancy, histoplasmosis, etc, may be made. Any presumptive radiologic diagnosis of TB must be confirmed by the isolation of *M. tuberculosis* in the sputum or lung tissue.

Microscopic examination of sputum, blood, pleural fluid, cerebrospinal fluid (CSF), pus, or body tissues by biopsy may reveal the tubercle bacilli. Culturing the sample has traditionally taken several weeks (usually 4 to 6) because of the organism's slow growth. As a result, research into the development of genetic and immunologic probes for the rapid but reliable identification of TB has resulted in exciting new test techniques. Nucleic acid probes have been developed that require 2 weeks' incubation period. However, newer DNA target amplification using polymerase chain reaction (PCR) technology has dramatically decreased the time needed to obtain results. These DNA probes, for example, the Gen-Probe *M. tuberculosis* Direct Test (MTDT) and Roche Amplicor *M. tuberculosis* Test, are highly sensitive and specific, and require less than 24 hours for results (Lama & Frohman, 1998). Enzyme-linked immunosorbent assay (ELISA) for the measurement of IgG to antigens of *M. tuberculosis* in serum is rapid and simple, and may help expedite the diagnosis of complicated cases (Amicosante et al, 1999).

Mycolic acids are part of all mycobacterium cells. Each species contains different amounts and types. High-performance liquid chromatography (HPLC) is a method used to identify *M. tuberculosis* by its mycolic acid pattern. The technique requires only a couple of hours, but still must have sufficient cells (2 to 3 weeks' growth) to identify the organism (Good & Mastro, 1989). The equipment required is too costly for routine use (Fadda & Sanguinetti, 1998).

Systemic

Pulmonary TB

Pulmonary TB is suspected in a patient with chronic productive cough, hemoptysis, and chest pain. Auscultation of the chest may reveal rales over the affected area. Tuberculin skin testing should be positive. Chest radiography should be abnormal. Definitive diagnosis is obtained via smear and culture of sputum. PCR testing may be performed. If necessary, bronchoscopy or lung biopsy may be performed.

Extrapulmonary TB

Pleural TB may occur with or without pulmonary TB. It may be diagnosed by pleuritic chest pain and evidence of pleuritic effusion on chest x-ray. A positive PPD, and identification of the mycobacterium via culture of the pleuritic fluid will aid in the diagnosis.

Miliary TB is characterized by persistent fever and may involve many organs. Chest x-rays are often normal, and skin testing is often negative. There may be a mild anemia and mild elevation of alkaline phosphatase, but physical examination is often unrevealing. Diagnosis is difficult, and may require blood cultures or liver or bone marrow needle biopsy.

If TB meningitis is present, the characteristic symptoms of headache and altered consciousness are present. Skin testing is usually positive. Laboratory analysis of the CSF will reveal increased protein, decreased glucose, decreased chloride, and pleocytosis. Culture of the CSF will reveal *M. tuberculosis.*

Lymphatic TB is characterized by multiple granulomatous lymphadenitis on physical examination. The tuberculin skin test is usually strongly positive. Culture of the pus from a node or biopsy of the node will reveal *M. tuberculosis.* Bone and joint TB may be diagnosed by positive skin testing and confirmed by culture of pus from abscesses. Radiographic examination of the vertebrae and other joints will reveal decreased joint spaces and bone damage.

Genitourinary TB may present in a multitude of ways. Diagnosis relies on physical examination (pelvic, prostate), as well as potential laparoscopy, endometrium biopsy, and examination and culture of the urine. Peritoneal TB may be diagnosed by the presence of a positive PPD, ascites (serous fluid–filled peritoneal cavity), and in the fibroadhesive form, may require stool cultures, digestive tract x-rays, laparoscopy or laparotomy, abdominal sonograms, or computerized tomography (CT).

Other forms of extrapulmonary TB require additional testing. Pericardial TB calls for an electrocardiogram, and possible pericardial puncture. Suspected tuberculomas (TB granulomas) of the brain may necessitate a variety of brain scans (CT and magnetic resonance imaging). Suspected dermatologic involvement may require skin biopsy.

Ocular

A good history, both medical and ocular, as well as thorough ocular examination, will reveal any suspected manifestations of TB. Choroiditis may present as a blurry, painful, photophobic eye with the complaint of floaters. Sheathing of retinal vessels may be seen. In the case of choroidal or retinal manifestations, fluorescein and/or indocyanine green angiography may be necessary to determine the extent of the chorioretinal involvement, capillary closure, and existence of neovascularization. Anterior uveitis (unilateral or bilateral) may present with a red, painful, photophobic, tearing eye, if acute. Acuity is variably affected. Chronic cases have fewer symptoms.

Conjunctivitis may present as a unilateral red eye, possible foreign-body sensation, and a palpebral nodule, with ipsilateral lymphadenopathy. Phlyctenular disease, unilateral or bilateral, presents with tearing, discomfort or pain, and photophobia. Corneal phlyctenulosis will cause more severe symptoms than conjunctival involvement alone. Unilateral interstitial keratitis acutely presents as a tearing, photophobic, red eye. In inactive cases, the patient may be unaware of past red eyes or current corneal scarring.

Scleritis will produce a painful, diffusely or sectorally red eye. Tearing, photophobia, and decreased vision may occur. Toxic optic neuropathy may be diagnosed by decreased visual acuity, visual field defects—central or peripheral, and abnormal green color vision.

Suspected ocular manifestations of TB require a systemic TB workup (Tables 42–3 and 42–4). At minimum, a tuberculin skin test should be performed. If positive, or if the clinician has a high index of suspicion, further testing should be done. A chest x-ray is mandated, with smears, cultures, and PCR testing of bodily fluids or tissues performed as needed.

Ocular TB testing may include histopathologic examination of ocular tissues (eg, conjunctival scrapping or chorioretinal biopsy). Purulent discharge from conjunctivitis or scleritis may be cultured, as may the aqueous and vitreous. PCR testing may be run on ocular fluids (Bowyer et al, 1999; Gupta et al, 1998).

TREATMENT AND MANAGEMENT

Combination therapy for active TB is required to avoid drug resistance problems (Table 42–5). Chemotherapy may last longer than 1 year, although multiple drug regimens have shortened treatment times. Nonadherence to drug regimens has contributed to relapses, acquired resistance, and transmission of TB. To address this issue, city departments of health have implemented an outpatient strategy of directly observed therapy (DOT) under the supervision of a healthcare provider (Chaulk & Kazandjian, 1998). This has been accomplished by dose adjustments from daily to twice weekly. Anti-TB drugs must be used with caution in patients with other conditions (eg, liver or kidney dysfunction, gout, diabetes, pregnancy) because of their potentially serious side effects. The most serious and disturbing new challenge in TB today is MDR-TB. This entity has created much alarm in the health community, and has prompted the CDC to change drug regimen recommendations.

Systemic

Pulmonary TB

The first-line medications commonly used are isoniazid (INH), rifampin (RIF), pyrazinamide (PZA), ethambutol (EMB), and streptomycin (SM). Because of potential toxic side effects, baseline tests may be recommended prior to starting therapy. These may include liver and kidney function tests, complete blood count, audiometry, and visual acuity testing. INH, RIF, and PZA each may induce hepatitis. INH increases urinary excretion of pyroxidine. This may lead to pellagra (a disorder caused by a deficiency of niacin), particularly in malnourished, pregnant, uremic, or diabetic patients. Therefore, these patients are often given supplemental daily pyroxidine. Gastrointestinal upset can occur with RIF and PZA. PZA may also cause hyperuricemia. EMB may cause optic neuropathy; therefore its use requires ocular monitoring. SM may alter hearing and vestibular function, and may be toxic to the kidney. Hypersensitivity reactions may occur with any of the drugs. Monthly monitoring for toxic side effects is extremely important.

In the face of acquired drug resistance, second-line medications may be necessary. These include fluoroquinolones, ethionamide, cyclosporine, para-aminosalicylate, capreomycin, kanamycin, and amikacin. Although the fluoroquinolones have minimal side effects, the other second-line medications may cause serious toxic side effects, requiring routine monitoring and possibly precluding their use.

The CDC-recommended drug regimens for TB in HIV-negative or HIV-positive adults or children are usually the same with two exceptions. Drug doses in children are lower, and therapy lasts longer in HIV-positive patients (usually a minimum of 9 months versus the standard minimum of 6 months). There are several different options in terms of drug combinations and length of therapy. Traditionally, INH and RIF are utilized, along with a third medication (PZA, EMB, or SM) in order to shorten the duration of the therapeutic regimen. In response to the rise of MDR-TB, the CDC recommendation is to initiate four-drug therapy routinely with INH, RIF, PZA, and EMB or SM. This

TABLE 42–5. TREATMENT AND MANAGEMENT OF TUBERCULOSIS

SYSTEMIC: PULMONARY AND EXTRAPULMONARY TB[a]

First-line medications

Therapy regimen for minimum 6 months (standard), minimum 9 months (HIV/AIDS and extrapulmonary TB), up to 18–24 months (MDR-TB)

Doses listed below are for adults; pediatric doses are similar or lower

- Isoniazid (INH) 5–10 mg/kg/day (max 300 mg/day) or 15 mg/kg (max 900 mg) twice weekly (consider adding pyridoxine 10–50 mg/day) *plus*
- Rifampin (RIF) 10 mg/kg/day (max 600 mg/day) or 10 mg/kg/day (max 600 mg) twice weekly *plus*
- Pyrazinamide (PZA) 15–30 mg/kg/day (max 2 g/day) or 50–70 mg/kg (max 4 g) twice weekly *plus*
- Ethambutol (EMB) 15–25 mg/kg/day (max 2.5 g/day) or 50 mg/kg (max 2.5 g) twice weekly *or*
- Streptomycin (SM) 15 mg/kg/day (max 1 g/day) or 25–30 mg/kg (max 1.5 g) twice weekly

Second-line medications

Used in case of hypersensitivity reaction or multidrug resistance

- Fluoroquinolones
  - Ciprofloxacin 500–750 mg
  - Ofloxacin 300–800 mg
- Ethionamide 500–1000 mg
- Cycloserine 250–1000 mg (pyridoxine 150 mg/day recommended adjunct therapy)
- Para-aminosalicylate 10–12 g
- Capreomycin 15 mg/kg
- Kanamycin 15 mg/kg
- Amikacin 15 mg/kg

Experimental medications

- Rifamycins
- Fluoroquinolones
- Nitroimidazoles
- Adjuvant cytokines—IL-2, IFN-gamma, IL-12, granulocyte-macrophage colony-stimulating factor (GM-CSF)

Other

- Occasional oral corticosteroid use
- Rare surgical intervention

OCULAR TB[b]

Anterior uveitis

- Topical steroids (e.g., 1.0% prednisolone acetate q1h to qid)
- Cycloplegics (e.g., 1.0% cyclopentolate, 2% or 5% homatropine, or 0.25% scopolamine bid to tid)

Choroiditis with or without retinal vasculitis

- Photocoagulation may be necessary if widespread capillary dropout or neovascularization occurs

Tubercles, granulomas

- Systemic treatment only

Conjunctivitis

- Warm compresses
- Artificial tears

Phlyctenular keratoconjunctivitis

- Topical steroids (e.g., 1.0% prednisolone acetate q2h to qid depending on severity) with rapid taper
- Broad-spectrum antibiotic if secondary bacterial infection exists

Interstitial keratitis

Acute:

- Topical steroids (e.g., 1.0% prednisolone acetate q1h to qid with slow taper)
- Topical cycloplegics (e.g., 5% homatropine bid to tid)

Inactive:

- Consider corneal transplant surgery if central cornea involved

Scleritis

- NSAIDs (e.g., ibuprofen 400–600 mg PO qid or indomethacin 25 mg PO tid × 1 week)
- Oral prednisone 60–80 mg qd with slow taper

Note: Oral steroid treatment requires concurrent systemic anti-TB treatment

Optic neuropathy secondary to EMB

- Reversible with early prompt discontinuation of EMB

[a]Directly observed therapy is recommended.

[b]Always start with systemic treatment.

Abbreviations: bid, twice a day; h, hour; NSAIDs, nonsteroidal anti-inflammatory drugs; PO, orally; q, each, every; qid, four times daily; tid, three times a day.

initial four-drug regimen may be altered after drug susceptibility testing has been done.

When MDR-TB is suspected in a patient, the four-drug regimen should be instituted along with one or two additional second-line anti-TB drugs. Testing must be done to ensure that the resistant strain is susceptible to at least three of the medications. The drug regimen must be lengthened to as long as 18 to 24 months. New experimental anti-TB medications are under investigation to simplify drug regimens and to aid in the treatment of drug-resistant TB. These include the rifamycin, fluoroquinolone, and nitroimidazole families; as well as adjuvant therapy with immune boosters called cytokines. These show real promise in shortening the duration of TB treatment and overcoming drug resistance. Other treatment research includes drugs that attack TB enzymes and disrupt TB DNA transcription and TB genetic modification (Schraufnagel, 1999).

Treatment during pregnancy is essential with a few provisos. SM may cause congenital deafness and therefore should be avoided, as should PZA, since its effects on the developing fetus are uncertain. With the recommended four-drug regimen now unavailable (two of the available five anti-TB drugs have been eliminated due to teratogenicity), treatment must be extended for 9 months. Despite the presence of these drugs in breast milk, the concentrations are so low they will cause neither adverse nor therapeutic effects on a nursing infant.

Extrapulmonary TB

Extrapulmonary TB follows the same treatment regimens as pulmonary TB, although the duration of therapy may be extended to 9 months, with occasional corticosteroid use and rare surgical intervention.

Ocular

Ocular manifestations of TB are treated with standard systemic anti-TB regimens, along with ocular medications when indicated (Table 42–5). Anterior uveitis requires topical corticosteroids and cycloplegics. Chorioretinal involvement may require pan or sector retinal photocoagulation to treat or prevent neovascularization.

Conjunctivitis is treated with warm compresses and artificial tears. Phlyctenular keratoconjunctivitis is typically treated with topical steroids (with taper), and topical antibiotics for secondary infections. Acute interstitial keratitis may be managed with topical steroids (with slow taper) and cycloplegics. Corneal transplant surgery should be considered in inactive disease with central corneal scarring.

Scleritis calls for systemic medications—nonsteroidal anti-inflammatory drugs (NSAIDs) or oral steroids. Oral corticosteroids, given in isolation to control severe ocular inflammation, may cause a reactivation of latent infection, and therefore should only be given after anti-TB therapy has been instituted. Toxic optic neuropathy due to EMB is treated by immediate replacement of the medication. Normal visual functioning returns if the drug is discontinued early enough.

Prevention

Vaccination

Preventing the transmission or reactivation of TB involves many factors (Table 42–6). Vaccination has long been employed throughout the world to combat TB.

TABLE 42–6. PREVENTION OF TUBERCULOSIS
Vaccination
Bacille Calmette-Guērin (BCG) vaccine not recommended
Other vaccines still experimental
Ventilation and Housing
Good ventilation, with increased daylight, and no recirculation of air
Negative pressure hospital rooms with 6 air changes per hour
Ultraviolet irradiation
Surgical masks have questionable efficacy
Screening
Purified protein derivative (PPD) testing and chest x-rays of certain populations:
HIV/AIDS patients
Persons in close contact with suspected or known TB patients
Persons with medical conditions known to increase risk of contracting TB after exposure
Alcohol or intravenous (IV) drug abusers
Foreign-born persons from countries with high TB prevalence
Medically underserved persons
Residents of long-term facilities (e.g., correctional facilities, mental institutions, nursing homes)
Healthcare workers in repeated contact with high-risk or infected patients
Prophylactic Therapy
Usually isoniazid (INH) for 6–12 months although shorter regimens are being investigated
Directly observed therapy recommended
Recommended for certain populations:
(+) PPD $\geq$ 5 mm *plus* Close recent TB contact *or*
Suspected or definitive HIV infection *or*
Radiographic evidence of old pulmonary TB
(+) PPD $\geq$ 10 mm *plus* Other high-risk factors:
Recent PPD conversion *or*
HIV (−) IV drug abusers *or*
Concurrent medical conditions increasing TB risk or
$\leq$ 35 years and part of high-incidence group:
Foreign-born in high-TB-prevalence countries *or*
Low-income medically underserved *or*
Resident of long-term-care facilities
(+) PPD $\geq$ 15 mm *plus* $\leq$ 35 years with no risk factors, and of a low-incidence group

Unfortunately, the current available vaccine, bacille Calmette-Guérin (BCG), has variable reported protective efficacy. Despite this, there is widespread use of BCG, particularly in countries where TB is highly prevalent. In the United States, TB is not considered a large enough health hazard to warrant implementation of a nationwide vaccination program. Resulting in a positive skin test, BCG vaccination complicates the diagnosis of TB. Derived from in vitro attenuation of *M. bovis*, BCG is a live vaccine, and therefore should be avoided in immunosuppressed patients due to the risk of adverse reactions. Newer vaccines, including DNA, recombinant, auxotrophic, and subunit vaccines, are under investigation (Orme, 1999a).

Ventilation and Housing

Improved ventilation with increased available daylight in public housing and institutions (e.g., correctional facilities, mental health facilities) is important in decreasing the risk of TB transmission. Hospitals should isolate actively infectious TB patients in negative pressure rooms with six air changes per hour. Air should not be recirculated in any facility treating TB patients. Although these ventilation issues are crucial, they are also costly to institutions that may require significant remodeling in order to meet these standards. Instituting ultraviolet irradiation may be less costly and still quite effective (Iseman, 1992).

Teaching infected patients to cover their mouths when coughing or sneezing is important. Due to the minute size of the aerosolized TB-infected droplets, common surgical masking devices often are not particularly effective in preventing transmission. Disposable particulate respirators have been recommended in the past, but implementation has been impractical.

Screening

Screening for TB through tuberculin skin testing and chest x-rays for positive reactors are key weapons in the fight against TB. The following populations should be screened: HIV-positive patients, those in close contact with suspected or known TB patients, persons with medical conditions known to increase the risk of contracting TB after exposure, alcohol and/or intravenous drug abusers, persons from high-prevalence-TB countries, medically underserved persons, residents of long-term care facilities, and healthcare workers in repeated contact with high-risk or infected populations.

Preventive or Prophylactic Therapy

The goal of prophylactic therapy is to prevent reactivation of a latent infection. INH has been found to decrease the incidence of reactivation by 54 to 88% (Levin et al, 1993). The criteria for preventive TB therapy are determined by age, risk factors, and incidence group.

Therapy is recommended for persons of all ages with a positive PPD (5 mm or more) plus close recent TB contact, concurrent suspected or definitive HIV infection, or evidence of old TB on chest x-ray. Treatment is also recommended for patients of all ages with a positive PPD (10 mm or more) plus a high-risk factor. High-risk factors include recent PPD conversion, HIV-negative intravenous substance abuse, or concurrent medical conditions known to increase the risk of TB. Patients with a positive PPD (10 mm or more), no known high-risk factors, but part of a high-incidence group (foreign-born from a high-prevalence country, low-income medically underserved, or resident of long-term-care institution) are candidates for therapy. Patients with a positive PPD ($\geq$ 15 mm or greater), no risk factors, belonging to a low-incidence group, should be treated if younger than 35 years of age.

Standard prophylaxis is INH therapy for 6 to 12 months. Monthly monitoring is key to diagnosing adverse drug effects. Hepatotoxicity is more common in those 35 years and older. If the TB is INH-resistant, rifampin may be used instead. Recent clinical trials suggest that shorter preventative regimens, in HIV-positive patients, may be efficacious and may improve adherence to the treatment protocol (Nolan, 1999).

CONCLUSION

The resurgence of tuberculosis in the mid-1980s, particularly in the form of multidrug-resistant TB, was extremely troubling. Although the rate of tuberculosis cases has been dropping since the early 1990s, TB is not a vanishing disease. Public education, widespread screening (especially of high-risk groups), treatment, and directly observed therapy are crucial to the eradication of this ancient disease. Eyecare practitioners should be alert and suspicious when confronted with an apparently idiopathic uveitis, particularly if in a patient at high risk for TB. The vigilance of all healthcare providers is necessary to successfully combat this disease.

REFERENCES

Aclimandos WA, Kerr-Muir M. Tuberculous keratoconjunctivitis. *Br J Ophthalmol.* 1992;76:175–176.

Alangaden GJ, Lerner SA. The clinical use of fluoroquinolones for the treatment of mycobacterial diseases. *Clin Infect Dis.* 1997;25:1213–1221.

Amicosante M, Houde M, Guaraldi G, Saltini C. Sensitivity and specificity of a multi-antigen ELISA test for the serological diagnosis of tuberculosis. *Int J Tuberc Lung Dis.* 1999;3:736–740.

Bastian I, Colebunders R. Treatment and prevention of multidrug resistant tuberculosis. *Drugs.* 1999;58:633–661.

Beck-Sagué C, et al. Hospital outbreak of multidrug-resistant *Mycobacterium tuberculosis* infections: Factors in transmission to staff and HIV-infected patients. *JAMA.* 1992; 268:1280–1286.

Binkin NJ, Vernon AA, Simone PM, et al. Tuberculosis prevention and control activities in the United States: An overview of the organization of tuberculosis services. *Int J Tuberc Lung Dis.* 1999;3:663–674.

Biswas J, Badrinath SS. Ocular morbidity in patients with active systemic tuberculosis. *Int Ophthalmol.* 1996;19:293–298.

Biswas J, Madhavan HN, Gopal L, Badrinath SS. Intraocular tuberculosis: Clinicopathologic study of five cases. *Retina.* 1995;15:461–468.

Blazquez EP, Rodriguez MM, Mendez Ramos MJ. Tuberculous choroiditis and acquired immunodeficiency syndrome. *Ann Ophthalmol.* 1994;26:50–54.

Bloch AB, et al. The epidemiology of tuberculosis in the United States: Implications for diagnosis and treatment. *Clin Chest Med.* 1989;10:297–313.

Bouza E, Merino P, Muñoz P, et al. Ocular tuberculosis: A prospective study in a general hospital. *Medicine.* 1997; 76:53–61.

Bowyer JD, Gormley PD, Seth R, et al. Choroidal tuberculosis diagnosed by polymerase chain reaction. *Ophthalmology.* 1999;106:290–294.

Braun MM, Coté TR, Rabkin CS. Trends in death with tuberculosis during the AIDS era. *JAMA.* 1993;269:2865–2868.

Brisson-Noel A, et al. Diagnosis of tuberculosis by DNA amplification in clinical practice evaluation. *Lancet.* 1991; 338:364–366.

Burgoyne CF, Verstraeten TC, Friberg TR. Tuberculin skin-test-induced uveitis in the absence of tuberculosis. *Graefes Arch Clin Exp Ophthalmol.* 1991;229:232–236.

Centers for Disease Control. Initial therapy for tuberculosis in the era of multidrug resistance. Recommendations of the Advisory Council for the Elimination of Tuberculosis. *MMWR.* 1993;42(no. RR-7):1–8.

Centers for Disease Control. National action plan to combat multidrug resistant tuberculosis; Meeting the challenge of multidrug resistant tuberculosis: Summary of a conference; Management of persons exposed to multidrug resistant tuberculosis. *MMWR.* 1992a;41(no. RR-11): 5–8, 49–57, 59–71.

Centers for Disease Control. Prevention and control of tuberculosis in U.S. communities with at-risk minority populations: Recommendations of the Advisory Council for the Elimination of Tuberculosis. Prevention and control of tuberculosis among homeless persons: Recommendations of the Advisory Council for the Elimination of Tuberculosis. *MMWR.* 1992b;41(no. RR-5):1–15.

Centers for Disease Control. Purified protein derivative (PPD)—tuberculin anergy and HIV infection: Guidelines for anergy testing and management of anergic persons at risk of tuberculosis. *MMWR.* 1991;40(no. RR-5):27–33.

Centers for Disease Control. Screening for tuberculosis and tuberculosis infection in high risk populations. *MMWR.* 1990a;39(no. RR-8):1–7.

Centers for Disease Control. The use of preventive therapy for tuberculosis infection in the United States: Recommendations of the Advisory Committee for the Elimination of Tuberculosis. *MMWR.* 1990b;39(no. RR-8):9–12.

Centers for Disease Control. Tuberculosis morbidity—United States, 1996. *MMWR.* 1997;46:695–699.

Chaulet P, Mulder D. Tuberculosis. In: Manson-Bahr PEC, Bell DR, eds. *Manson's Tropical Diseases.* London: Baillière-Tindall; 1987:987–997.

Chaulk CP, Kazandjian VA. Directly observed therapy for treatment completion of pulmonary tuberculosis: Consensus statement of the Public Health Tuberculosis Guidelines Panel. *JAMA.* 1998;279:943–948.

Comstock GW, O'Brien RJ. Tuberculosis. In: Evans AS, Brachman PS, eds. *Bacterial Infections of Humans: Epidemiology and Control.* New York: Plenum; 1990:745–771.

Daniel TM. Rapid diagnosis of tuberculosis: Laboratory techniques applicable in developing countries. *Rev Infect Dis.* 1989;11(suppl 2):S471–S478.

Daniel TM, Tripathy SP. Tuberculosis. In: Warren KS, Mahmoud AAF, eds. *Tropical and Geographical Medicine.* New York: McGraw-Hill; 1989:839–851.

Dannenberg AM. Immune mechanisms in the pathogenesis of pulmonary tuberculosis. *Rev Infect Dis.* 1989;11(suppl 2):S369–S378.

Dickensheets DL. Tuberculosis makes a comeback: Giving and interpreting the Mantoux test. *Postgrad Med.* 1989; 86:97–108.

Dooley SW, et al. Multidrug-resistant tuberculosis. *Ann Intern Med.* 1992;117:257–259.

Edlin BR, et al: An outbreak of multidrug-resistant tuberculosis among hospitalized patients with the acquired immunodeficiency syndrome. *N Engl J Med.* 1992;326: 1514–1521.

Fadda G, Sanguinetti M. Microbiology and diagnosis of tuberculosis. *Rays.* 1998;23:32–41.

Fine PEM. The BCG story: Lessons from the past and implications for the future. *Rev Infect Dis.* 1989;11(suppl 2):S353–S359.

Frankel RM, Boname ME. Detection of the new tuberculosis: Ocular examination as a diagnostic imperative. *J Am Optom Assoc.* 1994;65:472–479.

Frieden TR, et al. The emergence of drug-resistant tuberculosis in New York City. *New Engl J Med.* 1993;328:521–526.

Gladwin MT, Plorde JJ, Martin DR. Clinical application of the mycobacterium tuberculosis direct test: Case report, literature review, and proposed clinical algorithm. *Chest.* 1998;114:317–323.

Good RC. Serologic methods for diagnosing tuberculosis. *Ann Intern Med.* 1989;110:97–98.

Good RC, Mastro TD. The modern mycobacteriology laboratory: How it can help the clinician. *Clin Chest Med.* 1989;10:315–322.

Gross J, Gross FJ, Friedman AH. Tuberculosis. In: Tasman W, Jaeger EA, eds. *Duane's Clinical Ophthalmology.* Vol.5. Hagerstown, MD: Harper & Row; 1992:21–23.

Gupta V, Arora S, Gupta A, et al. Management of presumed intraocular tuberculosis: Possible role of the polymerase chain reaction. *Acta Ophthalmol Scand.* 1998;76:679–682.

Hamrick RM, Yeager H. Tuberculosis update. *Am Fam Physician.* 1988;38:205–213.

Holland SM. Cytokine therapy of mycobacterial infections. *Adv Intern Med.* 2000;45:431–452.

Hopewell PC. Impact of human immunodeficiency virus infection on the epidemiology, clinical features, management, and control of tuberculosis. *Clin Infect Dis.* 1992; 15:540–547.

Iseman MD. A leap of faith: What can we do to curtail intrainstitutional transmission of tuberculosis? *Ann Intern Med.* 1992;117:251–253.

Iseman MD. Drug-resistant tuberculosis: New threats from an old disease. *Postgrad Med.* 1989;86:109–114.

Iseman MD, Goble M. Treatment of tuberculosis. *Adv Intern Med.* 1988;33:253–266.

Iseman MD, Madsen LA. Drug-resistant tuberculosis. *Clin Chest Med.* 1989;10:341–353.

Jereb JA, et al. Tuberculosis morbidity in the United States: Final data, 1990. In: CDC surveillance summaries, December 1991. *MMWR.* 1991;40(SS-3):23–27.

Johnson MP, et al. Tuberculin skin test reactivity among adults infected with human immunodeficiency virus. *J Infect Dis.* 1992;166:194–198.

Kim JY, Carroll CP, Opremcak EM. Antibiotic-resistant tuberculosis choroiditis. *Am J Ophthalmol.* 1993;115:259–261.

Kochi A. The global tuberculosis situation and the new control strategy of the World Health Organization. *Tubercle.* 1991;72:1–6.

Lama P, Frohman L. Annual review of systemic disease—1997-II. *J Neuro-Ophthalmol.* 1998;18:127–142.

Levin AC, Gums JG, Grauer K. Tuberculosis: The primary care physician's role in eradication. *Postgrad Med.* 1993; 93:46–60.

Lordi GM, Reichman LB. Treatment of tuberculosis. *Am Fam Physician.* 1991;44:219–224.

Mansour AM, Haymond R. Choroidal tuberculomas without evidence of extraocular tuberculosis. *Graefes Arch Clin Exp Ophthalmol.* 1990;228:382–385.

McCray E, Weinbaum CM, Braden CR, Onorato IM. The epidemiology of tuberculosis in the United States. *Clin Chest Med.* 1997;18:99–113.

Near KA, Lefford MJ. Use of serum antibody and lysozyme levels for diagnosis of leprosy and tuberculosis. *J Clin Microbiol.* 1992;30:1105–1110.

Nolan CM. Community-wide implementation of targeted testing for and treatment of latent tuberculosis infection. *Clin Infect Dis.* 1999;29:880–887.

Orme IM. Beyond BCG: The potential for a more effective TB vaccine. *Mol Med Today.* 1999a;5:487–492.

Orme IM. New vaccines against tuberculosis. The status of current research. *Infect Dis Clin North Am.* 1999b;13:169–185.

Palittapongarnpim P, et al. DNA fragment length polymorphism analysis of *Mycobacterium tuberculosis* isolates by arbitrarily primed polymerase chain reaction. *J Infect Dis.* 1993;167:975–978.

Pearson ML, et al. Nosocomial transmission of multidrug-resistant *Mycobacterium tuberculosis. Ann Intern Med.* 1992; 117:191–196.

Perenti F. New experimental drugs for the treatment of tuberculosis. *Rev Infect Dis.* 1989;11(suppl 2):S479–S483.

Pérez-Stable EJ, Hopewell PC. Current tuberculosis regimens: Choosing the right one for your patient. *Clin Chest Med.* 1989;10:323–339.

Pitchenik AE, Fertel D, Bloch AB. Mycobacterial disease: Epidemiology, diagnosis, treatment, and prevention. *Clin Chest Med.* 1988;9:425–441.

Psilas K, et al. Antituberculosis therapy in the treatment of peripheral uveitis. *Ann Ophthalmol.* 1991;23:254–258.

Pust RE. Tuberculosis in the 1990s: Resurgence, regimens, and resources. *South Med J.* 1992;85:584–593.

Quinn TC. Interactions of the human immunodeficiency virus and tuberculosis and the implications for BCG vaccination. *Rev Infect Dis.* 1989;11(suppl 2):S379–S384.

Regill CD, et al. Ocular tuberculosis. *JAMA.* 1991; 266:1490.

Rieder HL, et al. Tuberculosis in the United States. *JAMA.* 1989;262:385–389.

Rieder HL, Snider DE, Cauthen GM. Extrapulmonary tuberculosis in the United States. *Am Rev Respir Dis.* 1990; 141:347–351.

Rosen PH, Spalton DJ, Graham EM. Intraocular tuberculosis. *Eye.* 1990;4:486–492.

Schraufnagel DE. Tuberculosis treatment for the beginning of the next century. *Int J Tuberc Lung Dis.* 1999;3:651–662.

Small PM, et al. Treatment of tuberculosis in patients with advanced human immunodeficiency virus infection. *N Engl J Med.* 1991;324:289–294.

Smith MHD. Tuberculosis in children and adolescents. *Clin Chest Med.* 1989;10:381–395.

Stead WW. The origin and erratic global spread of tuberculosis: How the past explains the present and is the key to the future. *Clin Chest Med.* 1997;18:65–77.

Stead WW. Pathogenesis of tuberculosis: Clinical and epidemiologic perspective. *Rev Infect Dis.* 1989a;11(suppl 2):S366–S368.

Stead WW. Special problems in tuberculosis: Tuberculosis in the elderly, and in residents of nursing homes, correctional facilities, long-term care hospitals, mental hospitals, shelters for the homeless, and jails. *Clin Chest Med.* 1989b; 10:397–405.

Stead WW, et al. Racial differences in susceptibility to infection by *Mycobacterium tuberculosis. N Engl J Med.* 1990;322: 422–427.

Stead WW, Dutt AK. Tuberculosis in elderly persons. *Ann Rev Med.* 1991;42:267–276.

Sudre P, ten Dam G, Kochi A. Tuberculosis: A global overview of the situation today. *Bull World Health Organ.* 1992;70:149–159.

Telenti A. Genetics of drug resistance in tuberculosis. *Clin Chest Med.* 1997;18:55–64.

Trebucq A. Should ethambutol be recommended for routine treatment of tuberculosis in children? A review of the literature. *Int J Tuberc Lung Dis.* 1997;1:12–15.

Van Scoy RE, Wilkowske CJ. Antituberculous agents. *Mayo Clin Proc.* 1992;67:179–187.

Welton TH, Townsend JC, Anderson SF, et al: Presumed ocular tuberculosis in an AIDS patient. *J Am Optom Assoc.* 1996;67:350–357.

Wolfensberger TJ, Piguet B, Herbort CP. Indocyanine green angiographic features in tuberculous chorioretinitis. *Am J Ophthalmol.* 1999;127:350–353.

Žorić LD, Žorić DLJ, Žorić DM. Bilateral tuberculous abscesses on the face (eyelids) of a child. *Am J Ophthalmol.* 1996;121:717–718.

Chapter 43

LYME DISEASE

Kelly H. Thomann

Lyme disease, a multisystem, multistage, inflammatory disease, has now been clinically recognized for approximately 25 years. The number of annually reported cases in the United States has increased 25 times since national surveillance began in 1982. The disease is characterized by early and late manifestations that primarily involve the skin, nervous system, joints, and heart. The skin lesion, erythema migrans, is a clinical marker for early diagnosis and is present in almost 90% of individuals with Lyme disease. Most cases of Lyme disease can be successfully treated with antibiotics when diagnosed early. Recent research has focused on serology, treatment, and prevention. In 1998, a recombinant outer-surface protein A (rOsp-A) vaccine (LYMErix) against Lyme disease became commercially available to persons between the ages of 15 and 70. Current recommendations for its use are based upon a combination of community and individual risk.

EPIDEMIOLOGY

Lyme disease is the leading cause of vector-borne infection in the United States. In 1998, a total of 16,801 cases were reported to the CDC, representing the highest number since reporting began. Over the past 10 years, 90% of the cases of Lyme disease in the United States occurred in 10 states (Table 43–1). The national map (Figure 43–1), diagrammed with county-specific data from 1994 to 1997 gathered from the CDC, shows a clear pattern of Lyme disease risk with the greatest concentration of cases occurring in the Northeast and upper Midwest regions of the United States. Lyme vaccine prescribers utilize this risk map to help determine if a person should be immunized.

Systemic

The erythema migrans lesion is present in up to 90% of patients with Lyme disease and is virtually specific

TABLE 43–1. DISTRIBUTION OF 90% OF CASES OF LYME DISEASE OVER THE PAST 10 YEARS

State	Annual Incidence per 100,000 Persons
Connecticut	54.2
Rhode Island	37.5
New York	21.6
New Jersey	16.9
Delaware	14.0
Pennsylvania	12.3
Wisconsin	9.3
Maryland	6.8
Massachusetts	4.5
Minnesota	3.8

Adapted from Centers for Disease Control and Prevention. Recommendations and Reports series, June 4. MMWR. *1999;48(RR07):21–24.*

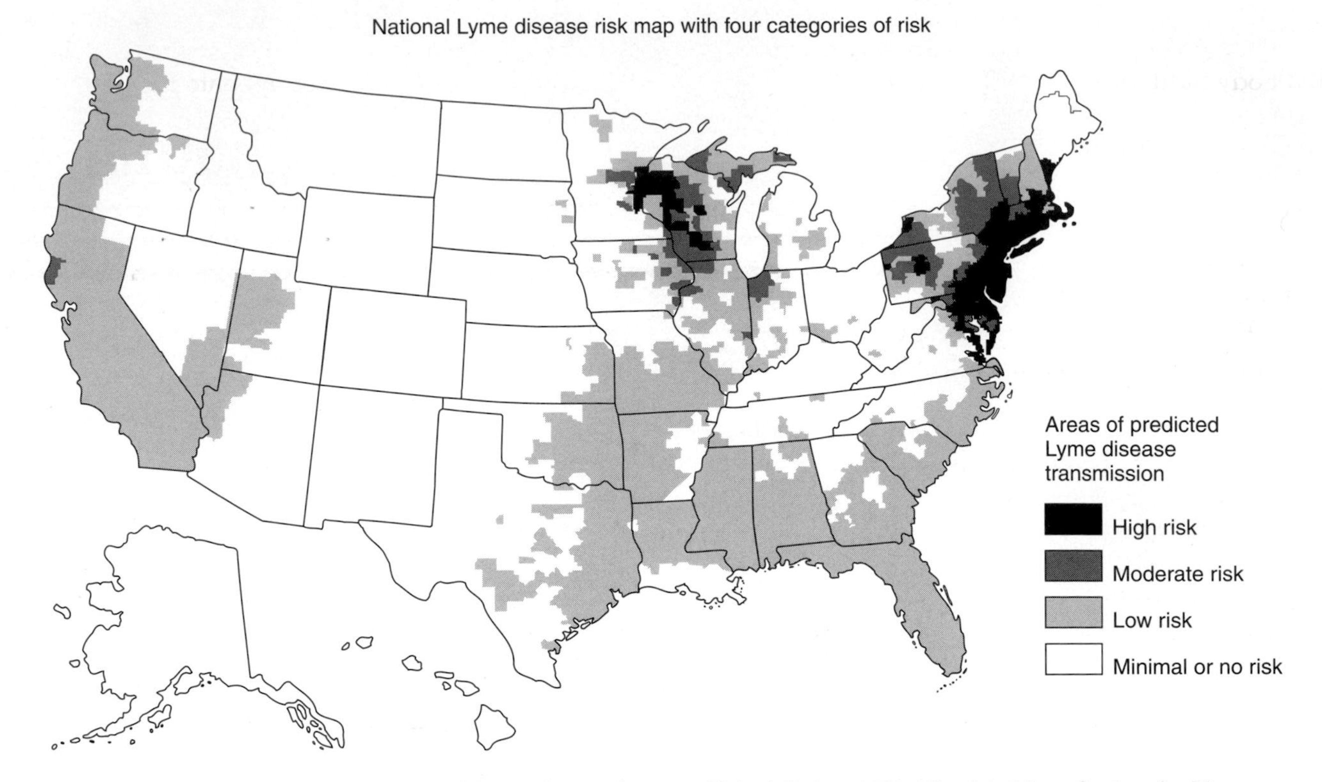

Figure 43–1. Number of reported cases of Lyme disease, by state, United States, 1996. (*Reprinted from Centers for Disease Control. Lyme disease—United States, 1996.* MMWR. *1997;46:531–535.*)

for diagnosis. According to Nadelman (1996), the most common symptoms associated with erythema migrans include fatigue (54%), myalgia (44%), arthralgia (44%), headache (42%), fever and/or chills (39%), and stiff neck (35%).

Carditis develops in 4 to 10% of patients not treated for Lyme disease. However, the incidence of carditis is less than 1% in the United States and less than 4% in Europe for patients who were treated with antibiotics for erythema migrans. Recent reports have also shown a reduced incidence of neurologic complications from Lyme disease. It is now thought that less than 10% of cases of Lyme disease have neurologic complications. Rheumatologic manifestations of Lyme disease can occur in up to 50% of untreated patients, but appear to be rare in those who are adequately treated with antibiotic therapy.

Ocular

Follicular conjunctivitis occurs in approximately 5 to 11% of patients with early Lyme disease. Every part of the eye can be involved in disseminated Lyme disease; however, these manifestations are not common.

PATHOPHYSIOLOGY/DISEASE PROCESS

Systemic

The Organism

The pathogenic organism responsible for Lyme disease remained unknown until 1982, when a spirochete belonging to the *Borrelia* family was isolated by Willy Burgdorfer, and thus named *Borrelia burgdorferi.* Helically shaped, motile spirochetes often cause diseases with similar features.

Transmission

Ixodes ticks are the major vectors for *B. burgdorferi. Ixodes scapularis* (also known as the black-legged or deer tick) is the main vector in the eastern United States, and *Ixodes pacificus* (the western black-legged tick) in the western United States. The white-footed mouse is the most important reservoir of *B. burgdorferi,* whereas deer are the principal maintenance hosts for adult black-legged ticks. The expanding deer population has been linked to the spread of the *Ixodes* ticks and Lyme disease in endemic regions.

Ticks are arachnids and are considered to be obligate ectoparasites, dependent upon a host's blood and body fluid for survival. Ticks feed on blood by insertion of their mouth parts into the skin of the host. The feeding takes several days, over which time the tick slowly enlarges. The tick life cycle follows a seasonal pattern with four developmental stages over a 2-year cycle (Figure 43–2). The life cycle begins when an adult female tick lays 1000 to 8000 eggs while sequestered in leaf or brush litter. The eggs hatch after a period of 8 to 135 days (depending upon the species) and become larvae. The larvae feed on a small animal (such as the white-footed mouse) for 3 to 9 days and then detach, molt, and become nymphs. Nymphs are about the size of a pinhead, do not have gender specificity, and are lacking the genital apertures of the adult tick. Twelve to thirty percent are infected with *Borrelia burgdorferi.* Nymphs feed once in the following spring or early summer, detach, and molt into adult ticks late in the summer. Adult ticks are slightly larger in size than a pinhead, have male/female sexual characteristics, and 28 to 65% are infected with *B. burgdorferi* in highly endemic areas. The male and female adult ticks seek a blood meal in the autumn. They attach and engorge completely, and then either copulate while engorging or after dropping from the host. The female adult drops her eggs a few weeks later and the cycle begins again.

At each stage of the life cycle, unfed ticks are attracted to sources of blood meals through the detection of host carbon dioxide and body heat by chemosensitive structures on their front legs. The ticks wait, poised on grass or foliage with their front legs uplifted, waving, as if to "sniff" the hosts passing nearby. Upon chemodetection of host carbon dioxide, the ticks crawl (they do not fly) onto the host.

White-tailed deer are not involved in the spirochete life cycle but are the preferred host for adult ticks. The prevalence of Lyme disease is most closely associated with the deer population, but many other animals also serve as hosts, the white-footed mouse in particular, but also birds and domestic animals, including dogs, cats, horses, and cattle. During any stage the tick can feed on humans (Figure 43–3) and transmit the disease. Because the feedings occur from spring to autumn, Lyme disease is typically noted during these seasons. However, most cases occur in late spring and early summer. Nymphs are responsible for transmission of almost 90% of cases of Lyme disease. Although fewer nymphs are infected by *B. burgdorferi* than adult ticks, nymphs are more numerous, more likely to go unnoticed when attached to a host, and found during the late spring/summer months when individuals are out of doors with minimal clothing. Snow and temperatures less than 45° inhibit adult tick activity; however, warm spells can reactivate them.

Lyme disease is rarely transmitted unless the tick has been attached to the host for at least 36 to 48 hours. Therefore, there is a grace period during which, if a tick is found and removed promptly, the likelihood of acquiring the disease is small.

Course of the Disease

The pathologic mechanism for the multisystemic involvement of Lyme disease includes direct spirochetal invasion of tissue, vessel inflammation and perivascular

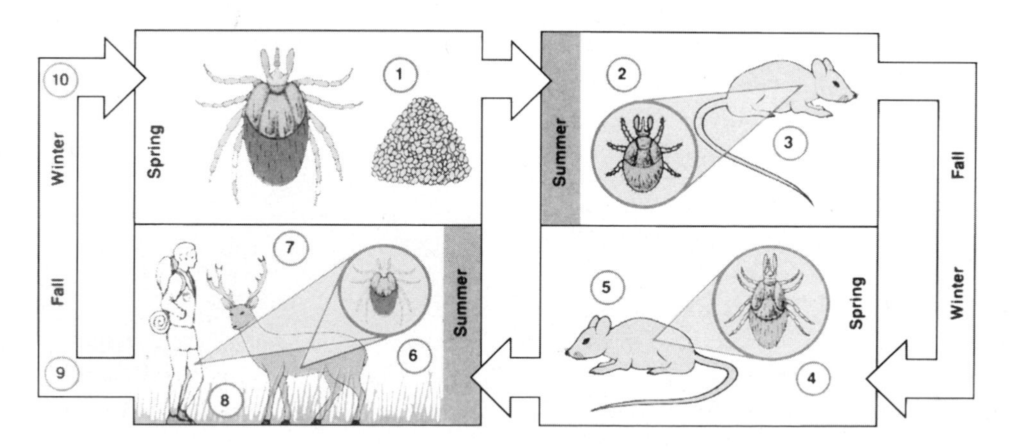

Figure 43–2. Tick life cycle. (*Reprinted with permission from Schlesinger PA. Lyme disease: Prevention and intervention.* Hosp Med. *1989; 25:93.*)

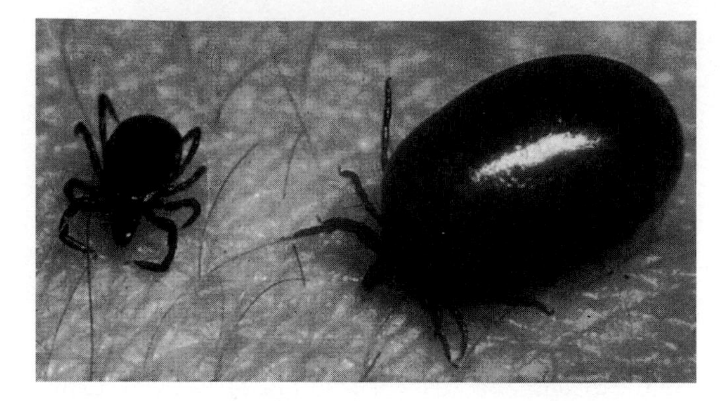

Figure 43–3. Female *Ixodes scapularis* tick in the unengorged and engorged states.

infiltration, and host immunologic reaction. Lyme disease can be broken into three stages, loosely defined by the duration of infection. These stages have been termed early (localized) infection, early disseminated infection, and late disseminated disease (Table 43–2). Early infection occurs days to weeks after the tick bite, and the erythema migrans lesion (Figures 43–4 to 43–7) can be found in almost 90% of cases. The lesion will often be located where the tick commonly attaches: the axilla, thigh, groin, buttocks, and where tight-fitting clothing begins. It can be variable in size and shape (circular, oval, or triangular). It may be uniform in color (however a central clearing or darkening may be noted), and it can be visualized more readily under natural illumination. Only about one half of the erythema migrans lesions have the classic "bulls eye" appearance with central clearing (Figure 43–4), and atypical lesions are also common (Figures 43–5 to 43–7). Early localized infection is also characterized by a flu-like illness with common complaints of fatigue, myalgia, arthralgia, headache, fever and/or chills, and stiff neck.

> The erythema migrans lesion, although easily overlooked, can be found in almost all patients with Lyme disease.

Early disseminated disease occurs days to weeks after infection as the spirochetes disseminate from the site of inoculation through cutaneous, lymphatic, and blood-borne routes. Patients may develop multiple or secondary asymptomatic erythema migrans lesions after hematogenous spread of the spirochetes. Neurologic manifestations of early disseminated Lyme disease

TABLE 43–2. SYSTEMIC MANIFESTATIONS OF LYME DISEASE

Early Localized Infection
- Erythema migrans lesion (present in over 80% of individuals with Lyme disease)
- Complaints of fatigue, myalgia, arthralgia, headache, fever and/or chills (flu-like symptoms), stiff neck

Early Disseminated Infection
- Dermatologic
  - Multiple or secondary erythema migrans lesions
- Nervous system disease
  - Lymphocytic meningitis
  - Cranial neuropathy (seventh-nerve palsy most common)
  - Peripheral neuropathy
  - Radiculoneuritis
- Musculoskeletal disease
  - Migrating joint and muscle pains with or without swelling
- Cardiac disease
  - Myocarditis (rare)
  - Transient atrioventricular block (rare)
- General
  - Malaise, fatigue, regional or generalized lymphadenopathy

Late Disseminated Infection
- Dermatologic
  - Acrodermatitis chronicum atrophicans (found primarily in Europe)
- Neurologic
  - Encephalitis, axonal polyneuropathy, leukoencephalopathy
- Rheumatologic
  - Arthritis (prolonged attacks, chronic pain)

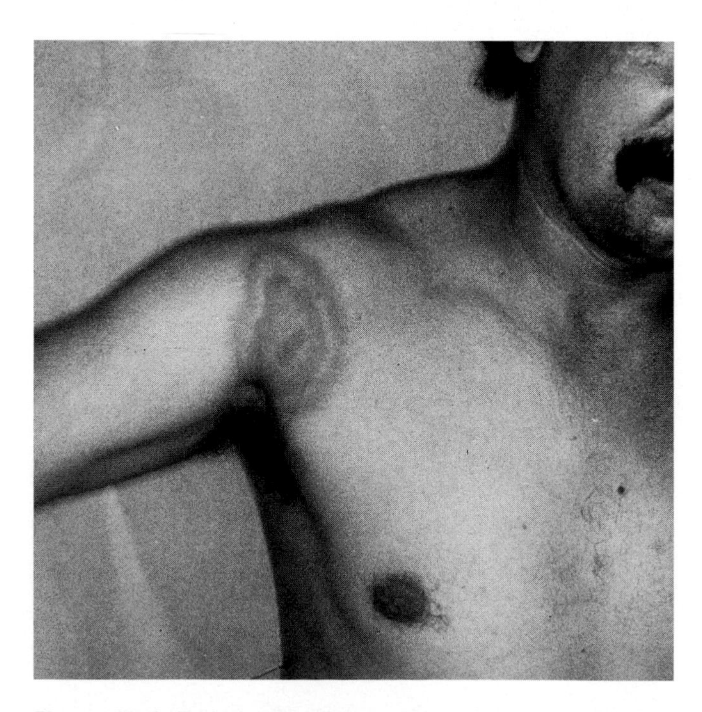

Figure 43–4. Typical expanding erythema migrans lesion, with "bull's eye" central clearing.

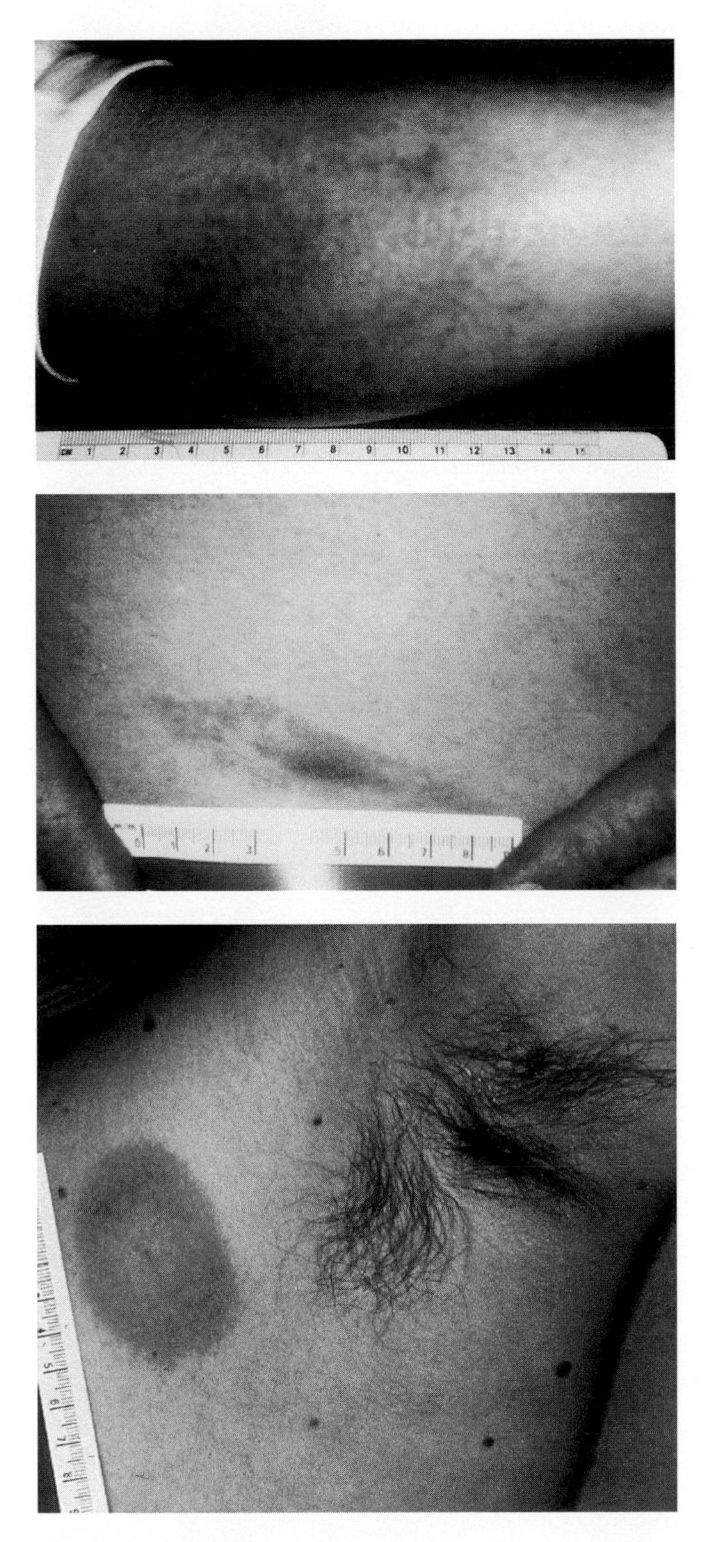

Figures 43–5 to 43–7. Erythema migrans lesions may also present with varying appearances.

include lymphocytic meningitis (with symptoms of neck pain and/or stiffness), cranial neuropathy (facial nerve palsy, most common), and radiculoneuritis. Early reports had indicated that neurologic disease was found in up to 20% of untreated cases, although more recent data consistently have found the incidence to be only as high as 10%. Cardiac manifestations (fluctuating degrees of atrioventricular conduction defects or tachyarrhythmias) probably occur less than previously reported. Symptoms may include lightheadedness, syncope, dyspnea, palpitations, and/or chest pain. Intermittent attacks of migratory monoarthritis or asymmetric oligoarthritis may occur in untreated patients days to several months after infection. Migratory joint and muscle pain with or without swelling are most commonly reported.

Late disseminated disease occurs weeks to months after infection. The most common sign of Lyme arthritis is intermittent swelling or pain of large weight-bearing joints, most commonly the knee. Chronic neurologic manifestations have also been recognized in late disseminated Lyme disease, and are often associated with a mild, low-grade reversible inflammatory process in the central nervous system. Subacute encephalitis is the most common chronic manifestation. It often affects memory, mood, and sleep and may cause subtle cognitive dysfunction. Polyneuropathy may cause paresthesias, and less commonly, radicular pain. Acrodermatitis chronicum atrophicans, rare in the United States, but well documented in Europe, is a secondary dermatologic lesion that can develop insidiously in a distal extremity. It is characterized by a swollen bluish-red lesion, which ultimately atrophies. A sensory neuropathy can also be associated with the skin lesion.

Despite isolated reports to the contrary, Nadelman, Herman, and Wormser (1997) confirmed that no causal relationship exists between untreated Lyme disease and multiple sclerosis, amyotrophic lateral sclerosis, or Alzheimer disease. The risk of transplacental transmission of *B. burgdorferi* appears to be minimal when appropriate antibiotics are prescribed in pregnant women with Lyme disease. To date, there are no data to support a congenital Lyme syndrome.

Ocular

A myriad of ocular complications from Lyme disease have been documented, involving virtually all parts of the eye (Table 43–3). Overall, however, ocular manifestations are not common in Lyme disease. A nonspecific, self-resolving follicular conjunctivitis is the most common ocular manifestation in early infection. Patients typically complain of photophobia. Periorbital edema and episcleritis may also be present.

Aside from conjunctivitis, most of the ocular findings in Lyme disease occur during the early and late disseminated stages of the disease, caused by either direct spirochetal invasion of tissue, or secondary to the host's immune response. The most common findings are pars planitis with posterior synechiae and granulomatous anterior uveitis. Keratitis is a rare finding in untreated late disseminated disease. It consists of bilateral scattered hazy infiltrates in the superficial and deep stroma. The visual axis is typically spared and corneal neovascularization is infrequent. The neuro-ophthalmic complications of Lyme disease include palsies of cranial nerves 3, 4, and 6 along with pupil abnormalities. Both unilateral and bilateral disc edema (Figure 43–8) can also occur.

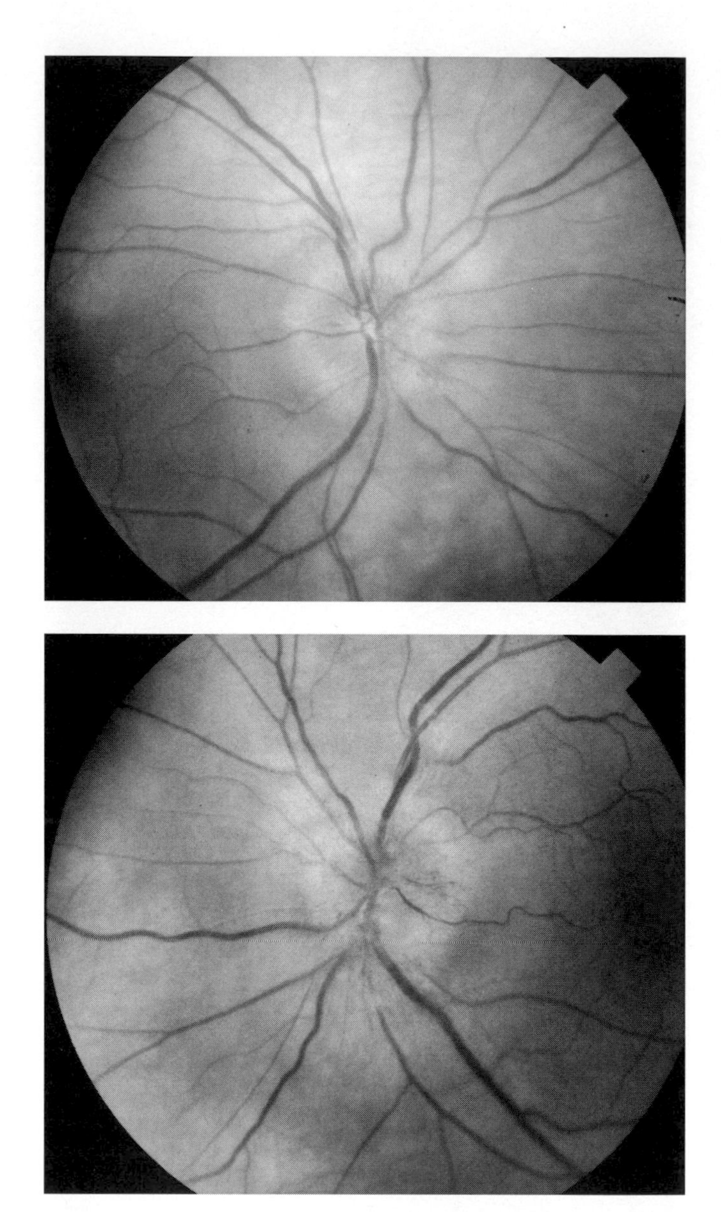

Figure 43–8. Bilateral disc edema in a patient with untreated late disseminated Lyme disease.

DIAGNOSIS

The surveillance definition for Lyme disease (Table 43–4) was developed by the Centers for Disease Control and Prevention in the United States for reporting and tracking purposes in 1991. Although it is not always appropriate for clinical diagnosis, it has proven to be helpful as a practice guideline. Diagnosis typically is defined by clinical findings, and treatment often is justified in early disease solely on the basis of objective signs and known exposure.

In the presence of an erythema migrans lesion, serologic testing for Lyme disease is not recommended, nor is the use of serologic testing recommended for screening or follow-up purposes. Serologic testing, however, can provide valuable information, especially in disseminated disease. Lyme serology is indirect, and only measures antibody response to the infection; therefore these methods only indicate exposure, not active infection.

TABLE 43–3. OCULAR MANIFESTATIONS OF LYME DISEASE

Early Infection

- Conjunctivitis
- Photophobia
- Episcleritis
- Periorbital edema

Disseminated Infection

- Keratitis
- Uveitis (nongranulomatous and granulomatous)
- Pars planitis
- Vitreitis
- Choroiditis
- Retinitis
- Endophthalmitis
- Panophthalmitis
- Neuroretinitis
- Optic nerve edema
- Papilledema
- Orbital myositis
- Blepharospasm
- Cranial nerve 3, 4, 6, or 7 palsy
- Pupil abnormalities (Horner syndrome and Argyll-Robertson-like pupils)

Systemic

Diagnosis of Lyme disease is straightforward when the erythema migrans lesion is present. However, the erythema migrans lesion can be difficult to identify, and a thorough physical examination is often necessary. In addition, many rashes can be misdiagnosed as ery-

TABLE 43–4. CENTERS FOR DISEASE CONTROL AND PREVENTION DIAGNOSTIC CRITERIA FOR LYME DISEASE

Clinical Case Definition
- Erythema migrans lesion

OR

- At least one late manifestation (as defined below) and laboratory confirmation

Laboratory Criteria for Diagnosis (must have one)
- Isolation of *Borrelia burgdorferi* from clinical specimen
- Demonstration of diagnostic levels of IgM and IgG antibodies to the spirochete in serum or CSF
- Significant change in IgM or IgG antibody response to *B. burgdorferi* in paired acute and convalescent serum samples

Definition of Late Manifestations
Musculoskeletal system
- Recurrent, brief attacks of objective joint swelling in one or a few joints, sometimes followed by chronic arthritis in one or a few joints
- Chronic progressive arthritis not preceded by brief attacks and chronic symmetric polyarthritis, arthralgia, myalgia, or fibromyalgia alone is NOT a criterion for musculoskeletal involvement

Nervous system
- Lymphocytic meningitis
- Cranial neuritis (especially facial palsy)
- Radiculoneuropathy
- Encephalomyelitis (must be confirmed by identification of antibody production in the CSF)
- Headache, fatigue, paresthesisa, or mild stiff neck alone is NOT a criterion for neurologic involvement

Cardiovascular system
- Acute-onset, high-grade atrioventricular conduction defects that resolve in days to weeks and are sometimes associated with myocarditis
- Palpitations, bradycardia, bundle branch block, or myocarditis alone is NOT a criterion for cardiovascular involvement

Adapted from Centers for Disease Control and Prevention. Case definition for public health surveillance. MMWR. *1990;39(RR-13):19–21.*

thema migrans (eg, insect bites). In straightforward cases, serology is not indicated to diagnose or assess efficacy of treatment. Patients who remove a tick from their body should not be treated for Lyme disease unless the erythema migrans lesion becomes evident or there is strong clinical evidence and serologic confirmation. However, some cases of highly probable Lyme disease may be treated prior to serologic confirmation.

Patients who do not recall a tick bite or EM lesion, with signs and symptoms consistent with Lyme disease, should have serologic testing (Table 43–5). The enzyme-linked immunosorbent assay (ELISA) and indirect immunofluorescence antibody (IFA) test are the most commonly utilized methods to detect specific antibodies against *B. burgdorferi* in the blood. IgM antibodies appear first, during the first 4 to 6 weeks of the disease, their presence indicating recent infection. IgG antibodies usually present 6 weeks after the onset of the disease, and may persist for months to years. A specimen that is negative through sensitive ELISA or IFA testing need not be tested further unless the disease is strongly suspected. In cases where Lyme disease is highly suspected, without erythema migrans, acute and convalescent phase serum samples should be tested and compared. Seroconversion is indicative of infection. In some of these cases, treatment should be initiated even without seroconversion. Specimens that are found to be positive or equivocal with ELISA or IFA testing next should have immunoblot (Western blot) testing to detect IgM or IgG antibodies to *B. burgdorferi* antigens that have been separated by electrophoresis. If immunoblot testing is negative, then IFA and ELISA probably were falsely positive. A positive IgG immunoblot test is necessary to support the diagnosis of Lyme disease in a patient who has been symptomatic for longer than 1 month. Sequential testing is not indicated if little or no clinical evidence is present to support the diagnosis of Lyme disease. Serology does not play a role in measuring the response to treatment since IgM and IgG antibodies persist in serum for years after recovery. In recent years, Lyme serology has been overused on patients who present with vague symptoms, without clear clinical evidence of Lyme disease.

Serology is less useful during early Lyme disease because it takes approximately 4 weeks for an individual to produce detectable IgM antibody against *B. burgdorferi.* This response peaks 6 to 8 weeks after onset of the illness, and declines to the normal range within 4 to 6 months in most patients. IgG antibody increases 6 to 8 weeks after onset of illness, peaks after 4 to 6 months, and remains elevated indefinitely in patients with continued infection. Therefore, untreated patients in later stages of the disease should show increased IgG levels. ELISA and IFA serology are 86 to

TABLE 43–5. LYME DISEASE SEROLOGY: APPROXIMATE REFERENCE RANGES[a]

ELISA
<1.0 = negative
0.85–1.25 = equivocal
>1.0 = positive

IFA IgG/IgM
IgG
<1:16 = negative
1:16–1:32 = equivocal
<1:32 = evidence of past or current infection

IgM
If any present, is considered positive

Western Blot
≤ 5 bands = normal

[a]Values differ according to laboratory.

TABLE 43–6. TREATMENT OF LYME BORRELIOSIS[a, b]

Antimicrobial	Duration (days)[c]	Comments
Erythema Migrans (EM)		
		Amoxicillin, cefuroxime, doxycycline probably equally effective; failure rate <5%; no evidence that intravenous ceftriaxone is advantageous in "disseminated" early disease
Doxycycline[b]	14	Covers human granulocyte ehrlichiosis (HGE); risk of photosensitivity
Amoxicillin	14	Not active against HGE
Cefuroxime axetil	14	Useful when cellulitis cannot be distinguished from EM; alternative for some penicillin-allergic patients; most expensive; not active against HGE
Phenoxymethylpenicillin (penicillin V)	14	Not active against HGE
Tetracycline[b]	14	Covers HGE; risk of photosensitivity
Azithromycin	7–10	Second-line choice, more failures than with amoxicillin; not active against HGE
Borrelial Lymphocytoma		
First-line EM regimen[b]	14	
Acrodermatitis Chronica Atrophicans		
First-line oral EM regimen[b]	21–28	Evaluation for neuropathy prudent; intravenous antibiotics (see below) may be effective, but advantages over oral therapy not established
Carditis		
First-line oral EM regimen[b]	14	For primary heart block
Ceftriaxone	14	For advanced heart block; no proof that intravenous more effective than oral
Facial Nerve Palsy		
First-line oral EM[b] regimen	14–28	No clinical trials; treatment does not shorten course; perform lumbar puncture if clinical signs exist
Meningitis		
Ceftriaxone	14	
Cefotaxime	14	
Penicillin G	14	
Doxycycline	14–28	Equivalence to IV penicillin requires confirmation
Radiculoneuritis		
Meningitis regimen[b]	See above	Concomitant meningitis frequent
Peripheral Neuropathy		
Meningitis regimen[b]	See above	

100% sensitive for late Lyme disease, and therefore remain the tests of choice.

Problems with current serology (ELISA, IFA) include serovariability and false-negative and false-positive results. Serovariability occurs when a sample of serum tests negative at one lab and positive at another. False-negative serology may be found in early Lyme disease before a full antibody response has occurred, if antibiotics were used that curtailed the immune response, or if the patient is immunosuppressed. False-positive serology can occur with syphilis, pinta, yaws, leptospirosis, autoimmune diseases (eg, juvenile rheumatoid arthritis, rheumatoid arthritis, systemic lupus erythematosus), and other infectious diseases (eg, mononucleosis, malaria, subacute bacterial endocarditis). Tests to rule out inflammatory conditions or syphilis are recommended if the diagnosis is questionable. The rapid plasma reagin (RPR) test is superior to the fluorescent treponemal antibody-absorption (FTA-ABS) test for differentiation from syphilis. Cross-reactivity of Lyme IFA and syphilis FTA-ABS may occur. RPR and Venereal Disease Research Laboratory (VDRL) testing should not give false-positive results. If these tests are positive, then the diagnosis of syphilis rather than (or concurrent with) Lyme disease should be made. Polymerase chain reaction (PCR) testing is another serologic modality that identifies the DNA of the spirochetes in the blood, spinal fluid, skin, and other tissue. However, PCR is not available routinely, and there is poor interlaboratory reliability. Contamination of the sample can lead to false-positives and since the DNA can be amplified with dead spirochetes, positive results do not always correlate with active infection.

Co-infection is a more recent dilemma encountered with Lyme disease. *I. scapularis* ticks can carry several infections that can be transmitted separately or simultaneously along with *B. burgdorferi.* Possible co-infections include *Babesia microti* (a parasite that causes

TABLE 43–6. TREATMENT OF LYME BORRELIOSIS[a, b] *(continued)*

Antimicrobial	Duration (days)[c]	Comments
Encephalomyelitis		Up to 6 weeks of therapy recommended by one expert panel, but no data available
Ceftriaxone	14–28	
Cefotaxime	14–28	
Penicillin G	14–28	
Chronic Encephalopathy		
Ceftriaxone	14–28	
Cefotaxime	14–28	
Penicillin G	14–28	
Arthritis		Oral therapy as effective as intravenous; some patients treated orally develop neurological disease; role of synovial fluid PCR to determine duration of treatment unclear; no comparison studies with shorter course of therapy
Doxycycline[b]	28	
Amoxicillin	28	
Ceftriaxone	14	
Lyme Borreliosis in Pregnancy[b]		No comparison trials; treatment duration should be appropriate for individual manifestation of Lyme borreliosis (see above)
Penicillin G		
Ceftriaxone		
Amoxicillin		
Asymptomatic Tick Bite		
None		Efficacy of prophylaxis not proven; risk of adverse effects for 10-day regimens studied comparable to risk of contracting Lyme borreliosis For pregnant women with tick bites, either a 10-day course of amoxicillin or no treatment options; no studies have been done in this population

[a]Few regimens studied in published trials in children; selection of amoxicillin in preference to penicillin V, or doxycycline to tetracycline is based upon convenience (decreased dosing) and theoretical concerns (higher attainable levels) and not upon comparison studies.
[b]Pregnant or lactating women, and children under 9 years old should not receive tetracyclines; tetracyclines are the only antimicrobial agents known to be effective against HGE agent. Pediatric dose should not exceed maximum adult dose.
[c]Limited data available on treatment duration; studies comparing treatment duration in EM showed no outcome differences, and duration of treatment for EM ranging from 10 to 30 days has been recommended. In one study of objective late Lyme disease (mostly arthritis) there was no difference in outcome with 14 or 28 days of ceftriaxone.
Reprinted with permission from Nadelman RB, Wormser GP. Lyme borreliosis. Lancet. *1998;352:563.*

a malaria-like disease) and the rickettsial agent causing human granulocytic ehrlichiosis. Co-infection may alter the clinical presentation of Lyme disease and response to treatment. When clinical features that are not suggestive of Lyme disease, such as thrombocytopenia or leukopenia, are present in an individual highly suspicious for Lyme disease, co-infection may exist.

Ocular

A patient with or without diagnosed Lyme disease may present to an eyecare practitioner with ocular manifestations of the disease. Clinicians should be aware of the systemic findings associated with Lyme disease, in order to elicit the proper history that may lead to diagnosis. However, most ocular manifestations of Lyme disease are not common. For the patient with known Lyme disease, the clinician should be aware of the possible ocular manifestations (Table 43–3). Diagnosis of ocular manifestations can be made through routine eye examination. Referral to the appropriate physician (internist, infectious disease specialist, rheumatologist, neurologist) and serologic testing may also be warranted.

TREATMENT AND MANAGEMENT

Overdiagnosis and misdiagnosis of Lyme disease have become more common in recent years. Many patients with nonspecific symptoms have been treated for Lyme disease without true clinical or serologic evidence of infection.

Systemic

Early Lyme disease can be successfully treated with oral antibiotics (Table 43–6), and the majority of cases treated early do not exhibit late complications. The recommended course of oral antibiotic therapy is 10 to 21 days.

> Most cases of early Lyme disease can be treated successfully with antibiotics.

Most of the late manifestations of Lyme disease are treated with intravenous antibiotics (Table 43–6), with the exception of arthritis. Lyme arthritis is usually successfully treated by oral antibiotics; however, intravenous antibiotics are utilized in refractory cases. If Lyme meningitis or encephalitis is suspected, a lumbar puncture is recommended. If the cerebral spinal fluid is normal, oral antibiotics may be prescribed, but if the CSF is positive for Lyme, then high-dose parenteral antibiotics are recommended.

"Post-Lyme syndrome" can occur following adequate treatment for erythema migrans, in which the patient experiences recurrent arthralgias, myalgias, neck pain, and headache. The pathogenesis of this syndrome is not known, but it usually self-resolves within 6 months. Treatment is not recommended; however, many patients with this syndrome are incorrectly treated with IV antibiotics. Chronic fatigue syndrome or fibromyalgia is often confused with this entity.

Ocular

The ocular complications of Lyme disease can be treated with standard ocular therapy, along with systemic or IV antibiotics. Follicular conjunctivitis and episcleritis, which may be present during early disease, are typically self-limiting and do not require treatment. Uveitis and other ocular inflammations can be treated with steroids and cycloplegic agents. Topical steroids are used to treat keratitis, which may rarely occur during late disseminated disease. Standard Lyme antibiotic therapy (Table 43–6) is essential in the management of all ocular complications.

Prevention

Lyme Vaccination

The LYMErix vaccine became commercially available in 1998 to persons between the ages of 15 and 70. This vaccine contains the rOsp-A antigen, which is cultured from *B. burgdorferi.* rOsp-A is one of the lipoproteins that has been identified in the genome of the spirochete. The immunized individual mounts an antibody response to the rOsp-A antigen, which in turn neutralizes the spirochete as it enters the body. The vaccine-induced antibody may enter the gut of the tick while it is feeding on the immunized host and kill the spirochete prior to transmission or this may occur after the spirochete enters the immunized host.

The current CDC Lyme disease vaccine recommendations are listed in Table 43–7. The decision regarding who should receive the vaccine should be based upon an assessment of the person's risk as determined by activities and behaviors relating to tick exposure in an endemic area. The vaccine is administered in three doses. The initial vaccination should coincide with the spring Lyme season. The second dose is administered 1 month after the first, and the third 1 year after the first. Further information and research are still necessary regarding Lyme vaccination. Research is ongoing to determine the efficacy of vaccinating children. The duration of immunity is currently not known; therefore, the need and frequency of booster immunizations must be determined. Alterations in the sequence and structure of proteins in the

TABLE 43–7. CDC ADVISORY COMMITTEE RECOMMENDATIONS FOR IMMUNIZATION PRACTICES REGARDING LYMErix VACCINE

Persons who reside, work, or recreate in areas of high or moderate risk	
Persons between the age of 15–70 years:	
With frequent or prolonged exposure to tick infested areas	1
With some exposure (infrequent, not prolonged) to tick-infested habitat	2
Exposure is minimal or none	3
Persons who reside, work, or recreate in areas of low or no risk	3
Travelers to areas of high or moderate risk:	
Between 15–70 years with frequent or prolonged exposure	1
Children <15 years	3
Pregnant women	3
Persons with immunodeficiency[a]	
Persons with musculoskeletal disease[b]	
Persons with previous history of Lyme disease	
Between 15–70 years with previous uncomplicated Lyme disease who are at continued risk	1
Persons with treatment-resistant Lyme arthritis	3
Persons with chronic joing or neurologic illness related to Lyme disease and persons with second- or third-degree atrioventricular block[a]	

1 = vaccine should be considered;
2 = vaccine may be considered;
3 = vaccine not recommended.
[a]No available data.
[b]Limited available data.
Adapted from centers for Disease Control and Prevention. Recommendations and Reports series, June 04. MMWR. *1999; 48(RR07): 1–17.*

spirochete antigen may make the rOsp-A antibody ineffective in future *B. burgdorferi* strains.

Other Preventive Measures

Avoidance of the tick habitat is one obvious, but necessary precautionary recommendation. Ticks favor a moist, shaded environment, especially one that is provided by leaf litter and low-lying vegetation in a wooded, brushy, or overgrown grassy habitat. Both deer and rodent hosts must be abundant in these areas in order to maintain the tick cycle.

Personal protection habits also should become routine, especially for persons living in a Lyme-endemic area. Lightly colored clothing helps to identify ticks prior to attaching to the skin. Long-sleeve shirts and pants tucked into socks or boots are advised when individuals are hiking or working in brushy, overgrown areas. High rubber boots also are helpful because ticks usually are found low to the ground. Insect repellent containing DEET (n,n-diethyl-m-toluamide) can be applied to clothes and exposed skin. Permethrin, which kills ticks on contact, can be applied to clothing prior to outdoor activities. Individuals who live in a tick-endemic area should perform nightly tick checks on themselves and all children after outdoor activity. If a tick is found, it should be removed with fine-tipped tweezers. Petroleum jelly, hot matches, nail polish, and other products are not recommended to assist in tick removal. The tick should be grasped firmly as close to the skin as possible and removed with a steady motion. Often, the tick mouthparts may remain attached to the skin; however, since they do not contain the spirochete, it is unlikely the disease will still be transmitted. The area should be cleaned with an antiseptic.

Reduction of the tick habitat is another preventive measure utilized to reduce the likelihood of exposure to Lyme disease. This can be accomplished by removal of leaf litter, brush, and woodpiles that are near houses and yards. Pesticides can reduce tick populations when applied to yards and property. The effectiveness of deer feeding stations with pesticide applicators to kill the ticks on the deer is currently being evaluated. Reducing the deer population in endemic areas does not seem to be a solution because the ticks will most likely find other alternative hosts.

Early treatment intervention is an important means of preventing the morbidity and cost of treating complicated and late-stage Lyme disease. If the erythema migrans lesion is identified on an individual, treatment should be initiated promptly. Persons who remove a tick from their body should seek prompt medical attention if any signs or symptoms of early Lyme disease develop over the ensuing days or weeks.

CONCLUSION

Lyme disease is now a household word in endemic areas. This disease is often over diagnosed, especially in persons with ill-defined symptoms. Yet many actual cases of Lyme disease probably continue to go unreported to the CDC. Our knowledge of the disease has grown tremendously in the past 25 years. We now know that the erythema migrans lesion is present in up to 90% of cases of early Lyme disease and early identification of this lesion along with prompt antibiotic therapy can successfully treat most cases of Lyme disease. A vaccine for Lyme disease is now commercially available to persons between the ages of 15 and 70 years. Studies are currently underway regarding the use of the vaccination in children. Despite our growing knowledge of Lyme disease, many persons living in endemic areas still do not follow simple precautionary methods to avoid tick exposure. Hopefully, continued public education will help to increase awareness about prevention of Lyme disease.

REFERENCES

American Academy of Pediatrics, Committee on Infectious Diseases. Prevention of Lyme disease. *Pediatrics.* 2000; 105:142–147.

Balcer LJ, Winterkorn MS, Galetta SL. Neuro-ophthalmic manifestations of Lyme disease. *J Neuroophthalmol.* 1997; 17:108–121.

Brown SL, Hansen SL, Langone JJ. Role of serology in the diagnosis of Lyme disease. *JAMA.* 1999;282:62–66.

Evans J. Lyme disease. *Curr Opin Rheumatol.* 1999;11:281–288.

Frohman L, Lama P. Annual update of systemic disease—1999: Emerging and re-emerging infections (Part II). *J Neuroophthalmol.* 2000;20:48–58.

Hilton E, et al. Seroprevalence and seroconversion for tick-borne diseases in a high-risk population in the northeast United States. *Am J Med.* 1999;106:404–409.

Huppertz H, Munchmeier D, Lieb W. Ocular manifestations in children and adolescents with Lyme arthritis. *Br J Ophthalmol.* 1999;83:1149–1152.

Karma A, Mikkila H. Ocular manifestations and treatment of Lyme disease. *Curr Opin Ophthalmol. 1996;7:7–12.*

Lesser RL. Ocular manifestations of Lyme disease. *Am J Med.* 1995;98 (suppl 4A):60S–62S.

Meltzer MI, Dennis DT, Orloski KA. The cost effectiveness of vaccinating against Lyme disease. *Emerg Infect Dis.* 1999; 5:321–328.

Mikkila H, Karma A, Viljanen M, Seppala I. The laboratory diagnosis of ocular Lyme borreliosis. *Graefes Arch Clin Exp Ophthalmol.* 1999;237:225–230.

Mikkila H, Seppala I, Leirisalo-Repo M, et al. The etiology of uveitis: The role of infections with special reference to Lyme borreliosis. *Acta Ophthalmol Scand.* 1997;75:716–719.

Mikkila HO, Seppala IT, Viljanen MK, et al. The expanding clinical spectrum of ocular Lyme borreliosis. *Ophthalmology.* 2000;107:581–587.

Miyashiro MJ, Yee RW, Patel G, Ruiz RS. Lyme disease associated with unilateral interstitial keratitis. *Cornea.* 1999; 18:115–116.

Nadelman RB, Herman E, Wormser GP. Screening for Lyme disease in hospitalized psychiatric patients: Prospective serosurvey in an endemic area. *Mt Sinai J Med.* 1997; 64:409–412.

Nadelman RB, Nowakowski J, Forseter G, et al. The clinical spectrum of early Lyme borreliosis in patients with culture-confirmed erythema migrans. *Am J Med.* 1996;100: 502–508.

Nadelman RB, Wormser GP. Lyme borreliosis. *Lancet.* 1998; 352:557–565.

Rahn DW, Felz MW. Lyme disease update. Current aproach to early, disseminated, and late disease. *Postgrad Med.* 1998; 103:51–64.

Recommendations for the use of Lyme disease vaccine. Recommendations of the Advisory Committee on Immunization Practices (ACIP). *MMWR Morb Mortal Wkly Rep.* 1999; 48 (RR-7):1–17.

Schwartz GS, Harrison AR, Holland EJ. Etiology of immune stromal (interstitial) keratitis. *Cornea.* 1998:17:278–281.

Sigal LH, et al. A vaccine consisting of recombinant *Borrelia burgdorferi* outer-surface protein A to prevent Lyme disease. *N Eng J Med.* 1998;339:216–222.

Steigbigel RT, Benach JL. Immunization against Lyme disease—An important first step. The *N Engl J Med.* 1998; 339. Editorial.

Verdon ME, Sigal LH. Recognition and management of Lyme disease. *Am Fam Physician.* 1997;56:427–442.

Wormser GP. Vaccination as a modality to prevent Lyme disease. A status report. *Infect Dis Clin North Am.* 1999; 13:135–148.

Wormser GP, Aguero-Rosenfeld ME, Nadelman RB. Lyme disease serology, problems and opportunities. *JAMA.* 1999; 282: 79–80.

Zaidman GW. The ocular manifestations of Lyme disease. *Int Ophthalmol Clin.* 1997;37:13–28.

Chapter 44

SYPHILIS

Kelly H. Thomann

Syphilis is a slowly evolving chronic infection caused by the spirochete *Treponema pallidum,* which can affect any system in the body. It has been called many names, and at one time was dubbed the "great pox," because it occurred in epidemic proportions in 15th-century Europe. Many people once attributed the spread of syphilis to the return of Christopher Columbus' expedition to Europe from the New World, where it was acquired in the West Indies. However, current evidence now suggests that the disease was actually present in Europe prior to this time but increased to epidemic proportions as a result of the movement of troops during the French and Spanish wars. Henry the VIII, Napoleon Bonaparte, Ludwig von Beethoven, and Florence Nightingale are just a few individuals who, throughout the past centuries, were believed to have had syphilis influence their lives. In the 1950s, penicillin treatment and preventative health programs helped lead to a significant decrease in its prevalence. From 1986 to 1990, there was a dramatic upswing in the number of cases of syphilis. However, this trend reversed, and in 1998 the lowest number of cases of syphilis were reported since tracking began in 1941. Ocular manifestations of syphilis are vast, and affect every part of the eye. The diversity of its effects explains why this disease has often been called "the great imitator."

EPIDEMIOLOGY

Systemic

In the early 1900s, syphilis was a major public health problem, and a significant cause of morbidity and mortality. Its incidence peaked around the time of World War II, reaching 75 cases per 100,000 persons in 1946. However, largely due to penicillin treatment, the number of cases dropped dramatically, to 4 per 100,000 persons in 1956. Between 1970 and 2000 the incidence of syphilis has followed cyclical trends. Beginning in the late 1970s to mid-1980s the incidence rose steadily, probably reflecting changes in sexual behavior, with a disproportionate increase in homosexual men. In 1986 the number of cases declined again, most likely because newfound public awareness of HIV led to changes in sexual behavior. However, between 1985 and 1990 there was a 75% increase in syphilis cases, rising to 20 per 100,000 persons in 1990. This increase was particularly evident in African-American males and females, rising 126 and 231%, respectively, from 1985 to 1990. In 1998, the number of cases of syphilis reported to the Centers for Disease Control and Prevention (CDC) was 6993. This represents the lowest number since reporting began in 1941, and an 86% reduction from the high in 1990. However, a disproportionate rate still exists in the southern United States and among non-Hispanic blacks.

Syphilis most commonly affects the 15- to 30-year age group. Approximately one-third of individuals exposed to infectious syphilis will acquire the disease. Virtually all patients with untreated primary syphilis will go on to the secondary stage, and 30% of patients with untreated secondary syphilis will go on to the tertiary stage. The disease will remain latent in the remainder of those with untreated secondary syphilis. Of those with tertiary syphilis, 10% will have cardiovascular complications, 15% will go on to have dermatologic involvement, and 10% will have neurosyphilis.

In 1998, 801 cases of congenital syphilis were reported to the CDC, representing a rate of 20.6 per 100,000 live births. This is a sharp reduction from the peak of 107.3 per 100,000 live births in 1991.

Ocular

Ocular involvement occurs in about 5% of untreated cases of secondary syphilis. Uveitis is the most common ocular manifestation of syphilis, and Moore (1931) reported that 4.6% of patients with secondary syphilis and 9% of patients with recurrent secondary syphilis get uveitis. Schlaegel and Kao (1982) reviewed the cases of presumptive syphilitic uveitis from 1970 to 1980 seen in their clinic and found that syphilis accounted for 1.1% of all uveitis cases. If the disease progresses to neurosyphilis, ocular involvement will occur in 10%. Hooshmand (1972) investigated ocular complications of neurosyphilis and found that of 241 cases, 44.8% had pupil abnormalities (Argyll Robertson pupil the most common), 12% had chorioretinitis, 4.6% had blepharoptosis, and 4.6% had optic atrophy.

PATHOPHYSIOLOGY/DISEASE PROCESS

Systemic

The Organism

Treponema pallidum is a delicate, spiral-shaped, motile spirochete that requires a warm, moist environment to survive and whose only host is humans. Its shape enables it to move by rotating, allowing rapid penetration into mucous membranes. It is too narrow to be seen with light microscopy, but its unique shape and movement allow it to be identified by dark-field microscopy.

Transmission

Transmission of *T. pallidum* primarily occurs through sexual contact, although it may also be transmitted, less frequently, via transfusion of infected blood (rare today), perinatally, and through needle sharing. The organism enters the blood through breaks in abraded areas of skin. Once it is within the tissue, it replicates locally and disseminates via the lymphatic system and bloodstream to produce systemic infection. The initial incubation period is from 9 to 90 days, with an average time of 3 weeks.

Course of the Disease

The natural history of syphilis reflects the interaction between the spirochete and the immune response of the infected individual. The first response to infection is the local infiltration of polymorphonuclear leukocytes at the site of inoculation. This leads to a cutaneous ulceration and infiltration of the lesion by lymphocytes and plasma cells. Local factors heal the lesion, but there are treponemas still present that are able to disseminate through the bloodstream, leading to the next stage of syphilis, secondary disease. The host response in this stage leads to cutaneous lesions consisting of lymphocytes and perivascular plasma cell infiltrates. Chronic inflammatory response is responsible for the tertiary stage of the disease, characterized by perivascular infiltration, which leads to obliterative endarteritis.

The course of syphilis has classically been broken into primary, secondary, latent, and tertiary stages. These most often overlap; therefore it is often easier to describe the stages of syphilis as early or late. Early disease includes primary, secondary, and early latency; late disease includes late latency and tertiary syphilis. Syphilis can also be acquired congenitally.

Primary Syphilis

Primary syphilis (Table 44–1) is characterized by the presence of a chancre at the site of treponema penetration and inoculation. The primary chancre, which may consist of one or multiple lesions, is described as a painless red papule varying in size from 0.5 to 1 cm. Within a few days of appearance its margins indurate and may become covered with a yellow or gray exudate. Because the lesion appears at the site of inoculation, it is most frequently found in genital, perineal, anal, or oral areas, although it may occur anywhere and go unnoticed if not on an exposed part of the body. The chancre will heal spontaneously in 3 to 8 weeks if untreated. It is an erosion, not an ulcer, and it therefore heals without leaving a scar. A bilateral regional lymphadenopathy may accompany the chancre.

Secondary Syphilis

Disseminated syphilis more accurately describes the secondary stage, because it is characterized by widespread dermatologic and systemic findings (Table 44–1) due to the hematogenous spread of *T. pallidum* from the primary chancre. It occurs 4 to 10 weeks after primary manifestations.

TABLE 44–1. SYSTEMIC MANIFESTATIONS OF PRIMARY AND SECONDARY SYPHILIS

Primary Syphilis
- Chancre
- Generalized lymphadenopathy

Secondary Syphilis
- **Skin**
  Early rash: macular syphilis (roseola syphilitica)
  Later rash: papular, maculopapular, or papulosquamous lesions
  Condylomata lata
  Mucous membrane lesions, especially mucous patches
  Alopecia of eyebrows, scalp, beard
- **General**
  Headache
  Lymphadenopathy
  Pruritus
  Fever
  Malaise
  Weight loss
  Arthralgia
- **Mouth/Throat**
  Tonsilitis
  Pharyngitis
  Mucous membrane lesions/mucous patches
  Ulcers/erosions
- **Genital**
  Chancre
  Condylomata lata
  Mucous patches
- **Central Nervous System**
  CSF abnormalities
  Meningismus (pain in the meningocortical region of the brain)
  Meningitis
  Cranial nerve II–IV and VI–VIII abnormalities
- **Skeletal/Joint**
  Periostitis of the skull, tibia, sternum, ribs
- **Renal (rare)**
  Glomerulonephritis
  Nephrotic syndrome
- **Gastrointestinal (rare)**
  Invasion of intestinal wall
- **Liver (rare)**
  Hepatitis

The skin manifestations of secondary syphilis are numerous and occur in almost all patients. A symmetrical, papular rash involving the entire trunk and extremities is a common finding in early secondary syphilis. It is most prominent on the palms of the hands and soles of the feet. When it first appears, the lesions usually consist of rounded, indistinct macules less than 1 cm in size, with a light pink to rose color. The rash may resolve or the lesions may go on to become scaly, reddish brown papules or maculopapules (described as a "raw ham" appearance) varying in size from 0.5 to 2 cm.

Condylomata lata skin lesions will be found in 20% of patients with secondary syphilis. These are large, relatively broad and flat, pale to grayish papules found in the folds of moist, warm locations, such as the vulva, anal area, scrotum, or perineum. They may become hypertrophic and protrude above the skin surface in some cases.

Mucous membrane lesions, which are small, superficial ulcerated areas with gray borders, frequently accompany cutaneous manifestations. They commonly occur in the tonsils and adjacent oropharynx, causing symptoms of sore throat, diffuse pharyngitis, tonsillitis, or laryngitis. Mucous patches are found in one third of patients with mucous lesions, usually in the late secondary stage. These are flat, grayish, rounded erosions covered by a membrane in the mouth or genital areas.

Alopecia of the scalp, eyebrows, eyelashes, and beard may occur, possibly as the only manifestation of this stage. This loss of hair may be diffuse or occur in a patchy distribution, causing a "moth-eaten" appearance at the involved area.

General systemic manifestations of disseminated syphilis occur in about one half of the patients as flu-like symptoms with malaise, low-grade fever, and diffuse painless lymphadenopathy. Less common symptoms include headache and arthralgia.

Bone involvement or periostitis (an inflammation of the periosteum of the bone) frequently involves the skull, tibia, sternum, and ribs, rarely becoming symptomatic. Other system involvement includes the liver, kidney, intestines, and joints (Table 44–1).

Neurological manifestations may appear late in this stage. Asymptomatic abnormalities in cerebral spinal fluid will be found in 32% of patients. A small percent will go on to have symptoms including meningitis with headache and mental changes. Cranial nerves II through IV and VI through VIII may be affected. Spinal cord or nerve root involvement may lead to tingling, weakness, and hyporeflexia.

Latent Syphilis

Untreated secondary syphilis persists 4 to 8 weeks before the patient becomes symptom and lesion free, entering the latent period. The CDC defines early latency as the first year of the latent period. During this time the patient is still considered infectious and may have a relapse back to secondary manifestations at any time. Late latency is defined as greater than 1 year after secondary syphilis. Relapse rarely occurs during this time, and the patient is considered to be noninfectious. However, pregnant women may infect the fetus during any stage of the disease.

Tertiary Syphilis

Tertiary syphilis is divided into benign late syphilis, cardiovascular syphilis, and late neurosyphilis. Cardiovascular and late neurosyphilis are the most damaging stages. Manifestations of tertiary syphilis are less frequently encountered today, probably due to antibiotic therapy for other illnesses that inadvertently treat syphilis.

Benign late syphilis involves nonvital structures. Although it is classified as "benign," the chronic destruction of this stage can lead to devastating consequences. This stage is characterized by the presence of gummas, which are localized, soft granulomas, best described as having a "gummy" consistency. Gummas represent a chronic maximum inflammatory response to a few spirochetes causing the slow destruction of tissue, eventually leading to fibrosis of the affected area. These present most commonly as isolated lesions of the skin and subcutaneous tissue, usually located on the face, neck, and extremities. They may persist several years if untreated. They may also occur in bones, commonly the tibia, fibula, clavicles, and skull, causing pain and swelling, and ultimately leading to the destruction of cartilage. Gummas may also be found in other organs (Table 44–2).

Cardiovascular tertiary syphilis results from perivascular infiltration that leads to obliterative endarteritis and ischemia. The destruction of elastic blood vessel walls can lead to medial necrosis with aneurysm formation. These effects are primarily found at the vaso vasorum of the ascending aorta, with aortic aneurysm, aortic regurgitation, and coronary artery stenosis the most common manifestations. Most of these patients are asymptomatic; however, clinical signs of cardiovascular disease may occur 10 to 40 years after primary infection.

Neurosyphilis is not actually a separate stage of the disease but a collection of syndromes spanning all stages of syphilis. However, its most devastating effects are found in tertiary syphilis; therefore it is usually classified as occurring in this stage. *Treponema pallidum* can invade the nervous system early in the disease course and cause changes in cerebrospinal fluid. These may be detected by laboratory tests, but the patient will usually be asymptomatic. However, acute syphilitic meningitis with fever, headache, stiff neck, and vomiting may occur less than 1 year after primary infection, and can be associated with acute hydrocephalus and cranial-nerve palsies. The patient with asymptomatic neurosyphilis may progress to late neurosyphilis. Symptomatic late neurosyphilis occurs after widespread damage to neuronal tissue in the brain and spinal cord, and is further broken down into meningovascular disease and parenchymal disease. These are not distinct categories, because vascular and parenchymous manifestations may occur at any time, and overlap.

TABLE 44–2. SYSTEMIC MANIFESTATIONS OF TERTIARY SYPHILIS

Benign Late Syphilis
- Gummas of skin (common); skeletal system (common); upper respiratory tract, mouth, and tongue; lower respiratory tract; digestive system; genitourinary system; breasts

Cardiovascular Syphilis
- Aortic aneurysm
- Aortic regurgitation
- Coronary artery disease
- Aortic valve insufficiency
- Any of above may lead to myocardial infarction, congestive heart failure, strokes, or seizures

Late Neurosyphilis
- **Meningovascular**
  - Cerebrovascular
    - Strokes with signs and symptoms pertaining to the vessel distribution affected
    - Seizures
  - Syphilis of the spinal cord
    - Syphilitic meningomyelitis: weakness and paresthesia of the legs progressing to paraparesis or paraplegia; urinary and fecal incontinence; sensory disturbance of the legs
    - Spinal vascular syphilis (rare): transection of the spinal cord at the thoracic level with accompanying signs and symptoms
- **Parenchymal**
  - General paresis
    - Personality changes
    - Speech disturbances
    - Tremor of tongue, face, hands
    - Hyper- or hypoactive reflexes
    - Expressionless face
    - Impaired handwriting
  - Tabes dorsalis
    - Lightning pains
    - Wasting
    - General paresis
    - Sensory disturbances
    - Loss of reflexes
    - Ataxia/broad-based gait
    - Bladder/bowel incontinence
    - Cranial nerve II–VIII palsy
    - Peripheral neuropathy
    - Visceral crises (gastric crises with intense epigastric pain, nausea, and vomiting)

Meningovascular syphilis is the result of chronic meningitis. Cerebrovascular involvement primarily manifests as strokes or seizures secondary to cerebrovascular occlusion with signs and symptoms as they relate to the particular vessel affected. Most of these patients are between the ages of 30 and 50; therefore syphilis should be considered when cerebrovascular accidents occur in a young adult. Meningovascular neurosyphilis of the spinal cord is considered separately because it presents with a different clinical picture. It occurs more than 20 years after primary infection and can be broken into syphilitic meningomyelitis, which is most commonly found, and spinal vascular syphilis (also called acute syphilitic transverse myelitis), which is rarely encountered. Syphilitic meningomyelitis has a gradual onset, beginning as weakness and paresthesia of the legs that may progress to parapareses or paraplegia. Urinary and fecal incontinence may occur, along with variable sensory disorders of the legs. Spinal vascular syphilis has an abrupt onset with signs and symptoms associated with transection of the spinal cord, usually at the thoracic level.

General paresis and tabes dorsalis are the most common manifestations of parenchymal disease, although rarely encountered today because of the use of antibiotics. General paresis can occur secondary to meningoencephalitis with direct invasion of the cerebrum by *T. pallidum.* It usually develops 15 to 20 years after primary infection and can lead to death if untreated. It is a chronic, dementing illness with psychiatric and neurologic manifestations. Tabes dorsales occurs about 20 years after the latent period and is caused by degeneration of the dorsal columns of the spinal cord and sensory nerve trunks. The classic clinical presentation includes lightning pains, paresthesia, decreased deep tendon reflexes, and abnormal pupils.

Congenital Syphilis

Maternal syphilis can adversely affect the birth of the child in many ways. Premature birth, spontaneous abortion, stillbirth, and nonimmune hydrops (abnormal serous fluid accumulation in tissues of body cavities) may occur, or the infant can be born with congenital syphilis. This is broken into early and late disease. The disease can be transmitted to an infant in two ways, most frequently through transplacental passage of *T. pallidum,* or rarely, through contact with genital lesions during the birth process. The risk of fetal infection is related directly to the stage of maternal syphilis at the time of pregnancy and the stage of pregnancy when the fetus is infected. Fetal transmission may be as high as 100% if the mother has primary or secondary syphilis. The risk of transmission is 40% when the mother is in the early latent stage, and this decreases to 10% when in the late latent stage. Fetal damage can be prevented with maternal treatment prior to the 16th week of gestation, and fetal infection usually does not occur before the 10th week of gestation. The most severely affected at birth are usually infected after the 23rd week of gestation.

Early Congenital Syphilis. Clinical manifestations appear within 3 months to the first 2 years of life in early congenital syphilis, because many treponemas are present and undergoing extensive multiplication. The typical clinical presentation is a healthy infant at birth who becomes ill several months later. The baby may also be small for gestational age. Clinical signs may include mucous patches and mucocutaneous lesions, similar to those found in secondary syphilis. A bilateral maculopapular rash, at first appearing red with oval lesions, later turning coppery brown with superficial desquamation or scaling, may be present. Vesicles and bullae are most commonly found on the palms of the hands and soles of the feet, but also may be found on the palate, perineum, and intertriginous (oppositional) body surfaces. These destructive eruptions are also called pemphigus syphiliticus, and are characterized by erythema and blister formation with eventual crusting. The blister fluid is highly contagious. These may heal and result in rhagades (scars or fissures in areas lesions were previously present). Also evident may be "snuffles" (a profuse whitish mucous nasal discharge, which is highly infectious, caused by the invasion of the nasal mucosa by *T. pallidum*); enlarged liver and spleen; and generalized lymphadenopathy.

Skeletal system involvement can be prominent and cause osteochondritis (inflammation of the cartilage and bone), periostitis, or osteitis (inflammation of the bones), especially the metaphyses of the long bones. Lesions will be painful, multiple, and symmetric, occurring in the lower limbs more often than upper extremities. The pain may be so severe that it inhibits movement and produces Parrott syphilitic pseudoparalysis, in which the child appears to be paralyzed. Other organ system involvement is listed in Table 44–3.

Late Congenital Syphilis. Fewer organisms are present at birth in late congenital syphilis; therefore obvious clinical manifestations are not yet apparent. If the ongoing inflammation continues for 6 to 12 months, the disease enters the latency stage. Beyond the age of 2 years, late congenital syphilis can manifest as clinically evident malformations affecting numerous body systems as a result of the scarring from chronic inflammation.

The teeth are prominently affected in late congenital syphilis. Hutchinson teeth are small, widely spaced permanent upper incisors with notching, thinning, and discoloration of the enamel caused by the vasculitis and subsequent inflammatory response to the infection in the developing permanent tooth bud prior to birth. Similar findings may also occur in the upper, lower, and lateral incisors. The canine teeth may be hypoplastic and poorly enameled. The surface of the 6-year molars may be underdeveloped with many small cusps arranged in a circle; these are known as

TABLE 44–3. SYSTEMIC MANIFESTATIONS OF CONGENITAL SYPHILIS

Early Congenital Syphilis

- **General**
  - Small for gestational age
  - Snuffles
  - Enlarged liver and spleen
  - Generalized lymphadenopathy
- **Cutaneous Lesions**
  - Mucous patches
  - Mucocutaneous lesions
  - Pemphigus syphiliticus (vesicles and bullae)
  - Maculopapular rash
  - Rhagades (linear scars radiating from body orifices such as mouth, nostril, and anus) resulting from mucous patches and condylomata lata
- **Skeletal**
  - Osteochondritis
  - Periostitis
  - Osteitis
  - Parrott syphilitic pseudoparalysis
- **Hematologic**
  - Anemia
  - Leukocytosis
  - Leukopenia
  - Thrombocytopenia
- **Throat/Esophagus**
  - Laryngitis
  - Hoarse aphonia
- **Neurosyphilis**
  - CSF abnormalities: pleocytosis, increased protein
  - Acute syphilitic leptomeningitis: meningismus, vomiting bulging fontanelle
  - Untreated neurosyphilis can lead to chronic meningovascular syphilis with progressive hydrocephalus, cranial nerve palsies, cerebral infarction, secondary endarteritis
- **Renal**
  - Nephrotic syndrome
  - Subacute glomerulonephritis
- **Other (uncommon)**
  - Pneumonia alba (syphilitic pneumonia)
  - Myocarditis
  - Pancreatitis
  - Fibrosis of GI tract

Late Congenital Syphilis

- **Dental**
  - Hutchinson teeth
  - Small, poorly enameled teeth
  - Mulberry molars
  - Prone to tooth decay
- **Hutchinson Triad**
  - Defective teeth, interstitial keratitis, eighth-nerve deafness
- **Skeletal System**
  - Periostitis leading frontal bossing, squaring of cranium, saber shins, Higouménakis sign
  - Clutton joints: caused by inflammatory lesions; painless symmetrical synovitis and hydroarthritis of the knees and sometimes elbow without involvement of adjacent bones
  - Saddle nose
  - Short maxilla with high palatal arch due to nasal chondritis
- **Central Nervous System**
  - Meningitis
  - Meningovascular syphilis causing arteritis and occlusion of cerebral arteries with accompanying signs and symptoms
  - Paresis (similar to that seen in adults with tertiary syphilis)
  - Tabes dorsalis (rare, similar to that seen in adults with tertiary syphilis)

"mulberry molars." The teeth of these children are also prone to decay due to defective enamelization.

The Hutchinson triad, another well-known manifestation of congenital syphilis, includes defective teeth, interstitial keratitis, and eighth-nerve deafness. Nerve deafness and vertigo are caused by osteochondritis of the otic capsule, leading to cochlear degeneration and fibrous adhesions. Nerve deafness is a very specific finding of congenital syphilis.

The skeletal system may be adversely affected in late congenital syphilis. Periostitis of the frontal bone may lead to rounding of the bone ("frontal bossing"), and involvement of the parietal bone may cause squaring of the cranium. Periostitis of the tibia may lead to a marked convexity or bowing and is known as "saber shins." Periostitis of the clavicle can cause sternoclavicular thickening (Higouménakis sign). Chronic syphilitic rhinitis may lead to a short maxilla with a high palatal arch. Inflammation of the nasal cartilage can lead to destruction of the underlying bone and result in a saddle nose.

Congenital neurosyphilis is rare today because most children are treated prior to the serious consequences of nervous system involvement. Congenital neurosyphilis presumably follows the same course as neurosyphilis in adults. Meningitis can occur from 3 to 12 months of age and may or may not cause symptoms. Meningovascular neurosyphilis can occur in the first 2 years of life, and paresis or tabes dorsalis can manifest from about 6 to 21 years of age (Table 44–3).

HIV and Syphilis

When *T. pallidum* infects the body, the healthy host mounts both a humoral and cell-mediated immune response, and recovery without medications can occur in many patients. However, with HIV infection, the host response is not competent to combat the infection, creating the scene for greater severity and more frequent late complications. Neurosyphilis is the most serious consequence of syphilis, with or without concurrent HIV infection. However, due to the dysfunctional immune response in the HIV patient, rapid progression from the primary stage through neurosyphilis seems to occur more frequently both with and without adequate treatment. It has also been shown that patients who have syphilis have an increased risk of transmission and acquisition of HIV infection. A genital ulcer probably acts as an entry point for HIV transmission.

Ocular

There is no pathognomonic scenario for the ocular manifestations of syphilis. Ocular involvement is rarely encountered earlier than 6 months following the primary chancre, and is frequently found in secondary and tertiary syphilis. Anterior uveitis (Figure 44–1) is the most common ocular complication in secondary syphilis (Table 44–4). Chorioretinitis, with varying presentations, and retinal vasculitis are also common. The chorioretinitis may be diffuse or focal (Figure 44–2) (posterior pole more often than periphery), with acute vitreal inflammation usually accompanying it. One or both optic nerves may become swollen from various mechanisms with syphilis as the underlying cause. Retinal vascular lesions include angiospasm, artery or vein occlusion, and aneurysm formation. Retinal vasculitis affects the arterial supply more often, but periphlebitis and inflammation of both vessels have also been reported.

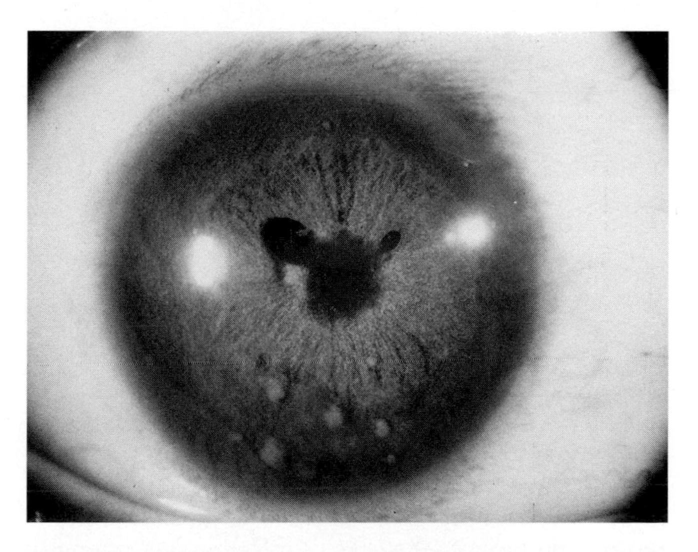

Figure 44–1. Bilateral uveitis with extensive posterior synechiae and inflammatory nodules of the iris in a patient with a positive VDRL and FTA-ABS. (*Reprinted with permission from Margo CE, Hamed LM. Ocular syphilis.* Surv Ophthalmol. *1992;37:211.*)

Ocular complications of late syphilis are typically found in older populations, often those who do not receive regular medical attention. In these cases, diagnosis is usually made by exclusion in a patient with positive treponemal serology. According to Schlaegel (1969), tertiary syphilis should be suspected in any patient with an unexplained pupillary abnormality, optic atrophy or neuritis, dislocated lens not related to other etiologies, apparent retinitis pigmentosa, or uveitis that is unresponsive to conventional therapy. Argyll Robertson pupils (unequal, irregular, and profoundly miotic pupils with a light-near dissociation) are most common; however, tonic pupils may also be found. The tonic pupils found in syphilis could be confused with Adie tonic pupils, but patient characteristics will help differentiate the two. Adie tonic pupils are found more commonly in females than males, and unilateral more often than bilateral, with a mean age of onset of 32 years; they are usually associated with decreased deep tendon reflexes. Syphilitic tonic pupils occur more frequently in males, are always bilateral, have a mean age of detection of 57, and usually do not have decreased deep tendon reflexes. Other common findings include retinal vascular lesions and keratitis (Table 44–4).

Ocular disorders such as uveitis, papillitis, vitritis, optic neuritis, and retinitis are among the more prominent manifestations of syphilis in the HIV-infected individual. These are more often bilateral and follow a more aggressive course.

Ocular manifestations of congenital syphilis are similar to those in adults with secondary syphilis (Table 44–4). Acute anterior uveitis with a secondary cataract is most common. Also, syphilis should be included in the differential diagnosis of any childhood case of chorioretinitis. The "salt-and-pepper" appearance of the retina is a classic finding. Secondary glaucoma is also commonly associated with early congenital syphilis. Interstitial keratitis is the most common late manifestation of syphilis, and can occur between the ages of 5 and 20 (Figure 44–3). After resolution, corneal opacification and ghost vessels (Figure 44–4) remain as permanent complications. Optic neuritis may also be found in late congenital syphilis.

DIAGNOSIS

Systemic

Primary Syphilis

Diagnosis of primary syphilis is based upon the presence of a syphilitic chancre and positive laboratory tests. Differential diagnoses of the syphilitic chancre/

TABLE 44–4. OCULAR MANIFESTATIONS OF SYPHILIS

Primary Syphilis
- Chancre of the eyelid or conjunctiva (rare)

Secondary Syphilis
- Conjunctivitis
- Interstitial keratitis
- Episcleritis
- Scleritis
- Iris capillary abnormalities
  - Iritis roseata—a collection of small, dilated capillaries present on the surface of the iris
  - Iritis papulosa—the roseata lesions increase in size and become papule-like
  - Iritis nodosa—the papulosa areas become larger and form yellow-red nodules
- Anterior uveitis
  - Acute or chronic
  - Recurrent
  - Nongranulomatous or granulomatous
- Postinflammatory iris atrophy
- Vitritis
- Posterior uveitis
  - Retinitis
  - Retinal pigment epitheliitis
  - Retinal vasculitis
  - Necrotizing retinitis
  - Choroiditis
  - Serous retinal detachment
  - Exudative retinal detachment
  - Uveal effusion
- Optic nerve involvement
  - Optic neuritis
  - Papillitis
  - Perineuritis
  - Neuroretinitis
  - Optic atrophy
  - Papilledema secondary to increased ICP from meningitis or meningoencephalitis
- Pupil abnormalities
  - Argyll Robertson pupils
  - Tonic pupils
- Vasculitis
  - Arteriolitis
  - Retinal periarteritis
  - Subretinal neovascularization
  - Retinal necrosis
  - Central retinal artery and/or central retinal vein occlusion
- Retinal involvement
  - Macula edema
  - Stellate maculopathy
  - Disciform macular detachment

Tertiary Syphilis
- Pupil abnormalities
  - Argyll Robertson pupils
  - Tonic pupils
- Keratitis
- Cataracts
- Lens dislocation
- Retinitis
- Optic neuritis
- Descending optic atrophy
- Optic atrophy secondary to chronic disc edema
- Papilledema due to meningitis or meningoencephalitis
- Perineuritis
- Gumma of the lids, conjunctiva, cornea, sclera, iris, ciliary body, orbit, optic nerve, superior orbital fissure

Neurosyphilis
- Pupil abnormalities
  - Argyll Robertson pupils
  - Tonic pupils
  - Dilated pupils fixed to both light and near stimuli
- Chorioretinitis
- Blepharoptosis
- Optic atrophy
- Cranial nerve palsies (3, 4, 6)
- Arteritis with stroke-like effects to any part of the ocular pathways

Congenital Syphilis
- Early
  - Salt-and-pepper chorioretinitis
  - Uveitis
  - Secondary glaucoma
  - Cataracts
  - Chancre of eyelid
  - Any manifestation of secondary syphilis
- Late
  - Interstitial keratitis/corneal opacities
  - Pupil abnormalities
  - Optic atrophy
  - Secondary glaucoma

genital ulcers are listed in Table 44–5. The surest way to diagnose primary syphilis is through dark-field microscopy. This uses a sample from either a chancre or lymph node to identify *T. pallidum.* Identification is based on the movement and shape of the spirochete. If positive, it is the only test needed to diagnose the disease. If negative, syphilis is not ruled out, and further testing is required.

Serological testing for syphilis is divided into nontreponemal and treponemal tests (Table 44–6). Nontreponemal (also called reaginic) tests measure antibody against a cardiolipin–lecithin cholesterol antigen known as reagin, which results from interaction of *T. pallidum* with host tissue. The venereal disease research laboratory (VDRL) and rapid plasma reagin (RPR) are the most frequently used reaginic tests, and are most useful as screening tests. These tests usually become positive within 4 to 8 weeks of infection and after 4 to 7 days of chancre appearance. However, they may be negative in 13 to 41% of patients with primary syphilis. Titers fall at a rate related to the duration of infection prior to treatment. Treatment within 6 months usually

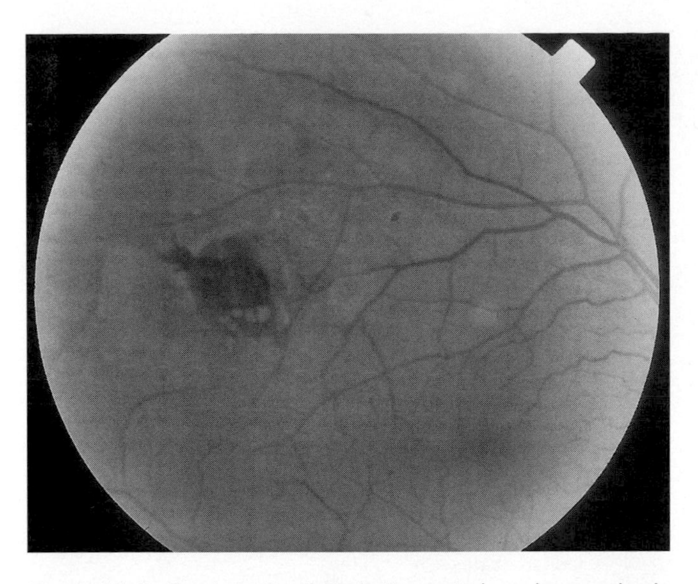

Figure 44–2. Focal chorioretinitis in the posterior pole occurring in secondary syphilis.

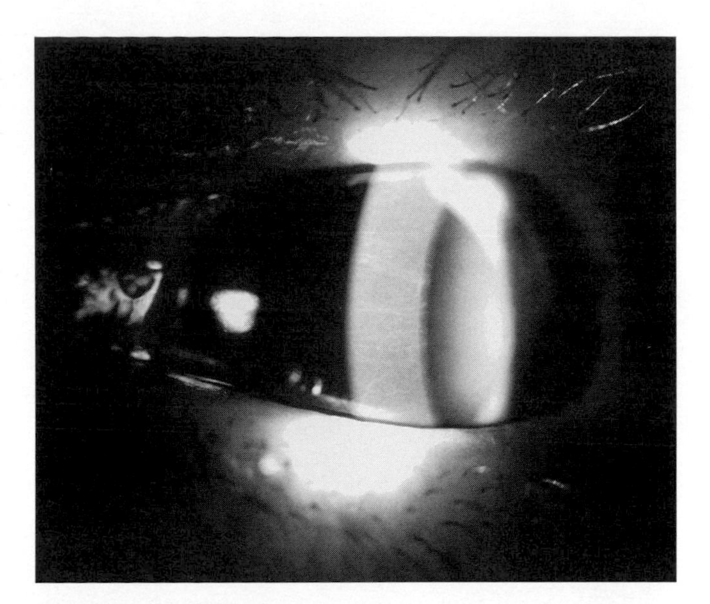

Figure 44–4. Ghost vessels secondary to interstitial keratitis in a patient with congenital syphilis.

causes the patient to become seronegative in 12 months. However, it may take 2 years for later infection to seroconvert after treatment and it may never occur after treatment of late syphilis. One drawback to reaginic tests is that they are nonspecific; therefore other stimulants of antigens can give false-positive test results (eg, autoimmune disease, Lyme disease, other acute or chronic infections). Therefore, positive reaginic tests must be confirmed with treponemal serology.

Treponemal tests detect specific treponemal antibodies, and once positive remain so for life. The most common treponemal tests include fluorescent treponemal antibody test (FTA-ABS), microhemagglutination *T. pallidum* assay (MHA-TP), and hemagglutination treponemal test for syphilis (HATTS). Treponemal tests are not used initially to diagnose primary syphilis because they are more expensive, have a 20% false-negative rate, and will be positive even in a patient who currently does not have the disease but was previously successfully treated for it. If dark-field microscopy is not available, diagnosis of syphilis is made by screening with nontreponemal tests and confirmation with treponemal tests.

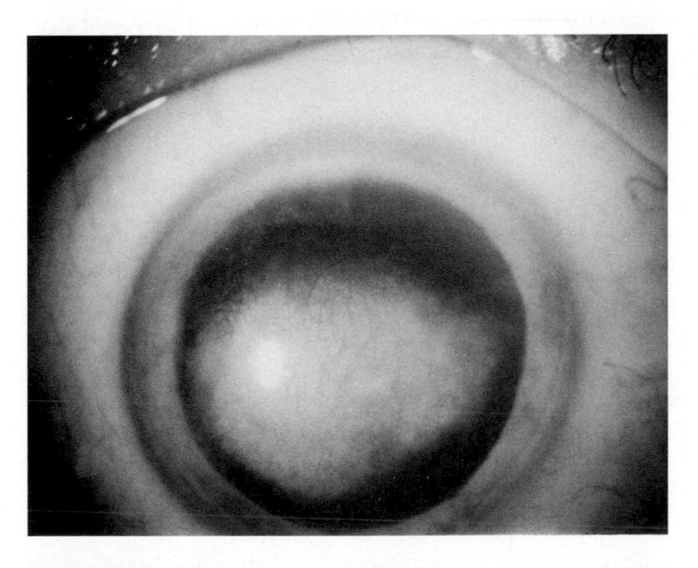

Figure 44–3. Late-onset interstitial keratitis in a patient with congenital syphilis. (*Reprinted with permission from Margo CE, Hamed LM. Ocular syphilis.* Surv Ophthalmol. *1992;37:211.*)

Secondary Syphilis

The diagnosis of secondary syphilis is made based upon clinical suspicion of the disease and supporting serology (Table 44–6). The rash found in this stage is the most prominent feature, present 75 to 100% of the time. The patient may also have flu-like symptoms or other clinical manifestations. Table 44–5 lists differential diagnoses of some of the more prominent manifestations of secondary syphilis.

Sensitivity is almost 100% for nontreponemal and treponemal tests in untreated secondary syphilis. Reaginic testing can be unreliable in extremely active cases due to excessive antibody production that blocks agglutination and gives a false-negative result. This

> The rash in secondary syphilis is present in most cases; both nontreponemal and treponemal tests will be positive in secondary syphilis.

TABLE 44–5. DIFFERENTIAL DIAGNOSES IN SYPHILIS

Stage	Manifestation	Differential Diagnoses
Primary	Chancre/genital ulcer	• Herpes simplex virus • *Haemophilus ducreyi* • Streptococci • Staphylococci • *Candida* • Chancroid • Lymphogranuloma venereum
Secondary	Rash	• Pityriasis rosea • Tinea corporis • Erythema multiforme • Psoriasis • Stevens–Johnson syndrome • Viral exanthem • Drug eruption • Seborrheic dermatitis • Lichen planus • Granuloma annulare • Scabies
	Condylomata latum	• Venereal warts • Condyloma acuminatum
	Mucous membrane lesions	• Mucosal lesions in orogenital herpes • Aphthous ulcer in Behçet syndrome • Stevens–Johnson syndrome
	Lymphadenopathy/fever	• HIV infection • Infectious mononucleosis • Other viral syndromes • Lymphoma
Tertiary	Gummas	• Mass lesions in tuberculosis, sarcoidosis, malignancy, leprosy, deep mycoses, lymphoblastoma

has been called the "prozone phenomenon," and may also be found in patients with concurrent HIV infection. Nontreponemal testing will usually be positive during this stage. About 30% of persons will have cerebrospinal fluid pleocytosis with increased protein, although most of these patients will have no clinical signs of central nervous system involvement. Some controversy exists as to the usefulness of CSF (colony-stimulating factor) evaluation in syphilis. CSF cell count and glucose level are nonspecific and cannot be

TABLE 44–6. SEROLOGY FOR SYPHILIS IN EACH STAGE OF THE DISEASE

Syphilis Stage	Nontreponemal Tests	Treponemal Tests
Primary	Positive after 4–8 weeks but up to 41% false negatives	Positive earlier than nontreponemal tests but up to 20% false negatives
Secondary	Almost always positive except with prozone phenomenon	Almost always positive; false positives possible
Latent	Usually positive	Almost always positive
Tertiary	May be positive or negative; becomes negative with time and treatment	Always positive, even if adequately treated; some false positives possible
Neurosyphilis	May be negative or weakly positive	Always positive, even if adequately treated; some false positives possible
Early congenital	Positive; role in congenital syphilis is to monitor antibody titer (can be positive due to passive transfer from mother; increasing titer implies active disease in the infant)	Always positive; may be false positive from passive transfer of antibodies from mother
Late congenital	May be negative or weakly positive	Always positive

used to diagnose neurosyphilis, but they may be the best indicator of disease activity. A normal cell count indicates inactive disease. Protein count greater than 45 mg/dL is consistent with active disease.

Latent Syphilis

Latent syphilis is difficult to diagnose because patients are asymptomatic and may not recall the manifestations of the primary or secondary stages that occurred previously. Often, latent syphilis is discovered inadvertently through premarital or prenatal screening. In latent syphilis, treponemal serology will be positive. Nontreponemal tests may be positive but decrease with time, and therefore can also be negative.

Controversy exists regarding the need for lumbar puncture in latent syphilis. Many currently believe the risk involved outweighs the benefits of the test. However, it is indicated when any neurological signs or symptoms are present, or in patients who have concurrent HIV infection (see "HIV and Syphilis" later in the chapter).

Tertiary Syphilis

Gummas are the presenting manifestations of benign tertiary syphilis, with the majority occurring in the skin and skeletal system. Nontreponemal and treponemal tests will usually be positive in this stage (Table 44–6). Active neurosyphilis is at best extremely difficult to diagnose. It is based on serology, after other possible disease mechanisms have been ruled out. The prozone phenomenon may also occur in tertiary syphilis; therefore a negative result with nontreponemal testing in a highly suspicious case also warrants treponemal testing or nontreponemal testing with diluted titers. The modern CSF VDRL should be the standard test for active neurosyphilis because it provides greater information than other tests. CSF pleocytosis can be indicative of neurosyphilis activity and in most cases protein will be elevated. Many recommend a CSF examination with VDRL testing in any patient with untreated syphilis whose duration is longer than 1 year and any patient with neurologic symptoms and syphilis. Positive CSF VDRL should be followed by FTA-ABS. If both are positive, they rule out a biologically false positive CSF VDRL.

Congenital Syphilis

It is vital that all pregnant women be tested for syphilis, and treated if positive to avoid the often devastating effects of congenital syphilis. Many experts feel that female patients at risk for syphilis should be tested early in the pregnancy, in the third trimester, and again at delivery. Using the 1990 CDC definition for congenital syphilis, any infant born to a woman with a history of untreated or inadequately treated syphilis with or without serologic confirmation is presumed to have congenital syphilis and treated as such. When this definition is not applied, diagnosis of the asymptomatic infant can be difficult because there is a passive transfer of IgG antibodies in utero and therefore false positives can occur in infants who are not infected. If not treated, the infant with positive serology must be followed over the first 3 months of life to determine if the serology titers increase or decrease. If the VDRL becomes more reactive (the titer increases), it indicates active infection, and a positive test beyond 12 to 15 months also confirms congenital syphilis. If the infant is not infected, the VDRL and FTA-ABS will eventually decrease and return to negative. Diagnosis is definitively made when the level of the nontreponemal test is fourfold or greater than the mother's serum. A probable diagnosis can be made when the infant has a reactive nontreponemal test with clinical manifestations of the disease.

Dark-field microscopy can also be used to establish the diagnosis of congenital syphilis. However, if the spirochete cannot be identified, it does not rule out infection with the disease, and serology must be used to make the diagnosis.

Polymerase chain reaction (PCR) has been shown to be highly sensitive and specific in the early detection of congenital syphilis. It holds promise for the future; however, it is not widely available at this time. Tests that specifically detect IgM antibodies (such as the FTA-ABS IgM) also are promising because IgM antibodies do not cross the placenta from the mother's blood, leading to increased accuracy in the detection of congenital infection.

HIV and Syphilis

Serologic tests for syphilis may give exaggerated results with concurrent HIV infection, and may not be as reliable as they are in other cases. Very high reaginic titers can be found when the host response is severely immunocompromised. Paradoxically, the prozone phenomenon may cause serology to appear negative in secondary syphilis because of a severely immunocompromised host in late HIV disease. In these cases, the lab must be requested to do serial dilutions on the serum. Dark-field microscopy may be more valuable in these patients because it actually detects the presence of spirochetes. All patients with HIV and syphilis should have a CSF evaluation because of the increased frequency of neurosyphilis complications. Most clinicians will suspect concurrent HIV infection if syphilis is diagnosed; therefore it is recommended that all patients with syphilis should be tested for HIV, and that all patients positive for HIV should be tested for syphilis.

Ocular

Once a specific ocular disorder is diagnosed, the examiner must consider syphilis in the differential (Table 44–7) according to the particular manifestation, its presentation, the age of the patient, and health status along with systemic signs and symptoms. Prompt diagnosis is important because delay may lead to irreversible vision loss that was potentially treatable. The patient may need to be questioned regarding the presence of a genital chancre, a rash, or any of the other systemic manifestations. Because almost all ocular manifestations occur in secondary or tertiary syphilis, treponemal and nontreponemal tests should both be positive. However, the reactivity of nontreponemal tests decrease with time, or the prozone phenomenon may give false negatives. Tamesis and Foster (1990) found that only 68% of patients with ocular syphilis had positive VDRL versus 100% with FTA-ABS. Therefore, if the clinician is highly suspicious of syphilis, treponemal testing must be done, because ocular syphilis cannot be excluded through nontreponemal serology. Because the eye is an extension of the nervous system, the CDC recommends CSF evaluation on all patients with ocular syphilis; however, the results are often negative.

TABLE 44–7. OCULAR DIFFERENTIAL DIAGNOSES OF THE MORE COMMON OCULAR MANIFESTATIONS IN SYPHILIS

Ocular Manifestation	Differential Diagnoses
Interstitial keratitis	• Cogan syndrome • Lyme disease • Tuberculosis • Leprosy • Viral interstitial keratitis • Drug-induced
Uveitis	• Sarcoid • Collagen vascular diseases • Toxoplasmosis • Tuberculosis • Idiopathic • Vogt–Koyanagi–Harada disease • Coccidioidomycosis • Histoplasmosis • Toxocariasis • Lyme disease • Cytomegalovirus • HLA-B27 syndromes
Optic neuropathy	• Lyme disease • Sarcoidosis • Tuberculosis • Neoplasm (leukemia, lymphoma) • Cryptococcal meningitis (in HIV) • Systemic lupus erythematosus • Toxic conditions • Nutritional • Leber hereditary optic neuropathy
Chorioretinitis	• Pigmented paravenous retinochoroidal atrophy • Rubella retinopathy • Retinitis pigmentosa variants
Pupil abnormality (Argyll Robertson)	• Pseudotabes pituitaria • Pseudotabes diabetica • Third cranial nerve misdirection • Systemic amyloid • Myotonic dystrophy • Chronic alcoholism • Neurosarcoidosis • Encephalitis • Herpes zoster • Midbrain tumor

TREATMENT AND MANAGEMENT

Systemic

Penicillin has long been known to be the standard treatment for all stages of syphilis. *Treponema pallidum* is most sensitive to this antibiotic, and remarkably, has not developed resistance over time. The goals of treatment are to eliminate the signs and symptoms, prevent transmission to others, and prevent the severe late sequelae of the disease. The CDC has set standards for each of the stages; however, it is almost impossible to establish a standard treatment because so many variables exist in syphilis. Most clinicians agree with the CDC protocols, but some prefer more aggressive amounts of penicillin in certain cases. Intramuscular injection is generally preferred as opposed to oral dosage primarily because it increases patient compliance. The Jarisch–Herxheimer reaction is a self-limited side effect to penicillin that occurs in some patients. When penicillin is administered, the sudden liberation of antigens or endotoxin from the spirochete causes a local anaphylactic reaction. Symptoms include fever, chills, diaphoresis, myalgia, headache, tachycardia, mild hypertension, and increased rate of respiration. It usually resolves within 24 hours and supportive care (bedrest, analgesics, antipyretics) alone is recommended. Patients should be advised of this reaction before treatment is begun. Current management of syphilis should include counseling and testing for concurrent HIV infection. The treatment of neurosyphilis is controversial because penicillin does not penetrate inflamed meninges well. Recommendations include high-dose penicillin G (Table 44–8).

It is recommended that treatment of congenital syphilis be started, even if the diagnosis is not definite. Also, any infant with the diagnosis of congenital syphilis should have radiography of the long bones, because metaphyseal changes are found in 95% of infants at the time of diagnosis. Cerebral spinal fluid ex-

TABLE 44–8. TREATMENT AND MANAGEMENT OF SYPHILIS

Primary, Secondary, and Early Latent Syphilis
- Procaine penicillin G. 600,000 U IM daily for 10–14 days
- Contraindications: Penicillin allergies
- Follow-up: Re-examination clinically and serologically at 3 and 6 months; if nontreponemal titers have not declined fourfold by 3 months with primary or secondary syphilis, or 6 months with early latent syphilis or if signs or symptoms persist and reinfection ruled out, should have CSF examination and be retreated appropriately; all patients should be counseled and encouraged to have HIV testing

Primary, Secondary, and Early Latent with Allergy to Penicillin
- Doxycyline, 100 mg PO bid for 14 days or tetracycline, 500 mg PO qid for 14 days
- Contraindications: Pregnancy
- Follow-up: See above

Late Latent and Tertiary (Gummatous and Cardiovascular)
- Procaine penicillin 600,000 U IM daily for 17–21 days
- Alternative regimen: Benzathine penicillin G, 7.2 million units total, administered as 3 doses of 2.4 million units IM, given 1 week apart for 3 consecutive weeks
- Contraindication: Penicillin allergy
- Follow-up: These patients all should have thorough clinical examination and CSF evaluation is strongly recommended; if CSF reveals findings consistent with neurosyphilis, treat as such

Late Latent and Tertiary with Allergy to Penicillin
- Doxycyline, 200 mg PO bid for 4 weeks
- Contraindication: Pregnancy
- Follow-up: Quantitative nontreponemal tests repeated at 6 and 12 months; if titers increase fourfold or initially high titer fails to decrease or patient shows signs or symptoms attributable to syphilis, patient should be evaluated for neurosyphilis and treated appropriately; HIV testing and counseling indicated

Neurosyphilis and Ocular Syphilis
- Procaine penicillin 1.8–2.4 million U IM daily and probenicid 500 mg PO qid for 17–21 days
- Alternative regimen: Aqueous crystalline penicillin G, 18–24 million units administered 3–4 million units every 4 hours IV, for 17–21 days
- Adjunctive cycloplegics, oral/topical steroids are used when indicated for ocular complications
- Contraindications: Penicillin allergy: These patients should have skin tested and desensitized and managed by expert in syphilis treatment
- Follow-up: Many recommend benzathine penicillin G, 2.5 million units IM weekly for 3 doses after completion of neurosyphilis treatment regimens; follow up: CSF examination repeated every 6 months until cell count normal; if it has not decreased at 6 months, or not normal by 2 years, retreatment strongly indicated; HIV testing and counseling indicated

Syphilis in Pregnancy
- Follow the penicillin regimen appropriate for the stage of syphilis
- Contraindications: Penicillin allergy patients should be skin tested and treated or desensitized

  Women treated in the second half of pregnancy are at risk for Herxheimer reaction, which may cause premature labor and/or fetal distress
- Monthly follow-up mandatory so retreatment can be given if needed; HIV counseling and testing indicated

Congenital Syphilis
- Procaine penicillin 50,000 U/kg IM daily for 10–14 days
- Follow-up: Seropositive untreated infants must be followed closely at 1, 2, 3, 6, and 12 months; if not infected, antibody titers must be decreasing by 3 months of age and have disappeared by 6 months; if titers stable or increasing, infant must be treated
- Treated infants: Nontreponemal titers should disappear by 6 months; infants with CSF pleocytosis should be reexamined every 6 months or until cell count normal; if cell count abnormal after 2 years or no downward trend present, treatment should be reinstituted; if CSF VDRL still reactive at 6 months, retreatment is indicated

amination, complete blood count including platelet count, and urinalysis should also be performed.

The CDC does not recommend any alterations from standard treatment for those concurrently infected with HIV, although some advocate more extensive dosage regimen. Serology to follow treatment of syphilis in HIV patients may be difficult because of the alterations in the test results. In order to provide long-range care, follow-up must include careful clinical evaluation and repeated CSF examinations if abnormalities were detected. Some have recommended maintenance doses of penicillin; however, it is generally accepted that rigorous follow-up is more efficacious. More studies are needed to determine optimum treatment of HIV patients with concurrent syphilis. Some vaccinations have been implicated in causing relapse to secondary syphilis in HIV patients, and it has been recommended that any unnecessary vaccination be avoided.

Ocular

Most experts recommend using the CDC standards for neurosyphilis to treat the ocular manifestations (Table 44–8), even if the CSF examination is negative. Treatment of ocular syphilis may need to be prolonged in order to eradicate the disease because penicillin does not penetrate the eye very well. The Jarisch–Herxheimer reaction often occurs and may exacerbate the eye inflammation. Systemic corticosteroids can help to control this reaction. Anterior segment complications (acute interstitial keratitis, uveitis) may be treated adjunctively with cycloplegics or topical steroids, when indicated. Use of antibiotics are indicated in congenital syphilis; however, this type of keratitis does not respond to them, therefore topical steroids are needed to prevent vision loss.

CONCLUSION

Syphilis has been a known clinical entity for many centuries. It has undergone several evolutions, and its incidence has followed cyclical trends. Sir William Osler is often quoted as saying, "Know syphilis in all its manifestations and relations, and all other things clinical will be added unto you." This is especially true as it pertains to eyecare practitioners, because knowledge of ocular syphilis provides a wealth of information regarding ocular disease.

REFERENCES

Alexander LL. Sexually transmitted diseases: Perspectives on this growing epidemic. *Nurse Practitioner.* 1992;17:31–42.

Ampel NM. Plagues—what's past is present: Thoughts on the origin and history of new infectious diseases. *Rev Infect Dis.* 1990;13:658–665.

Arruga J, Valentines J, Mauri F, et al. Neuroretinitis in acquired syphilis. *Ophthalmology.* 1985;92:262–270.

Augenbraun MH, Rolfs R. Treatment of syphilis, 1998: Nonpregnant adults. *Clin Infect Dis.* 1999;28(suppl 1):S21–28.

Bos JD. Fluorescent treponemal antibody-absorption (FTA-ABS) test. *Int J Dermatol.* 1982;21:125–130.

Brown TJ, Yen-Moore A, Tyring SK. An overview of sexually transmitted diseases. Part I. *J Am Acad Dermatol.* 1999; 41:511–529.

Buckley HB. Syphilis: A review and update of this "new" infection of the '90s. *Nurse Practitioner.* 1992;17:25–32.

Centers for Disease Control. Primary and secondary syphilis—United States, 1998. *MMWR.* 1999;48:873–878.

Centers for Disease Control. Summary of notifiable diseases, United States. *MMWR.* 1999;47.

Centers for Disease Control. Congenital syphilis—United States, 1998. *MMWR.* 1999;48:757–761.

Centers for Disease Control. 1989 sexually transmitted diseases treatment guidelines. *MMWR.* 1989;38(S-8):5–13.

Clinical Effectiveness Group. National guidelines for the management of early syphilis *Sex Trans Inf.* 1999; 75 (suppl 1):529–533.

Clinical Effectiveness Group. National guidelines for the management of late syphilis. *Sex Trans Inf.* 1999;75 (suppl 1):534–537.

Crouch ER, Goldberg MF. Retinal periarteritis secondary to syphilis. *Arch Ophthalmol.* 1975;93:384–387.

DeLuise VP, Clark SW, Smith JL. Syphilitic retinal detachment and uveal effusion. *Am J Ophthalmol.* 1982; 94:757–761.

Deschenes J, Seamone C, Baines M. Acquired ocular syphilis: Diagnosis and treatment. *Ann Ophthalmol.* 1992;24:134–138.

Deschenes J, Seamone C, Baines M. The ocular manifestations of sexually transmitted diseases. *Can J Ophthalmol.* 1990;25:177–185.

Drusin LM. Syphilis: Clinical manifestations, diagnosis, and treatment. *Urol Clin North Am.* 1984;11:121–131.

Farnes SW, Setness PA. Serologic tests for syphilis. *Postgrad Med.* 1990;87:37–46.

Feder HM, Manthous C. The asymptomatic patient with a positive VDRL test. *Am Fam Practitioner.* 1988;37:185–190.

Fitzgerald TJ. Pathogenesis and immunology of *Treponema pallidum. Annu Rev Microbiol.* 1981;35:29–54.

Fletcher WA, Sharpe JA. Tonic pupils in neurosyphilis. *Neurology.* 1986;36:188–192.

Frohman L, Lama P. Annual update of systemic disease—1999: Emerging and re-emerging infections (Part II). *J Neuroophthalmol.* 2000;20:48–58.

Gregory N. Clinical problems of syphilis in the presence of HIV. *Clin Dermatol.* 1991;9:71–74.

Hart G. Syphilis tests in diagnostic and therapeutic decision making. *Ann Int Med.* 1986;104:368–376.

Hook EW, Marra CM. Acquired syphilis in adults. *N Engl J Med.* 1992;326:1060–1069.

Hooshmand H, Escobar MR, Kopf SW. Neurosyphilis: A study of 241 patients. *JAMA.* 1972;219:726–730.

Hutchinson CM, Hook EW. Syphilis in adults. *Med Clin North Am.* 1990;74:1389–1416.

Jordan KG. Modern neurosyphilis—a critical analysis. *West J Med.* 1988;149:47–57.

Kirchner JT. Syphilis—an STD on the increase. *Am Fam Practitioner.* 1991;44:843–857.

Larsen SA. Syphilis. *Clin Lab Med.* 1989;9:545–557.

Levy JH, Liss RA, Maguire AM. Neurosyphilis and ocular syphilis in patients with concurrent human immunodeficiency virus infection. *Retina.* 1989;9:175–180.

Lowhagen G. Syphilis: Test procedures and therapeutic strategies. *Semin Dermatol.* 1990;9:152–159.

Margo CE, Hamed LM. Ocular syphilis. *Surv Ophthalmol.* 1992;37:203–220.

Martin NF, Fitzgerald CR. Cystoid macular edema as the primary sign of neurosyphilis. *Am J Ophthalmol.* 1979;88:28–31.

Melvin SY. Syphilis, resurgence of an old disease. *Primary Care.* 1990;17:47–58.

Mendelsohn AD, Jampol LM. Syphilitic retinitis, a cause of necrotizing retinitis. *Retina.* 1984;4:221–224.

Moore JE. Syphilitic iritis. *Am J Ophthamol.* 1931;14:110–126.

Morgan CM, Webb RM, O'Connor GR. Atypical syphilitic chorioretinitis and vasculitis. *Retina.* 1984;4:225–231.

Musher DM. Syphilis, neurosyphilis, penicillin, and AIDS. *J Infect Dis.* 1991;163:1201–1602.

Musher DM. Syphilis. *Pediatr Infect Dis J.* 1990;9:768–769.

Musher DM. Syphilis. *Infect Dis Clin North Am.* 1987;1:83–95.

Musher DM, Hamill RJ, Baughn RE. Effect of human immunodeficiency virus (HIV) infection on the course of syphilis and on the response to treatment. *Ann Int Med.* 1990;113:872–881.

Poitevin M, Bolgert M. Syphilis in 1986. *J Clin Neuro-ophthalmol.* 1987;7:11–16.

Ross WH, Sutton HF. Acquired syphilitic uveitis. *Arch Ophthalmol.* 1980;98:496–498.

Ruder AJ, Halverson KD, Austin JK, Jones WL. Neurosyphilis with associated retinitis. *J Am Optom Assoc.* 1993; 64:245–249.

Rush JA, Ryan EJ. Syphilitic optic perineuritis. *Am J Ophthalmol.* 1981;91:404–406.

Sacks JG, Osher RH, Elconin H. Progressive visual loss in syphilitic optic atrophy. *J Clin Neuro-ophthalmol.* 1983;3:5–8.

Sanchez PJ. Congenital syphilis. *Adv Pediatr Infect Dis.* 1992; 7:161–180.

Schlaegel TF. *Essentials of Uveitis.* Boston: Little, Brown; 1969:84–89.

Schlaegel TF, Kao SF. A review (1970–1980) of 28 presumptive cases of syphilitic uveitis. *Am J Ophthalmol.* 1982; 93:411–414.

Singh AE, Romanowski B. Syphilis: Review with emphasis on clinical, epidemiologic, and some biologic features. *Clin Microbiol Rev.* 1999;2:187–209.

Spoor TC, Wynn P, Hartel WC, Bryan CS. Ocular syphilis, acute and chronic. *J Clin Neuro-ophthalmol.* 1983;3:197–203.

Tamesis RR, Foster S. Ocular syphilis. *Ophthalmology.* 1990; 97:1281–1287.

Toshniwal P. Optic perineuritis with secondary syphilis. *J Clin Neuro-ophthalmol.* 1987;7:6–10.

Tramont EC. Controversies regarding the natural history and treatment of syphilis in HIV disease. *AIDS Clin Rev.* 1991:97–107.

Tramont EC. Syphilis: From Beethoven to HIV. *Mt Sinai J Med.* 1990;57:192–196.

Wellington Belin M, Baltch AL, Hay PB. Secondary syphilitic uveitis. *Am J Ophthalmol.* 1981;92:210–214.

Wicher K, Horowitz HW, Wicher V. Laboratory methods of diagnosis of syphilis for the beginning of the third millenium. *Microbes Infect.* 1999;1:1035–1049.

Wooldridge WE. Syphilis, a new visit from an old enemy. *Postgrad Med.* 1991;89:193–202.

Zenker PN, Rolfs RT. Treatment of syphilis, 1989. *Rev Infect Dis.* 1990;12(suppl 6):S590–S608.

Chapter 45

HIV AND AIDS

Connie L. Chronister, David C. Bright, David S. Altenderfer

Human immunodeficiency virus (HIV) infection and acquired immune deficiency syndrome (AIDS) continue to be global problems. The international HIV infection rate is over 40 million with approximately 10 new cases every minute. AIDS is now the second leading cause of death in the United States among people aged 25 to 44 years.

HIV-1 (the most prevalent serotype) evolved with the *Pan troglodytes troglodytes* subspecies of chimpanzee in Africa, being present in that subspecies for centuries without causing disease. Over centuries, multiple viral mutations plus sporadic transmission to humans set the stage for epidemic spread. Most likely the virus was transmitted to humans by contamination of a person's open wound during butchering of chimpanzees for human consumption. Not until social and demographic conditions changed did the virus move from rural to urban areas and an epidemic emerge. Factors contributing to viral spread included migration to urban areas, breakup of family units due to the migratory nature of employment, access to commercial sex workers, and contamination of the blood supply. The availability and ease of air travel allowed the transmission of HIV-1 from Africa to Europe and the North American continent during the late 1970s.

Since its discovery in 1981, the treatment of HIV infection and AIDS has dramatically changed with the development of new antiretroviral medications. Clinicians have utilized highly active antiretroviral treatment (HAART) regimens that have improved the health, well-being, and longevity of HIV-infected patients. HAART has reduced the risk of many opportunistic infections and malignancies and has improved immunity. This has resulted in a major impact on the management of HIV. The study of HIV infection and AIDS is changing so rapidly that current literature must be constantly monitored to stay fully informed about the condition.

EPIDEMIOLOGY

Systemic

The most recent data (June 2000) from the United Nations Programme on HIV/AIDS (UNAIDS) now estimates that more than 40 million persons are infected with the human immunodeficiency virus (HIV) worldwide. About 16.3 million people had died of AIDS by the end of 1999. More than 70% of HIV-positive people live in sub-Saharan Africa, a region that contains only 10% of the world's population. UNAIDS further estimates that 5.6 million people were infected with HIV in 1999 alone. At least 95% of both infections and deaths are in the developing world, impacting adults in their peak productive years and leaving a trail of personal tragedy, disrupted social networks, and lost productivity.

Throughout the 1990s in the United States, the number of new HIV infections is believed to be holding at about 40,000 per year. The first cases were reported in 1981 among previously healthy homosexual men. Other groups affected were hemophiliacs, Haitian immigrants, blood transfusion recipients, and intravenous drug users. Today, new cases of HIV infection in the United States result primarily from injection-drug use and heterosexual contact. Minority populations are disproportionately represented among new cases. Through June 1999, 711,344 cumulative cases of AIDS and 420,201 AIDS-related deaths had been reported to the Centers for Disease Control and Prevention.

Ocular

Since 1983 when Holland and associates reported eye changes in AIDS patients, ocular findings are seen in the majority of patients with AIDS. Ocular sequelae have been reported in 73 to 100% of AIDS patients.

PATHOPHYSIOLOGY/DISEASE PROCESS

The Organism—Infection and Viral Replication

The human immunodeficiency virus is a member of the Lentivirinae ("slow virus") family of retroviruses. HIV binds a specific region of its envelope with the CD4+ glycoprotein molecule on the surface of its targeted host cell. The CD4+ membrane antigen acts as a high-affinity receptor on the HIV host cells, which include T helper cells (CD4+ cells) and monocyte-derived macrophages, both of which bear the surface CD4+ molecules. T helper cells, with abundant CD4+ molecules, are a major target for infection by HIV-1. In addition to CD4+ receptors, HIV-1 also binds to chemokine receptor sites present on host cells. Following binding at two separate molecular sites, HIV is fused with its host cell and releases its genetic material in the form of RNA (the "genome") into the nucleus of the host cell.

Viral replication begins with the transformation of viral RNA into DNA compatible with the host cell's DNA. This critical replication step involves virus-associated reverse transcriptase. This retrograde process of conversion of RNA into DNA is known as reverse transcription, hence the name "retrovirus" to describe viruses of this particular group. The newly produced DNA ("proviral DNA") is then integrated into the host cell's genetic material by a second viral enzyme, integrase. If the CD4+ cell is "resting" (nonactivated), proviral DNA will not replicate. If the immune system is chronically activated as is typical in HIV-1 infection, both messenger RNA and new viral genomes are produced. Multiple mechanisms have been proposed for the chronic immune hyperactivity in HIV-1 infection, including autoimmune phenomena, overproduction of various cytokines by B cells, and activation by various gene products of different viruses. Viral genes for HIV-1 structural elements, HIV-1 enzymes, and HIV-1 exterior protein coats direct the production of these elements, which are assembled into new viral offspring ("progeny") that bud from the host cell. Following budding, a third viral enzyme, protease, snips the unwieldy strings of proteins into properly sized units and renders them infectious, able to infect new host cells.

The development of polymerase chain reaction (PCR) technology in the late 1980s enabled the analysis of target DNA existing in very tiny amounts of plasma and improved the study of many viral infections. PCR technology has provided researchers with profound insight into the dynamics of HIV-1 replication and infection. It is now known that HIV-1 replicates at a staggering rate, with typically 10 to 100 billion new viruses being produced daily in the absence of therapy. A single infected cell is making about 3000 to 4000 viruses at any one point in time. The turnover of both cell-free viruses and infected T cells is similarly staggering, with upwards of 30% of both types being turned over daily. There is no latent period in which HIV-1 becomes dormant; HIV-1 replication levels off at a "set point" within several months after initial infection. This "set point" may or may not remain stable over time. However, HIV-1 continually replicates in lymphatic tissue throughout the course of the disease. Though 10 billion or more virions are produced daily, the vast majority are noninfectious, presumably because of errors in reverse transcription or their inactivation by the immune system.

"Viral load" is the number of HIV-1 RNA molecules per milliliter of plasma. Viral load is measured in log units rather than numbers. The value of 3.0 logs of HIV RNA/mL is equivalent to 1000 RNA particles (10 to the third power); the value of 5.0 logs is equivalent to 100,000 particles. The difference between 3.0 logs and 5.0 logs is only 2.0 log units, but the difference between 1000 and 100,000 is 100-fold. When viral load is expressed in log units, it is critical to remember changes of 10-fold (1.0 log), 100-fold (2.0 log), or 1000-fold (3.0 log), rather than two or three times larger or smaller. For example, consider a patient who experiences a drop from 4.43 logs (27,141 copies) to 3.27 logs (1,872 copies). This seemingly small reduction of 1.16 log units is actually greater than a 10-fold reduction in viral load.

Viral load is measured by one of three techniques (Table 45–1). Most tests of viral load previously had sensitivity limits of either 400 or 500 copies of HIV-1

TABLE 45–1. VIRAL LOAD TESTS

Amplicor HIV Monitor
- *Methodology:* measures HIV-1 RNA by quantitative competitive reverse transcriptase polymerase chain reaction (QC-PCR)
- *How it works:* utilizes a target amplification methodology in which amplified RNA products of test plasma are compared to amplified products of an internal standard

Quantiplex HIV RNA bDNA
- *Methodology:* measures viral load by branched DNA (bDNA)
- *How it works:* utilizes signal amplification, which measures the amplified signal from target HIV DNA, rather than the amplified target itself, as is done with QC-PCR

Nuclisens HIV-1 QT
- *Methodology:* nucleic acid-based amplification (NASBA)
- *How it works:* utilizes nucleic acid-based amplification, similar to QC-PCR, but is used infrequently in the United States

> Viral load is defined as the number of HIV-1 RNA molecules per milliliter of plasma.

RNA per milliliter of plasma, but more sensitive versions of these tests have become available, with limits of 50 copies or less. When the designation "below the limit of quantitation" (BLQ) is utilized, it reflects a situation in which the patient's measured viral load is lower than the lowest viral load that can be precisely (or reproducibly) measured.

Transmission

The most common mode of HIV-1 transmission resulting in primary infection is through sexual contact at the genital mucosa. Breaks in the mucosal barrier and increased inflammation caused by genital ulcer disease (chancroid, herpes simplex), cervicitis, or urethritis increase the risk of acquiring HIV-1 infection. Tissue dendritic cells (Langerhans cells) are the first cells to be contacted and infected by HIV-1. These Langerhans cells then fuse with CD4+ lymphocytes (T helper cells) and are transported to regional lymph nodes. With immune activation of CD4+ lymphocytes, HIV-1 infection then spreads to other CD4+ lymphocytes that enter the bloodstream and widely disseminate. With dissemination, there is seeding of lymphoid organs and trapping of HIV-1 by follicular dendritic cells (FDCs). Plasma viremia rises rapidly, as high as 1 million HIV-1 RNA molecules per milliliter. This viremia later levels off, most likely because of HIV-1–specific immune responses consisting of cytotoxic T lymphocytes (CD8+ cells) specific for HIV-1. Neutralizing antibodies generated in response to HIV-1 are usually not seen until weeks to months after the reduction in levels of replicating virus in plasma.

> The average CD4+ count is approximately 1000 cells/mm^3 (range 600 to 1500).

Progression

The viral load in the plasma represents ongoing viral replication from recently infected lymphocytes present within peripheral lymphatic tissue (including lymph nodes and spleen), which continually releases HIV into the bloodstream. Depending on the level of viral replication, patients will develop manifestations of progressive immunodeficiency over a wide range of years following primary infection with HIV-1. A higher viral load has been correlated with more rapid progression to clinical AIDS and death. CD4+ counts, which average about 1000 cells/mm^3 (range 600 to 1500), drop progressively in HIV infection and provide an estimate of the immunologic health of the patient. Cell-mediated immunity is critical for immunologic protection against various infectious processes and involves memory CD4+ cells that are able to recognize specific pathogens. With the progressive loss of CD4+ cells to less than 200 cells/mm^3, the patient becomes vulnerable to opportunistic pathogens that would be otherwise controlled by cell-mediated defenses. The average time of progression to AIDS after initial infection is approximately 10 to 11 years in the absence of antiretroviral therapy. Prognosis for survival in HIV-1–infected individuals is presently correlated to both the CD4+ counts as well as the viral load.

The exact mechanism of CD4+ cell destruction in HIV-1 infection is not completely understood. A variety of differing hypotheses have been presented, and the ultimate mechanism will likely be multifactorial. It is known that HIV-1 is trapped by the FDCs in the germinal cells of lymph nodes; this results in both continuous immune stimulation as well as constant exposure of HIV-1 to uninfected CD4+ cells residing in or circulating through the lymph nodes. HIV-1 is able to progressively disrupt and destroy the FDC network, which serves as both antigen repository and the major antigen-presenting cell network for B- and T-cell interaction with antigens. Other mechanisms include direct or indirect killing of infected CD4+ cells by CD8+ cytotoxic lymphocytes, exaggerated apoptosis (programmed cell death), syncytia formation (aggregations of uninfected but useless CD4+ cells), and HIV-1-infection–induced "exhaustion" of CD4+ cell production.

During the process of viral replication—specifically, during the transcription of RNA into DNA—errors frequently occur in the genetic makeup of the virus. The error-prone nature of reverse transcriptase and the lack of a self-correcting ability during reverse transcription result in a variety of mutations. Each mutation in either the reverse transcriptase or protease gene consists of a substitution of one nucleotide for another. As a result, future generations of virus will have amino acid substitutions in either reverse transcriptase or protease enzymes. Many mutations have little or no effect on the hardiness of HIV-1, while some may actually weaken its infectivity or replicative ability. Other mutations may confer a survival advantage to HIV-1, giving it the ability to resist certain antiretroviral drugs.

Each cycle of viral replication results in the production of at least one mutation per genome, with as many as 10,000 to 100,000 mutations at each site in the HIV genome each day. Considering the immense productivity of HIV-1 with the potential for a large number of possible mutations, it is likely that many HIV-1–infected individuals, prior to the initiation of any antiretroviral therapy, may have subgroups ("quasi-species") of HIV-1 already resistant to one or more anti-HIV drugs. Mutations that provide strains of HIV-1 with a survival advantage over drugs targeted for their destruction may allow that mutant strain to dominate, in a Darwinian "survival of the fittest." This situation most likely occurs when the drug regimen utilized for therapy is unable to fully inhibit HIV-1 replication; the resulting evolutionary pressure selects for the emergence of resistant viral strains.

Until the mid-1990s, when more antiretroviral drugs became available, therapy for HIV-1 infection consisted of treatment with a single drug (monotherapy) that was switched to the latest or newest drug when the patient's CD4+ count or health status declined. This strategy of "sequential monotherapy" was only effective for short periods of time because of the development of HIV-1 resistant to antiretroviral drugs. To compound the problem, HIV-1 can develop both primary and secondary mutations upon exposure to antiretroviral drugs.

A primary mutation usually develops soon after exposure to a drug unable to adequately suppress viral replication and typically impairs binding of the drug to the HIV-1 site for interaction. Primary mutations result in an increase in the amount of drug needed to inhibit the targeted viral enzyme (either reverse transcriptase or protease).

Secondary mutations typically develop slowly, over a period of months, and may increase the level of resistance by improving the fitness of viruses carrying primary mutations. Secondary mutations result if HIV-1 is allowed to continue replicating in the presence of a drug (or drugs) unable to fully suppress viral replication. Secondary mutations are also able to confer cross-resistance to other antiretroviral drugs in the same drug class without prior exposure. This phenomenon is particularly critical for protease inhibitors, in which secondary mutations accumulate and confer widespread cross-resistance between members of this drug class.

Course of the Disease

There are three distinct stages of HIV infection and disease manifestation: initial, chronic, and final (or crisis) stage. The early phase occurs when a person is newly infected with HIV. Upon initial infection with HIV a person may have no clinical symptoms at all. More commonly, an influenza-like illness develops, referred to as an acute retroviral syndrome. The person fully recovers from this illness within weeks and feels well again. However, the infection is nonetheless present and slowly taking hold within the person's immune system. Shortly after infection, the body mounts an immune response. At this point the person is HIV-positive (HIV+), having produced an antibody to HIV. Although this response seems to temporarily combat the infection, it is typically not sufficient to fully clear the infection. The antibody titers are too low and lack the heterogeneity necessary to destroy genetic variations of the replicating virus. Thus, HIV begins its insidious course of destruction.

> There are three distinct stages of HIV infection and disease: Initial—new infection with HIV. Chronic—period when most people are healthy, and only minor pathological changes are present and can be measured. Crisis—frank diagnosis of AIDS.

The next stage of HIV disease is the chronic phase, typically lasting years. The average time from initial infection to clinical manifestations of problems associated with HIV disease is 10 years without treatment. During this phase most people are reasonably healthy and feel well, but minor pathological changes are present and can be measured. These changes usually manifest as minor immune dysfunctions, abnormal blood studies, and/or minor constitutional problems. Previously, it was thought that in this stage of infection, also referred to as the "latent period," HIV was dormant. However, studies have shown that there is progressive deterioration of the immune system during the chronic stage, with ongoing replication of the virus.

Patients in the crisis stage of HIV infection have a frank diagnosis of AIDS. The final phase may last months or years depending on the overall health of the patient and response to the various treatments. Most patients do not feel well. The CD4+ cell counts are far below the normal range, usually falling to 200 cells/mm^3 and below. Pronounced clinical manifestations develop and life-threatening opportunistic infections, diseases, and other problems emerge. Eventually, patients in the crisis stage die as a result of diseases that the body can no longer fight and therapies cannot control.

SYSTEMIC HIV DISEASE

Diagnosis

Primary HIV Disease

Screening tests have been designed to detect the presence of antibodies towards the virus. These antibodies take from 6 weeks to 6 months to develop in over 95% of infected individuals. Therefore, a negative screening test should be rechecked in 6 months to rule out previous exposure.

> Negative screening tests should always be rechecked in 6 months to rule out previous HIV exposure.

Testing for the HIV is targeted at detection of antibodies. The two main initial screening tests are the enzyme-linked immunosorbent assay (ELISA) and the enzyme immunoassay (EIA). A newer screening test, which may replace these, is the HIV RNA test, or viral load, which is currently being used for the evaluation of when to initiate treatment. A positive test result must be confirmed with a Western blot test. After a patient has been diagnosed with HIV, he or she must be routinely monitored with a CD4+ count as well as an HIV RNA viral load.

AIDS

In 1993 the Centers for Disease Control and Prevention established new criteria for the definitive diagnosis of AIDS (Tables 45–2, 45–3, 45–4, and 45–5). These criteria include several different categories to reflect the progression of the HIV disease. The AIDS-defining diseases and conditions vary depending on the laboratory evidence of HIV infection that exists. The criteria are very restrictive when little laboratory evidence of HIV infection exists and expand in scope as the laboratory evidence is confirmed.

A positive diagnosis of AIDS can be made on the basis of three different categories of clinical findings:

- The manifestation of an indicator disease without laboratory confirmation of HIV infection (assuming the patient has no other condition that would contribute to the indicator disease).
- The manifestation of an indicator disease with laboratory confirmation of HIV infection whether or not other diseases or conditions related to immunodeficiency are present.
- Laboratory confirmation of HIV infection and a CD4+ count of less than 200 cells/mm^3 whether or not other indicator diseases are present.

All newly diagnosed cases of AIDS must be reported to the CDC.

TABLE 45–2. CDC DIAGNOSTIC CRITERIA FOR A CASE OF AIDS[a]

CD4+ Cell Counts	Clinical Categories		
≥ 500/mm^3	A1	B1	**C1**
200–499/mm^3	A2	B2	**C2**
<200/mm^3	**A3**	**B3**	**C3**

Bold categories A3, B3, C1, C2, and C3 represent reportable cases of AIDS.
[a] 1993 CDC classification system for HIV infection and expanded AIDS surveillance case definition for adolescents and adults. Refer to clinical categories A–C (Tables 45–2 to 45–4). A case of AIDS in an adolescent or adult is diagnosed based upon the clinical category of a patient and/or the CD4+ count in an HIV-infected individual. A diagnosis of AIDS linked to CD4+ alone is not a marker for HIV infection or AIDS. HIV infection must be assured before reporting a case of AIDS to the CDC. HIV infection is defined as repeatedly reactive screening tests to HIV-1 antibody (e.g., EIA) with specific HIV antibody identified by use of supplemental tests (e.g., Western blot, immunofluorescence assay). Other methods of HIV-1 diagnosis include virus isolation, antigen detection, and detection of HIV genetic material (DNA or RNA) by PCR.
Adapted from Centers for Disease Control and Prevention. 1993 revised classification system for HIV infection and expanded surveillance case definition for AIDS among adolescents and adults. MMWR. *1992;41 (No. RR-17).*

TABLE 45–3. CDC CLINICAL CATEGORY A CONDITIONS OF HIV-INFECTED ADOLESCENTS AND ADULTS[a]

Asymptomatic HIV infection
Persistent generalized lymphadenopathy
Acute (primary) HIV infection with accompanying illness or history of acute HIV infection

[a]Category A is defined as one or more of the above conditions. However, conditions listed in categories B or C must not have occurred.
Adapted from Centers for Disease Control and Prevention. 1993 revised classification system for HIV infection and expanded surveillance case definition for AIDS among adolescents and adults. MMWR. *1992;41(No. RR-17).*

TABLE 45–4. CDC CLINICAL CATEGORY B CONDITIONS OF HIV-INFECTED ADOLESCENTS AND ADULTS[a]

Bacillary angiomatosis
Candidiasis, oropharyngeal (thrush)
Candidiasis, vulvovaginal; persistent, frequent, or poorly responsive to therapy
Cervical dysplasia (moderate or severe)/carcinoma in situ
Constitutional symptoms, such as fever (38.5°C) or diarrhea (lasting >1 month)
Hairy leukoplakia, oral
Herpes zoster (shingles), involving at least two distinct episodes or more than one dermatome
Idiopathic thrombocytopenia purpura
Listeriosis
Pelvic inflammatory disease, particularly if complicated by tubo-ovarian abscess
Peripheral neuropathy

[a]Symptomatic conditions that are not included among conditions listed in clinical category C and which meet at least one of the following criteria: the conditions are attributed to HIV infections and/or are indicative of a defect in cell-mediated immunity; or the conditions are considered by physicians to have a clinical course or management that is complicated by HIV infection. The above are examples of these conditions, but are not exhaustive.

Adapted from Centers for Disease Control and Prevention. 1993 revised classification system for HIV infection and expanded surveillance case definition for AIDS among adolescents and adults. MMWR. *1992;41(No. RR-17).*

TREATMENT AND MANAGEMENT

There is no cure for AIDS. The ideal therapy against HIV is a vaccine to protect a person from becoming infected. Acquired immunity via vaccination enables the body to mount a virocidal response before the infection is established. Researchers have thus far been unable to develop an effective vaccine against HIV. The major obstacle is the multitude of genetic variations that HIV produces as it replicates. Therefore, in order to be effective, an HIV vaccine must be capable of mounting a multiple immune response to protect against viral heterogeneity.

> Current HIV management protocols include treatment with a combination of antiretroviral drugs, opportunistic disease prophylaxis, and prompt, aggressive treatment of any problems that arise.

Current management protocols include treatment of primary HIV disease with a combination of antiretroviral drugs, prophylaxis against opportunistic diseases, and prompt, aggressive treatment of any problems that arise. Medical therapy has been particularly challenging because HIV, like other viruses, depends on the internal metabolism of an infected cell for replication. Inhibiting cellular processes with medications often causes damage to the host cell as well as others that are not infected. Additionally, because patients with HIV disease are on multiple medications, close monitoring for drug interactive side effects is required.

A frequently overlooked aspect of HIV care is the psychosocial needs of the patient. HIV-infected patients may suffer loss of independence (physical, financial), rejection (family, employment, housing), depression, prejudice, and other personal and social problems. Sensitivity to these issues and knowledge of community resources are integral components to successful HIV management, and may greatly enhance the quality of life for HIV patients.

TABLE 45–5. CDC CLINICAL CATEGORY C CONDITIONS OF HIV-INFECTED ADOLESCENTS AND ADULTS[a]

Candidiasis of bronchi, trachea, or lungs
Candidiasis, esophageal
Cervical cancer, invasive
Coccidioidomycosis, disseminated or extrapulmonary
Cryptococcosis, extrapulmonary
Cryptosporidiosis, chronic intestinal (>1 month duration)
Cytomegalovirus disease (other than liver, spleen, or nodes)
Cytomegalovirus retinitis (with loss of vision)
HIV encephalopathy
Herpes simplex: chronic ulcer(s) (>1 month duration); or bronchitis, pneumonitis, or esophagitis
Histoplasmosis, disseminated or extrapulmonary
Isopsoriasis, chronic intestinal (>1 month duration)
Kaposi sarcoma
Lymphoma, Burkitt (or equivalent term)
Lymphoma, immunoblastic (or equivalent term)
Lymphoma, primary in brain
Mycobacterium-avium complex of *M. kansasii,* disseminate or extrapulmonary
Mycobacterium tuberculosis, any site (pulmonary or extrapulmonary)
Mycobacterium, other species or unidentified species, disseminated or extrapulmonary
Pneumocystis carinii pneumonia
Pneumonia, recurrent
Progressive multifocal leukoencephalopathy
Salmonella septicemia, recurrent
Toxoplasmosis of the brain
Wasting syndrome due to HIV

[a]Category C includes any conditions listed in the 1987 surveillance case definition for AIDS. The conditions in clinical category C are strongly associated with severe immunodeficiency, occur frequently in HIV-infected individuals, and cause serious morbidity and mortality.

Adapted from Centers for Disease Control and Prevention. 1993 revised classification system for HIV infection and expanded surveillance case definition for AIDS among adolescents and adults. MMWR. *1992;41(No. RR-17).*

Antiretroviral Therapy

Antiretroviral drugs specifically target viral enzymes necessary for viral replication. The two HIV-1–associated enzymes are reverse transcriptase and protease. With the potential for viral mutations being very likely caused by high viral replication rates and susceptibility to errors, researchers have determined that combinations of different antiretroviral drugs are best able to reduce viral replication to very low levels. The lower the level of replication, the less the likelihood of mutations developing. "Convergent therapy" utilizes drugs from the same class that target the same viral enzyme, whereas "divergent therapy" combines drugs that target different enzymes. The combination of both convergent and divergent therapy is now the cornerstone of current anti-HIV-1 drug regimens, known as highly active antiretroviral therapy, or HAART. Traditional regimens of HAART selected two drugs targeting viral reverse transcriptase and a single drug targeting viral protease. More recent versions of HAART utilize three drugs targeted at reverse transcriptase. It has been determined by multiple studies that viral load plus CD4+ count are predictors of progression to both AIDS and death, and that changes in both markers predict the response to antiretroviral therapy.

There are currently two distinct groups of anti-HIV-1 drugs targeted at different viral enzymes: reverse transcriptase inhibitors and protease inhibitors. The reverse transcriptase group has two subgroups: nucleoside analogue reverse transcriptase inhibitors (NRTIs) and nonnucleoside analogue reverse transcriptase inhibitors (NNRTIs) (Table 45–6).

Nucleoside Reverse Transcriptase Inhibitors

Nucleoside inhibitors of reverse transcriptase (NRTIs) cause a termination of the DNA chain. The expected reduction in viral load with a single NRTI is 0.5 to 1.0

TABLE 45–6. ANTIRETROVIRAL DRUGS

Nucleoside Reverse Transcriptase Inhibitors (NRTIs)

Zidovudine (ZDV) (Retrovir)
- *Dose:* 300 mg bid, with or without food
- *Side effects:* anemia, neutropenia; nausea, vomiting, headache, myalgia

Didanosine (ddI) (Videx)
- *Dose:* 200 mg bid (>60 kg) or 125 mg bid (<60 kg), prior to meals; 400 mg qd (>60 kg), prior to meal [as of November 1999]
- *Side effects:* pancreatitis; diarrhea and GI upset; peripheral neuropathy

Zalcitabine (ddC) (Hivid)
- *Dose:* 0.75 mg tid, with or without meals
- *Side effects:* peripheral neuropathy; skin rash, aphthous oral stomatitis

Stavudine (d4T) (Zerit)
- *Dose:* 40 mg bid (>60 kg) or 30 mg bid (<60 kg) with or without food
- *Side effects:* peripheral neuropathy; elevated liver function tests (LFTs)

Lamivudine (3TC) (Epivir)
- *Dose:* 150 mg bid, with or without food
- *Side effects:* headache, malaise, fatigue, nausea, anorexia, rash, cough

Abacavir (Ziagen)
- *Dose:* 300 mg bid, with or without food
- *Side effects:* hypersensitivity; headache, nausea, vomiting, malaise

Zidovudine/lamivudine (Combivir)
- *Dose:* 300 mg ZDV plus 150 mg 3TC, bid, with or without food
- *Side effects:* anemia, neutropenia; nausea, vomiting, headache, myalgia

Nonnucleoside Reverse Transcriptase Inhibitors (NNRTIs)

Nevirapine (Viramune)
- *Dose:* 200 mg qd for 2 weeks, then 200 mg bid, with or without food
- *Side effects:* skin rash; fever, nausea, headache, abnormal LFTs

Delavirdine (Rescriptor)
- *Dose:* 400 mg tid, with or without food
- *Side effects:* skin rash; abnormal LFTs, GI toxicity, pruritis

Efavirenz (Sustiva)
- *Dose:* 600 mg qhs
- *Side effects:* Central nervous system (CNS) effects (depressive or stimulatory); skin rash; teratogenicity

Protease Inhibitors (PIs)

Saquinavir (hard gel) (Invirase)
- *Dose:* 600 mg tid, with high-fat, high-calorie meal
- *Side effects:* diarrhea, abdominal pain, nausea, rash

Saquinavir (soft gel) (Fortovase)
- *Dose:* 1200 mg tid, with high-fat, high-calorie meal
- *Side effects:* diarrhea, abdominal discomfort, nausea

Ritonavir (Norvir)
- *Dose:* 600 mg bid, with food
- *Side effects:* nausea, vomiting, diarrhea, taste perversion, paresthesias, asthenia

Indinavir (Crixivan)
- *Dose:* 800 mg tid, before meals or with a low-protein, low-fat snack
- *Side effects:* renal stones; GI upset, asthenia, fatigue, headache

Nelfinavir (Viracept)
- *Dose:* 750 mg tid, with food; 1250 mg bid, with food [as of November 1999]
- *Side effects:* diarrhea

Amprenavir (Agenerase)
- *Dose:* 1200 mg bid, with or without food
- *Side effects:* nausea, diarrhea, headache, rash

Abbreviations: bid, twice a day; qd, every day; qhs, every hour of sleep; tid, three times a day

log unit, but is not durable; with 2 NRTIs in combination, the viral load reduction is approximately 1.0 log, and is durable for over 1 year (see Table 45–6).

Zidovudine. The first NRTI to be approved for use was azidothymidine or zidovudine (AZT, ZDV). It received FDA approval in 1987, and was the only anti-HIV-1 drug available for several years. It is currently used with one or more other NRTIs as well as either an NNRTI or protease inhibitor. The average wholesale price for 1 year of zidovudine therapy is approximately $3488. At least 10% of patients on zidovudine experience granulocytopenia and anemia, both of which develop within 4 to 8 weeks of therapy initiation. Incidence and severity of anemia and neutropenia are related to both dosage as well as severity of HIV-1 infection. Other more common toxicities develop soon after therapy initiation and include nausea, vomiting, severe headaches, and myalgia.

The AIDS Clinical Trials Group (ACTG) and other agencies performed clinical trials of zidovudine monotherapy. No study determined any benefits in improved survival with ZDV monotherapy, but definite reductions in AIDS-defining events and clinical disease progression were noted in some, but not all, clinical trials. Zidovudine monotherapy is not effective as the sole, long-term treatment in asymptomatic HIV infection, and it has short-lived benefits for patients in later stages of disease.

When newer NRTIs became available, dual-NRTI therapy (zidovudine with a second NRTI) was compared to ZDV monotherapy. Three large clinical trials demonstrated improvements in CD4+ counts, clinical disease progression, and survival with dual-NRTI therapy compared to NRTI monotherapy. Treatment was most effective in patients naive to all therapy. These trials radically influenced the management of HIV-1 disease in 1995. After 1995, with the increasing availability of both NNRTIs and protease inhibitors, combination therapy using two NRTIs as the backbone in HAART regimens became the standard of care. Zidovudine is probably more utilized than any other NRTI in combination therapy at this time because of its long history as well as physician experience with it.

Didanosine. The second NRTI to be approved by the FDA (in 1991) was didanosine (ddI). The average wholesale cost of therapy for 1 year is approximately $2472. As a result of the complexity of dosing regimens, didanosine is less widely utilized than zidovudine. However, its toxicity profile differs significantly from that of zidovudine and offers advantages to patients experiencing neutropenia or anemia related to ZDV therapy. The most critical toxicity of didanosine is pancreatitis, ranging from 29% (high doses in phase I trials) to 0.6% or less using current dosing regimens (more recent clinical trials). Pancreatitis presents with vague abdominal pain, nausea, and vomiting. The risk of pancreatitis correlates with a previous history of pancreatitis and advanced HIV-1 disease, although it can occur with approved doses at any time during therapy. Other toxicities include diarrhea and gastrointestinal upset (which are relatively common) and peripheral neuropathy, which is more common in advanced HIV-1 disease. An unusual form of retinal pigment atrophy has been observed in 7% of children during phase I and II trials, presenting in the retinal midperiphery. No subsequent reports of retinal pigmentary changes have appeared in either adult or pediatric populations.

Didanosine does not possess the same in vitro potency of zidovudine, but it allows better tolerance from a hematologic standpoint. Patients on previous ZDV monotherapy experienced less clinical disease progression with a switch to ddI monotherapy. Didanosine has been utilized in many trials of dual-NRTI therapy, typically combined with either zidovudine or stavudine (d4T). Didanosine has also been combined with hydroxyurea, which acts to reduce the intracellular concentrations of endogenous nucleosides. This allows ddI to perform more efficiently, since its competition for binding with nucleosides is enhanced.

At this time, didanosine is a valuable member of the NRTI family. It is utilized less frequently than ZDV, mainly due to the frequent side effect of nausea and the complexities of its dosing regimen. Once-daily doses of didanosine have been combined with stavudine (bid) and once-daily nevirapine in recent clinical trials, which allows simplified regimens for improved patient adherence and acceptance. With a recent approval for once-daily dosing, ddI may be more frequently utilized in the future, especially as clinicians strive to simplify regimens for improved compliance and patient acceptance.

Zalcitabine. Zalcitabine (ddC) was the third NRTI approved for management of HIV-1 infection. It received FDA approval in 1992, and was originally specified for use only in combination with zidovudine. Average wholesale cost of therapy for 1 year is approximately $2580.

The primary toxicity of ddC is dose-dependent peripheral neuropathy. The most recent toxicity data determined that peripheral neuropathy occurs at a frequency of 28.3%. Peripheral neuropathy is characterized as symmetric painful burning or numbness, which primarily involves the feet. Other toxicities associated with zalcitabine therapy include maculopapular skin rash and aphthous oral stomatitis, occurring at frequencies of 3% or less.

Large clinical trials comparing ddC to either ZDV or ddI in treatment-experienced patients did not determine any significant advantage of a switch to ddC in terms of either disease progression or survival. A combination of ZDV with ddC was evaluated to provide greater antiviral efficacy with nonoverlapping toxicity profiles, but the ZDV/ddC combination provided only modest increases in CD4+ counts and inconsistent benefits in slowing disease progression. Despite equivocal findings and equivocal benefits, ddC was the first anti-HIV-1 drug to be approved under the FDA accelerated approval process. Currently, ddC is rarely utilized in combination therapy (less than 20% of the time) because of its marginal efficacy and frequent side effects.

Stavudine. Stavudine (d4T) was the fourth NRTI to be granted FDA approval (1994) for HIV-1 infection. Wholesale costs of therapy for 1 year are $3225 and $3110 for high- and low-dose regimens, respectively.

The major toxicity of stavudine is peripheral neuropathy, which is dose-related and is usually reversible on dose reduction or discontinuation of therapy. Manufacturer studies determined that neuropathy occurred in up to 24% of patients, being significantly correlated with both prior neuropathy and lower CD4+ counts at baseline. Stavudine is otherwise well tolerated; infrequently reported toxicities include abnormal liver function tests (13% or less) and anemia, gastrointestinal disturbances, rash, and myalgia, all at frequencies of 5% or less.

Stavudine possesses antiretroviral activity equal to that of ZDV and is either additive or synergistic with other NRTIs. Concerns exist regarding the potentially negative impact of either simultaneous or prior ZDV treatment. Coadministration of ZDV with d4T is not recommended at this time.

Stavudine monotherapy resulted in increases in CD4+ counts as well as moderate reductions in viral load in its early clinical trials. Stavudine has also slowed clinical progression of the disease in patients previously treated with ZDV. It also resulted in more peripheral neuropathy but less myelosuppression and GI upset. Stavudine is most often combined with either ddI or with lamivudine (3TC), and either combination is often used as the dual-NRTI backbone in triple- or quadruple-HAART regimens. Stavudine is often a first choice of NRTIs, because of its potency and general tolerability. It is also frequently utilized as an alternative to ZDV in patients unable to tolerate the latter drug because of either myelotoxicity and/or GI upset.

Lamivudine. Lamivudine (3TC) was the fifth NRTI drug to be approved for HIV-1 infection. Lamivudine was approved in 1995, specifically for use in combination with zidovudine. Since that time, it has also been utilized in combination with stavudine in dual-NRTI combination therapy and with zidovudine and abacavir in triple-NRTI combination therapy, as well as in PI- and NNRTI-based HAART regimens. Wholesale cost of lamivudine therapy for 1 year is approximately $2985. Lamivudine is also available in a fixed-combination form with zidovudine as Combivir with an approximate 1-year wholesale cost of $6473.

Isolation or evaluation of side effects caused by lamivudine has not been possible since the drug has never been tested as long-term monotherapy in any patient group because of exceptionally rapid development of resistance. All commonly reported toxicities associated with zidovudine therapy were slightly more frequent in patients taking zidovudine plus lamivudine. Toxicities included headache, malaise or fatigue, nausea, anorexia, dizziness, nasal signs and symptoms, rash, cough, and musculoskeletal pain.

Unlike other antiretroviral drugs in the NRTI class, lamivudine monotherapy results in the development of a specific mutation in HIV-1 within 8 to 12 weeks of therapy initiation. This mutation confers up to 1000-fold resistance to lamivudine. Lamivudine is unique in the development of rapid resistance among NRTIs; HIV-1 develops resistance mutations to other NRTIs in a stepwise fashion over many months (zidovudine or abacavir) or to small degrees (didanosine, zalcitabine, or stavudine).

Three large trials (Eron et al, 1995; Katlama et al, 1996; Staszewski et al, 1996) compared ZDV monotherapy to a ZDV/3TC combination and determined that treatment with the combination resulted in significant increases in CD4+ counts, reduced viral loads, and reduced disease progression. These three trials caused the ZDV/3TC combination to become the most frequently prescribed antiretroviral drug combination prior to the availability of protease inhibitors in 1996.

Lamivudine is most often combined with either ZDV or d4T. The combination of ZDV with 3TC in Combivir is particularly attractive, since it reduces the heavy pill burden of many HIV-1–infected patients, providing a simplified regimen of two pills per day as the NRTI backbone of many HAART regimens. Additionally, Combivir performed equally well or better than the separate forms of ZDV and 3TC when utilized with protease inhibitors. Improved patient compliance because of a simplified regimen was a likely factor associated with its improved performance.

Abacavir. Abacavir is the most recently available NRTI, having received FDA approval in December 1998. The estimated wholesale cost of therapy for 1 year is approximately $3450. Toxicities of abacavir are similar to those seen with zidovudine and lamivudine, and typically consist of headache, nausea, vomiting, and malaise. A unique hypersensitivity reaction has been reported with abacavir therapy, typically occurring within 6 weeks of initiation of therapy. Patients report nonspecific flu-like symptoms, including malaise, abdominal cramping, and nausea, which worsen with continued therapy and resolve within 1 to 2 days of discontinuation of abacavir therapy. After resuming abacavir therapy, severe and fatal hypersensitivity reactions have occurred. The frequency of hypersensitivity reactions in patients on abacavir therapy is about 5%. Abacavir should not be resumed as part of any HAART regimen in any patient experiencing this unique hypersensitivity reaction.

Since abacavir is the newest NRTI, concerns have arisen regarding its resistance profile and its value if added to an ongoing antiviral drug regimen. Similar to lamivudine, monotherapy with abacavir results in a mutation, but resistance to abacavir is relatively modest, four- to eight fold compared with the up to 1000-fold resistance observed with lamivudine monotherapy. Interestingly, many patients with the mutation still achieve good antiviral effects while taking abacavir in combination therapy, potentially caused by the slow development of abacavir resistance. The ultimate role of abacavir resistance remains to be determined in future clinical trials.

Abacavir has potency equal to that of ZDV when tested in vitro. It has been studied in combination with all FDA-approved protease inhibitors, providing significant reductions in viral load and increases in CD4+ counts resulting from all combinations evaluated. The largest study of abacavir to date (Staszewski et al, 1999a) has found durable antiviral efficacy of an abacavir/ZDV/3TC combination compared to an indinavir/ZDV/3TC combination for patients with baseline viral loads between 50,000 and 100,000 copies/mL. However, for patients entering the study with over 100,000 copies of HIV-1 RNA at baseline, results were significantly poorer than with the protease inhibitor–containing combination regimen.

The ultimate role of abacavir needs to be evaluated in further clinical trials. Its use in a triple-NRTI regimen (with Combivir) is interesting and holds promise as a potential form of HAART, consisting of only four pills per day in a patient-friendly regimen. Short-term data from a study comparing the efficacy of remaining on a successful PI-based HAART regimen or switching to a simplified abacavir/ZDV/3TC are tantalizing, since both cohorts have maintained similar virologic suppression; however, long-term data are needed. Data about the efficacy of abacavir combined with other NRTIs, NNRTIs, or protease inhibitors are sparse at this time, and more clinical trials are clearly required.

Nonnucleoside Reverse Transcriptase Inhibitors

Nonnucleoside reverse transcriptase inhibitors (NNRTIs) act to inhibit reverse transcriptase by binding in a specific locus or pocket, adjacent to the active site of the RT enzyme, which apparently disrupts the enzyme's catalytic site and may potentially distort the enzyme's shape and function. In contrast to NRTIs, they do not bind to viral DNA and do not directly inhibit DNA chain lengthening (see Table 45–6).

Nevirapine. Nevirapine was the first nonnucleoside reverse transcriptase inhibitor to be approved for antiretroviral therapy, in 1996. Because of the high frequency of skin rash occurring early in therapy (in up to 20% or more of patients), nevirapine requires a gradual dose-escalation strategy when treatment is begun. Less frequently reported side effects include fever, nausea, headache, and abnormal liver function tests. The average wholesale cost of 1 year's therapy is approximately $3041.

Nevirapine is a potent inhibitor of HIV-1 replication and possesses rapid oral absorption. Early clinical trials detected significant reductions in HIV-1 RNA plasma after only 2 weeks of nevirapine monotherapy, but antiviral efficacy was lost within 12 weeks because of rapidly developing viral resistance.

Nevirapine should never be utilized in combination with drugs unable to achieve profound suppression of viral load because a resistant virus will inevitably develop during the course of therapy. Because of the speed with which resistance develops, as well as the likelihood of cross-resistance to other available NNRTI agents, nevirapine is a tricky drug, the use of which demands close patient follow-up as well as adherence. Many patients have done well while taking nevirapine and continue on nevirapine-based regimens. However, with its high potency and once-daily dosing, efavirenz has been considered the preferred agent in this drug class.

Delavirdine. Delavirdine was the second NNRTI to be granted FDA approval for management of HIV-1 infection (in 1997). Wholesale cost of therapy for 1 year is approximately $2781.

Delavirdine and nevirapine both cause skin rash during treatment initiation. Delavirdine commonly causes rash during the first 1 to 3 weeks of therapy, but the frequency is less than that observed with nevirapine, and dose escalation is not useful in reducing the risk of delavirdine-induced skin rash. Other less frequently observed toxicities of moderate or severe intensity include abnormal liver function tests, gastrointestinal toxicity, and pruritis. HIV-1 develops resistance to delavirdine through a small number of mutations.

Early trials that combined delavirdine with single or double NRTIs were able to demonstrate only modest increases in CD4+ counts and reductions in viral load. Potentially the greatest use for delavirdine at this time may be as an enhancer of bioavailability of various protease inhibitors, rather than as a single NNRTI in a HAART regimen. Delavirdine possesses cross-resistance with efavirenz, and with nevirapine to a lesser degree, because of a single mutation. Patients previously treated with either efavirenz or nevirapine may not benefit from a switch to delavirdine therapy. At this time, delavirdine seems to be a "bridesmaid" drug, and is infrequently utilized, at least partly because of its lesser potency plus a very large pill burden, compared to both nevirapine and efavirenz.

Efavirenz. Efavirenz is the newest NNRTI for anti-HIV-1 therapy, receiving its FDA approval in September 1998. As a consequence of its long serum half-life, efavirenz is the only FDA-approved NNRTI given once a day. The wholesale cost for 1 year of therapy in adult patients is approximately $3997.

More than 50% of patients initiating efavirenz therapy experience central nervous system (CNS) side effects. Depressive effects include dizziness (most common), as well as stupor, vivid dreams, or feeling "disconnected." Stimulatory effects include agitation and insomnia. Other reported effects are confusion, abnormal thinking, impaired concentration, amnesia, hallucinations, and/or euphoria. CNS effects typically occur during the first few weeks of treatment, and may be lessened by taking efavirenz at bedtime. A mild-to-moderate skin rash typically occurs in the first few weeks of therapy, although it is less severe than with other NNRTIs. Since efavirenz is potentially teratogenic, its use by pregnant women is not recommended.

Cross-resistance between the three members of the NNRTI class is of considerable concern. Since each NNRTI binds in the same pocket, resistance to one NNRTI confers cross-resistance to other NNRTIs, despite the unique chemical structure of each agent. No NNRTI should be administered as monotherapy, added to any failing regimen, or included in a combination regimen incapable of adequately suppressing viral replication. When efavirenz therapy is initiated, it should be utilized in combination with at least one other antiretroviral agent to which the patient has not been previously exposed.

Efavirenz has been combined with other antiretroviral agents in company-sponsored clinical trials. Both the suppression of viral replication and the improvements in immune function have been very impressive in most trials thus far. In the largest study of efavirenz to date (Staszewski et al, 1999b), an efavirenz/ZDV/3TC combination was as effective as an indinavir/ZDV/3TC combination in treatment-naive patients. Prior to the study, it was assumed that PI-based HAART was the most potent combination available, and that NNRTI-based combinations were unlikely to provide acceptable viral suppression for patients with high viral loads. The addition of efavirenz has also been beneficial to treatment-experienced patients, providing that the NRTI components of the regimen are either amplified or switched to new drugs at the time of adding efavirenz.

Since efavirenz is a relatively new drug, few studies provide information about the long-term durability of regimens containing efavirenz that are comparable to PI-containing HAART regimens. However, the impressive performance of this newest NNRTI bodes well for anti-HIV-1 treatment in the future.

Protease Inhibitors

Unlike reverse transcriptase inhibitors, drugs inhibiting the protease enzyme act at both a different stage in the viral life cycle as well as at a different site. They do not prevent viral replication, but render new HIV-1 progeny noninfectious (Table 45–6).

Protease inhibitors (PIs) are complicated and difficult drugs for a number of reasons: (1) they are expensive to synthesize and manufacture; (2) they are both inducers and inhibitors (to varying degrees) of a liver enzyme; (3) they are often highly protein-bound, thus reducing plasma drug levels; (4) they frequently have complex dietary and scheduling requirements for administration; (5) broad cross-resistance exists between members of the PI family; (6) they frequently cause adverse side effects; (7) dosing often results in sizeable daily pill burdens; and (8) strict adherence to an unforgiving PI regimen is absolutely mandatory. Despite the complexities of PI-based HAART, the availability of protease inhibitors in 1996 to 1997 marked an immense change in the management of HIV-1 infection, with many individuals experiencing significant improvements in health status previously unknown in HIV-1 disease.

Saquinavir. Saquinavir was the first protease inhibitor to be approved by the FDA for HIV-1 infection. The hard-gel capsule formulation received its approval in December 1995. The wholesale cost of 1 year of therapy with saquinavir hard-gel capsules (HGCs) is approximately $7143. Adverse events from saquinavir-HGC therapy are typically mild, consisting of diarrhea, abdominal discomfort, nausea, flatulence, and rash. Moderate or more severe adverse events (diarrhea, abdominal pain, or nausea) are observed infrequently. Because of its exceptionally low oral bioavailability—4% when administered with a high-fat, high-calorie meal—saquinavir-HGC has been used less frequently than other protease inhibitors.

A soft-gel capsule (SGC) formulation of saquinavir received FDA approval in November 1997, and has considerably higher oral bioavailability (12 to 15%) than the hard-gel formulation. According to the manufacturer, saquinavir-HGC will be phased out over time and completely replaced by saquinavir-SGC at a 1-year wholesale cost of $7152.

Because of its greater potency, toxicities related to saquinavir-SGC occur more frequently than with saquinavir-HGC. Moderate or more severe adverse events (diarrhea, abdominal discomfort, and nausea) occur at frequencies of 20% or less. Both hard-gel and soft-gel formulations of saquinavir must be taken with a high-fat, high-calorie meal, which enhances the drug's bioavailability.

Although saquinavir is potent in vitro, saquinavir-HGC monotherapy provided only modest reductions in viral load or increases in CD4+ cell counts. The addition of saquinavir-HGC to an ongoing NRTI regimen in heavily pretreated patients provided only modest results. The subsequent use of ritonavir (see below) to inhibit the enzymatic degradation of saquinavir-HGC was successful in achieving higher plasma levels of saquinavir, as well as both improvements in CD4+ counts and reductions in viral load. For patients failing other PI-based HAART regimens (most notably those taking nelfinavir), a switch to a saquinavir-HGC/ritonavir combination has been variably successful as salvage therapy. The greatest benefits were derived when the failing regimen was identified promptly after therapy initiation, viral loads were still low, and patients were promptly switched to the salvage regimen.

The soft-gel formulation of saquinavir has been found to be as effective as other protease inhibitors when combined with two NRTIs, and considerably more effective than the hard-gel formulation. Saquinavir-SGC combined with ZDV/3TC provides reductions in viral load and increases in CD4+ cell counts comparable to other PI-based HAART. Triple-drug HAART combinations based on saquinavir-HGC and saquinavir-SGC have been compared for antiretroviral efficacy. Over 80% of patients who received soft-gel–based combinations were below the level of quantitation compared to no more than 43% of patients who received hard-gel–based combinations. Until the introduction of a soft-gel capsule, saquinavir was the least used of the PIs because of its poor bioavailability. When two other PIs were granted FDA approval within 4 months, the more potent drugs were quickly favored over saquinavir-HGC. Saquinavir-SGC has proven to be similar in potency to the other PIs, and only this soft-gel formulation is regularly utilized as a single PI in HAART regimens.

Ritonavir. Ritonavir was the second PI approved for anti-HIV-1 treatment, in March 1996. Ritonavir is available as capsules or in a liquid formulation. The average wholesale cost of therapy for 1 year is approximately $8125. Its exceptional potency compared to saquinavir-HGC plus its twice-daily dosing regimen made it the first potent PI in the early days of PI therapy.

Ritonavir is a difficult drug to use. It is frequently very toxic for many patients, resulting in severe nausea, vomiting, and diarrhea during the early stages of therapy. Even with ritonavir dose escalation over the first 4 days of therapy, GI toxicities are very common—particularly for treatment-naive patients initiating ritonavir simultaneously with ZDV. Ritonavir's side effects may be reduced when administered with food, particularly with a high-fat meal. Taste disturbances are very common with the foul-tasting liquid formulation. Other toxicities include headaches, circumoral paresthesias, asthenia (loss of strength and energy), and fatigue. Ritonavir is the least tolerated PI; up to 17% of patients discontinue the drug within the first few weeks of therapy.

In addition to frequent toxicities, ritonavir interacts potently with a liver enzyme, resulting in extremely high levels of many drugs that the liver would normally metabolize. Twenty-five individual drugs (including sedatives, hypnotics, and cardiac drugs) are contraindicated with ritonavir therapy, as a result of dangerous or fatal drug levels caused by reduced metabolism. However, ritonavir's inhibition of the liver's metabolism of other PIs (particularly saquinavir and indinavir) is being utilized to provide more patient-friendly dosing regimens. Small doses of ritonavir result in significantly increased plasma levels of the paired PI, allowing either reduced strength or less frequent dosing. It has been also found that the addition of ritonavir to NRTI regimens has led to reduced AIDS-related deaths, profound reductions in viral load, and improvements in immunologic function.

In summary, ritonavir is a very effective agent, but it is the most difficult PI to utilize, because of its toxicity and complex metabolic interactions. Another drawback is its similar resistance pattern to indinavir and other PIs. However, the use of low-dose ritonavir has been beneficial, both as salvage therapy (particularly combined with saquinavir-HGC) as well as dual-PI therapy (combined with indinavir or either form of saquinavir), which allows simpler dosing and potentially fewer PI-related toxicities.

Indinavir. Indinavir was the third PI to become available for HIV-1 treatment. Its FDA approval in March 1996 was achieved in the shortest time (to date) for any drug approval. Wholesale cost of 1 year of therapy is approximately $5475.

Its primary toxic effect is nephrolithiasis because of its poor water solubility. Nephrolithiasis, including flank pain with or without hematuria, has been reported in up to 8% of individuals taking indinavir. The most frequently observed toxicities related to indinavir therapy include GI upset (abdominal pain, nausea, diarrhea, and vomiting), asthenia, fatigue, and headache, which may diminish over time. Dosing requirements with indinavir are quite complex, since oral absorption is considerably better when the drug is administered without a high-fat meal. It is recommended that it should be taken either before a full meal or with a low-protein, low-fat snack. It is also critical that the patient drink at least 48 ounces of water daily to maintain good hydration and reduce the risk of kidney stones.

Indinavir, either alone or in combination with single NRTIs, provides potent antiviral activity, and the highest tolerable doses of indinavir have resulted in both profound reductions in viral load as well as much slower development of indinavir-resistant strains of HIV-1. It is critical that indinavir (and PIs in general) be given in doses sufficient to provide optimal antiviral activity, since the development of resistance mutations occurs much more slowly when antiviral activity is optimal.

Two major studies evaluated the impact of indinavir-based HAART. One study (Currier et al, 1998) determined a rate of AIDS progression or death of 11% for patients on ZDV/3TC compared to a rate of 6% for patients on indinavir/ZDV/3TC; the mean CD4+ count at study enrollment was 87 cells/mm^3. Additionally, patients on the triple combination had lower incidence rates for several common opportunistic infections. The other study (Gulick et al, 1998) compared an indinavir/ZDV/3TC combination to indinavir monotherapy or ZDV/3TC. Marked reductions in viral load as well as increases in CD4+ cell counts were durable to 100 weeks in 78% of patients starting on the triple combination at the study's onset. Patients in the other two study arms added drugs sufficient to continue with triple therapy, but did not achieve either antiviral efficacy or immunologic improvements seen in the triple-combination cohort. As a result of both studies, combination therapy with two NRTIs plus a single PI became the standard of care in 1997. Indinavir has also been combined with other NRTI pairs, including ddI/d4T and d4T/3TC, as well as each of the currently available NNRTIs.

Currently, indinavir is probably the most widely used PI because of its lower wholesale cost as well as its exceptional potency and relatively well-tolerated toxicities. However, difficult dosing regimens with regard to meals and the need for continued hydration have made it a complicated medication to administer. The combination of low doses of ritonavir with indinavir results in reduced doses of indinavir, thus eliminating meal restrictions and fluid-intake requirements. With this combination there is the potential for more patient-friendly regimens with simpler dosing (twice daily) and possibly less indinavir-related toxicities; however, more clinical trials are warranted.

Nelfinavir. Nelfinavir was the fourth PI to gain FDA approval, in March 1997. Wholesale cost is approximately $6780 for 1 year of therapy. In November 1999, the FDA approved a twice-daily regimen with standard doses of d4T/3TC.

The primary side effect of nelfinavir is mild-to-moderate diarrhea. The recent data leading to the twice-daily FDA approval determined moderate-to-severe diarrhea at a frequency no higher than 18%. Clinical experience with nelfinavir suggests that diarrhea is actually an increased number of bowel movements rather than watery stool, and although it does not markedly interfere with activities of daily life, it is experienced by up to 40% of patients. Over-the-counter antidiarrheal preparations (loperamide) are usually able to control these symptoms adequately. Nelfinavir may be the best-tolerated PI currently available, because of its side-effect profile. It is a less potent inhibitor of the liver enzyme that metabolizes it than is ritonavir or indinavir, and consequently it is less difficult to administer.

Nelfinavir has good oral bioavailability. Clinical trials have combined nelfinavir with ZDV/3TC, as well as ddI/d4T, d4T/nevirapine, d4T/3TC, and efavirenz. As is typical with PI-based combination therapy, patients who were naive to PI therapy demonstrated the best antiviral efficacy and immunologic improvements. Since nelfinavir is a newer PI, there are fewer published long-term clinical trial data for this drug than for the older PIs.

Varying degrees of cross-resistance exist between all drugs of the PI class because of the development of overlapping secondary mutations that occur in a stepwise fashion over months of incompletely suppressive antiretroviral therapy. Primary mutations also occur soon after therapy initiation and tend to be unique to each PI. Reports about HIV-1 resistance to nelfinavir have emphasized a unique mutation that did not occur with other PIs currently in use. HIV-1 strains resistant to other PIs were found to be susceptible to nelfinavir, while HIV-1 strains resistant to nelfinavir retained their susceptibility to other PIs, particularly ritonavir and saquinavir. Patients developing resistance to nelfinavir may benefit from a switch to the combination of ritonavir/saquinavir-HGC, provided that NRTI agents are also changed at the time of the switch.

Amprenavir. Amprenavir is the fifth PI for HIV-1 infection, receiving its FDA approval in April 1999. Amprenavir has a long half-life, which allows twice-daily dosing. Toxicities reported with amprenavir therapy include rash, nausea, diarrhea, and headache, all of which have been mild. Gastrointestinal disturbances are the most commonly reported side effects. Since amprenavir has a sulfonamide-based structure, its use is contraindicated in sulfonamide-allergic patients.

Similar to other PIs (and NNRTIs), amprenavir is metabolized by the same liver enzyme and it will potentially interact with other PIs and other drugs. The degree of this liver enzyme's influence on amprenavir has yet to be determined definitively at this time. Amprenavir is either synergistic or additive with most NRTIs and other PIs. A number of small studies have combined amprenavir with various NRTI combinations or other protease inhibitors. The largest trial to date (Goodgame et al, 1999) evaluated the triple combination of amprenavir with ZDV/3TC and found antiviral efficacy and immunologic improvements similar to those achieved with other PI-based HAART regimens.

Since all studies of amprenavir report data of no more than 48 weeks, it would be premature to attempt to rank amprenavir's anti-HIV-1 efficacy against that of the other PIs or NNRTIs. However, its relatively mild side-effect profile and a twice-daily regimen indicate that amprenavir will likely be a useful addition to the anti-HIV armamentarium of drugs in the future.

Despite the tremendous promise of PI-based HAART regimens, some major long-term side effects associated with therapy have been described. Reports of unusual changes in body fat composition have appeared within the past 2 years. Most patients experiencing "lipodystrophy" have taken either indinavir or the ritonavir/saquinavir-HGC combination, implying a possible cause–effect relationship. However, more recent reports have described similar changes in patients *never* treated with PIs. The changes in body habitus are extremely varied. Peripheral changes include depletion of fat from extremities (particularly the limbs) as well as buttocks, plus concurrent venomegaly in the affected extremities. "Buffalo hump," a "horse collar" redistribution of fat in the neck and shoulder areas, has been reported. Deep abdominal fat accumulation or visceral adiposity has also been described. Approximately 35 to 50% in patients treated with PIs for more than 3 years experience these body changes. Considerably more study is needed in order to gain a complete understanding of the underlying mechanisms related to these metabolic abnormalities and whether some drug classes are likelier to result in these disfiguring presentations. In addition to fat redistribution, less frequent occurrences of diabetes mellitus have been reported, primarily in patients treated with PIs.

Recommendations for Initiation of Antiretroviral Therapy

Previously, the International AIDS Society — USA Panel urged treatment of HIV-1 infection in any patient with established (chronic) infection and confirmed plasma HIV-1 RNA viral load greater than 5000 to 10,000 copies/mL. (The range in values of 5000 for bDNA and 10,000 for QC-PCR depends on the measurement technique.) The stringency of their earlier recommendations should be contrasted with their most recent guidelines. They now recommend therapy for patients with confirmed plasma HIV-1 RNA level above 30,000 copies/mL, irrespective of CD4+ cell count, and for patients with CD4+ counts less than 350 cells/mm^3, irrespective of HIV-1 RNA level. They additionally recommend treatment for patients with both plasma HIV-1 RNA level in the range of 5000 to 30,000 copies/mL and CD4+ cell count ranging between 350 and 500 cells/mm^3. Patients with CD4+ counts greater than 500 cells/mm^3 and viral loads ranging between 5000 and 30,000 copies should consider initiating therapy, because of the risks of progression at higher viral loads. Treatment recommendations are not different for women. The Panel on Clinical Practices for Treatment of HIV Infection has proposed a differing set of recommendations. [This panel was convened by the U.S. Department of Health and Human Services (DHHS) and the Henry J. Kaiser Family Foundation.] The DHHS panel urges treatment of any patient with symptomatic HIV-1 infection, while asymptomatic patients with CD4+ counts less than 500 cells/mm^3 and viral loads greater than 10,000 (bDNA) or 20,000 (QC-PCR) should be offered treatment. The rationale for treatment considers the value of improving long-term survival, but must acknowledge the patient's willingness to accept therapy. However, patients who are asymptomatic with CD4+ counts *over* 500 and viral loads *under* 10,000 (bDNA) or 20,000 (QC-PCR) may either be treated or followed.

Rationale for Early Initiation of Treatment

There are a number of good reasons for initiating antiretroviral therapy earlier rather than later in chronic HIV-1 infection.

1. It is easier to achieve profound reductions in viral load when baseline, pretreatment viral loads are lower rather than higher and CD4+ counts are higher. Rebound of viral load during therapy is also less likely in those patients initiating therapy early (with lower viral load and higher CD4+ counts).
2. The viral load must be suppressed as completely as possible, since the viral load nadir achieved is directly correlated with the durability of therapy.
3. Incomplete suppression of viral replication allows for selection of mutations leading to drug resistance; conversely, completely suppressive therapy allows minimal to no viral mutations and resistance.
4. Immune recovery is more likely in those patients starting therapy with less advanced HIV-1 infection. Patients initiating therapy with a nadir CD4+ count less than 50 cells/mm^3 had almost a threefold higher risk of disease progression than patients initiating therapy with CD4+ counts greater than 150 cells/mm^3.
5. Medication toxicities are usually less severe and tolerated better by healthier patients.
6. HAART regimens are now more patient-friendly, particularly with the better-tolerated NNRTIs allowing twice- or once-daily dosing. Triple-NRTI HAART (abacavir/ZDV/3TC) and NNRTI-based HAART regimens are as efficacious as PI-based HAART regimens when the viral load is moderately elevated. Dual-PI combinations (with ritonavir promoting better drug levels of the partner PI) may allow less toxicity, fewer dietary restrictions, and more convenient dosing.

Rationale for Later Initiation of Treatment

There are likewise several compelling reasons for initiating therapy later rather than earlier.

1. Even though clinical trials of PI-based HAART regimens have demonstrated marked reductions in morbidity and mortality, they have been undertaken in later-stage AIDS rather than in earlier infection.
2. There are no large, controlled trials demonstrating improvements in morbidity and mortality from early initiation of HAART for patients with CD4+ counts in the range of 200 to 350 cells/mm^3. The last trial of PI-based HAART had patients enrolled with a mean CD4+ count at baseline of 87 cells/mm^3. One must look prior to 1995 for trials comparing single- to dual NRTI therapy to demonstrate changes in morbidity and mortality for patients starting therapy with CD4+ counts in the range of 200 to 350.
3. HAART regimens, even when simplified with once- or twice-daily dosing, remain unforgiving of lapses in therapy adherence that allow for the development of resistant HIV-1 strains, and thus narrow future choices for alternative drugs for therapy switches or salvage regimens.
4. Because of cross-resistance patterns in all three drug classes (NRTI, NNRTI, and PI) plus considerations of toxicity and/or food–drug interactions, realistically there are two or at most three sequential drug regimens available for any patient.
5. There is no evidence of preservation of specific anti-HIV-1 cytolytic activity able to control HIV-1 replication (by HIV-1–specific CD4+ and CD8+ cells) resulting from early initiation of treatment in chronically infected individuals. There are sporadic reports of retained anti-HIV-1 cytolytic activity in patients treated soon after primary infection.
6. Failure rates of HAART are as high as 60% in real-life clinical settings. Failure may be due to subtherapeutic drug concentrations (incomplete adherence, variability in pharmacokinetics), drug toxicity, advanced HIV-1 disease, and/or viral resistance.
7. Concerns about the long-term effects of fat redistribution and metabolic abnormalities (diabetes mellitus, hypercholesterolemia) remain unanswered at this time.
8. Since new drugs are in development, with the potential for both greater potency and less toxicity, waiting may be appropriate, given the high likelihood of treatment failure and exhaustion of available drugs.

There is no clear-cut "best" time to initiate HAART. When HAART is initiated, it is a decision to be made by both physician and patient in collaboration. Factors to be considered include high costs, risks of cross-resistance within protease inhibitor and NNRTI drug classes, very rapid development of resistance with less than optimal viral suppression, daunting and complex treatment regimens, negative impact on daily life, large pill burdens, and associated drug-related toxicities. Before starting any regimen, the patient must be advised about the importance of strict adherence, since HAART regimens are unforgiving of nonadherence. The risk of developing drug-resistant viral strains because of incomplete viral suppression is significant; nonadherence increases this risk markedly, as well as narrowing the choice of alternative drugs if the first HAART regimen fails. Tailoring the regimen, when possible, to the patient's schedule and needs is mandatory. The first HAART regimen will be the "best shot." Subsequent HAART regimens never work as well in treatment-experienced patients as they do in treatment-naive patients; patients are treatment-naive one time only.

Structure of Highly Active Antiretroviral Therapy

Highly active antiretroviral therapy has become the cornerstone of HIV-1 management in the late 1990s. Based on the earliest clinical trials of PIs, HAART was originally considered to be a combination of a potent PI (indinavir, ritonavir, nelfinavir, or saquinavir-SGC) plus two compatible NRTIs. The most commonly utilized NRTI pairs are ZDV/3TC and d4T/3TC; less frequently utilized pairs are ddI/d4T, ZDV/ddI, and ZDV/ddC. After study, efavirenz coupled with ZDV/3TC became an additional HAART combination in 1999. Less frequently utilized HAART combinations may also include nevirapine plus two NRTIs, two protease inhibitors (typically ritonavir/saquinavir-HGC) with one or two NRTIs, a single protease inhibitor plus one NNRTI with or without one or two NRTIs, or three NRTIs (abacavir plus ZDV/3TC). These HAART recommendations from the International AIDS Society—USA Panel differ somewhat from those of the DHHS—Kaiser Family Foundation Panel listed in Table 45–7.

TABLE 45–7. COMPONENTS OF HAART REGIMENS: DHHS–KAISER FAMILY PANEL RECOMMENDATIONS

Preferred
- Strong evidence of clinical benefit and/or sustained viral suppression
- One choice each from column A and column B (drugs are listed in random order)

Column A	Column B
Indinavir	ZDV + 3TC
Nelfinavir	d4T + 3TC
Ritonavir	ddI + d4T
Saquinavir-SGC	ZDV + ddI
Ritonavir + saquinavir-SGC or -HGC	ZDV + ddC
Efavirenz	

Alternative
- Data inadequate or regimen less likely to provide viral suppression
- One of the following:
  - Amprenavir + 2 NRTIs from Column B, above *OR*
  - Nevirapine + 2 NRTIs from Column B, above *OR*
  - Abacavir + ZDV + 3TC *OR*
  - Delavirdine + 2 NRTIs from Column B, above

Not Generally Recommended
- Viral suppression not sustained in most patients
- One of the following:
  - 2 NRTIs from Column B, above *OR*
  - Saquinavir-HGC plus 2 NRTIs from Column B, above

Not Recommended
- Insufficient viral suppression and/or overlapping toxicities
- All monotherapies (any drug class):
  - d4T + ZDV
  - ddC + ddI
  - ddC + d4T
  - ddC + 3TC

There are several principles to consider when selecting an initial antiretroviral regimen:

1. Since fully one half or more of regimens will fail, the first regimen should allow opportunities for rescue or salvage therapy with the subsequent regimen(s).
2. In untreated patients with advanced disease (low CD4+ count plus very high viral load), treatment potency is the main concern. Physicians often utilize two protease inhibitors combined with two NRTIs for additional antiviral efficacy. The combination of a single PI, a single NNRTI, plus two NRTIs is also possible but less frequently utilized or studied.
3. For patients with early disease, the choices of drugs are broader and allow more flexibility in structure of the regimen.
4. Factors that have a significant impact on patient acceptance include the total number of pills to be taken, frequency of administration, dosing requirements around meals and other medications, drug interactions (with other medications taken for HIV-related or unrelated conditions), side effects and tolerability, and potential for long-term side effects. The "forgiving" nature of drugs should be considered, both in terms of pharmacokinetics (once or twice daily) and resistance (slower development of resistance or cross-resistance).

PI-based triple combinations have been the most studied of HAART regimens, because of the sequence in which the medications were approved by the FDA.

As previously discussed, PI-based HAART regimens are able to reduce morbidity and mortality, are durable, and are able to provide some degree of immune reconstitution. The genetic barriers for developing resistance to PIs are higher than for NNRTIs. However, PI-based regimens are generally the most complex, least patient-friendly, most difficult to schedule (due to food and drug interactions), and most toxic with the greatest number of side effects. Finally, PI-based HAART regimens have the highest pill burdens of all combination regimens and have the potential for cross-resistance between different members of the PI class (see Table 45–6).

Dual-PI–based combinations utilizing standard doses are typically considered as initial therapy for patients with high viral loads. However, small doses ("baby doses") of ritonavir are able to exploit the pharmacokinetics of the fellow PI, resulting in decreased pill burdens and simplified dosing requirements. The most frequently utilized combination is ritonavir/saquinavir, but ritonavir/indinavir or nelfinavir/saquinavir pairings hold promise in providing patient-friendly regimens. The potential for greater cross-resistance among the PI drugs needs to be evaluated in clinical trials of dual-PI therapy.

HAART regimens based on a single NNRTI with two NRTIs are becoming increasingly popular. The primary advantage is a well-tolerated, simple regimen that is felt to be equivalent to the most potent PI-based HAART regimens, while sparing the protease inhibitor drug class for later use. Smaller pill burdens and no food restrictions contribute to improved patient acceptance of these regimens. There is a potential for better adherence and a more durable antiviral response as a result. Other benefits thus far have been no reports of fat redistribution syndromes as well as the general efficacy of protease inhibitors used subsequently for patients initially treated with NNRTI-based HAART. There are less data demonstrating the long-term efficacy of NNRTI-based regimens compared to PI-based regimens. Final analysis of outcomes from the DuPont 006 study may resolve the issue of durability of NNRTI-based regimens. Possibly the greatest concerns with NNRTI-based HAART regimens are their efficacy in late-stage AIDS as well as the inability to utilize other NNRTIs with development of resistance to the initial NNRTI selected (Table 45–8).

Triple-NRTI regimens have been the least studied of triple-drug combinations thus far. Data from the CNA3005 study have demonstrated similar efficacy of abacavir/ZDV/3TC to indinavir/ZDV/3TC for patients with moderately elevated viral loads. However, for patients with greater than 100,000 copies/mL at study entry, the triple-NRTI combination was less efficacious, in both the CNA3005 and Atlantic studies. Triple-NRTI regimens are generally simple and well tolerated; they additionally allow deferral of both PIs and NNRTIs for later treatment options. Unfortunately, there are insufficient data at this time about their durability and efficacy in late-stage AIDS (Table 45–7).

TABLE 45–8. PROS AND CONS OF VARIOUS HAART REGIMENS

PI Plus two NRTIs	
Pro: Standard of care Long-term data Durable and potent Improved survival	Con: Complex dosing regimens PI cross-resistance Toxicities Intolerance
NNRTI Plus two NRTIs	
Pro: Simple regimens Well-tolerated Efavirenz as potent as PI in HAART Preserves PIs for later treatment	Con: Cross-resistance No survival advantage yet Not all NNRTIs equipotent Efficacy with high viral load? Efficacy in late-stage disease?
NRTI-Based	
Pro: Simple, well-tolerated Preserves NNRTIs for later treatment Preserves PIs for later treatment	Con: Efficacy with high viral load? Efficacy in late-stage disease? Unknown durability

The dual-NRTI components of HAART regimens all possess advantages (simplicity and tolerability) and disadvantages (side effects and resistance). The ZDV/3TC pairing has the smallest pill burden but somewhat difficult side effects, and significant concerns exist about cross-resistance to other NRTIs with long-term therapy. The d4T/3TC combination is the best tolerated, but the subsequent efficacy of d4T following ZDV therapy remains a matter of concern to some clinicians. The ZDV/ddI regimen is well studied from the pre-HAART era, but toxicities of both medications can be difficult for the patient. The ddI/d4T combination allows use of hydroxyurea and may have greater durability than other NRTI pairs, but peripheral neuropathy from both drugs as well as GI toxicity from ddI are sometimes difficult. Finally, the abacavir/3TC combination may well the most potent NRTI combination in vitro. It is both simple and well tolerated, but has been studied the least. However, the hypersensitivity reaction to abacavir is of concern.

Follow-Up with Antiretroviral Therapy

Consistent and regular follow-up with viral load testing is absolutely mandatory to evaluate the initial success of the HAART regimen. Monitoring viral load determines the initial success of the regimen, evaluates its stability and durability, and can promptly detect a regimen that is not performing as hoped. Other critical factors for follow-up include falling CD4+ counts or intolerance of drugs caused by toxicity. Changes made promptly in a failing regimen (defined as any detectable viral load after 16 weeks or more of therapy) frequently allow continuation of undetectable viral loads following the failure of a prior HAART regimen. When the regimen is changed, it should be switched to drugs with minimal cross-resistance potential to PIs as well as to NRTIs to which the patient has not been exposed.

The primary goal of anti-HIV-1 therapy at this time is to drive viral replication to such a low level that mutations in HIV-associated enzymes (reverse transcriptase, protease) will be unlikely to develop or will not occur at all. Durable viral load suppression over long periods of time has not allowed the development of resistance-conferring mutations. With the loss of viral suppression, the risk for development of multiple mutations increases, as does the difficulty of selecting alternative drugs for treatment. If possible, resistance should be avoided by preventing it in the first place. A detectable viral load in a patient with a previously undetectable viral load is a very important finding suggesting resistance, but other factors (including poor adherence and insufficient drug levels from absorption) must be evaluated to determine if the rising viral load is actually due to resistance.

If a patient is failing with a previously successful PI-based HAART regimen, the drugs should be switched at the time of a confirmed virologic failure due to resistance, since early changes have been correlated with greater chances of future success with subsequent regimens. A favored strategy is the use of a ritonavir/saquinavir combination for patients who have failed with the first PI-based regimen. Patients taking nelfinavir have had the best results with a switch to a ritonavir/saquinavir combination. Recent data indicate higher rates of success with a switch to other drugs with reduced potential for cross-resistance *plus* the addition of a drug from a completely new class of agents (typically an NNRTI), which gives many patients a realistic "second shot" at HAART. This latter approach may also be helpful for patients with probable resistance to multiple NRTIs, in that resistance to the entire NRTI class is now understood. ZDV-experienced patients may have a blunted response to subsequent NRTI therapy.

The ultimate role of resistance testing in patient management remains to be defined, but small clinical studies have suggested that evaluation of potential resistance *prior* to switching medications is of value and is correlated with greater and more durable viral suppression after changes in medications. Two different methodologies are available for analysis of resistance. *Genotypic analysis* is able to detect resistance mutations in either reverse transcriptase- or protease-encoding genomes. However, only the predominant mutation or mutations are detected because of their increased presence, whereas mutations occurring at lesser frequencies may not be detected at all. *Phenotypic analysis* does not detect specific mutations but rather analyzes the efficacy of varying drugs (NRTIs, NNRTIs, and PIs) against HIV-1. As both types of tests become increasingly available, they likely will be of value to patients experiencing treatment failure with the initial HAART regimen. The value of resistance testing in heavily pretreated patients remains to be evaluated.

Additional Strategies with Antiretroviral Therapy

The concept of treatment utilized in cancer therapy is known as "induction–maintenance" therapy, in which a very potent regimen is followed by a maintenance regimen of lesser strength and toxicity. Because of the impressive performance of indinavir-containing three-drug regimens, this concept was borrowed for treatment-naive patients achieving profound reductions in viral load. Studies have evaluated whether switching to maintenance with a simplified regimen after 12 to 16 weeks of induction therapy was as efficacious in maintaining viral suppression as remaining on the induction regimen. In all studies, more patients on maintenance therapy experienced viral load rebounds than did those patients continuing with the induction combination regimen. These results do not doom the concept of maintenance therapy outright, since many patients on maintenance regimens were able to maintain viral loads below detection. Probable reasons for the lackluster results of these trials relate to the inadequate duration of the induction period as well as the insufficient potency of the maintenance regimen. An ongoing trial is evaluating a considerably longer induction period (9 months) with a more potent regimen of five drugs. Short-term results (no longer than 3 months) have determined that a majority of patients are able to maintain adequate viral suppression.

The possibility of simplifying a HAART regimen has led researchers to design trials of patients successfully taking PI-based HAART regimens who were switched to simpler, but no less potent regimens containing either an NNRTI (primarily nevirapine) or abacavir with two NRTIs. Although only short-term results are available (no longer than 48 weeks), most patients switched have been able to maintain adequate viral suppression, using patient-friendly regimens. The critical difference between these simplification trials and the previously described induction–maintenance trials has been in the change to an equipotent, but simpler regimen. Long-term data and durability evaluations are clearly needed.

The prevention of HIV-1 transmission from mother to infant is obviously of critical importance if HIV infection is to be controlled worldwide. ACTG 076 demonstrated the benefits of a ZDV regimen delivered to the mother before and after delivery, as well as ZDV delivery to the infant postnatally. Though both expensive and cumbersome, the use of zidovudine was able to reduce transmission to the infant by about two thirds. Two recent trials evaluated the use of zidovudine therapy initiated at 36 weeks' gestation and continued until delivery. Up to 50% reduction in transmission was achieved. A separate trial compared nevirapine and zidovudine. The nevirapine arm provided a single oral dose of 200 mg to the mother at onset of labor and 2 mg/kg to infants within 72 hours of birth. The zidovudine arm provided 600 mg orally to the mother at onset of labor and 300 mg every 3 hours until delivery; infants received 4 mg/kg orally twice daily for 7 days after birth. Nevirapine therapy resulted in less HIV-1 infection than did the zidovudine regimen; overall, the risk of HIV-1 infection was reduced by almost 50%.

As HIV-infected individuals were treated with increasingly available and diverse NRTIs from 1987 to 1995, survival trends improved for both longer AIDS-free life and reduced mortality. However, the impact of protease inhibitor–based combination therapy has resulted in astonishing improvements in survival, with up to a 5.7-fold reduction in mortality by March 1998. Many patients facing imminent death have become survivors, returning to life like Lazarus and facing new challenges in the arenas of employment and social life.

The glowing success rates of 70 to 90% seen in controlled clinical trials of HAART stand in contrast to the many failures of HAART regimens. Environments of clinical trials usually differ from real-life clinical settings in many ways. Individuals enrolled in clinical trials are very often treatment-naive, free of underlying conditions that could exacerbate drug toxicities, possibly more proactive about their therapy, and often followed more diligently by researchers and support staff. Real-life patients, in contrast, frequently have been on sequential NRTI monotherapy as well as the equivalent of PI monotherapy and are likely have cross-resistance to many drugs. These patients may also frequently be nonadherent with complicated regimens, which typically consist of 20 or more pills devoted just to HAART on a daily basis. Adherence with HAART regimens is directly correlated with successful virologic control. Considering the difficulty of adherence with demanding, unforgiving regimens, it is not surprising that failure rates are so high.

Even with the success story of HAART, concerns exist about the long-term durability and efficacy of these regimens. Very few studies have evaluated patients on HAART for more than 2 years. The study with the longest follow-up to date is Merck 035, which has followed patients on indinavir/ZDV/3TC to 148 weeks. Researchers are now finding that HAART regimens will maintain their efficacy and durability when viral loads are reduced to less than 50 copies/mL, using the most sophisticated QC-PCR technology. To achieve truly durable benefits from HAART regimens, physicians will need to be ever more vigilant with measurements of viral load, and patients will likewise need to be completely adherent to drug regimens in order to maximize their potential.

There is clearly a continuing need for new drugs to manage HIV-1 infection. Drugs requiring a once-daily administration will be helpful to simplify regimens for patients. Modifications of pharmacokinetics to promote simpler dosing regimens as well as fewer drug–drug or drug–food interactions are also needed. New drugs targeted to either reverse transcriptase or protease are needed, but with differing resistance profiles than those currently available. Heavily pretreated patients, with prior failure of one or more HAART regimens, have limited options for further treatment and clearly would benefit from medications that have limited or no cross-resistance potential. Much work is currently concentrated on developing agents that attack other sites for potential drug intervention in the HIV-1 viral life cycle.

SYSTEMIC HIV-RELATED DISEASES AND OPPORTUNISTIC INFECTIONS

It is impossible to inventory the myriad systemic problems encountered in HIV disease because patients' immune systems are often so compromised that virtually any type of infection is possible. The CDC has classified the disease into three clinical categories for adolescents and adults. These classifications include: (1) general manifestations of HIV disease (Tables 45–2 through 45–5, clinical category A), (2) symptomatic conditions that contribute to or are complicated by HIV infection (Tables 45–2 through 45–5, clinical category B), and (3) those that are associated with severe immunodeficiency and occur frequently in persons with HIV infection (Tables 45–2 through 45–5, clinical category C). Brief descriptions of some of the more common systemic disorders and opportunistic infections (OIs) follow.

AIDS Dementia Complex

AIDS dementia complex (ADC) (also refered to as HIV encephalopathy) is one of several HIV-induced conditions affecting the central nervous system (CNS) of individuals with AIDS. Other related conditions include vacuolar myelopathy and peripheral neuropathies.

The incidence of ADC is between 30 and 60% in untreated AIDS patients. Typically it occurs with a CD4+ cell count less than 200 cells/mm^3, although it can present as the initial manifestation of HIV infection. Since the initiation of antiretroviral therapy the prevalence has declined steadily to 20% of AIDS patients on HAART.

ADC affects the cognitive, behavioral, and motor function of affected individuals, as demonstrated by the insidious onset of reduced work productivity, reduced concentration, an overall mental slowness, reduced libido, and forgetfulness. As the symptoms worsen, the patients often become apathetic and withdraw from social activities. Motor problems also develop including imbalance, clumsiness, and weakness. As the condition progresses, severe memory loss, language impairment, and eventual decline into a vegetative state may occur. Death ensues within a few months.

The pathogenesis is not clearly defined although several possibilities have been postulated. The CNS is infiltrated by HIV-infected mononuclear cells, which secrete neurotoxic factors, several of which have been identified. These may cause malfunction and destruction of the CNS. Several groups have also reported the infection of astrocytes and neurons by HIV. This may lead to an alteration in neurotransmitter release. In addition, an increase in excitatory amino acids and free intracellular calcium has been observed. Several recent studies have found that a lower incidence of ADC is seen in AIDS patients with Kaposi's sarcoma. The exact mechanism responsible for this is not yet fully understood.

Treatment with AZT and other antiretroviral agents greatly improves the prognosis of the condition and in some cases can completely restore cognitive functions.

Kaposi Sarcoma

Kaposi sarcoma (KS) is the most commonly diagnosed malignancy in AIDS. The lesions are characterized pathohistologically by spindle-shaped and infiltrative cells, neovascularization, and edema. Previous to the AIDS epidemic, KS was a rare, benign lesion primarily affecting older Jewish, eastern European, and Mediterranean men. Initially, KS was seen in nearly 40% of AIDS patients. However, the incidence has decreased over the past several years, and KS is now found in approximately 15% of newly diagnosed cases. Potent antiretroviral drug combinations that suppress HIV replication are responsible for this reduction in the frequency of KS in HIV-infected persons. It is important to note, however, that although the incidence of KS has declined, an increasing number of AIDS deaths are directly caused by KS.

The etiology of KS remains unclear, but evidence suggests that alterations in immunosuppression and immune activation, in conjunction with sexually transmitted infectious agents, may play a role. An initial event, such as infection with human herpesvirus 8 (HHV-8) (also referred to as the KS herpesvirus [KS HV]), may lead to a transformation of normal cells, leading ultimately to malignancy. Recently HHV-8–like DNA was isolated from both KS lesions and in KS-derived cell cultures. The mechanism of transmission of HHV-8 is unknown. Although epidemiological evidence suggests that sexual transmission is likely in men who have sex with men, it may occur in heterosexuals as well. Other suspected etiological agents for KS include cytomegalovirus (CMV), hepatitis B virus (HBV), human herpesvirus 6 (HHV-6), human papillomavirus 16 (HPV-16), HIV, and *Mycoplasma penetrans.*

Increasing evidence also indicates that circulating growth factors may play a crucial role in the pathogenesis of AIDS-related KS. Other evidence suggests that KS may not be a malignancy at all but rather an angiogenic disorder with enhanced cellular proliferation in response to these circulating growth factors. Currently, drug trials are underway on several antiangiogenic substances.

Kaposi's sarcoma in an individual less than 60 years of age, or in conjunction with evidence of HIV infection, is a strong indicator for AIDS. Most often initially involving the skin, KS lesions appear as nodules or plaques, red to purple in color, that can appear in several locations simultaneously, often with edema. Other areas affected include the lymph nodes, oral cavity, gastrointestinal tract, pulmonary tract, and ocular structures.

The natural course of the disease can be quite variable and KS can be fatal. None of the therapeutic approaches are curative, and many are, in fact, immunosuppressive. Most recently, HAART has reduced the incidence of KS in individuals with AIDS by restoring the natural functioning of the immune system.

Pneumocystis carinii Pneumonia

The opportunistic fungus *Pneumocystis carinii* is a ubiquitous organism, found in the environment as well as the lungs of healthy humans and animals. It is estimated that most healthy children have been exposed to *P. carinii* by the age of 4 years. *P. carinii* pneumonia (PCP) occurs in immunosuppressed individuals and malnourished infants; it is the most common opportunistic infection in AIDS.

The symptoms of PCP include dyspnea, nonproductive cough, and fever. Extrapulmonary lesions occur only rarely in the lymph nodes, spleen, liver, ocular structures, and bone marrow. Untreated, PCP invariably leads to death.

> *Pneumocystis carinii* pneumonia (PCP) is the most common opportunistic infection in AIDS.

Adults and adolescents with HIV infection (including pregnant women and those on HAART) should receive prophylaxis against PCP if they have a CD4+ count less than 200 cells/mm^3. Others who should be considered for PCP prophylaxis include persons who have a T-lymphocyte percentage less than 14% or a history of an AIDS-defining illness.

Trimethoprim-sulfamethoxazole (TMP-SMZ) is the preferred prophylactic agent. If TMP-SMZ cannot be tolerated, alternative prophylactic regimes can include dapsone, dapsone plus pyrimethamine plus leucovorin, aerosolized pentamidine, and atovaquone.

The recommended therapy for active PCP is TMP-SMZ. Alternatives include pentamidine, trimetrexate with folic acid, trimethoprim with dapsone, atovaquone, and primaquine with clindamycin.

Tuberculosis

Tuberculosis (TB) affects upward of 35% of HIV-infected patients. Although pulmonary TB is not by itself an indicator disease of AIDS, disseminated TB is an AIDS-defining disease. Most cases of TB are still treatable; however, resistant and fatal strains are developing.

> Activities and occupations such as volunteer work or employment in healthcare facilities, correctional institutions, and shelters for the homeless might increase the likelihood of exposure to TB for HIV-positive individuals.

HIV-positive persons should be advised that certain activities and occupations, such as volunteer work or employment in healthcare facilities, correctional institutions, and shelters for the homeless, might increase the likelihood of exposure to TB. Those at risk of developing TB, or with CD4+ cell counts less than 75 cells/mm^3, should receive prophylaxis with isoniazid and pyridoxine, refabutin and pyrazinamide, or rifampin and pyrazinamide.

Mycobacterium avium-intracellulare Complex

Mycobacterium avium-intracellulare complex (MAC) refers to a family of very similar mycobacterial organisms, *M. avium* and *M. intracellulare,* which are ubiquitous in soil, food, and water. In nonimmunocompromised individuals, MAC causes respiratory tract infection. However, in patients with AIDS, MAC causes a more disseminated disease affecting almost any organ system, especially those with many mononuclear phagocytes (eg, the liver, spleen, and bone marrow). Disseminated MAC is a serious infectious disease, affecting up to 40% of AIDS patients, and typically occurs with CD4+ cell counts less than 50 cells/mm^3.

MAC generally affects individuals late in the disease and presents with symptoms including fever, chills, night sweats, swollen glands, abdominal pain, diarrhea, weight loss, and overall weakness. MAC usually affects the intestines and inner organs first. Swelling and inflammation also occur.

Adults and adolescents with HIV infection and CD4+ cell counts less than 50 cells/mm^3 should receive chemoprophylaxis against disseminated MAC disease. Clarithromycin or azithromycin is the preferred agent for MAC prophylaxis; rifabutin is used as an alternative. With the advent of HAART it is now reasonable to consider discontinuing MAC prophylaxis in patients with a sustained (e.g., more than 3 to 6 months) CD4+ cell count greater than 100 cells/mm^3 and sustained suppression of HIV plasma RNA.

Treatment of disseminated MAC disease consists of either clarithromycin or azithromycin in combination with at least one other drug (ie, ethambutol or rifabutin). Breakthrough disease is observed in patients on HAART with CD4+ counts greater than 100 cells/mm^3 and low viral loads who have discontinued treatment for disseminated MAC. For this reason, all patients with a history of disseminated MAC disease should continue full therapeutic antimycobacterial therapy for life.

> All patients with a history of disseminated MAC disease should continue full therapeutic antimycobacterial therapy for life, regardless of their CD4+ counts.

Cytomegalovirus Disease

Cytomegalovirus (CMV) is a ubiquitous DNA herpesvirus found in upward of 85% of the general population. Most individuals are infected before the age of 3. CMV is present in nearly all body fluids and is transmitted via mother's milk, semen and vaginal fluids, urine, saliva, tears, tissue transplantation, and exposure to blood and blood products. The immune system of an immunocompetent individual does not prevent CMV from infecting the body, but it does inactivate the virus to a dormant state throughout the life span of the individual. CMV has a limited cellular distribution in normal individuals and is found only in the ductal epithelium of salivary glands, mucosal epithelium and submucosal endothelium in the intestine, bile duct epithelium, and alveolar and bronchial epithelial cells. CD4+ cells seem to play an important role in controlling CMV replication, which could explain the resurgence of CMV as an OI associated with AIDS.

Unchecked by a weakened immune system in individuals with AIDS, CMV attacks several areas of the body. The area most often affected is the retina. The optic nerve is involved in up to 5% of patients. The lungs, CNS, gastrointestinal system, esophagus, liver, adrenal glands, and kidneys are also affected. This generally occurs after the CD4+ cell count is less than 100 cells/mm^3.

HIV-positive individuals should be counseled to always use sexual protection and maintain proper hygiene when handling any bodily fluid, including baby diapers. Prophylaxis with oral ganciclovir should be considered for all HIV-infected adults and adolescents who are CMV seropositive and who have a CD4+ count of less than 50 cells/mm^3. Acyclovir has been shown to be ineffective prophylactically against CMV, and valacyclovir is associated with an increased rate of mortality when used prophylactically.

> To avoid exposure to CMV, HIV-positive individuals should always use sexual protection and maintain proper hygiene when handling any bodily fluid, as well as baby diapers.

Since active CMV infection is not cured with the currently available antiviral agents, maintenance therapy is required. Therapies include parenteral or oral ganciclovir, parenteral foscarnet, alone or in combination with ganciclovir, and parenteral cidofovir. Oral ganciclovir is currently under investigation for use in children. Recent clinical evidence indicates that those individuals on HAART who show a rise in their CD4+ cell count may also demonstrate a sustained recovery of immune function allowing for the effective control of OIs. Many of these individuals have been removed from CMV maintenance therapy without recurrence of the disease.

HIV Wasting Syndrome

HIV wasting syndrome is a common problem among individuals infected with HIV. It is an unintended and progressive weight loss accompanied by weakness, fever, nutritional deficiencies, and diarrhea. The syndrome often diminishes the quality of life, exacerbates other illnesses, and can increase the risk of death. The wasting experienced can be secondary to the HIV infection itself, but it is also associated with other OIs and cancers.

HIV wasting syndrome is diagnosed when individuals have lost more than 10% of their body weight, experience fevers lasting longer than 1 month, and experience diarrhea for a period exceeding 1 month, without any other identifiable etiological mechanism. Most individuals with advanced disease experience some degree of wasting. The exact etiology of the syndrome is not known. However, evidence suggest that inadequate dietary intake secondary to nausea, malabsorption of nutrients, abnormalities in metabolism and energy expenditure, and secondary opportunistic infections are responsible. Therapy includes appetite stimulants such as megestrol and dronabinol, anabolic agents such as serostim, cytokine inhibitors such as thalidomide, and hormones such as testosterone and oxymethalone.

Syphilis

Treponema pallidum infection in individuals with AIDS often progresses quickly to neurosyphilis. For this reason, all individuals with AIDS should be tested for syphilis and all those who are seropositive for *T. pallidum* should immediately be treated as if they have neurosyphilis.

The treatment of choice for neurosyphilis in patients with AIDS is intravenous aqueous penicillin G. The treatment is repeated if the symptoms persist or recur.

Toxoplasmosis

Toxoplasmosis is one of the most common infections in humans in the world today. Infection of the brain with *Toxoplasma gondii* is an AIDS-defining disease and the most common opportunistic infection of the CNS. It is associated with profound morbidity and death in as many as 35% of cases. HIV-infected persons should be tested for IgG antibody to *Toxoplasma* soon after diagnosis of HIV infection to detect latent infection with *T. gondii.*

To prevent exposure all HIV-infected persons should be counseled not to eat raw or undercooked meat. They should wash their hands after gardening or other contact with soil. In addition, they should wash fruit and vegetables carefully. Cat boxes should be cleaned daily by a non-HIV-infected person if possible.

> To prevent exposure to toxoplasmosis, all HIV-infected persons should be counseled not to eat raw or undercooked meat. They should wash their hands after gardening or other contact with soil. In addition, they should wash fruit and vegetables carefully. A non-HIV-infected person should clean cat boxes daily if possible.

Toxoplasmosis seropositive patients with CD4+ counts less than 100 cells/mm^3 should receive prophylaxis with TMP-SMZ or dapsone-pyrimethamine against toxoplasmosis. Use of HAART may alter recommendations for prophylaxis.

OCULAR HIV-RELATED DISEASES AND OPPORTUNISTIC INFECTIONS

The literature continues to evolve regarding the ocular sequelae of HIV infection. HIV manifests as a direct infection of the eye, and as a cause of secondary opportunistic infections (OIs) and malignancies. HIV causes anterior segment and adnexal eye disease (orbit, lids, conjunctiva, and cornea), as well as internal eye disease of the anterior chamber (iris and ciliary body) and posterior segment (retina, choroid, optic nerve, and visual pathway). The effects of HIV may manifest as inflammatory reactions, vascular disorders, OIs, neoplasms, or neuro-ophthalmic disorders. HIV has been isolated in the following ocular fluids and tissues: tears, conjunctiva, cornea, aqueous, vitreous, and retina. The effects of HAART on the ocular manifestations of HIV infection are just beginning to appear in the literature. It is impossible to inventory the varied ocular problems encountered in HIV disease. Therefore, brief descriptions of some of the more common ocular disorders and OIs follow.

Adnexal and Anterior Segment Disorders

Keratoconjunctivitis Sicca

Among the common adnexal and anterior segment disorders (Table 45–9) in HIV-infected patients is dry eye syndrome or keratoconjunctivitis sicca (KCS). Approximately 17 to 20% of HIV-infected patients develop KCS during the course of their illness. This is far greater than the incidence rate of less than 1% in the general population. A recent study by Gritz and associates (1997), reported that the presence of KCS and the level of immunosuppression did not appear to affect the ocular flora in patients with AIDS. Studies have also failed to report an association of dry eye to the CD4+ count or to the severity of HIV disease.

TABLE 45–9. OCULAR ADNEXAL AND ANTERIOR SEGMENT MANIFESTATIONS OF HIV

Location	Problem	Frequency
Adnexa/orbit	Molluscum contagiosum	C
	Herpes zoster ophthalmicus	C
	Kaposi sarcoma	C
	Orbital lymphoma	R
Conjunctiva	Microvasculopathy	VC
	Kaposi sarcoma	C
Cornea	Keratoconjunctivitis sicca	VC
	Herpes zoster keratitis	R
	Herpes simplex keratitis	R
	Microsporidial keratitis	R
Anterior chamber	Primary HIV-related uveitis	R-C

VC = very common (>25%); C = common (10–25%); R = rare (<10%).

KCS in HIV-infected patients should be managed with ocular topical lubricants, bland ophthalmic ointments, and punctal occlusion. HIV-infected patients who develop microbial keratitis can be more difficult to treat, and the potential for complications is greater than that seen in the non-HIV population. Therefore, these patients should be closely followed and carefully educated about the potential for corneal complications secondary to dry eye.

Conjunctival Microvasculopathy

Conjunctival microvasculopathy has been reported in 70 to 80% of HIV-positive patients. Slit-lamp evidence of conjunctival microvasculopathy includes perilimbal segmental vascular dilation and narrowing, comma-shaped vascular fragments, microaneurysm formation, and "sludging" of the blood column (Figure 45–1). The microvasculopathy appears to be noninfectious and asymptomatic in nature. It may be related to the microvascular changes seen in HIV retinopathy. No treatment for conjunctival microvasculopathy has been reported in the literature.

> Conjunctival microvasculopathy has been reported in 70 to 80% of HIV-positive patients.

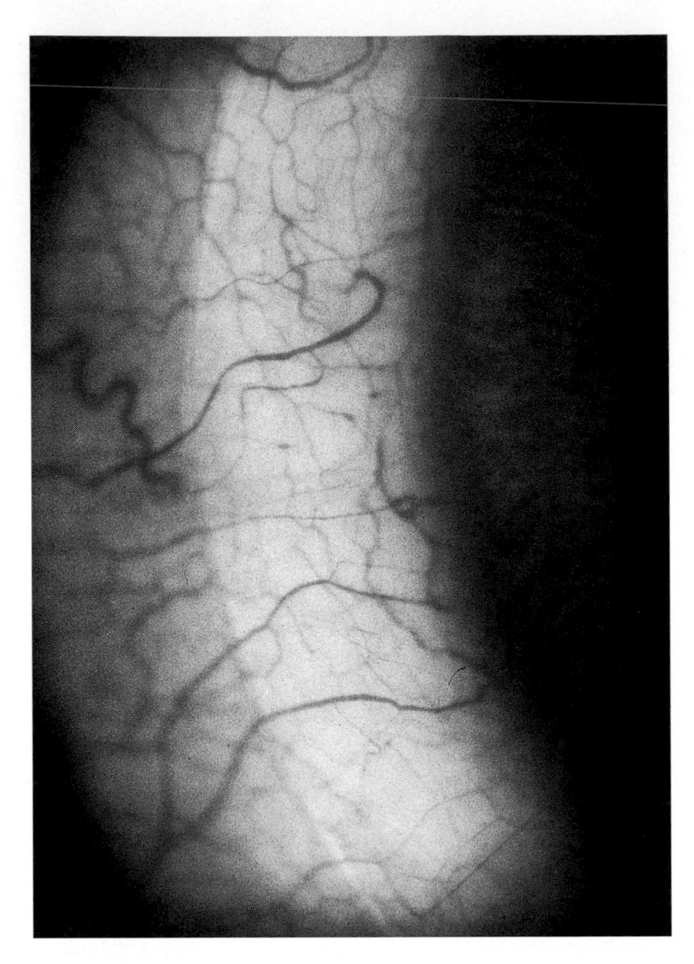

Figure 45–1. Conjunctival microvasculopathy in an HIV-infected patient demonstrating the perilimbal segmental vascular irregularities with sludging of the blood column.

Molluscum Contagiosum

Molluscum contagiosum is a poxvirus that can cause wart-like lesions of the lids and lid margin. It has been reported in up to 5% of HIV-infected patients (Figure 45–2). It is more common, severe and recurrent in HIV-infected patients than in non-HIV-infected patients. It can also cause follicular conjunctivitis and superficial keratitis secondary to toxic reactions to molluscum contagiosum involving the eyelid margins. Treatment of molluscum includes cryotherapy, curettage, and surgical excision and incision. It has been recently reported that HAART has improved disseminated molluscum contagiosum with facial lesions.

Herpes Zoster Ophthalmicus

Reactivation of the herpes zoster virus (HZV) ordinarily occurs in immunocompetent persons older than 60 years of age, presenting as either shingles or herpes zoster ophthalmicus (HZO). However, in HIV disease, reactivation may be seen in younger persons (less than 40 years of age) due to immunosuppression. Approximately 5 to 15% of HIV-positive patients develop HZO.

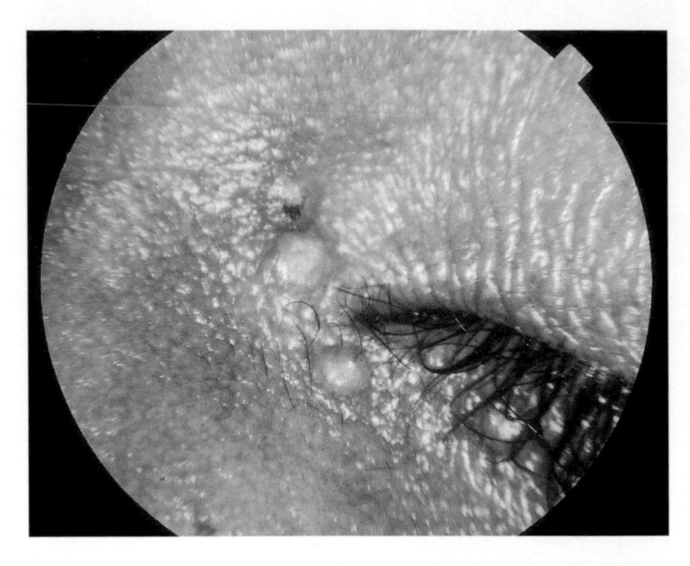

Figure 45–2. Molluscum contagiosum located nasal to the left upper and lower lids of an HIV-positive patient.

HZO in HIV disease presents with the classic vesicular eruptions corresponding to the ophthalmic division of the trigeminal nerve. Studies suggest that HIV-infected patients with HZO may have a high rate of painful and/or sight-threatening complications. A study by Margolis and colleagues (1991) reported low incidence of stromal keratitis, but the infectious epithelial keratitis was more common, particularly devastating, and difficult to manage.

> Persons under 40 years who present with HZO should be referred for a complete medical work-up to rule out HIV disease as the trigger for the HZV reactivation.

Treatment of HZO includes analgesics for pain and oral systemic antivirals such as 600 to 800 mg of oral acyclovir qid for 10 days. Valacyclovir and famciclovir are newer forms of acyclovir and can be used to systemically treat the HZV. Treatment for HIV-infected patients often requires an initial IV dose of acyclovir followed by an oral maintenance regimen of acyclovir or famciclovir for the prevention of recurrence. Uveitis and other ocular inflammations (e.g., stromal infiltrates) are treated with steroids and cycloplegics.

Corneal lesions must be watched closely for secondary bacterial infection and treated with topical antibiotics if necessary. The vesicular skin lesions should be treated with topical acyclovir ointment and antibiotics if necessary. The patient should keep the lesions clean and medicated. Early aggressive treatment with oral antivirals is the best approach to prevent postherpetic pain. Patients with HIV disease may require longer, more aggressive therapy than immunocompetent persons.

Persons under the age of 40 years who present with HZO should be referred for a complete medical workup to rule out HIV disease as the trigger for the HZV reactivation.

Herpes Simplex Keratitis

The incidence and clinical course of herpes simplex virus (HSV) keratitis is similar in both HIV-positive and HIV-negative persons. However, the recurrence rate of HSV keratitis is greater in the HIV-positive person. HSV keratitis in HIV-infected patients can be a difficult management dilemma. HIV-infected patients who develop HSV keratitis can be more resistant to treatment and often require topical antiviral treatment with trifluridine (Viroptic i gtt q2h) along with oral acyclovir (400 mg 5 times a day) or famciclovir (125 to 500 mg tid). Vidarabine (Vira-A) ophthalmic ointment can be given at bedtime to protect the cornea while the patient sleeps. Long-term therapy with oral antivirals may be necessary to prevent recurrence of herpes simplex keratitis.

Microsporidial Keratitis

Microsporidia are small obligate intracellular protozoal parasites that have been reported in HIV-infected patients. These parasites have been isolated from conjunctival and corneal scrapings as the cause of keratitis in HIV-infected patients. They are most commonly seen in patients with decreased CD4+ cell counts. Schwartz and co-workers (1993) reported a CD4+ count of 2 to 50 cells/mm^3, indicating that ocular microsporidiasis occurs in patients with advanced AIDS.

Symptoms of microsporidial infection include foreign-body sensation, light sensitivity, conjunctival hyperemia, and tearing. Slit-lamp evaluation of the cornea reveals diffuse coarse white infiltrates and erosions of the corneal epithelium. The lesions are variable in size and confined mostly to the epithelial layer (Figure 45–3). The organism can be difficult to detect and requires special culturing and specimen collection via conjunctival and corneal scrapings. Thus, HIV-infected patients who exhibit coarse white infiltrates and erosions of the corneal epithelium should be carefully cultured for microsporidia. Treatment is very difficult. Medication options include oral itraconazole, topical fumagillin, and oral albendazole.

> HIV-infected patients who exhibit coarse white infiltrates and erosions of the corneal epithelium should be carefully cultured for microsporidia.

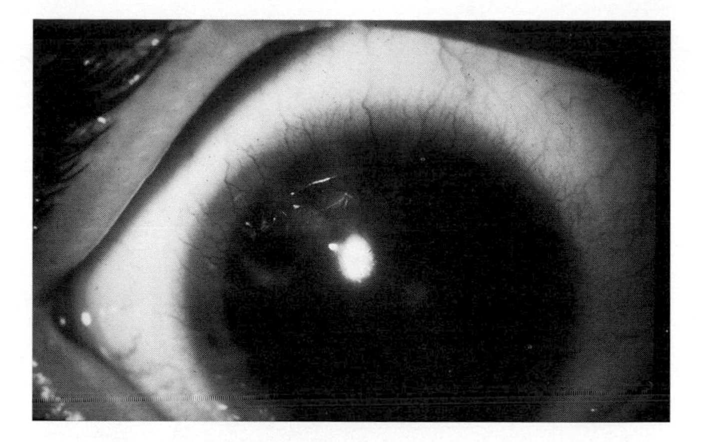

Figure 45–3. Microsporidial keratoconjunctivitis with characteristic granular corneal epithelial infiltrates. (*Courtesy of Drs. J. Shovlin and G. Rossenwasser.*)

Uveitis

Uveitis may present in HIV-positive patients without any apparent etiology other than HIV itself. It also may occur secondary to ocular OIs. Possible etiologic organisms include CMV, HZV, TB, syphilis, toxoplasmosis, cryptococci, and MAC. Therefore, management of uveitis in an HIV-infected individual lies in the treatment of the underlying OI, if present. In addition, rifambutin, cidofovir, ritonavir, indinavir, and rindinavir-saquinavir have been implicated as causes of anterior uveitis.

> Management of uveitis in an HIV-infected individual involves the treatment of the underlying OI, if present.

Kaposi Sarcoma

Approximately 20% of HIV-infected patients with systemic Kaposi sarcoma (KS) have ocular involvement. Ocular KS presents as tumor foci on the conjunctiva and eyelids (Figure 45–4). The eyelids are affected much more often than the conjunctiva. Lesions are painless and slow-growing and other than the cosmetic concerns, many patients remain asymptomatic. Ocular involvement can include loss of lashes, disruption of the lid margin, local irritation, trichiasis, ptosis, infection, recurrent hemorrhage, and rarely, visual obstruction. Current therapeutic options are not curative, and in fact many are immunosuppressive.

> Approximately 20% of HIV-infected patients with systemic Kaposi sarcoma (KS) have ocular involvement.

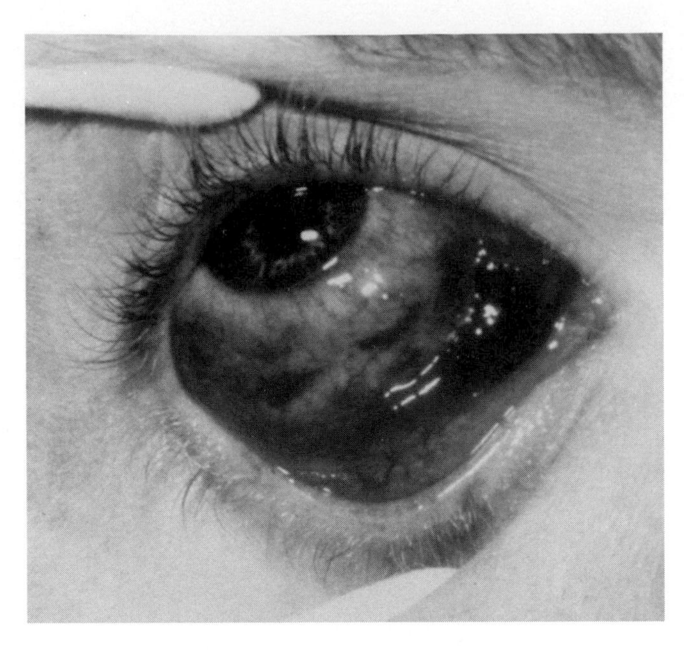

Figure 45–4. Kaposi sarcoma of the eyelid and conjunctiva. (*Courtesy of Dr. Brian DenBeste.*)

Other types of adnexal and orbital tumors are rare in HIV-infected patients. Orbital lymphoma is found in only 1% of AIDS patients.

Posterior Segment Disorders

HIV Retinopathy

Among posterior segment disorders (Table 45–10), microvascular retinal disease is the most common ocular manifestation of HIV infection. HIV retinopathy most commonly presents as cotton-wool spots, but also can manifest as intraretinal hemorrhages (Figure 45–5). Cotton-wool spots have been reported in 28 to 92% of patients with AIDS, whereas intraretinal hemorrhages have been reported in 0 to 54% of patients with AIDS.

> Microvascular retinal disease is the most common ocular manifestation of HIV infection.

Fluorescein angiographic studies suggest that HIV retinopathy may be more common than is noted with traditional fundus examination.

> Fluorescein angiographic studies suggest that HIV retinopathy may be more common than is noted with traditional fundus examination.

TABLE 45–10. OCULAR POSTERIOR SEGMENT AND NEURO-OPHTHALMIC MANIFESTATIONS OF HIV

Location	Problem	Frequency
Retina/choroid	HIV retinopathy	VC
	CMV retinitis	VC
	VZV retinitis	R
	Toxoplasmosis retinochoroiditis	R
	Choroidal pneumocystosis	R
	Cryptococcus sp. chorioretinitis	R
	Histoplasmosis chorioretinitis	R
	Candida sp. chrorioretinitis	R
	Syphilitic retinitis	R-C
	Tubercular choroiditis	R
	MAC choroiditis	R
Cranial nerves	Palsies	R-C
	Optic neuropathy	C
	Papilledema	R
Extraocular muscles	Abnormal saccades	VC
	Abnormal pursuits	R-C
Visual pathways	Visual field defects	R

VC = very common (>25%); C = common (10–25%); R = rare (<10%).

HIV retinopathy has been associated with the degree of immunodeficiency and thus has been correlated with declining CD4+ counts. Patients that present with HIV retinopathy should be followed closely as it could be a sign of disease progression and the microvasculopathy could allow retinal opportunistic infections to access and infect the retina. Pivetti-Pezzi and associates (1997) suggested an association between early administration of antiretrovirals and a significant reduction of the prevalence of HIV retinopathy (especially cotton-wool spots). It is theorized that early inhibition of HIV replication may play a protective role in the retina, thus preventing retinal dysfunction and opportunistic infections.

> Patients that present with HIV retinopathy should be followed closely as it could be a sign of disease progression and the microvasculopathy could allow retinal opportunistic infections to access and infect the retina.

Cytomegalovirus Retinitis

CMV retinitis is the most common sight-threatening opportunistic infection in AIDS, occurring in 20 to 40% of patients. CMV retinitis does not generally present

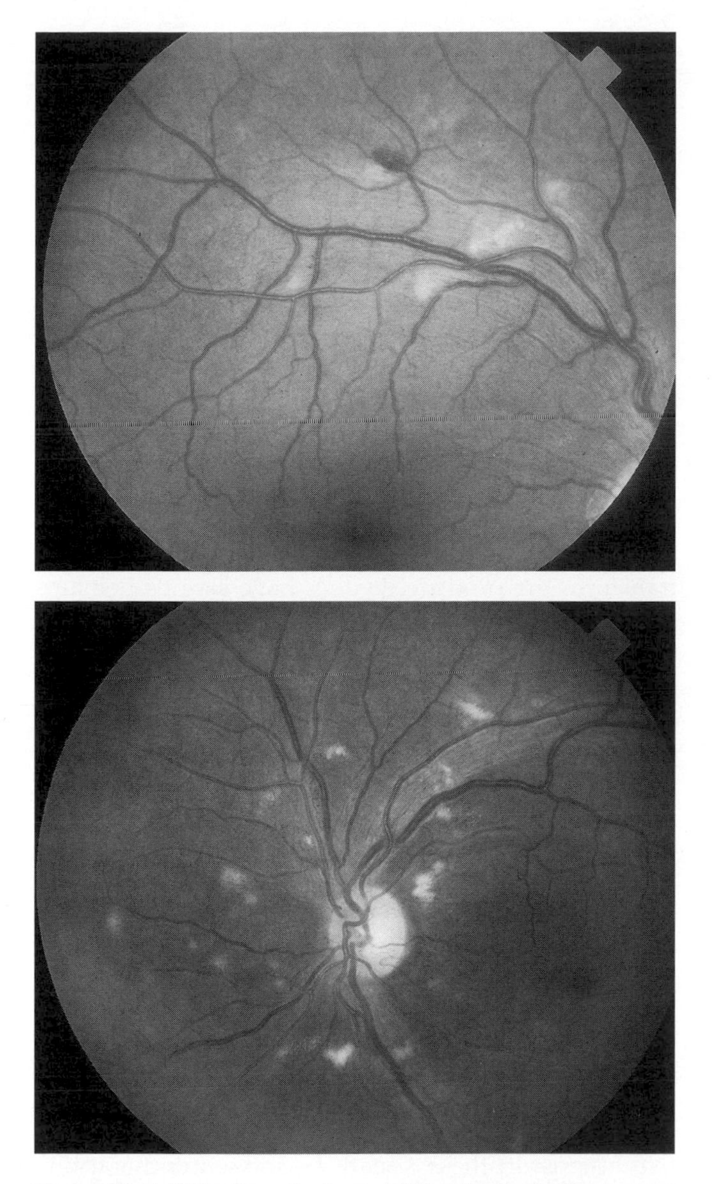

Figure 45–5. HIV retinopathy in an AIDS patient with CD4+ count of 10 cells/mm^3. Both eyes have the typical cotton-wool spots, and the right eye also has one hemorrhage. The patient died 6 months later.

until late in the course of AIDS and after the CD4+ cell count is less than 50 cells/mm^3 or when the CD4+/CD8+ cell ratio is less than 0.11. Thus, CMV retinitis is considered to indicate the failure of the present treatment regimen and to be a negative prognostic indicator of survival.

Initially, CMV is thought to gain access to the retina via microangiopathic disturbances that affect the blood–retina barrier and directly via the optic nerve. Initially, cells in the inner retinal layers are affected, although the virus has been isolated in all layers of the retina and in RPE cells. Replication occurs in the RPE cells and glial cells; it does not appear to occur in the neurosensory retina.

> CMV retinitis is the most common sight-threatening opportunistic infection in AIDS, occurring in 20 to 40% of patients.

Retinitis subsequently occurs as a result of CMV replication and resultant inflammation. CMV disease represents a systemic infection, and therefore the retinitis may present either unilaterally or bilaterally. Ophthalmoscopy reveals irregular yellow-to-white flat granular lesions along the vascular arcades and near the optic nerve head (Figure 45–6). The lesions, which represent areas of retinal necrosis and edema, are initially noted usually in the posterior pole. With progression of the disease via intercellular transmission, the lesions may hemorrhage and extend to cover the entire retina. The Bruch membrane prevents penetration of the virus into the choroid. Inflammatory cells migrate into retinal tissue and subretinal fluid collects, producing elevation and a hazy and grayish-white appearance to the lesions. This opacification is due to the edema and tissue necrosis, which affect retinal transparency. Areas of retinal necrosis are eventually replaced by mottling and clumping of the RPE and scarring. In addition, areas of vascular occlusion and nonperfusion develop, further compromising the retinal tissue. Untreated, CMV retinitis is progressive and eventually results in retinal detachment (Figure 45–7) and blindness. Both rhegmatogenous and nonrhegmatogenous retinal detachments are possible. The nonrhegmatogenous retinal detachments occur posteriorly as a result of the exudative process, whereas the rhegmatogenous retinal detachments occur in the periph-

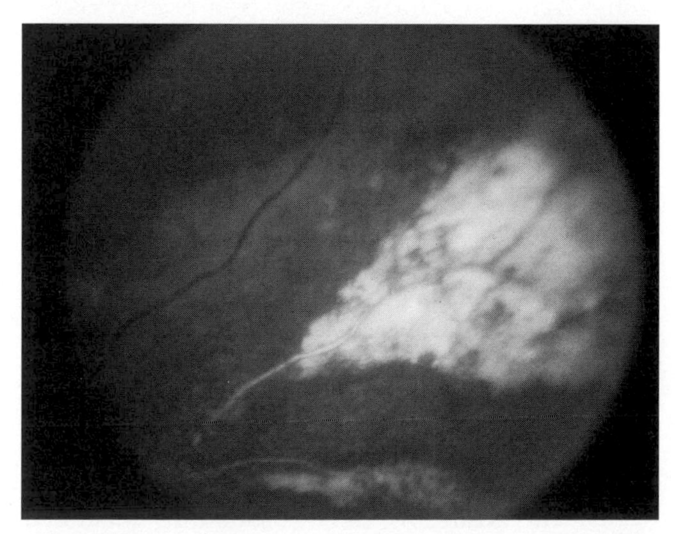

Figure 45–6. Granular CMV retinitis. Note the retinal vascular sheathing as well as the granular retinal necrosis characteristic of this form of CMV retinitis.

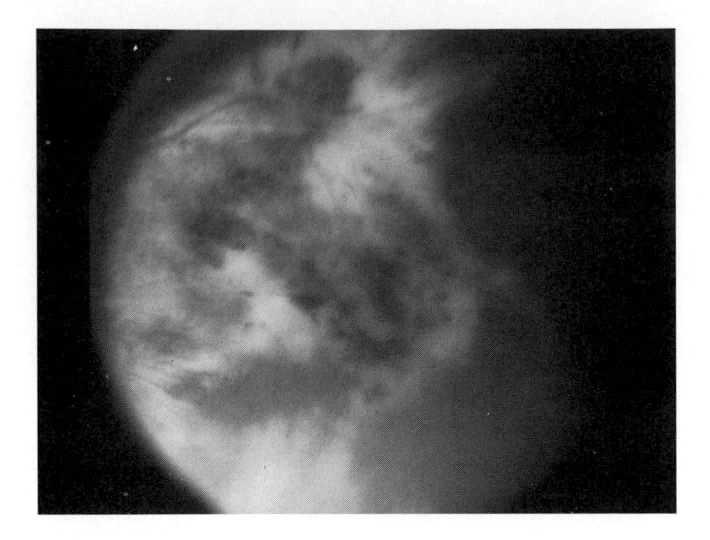

Figure 45–7. Hemorrhagic CMV retinitis. Note the extensive hemorrhaging and full-thickness necrosis.

ery at areas of thinning and atrophy associated with healing. Because of the compromised immune response, CMV vitreitis and uveitis are seldom seen.

Two main variants of CMV retinitis have been described, the so-called edematous variant and the granular variant. The most common is the classic edematous variant, the "pizza pie" or "ketchup and cottage cheese" presentation. Areas of edema and intraretinal hemorrhages and vasculitis mark this form. The less common granular variant consists of grainy opacifications in the periphery that are less dense, more transparent, and associated with minimal hemorrhage.

Depending on the area(s) of the retina and optic nerve initially affected, patients may be asymptomatic, or may complain of floaters, photopsia, blurred vision, metamorphopsia, or restriction of field of vision. Complaints of pain, photophobia, and injection are uncommon. Left untreated, complete retinal destruction will result within several months.

Diagnosis of CMV retinitis is based on funduscopic appearance, although laboratory testing, including biopsy, serologic and viral genome studies, and viral culturing, is also possible. However, these laboratory tests do not routinely provide information useful in the determination of a clinical diagnosis. CMV retinitis must be differentiated from myelinated nerve fibers, cotton-wool spots, toxoplasmic retinochoroiditis, herpes simplex retinitis, candidal endophthalmitis, herpes zoster retinitis, syphilitic retinitis, diabetic and hypertensive retinopathy, retinal vein occlusion, and neoplasm.

Patients with CMV retinitis should be monitored every 2 to 4 weeks; those patients with sight-threatening disease (lesions within one disc diameter of the disc or three disc diameters of the fovea) should be followed more closely. Serial photography and visual field testing are required to document both the progression of the disease and the determination of the efficacy of treatment.

Direct treatment of CMV retinitis relies most commonly on the virustatic agents ganciclovir, foscarnet, and cidofovir. All are administered via an indwelling catheter, although because of its serious nephrotoxic side effects cidofovir is used less frequently. The drugs are initially given in an induction dose, followed by a maintenance protocol. The drugs usually show a positive response within 3 weeks of treatment in 80 to 100% of patients. Ganciclovir is most often the first drug of choice. Ganciclovir is a prodrug that is activated after phosphorylation by the virus and acts by inhibiting the synthesis of CMV DNA. Resistance can occur in viral mutants that are unable to transform the prodrug. It does have serious hematological side effects that must be controlled with the concomitant use of granulocyte-macrophage colony-stimulating factor (GM-CSF). Valganciclovir is an oral prodrug that is rapidly converted to ganciclovir and provides systemic therapeutic levels similar to those obtained via infusion.

Ganciclovir ophthalmic implants contain 4.5 mg of ganciclovir that is released at the rate 1 to 2 μg/hour. Surgical complications can occur and patients receiving the ganciclovir implant as sole therapy are at risk for the development of systemic CMV and retinitis in the contralateral eye. As a result, the implant is only used in those with immediate sight-threatening disease and in conjunction with systemic therapy.

Despite treatment, patients with CMV retinitis often experience relapses of the disease. New areas of inflammation are seen at the borders of previously inactive lesions. In these situations, induction therapy is reinitiated with the same or a different drug. In some refractory situations, the therapy remains ineffective through two or more cycles of induction-maintenance therapy. This may occur because of the deterioration of immune function associated with HIV infection, or increased viral resistance to the drugs. These patients often benefit from induction with combination therapy.

Vitravene (fomivirsen), a newer drug, is an antisense molecule with complementary nucleotides that bind to a specific sequence of nucleotides in viral mRNA. This binding prevents the translation of the mRNA into viral proteins. Vitravene must be injected intravitreally, however, and may be associated with secondary endophthalmitis and retinal detachment.

Most recently, studies have found that patients with CMV retinitis on HAART were able to stop their conventional anti-CMV medications without progression of the retinitis. The restored immune system was able to control the CMV infection without the aid of other therapeutic agents.

Previous to the use of HAART, specific CMV-directed antiviral therapy garnered patients only a marginally better long-term prognosis. However, with the newer antiretroviral therapeutics and their ability to raise the CD4+ cell counts, the incidence of CMV retinitis is declining rapidly. In certain instances, CMV retinitis may be observed in individuals with higher than expected (for CMV retinitis) CD4+ cell counts shortly after the initiation of HAART. At first, the therapy increases the population of memory nonimmunocompetent CD4+ cells, allowing for a relapse of CMV retinitis in patients with CD4+ cell counts of 50 to 100 cells/mm^3. These individuals, unlike patients with CMV retinitis and CD4+ cell counts less than 50 cells/mm^3, may also experience anterior uveitis, cataract, vitritis, cystoid macular edema, epiretinal membrane formation, and disc edema. This is thought to occur because the recovery has been substantial enough to allow ocular inflammatory reactions to occur, although the recovery is still not sufficient to mount a reaction against the CMV. Eventually, the population of naive immunocompetent CD4+ cells is increased sufficiently to control the CMV retinitis.

> CMV retinitis is considered to indicate the failure of the present treatment regimen and to be a negative prognostic indicator of survival.

Direct treatment of CMV retinitis is dependent upon several factors. The size and location of the lesions must be weighed against the side effects associated with anti-CMV therapies, although large lesions or sight-threatening lesions are always treated. Because of the hope afforded recently by HAART, patients may opt to forego treatment in favor of quality-of-life issues.

Varicella-Zoster Virus Retinitis

Varicella-zoster virus (VZV) retinitis occurs in less than 1% of patients with HIV infection. VZV retinitis presents either as acute retinal necrosis (ARN) syndrome or progressive outer retinal necrosis (PORN) syndrome. ARN is associated with peripheral necrotizing retinitis, with multiple scalloped lesions, that coalesce. There is little retinal hemorrhage, and the lesions respond to treatment with intravenous acyclovir. Traditionally, long-term therapy with acyclovir is required to prevent recurrence.

PORN, a second form of VZV retinitis, occurs in profoundly immunocompromised AIDS patients (Figure 45–8). PORN is usually seen in patients with CD4+ counts less than 50 cells/mm^3 (in contrast to ARN, which can occur at any CD4+ count). The fundus appearance of PORN differs from ARN. It clinically presents as multiple deep yellowish retinal lesions with extensive posterior pole involvement. These lesions coalesce and rapidly progress to result in extensive retinal necrosis and vision loss. The response to treatment with IV acyclovir is poor. HAART may have a profound effect on the recurrence of ARN and PORN.

Ocular Toxoplasmosis

In studies of patients in the United States, it was found that 1 to 2% of patients with AIDS develop ocular toxoplasmosis. Toxoplasmic infection in patients with

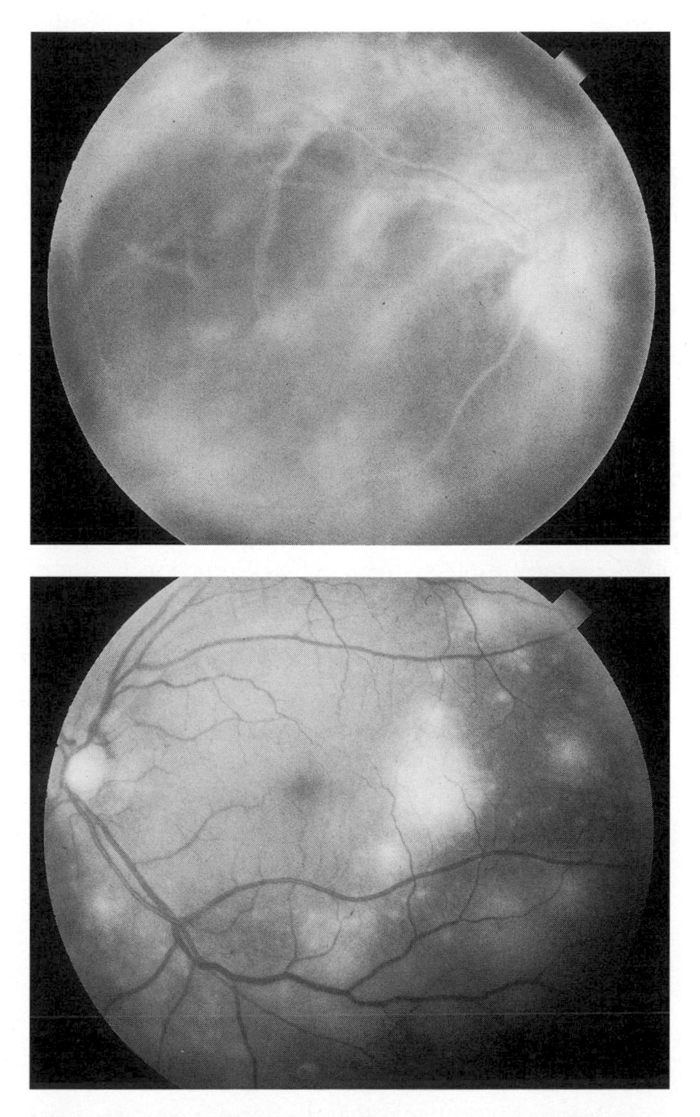

Figure 45–8. Progressive outer retinal necrosis in an AIDS patient that resulted in severe necrosis, retinal detachment, and severe visual loss in the right eye, and multiple deep retinal lesions in the left eye that coalesced.

AIDS is generally associated with CD4+ counts under 100 cells/mm^3. In AIDS patients, ocular toxoplasmosis has varying presentations. It can present as a focal necrotizing retinitis or as a diffuse multifocal necrotizing retinitis that may be bilateral.

Ocular toxoplasmosis responds well to pyrimethamine, sulfadiazine, and/or clindamycin. Maintenance therapy is often required to prevent relapse of the disease, and prophylaxis is often used to prevent infection. *Toxoplasma*-seropositive patients who have a CD4+ count of under 100 cells/mm^3 should be administered prophylaxis against toxoplasmic encephalitis (TE). Limited data suggest that discontinuation of prophylaxis in patients whose CD4+ counts increase to more than 100 cells/mm^3 in response to HAART is associated with a low risk of TE. However, the numbers of patients who have been evaluated are insufficient to recommend routine discontinuation of prophylaxis in such patients.

Fungal Infections

Pneumocystis carinii infection can disseminate and cause pneumocystic choroidopathy. This infection occurs in less than 1% of AIDS patients. Multiple yellow-white subretinal plaques located in the posterior pole characterize the disease. Vitreal cells are not seen in choroidal pneumocystosis, most likely because the infection does not reach the retina. Serous retinal detachments over the choroidal lesions have been reported.

Choroidal pneumocystosis is most often seen in patients utilizing PCP prophylaxis in the form of aerosolized pentamidine. The aerosolized pentamidine does not have systemic absorption and thus allows extrapulmonary (e.g., ocular) infection to occur. Extrapulmonary infections respond to IV TMP-SMX or IV pentamidine. Utilization of oral pentamidine is helping to prevent extrapulmonary infection.

Candidal chorioretinitis has been reported in less than 1% of AIDS patients. Although oral and esophageal candiasis is relatively common in HIV-infected patients, the eye is usually spared infection. *Histoplasma capsulatum* and cryptococci have also been reported to cause chorioretinitis in AIDS patients.

Bacterial Infections

Syphilis, caused by *Treponema pallidum,* is the most common bacterial infection in AIDS patients. It can infect the retina, as well as cause uveitis and neuro-ophthalmic lesions. Syphilis can occur at any stage of HIV infection although neurosyphilis presents earlier in HIV-infected patients than in non-HIV-infected patients. Syphilis in AIDS patients should be treated with traditional antibiotics for syphilis. These patients often require higher doses of antibiotics with a more prolonged therapy.

Syphilis, caused by *Treponema pallidum,* is the most common bacterial infection in AIDS patients.

Mycobacterium-avium complex (MAC) causes choroidal infection in association with bacteremia. It usually occurs in patients with CD4+ counts under 100 cells/mm^3. In many instances, choroidal infection is not detected clinically, but autopsy studies have shown mycobacterial infection of the choroid.

Mycobacterium tuberculosis is a common cause of pulmonary infection in HIV-infected patients. Extrapulmonary tuberculosis of the choroid (tubercular choroiditis) is rare. It causes multiple yellowish choroidal infiltrates and a vitritis. Treatment includes isoniazid, rifampin, and pyrazinamide.

Neuro-Ophthalmic Manifestations

Neuro-ophthalmic manifestations (Table 45–10) reported in HIV-infected patients are caused by OIs or directly by HIV infection of the nervous system. According to Jabs and Quinn (1996), 50% of neuro-ophthalmic manifestations are due to cryptococcal meningitis. Cryptococci have been reported to cause cranial nerve palsies, papilledema, optic neuropathy, and hemianopsia. *Cryptococcus neoformans* infection, although very rare, has caused vision loss due to optic neuropathy. Numerous opportunistic infections have been reported to cause neuro-ophthalmic complications.

Neuro-ophthalmic manifestations reported in HIV-infected patients are caused by OIs or directly by HIV infection of the nervous system.

HIV infection of the nervous system has been reported. Ocular motility defects such as slowed saccades, abnormal pursuits, and poor fixation abilities appear to be related to HIV infection of the central nervous system. Visual field defects related to HIV infection of the retina have also been reported.

Management of Ocular Manifestations

Management protocols for patients with ocular manifestations of HIV disease generally link the frequency of eye examinations to the CD4+ count as follows:

CD4+ Count (cells/mm^3)	Frequency of Eye Exam
Unknown, or at diagnosis	Baseline, follow as appropriate
200–500	6–12 months[a]
<200	2–6 months[a]
New symptom	Stat, follow as appropriate

[a]Frequency of examination depends on overall patient health.

INFECTION CONTROL PROCEDURES RECOMMENDED BY THE CDC*

Shortly after HIV was isolated in tears, the CDC published recommendations for the prevention of possible transmission of HIV from tears. To date, the CDC has not updated its recommendations from 1986. These recommendations have been utilized by eyecare practitioners and remain the most effective "in office" infection control procedures. These recommendations are utilized by the Occupational Health and Safety Administration (OSHA) and should be adhered to whenever possible. The following precautions are judged suitable to prevent the spread of HIV and other microbial pathogens that might be present in tears.

Handwashing

Practitioners should wash their hands before and after any patient encounter. If contact with tears occurs during a procedure, the hands should be washed immediately.

Gloves

If the examiner is going to come into contact with bodily fluids that require universal precautions, such as blood, ear secretions, semen, or cerebral spinal fluid, gloves must always be worn. Tears are a bodily fluid that do not require universal precautions. Thus, OSHA does not require gloves for contact with the tear film. If the examiner has a break in the integrity of their skin and contact with tears is anticipated, gloves should be worn. Handwashing is necessary before gloving and after the gloves are removed.

Instrument Disinfection

Instruments that come into contact with the external surfaces of the eye or the tear film should be wiped clean and then disinfected by a 5- to 10-minute soak in one of the following:

1. 3% hydrogen peroxide
2. Fresh solution containing 5000 parts per million (mg/L) free available chlorine—a 1/10 dilution of household bleach (sodium hypochlorite)
3. 70% ethanol
4. 70% isopropyl alcohol

The device should be thoroughly rinsed and dried before use. Further studies have shown that alcohol soaking may damage tonometer tips and is thus not recommended for tonometer tips. The manufacturer of the eye contact devices should be consulted before using the above CDC recommendations because damage to the devices can occur. Although not recommended by the CDC, many hospital-level disinfectants are available and effective against HIV. These should be used with caution on eye contact devices because any residual disinfectant left on the device could cause severe chemical ocular burns.

Contact Lenses

Contact lenses used in trial fittings should be disinfected between each fitting by one of the following regimens:

1. Hard lenses. Use commercially available hydrogen peroxide contact lens disinfecting systems currently approved for soft lenses. Alternately, most trial hard lenses can be treated with standard heat disinfection for soft lenses (78° to 80° C or 172° to 176° F) for 10 minutes. Practitioners should check with hard lens suppliers to ascertain which lenses can be safely heat-treated.
2. Rigid gas permeable (RGP) lenses. RGP trial lenses can be disinfected using commercially available hydrogen peroxide systems. RGP lenses warp if heat-treated.
3. Soft lenses. Soft trial fitting lenses can be disinfected using commercially available hydrogen peroxide systems. Some soft lenses have also been approved for heat disinfection. Other than hydrogen peroxide, the chemical disinfectants used in standard contact lens solutions have not yet been approved by the FDA for deactivation of HIV. Most cold chemical disinfectants do deactivate herpes simplex virus, which is a larger enveloped virus similar to HIV, but they have not yet been approved by the CDC.

To date, there have been no reported cases of transmission of HIV via eye examination or contact lens fitting. Table 45–11 lists other recommendations for HIV-infected patients and contact lens wear.

CONCLUSION

Since their discovery in 1981, HIV infection and AIDS have dramatically altered the face of the healthcare industry. During this time period the treatment of HIV and AIDS has also changed dramatically with the development of new antiretroviral medications, offering hope to hundreds of thousands of individuals who would have been assured of death only 10 years ago.

Current management protocols include treatment of primary HIV disease with a combination of anti-

*Reprinted with permission from Chronister CL: Viral infections and the immunocompromised patient. In: Silbert J, ed. *Anterior Segment Complications of Contact Lens Wear,* 2nd ed. Boston: Butterworth-Heinemann; 2000:214.

TABLE 45–11. CONSIDERATIONS FOR CONTACT LENS WEAR IN HIV-INFECTED PATIENTS

Some general comments regarding contact lens wear in HIV-infected patients. Since the corneal ulcerations, although somewhat rare, tend to be more severe and difficult to treat, HIV-infected patients that choose to wear contact lenses should strictly adhere to some precautions:

1. Extended wear should be contraindicated in HIV-infected patients. The risk of contact-lens-induced keratitis due to extended wear is greater in the non-HIV population. Although not researched, one would assume that the same would apply to the HIV-infected population
2. Daily wear disposable lenses would be a good alternative to allow for minimal exposure to possible pathogens. This would reduce the disinfection concerns.
3. Careful disinfection of the contact lenses is extremely important for HIV-infected patients. Again, their risk of more severe infection would necessitate careful disinfection techniques.
4. Careful cleaning of contact lens cases is important. A clean lens in a dirty case certainly requires no further explanation.
5. Careful and more numerous contact lens follow-up visits for HIV-infected patients are necessary.
6. Careful patient education about the possibility of dry eye syndrome and other ocular pathogens is important.
7. Under no circumstance should patients share their contact lenses with other individuals—even with careful disinfection.

Reprinted with permission from Chronister CL: Viral infections and the immunocompromised patient. In: Silbert J ed. Anterior Segment Complications of Contact Lens Wear, *2nd ed. Boston: Butterworth-Heinemann; 2000:214.*

retroviral drugs, prophylaxis against opportunistic diseases, and prompt, aggressive treatment of any problems that arise. This has lengthened the chronic stage of HIV infection, affording many HIV-positive persons an increasing number of years of reasonably good health.

In this same time period the ocular sequelae experienced by HIV-positive individuals have also changed. In the past several years decreases in the prevalence of many ocular infections have been observed. However, it is imperative to remember that ocular anomalies and opportunistic infections may be the initial manifestation of active HIV infection. In addition, the presence of opportunistic infections in an HIV-positive individual may indicate the failure of the current treatment regimen and resultant immune failure. Treatment of these OIs requires aggressive, often altered treatment regimens.

The myriad of problems that arise with HIV infection and disease are multisystemic; therefore, a team approach is required to ensure coordination of all aspects of patient care. Given that there are so many ocular manifestations of HIV infection, optometry is an important member of the multidisciplinary team, providing eyecare and appropriate treatment for HIV-infected individuals, as well as education for both patients and healthcare providers alike.

REFERENCES

Ablashi DV, Sturzenegger S, Hunter EA, et al. Presence of HTLV-III in tears and cells from the eyes of AIDS patients. *J Exp Pathol.* 1987;3:693–703.

Abrams DI, Goldman AI, Launer C, et al. A comparative trial of didanosine or zalcitabine after treatment with zidovudine in patients with human immunodeficiency virus infection. *N Engl J Med.* 1994;330:657–662.

Akduman L, Pepose JS. Anterior segment manifestations of acquired immunodeficiency syndrome. *Semin Ophthalmol.* 1995;10:111–118.

Autran B, Carcelain G, Li TS, et al. Positive effects of combined antiretroviral therapy on $CD4^+$ T cell homeostasis and function in advanced HIV disease. *Science.* 1997;227:112–116.

Balzarini J, Herdewijn P, De Clercq E. Differential patterns of intracellular metabolism of 2′,3′-didehydro-2′,3′-dideoxythymidine and 3′-azido-2′,3′-dideoxythymidine, two potent anti-human immunodeficiency virus compounds. *J Biol Chem.* 1989;264:6127–6133.

Bardenstein DS, Elmets C. Hyperfocal cryotherapy of multiple molluscum contagiosum lesions in patients with the acquired immune deficiency syndrome. *Ophthalmology.* 1995;102:1031–1034.

Bartlett JD, Jaanus SD, Ross RN. *Clinical Ocular Pharmacology.* 3rd ed. (Pocket Companion). Boston: Butterworth-Heinemann; 1997.

Barry M, Mulcahy F, Merry C, et al. Pharmacokinetics and potential interactions amongst antiretroviral agents used to treat patients with HIV infection. *Clin Pharmacokinet.* 1999;36:289–304.

Baxter JD, Mayers DL, Wentworth DN, et al. A pilot study of the short-term effects of antiretroviral management based on plasma genotypic antiretroviral resistance testing (GART) in patients failing antiretroviral therapy. Abstracts of the 6th Conference on Retroviruses and Opportunistic Infections, 1999; abstract LB8.

Benet LZ, Kroetz DL, Sheiner LB. Pharmacokinetics: The dynamics of drug absorption, distribution, and elimination. In: Hardman JG, Limbird LE, eds. *Goodman & Gilman's The Pharmacological Basis of Therapeutics.* 9th ed. New York: McGraw-Hill; 1996:3–27.

Bisset LR, Cone RW, Huber W, et al. Highly active antiretroviral therapy during early HIV infection reverses T-cell activation and maturation abnormalities. Swiss HIV Cohort Study. *AIDS.* 1998;12:215–223.

Blumenkranz MS, Culbertson WW, Clarkson JG, et al. Treatment of the acute retinal necrosis syndrome with intravenous acyclovir. *Ophthalmology.* 1986;93:296–300.

Brinkman K, Smeitink JA, Romijn JA, et al. Mitochondrial toxicity induced by nucleoside-analogue reverse-transcriptase inhibitors is a key factor in the pathogenesis of antiretroviral-therapy-related lipodystrophy. *Lancet.* 1999;354:1112–1115.

British HIV Association. British HIV Association (BHIVA) Guidelines for the Treatment of HIV Disease with Antiretroviral Therapy. Consultation draft number 2:30/04, April 1999.

Brun SC, Jakobiec FA. Kaposi's sarcoma of the ocular adnexa. *Int Ophthalmol Clin.* 1997;37:25–33.

Bryan RT. Microsporidiosis: An AIDS-related opportunistic infection. *Clin Infect Dis.* 1995;21(suppl 1):S62–S65.

Burd EM, Pulido JS, Puro DG, et al. Replication of human cytomegalovirus in human retinal glial cells. *IOVS.* 1996; 37:1957–1966.

Calista D, Boschini A, Landi G. Resolution of disseminated molluscum contagiosum with highly active anti-retroviral therapy (HAART) in patients with AIDS. *Eur J Dermatol.* 1999;9:211–213.

Cameron DW, Heath-Chiozzi M, Danner S, et al. Randomised placebo-controlled trial of ritonavir in advanced HIV-1 disease. Advanced HIV Disease Ritonavir Study Group. *Lancet.* 1998;351:543–549.

Cameron DW, Japour AJ, Xu Y, et al. Ritonavir and saquinavir combination therapy for the treatment of HIV infection. *AIDS.* 1999;13:213–224.

Carpenter CCJ, Cooper DA, Fischl MA, et al. Antiretroviral therapy in adults. Updated recommendations for the International AIDS Society—USA Panel. *JAMA.* 2000; 283:381–390.

Carpenter CCJ, Fischl MA, Hammer SM, et al. Antiretroviral therapy for HIV infection in 1998. Updated recommendations of the International AIDS Society—USA Panel. *JAMA.* 1998;280:78–86.

Carr A, et al. Trimethoprim-sulfamethoxazole appears more effective than aerosolized pentamidine as secondary prophylaxis against *Pneumocystis carinii* pneumonia in patients with AIDS. *AIDS.* 1992;6:165–171.

Carr A, Samaras K, Burton S, et al. A syndrome of peripheral lipodystrophy, hyperlipidaemia and insulin resistance in patients receiving HIV protease inhibitors. *AIDS.* 1998; 12:F51–F58.

Carr A, Samaras K, Thorisdottir A, et al. Diagnosis, prediction, and natural course of HIV-1 protease-inhibitor-associated lipodystrophy, hyperlipidaemia, and diabetes mellitus: A cohort study. *Lancet.* 1999;353:2093–2099.

Carter JB, Hamill RJ, Matoba AY. Bilateral syphilitic optic neuritis in a patient with a positive test for HIV. *Arch Ophthalmol.* 1987;105:1485–1486.

Cassoux N, Bodaghi B, LeHoang P. Ocular manifestations of AIDS. In: *Ocular Inflammation: Basic and Clinical Concepts.* BenEzra D, ed. Jerusalem: Martin Dunitz; 1999:427–449.

Centers for Disease Control. Guidelines for the prevention of opportunistic infections in persons infected with human immunodeficiency virus. *MMWR.* 1999;48(no. RR-10).

Centers for Disease Control. Guidelines for the prevention of opportunistic infections in persons infected with human immunodeficiency virus. *MMWR.* 1997;46,(no. RR-12).

Centers for Disease Control. Recommendations for prevention of possible transmission of human T-lymphocyte virus type III/lymphadenopathy-associated virus from tears. *MMWR.* 1985;34:533–537.

Centers for Disease Control and Prevention. Update: Trends in AIDS incidence, deaths, and prevalence—United States, 1996. *MMWR.* 1997;46:165–192.

Centers for Disease Control and Prevention. Report of the NIH Panel to Define Principles of Therapy of HIV Infection and Guidelines for the Use of Antiretroviral Agents in HIV-Infected Adults and Adolescents. *MMWR.* 1998; 47(RR-5):1–83.

Chaisson RE. Treatment of *Mycobacterium–avium* complex (MAC) in the era of potent antiretroviral therapy. *TAGline.* 1999;6. *www.aidsinfonyc.org/tag/taglines/9911.html.*

Chronister CL. Dry eye in an HIV-infected female. *Clin Eye Vision Care.* 1992;4:61–63.

Chronister CL. Review of external ocular disease associated with AIDS and HIV infection. *Optom Vis Sci.* 1996;73:225–230.

Chronister CL. Serologic confirmation of HIV infection. *Optom Vis Sci.* 1995;72:299–301.

Chronister CL. Viral infections and the immunocompromised patient. In: Silbert J, ed. *Anterior Segment Complications of Contact Lens Wear.* 2nd ed. Boston: Butterworth-Heinemann; 2000.

Chronister CL, Gurwood AS.Type 2 diabetes in association with HIV-1 protease inhibitors in HIV-infected patients. *J Am Optom Assoc.* 1998;69:695–698.

Chronister CL, Russo P. Effects of disinfecting solutions on tonometer tips. *Optom Vis Sci.* 1990;67:818–821.

Clough LA, D'Agata E, Raffanti S, et al. Factors that predict incomplete virological response to protease inhibitor-based antiretroviral therapy. *Clin Infect Dis.* 1999;29:75–81.

Cochereau-Massin I, et al. Ocular toxoplasmosis in human immunodeficiency virus infected patients. *Am J Opthalmol.* 1992;114:130–135.

Coffin J. HIV population dynamics in vivo: Implications for genetic variation, pathogenesis, and therapy. *Science.* 1995; 267:483–489.

Cohen DB, Glasgow BJ. Bilateral optic nerve cryptococcosis in sudden blindness in patients with acquired immune deficiency syndrome. *Ophthalmology.* 1993;100:1689–1694.

Cohen C, Mogyoros M, Sands M, et al. TIDBID study: Fortovase-TM (FTV) TID regimen compared to FTV BID or FTV + NFV BID regimens in HIV-1-infected patients. Abstracts of the 39th ICAAC, 1999; abstract 508.

Cohen OJ, Fauci AS. Transmission of drug-resistant strains of HIV-1: Unfortunate, but inevitable. *Lancet.* 1999; 354: 697–698.

Cohen Stuart JW, Schuurman R, Burger DM, et al. Randomized trial comparing saquinavir soft gel capsules versus indinavir as part of triple therapy (CHEESE study). *AIDS.* 1999;13:F53–F58.

Cole EL, Meisler DM, Calabrese LH, et al. Herpes zoster ophthalmicus and acquired immune deficiency syndrome. *Arch Ophthalmol.* 1984;102:1027–1029.

Collier AC, Coombs RW, Schoenfeld DA, et al. Treatment of human immunodeficiency virus infection with saquinavir, zidovudine, and zalcitabine. AIDS Clinical Trials Group protocol 229. *N Engl J Med.* 1996;334:1011–1017.

Condra JH. Resisting resistance: Maximizing the durability of antiretroviral therapy. *Ann Intern Med.* 1998;128: 951–954.

Connor EM, Sperling RS, Gelber R, et al. Reduction of maternal-infant transmission of human immunodeficiency virus type 1 with zidovudine treatment. Pediatric AIDS

Clinical Trials Group Protocol 076 Study Group. *N Engl J Med.* 1994;331:1173–1180.

Couderec LJ, D'Agay MF, Danon F, et al. Sicca complex and infection with human immunodeficiency virus. *Arch Intern Med.* 1987;147:898–901.

Crumpacker CS. Ganciclovir. *N Engl J Med.* 1996;335:721–729.

Cunningham ET, Margolis TP. Ocular manifestations of HIV infection. *N Engl J Med.* 1998;339:236–244.

Currie J, Benson E, Ramsden B, et al. Eye movement abnormalities as a predictor of the acquired immunodeficiency syndrome dementia complex. *Arch Neurol.* 1988;45: 949–953.

Currier JS, Williams PL, Grimes JM, et al. Incidence rates and risk factors for opportunistic infections in a phase III trial comparing indinavir + ZDV + 3TC to ZDV + 3TC. The ACTG 320 Study Team. Abstracts of the 5th Conference on Retroviruses and Opportunistic Infections, 1998; abstract 257.

Daluge SM, Good SS, Faletto MB, et al. 1592U89, a novel carbocyclic nucleoside analog with potent, selective anti-human immunodeficiency virus activity. *Antimicrob Agents Chemother.* 1997;41:1082–1093.

Danner SA. Zidovudine: Anno 1995. *Adv Exp Med Biol.* 1996; 394:225–243.

D'Aquila RT, Hughes MD, Johnson VA, et al. Nevirapine, zidovudine, and didanosine compared with zidovudine and didanosine in patients with HIV-1 infection. A randomized, double-blind, placebo controlled trial. National Institute of Allergy and Infectious Diseases AIDS Clinical Trials Group Protocol 241 Investigators. *Ann Intern Med.* 1996;124:1019–1030.

Davey RT Jr, Chaitt DG, Reed GF, et al. Randomized, controlled phase I/II trial of combination therapy with delavirdine (U-90152S) and conventional nucleosides in human immunodeficiency virus type 1-infected patients. *Antimicrob Agents Chemother.* 1996;40:1657–1664.

Davis J. Human immunodeficiency virus-related uveitis. *Curr Opin Ophthalmol.* 1991;2:471–479.

Davis JL, Nussenblatt RB, Bachman DM, et al. Endogenous bacterial retinitis in AIDS. *Am J Ophthalmol.* 1989;107: 613–623.

Decker CJ, Laitinen LM, Bridson GW, et al. Metabolism of amprenavir in liver microsomes: Role of CYP3A4 inhibition for drug interactions. *J Pharm Sci.* 1998;87:803–807.

De Clerck LS, Couttenye MM, De Broe ME, Stevens WJ. Acquired immunodeficiency syndrome mimicking Sjögren's syndrome and systemic lupus erythematosus. *Arthritis Rheum.* 1988;31:272–275.

Deeks SG, Volberding PA. Antiretroviral therapy. In: Sande MA, Volberding PA, eds. *The Medical Management of AIDS.* 6th ed. Philadelphia: WB Saunders; 1999:97–115.

Delta Coordinating Committee. Delta: A randomised double-blind controlled trial comparing combinations of zidovudine plus didanosine or zalcitabine with zidovudine alone in HIV-infected individuals. *Lancet.* 1996;348:283–291.

Deminie CA, Bechtold CM, Stock D, et al. Evaluation of reverse transcriptase and protease inhibitors in two-drug combinations against human immunodeficiency virus replication. *Antimicrob Agents Chemother.* 1996;40:1346–1351.

Detrick B, Rhame J, Wang Y, et al. Cytomegalovirus replication in human retinal pigment epithelial cells. *IOVS.* 1996; 37:814–825.

Diesenhouse MC, Wilson LA, Corrent GF, et al. Treatment of microsporidial keratoconjunctivitis with topical fumagillin. *Am J Ophthal.* 1993;115:293–298.

Drew WL, Miner RC, Busch DF, et al. Prevalence of resistance in patients receiving ganciclovir for serious cytomegalovirus infection. *J Infect Dis.* 1991;163:716–719.

Dugel PU, Gill PS, Frangieh GT, Rao NA. Ocular adnexal Kaposi's sarcoma in acquired immunodeficiency syndrome. *Am J Ophthalmol.* 1990;110:500–503.

Durant J, Clevenbergh P, Halfon P, et al. Drug-resistance genotyping in HIV-1 therapy: The VIRADAPT randomised controlled trial. *Lancet.* 1999;353:2195–2199.

Engstrom RE Jr, Holland GN, Hardy WD, Meiselman HJ. Hemorheologic abnormalities in patients with human immunodeficiency virus infection and ophthalmic microvasculopathy. *Am J Ophthalmol.* 1990;109:153–161.

Eron JJ, Benoit SL, Jemsek J, et al. Treatment with lamivudine, zidovudine, or both in HIV-1 positive patients with 200 to 500 CD4+ cells per cubic millimeter. North American HIV Working Party. *N Engl J Med.* 1995;333:1662–1669.

Farthing C, Mess T, Ried C, et al. Ritonavir, saquinavir, and nevirapine as a salvage regimen for indinavir or ritonavir resistance. International Conference on AIDS, 1998; abstract 22356.

Fauci AS. Host factors and the pathogenesis of HIV-induced disease. *Nature.* 1996;384:529–534.

Fauci AS. Multifactorial nature of human immunodeficiency virus disease: Implications for therapy. *Science.* 1993; 262:1011–1018.

Fauci AS. The AIDS epidemic—Considerations for the 21st century. *N Engl J Med.* 1999;341:1046–1050.

Finzi D, Hermankova M, Pierson T, et al. Identification of a reservoir for HIV-1 in patients on highly active antiretroviral therapy. *Science.* 1997;278:1295–1300.

Fischl MA, Olson RM, Follansbee SE, et al. Zalcitabine compared with zidovudine in patients with advanced HIV-1 infection who received previous zidovudine therapy. *Ann Intern Med.* 1993;118:762–769.

Fischl MA, Stanley K, Collier AC, et al. Combination and monotherapy with zidovudine and zalcitabine in patients with advanced HIV disease. The NIAID AIDS Clinical Trials Group. *Ann Intern Med.* 1995;122:24–32.

Fleming TR, DeMets DL. Surrogate endpoints in clinical trials: Are we being misled? *Ann Intern Med.* 1996; 125:605–613.

Flexner C, Hendrix C. Antiretroviral therapy. In: DeVita VT Jr, Hellman S, Rosenberg SA, eds. *AIDS. Etiology, Diagnosis, Treatment and Prevention.* 4th ed. Philadelphia: Lippincott-Raven; 1997:479–493.

Forster DJ, et al. Rapidly progressive outer retinal necrosis in the acquired immunodeficiency syndrome. *Am J Ophthalmol.* 1990;110:341–348.

Foster RE, et al. Presumed *Pneumocystis carinii* choroiditis: Unifocal presentation, regression with intravenous pentamidine, and choroiditis recurrence. *Ophthalmology.* 1991; 98:1360.

Fournier S, Delphus S, et al: Anterior uveitis in HIV-infected patients. 3 cases in patients treated with an antiprotease. *Presse Med.* 1998;18:844–848.

Freeman WR, Chen A, Henderly DE, et al. Prevalence and significance of acquired immunodeficiency syndrome-related retinal microvasculopathy. *Am J Ophthalmol.* 1989; 107:863–867.

Friedberg DN, Stenson SM, Orenstein JM, et al. Microsporidial keratoconjunctivitis in acquired immunodeficiency syndrome. *Arch Ophthalmol.* 1990;108:504–508.

Friedland GH, Pollard R, Griffith B, et al. Efficacy and safety of delavirdine mesylate with zidovudine and didanosine compared with two-drug combinations of these agents in persons with HIV disease with CD4 counts of 100 to 500 cells/mm^3 (ACTG 261). ACTG 261 Team. *J Acquir Immune Defic Syndr Hum Retrovirol.* 1999;21:281–292.

Fujikawa LS, Salahuddin SZ, Ablashi D, et al. Human T-cell leukemia/lymphotropic virus type III in the conjunctival epithelium of a patient with AIDS. *Am J Ophthalmol.* 1985;100:507–509.

Gallant JE, Chaisson RE, Keruly JC, et al. Stavudine in zidovudine (ZDV)-experienced compared with ZDV-naive patients. *AIDS.* 1999;13:225–229.

Gao EK, Yu XH, Lin CP, et al. Intraocular viral replication after systemic murine cytomegalovirus infection requires immunosuppression. *IOVS.* 1995;36:2322–2327.

Gao F, Bailes E, Robertson D, et al. Origin of HIV-1 in the chimpanzee *Pan troglodytes troglodytes. Nature.* 1999;397: 436–441.

Garcia F, Knobel H, Sambeat MA, et al. An open randomized study comparing d4T plus ddI and nevirapine (QD) vs. d4T plus ddI and nevirapine (BID) in antiretroviral naive chronic HIV-1 infected patients in very early stages (Spanish SCAN Study). Abstracts of the 6th Conference on Retroviruses and Opportunistic Infections, 1999; abstract 628.

Geleziunas R, Greene WC. Molecular insights into HIV-1 infection and pathogenesis. In: Sande MA, Volberding PA, eds. *The Medical Management of AIDS.* 6th ed. Philadelphia: WB Saunders; 1999:23–39.

Gill PS, Tulpule A, Espina BM, et al. Paclitaxel is safe and effective in the treatment of advanced AIDS-related Kaposi's sarcoma. *J Clin Oncol.* 1999;17:1876–1883.

Goodgame J, Hanson C, Vafidis I, et al. Amprenavir (141W94, APV)/3TC/ZDV exerts durable antiviral activity in HIV-1-infected antiretroviral therapy naive subjects through 48 weeks of therapy. Abstracts of the 39th ICAAC, 1999; abstract 509.

Gottlieb M, Peterson D, Adler M, et al. Comparison of safety and efficacy of two doses of stavudine (Zerit, d4T) in a large simple trial in the US Parallel Track Program. Abstracts of the 35th ICAAC, 1995; abstract I-171.

Gottlieb MS, Schroff R, Schanker HM, et al. *Pneumocystis carinii* pneumonia and mucosal candidiasis in previously healthy homosexual men: Evidence of a new acquired cellular immunodeficiency. *N Engl J Med.* 1981;305:1425–1431.

Grant RM, Saag MS. Laboratory testing for HIV-1. In: Sande MA, Volberding PA, eds. *The Medical Management of AIDS.* 6th ed. Philadelphia: WB Saunders; 1999:43–65.

Green S, Para MF, Daly PW, et al. Interim analysis of plasma viral burden reductions and CD4 increases in HIV-1 infected patients with Rescriptor (DLV) + Retrovir (ZDV) + Epivir (3TC). International Conference on AIDS, 1998; abstract 12219.

Grier SA, Libera S, Klauss V, Goebel FD. Sicca syndrome in patients infected with the human immunodeficiency virus. *Ophthalmology.* 1995;102:1319–1324.

Gritz DC, Scott TJ, Sedo SF, et al. Ocular flora of patients with AIDS compared with those of HIV-negative patients. *Cornea.* 1997;16:400–405.

Guay LA, Musoke P, Fleming T, et al. Intrapartum and neonatal single-dose nevirapine compared with zidovudine for prevention of mother-to-child transmission of HIV-1 in Kampala, Uganda: HIVNET 012 randomised trial. *Lancet.* 1999;354:795–802.

Gulick RM, Mellors JW, Havlir D, et al. Simultaneous vs sequential initiation of therapy with indinavir, zidovudine, and lamivudine for HIV-1 infection. 100-week follow-up. *JAMA.* 1998;280:35–41.

Gulick RM, Mellors J, Havlir D, et al. Treatment with indinavir (IDV), zidovudine (ZDV), and lamivudine (3TC): three-year follow-up. Abstracts of the 6th Conference on Retroviruses and Opportunistic Infections, 1999; abstract 388.

Hall CS, Raines CP, Barnett SH, et al. Efficacy of salvage therapy containing ritonavir and saquinavir after failure of single protease inhibitor-containing regimens. *AIDS.* 1999; 13:1207–1212.

Hamed LM, Schatz NJ, Galetta SL. Brainstem ocular motility defects in AIDS. *Am J Ophthalmol.* 1988;106:437–442.

Hammer SM, Katzenstein DA, Hughes MD, et al. A trial comparing nucleoside monotherapy with combination therapy in HIV-infected adults with CD4 cell counts from 200 to 500 per cubic millimeter. The AIDS Clinical Trials Group Study 175 Study Team. *N Engl J Med.* 1996;335:1081–1090.

Hammer SM, Squires KE, Hughes MD, et al. A controlled trial of two nucleoside analogues plus indinavir in persons with human immunodeficiency virus infection and CD4 cell counts of 200 per cubic millimeter or less. The AIDS Clinical Trials Group 320 Study Team. *N Engl J Med.* 1997; 337:725–733.

Hammer SM, Yeni P. Antiretroviral therapy: Where are we? *AIDS.* 1998;12(suppl A):S181–S188.

Hardy D, Spector S, Polsky B, et al. Combination ganciclovir and granulocyte-macrophage colony stimulating factor in the treatment of cytomegalovirus retinitis in AIDS patients. *Eur J Clin Microbiol Infect Dis.* 1994;13(suppl 2):S34–S40.

Havlir DV, Marschner IC, Hirsch MS, et al. Maintenance antiretroviral therapies in HIV-1infected subjects with undetectable plasma RNA after triple-drug therapy. The AIDS Clinical Trials Group Study 343 Team. *N Engl J Med.* 1998; 339:1261–1268.

Haynes BF, Pantaleo G, Fauci AS. Toward an understanding of the correlates of protective immunity to HIV infection. *Science.* 1996;271:324–328.

Hecht FM, Chesney MA. Adherence to HIV therapy. In: Deeks SG, Volberding PA, eds. *The Medical Management of AIDS.* 6th ed. Philadelphia: WB Saunders; 1999:117–121.

Hellerstein M, Hanley MB, Cesar D, et al. Directly measured kinetics of circulating T lymphocytes in normal and HIV-1-infected humans. *Nat Med.* 1999;5:83–89.

Hemandy RK. Microbial keratitis in patients infected with human immunodeficiency virus. *Ophthalmology.* 1995;102: 1026–1030.

Henrard DR, Phillips JF, Muenz LR, et al. Natural history of HIV-1 cell-free viremia. *JAMA.* 1995;274:554–558.

Henry K, Shaeffer M, Ross RL, et al. Response to Combivir[R] and abacavir given BID to nucleoside experienced patients is not affected by the presence of the M184V mutations. Abstracts of the 6th Conference on Retroviruses and Opportunistic Infections, 1999; abstract 132.

Hertogs K, Mellors JW, Schel P, et al. Patterns of cross-resistance among protease inhibitors in 483 clinical HIV-1 isolates. Abstracts of the 5th Conference on Retroviruses and Opportunistic Infections, 1998; abstract 395.

Hirsch MS, Conway B, D'Aquila RT, et al. Antiretroviral drug resistance testing in adults with HIV infection: Implications for clinical management. International AIDS Society—USA Panel. *JAMA.* 1998;279:1984–1991.

HIV/AIDS Surveillance Report. vol. 11, no. 1. Atlanta: Centers for Disease Control and Prevention:1999:1–43.

Ho DD, Newmann AU, Perelson AS, et al. Rapid turnover of plasma virions and CD4 lymphocytes in HIV-1 infection. *Nature.* 1995;373:123–126.

Hodge WG, Margolis TP: Herpes simplex virus keratitis among patients who are positive or negative for human immunodeficiency virus: An epidemiologic study. *Ophthalmology.* 1997;104:120–124.

Hodge WG, Seiff SR, Margolis TP. Ocular opportunistic infection incidences among patients who are HIV positive compared to patients who are HIV negative. *Ophthalmology.* 1998;105:895–900.

Hogg RS, Heath KV, Yip B, et al. Improved survival among HIV-infected individuals following initiation of antiretroviral therapy. *JAMA.* 1998;279:450–454.

Holder D, Shivaprakash M, Schleif WA, et al. Two-year durability of HIV-1 load suppression in patients treated with indinavir who experience virus load declines to <500 vRNA copies/mL. International Conference on AIDS, 1998; abstract 12279.

Holland GN. Acquired immunodeficiency syndrome and ophthalmology: The first decade. *Am J Ophthalmol.* 1992; 114:86–95.

Holland GN, Buhles WC Jr, Mastre B, et al. A controlled retrospective study of ganciclovir treatment for cytomegalovirus retinopathy. Use of a standardized system for the assessment of disease outcome. UCLA CMV Retinopathy Study Group, *Arch Ophthalmol.* 1989;107:1759–1766.

Holland GN, Engstrom KRE, Glasgow BJ, et al. Ocular toxoplasmosis in patients with the acquired immunodeficiency syndrome. *Am J Ophthalmol.* 1088;106:653–657.

Holland GN, Pepose JS, Pettit JH, et al. Acquired immune deficiency syndrome: Ocular manifestations. *Ophthalmology.* 1983;90:859–873.

Jabs DA, Green WR, Fox R, et al. Ocular manifestations of acquired immune deficiency syndrome. *Ophthalmology.* 1989;96:1092–1099.

Jabs DA, Quinn TC. Acquired immunodeficiency syndrome. In: Pepose JS, Holland GN, Wilhelmus KR, eds. *Ocular Infection and Immunity.* St. Louis: Mosby; 1996.

Jabs DA, Schachat AP, Liss R, et al. Presumed varicella zoster retinitis in immunocompromised patients. *Retina.* 1987; 7:9–13.

Jacobs DS, Pilero PJ, Kuperwaser MG, et al. Acute uveitis associated with rifabutin use in patients with human immunodeficiency virus infection. *Am J Ophthalmol.* 1994; 118:716–722.

Jarvis B, Faulds D. Nelfinavir. A review of its therapeutic efficacy in HIV infection. *Drugs.* 1998;56:147–167.

Jeffrey S, Baker D, Tritch R, et al. A resistance and cross resistance profile for SUSTIVA (efavirenz, DMP 266). Abstracts of the 5th Conference on Retroviruses and Opportunistic Infections, 1998; abstract 702.

The Johns Hopkins University Division of Infectious Diseases and AIDS Service. Treatment of sexually transmitted diseases by pathogen. Adapted from CDC 1998 Guidelines. *MMWR.* 1998;47(RR-1):1–116; and CID 1999;29 (suppl).

Jonjic S, Mutter W, Weiland F, et al. Site-restricted persistent cytomegalovirus infection after selective long-term depletion of $CD4^+$ T lymphocytes. *J Exp Med.* 1989;169:1199–1212.

Kahn J. The clinical use of didanosine. *Adv Exp Med Biol.* 1996;394:245–256.

Kahn JO, Walker BD. Current concepts: Acute human immunodeficiency virus type 1 infection. *N Engl J Med.* 1998; 339:33–39.

Katlama C, Ingrand D, Loveday C, et al. Safety and efficacy of lamivudine-zidovudine combination therapy in antiretroviral-naive patients. A randomized controlled comparison with zidovudine monotherapy. The Lamivudine European HIV Working Group. *JAMA.* 1996;276:118–125.

Katlama C, Valantin M-A, Matheron S, et al. Efficacy and tolerability of stavudine plus lamivudine in treatment-naive and treatment-experienced patients with HIV-1 infection. *Ann Intern Med.* 1998;129:525–531.

Kelleher D, Mellors J, Lederman M, et al. Activity of abacavir (1592, ABC) combined with protease inhibitors (PI) in therapy naive patients. International Conference on AIDS, 1998; abstract 12210.

Kempf DJ, Marsh KC, Denissen JF, et al. ABT-538 is a potent inhibitor of human immunodeficiency virus protease and has high oral bioavailability in humans. *Proc Nat Acad Sci USA.* 1995;92:2484–2488.

Kempf DJ, Marsh KC, Kumar G, et al. Pharmacokinetic enhancement of inhibitors of the human immunodeficiency virus protease by coadministration with ritonavir. *Antimicrob Agents Chemother.* 1997;41:654–660.

Kempf DJ, Marsh KC, Paul DA, et al. Antiviral and pharmacokinetic properties of C2 symmetric inhibitors of the human immunodeficiency virus type 1 protease. *Antimicrob Agents Chemother.* 1991;35:2209–2214.

Kempf DJ, Rode RA, Xu Y, et al. The duration of viral suppression during protease inhibitor therapy for HIV-1 infection is predicted by plasma HIV-1 RNA at the nadir. *AIDS.* 1998;12:F9–F14.

Kestelyn P, et al. Ophthalmic manifestations of infections with *Cryptococcus neoformans* in patients with the acquired immunodeficiency syndrome. *Am J Ophthalmol.* 1993;116: 721–727.

Kohn SR. Molluscum contagiosum in patients with acquired immunodeficiency syndrome. *Arch Ophthalmol.* 1987;105: 458. Letter.

Kopp JB, Miller KD, Mican JA, et al. Crystalluria and urinary tract abnormalities associated with indinavir. *Ann Intern Med.* 1997;127:119–125.

Kordossis T, Paikos S, Aroni K, et al. Prevalence of Sjögren's-like syndrome in a cohort of HIV-1 positive patients: Descriptive pathology and immunopathology. *Br J Rheumatol.* 1998;37:691–695.

Krogstad P, Wiznia A, Luzuriaga K, et al. Treatment of human immunodeficiency virus 1-infected infants and children with the protease inhibitor nelfinavir mesylate. *J Infect Dis.* 1999;28:1109–1118.

Kuppermann BD, et al. Correlation between CD4+ counts and prevalence of cytomegalovirus retinitis and human immunodeficiency virus-related noninfectious retinal vasculopathy in patients with acquired immunodeficiency syndrome. *Am J Ophthalmol.* 1993;115:575–582.

Kuritzkes DR, Marschner I, Johnson VA, et al. Lamivudine in combination with zidovudine, stavudine, or didanosine in patients with HIV-1 infection. A randomized, double-blind, placebo-controlled trial. National Institute of Allergy and Infectious Disease AIDS Clinical Trials Group Protocol 306 Investigators. *AIDS.* 1999;13:685–694.

Lau RKW, Goh BT, Estreich S, et al. Adult gonococcal keratoconjunctivitis with AIDS. *Br J Ophthalmol.* 1990; 74:52.

Lederman MM, Connick E, Landay A, et al. Immunologic responses associated with 12 weeks of combination antiretroviral therapy consisting of zidovudine, lamivudine, and ritonavir: Results of AIDS Clinical Trials Group Protocol 315. *J Infect Dis.* 1998;178:70–79.

Lee A, Chronister CL. Sarcoidosis-related anterior uveitis in a patient with human immunodeficiency virus. *J Am Optom Assoc.* 1999;70:384–390.

Leeds JM, Henry SP, Bistner S, et al. Pharmacokinetics of an antisense oligonucleotide injected intravitreally in monkeys. *Drug Metab Dispos.* 1998;26:670–675.

Lo JC, Mulligan K, Tai VW, et al. "Buffalo hump" in men with HIV-1 infection. *Lancet.* 1998;351:867–870.

Lori F. Hydroxyurea and HIV: 5 years later—from antiviral to immunemodulating effects. *AIDS.* 1999;13:1433–1442.

Lucca JA, Farris RL, Bielory L, Caputo AR. Keratoconjunctivitis sicca in male patients infected with human immunodeficiency virus type 1. *Ophthalmology.* 1990;97: 1008–1010.

Lucca JA, Kung JS, Farris RL. Keratoconjunctivitis sicca in female patient infected with human immunodeficiency virus. *CLAOJ.* 1994;20:49–51.

MacArthur RD, Kosmyna JM, Crane LR, et al. Sequencing of non-nucleoside reverse transcriptase inhibitors based on specific mutational patterns fails to lower plasma HIV-RNA levels in persons extensively pre-treated with antiretrovirals who are failing virologically on nevirapine-containing antiretroviral regimens. Program and Abstracts from the Seventh European Conference on Clinical Aspects and Treatment of HIV Infection, 1999; abstract 208.

Macher A, Rodriguez MM, Kaplan W, et al. Disseminated bilateral chorioretinitis due to *Histoplasma capsulatum* in a patient with the acquired immunodeficiency syndrome. *Ophthalmology.*1985;92:1159–1164.

Maguen E, Salz JJ, Nesburn AB. *Pseudomonas* corneal ulcer associated with rigid, gas-permeable, daily wear lenses in a patient infected with human immunodeficiency virus. *Am J Ophthalmol.* 1992;113:336–337.

Margolis TP, et al. Varicella-zoster virus retinitis in patients with the acquired immunodeficiency syndrome. *Am J Ophthalmol.* 1991;112:119–131.

Markowitz M, Conant M, Hurley A, et al. A preliminary evaluation of nelfinavir mesylate, an inhibitor of human immunodeficiency virus (HIV)-1 protease, to treat HIV infection. *J Infect Dis.* 1998;177:1533–1540.

Markowitz M, Saag M, Powderly WG, et al. A preliminary study of ritonavir, an inhibitor of HIV-1 protease, to treat HIV-1 infection. *N Engl J Med.* 1995;333:1534–1539.

Maugh TW III. AIDS death toll at new high despite advances. *Los Angeles Times.* 1999; November 24:A1,A26–27.

Mayers DL. Drug-resistant HIV-1: The virus strikes back. *JAMA.* 1998;279:2000–2004.

McAuthor J. Neurologic manifestations of AIDS, *Medicine.* 1987;66:407–437.

McLeish WM, Pulido JS, Holland S, et al. The ocular manifestations of syphilis in the human immunodeficiency virus type 1-infected host. *Ophthalmology.* 1990;97:196–203.

Mellors JW, Munoz A, Giorgi JV, et al. Plasma viral load and CD4+ lymphocytes as prognostic markers of HIV-1 infection. *Ann Intern Med.* 1997;126:946–954.

Mildvan D, Landay A, De Gruttola V, et al. An approach to the validation of markers for use in AIDS clinical trials. *Clin Infect Dis.* 1997;24:764–774.

Miller V, Mocroft A, Reiss P, et al. Relations among CD4 lymphocyte count nadir, antiretroviral therapy, and HIV-1 disease progression: Results from the EuroSIDA study. *Ann Intern Med.* 1999;130:570–577.

Miller V, Sturmer M, Staszewski S, et al. The M184V mutation in HIV-1 does not result in broad cross-resistance to nucleoside analogue RT inhibitors. *AIDS.* 1998;12:705–712.

Mitsuyasu RT, Skolnik PR, Cohen SR, et al. Activity of the soft gelatin formulation of saquinavir in combination therapy in antiretroviral-naive patients. NV15355 Study Team. *AIDS.* 1998;12:F103–F109.

Mocarski, ES. Cytomegalovirus biology and replication. In: Roizman B, Whitley RJ, Lopez C, eds. *The Human Herpesviruses.* New York: Raven Press: 1993:173–225.

Mocarski ES, Abenes GB, Manning WC, et al. Molecular genetic analysis of cytomegalovirus gene regulation in growth, persistence and latency. *Curr Top Microbiol Immunol.* 1990;154:47–74.

Mocroft A, Vella S, Benfield TL, et al. Changing patterns of mortality across Europe in patients infected with HIV-1. *Lancet.* 1998;352:1725–1730.

Mody GM, Hill JC, Meyers OL. Keratoconjunctivitis sicca in rheumatoid arthritis. *Clin Rheumatol.* 1988;7:237–241.

Montaner JSG, Rachlis A, Beaulieu R, et al. Safety profile of didanosine among patients with advanced HIV disease who are intolerant to or deteriorate despite zidovudine therapy: Results of the Canadian Open ddI Treatment Program. *J Acquir Immune Defic Syndr Hum Retrovirol.* 1994; 7:924–930.

Montaner JSG, Reiss P, Cooper D, et al. A randomized, double-blind trial comparing combinations of nevirapine, didanosine, and zidovudine for HIV-1 infected patients: The INCAS Trial. Italy, the Netherlands, Canada and Australia Study Group. *JAMA.* 1998;279:930–937.

Moore RD, Fortgang I, Keruly J, et al. Adverse events from drug therapy for human immunodeficiency virus disease. *Am J Med.* 1996;101:34–40.

Morinelli EN, et al. Infectious multifocal choroiditis in patients with acquired immunodeficiency syndrome. *Ophthalmology.* 1993;100:1014–1021.

Mullin SM, Jamjian CM, Spruance SL. Antiretroviral adverse effects and interactions: Clinical recognition and management. In: Sande MA, Volberding PA, eds. *The Medical Management of AIDS.* 6th ed. Philadelphia: WB Saunders; 1999:79–96.

Munoz V, Casado JL, Moreno A, et al. Persistent viral suppression after switching a protease inhibitor (PI)-containing regimen to a nonnucleoside reverse transcriptase inhibitor (NNRTI)-based therapy (BEGIN study). Abstracts of the 39th ICAAC, 1999; abstract 2195.

Murphy RL, Katlama C, Johnson V, et al. The Atlantic Study: A randomized, open-label trial comparing two protease inhibitor (PI)-sparing antiretroviral strategies versus a standard PI-containing regimen, 48 week data. Abstracts of the 39th ICAAC, 1999; abstract LB-22.

Murray HW, Squires KE, Weiss W, et al. Stavudine in patients with AIDS and AIDS-related complex: AIDS clinical trials group 089. *J Infect Dis.* 1995;171(suppl 2):S123–S130.

Musch, DC, Martin, DF, Gordon, JF, et al. Ganciclovir Implant Study Group. Treatment of cytomegalovirus retinitis with a sustained ganciclovir implant. *N Engl J Med.* 1997;337:83–90.

Myerson, D, Hackman, RC, Nelson, JA, et al. Widespread presence of histologically occult cytomegalovirus. *Hum Pathol.* 1984;15:1645–1658.

Nanda M, Pflugfelder SC, Holland S. Fulminant pseudomonal keratitis and scleritis in human immunodeficiency virus-infected patients. *Arch Ophthal.* 1991;109:503–505.

National Institutes of Allergy and Infectious Diseases. HIV wasting syndrome. 1997; *www.niaid.nih.gov/factsheets/hivwasting.htm.*

Neipel F, Fleckenstein B. The role of HHV-8 in Kaposi's sarcoma. *Sem Cancer Bio.* 1999;9:151–164.

Newsome DA, Green WR, Miller ED, et al. Microvascular aspects of acquired immune deficiency syndrome retinopathy. *Am J Ophthalmol.* 1984;98:590–601.

Nguyen N, Rimmer S, Katz B. Slowed saccades in the acquired immunodeficiency syndrome. *Am J Ophthalmol.* 1987;94:831–838.

O'Brien TR, Rosenberg PS, Yellin F, et al. Longitudinal HIV-1 RNA levels in a cohort of homosexual men. *J Acquir Immune Defic Syndr Hum Retrovirol.* 1998;18:155–161.

O'Brien WA, Hartigan PM, Daar ES, et al. Changes in plasma HIV RNA levels and CD4+ counts predict both response to antiretroviral therapy and therapeutic failure. The VA Cooperative Study Group on AIDS. *Ann Intern Med.* 1997;126:939–945.

Onofrey BE, Skorin L, Holdeman NR. *Ocular Therapeutics Handbook: A Clinical Manual.* Philadelphia: Lippincott-Raven; 1998.

Opravil M, Hirschel B, Lazzarin A, et al. Simplified maintenance therapy with abacavir + lamivudine + zidovudine in patients with long-term suppression of HIV-1 RNA. Abstracts of the 39th ICAAC, 1999; abstract 510.

Ortiz GM, Nixon DF, Trkola A, et al. HIV-1-specific immune responses in subjects who temporarily contain virus replication after discontinuation of highly active antiretroviral therapy. *J Clin Invest.* 1999;104(6):R13–R18.

Palella FJ Jr, Delaney KM, Moorman AC, et al. Declining morbidity and mortality among patients with advanced human immunodeficiency virus infection. *N Engl J Med.* 1998;338:853–860.

Palestine AG, Rodrigues MM, Macher AM, et al. Ophthalmic involvement in acquired immunodeficiency syndrome. *Ophthalmology.* 1984;91:1092–1099.

Panel on Clinical Practices for Treatment of HIV Infection. *Guidelines for the Use of Antiretroviral Agents in HIV-Infected Adults and Adolescents.* Department of Health and Human Services (DHHS) and the Henry J. Kaiser Family Foundation; 1999.

Park KL, Smith RE, Rao NA. Ocular manifestations of AIDS. *Curr Opin Ophthalmol.* 1995;6:82–87.

Parke DW, Font RL. Diffuse toxoplasmic retinochoroiditis in a patient with AIDS. *Arch Ophthalmol.* 1986;104:571–575.

Parrish CM, O'Day DM, Hoyle TC. Spontaneous fungal corneal ulcer as an ocular manifestation of AIDS. *Am J Ophthalmol.* 1987;104:302–303. Letter.

Passo MS, Rosenbaum JT. Ocular syphilis in patients with human immunodeficiency virus infection. *Am J Ophthalmol.* 1988;106:1–5.

Patick AK, Duran M, Cao Y, et al. Genotypic and phenotypic characterization of human immunodeficiency virus type 1 variants isolated from patients treated with the protease inhibitor nelfinavir. *Antimicrob Agents Chemother.* 1998; 42:2637–2644.

Pepose JS, Holland GN, Nestor MS, et al. Acquired immune deficiency syndrome: Pathogenic mechanisms of ocular diseases. *Ophthalmology.* 1985;92:472–484.

Pepose JS, Holland GN, Wilhelmus KR. *Ocular Infection and Immunity.* St. Louis: Mosby; 1996.

Perelson AS, Neumann AU, Markowitz M, et al. HIV-1 dynamics in vivo: Virion clearance rate, infected cell life-span, and viral generation time. *Science.* 1996;271:1582–1586.

Pialoux G, Raffi F, Brun-Vezinet F, et al. A randomized trial of three maintenance regimens given after three months of induction therapy with zidovudine, lamivudine, and indinavir in previously untreated HIV-1-infected patients. *N Engl J Med.* 1998;339:1269–1276.

Pivetti-Pezzi, Accorinti M, Ciapparoni V, et al. Antiretroviral therapy and HIV-related retinal microangiopathy. *AIDS.* 1997;11:1890–1891.

Pomerantz RJ, Kuritzkes R, Monte M, et al. Infection of the retina by human immunodeficiency virus type I. *N Engl J Med.* 1987;317:1643–1647.

Pozniak A. Surrogacy in HIV-1 clinical trials. *Lancet.* 1998; 351:536–537.

Quiceno JI, et al. Visual dysfunction without retinitis in patients with acquired immunodeficiency syndrome. *Am J Ophthalmol.* 1992;113:8–13.

Quinn TC. Global burden of the HIV pandemic. *Lancet.* 1996; 348(9020):99–106.

Quinnan GV Jr, et al. Herpesvirus infections in the acquired immune deficiency syndrome. *JAMA.* 1984;252:72–77.

Rabkin JG, Ferrando S. A 'second life' agenda: Psychiatric research issues raised by protease inhibitor treatments for people with the human immunodeficiency virus or the acquired immunodeficiency syndrome. *Arch Psychiatry.* 1997; 54:1049–1053.

Raboud JM, Montaner JS, Conway B, et al. Suppression of plasma viral load below 20 copies/ml is required to achieve a long-term response to therapy. *AIDS.* 1998;12:1619–1624.

Raffi F, Bonnet B, Esnault JL, et al. Switch from PI to once daily NNRTI in HIV-infected patients maintaining undetectable plasma loads on PI-containing regimens: The Maintavir Study. Abstracts of the 39th ICAAC, 1999; abstract 2198.

Reijers MHE, Weverling GJ, Jurriaans S, et al. Maintenance therapy after quadruple induction therapy in HIV-1 infected individuals: Amsterdam Duration of Antiretroviral Medication (ADAM) Study. *Lancet.* 1998;352:185–190.

Richman DD, Havlir D, Corbeil J, et al. Nevirapine resistance mutations of human immunodeficiency virus type I selected during therapy. *J Virol.* 1994;68:1660–1666.

Robinson MR, Udell IJ, Garber PF, et al. Molluscum contagiosum of the eyelids in patients with acquired immune deficiency syndrome. *Ophthalmology.* 1992;99:1745–1747.

Roche Valganciclovir Study Group. Valganciclovir vs IV ganciclovir as induction therapy for newly diagnosed cytomegalovirus retinitis: A randomized, controlled study. 7th Conference on Retroviruses and Opportunistic Infections, 2000.

Roseberger DF, Heinemann MH, et al. Uveitis associated with human immunodeficiency virus infection. *Am J Ophthalmol.* 1998;125:301–305.

Roseberger DF, Serdarevic ON, Erlandson RA, et al. Successful treatment of microsporidial keratoconjunctivitis with topical fumagillin in a patient with AIDS. *Cornea.* 1993;12:261–265.

Rosenberg PR, Uliss AE, Friedland GH, et al. Acquired immunodeficiency syndrome: Ocular manifestations in ambulatory patients. *Ophthalmology.* 1983;90:874–878.

Rosenberg PS. Scope of the AIDS epidemic in the US. *Science.* 1995;270:1372–1375.

Rosenwasser GOD, Greene WH. Simultaneous herpes simplex types 1 and 2 keratitis in acquired immunodeficiency syndrome. *Am J Ophthalmol.* 1992;113:102–103. Letter.

Rothenberg R, Woelfel M, Stoneburner R, et al. Survival with the acquired immunodeficiency syndrome. Experience with 5833 cases in New York City. *N Engl J Med.* 1987; 317:1297–1302.

Ruane PJ, Tam JT, Libraty DH, et al. Salvage therapy using ritonavir/saquinavir with a non-nucleoside reverse transcriptase inhibitor after prolonged failure with indinavir or ritonavir. International Conference on AIDS, 1998; abstract 32308.

Sadler BM, Hanson CD, Chittick GE, et al. Safety and pharmacokinetics of amprenavir (141W94), a human immunodeficiency virus (HIV) type 1 protease inhibitor, following oral administration of single doses to HIV-1 infected adults. *Antimicrob Agents Chemother.* 1999;43:1686–1692.

St. Clair MH, Millard J, Rooney J, et al. In vitro antiviral activity of 141W94 (VX-478) in combination with other antiretroviral agents. *Antiviral Res.* 1996;29:53–56.

Saint-Marc T, Partisani M, Poizot-Martin I, et al. A syndrome of peripheral fat wasting (lipodystrophy) in patients receiving long-term nucleoside analogue therapy. *AIDS.* 1999;13:1659–1667.

Sample PA, Plummer DJ, Mueller AJ, et al. Pattern of early visual field loss in HIV-infected patients. *Arch Ophthalmol.* 1999;117:755–760.

Santos C, Parker J, Dawson C, Ostler B. Bilateral fungal corneal ulcers in a patient with AIDS-related complex. *J Am Ophthalmol.* 1986;102:118–119.

Saravolatz LD, Winslow DL, Collins G, et al. Zidovudine alone or in combination with didanosine or zalcitabine in HIV-1 infected patients with the acquired immunodeficiency syndrome or fewer than 200 CD4 cells per cubic millimeter. Investigators for the Terry Beirn Community Programs for Clinical Research on AIDS [007]. *N Engl J Med.* 1996;335:1099–1106.

Schapiro JM, Winters MA, Stewart F, et al. The effect of high-dose saquinavir on viral load and CD4+ T-cell counts in HIV-infected patients. *Ann Intern Med.* 1996;124:1039–1050.

Schechter M, Struchiner CJ, Harrison LH. Protease inhibitors as initial therapy for individuals with an intermediate risk of HIV disease progression: Is more necessarily better? *AIDS.* 1999;13:97–102.

Schuurman R, Nijhuis M, van Leeuwen R, et al. Rapid changes in human immunodeficiency virus type 1 RNA load and appearance of drug-resistant virus populations in persons treated with lamivudine (3TC). *J Infect Dis.* 1995;171:1411–1419.

Schwartz DA, Visvesvara GS, Diesenhouse MC, et al. Pathologic features and immunofluorescent antibody demonstration of ocular micropsoridiosis (*Encephalitozoon hellem*) in seven patients with acquired immunodeficiency syndrome. *Am J Ophthalmol.* 1993;115:285–292.

Sellitti TP, et al. Association of herpes zoster ophthalmicus with acquired immunodeficiency syndrome and acute retinal necrosis. *Am J Ophthalmol.* 1993;116:297–301.

Shaefer M, Eron J, Yetzer E, et al. Combivir (lamivudine (3TC) 150 mg/zidovudine (ZDV) 300 mg) given BID plus a protease inhibitor (PI) compared to 3TC 150 mg BID and ZDV 200 mg TID plus a PI. International Conference on AIDS, 1998; abstract 12220.

Shaffer N, Chuachoowong R, Mock PA, et al. Short-course zidovudine for perinatal HIV-1 transmission in Bangkok, Thailand: A randomised controlled trial. Bangkok Collaborative Perinatal HIV Transmission Study Group. *Lancet.* 1999;353:773–780.

Shuler JD, Holland GN, Miles SA, et al. Kaposi sarcoma of the conjunctiva and eyelids associated with the acquired immunodeficiency syndrome. *Arch Ophthalmol.* 1989;107: 858–862.

Sneed SR, et al. *Pneumocystis carinii* chroroiditis in patients receiving inhaled pentamidine. *N Eng J Med.* 1990;322:936.

Sommadossi JP, Zhou XJ, Moore J, et al. Impairment of stavudine phosphorylation in patients receiving a combination of zidovudine and d4T (ACTG 290). The ACTG 290 Team. Abstracts of the 5th Conference on Retroviruses and Opportunistic Infections, 1999; abstract 03.

Soriano V, Barreiro P, Dona C, et al. Induction-maintenance (5-3 drugs) in patients with high viral load. Program and Abstracts of the Seventh European Conference on Clinical Aspects and Treatment of HIV Infection, 1999; abstract 553.

Spruance SL, Pavia AT, Mellors JW, et al. Clinical efficacy of monotherapy with stavudine compared with zidovudine in HIV-infected, zidovudine-experienced patients. A randomized, double-blind, controlled study. The Bristol-Myers Squibb Stavudine/019 Study Group. *Ann Intern Med.* 1997;126:355–363.

Spruance SL, Pavia AT, Peterson D, et al. Didanosine compared with continuation of zidovudine in HIV-infected patients with signs of clinical deterioration while receiving zidovudine. A randomized, double-blind clinical trial. The Bristol-Myers Squibb AI454-010 Study Group. *Ann Intern Med.* 1994;120:360–368.

Staszewski S, Keiser P, Gathe J, et al. Comparison of antiviral response with abacavir/Combivir to indinavir/Combivir in therapy-naive adults at 48 weeks (CNA3005). Abstracts of the 39th ICAAC, 1999a; abstract 505.

Staszewski S, Loveday C, Picazo JJ, et al. Safety and efficacy of lamivudine-zidovudine combination therapy in zidovudine-experienced patients. A randomized controlled comparison with zidovudine monotherapy. The Lamivudine European HIV Working Group. *JAMA.* 1996;276: 111–117.

Staszewski S, Morales-Ramirez J, Tashima KT, et al. Efavirenz plus zidovudine and lamivudine, efavirenz plus indinavir, and indinavir plus zidovudine and lamivudine in the treatment of HIV-1 infection in adults. *N Engl J Med.* 1999b; 341:1865–1873.

Stoumbos VD, Klein ML. Syphilitic retinitis in a patient with acquired immunodeficiency syndrome-related complex. *Am J Ophthalmol.* 1987;103:103–104.

Studies of Ocular Complications of AIDS Research Group and the AIDS Clinical Trials Group. Mortality in patients with the acquired immunodeficiency syndrome treated with either foscarnet or ganciclovir for cytomegalovirus retinitis. *N Engl J Med.* 1992;326:213–220.

Studies of Ocular Complications of AIDS Research Group and the AIDS Clinical Trials Group. Studies of Ocular Complications of AIDS Foscarnet-Ganciclovir Cytomegalovirus Retinitis Trial, I: Rationale, design, and methods. *Control Clin Trials.* 1992;13:22–39.

Tebas P, Patick AK, Kane EM, et al. Virologic responses to a ritonavir/saquinavir-containing regimen in patients who had previously failed nelfinavir. *AIDS.* 1999;13:F23–F28.

Teich SA. Conjunctival microvascular changes in AIDS and AIDS-related complex. *Am J Ophthalmol.* 1987;103:332–333.

Thomas FP. HIV-1 Encephalopathy and AIDS dementia complex. *Neurology.* 1999;53:2032–2036.

Tschachler E, Berbstresser PR, Stingl G. HIV-related skin diseases. *Lancet.* 1996;348:659–663.

Verma N, Kearney J. Ocular manifestations of AIDS. *P N G Med J.* 1996;39:196–199.

Vrabec TR. Advances in the diagnosis and management of AIDS-related eye disease. *Curr Opin Ophthalmol.* 1998; 9:93–99.

Whitcup, SM. Cytomegalovirus retinitis in the era of highly active antiretroviral therapy. Clinical Conference. *JAMA.* 2000;283:653–657.

Whitcup SM, Butler KM, Caruso R, et al. Retinal toxicity in human immunodeficiency virus-infected children treated with 2′,3′-dideoxyinosine. *Am J Ophthalmol.* 1992;113:1–7.

Whitcup SM, Dastgheib K, Nussenblatt RB, et al. A clinicopathologic report of the retinal lesions associated with didanosine. *Am J Ophthalmol.* 1994;112:1594–1598.

Whitley RJ, Jacobson MA, Friedberg DN, et al. Guidelines for the treatment of cytomegalovirus diseases in patients with AIDS in the era of potent antiretroviral therapy. *Arch Int Med.* 1998;158:957–969.

Wiktor SZ, Ekpini E, Karon JM, et al. Short-course oral zidovudine for prevention of mother-to-child transmission of HIV-1 in Abidjan, Cote d'Ivoire: A randomised trial. *Lancet.* 1999;353:781–785.

Wilson R. Cytomegalovirus retinitis in AIDS. *J Am Optom Assoc.* 1992;63:49–58.

Wilson R. HIV and contact lens wear. *J Am Optom Assoc.* 1992; 63:13–15. Editorial.

Winward KE, Hamed LM, Glaser JS. The spectrum of optic nerve disease in human immunodeficiency virus infection. *Am J Ophthalmol.* 1989;107:373–380.

Workman C. Combining ritonavir (RTV) & indinavir (IDV) decreases IDV-associated urinary & renal adverse effects (AEs). Program and Abstracts of the Seventh European Conference on Clinical Aspects and Treatment of HIV Infection, 1999; abstract 116.

World Health Organization. HIV/AIDS: The global epidemic, December 1996. *Wkly Epidemiol Rec.* 1997;72:17–21.

Yarchoan R, Venzon DJ, Pluda JM, et al. CD4 count and the risk for death in patients infected with HIV receiving antiretroviral therapy. *Ann Intern Med.* 1991;115:184–189.

Young TL, Robin JB, Holland GN. Herpes simplex keratitis in patients with acquired immune deficiency syndrome. *Ophthalmology.* 1989;96:1476–1479.

Ypma-Wong MF, Fonzi WA, Sypherd PS. Fungus-specific translation elongation factor 3 gene present in *Pneumocystis carinii. Infect Immun.* 1992;60:4140–4145.

Chapter 46

HERPES SIMPLEX

Christine M. Dumestre

Herpes simplex virus (HSV) is one of the most common infectious agents known to humans. The word herpes, meaning "to creep" in Greek, was used to describe the spreading nature of the cutaneous lesions back in the time of Hippocrates in 400 BC. It remains latent in neurons of sensory ganglia after primary infection, allowing it to reactivate at any time during the life of the host.

HSV is divided into two different serotypes, type 1 (HSV-1) and type 2 (HSV-2). It can range in manifestations from asymptomatic infections and self-limiting "cold sores" to fatal encephalitis. HSV-1 is usually responsible for infections above the waist such as labial, oral, upper respiratory tract infections, eye infections, encephalitis, and some cases of generalized herpes simplex. HSV-2 is primarily responsible for infections affecting areas below the waist such as venereally transmitted genital herpes and infections affecting newborns via transmission through the mother's infected birth canal. However, HSV-1 and HSV-2 are not limited to these sites.

Ocular HSV, although commonly misdiagnosed, is the most common cause of severe ocular infection in the United States. Ocular herpes simplex infections are usually due to HSV-1, although HSV-2 can cause some cases of neonatal infection or be secondary to autoinoculation from genital herpes. HSV can cause blepharitis, conjunctivitis, keratitis, uveitis, and retinitis, depending on whether the infection is primary or recurrent.

EPIDEMIOLOGY

Systemic

HSV infections are found throughout the world with humans being the only known natural host. HSV-1 is generally acquired during early childhood years, whereas HSV-2 infection occurs predominantly in sexually active adolescents and young adults. After primary infection, the virus becomes latent in sensory ganglia. Recurrent infection occurs with both HSV-1 and HSV-2. Approximately 20 to 40% of the population experience recurrent labial herpes or "cold sores" from HSV-1. After a primary genital herpes infection (HSV-2), recurrence is approximately 60 to 80%. Up to 50 to 100% of the adult population has antibodies to HSV, indicating previous exposure to the virus.

Herpesvirus infections are among the most common opportunistic infections in persons infected with HIV. HSV-1 and HSV-2 are highly prevalent infections in HIV-seropositive persons. In the United States and Europe, 95% of homosexual men are seropositive for HSV-1, HSV-2, or both, and 40 to 60% of injection drug users are HSV-2-seropositive (Schacker et al, 1997). The degree of immunosuppression also appears to influence the reactivation rate and severity of the disease. Persons with lower CD4 cell counts appear to have larger and more persistent ulcerating lesions. Bagdades and associates (1992) showed that patients whose CD4 cell counts have fallen below 50×10^6/liter have a significantly higher risk of developing HSV ulceration.

Newborns are usually infected with HSV-2 from mothers with genital herpes. Dental and medical personnel are at increased risk of acquiring HSV from patients with oral or genital HSV infections. Also, wrestlers have acquired HSV from contact with superficial abrasions.

Ocular

Epidemiology of herpetic ocular disease has been less thoroughly investigated, although it is known to be the most common cause of corneal blindness. Ocular infection is primarily due to HSV-1, although HSV-2 can also be responsible. There are 500,000 cases of ocular HSV reported each year in the United States. The recurrence rate following initial herpetic keratitis is about 25% in 2 years. The most common cause of visual loss from HSV keratitis is from involvement of the corneal stroma, which occurs in 10 to 48% of recurrent HSV keratitis infections. Ocular involvement occurs in 20% of neonatal HSV infections.

Hodge and colleagues (1997) found no increase in the incidence of HSV keratitis among HIV-positive patients. However, he did find the recurrence rate of HSV keratitis to be 2.48 times greater than among non-HIV persons with HSV keratitis.

PATHOPHYSIOLOGY/DISEASE PROCESS

Systemic

The Organism

Herpes simplex virus is a member of the Herpesviridae family. It is a linear, double-stranded DNA virus with two serotypes, HSV-1 and HSV-2. Infection begins with the spread of virus from one person to another.

Transmission

Transmission occurs by direct contact with actively infected symptomatic or asymptomatic individuals, although those with active lesions are much more infectious. HSV-1 is usually transmitted through contact with oral secretions, and HSV-2 through contact with genital secretions. The virus enters the host through the mucosal surfaces or breaks in the skin. Upon entry, the virus infects localized epithelial cells and uses the cell for its own replication. Once replication is complete, the host cells are lysed, releasing replicated virions and causing a localized inflammatory response. This inflammatory response is what is seen in both the primary infection (although generally subclinical), and reactivation.

Course of the Disease

Primary HSV-1 infection is commonly acquired during childhood and is usually asymptomatic or may present as a nonspecific upper respiratory tract infection. Gingivostomatitis (inflammation of the gums and mouth) and pharyngitis (inflammation of the pharynx) are the most common clinical presentations of primary HSV-1 infection. The incubation period is 3 to 5 days, and patients may suffer from fever, malaise, myalgia, inability to eat, irritability, and cervical adenopathy. Signs include lesions or vesicles involving intraoral membranes, lips, and facial area (Figure 46–1). This

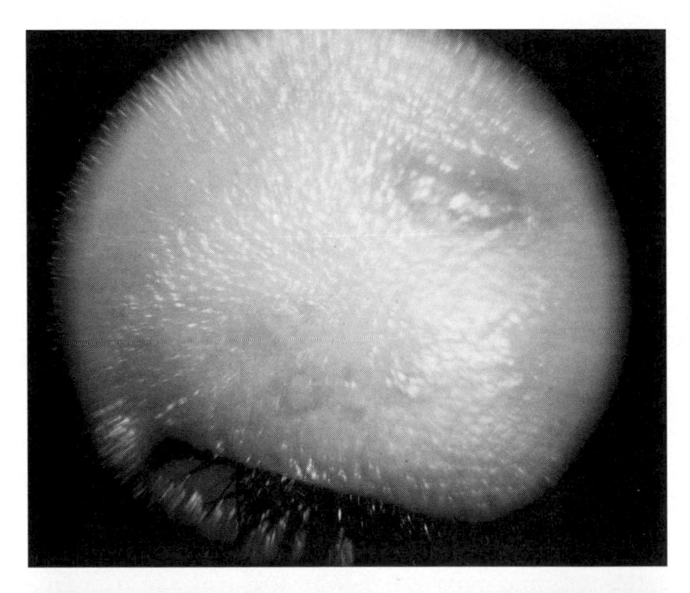

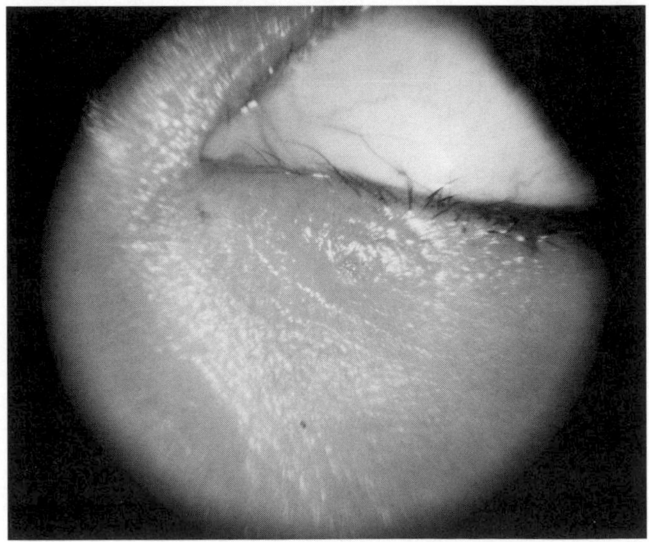

Figure 46–1. Recurrent ocular HSV infection with upper and lower lid vesicles. (*Courtesy of Susan P. Schuettenberg, OD.*)

acute primary infection is self-limiting and recovery is complete within 1 to 2 weeks.

Herpes simplex infection varies widely in severity and duration. Neonates as well as immunocompromised patients (eg, secondary to AIDS, chemotherapy, malnutrition) suffer more severe and prolonged HSV infections.

After primary infection, the virus is transported intraaxonally to the nerve cell bodies of regional ganglia, where it resides in a latent state. It remains controversial as to whether this latent state is one of no replication or one of very low continuous replication of the virus. The virus can remain latent for the lifetime of the host, or it can reactivate, causing recurrent infection. Reactivation occurs by virus transportation from the regional ganglia to the body surface along sensory nerves by anterograde axoplasmic transport. This leads to a recurrent infection of the same or neighboring site as that affected during primary infection. There are precipitating factors associated with HSV recurrence. These precipitating "trigger" factors include sun exposure, wind, fever, local trauma, menstruation, emotional stress, and decreased immunity.

Herpes labialis or "cold sores" is the most frequent clinical manifestation of recurrent HSV-1 infection. Reactivation of latent virus in the trigeminal nerve can produce intraoral mucosal ulcers, or more commonly a herpetic ulceration at the vermilion border of the lip known as the herpetic cold sore. Prodromal itching, tingling, or burning sensation is commonly described before the formation of vesicles on the lip border. Once the vesicles form, they progress to an ulcer, and then crust, and heal without scarring within a few days. Studies have shown that through asymptomatic viral shedding, persons can be infectious without the presence of the labialis lesion. However, the presence of the lesion makes the person far more infectious. Recurrent infections usually occur at the same site and are associated with precipitating factors such as stress, menstruation, fever, sun and wind exposure, direct trauma, and immunosuppression. Oral facial HSV infection is self-limiting in the immunocompetent, but may produce severe infection in the immunocompromised if left untreated.

HSV-2 infection is usually acquired by sexual contact via infected genitalia. It usually occurs in young adulthood as a primary infection, with an incubation period of 2 to 7 days. Genital herpes as a primary infection is associated with fever, malaise, headache, myalgia, and bilateral inguinal adenopathy. Pain and itching of genitalia develop into vesicular lesions and painful erythematous ulcers. Prodromal neuralgic type pain is sometimes described as radiating to the lower back and hips. Patients may also present with dysuria and vaginal or urethral discharge. Lesions of primary infection may last several weeks before completely healing. Recurrent genital herpes occurs from reactivation of HSV-2 in the sacral ganglia. HSV-2 genital infections have a recurrence rate of 80% within 12 months. Recurrent infections have a similar but milder course, and healing occurs within 5 to 10 days.

Primary oral or genital HSV can also cause a finger infection known as herpetic whitlow. This HSV infection is usually acquired by medical or dental personnel who are in contact with patients' active lesions. Signs and symptoms include abrupt onset of edema, erythema, and localized tenderness at the base of the cuticle in the infected finger. Fever and lymphadenitis are also not uncommon.

Visceral HSV infections are rare and most commonly seen in immunosuppressed patients. Immunodeficient patients are more likely to develop disseminated HSV infection involving visceral organs. Visceral HSV infections may include the esophageal mucosa, lungs, and liver (Table 46–1).

Herpes simplex meningitis is usually associated with primary genital herpes infection. The course of the disease is acute, self-limiting, and benign. Symptoms include headache, fever, and mild photophobia that lasts 2 to 7 days.

Although uncommon, HSV infections can spread from a peripheral site to the brain, causing HSV encephalitis. HSV is the most common etiology of acute sporadic viral encephalitis in the United States. It is usually associated with HSV-1. Symptoms include acute onset fever, headache, and neurological disturbances similar to those seen with temporal lobe dysfunction. There are no clinical signs indicative of herpetic etiology. Only the detection of HSV from brain biopsy is diagnostic. Untreated patients deteriorate rapidly, and mortality is as high as 60 to 80%.

Neonatal HSV infections are acquired by newborns from the infected birth canal of the mother during delivery. Most neonatal HSV infections are type 2. Infected newborns can present with self-limiting skin infections, conjunctivitis, or fatal disseminated disease with or without CNS involvement. Of those with CNS involvement, neurological sequelae include lethargy, cranial nerve palsies, and seizures. Untreated neonatal HSV disseminates and develops into CNS infection in 70% of cases, and results in death in 65% of cases.

Ocular

Ocular HSV infections usually present as recurrent infection and are primarily due to HSV-1. HSV-2 can sometimes cause ocular infection by secondary spread from genital herpes or as a part of widespread infection with neonatal HSV.

TABLE 46–1. SYSTEMIC MANIFESTATIONS OF HERPES SIMPLEX VIRUS (HSV)

	Symptoms	Signs
Oral Facial HSV		
1. Primary infection: gingivostomatitis and pharyngitis	• Fever, malaise, myalgia, inability to eat, irritability	• Lesions of hard and soft palate, gingiva, tongue, lip, facial area, and cervical adenopathy
2. Recurrent herpes labialis	• Itching, burning, or tingling on the mucocutaneous junction of the lip	• Vesicles that rupture to form an ulcer that will crust without scarring
Genital HSV		
1. Primary infection	• Fever, headache, malaise, myalgia, pain, itching, dysuria, vaginal and urethral discharge	• Lesions of external genitalia, form vesicles, pustules, to painful erythematous ulcers and tender inguinal adenopathy
2. Recurrent infection	• Same as above with a milder course	
Herpetic Whitlow	• Tenderness of infected finger and fever	• Abrupt onset of edema and erythema of finger and lymphadenitis
CNS HSV		
1. Encephalitis	• Acute onset of fever and focal neurological symptoms, especially temporal lobe	• No clinical signs upon which herpetic etiology can be established
2. Meningitis	• Acute onset of fever, headache, and mild photophobia	
Neonatal HSV	• Infection can be localized, disseminated, or involve the CNS	• Newborns often present with vesicles or conjunctivitis or neurological dysfunction such as seizures, CN palsies, and lethargy
Visceral HSV		
1. Esophagitis	• Dysphagia, substernal pain, and weight loss	• Ulcerations of esophagus seen with endoscopy
2. Pneumonitis	• Fever, cough, dyspnea	• Mucosal lesions or tracheobronchitis
3. Hepatitis	• Fever	• Abrupt elevations of bilirubin and serum transaminase

Ocular herpes can be acquired as a primary infection from contact with an infected individual, or it can be mechanically transferred to the eye from other HSV-infected sites on the same individual. More commonly, HSV infection is acquired affecting a nonocular site (skin or mouth), which later spreads to the eye by recurrent infection of the latent virus. Reactivation affecting the eye is usually in the form of a keratitis.

Although rare, HSV-1 can occur as a primary ocular infection. Primary ocular HSV infection is mainly associated with unilateral blepharitis and/or conjunctivitis (Figure 46–1). Patients can experience fever, malaise, and tenderness of preauricular nodes. Vesicles form on lids and lid margins, ulcerate within days, and heal without scarring. Conjunctivitis is acute and follicular, with the presence of mucoid discharge. Approximately 20% of primary ocular infections involve the cornea. Primary HSV is self-limited and lasts 2 to 3 weeks, although in the presence of keratitis it may last longer.

Recurrent ocular HSV infections occur by reactivation of latent virus from the trigeminal, superior cervical, or ciliary ganglion. The most common target of recurrent ocular HSV disease is the cornea, although the lids may also be affected. Epithelial keratitis begins with fine superficial punctate lesions caused by actively replicating virus. These fine lesions increase in size to form the classic dendritic ulcer with its characteristic branching and terminal end bulbs (Figure 46–2). Signs and symptoms include irritation, tearing, photophobia, blurred vision, and decreased corneal sensation. Dendritic ulcers usually heal spontaneously within 5 to 12 days, but can progress to larger, slower-healing geographic ulcers.

In cases of recurrent HSV infection, HSV particles may extend into the stroma, causing stromal keratitis (Figure 46–3). HSV stromal disease is thought to be due to a hypersensitivity reaction in response to viral particles that have settled into the stroma. Disciform keratitis is a round pattern of stromal edema, usually found under intact epithelium, which may heal after several months. Interstitial keratitis presents with areas of stromal infiltration from inflammatory cells and tends to be chronic and persistent. Complications from recurrent HSV stromal keratitis include vascularization, necrosis, scarring, stromal thinning, and perfora-

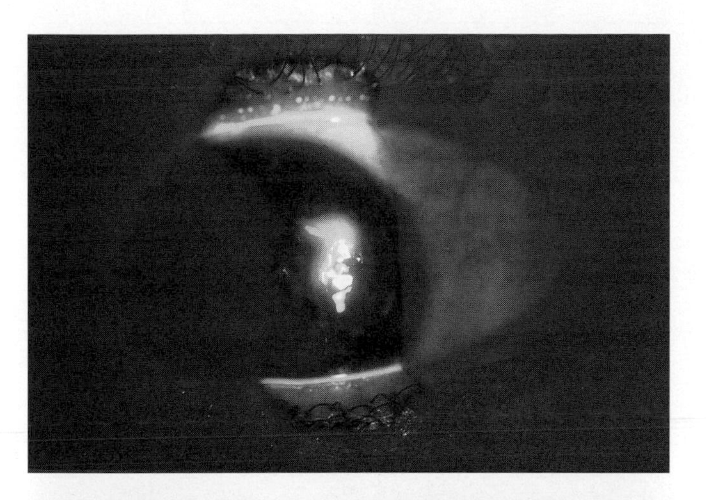

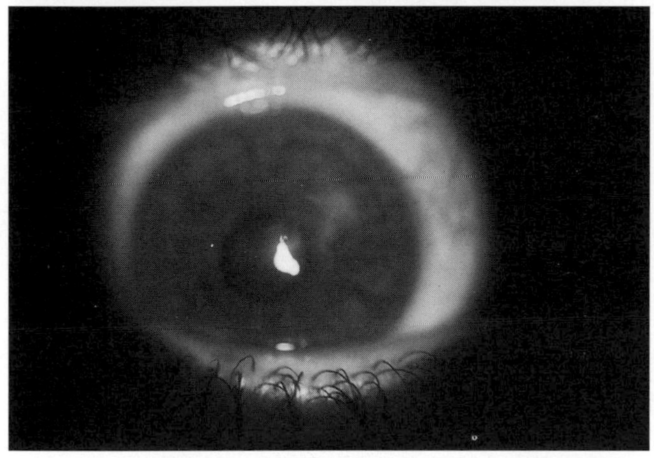

Figure 46–2. Classic appearance of HSV dendritic keratitis with characteristic branching, terminal end bulbs, and fluorescein stain pattern.

tion, which may result in blindness. Symptoms of stromal keratitis include photophobia, lacrimation, blurred vision, and variable pain, depending on the severity.

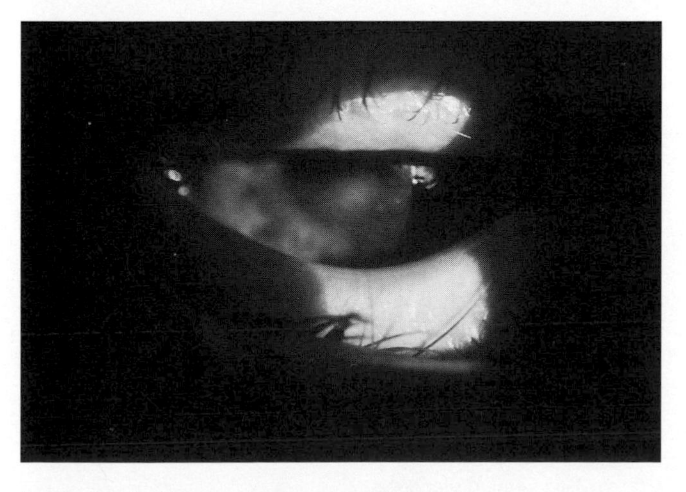

Figure 46–3. Herpes simplex stromal keratitis.

Postinfectious herpetic ulcers may follow epithelial or stromal disease and are known as metaherpetic or trophic ulcers. The ulcer is sterile and occurs due to basement membrane disruption, similar to recurrent corneal erosions. The ulcer is characterized as round with rolled edges from epithelial cells that cannot adhere well to the basement membrane. They can persist from weeks to months, and re-epithelialization is limited until basement membrane healing occurs. Symptoms are limited by decreased corneal sensation, but can involve tearing, foreign body sensation, and pain upon awakening.

Uveitis can occur as a sequela to stromal and endothelial inflammation or as a direct site of recurrent HSV infection. It can present as a mild to severe anterior chamber reaction. Secondary glaucoma may occur following uveitis.

Herpes simplex retinitis is the least common ocular manifestation of HSV infection, and is limited to neonates and immunocompromised patients (Table 46–2). It manifests as an acute retinal necrosis or a chorioretinitis.

DIAGNOSIS

Systemic

The diagnosis of HSV infection is usually based on clinical presentation, particularly the appearance of characteristic vesicular lesions (Tables 46–3 and 46–4). In addition, several laboratory methods are used in the diagnosis of HSV (Table 46–5). The "gold standard" or definitive diagnosis is made by isolating the virus itself in tissue cultures inoculated with vesicular scrapings or fluid. This method is expensive, time consuming, and not readily available. Another method is by

> Recurrent herpes labialis is the most frequent clinical manifestation of recurrent HSV-1 infection.

cytological examination of lesion scrapings with Giemsa stain for multinucleated epithelial giant cells or intranuclear eosinophilic inclusion bodies. This is a good, quick, in-office procedure used to confirm diagnosis, but is not very sensitive and cannot differentiate between HSV and varicella zoster. A variety of serological tests are available to detect HSV antibodies; however, these are only useful for the diagnosis of primary infection by documenting rising antibody titers. Currently, HSV antigen detection is being accomplished through the use of monoclonal antibodies.

TABLE 46–2. OCULAR MANIFESTATIONS OF HERPES SIMPLEX VIRUS (HSV)

	Symptoms	Signs
Blepharitis (usually with primary infection)	• Itching, irritation, and swelling of lids	• Unilateral, vesicles on lid and lid margins, which ulcerate, crust, and heal without scarring
Conjunctivitis (usually with primary infection)	• Redness, lacrimation, discharge	• Acute follicular conjunctivitis with preauricular lymphadenopathy; may be associated with lid or corneal involvement
Keratitis		
1. Epithelial keratitis	• Irritation, lacrimation, photophobia, blurred vision	• SPK, dendritic lesions, geographic ulcers, decreased corneal sensation
2. Stromal keratitis	• Photophobia, lacrimation, mild pain, blurred vision	• Stromal edema, stromal infiltration, vascularization, necrosis
3. Trophic ulcer	• Slight tearing, foreign body sensation, pain upon awakening, symptoms limited by decreased corneal sensation	• Loss of corneal sensation, round ulcer with rolled edges from epithelial cells that cannot adhere to damaged basement membrane
Uveitis	• Photophobia, pain, blurred vision	• Mild to severe anterior chamber reaction, ciliary injection, small KPs
Glaucoma		• Secondary glaucoma from uveitis
Retinitis		• Choroidal hemorrhage, exudates, fine vitreal opacities, retinal edema, narrowing of arterioles

TABLE 46–3. DIAGNOSIS OF SYSTEMIC HERPES SIMPLEX VIRUS (HSV)

	Clinical Correlates
Oral–Facial HSV	
Gingivostomatitis (primary infection)	• Presents between ages of 10 months and 3 years • Clinical presentation: fever, vesicular lesions on lips along gingiva, anterior tongue, and anterior hard palate • Child may refuse to eat secondary to discomfort • Lesions bleed easily and persist approximately 10 days
Recurrent herpes labialis	• Most frequent clinical manifestation of recurrent HSV-1 infection • Prodromal tingling, burning, and itching commonly described prior to appearance of the vesicle • Precipitating factors include sun exposure, wind, fever, local trauma, menstruation, emotional stress, and decreased immunity • Vesicles appear at the vermilion border of the lip, progress to ulcers and crust within 48 hours • Persist 8 to 10 days
Genital HSV	• Diagnosis based upon clinical presentation, appearance of characteristic lesions, and confirmed with detection of HSV antigen by enzyme immunoassay • Associated with fever, headaches, malaise, myalgia, aseptic meningitis, genital itching and pain, discharge, and inguinal adenopathy • Vesicles can become ulcers around genitalia and buttocks • Recurrent
CNS HSV	• Polymerase chain reaction from spinal fluid or brain biopsy is diagnostic • Tissue culture is not always useful because HSV only grows occasionally from CSF • Clinical presentation of acute illness with fever, malaise, irritability, and progressing to CNS involvement • CSF reveals pleocytosis, increased lymphocytes, neutrophils, and protein • Neurodiagnostic testing may reveal abnormal EEG • CT scan/ MRI may be useful in diagnosis

TABLE 46–4. DIFFERENTIAL DIAGNOSIS OF SYSTEMIC HERPES SIMPLEX VIRUS (HSV)

HSV Manifestation	Differential Diagnoses
Oral–Facial HSV	
Primary infection gingivostomatitis	Herpangina (enteroviral infection)
Recurrent herpes labialis	Stevens–Johnson syndrome (erythema multiforme) Impetigo
Genital HSV	Syphilic chancre Behçet syndrome Stevens–Johnson syndrome (erythema multiforme) Candidiasis
CNS HSV	
Encephalitis Meningitis	*Cryptococcus* *Listeria monocytogenes* Lyme disease Tuberculosis Bacterial endocarditis Meningococcal meningitis Toxoplasmosis Mumps virus Coxsackie virus Reyes syndrome Postinfluenza encephalitis Epstein–Barr virus Rubella Cytomegalovirus Adenovirus Measles virus Arbovirus Enterovirus

Commercially available HSV antigen detection tests (DuPont Herpchek) have shown to be rapid (4 hours) and similar in sensitivity to tissue cultures. This test has proven reliable in diagnosis of HSV infection of the skin, genitourinary system, and eyes.

Recently, molecular techniques such as polymerase chain reaction (PCR) have been used in the detection of HSV nucleic acids (DNA or RNA), rather than antibody or antigen detection. Polymerase chain reaction is highly specific and sensitive, allowing the detection of a single copy of DNA in a sample. Currently, it remains a rather labor-intensive and expensive test. Also, because of its extreme sensitivity, false-positives may be introduced because of poor technique or environmental contamination. However, further developments and improvements in PCR technology may make this test more attractive in the future.

TABLE 46–5. DIAGNOSTIC TESTS FOR HERPES SIMPLEX VIRUS (HSV)

Tzank smear: nonspecific cytological examination with Giemsa stain; cannot differentiate between HSV and varicella zoster.

Serum conversion: antibody detection; documenting rising antibody titers; valuable for detection of primary HSV.

Enzyme immunoassay (Herpchek): antigen detection; rapid, very sensitive, and specific, although antigen detection for HSV in CSF has been unsuccessful.

Polymerase chain reaction (PCR): HSV DNA detection; rapid, very sensitive, and specific; successful with samples containing small amount of virus such as CSF.

HSV tissue culture: "gold standard"; isolation of HSV in cell culture; takes 2 to 14 days for results.

TABLE 46–6. DIAGNOSIS OF OCULAR HERPES SIMPLEX VIRUS (HSV)

	Clinical Correlates
Blepharitis	• Vesicles adjacent to lid margin that ulcerate within days • Preauricular lymphadenopathy • Unilateral and does not respect dermatome
Conjunctivitis	• Acute, follicular conjunctivitis • Preauricular lymphadenopathy • Unilateral
Keratitis	
Epithelial	• Classic dendritic lesion: linear branching with terminal end bulbs with NaFl • Stains with rose bengal • Reduced corneal sensitivity • Unilateral • Recurrent • Positive HSV antigen detection by enzyme immunoassay done with atypical presentations of dendritic lesion
Stromal	• Stromal edema (disciform) or stromal infiltration (interstitial), vascularization, and necrosis • Reduced corneal sensitivity • Unilateral • Recurrent • Positive HSV antigen detection by enzyme immunoassay
Uveitis	• Anterior chamber reaction with small KPs • Unilateral and recurrent • Diagnosed by PCR from aqueous humor
Retinitis	• Diagnosed by PCR from vitreous sample (biopsy)

Ocular

Ocular HSV infection is usually diagnosed by clinical examination (Tables 46–6 and 46–7). The unilateral presence of lid vesicles with follicular conjunctivitis, dendritic or geographic ulcers, or disciform or interstitial keratitis can all indicate HSV ocular infection. The diagnosis of HSV keratitis can be made on the characteristic fluorescein staining appearance of the dendritic epithelial lesion with its branching nature and terminal

> HSV keratitis should be ruled out in any patient presenting with a unilateral red eye.

TABLE 46–7. DIFFERENTIAL DIAGNOSIS OF OCULAR HERPES SIMPLEX

Blepharitis	Herpes zoster Molluscum contagiosum Psoriasis
Conjunctivitis	Adenoviral Bacterial Allergic
Keratitis	
Epithelial	Recurrent corneal erosion Keratitis sicca Herpes zoster keratitis Superficial punctate keratitis Atopic/vernal keratoconjunctivitis Contact-lens-related pseudodendrites Superior limbic keratoconjunctivitis Thygeson superficial punctate keratopathy
Stromal	Syphylitic interstitial keratitis Herpes zoster interstitial keratitis Bacterial corneal ulcer
Uveitis	Herpes zoster Ankylosing spondylitis Lyme disease Reiter syndrome Posner–Schlossman syndrome Inflammatory bowel disease Behçet disease Varicella Trauma
Retinitis	Herpes zoster Toxoplasmosis Cytomegalovirus

end bulbs. Central epithelium is lost and stains with fluorescein, while the periphery of the lesion consists of infected cells and stains with rose bengal. HSV keratitis does not always present with a characteristic dendritic lesion; sometimes only a superficial punctate keratitis is noted. The history of recurrent disease, unilateral presentation, decreased corneal sensation, and the involvement of multiple corneal layers are all suggestive of HSV ocular infection. HSV ocular infection should always be ruled out with the presentation of a unilateral keratitis. Reduced corneal sensation can be tested and serve as a diagnostic tool for HSV keratitis. A cotton wisp used to touch the cornea can grossly qualify asymmetry in corneal sensation. There are also commercially available corneal sensation devices that can quantify corneal sensation. Reduced corneal sensation is noted in the eye with HSV even after the acute condition is resolved. Diagnosis is not always readily available by clinical examination; therefore, laboratory testing may be necessary. As mentioned previously, Herpchek is a reliable diagnostic test for detecting HSV antigen. Tear film swabs used with viral transport media (Herptran media) can be sent to hospitals or reference labs where Herpchek assay is readily available to confirm the diagnosis of HSV infectious keratitis. Polymerase chain reaction also provides rapid testing for HSV infections of the cornea, but is currently not as readily available as immunoassay testing. Because this method actually measures HSV DNA, it might become an indicator of how effective antivirals such as acyclovir are in the treatment of HSV. These laboratory tests are valuable to confirm the diagnosis, but treatment should be instituted upon clinical presentation. Necrotizing retinitis caused by HSV may be difficult to distinguish from other pathogens that cause retinitis such as *Toxoplasma gondii* and *Treponema pallidum.* In such cases, laboratory evaluation of intraocular fluid may be necessary for diagnosis.

TREATMENT AND MANAGEMENT

There are a number of antiviral agents available for the treatment of HSV infections. These agents are nucleoside derivatives that work by interfering with the synthesis of HSV DNA. They include idoxuridine, vidarabine, trifluridine, and acyclovir.

Systemic

The course of labial or genital herpetic infections is usually self-limiting and benign; however, complications do exist and can be quite severe. This holds especially true for the immunocompromised and the neonate. In severe and life-threatening cases, antiviral therapy becomes essential. Vidarabine and acyclovir (ACV) are both useful in treating systemic HSV infections. Intravenously they are effective in reducing mortality associated with HSV encephalitis and disseminated neonatal infection. Oral or intravenous ACV is effective against mucocutaneous HSV infections in immunocompromised patients, and can also prevent the frequency of reactivation. Oral ACV is also used to shorten the duration and symptoms of genital herpes as well as prophylactically to prevent genital HSV recurrence. Long-term treatment with oral ACV has been shown to prevent recurrences of genital HSV by 80% (Mertz et al, 1988) and orofacial HSV significantly. Topical ACV is available for use on genital herpes lesions and other localized external lesions (Table 46–8).

Along with antiviral therapy, preventative measures can also be used to reduce HSV infection. Sunblock on lips can be used to prevent recurrent labial herpes. Condoms should be used to prevent sexual transmission. Medical and dental workers should wear gloves when in contact with oral or genital secretions. Cesarean section delivery may be considered to avoid

TABLE 46–8. TREATMENT AND MANAGEMENT OF HERPES SIMPLEX VIRUS (HSV)

Systemic

- **Vidarabine (Vira–A)**
  15 mg/kg/d IV for 10 days
  Indication: Systemic treatment of HSV encephalitis
  Contraindication/side effect: May produce nausea, diarrhea, GI disturbance, bone marrow depression, CNS toxicity
- **Acyclovir (Zovirax)**
  Ointment: 5% cream applied 4–6 times a day for 10 days
  Oral: 200 mg tablets po 5 times a day for 2 weeks
  Intravenous: 5–10 mg/kg IV q8h for 5–7 days
  Indication: Topical ointment used for genital herpes lesions or immunosuppressed patients with localized external lesions
  Oral ACV used for treatment of genital herpes and also used prophylactically to prevent recurrence
  IV ACV is useful to treat immunocompromised patients, neonates, and patients with progressive cutaneous, CNS, or visceral dissemination of HSV infection
  Contraindication/side effect: Oral: nausea, headache, diarrhea, anorexia, leg pain, rash, renal dysfunction
  IV: local phlebitis, nausea, vomiting, hypotension, diaphoresis, renal toxicity, rash, headache, hematuria

Ocular

Conjunctivitis/blepharitis

- Supportive therapy
- Prophylactic antiviral or antiviral/antibiotic combination may be used

Epithelial/stromal keratitis and uveitis

- **Trifluridine (Viroptic)**
  1% solution 9 times a day for 2 weeks
  Indications: Topical treatment of HSV keratitis; currently drug of choice in U.S.
  Contraindication/side effects: Most toxic of the ocular agents used, may result in SPK, follicular conjunctivitis, punctal occlusion, thickening and keratinization of lid margins, meibomian gland pouting, ptosis, contact dermatitis
- **Idoxuridine (IDU)**
  1% solution q2h or 0.5% ointment 5 times a day for 2 weeks
  Indication: Topical treatment of HSV epithelial keratitis
  Contraindication/side effect: Toxicity due to adverse effect on host cells; may result in SPK, follicular conjunctivitis, lid margin thickening and keratinization, punctal occlusion, conjunctival cicatrization, corneal scarring, ptosis, contact dermatitis
- **Vidarabine (Vira–A)**
  3% ointment 5 times daily for 2 weeks
  Indication: Topical treatment of HSV epithelial keratitis
  Contraindication/side effects: Similar side effects to IDU, although less toxic
- **Acyclovir (Zovirax)**
  3% ointment 5 times daily for 2 weeks
  Indication: Topical ophthalmic ointment; not FDA approved in U.S.
  Contraindication/side effect: Almost no adverse side effects; occasional punctate keratitis, conjunctivitis
  Oral: 400 mg tablets PO 5 times a day for 2 weeks.
  Indication: Treatment of HSV epithelial and/or stromal keratitis in patients who have adverse reactions to topical antivirals
  Oral: 400 mg tablets PO bid for 1 year
  Indication: Patients with history of stromal keratitis to prevent recurrence
  Contraindications: Minimal, generally well tolerated
- **Debridement**
  Indication: Was once the only effective treatment of HSV epithelial keratitis and remains a safe, effective alternative to antiviral agents

Stromal herpetic disease and metaherpetic ulcer

- **Referral to corneal specialist**
- **Cycloplegics**
  5% homatropine tid
  Indication: Treatment of uveitis
- **Cortocosteroids**
  0.125–1% prednisolone acetate 2–4 times a day with tapering
  Indication: Treatment of stromal keratitis and uveitis
  Contraindication/side effect: Contraindicated for epithelial keratitis; complications include progression of epithelial infection, stromal ulceration, glaucoma, cataract, microbial superinfection, steroid dependence
- **Lubricants**
  Artificial tears IGTT qid to q2h for symptomatic relief
  Indication: Used in the treatment of metaherpetic or trophic ulcers
  Contraindication/side effect: None

Penetrating keratoplasty, if indicated

neonatal HSV in those infected with genital herpes. Antiviral treatment has no effect on viral latency.

Ocular

The three antiviral agents approved for the treatment of HSV ocular infection in the United States are idoxuridine (IDU) 0.5% ointment and 0.1% solution, vidarabine (Vira-A) 3% ointment, and trifluridine (Viroptic) 1% solution. ACV (Zovirax) 3% ointment has also shown to be quite effective in the treatment of ocular herpes, but is not commercially available in the United States. Idoxuridine and vidarabine are equally effective in treating epithelial keratitis. They both have poor corneal penetrance and therefore are not very effective in treating HSV stromal keratitis. Trifluridine is currently the drug of choice in the United States in the treatment of HSV epithelial keratitis. It is more potent and has better ocular penetration than idoxuridine or vidarabine. All three antiviral agents present with the common side effects of ocular toxicity, especially with long-term application. Toxicities include superficial punctate keratitis, lid margin thickening, narrowing of lacrimal puncta, follicular conjunctivitis, and contact dermatitis (Table 46–8).

Topical ACV is as effective, if not better, than other antiviral medications in the treatment of epithelial keratitis. ACV is more effective than other agents because the nature of its chemical structure makes it more specific in its action towards the virus. It is highly potent, less toxic to the ocular surface, and penetrates the cornea topically. One disadvantage of ACV is its greater potential in developing resistance. It therefore should be used with caution in those countries where it is available.

Treatment of ocular HSV depends on its presentation. It is necessary to establish which ocular structures are effected by the virus and whether the infection is primary or recurrent. The immune status of the patient is also contributory in deciding the mode of treatment.

Herpes simplex blepharoconjunctivitis is usually self-limiting and warrants no treatment. Some believe that antiviral therapy should be used prophylactically to prevent corneal involvement. Using an antiviral agent may shorten the course of the disease. Sometimes a combination antiviral and antibiotic ointment is used on lid vesicles to avoid secondary bacterial infection.

Herpes simplex epithelial disease (dendritic, geographic) is treated with antiviral medications to destroy the active virus that has invaded epithelial cells. Viroptic is the current treatment of choice (see Table 46–8 for specific dosages). Debridement was the sole mode of treatment prior to the availability of antiviral therapy. It is effective in removing infected epithelial cells and currently is used alone or in combination with antiviral therapy. Virus-laden cells have poor adherence to the basement membrane of the epithelium and are easily removed with a cotton-tip applicator. Regeneration of the surrounding noninfected epithelium promotes healing. Corticosteroids should not be used in the presence of an epithelial defect where there is active viral replication such as dendritic (epithelial) keratitis. This enhances viral replication and can lead to geographic ulceration.

Recently, a periocular vaccination for HSV dendritic keratitis has been investigated. The vaccine is an HSV recombinant glycoprotein D that is being examined for its ability to decrease HSV-induced recurrent dendritic keratitis. Nesburn and co-workers (1998) demonstrated that a periocular vaccination reduced HSV shedding and resulted in a significant decrease in recurrent HSV keratitis in latently infected rabbits. This supports the possible development of a therapeutic vaccine for ocular HSV-1 recurrence in humans in the future.

Stromal herpetic disease (disciform, interstitial keratitis) is more complicated to treat. Corticosteroids have been found helpful in the treatment of HSV stromal keratitis. According to the Herpetic Eye Disease Study, corticosteroid therapy reduces the risk of persistent or progressive stromal keratitis by 68%. Corticosteroids are used only with an intact epithelium. Their use is indicated when the keratitis is solely due to the host immunologic response, as in disciform (stromal) keratitis in which inflammation that is potentially destructive to the cornea can be suppressed. Disciform keratitis tends to be more responsive to steroids than interstitial keratitis. When corticosteroids are used to treat stromal keratitis, low dosages should be used with careful follow-up. An example would be 0.125 to 1% prednisolone acetate two to four times a day with tapering to avoid rebound inflammation, once the desired effect is achieved. The side effects of steroids include glaucoma, cataract, secondary microbial infection, and steroid dependence. One should also use an antiviral concurrently to prevent the reactivation of epithelial disease. In herpetic stromal disease, corticosteroids can potentially reduce pain, edema, scarring, and vascularization, and improve vision.

The Herpetic Eye Disease Study also examined the role of oral acyclovir in the treatment and prevention of HSV stromal keratitis. When comparing patients taking oral acyclovir (400 mg five times a day) concurrently with a topical steroid and trifluridine versus patients not taking oral acyclovir, no significant difference was found in the outcome of HSV stromal keratitis. Oral acyclovir also showed no value in the prevention of HSV stromal keratitis in patients with an already existing HSV epithelial keratitis. However, the Herpetic Eye Disease Study was successful in demonstrating that oral acyclovir had a significant effect in reducing recurrence. A 12-month treatment of oral acyclovir (400 mg bid) reduced the recurrence of HSV stromal keratitis by nearly half (45%). Therefore, prolonged acyclovir treatment should provide a clinical benefit in patients with a history of stromal keratitis because it may help reduce the likelihood of corneal scarring and vision loss associated with recurrent episodes. Oral acyclovir is a well-tolerated drug with minimal side effects and should be considered when treating HSV stromal keratitis, especially in patients with a history of recurrence. It can also be used as the primary antiviral agent in patients who might have adverse reactions to topical antivirals.

Metaherpetic or trophic ulcers are recurrent corneal erosions due to persistent epithelial defects caused by poor adherence to a damaged basement membrane from repeated HSV attacks; thus they can be easily distinguished from active herpes simplex lesions (through the history of corneal lesions). Antiviral agents do not help in these cases because there is no active viral replication. These ulcers are best managed with lubricating agents, patching, or bandage contact lenses to help promote reepithelialization. Referral to a corneal specialist may be indicated. Low-dose steroids may also be used. Close follow-up is necessary to avoid stromal thinning and to ensure that epithelial healing is taking place. Surgical treatment should be considered if medical treatment is unsuccessful. Conjunctival flaps are an alternative to provide a stable epithelial surface.

In severe cases of chronic ocular HSV infection where medical treatment has failed, penetrating keratoplasty may be necessary. Keratoplasty should be considered in patients who have corneal scarring, corneal perforation, or irreversible corneal edema. Corneal transplantation may preserve vision and/or the integrity of the eye. Corneal transplants are most successful when performed on a quiet nonactively infected eye. Recurrent ocular HSV infection can present itself even after corneal transplantation.

Whenever there is involvement of the anterior chamber (uveitis), in ocular HSV infection, cycloplegics are indicated. Corticosteroids may be used, but should be avoided if there is an epithelial defect or stromal ulceration. Antiviral treatment is also needed, preferably one that can penetrate into the anterior chamber, such as oral acyclovir or trifluridine.

Acute retinal necrosis and chorioretinitis caused by HSV are treated with intravitreal, intravenous, and/or oral ACV.

Immunocompromised patients who have ocular HSV infections in general should be treated more aggressively. Because of their immunodeficiency, the course of disease is generally longer and recurrent infections more frequent. Educating the patient on trigger factors and how to avoid them can be helpful. Some even recommend the use of oral ACV prophylactically to prevent recurrent episodes.

CONCLUSION

HSV, one of the most common infectious agents, is diverse in its clinical presentation and severity. Its benign manifestations are universal and felt by nearly everyone. Unfortunately, the more severe clinical consequences can be life- or sight-threatening. Prompt, appropriate treatment is imperative to help avoid a poor outcome.

REFERENCES

Alexander LJ. Diseases of the retina. In: Bartlett JD, Jaanus DS, eds. *Clinical Ocular Pharmacology.* Boston: Butterworth; 1984.

Arffa RC, ed. *Graysons Diseases of the Cornea.* 3rd ed. St. Louis: Mosby; 1991.

Bagdades EK, et al. Relationship between herpes simplex virus ulceration and CD4+ cell counts in patients with HIV infection. *AIDS.* 1992;6:1317–1320.

Baker DA, Pavan-Langston D, Gonik B, et al. Multicenter clinical evaluation of the DuPont Herpchek HSV ELISA, a new rapid diagnostic test for the direct detection of herpes simplex virus. *Adv Exp Med Bio.* 1990;263:71–76.

Barron BA, et al. Herpetic Eye Disease Study. A Controlled trial of oral acyclovir for herpes simplex stromal keratitis. *Ophthalmology.* 1994;101:1871–1882.

Barron BA, et al. A controlled trial of oral acyclovir for the prevention of stromal keratitis or iritis in patients with herpes simplex virus epithelial keratitis. The Epithelial Keratitis Trial. The Herpetic Eye Disease Study Group. *Arch Ophthalmol.* 1997;115:703–715.

Barron BA, et al. Acyclovir for the prevention of recurrent herpes simplex virus eye disease. The Herpetic Eye Disease Study Group. *N Engl J Med.* 1998;339:300–306.

Blodi MD, Frederick C, eds. *Herpes Simplex Infections of the Eye.* New York: Churchill Livingstone; 1984.

Catania, LJ. *Primary Care of the Anterior Segment.* Norwalk, CT: Appleton & Lange; 1988.

Collum L, Akhtar J, McGettrick P. Oral acyclovir in herpetic keratitis. *Trans Ophthalmol Soc UK.* 1985;104:629–632.

Corey L, Spear PG. Infections with herpes simplex virus. *N Engl J Med.* 1986;318:749–756.

Cullom DR, Chang B. *The Wills Eye Manual Office and Emergency Room Diagnosis and Treatment of Eye Disease.* Philadelphia: JB Lippincott; 1994.

Dascal A, Chan-Thim J, Morahan M, et al. Diagnosis of herpes simplex virus infection in a clinical setting by a direct antigen detection enzyme immunoassay kit. *J Clin Microbiol.* 1989;27:700–704.

Dawson CR. The herpetic eye study. *Arch Ophthamol.* 1990; 8:191–192.

Eggleston M. Therapy of ocular herpes simplex infections. *Infection Control.* 1987;8:294–296.

Evans AS, ed. *Viral Infections of Humans: Epidemiology and Control.* 3rd ed. New York: Plenum; 1989.

Falcon MG. Rational acyclovir therapy in herpetic eye disease. *Br J Ophthamol.* 1987;71:102–106.

Fingeret M, Casser L, Woodcome HT. *Atlas of Primary Eyecare Procedures.* Norwalk, CT: Appleton & Lange; 1990.

Glaser R, Gotlieb-Stematsky T. *Human Herpes Virus Infections: Clinical Aspects.* New York: Marcel Dekker; 1982.

Gordon JY. Pathogenesis and latency of herpes simplex virus type 1(HSV-1): An ophthamologist's view of the eye as a model for the study of virus–host relationship. *Adv Exp Med Biol.* 1990;278:205–209.

Ho M. Interferon as an agent against herpes simplex virus. *J Invest Dermatol.* 1990;95:158s–160s.

Hodge WG, et al. Herpes simplex virus keratitis among patients who are positive or negative for human immunodeficiency virus. *Ophthalmology.* 1997;104:120–124.

Knox MC, et al. Polymerase chain reaction–based assays of vitreous samples for the diagnosis of viral retinitis. *Ophthalmology.* 1998;105:37–45.

Kohl S. Herpes simplex virus. In: Feigin RD, Cherry JD (eds). *Textbook of Pediatric Infectious Diseases.* 4th ed. Philadelphia: WB Saunders; 1998.

Kowalski RP, et al. A comparison of enzyme immunoassay and polymerase chain reaction with the clinical examination for diagnosing ocular herpetic disease. *Ophthalmology.* 1993;100:530–533.

Langston D, Dunkel EC. A rapid clinical diagnostic test for herpes simplex infectious keratitis. *Am J Ophthamol.* 1989; 107:675–677.

Lee SF. Comparative laboratory diagnosis of experimental herpes simplex keratitis. *Am J Ophthamol.* 1990;109:8–12.

Leisegang TJ. Ocular herpes simplex infection: Pathogenesis and current therapy. *Mayo Clinic Proc.* 1988;63:1092–1105.

Mandell GL, Bennett JE, Dolin R. *Principles and Practice of Infectious Diseases.* New York: Churchill Livingstone; 1995.

Mannis MJ, Plotnick RD, Schwab IR, Newton RD. Herpes simplex dendritic keratitis after keratoplasty. *Am J Ophthamol.* 1991;111:480–484.

Mertz GJ, et al. Long-term acyclovir suppression of frequently recurring genital herpes simplex virus infection: A multicenter double-blind trial. *JAMA.* 1988;260:201–206.

Monnickendam MA. Herpes simplex virus ophthalmia. *Eye.* 1988;2:s56–s69.

Nesburn AB, et al. A therapeutic vaccine that reduces recurrent herpes simplex virus type 1 corneal disease. *Invest Ophthalmol Vis Sci.* 1998;39:1163–1170.

Pavan-Langston D. Herpes simplex virus ocular infections: Current concepts of acute, latent and reactivated disease. *Trans Am Ophthamol Soc.* 1990;88:727–793.

Pavan-Langston D, Dunkel EC. *Handbook of Ocular Drug Therapy and Ocular Side Effects of Systemic Drugs.* Boston: Little, Brown; 1991:158–181.

Pepose JS. External ocular herpes infections in immunodeficiency. *Curr Eye Res.* 1991;10:87–95.

Pepose JS. Herpes simplex keratitis: Role of viral infection versus immune response. *Surv Ophthamol.* 1991;35:345–352.

Rakel, RE. *Saunders Manual of Medical Practice.* Philadelphia: WB Saunders; 1996.

Roy FH. *Ocular Differential Diagnosis.* Baltimore: Williams & Wilkins; 1997.

Schacker T, et al. Herpes virus infections in human immunodeficiency virus–infected persons. In: DeVita VT, Hellman S, Rosenberg SA (eds). *AIDS: Biology, Diagnosis, Treatment and Prevention,* 4th ed. Philadelphia: Lippincott-Raven; 1997.

Sillis M. Clinical evaluation of enzyme immunoassay in rapid diagnosis of herpes simplex infection. *J Clin Pathol.* 1992;45:165–167.

Spruance SL, et al. Acyclovir prevents reactivation of herpes simplex labialis in skiers. *JAMA.* 1988;260:1597–1599.

Wilhelmus KR. Diagnosis and management of herpes simplex stromal keratitis. *Cornea.* 1987;6:286–291.

Wilhelmus KR, et al. Herpetic Eye Disease Study. A controlled trial of topical corticosteroids for herpes simplex stromal keratitis. *Ophthalmology.* 1994;101:1883–1896.

Yamamoto S, et al. Detection of herpes simplex virus DNA in human tear film by the polymerase chain reaction. *Am J Ophthalmol.* 1994;117:160–163.

Chapter 47

HERPES ZOSTER

Diane T. Adamczyk

Varicella zoster is a highly contagious virus that causes an infection, usually during childhood, known as varicella or chickenpox. It is characterized by a vesicular skin rash. Once the primary infection runs its course, the virus remains dormant in the sensory ganglia. Later in life the latent virus may reactivate as a secondary infection, herpes zoster (HZ) or shingles. The name is derived from the Greek words "herpein," which means to spread or to creep, and "zoster," which means girdle, zone, or sword belt.

Classically HZ manifests as a vesicular skin eruption along a dermatome or cranial nerve, with the potential for various complications, including painful postherpetic neuralgia (PHN). Most commonly, HZ affects the thoracic dermatome. Herpes zoster ophthalmicus (HZO) occurs when the virus affects the trigeminal nerve, specifically the ophthalmic division, with the potential for ocular complications.

EPIDEMIOLOGY

Systemic

Varicella/herpes zoster viral infection occurs worldwide. In the United States, almost all adults carry the HZ virus in a latent state, with serological evidence of a previous infection found in 95% (Liesegang, 1984).

In Western countries, the initial infection of varicella usually occurs in those younger than 15 years of age. In tropical or semitropical countries, varicella infection does not occur until an older age. This is particularly important in the development of congenital HZ, where the initial infection of varicella affects the pregnant woman, and subsequently the developing fetus.

In the United States, approximately 3 million cases of chickenpox occur per year, more commonly in the spring. Varicella results in approximately 100 deaths per year. Death occurs in 2 per 100,000 cases of healthy children, with more than a 15 times greater risk present in adults (Straus et al, 1988).

HZ has no sexual or seasonal predilection.

Blacks are one fourth less likely to have HZ than whites, when controlling for age, cancer, and demographic factors (Schmader et al, 1995). Since the occurrence of HZ is related to a decrease in an individual's cell-mediated immunity, those more frequently affected include the elderly, who experience a natural decline in immunity as a function of age, the immunocompromised, such as those with HIV/AIDS or cancer, and those undergoing immunosuppressive therapy, such as chemotherapy or radiation therapy, or chronic steroid use. HZ has a lifetime incidence of 10 to 20% (Stankus et al, 2000).

HZ usually affects those older than 50, with about 2.5 cases per 1000 from ages 20 to 49 years, 5 cases per 1000 for those 50 to 59, and 10 per 1000 for those 80 years and older (Hope-Simpson, 1965). There is an overall age-adjusted incidence of 130 cases per 100,000, with at least 300,000 cases per year occurring in the United States (Ragozzino et al, 1982). The chance of a patient experiencing a second attack of HZ is probably the same as a person of the same age, in the general population, experiencing a first attack. Up to 4% of patients with HZ have a second attack (Marsh, 1992).

HZ affects the thoracic region in over half of cases, followed by the cranial nerves in approximately 20% of cases, and then the cervical or lumbar region, with the sacral region least affected (Burgoon et al, 1957).

Postherpetic neuralgia (PHN) occurs in approximately 20% of HZ patients, with PHN affecting those 50 years and older 15 times more frequently (Stankus et al, 2000). PHN is found to affect 50% of those at 60 years and 75% of those at 70 (Watson & Evans, 1986). Cutaneous dissemination may occur in up to 26% of patients. Approximately half of these cases will have systemic involvement, that is, visceral (eg, pneumonitis) or neurologic (Straus et al, 1988).

Ocular

The range of involvement of the ophthalmic division of the trigeminal nerve varies from 8 to 56%, depending on the study. All or some of the branches of the ophthalmic division may be affected, with the frontal nerve (the supraorbital branch and then the supratrochlear) most commonly affected, followed by the nasociliary nerve. Occasionally the ophthalmic, along with the maxillary (second division), are involved, with all three divisions rarely affected (Edgerton, 1945).

Herpes zoster ophthalmicus (HZO) is almost always unilateral. Ocular complications may occur in 50 to 72% of the cases. In a series by Womack and Liesegang in 1983, ocular complications included lids (28% with only vesicle involvement and 13% with other lid involvement), cornea (55%), uveitis (43%), and postherpetic neuralgia (17%). Ophthalmoplegia may occur in up to one third of patients. In a study by Liesegang (1985), corneal involvement occurred in 65% of HZO patients. This involvement included punctate epithelial keratitis (51%), pseudodendrites (51%), corneal scarring (51%), anterior stromal infiltrates (41%), keratouveitis/endotheliitis (34%), neurotrophic keratitis (25%), mucous plaques (13%), exposure keratitis (11%), and disciform keratitis (10%).

PATHOPHYSIOLOGY/DISEASE PROCESS

Systemic

The Organism

The varicella zoster virus (human herpes virus 3) is a double-stranded DNA virus, surrounded by an envelope. Only one serotype for varicella exists, with the possibility of minor variations. In HZ, the virus can be isolated from the papules and clear vesicles up to 7 days after the rash, and longer in the immunosuppressed. The virus sheds up to 14 days. Crusted skin lesions do not contain any viable virus. The only natural host is humans.

Transmission

The primary infection of varicella occurs when the virus is spread by direct contact with a skin lesion of either varicella or herpes zoster, or is transmitted by inhaling infected airborne droplets (eg, from nasal or pharyngeal secretions). Varicella is highly contagious; however, moderately close contact must take place in order for transmission to occur. Transmission occurs in 61 to 87% of uninfected siblings, with less transmission occurring at school (Weller, 1983b). The incubation period is 14 to 17 days. The contagious period ranges from 2 days prior to the onset of the rash to the time the lesions are crusted in those immunocompetent, and slightly longer in the immunocompromised. Nonimmune individuals exposed to the virus are considered infectious for 10 to 21 days after exposure (Benenson, 1995; Lund, 1993).

Viral infection can occur only through enveloped virions, which are susceptible to physical or chemical agents. It is believed that the sensory ganglion is infected either through a hematogenous route or by the virus traveling from the skin to the nerves to the ganglion of the spinal or cranial nerves. It then remains in the ganglion in a latent state, unless reactivated.

> Nonimmune health care workers who are exposed to varicella-zoster virus should not work from day 10 after exposure to day 21, and nonimmune exposed children should be kept from school and/or public places at least 5 days after the rash erupts or until the vesicles dry.

HZ or shingles (the secondary infection) is a reactivation of the latent varicella virus. Effective regulatory mechanism and lack of susceptibility to trigger factors in HZ prevents frequent reactivation, as compared to herpes simplex (HS) (Straus, 1989). Viral reactivation is initiated when immunity is decreased. This occurs most commonly in a generally healthy elderly patient who has a normal age-related decrease in immunity. Reactivation also may occur with illnesses such as AIDS, tuberculosis, or syphilis; or chemotherapy, steroid use, irradiation, anticancer treatments, poisons, malignancy, physical or emotional trauma, stress, or surgery.

Although contact with a patient with varicella or HZ may result in HZ, it is unlikely, because lifelong immunity results from the initial infection. However, HZ may occur in a reexposed patient who, although previously infected with varicella, did not develop adequate immunity.

With reactivation, the virus replicates, follows the sensory nerve to the epidermis and dermis, accompanied by inflammation. Viral replication is greatest within the first 72 hours, and then decreases. HZ patients do not have infectious respiratory secretions and therefore are less contagious than varicella patients.

Course of the Disease

Varicella. Varicella is characterized by itching, fever, and vesicular skin lesions. The skin lesions affect the epidermis and heal within 2 weeks usually without scarring. The lesions initially present as macules with edema, followed by papules, and then vesicles with a surrounding red areolar area, and finally crusting, without sequelae. However, occasionally the lesions become pustular, punched out, painful ulcers. An uncomplicated, self-limiting course of varicella usually occurs in healthy children. Infants, adults, and immunocompromised individuals may be at increased risk for complications (eg, encephalitis, pneumonia, and death).

Herpes Zoster. With reactivation of the varicella virus, HZ manifestations may be categorized into prodromal, acute, and postherpetic phases (Table 47–1). The prodromal phase may precede the acute phase by hours to days.

The acute phase is characterized by grouped skin lesions that follow the affected dermatome (Figure 47–1) or cranial nerve, with the potential to affect adjacent areas. The lesions are usually unilateral and rarely bilateral. An occasional vesicle may affect an area other than the dermatome, possibly resulting from a hematogenous spread of the virus. Skin hypersensitivity (hyperesthesia) is usually present with the rash. Because both the dermis and epidermis are involved, scarring may result in HZ because of involvement of the deeper skin layers.

In mild cases, vesicles may not form, with only an erythematous maculopapule forming that resolves in 7 to 10 days. In severe cases the lesions may become gangrenous, sometimes taking weeks to heal. Generally, the cutaneous lesions are self-limiting, clearing within 1 to 3 weeks. The severity and duration is usually less in the young. Occasionally no skin lesions form, but reactivation occurs, with positive serologic evidence, which is called zoster sine herpete.

Accompanying the acute phase is an increase in the antibody titers of IgG, IgM, and IgA. These are present for 2 to 5 days after the skin rash, peaking at 2 to 3 weeks (Weller, 1983a). Also present is an acute inflammation that usually lasts 8 to 14 days, accompanied by pain. The acute pain may be the result of viral invasion to the nerve and from the associated inflammatory reaction. This inflammatory process may explain why pain is more common and severe in HZ than herpes simplex. The pain is often greater and lasts longer in the elderly. There is no apparent association with the skin lesions, and it may be brought on by simply touching the area.

A serious complication of HZ is postherpetic neuralgia, which affects the thoracic dermatome and the ophthalmic nerve most commonly. This is a persistent, boring pain that follows (usually 1 month after) the acute phase of the disease. PHN increases with age, and is rarely seen in those younger than 40 years. It may occur spontaneously or be precipitated by light touch or clothing. This unrelenting pain may result in mood changes, antisocial behavior, and severe depression or suicidal tendencies. It is not known if the depression is part of the disease process or a result of the severe pain. PHN resolves in 1 to 3 months in approximately half the patients. About 20% continue to suffer with PHN beyond a year.

Generally HZ is a self-limited disease. In those younger than 20 years, the course is usually less severe and of a shorter duration (approximately 2 weeks), than that seen in older patients (in which the disease may persist for months). After resolution, reduced sensitivity or numbness may continue over

TABLE 47–1. PHASES OF HERPES ZOSTER (SHINGLES)

Prodromal Phase	
Malaise	GI disturbance (eg, nausea)
Headache	Chills
Fever	Anorexia
Dysesthesia/hyperesthesia	Itch
Tingling	Increased skin temperature
Burning	Pain (deep, boring, sharp, lancing; constant or intermittent)
Redness	
Acute Phase	
Variable patterns of pain	
Hypersensitivity and decreasing dysesthesia	
Unilateral, grouped skin lesions, following a dermatome[a]	
Erythematous papules and edema (in 12–24 hours)	
Vesicular lesion, with erythematous base (in 72 hours), may have turbid yellow fluid or hemorrhagic changes	
Pustule, with less erythema (in 7–8 days)	
Crust (in 10–12 days)	
Crust falls off (in 14–21 days)	
Postherpetic Neuralgia	
Steady, boring, burning, lancing pain	
May be accompanied by insomnia, anorexia, lassitude, or depression	

[a]In part modified from Burgoon et al, 1957.

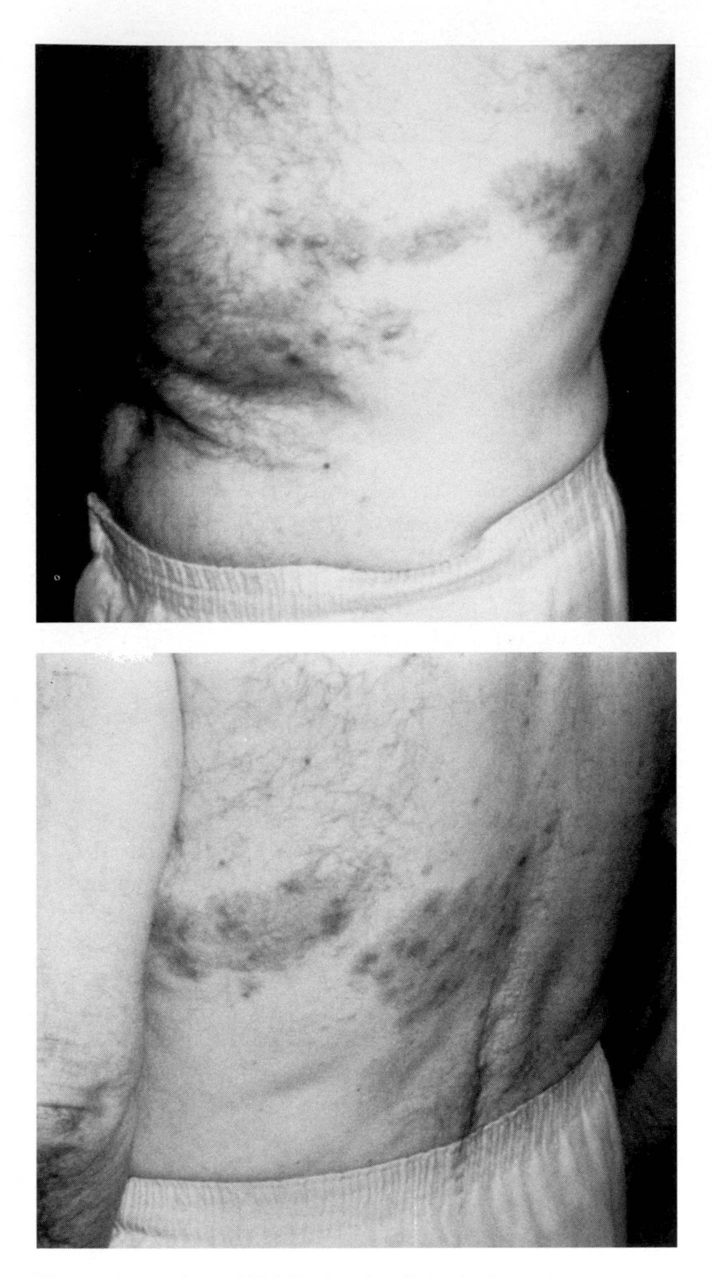

Figure 47–1. Acute HZ following the thoracic dermatome.

the affected areas, along with a tingling or painful sensation brought on by wind or cold air.

HZ is usually a localized disease. However simultaneous, multiple areas (eg, ophthalmic and thoracic) may rarely be involved (HZ generalisatus). Disseminated disease, which may include multisystemic involvement, increases with age, resulting from viral spread either through direct or hematogenous routes (Table 47–2). Rarely, dissemination may result in cerebral angiitis, myelitis, or meningoencephalitis, leading to death. In the immunosuppressed, HZ may occur more commonly, with severe skin dissemination and neurological complications.

TABLE 47–2. SYSTEMIC MANIFESTATIONS OF VARICELLA AND HERPES ZOSTER

Varicella (Chickenpox)
- Itch
- Fever
- Vesicular lesions
- Complications: encephalitis, pneumonia

Herpes Zoster (Shingles)
- Vesicular rash along a dermatome
- Fever
- Headache
- Depression
- Lymphadenopathy
- Mucous membrane lesions
- Complications
    - Visceral organs (rare)
        - Lungs—pneumonitis
        - Liver—hepatitis
        - Bladder—urinary retention
        - Heart—myocarditis, endocarditis
    - Central nervous system
        - Bell palsy
        - Myelitis (rare)
        - Meningoencephalitis (rare)
    - Vasculitis
        - Cerebral angiitis: stroke or contralateral hemiplegia (unique to HZO)
        - Segmental granulomatous arteritis (carotid or internal cerebral artery)
    - Skeleton—arthritis
    - Miscellaneous: delirium and hallucination

Ocular

Varicella. The primary infection of varicella may involve the ocular area. Ocular involvement may commonly include conjunctivitis along with other manifestations (Table 47–3).

Herpes Zoster. Herpes zoster ophthalmicus (HZO) results from a reactivation of the virus in the trigeminal/gasserian ganglion, affecting the ophthalmic division (Figure 47–2). This division may be more commonly affected because of the increased potential for it to be exposed to trauma. However, the nasociliary nerve of the ophthalmic division is often the site for the most serious ocular complications. HZO is classically characterized by unilateral skin lesions that do not cross the midline, accompanied by hyperesthesia and preauricular lymphadenopathy.

Viral dissemination occurs more commonly in HZO than any other HZ presentation. Viral spread may affect adjacent areas to the trigeminal ganglion such as the brainstem or carotid artery. Death may rarely result.

TABLE 47–3. OCULAR MANIFESTATIONS OF VARICELLA AND HERPES ZOSTER

Varicella

- Conjunctivitis
- Eyelid vesicular lesions
- Limbal/conjunctival vesicles
- Superficial punctate keratopathy
- Stromal disciform keratitis
- Rare: anterior uveitis, retinitis, secondary glaucoma, optic neuritis, cataract

Herpes Zoster

- **Ophthalmic division of the trigeminal nerve**[a]
  - Frontal nerve
    - Upper lid
    - Superior conjunctiva
    - Forehead
    - Midline of scalp
  - Lacrimal nerve
    - Lacrimal gland
    - Conjunctiva
    - Skin of the upper lid (external 1/3 of eyelid)
  - Nasociliary nerve
    - Choroid
    - Conjunctiva
    - Cornea
    - Lacrimal sac
    - Sclera
    - Iris
    - Skin of the lids (inner 1/3 of the upper lid)
    - Anterior and posterior ethmoid sinuses
    - Vesicle tip of the nose (Hutchinson sign)
- **Ocular complications**
  - Skin/lids
    - Skin lesions (papule, vesicle, pustule, crust)
    - Ptosis
    - Secondary staphylococcal aureus infection
    - Complications secondary to scarring: ectropion, entropion, punctal eversion, madarosis, poliosis, trichiasis, distichiasis, lagophthalmos, exposure keratitis, lid retraction, meibomian damage
  - Conjunctiva
    - Conjunctivitis (mucopurulent)
    - Mucous membrane lesions: conjunctiva, nose, and mouth
    - Conjunctival vesicles (associated pain, photophobia, lacrimation)
    - Petechial hemorrhages
    - Pseudomembrane (rare)
    - Symblepharon (rare)
- **Ocular complications (con't)**
  - Cornea, early
    - Punctate epithelial keratitis (first week)
    - Pseudodendrite (first 2 weeks)
  - Cornea, late
    - Anterior stromal infiltrates (1–3 weeks)
    - Mucous adherent plaques (any time, usually 8–12 weeks)
    - Sclerokeratitis (1–3 months) (rare)
    - Keratouveitis/endotheliitis (1–21 days) (may last days to years)
    - Serpiginous ulcerations (2–20 weeks) (rare)
    - Disciform keratitis (1–9 months)
    - Neurotrophic keratitis (3–21 days)
    - Exposure keratitis (anytime, usually 2–3 months)
    - Corneal scarring
  - Inflammation
    - Episcleritis
    - Iritis
    - Scleritis: (rare) diffuse or nodular
  - IOP
    - Hypotony
    - Acute and chronic glaucoma
  - Pupil
    - Pupil distortion
    - Horner syndrome
    - Light-near dissociation
  - EOM
    - Ophthalmoplegia—3rd (most common), 6th, or 4th nerve palsy
  - Retina/optic nerve (rare)
    - Acute retinal necrosis
    - Progressive outer retinal necrosis
    - Neuroretinitis
    - Vascular occlusion
    - Choroidal/retinal detachment
    - Choroiditis
    - Optic neuritis
    - Thrombophlebitis
  - Miscellaneous
    - Iris sector atrophy
    - Iris cyst formation
    - Hypopyon
    - Cataract
    - Sympathetic ophthalmia/phthisis bulbi (rare)
    - Heterochromia irides
    - Proptosis
    - Anterior chamber hemorrhage
    - Dacryoadenitis, canaliculitis

[a]When the maxillary division is affected, the skin and conjunctiva of the lower lid may be affected, along with other structures in this region.

Ocular structures are affected by HZ from direct viral invasion and replication into the eye, secondary inflammation, or autoimmune reactions. Ocular complications are not dependent on age and affect up to 70% of patients. They usually occur during or after the skin involvement, within the first 2 weeks. These complications may resolve without sequelae or may result in a poor visual outcome. Specific areas of ocular involvement or those unique to HZO will be described below (see Table 47–3).

Pain. Postherpetic neuralgia is common and especially severe in those affected by HZO. The elderly and those who have persistent, moderate to severe pain at presentation may be more inclined to PHN. However, PHN may still occur even in the absence of acute pain.

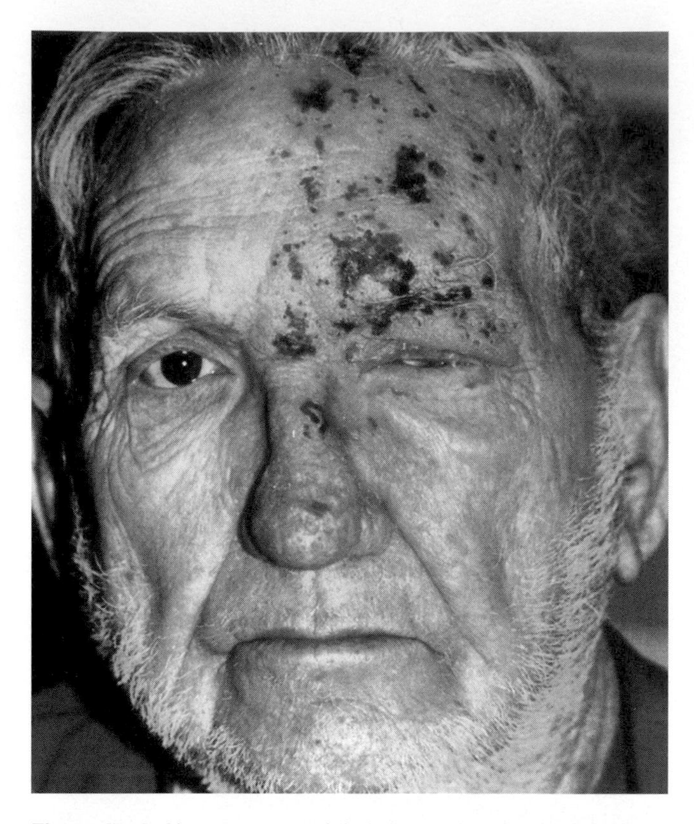

Figure 47–2. Herpes zoster ophthalmicus with a classic clinical presentation. *(Reprinted with permission from Looney B. Herpes zoster ophthalmicus.* Clin Eye Vision Care. *1997;9:204.)*

Skin/Lid. The vesicles found in HZO are usually smaller and more numerous than those found elsewhere (Figure 47–3). Although the lesions do not cross the midline, the edema may. An acute inflammation may accompany the skin lesions, along with a secondary staphylococcal aureus infection. A classic sign of nasociliary nerve involvement is Hutchinson sign (a vesicle at the tip of the nose).

Other lid involvement of HZ includes scarring, often more severe in this area, and ptosis. Lid scarring may result in a number of manifestations such as entropion, ectropion, exposure keratitis, and trichiasis, with a secondary epithelial keratopathy. Ptosis may occur secondary to the edema or from affected sympathetic innervation to the levator. Usually the ptosis is transient, but occasionally it may be permanent.

Conjunctiva. Conjunctivitis is a common ocular manifestation of HZO. It usually has a rapid resolution that does not require treatment.

Cornea. Corneal involvement is a frequent ocular manifestation of HZO. It is uncertain if the virus arrives via the lid margin, conjunctiva, or from the corneal nerves. Corneal complications may result from viral replication, denervation, lid abnormalities, decreased blink, abnormal tear film, hypoesthesia, neurotrophic damage, corneal exposure, and inflammation. Localized decreased corneal sensation is a hallmark of HZO. Many corneal manifestations will resolve without treatment or sequelae (Figure 47–4); others however, if left untreated, could potentially lead to vision loss.

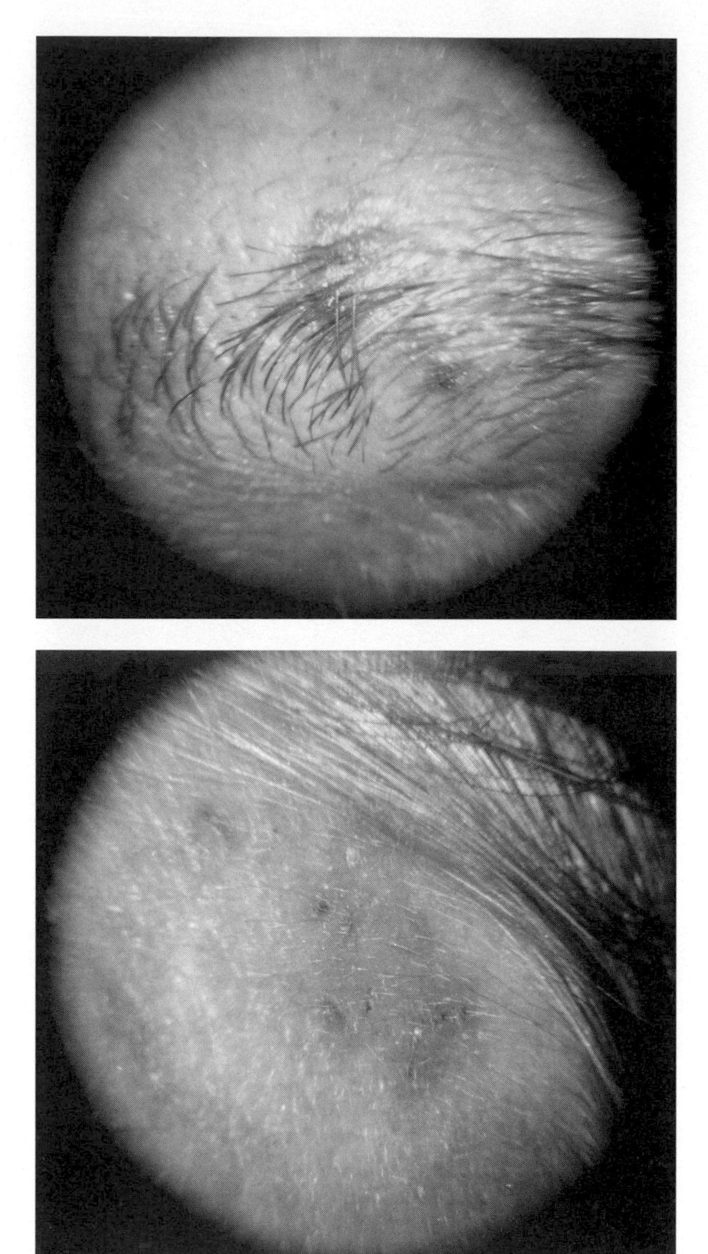

Figure 47–3. HZO affecting the frontal nerve of the ophthalmic division.

Corneal involvement may be divided into early (2 to 4 weeks) manifestations, which are generally self-limited; and late manifestations. Early involvement

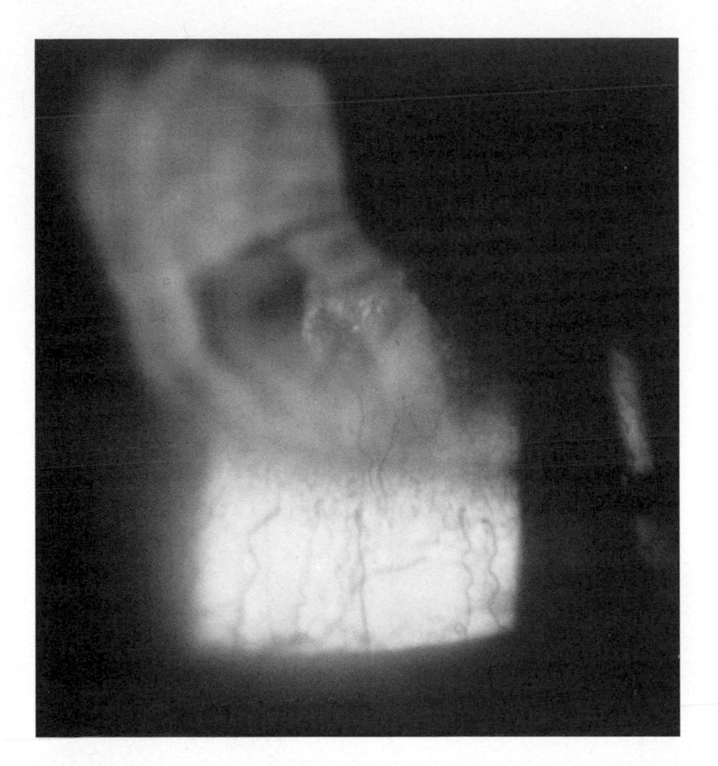

Figure 47–4. HZ corneal scar. (*Courtesy of Optometry Service, FDR VA Hospital, Montrose, NY.*)

may be the result of direct viral assault and its sequelae. Late involvement may reflect an immune reaction or an inflammatory response.

The following discussion of corneal complications is a compilation from Liesegang (1985) and Cobo (1988) (see Table 47–3). Early corneal manifestations include punctate epithelial keratitis (PEK) and zoster pseudodendrites (Figure 47–5). Both involve corneal epithelial cells, which are probably where viral replication occurs. Positive viral cultures still occur at this stage.

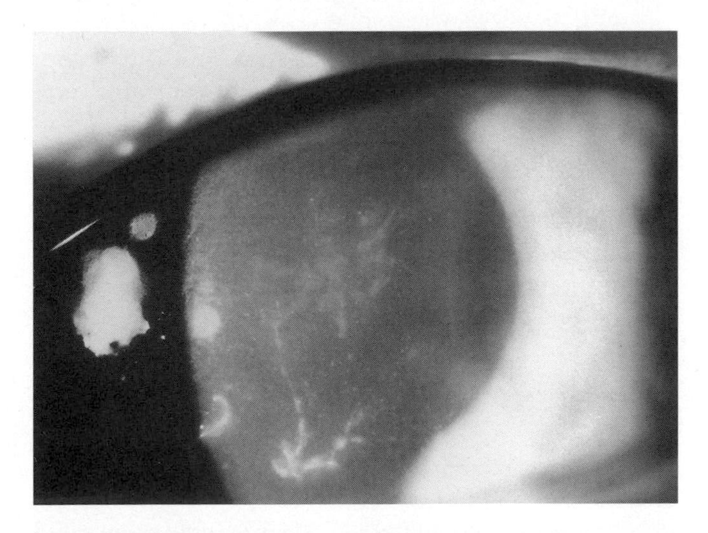

Figure 47–5. Pseudodendritic epithelial keratitis in HZO. *(Reprinted with permission from Looney B. Herpes zoster ophthalmicus.* Clin Eye Vision Care. *1997;9:204.)*

Punctate epithelial keratitis is an area of elevated, swollen epithelial cells, with or without stromal edema, which are usually multiple and peripherally located. PEK is self-limiting and is believed to be an early form of a pseudodendrite. The pseudodendrite is composed of peripherally located swollen epithelial cells, with a gray-white, dendritic pattern. Pseudodendrites are self-limited, usually resolving within days or up to a month.

Mucous adherent plaques are sometimes confused with the early zoster pseudodendrite. They may occur anywhere on the cornea, or can be found over the areas of chronic stromal inflammation. It is believed that tear film instability and epithelial changes play a role in their formation. No viruses are found in these self-limited lesions. They are flat to slightly elevated, gray-white plaques, sharply demarcated, and variable in size and configuration (e.g., linear or branched).

Anterior stromal infiltrates, which are an early form of stromal keratitis, also known as nummular keratitis, are often associated with a pseudodendrite or PEK. These lesions are located in the periphery, under the Bowman membrane, and are 1 to 2 mm in diameter. When the subepithelial infiltrates are limited to a sector of the cornea, a branch of the corneal nerve may be affected. They may follow a variable course, but usually resolve with minimal treatment. Nummular scars usually do not affect vision.

Disciform keratitis may result from stromal keratitis, weeks to months after the initial onset. It presents clinically as a focal, well-demarcated, mid to deep stromal infiltration, with localized stromal edema, located either centrally or peripherally. Disciform keratitis may lead to interstitial keratitis, with neovascularization and scarring.

Rarely will corneal involvement include serpiginous ulcers or sclerokeratitis. Serpiginous ulcers are crescent shaped, peripherally located, and can potentially lead to thinning and perforation.

Decreased corneal sensation is usually localized, may be brief or last months to years, and may lead to neurotrophic keratopathy. Neurotrophic keratopathy can lead to a pannus or scar formation, or an ulcer with the potential for decreased vision, perforation, or loss of the eye.

Inflammation and Intraocular Pressure. Inflammation, particularly of the anterior segment, is a common clinical manifestation of HZO. It may occur any time in the disease process. Iritis/iridocyclitis occurs in less than half the patients. It is associated with the classic signs and symptoms, and is usually mild and self-limited (in 6 to 12 months), with only the severe cases resulting in serious sequelae. The intraocular pressure may be either increased, from inflammation, debris, or synechiae, or decreased, from necrosis of the ciliary body. Pressure increases may manifest acutely or chronically, with glaucoma resulting from chronically increased intraocular pressure (IOP).

Pupil. Localized ischemic changes may result in pupil distortion. Sympathetic nerve and ciliary ganglion involvement may result in Horner syndrome or a light near dissociation pupil, respectively.

Extraocular Muscle. Extraocular muscle (EOM) involvement is generally seen in patients who are older than 40 years. It may occur at any time in the disease process, even weeks or months after the onset, but it usually takes place when the skin lesions scar. The patient may be asymptomatic or complain of diplopia. The third cranial nerve (total or partial involvement) is most frequently affected, followed by the sixth or the fourth nerves. It generally is self-limited, resolving in 2 months, although rarely it may be permanent.

Retina and Optic Nerve. Retinal and optic nerve manifestations of HZO are generally rare, with poor visual prognosis. Varicella zoster virus is a cause of acute retinal necrosis (ARN) syndrome (Browning et al, 1987; Culbertson et al, 1986) and progressive outer retinal necrosis (PORN).

DIAGNOSIS

The diagnosis of varicella/HZ is typically based on clinical presentation, specifically the characteristic skin lesions and their distribution, along with history and physical exam. See Table 47–4 for the differential diagnosis. Other tests, though less frequently used, may assist in the diagnosis. These include the Tzanck technique, a nonspecific test for herpetic infection, which stains material from the base of the vesicle; skin biopsy; viral culture (which is definitive, but slow); serum conversion; antibody titers; enzyme-linked immunosorbent assay (ELISA), used for serodiagnosis; fluorescein antibody membrane antigen (FAMA) test, used for serodiagnosis; serological tests; and immunofluorescent and immunoenzyme stains (see Table 47–5).

TABLE 47–4. DIFFERENTIAL DIAGNOSTIC CONSIDERATIONS: HERPES ZOSTER (SYSTEMIC AND OCULAR)

Herpes simplex
Impetigo
Rubeola
Bacterial infections with skin (vesicular/pustular) lesions
Mumps
Vaccinia

TABLE 47–5. DIAGNOSTIC TESTING FOR VARICELLA/HERPES ZOSTER

Tissue culture
Tzanck smear
Direct immunofluorescence
Polymerase chain reaction (PCR) (ocular use)
Assays/serologic tests:
Enzyme-linked immunosorbent assay (ELISA) (most common)
Radioimmunoassay (RIA)
Fluorescent antibody-to-membrane antigen (FAMA)
Latex agglutination
Indirect fluorescent antibody
Complement fixation

Systemic

A general physical exam, including chest x-ray and blood workup, should be a part of the management of a HZ patient. This will assist in ruling out any underlying systemic disease with associated decreased immunity. When dissemination has occurred, referral and workup by the appropriate specialist is recommended. In addition, HZ in a patient younger than 45 may indicate underlying HIV infection (Sandor et al, 1986).

Ocular

Diagnosis of specific ocular manifestations of HZ is made through a complete eye health evaluation. Corneal evaluation includes biomicroscopy and use of fluorescein and rose bengal dyes, along with testing for corneal anesthesia (eg, esthesiometer). Diagnostic features of specific corneal involvement is as follows.

PEK stains poorly with fluorescein or rose bengal. Pseudodendrites differ from the true dendrite of simplex, in that they are broader, without central ulceration and rounded raised borders. Consequently pseudodendrites do not stain with fluorescein and stain more with rose bengal. Herpes simplex stains centrally with fluorescein, in an area excavated, with no epithelium, and with rose bengal at the ulcer border. Mucous adherent plaques of HZ stain uniformly with rose bengal, but poorly with fluorescein.

TREATMENT AND MANAGEMENT

Table 47–6 summarizes varicella and HZ treatment and management.

In the United States, in 1995, a live attenuated varicella virus vaccine became available to immunize those who have not had chickenpox. By 13 years of

TABLE 47–6. TREATMENT AND MANAGEMENT OF VARICELLA AND HERPES ZOSTER

Varicella
- Vaccine
- Varicella-zoster immune globulin (prophylaxis)
- Supportive palliative care
- Isolation of patient
- Analgesics (avoid aspirin)
- Oral acyclovir (within 24 hours of rash)

Herpes Zoster
- Complete physical, if <45 years, rule out concurrent HIV infection
- **General therapies**
  - Acyclovir: 800 mg, 5 times/day, for 7–10 days; (within 72 hours of skin lesions)
    - Side effects: GI disturbances (nausea, vomiting, diarrhea), headache, bone marrow suppression, lethargy, seizure, transient increases serum creatinine, and nephrotoxicity.
    - If concurrent HIV infection, hospitalize for IV acyclovir
  - Famciclovir: 500 mg tid, for 7–10 days (within 72 hours of skin lesions)
    - Side effects: HA, nausea, vomiting, dizziness, abdominal pain
  - Valacyclovir: 1000 mg, tid for 7–10 days (within 72 hours of skin lesions)
    - Side effects: HA, nausea, vomiting, dizziness, abdominal pain
  - Steroid: Immunocompetent, <60 years: 60–80 mg/day, for 7–10 days, then taper over additional 2 weeks
    - Use with caution, questionable efficacy >60 years: treat concurrently with ACV, to decrease the risk of dissemination
    - Side effects: viral dissemination, cataracts, increased IOP, recurrences, prolonged disease, decreased immunity, risk of concurrent bacterial, fungal or herpes simplex disease, others
- **Skin lesions**
  - Cloth soaked with cool/warm water
  - Burow solution (5% aluminum acetate)
  - Calamine lotion
  - Silver nitrate 0.25%
  - Oral antihistamine
  - Topical antibiotic ointment
- **Acute pain**
  - ACV
  - Analgesics
  - Capsaicin cream (Zostrix)
  - Steroid
  - Nonsteroidal anti-inflammatory drugs
  - Narcotics
  - Antidepressants
  - Anticonvulsants
  - Unsubstantiated use: amantadine, cimetidine
  - Local anesthetics (e.g., stellate ganglion block)
- **Postherpetic neuralgia**
  - Steroid
  - Capsaicin cream (Zostrix)
  - Tricyclic antidepressants (e.g., amitriptyline HCl, 10 mg/d initial, increase to 50–75 mg/d prn)
  - Anticonvulsant: Gabapentin
  - Combination anticonvulsant and tricyclic antidepressant (e.g., amitriptyline HCl, 25 mg/d, plus carbamazepine 200 mg/d)
  - Local anesthetics (e.g., lidocaine (Xylocaine) patch, somatic or sympathetic block)
  - Surgery
- **Miscellaneous treatments**
  - Pain
    - Neuroaugmentation (e.g., ultrasound, acupuncture)
    - Neurosurgical procedures (e.g., neurectomy)
    - Cryoanalgesia (dry ice)
  - Other Potential antiviral agents
    - Sorivudine (BV-ara U)
    - Brivudin (bromovinyl deoxyuridine)
    - Cidofovir
- **Ocular treatment**
  - *Note*: concentration and frequency of topical agents are dependent on the severity of the disease, with topical ACV 3% prescribed 5 times per day
  - Lids
    - Trichiasis: cryotherapy
    - En/ectropion: lid surgery
    - Skin lesions/scarring: oral ACV
  - Cornea
    - Epithelial disease: topical and oral ACV
    - Punctate epithelial keratopathy: monitor
    - Pseudodendrite: monitor, oral ACV
    - Mucoid adherent plaques: monitor, topical steroids, lubricants, mucolytics (acetylcysteine)
    - Keratitis: oral and topical ACV; steroid
    - Stromal disease: monitor (e.g., anterior stromal infiltrates), steroids, oral ACV
    - Ulcer: steroid, topical ACV
    - Disciform keratopathy: steroid
    - Neurotrophic keratopathy: lubricants, mucolytic agents, soft contact lens, tape lids or for more severe cases; tarsorrhaphy, cyanoacrylate glue patch conjunctival flap or botulinous toxin-induced ptosis,(steroids should be avoided or used with caution), patient education
    - Exposure keratopathy: tarsorrhaphy, conjunctival flap
    - Corneal perforation: penetrating keratoplasty
    - Corneal scar: penetrating or lamellar keratoplasty
    - Patient education: monitor for redness, decreased vision, lack of corneal luster
  - Inflammation
    - Episcleritis: monitor, topical vasoconstrictor, steroid
    - Keratouveitis: topical ACV, steroid
    - Iritis: steroids, mydriatics
    - Secondary glaucoma: e.g., beta blocker, epinephrine; topical steroid
    - Scleritis: steroid, NSAIDs
    - Uveitis: oral ACV, steroid, cycloplegic
    - Optic neuritis: ACV, steroid
  - Ophthalmoplegia
    - Monitor
    - Persistent diplopia: prism or occlusion
    - Proptosis, contralateral hemiplegia: oral steroid
  - Retina
    - Acute retinal necrosis: IV ACV, steroids (oral prednisone), aspirin, laser photocoagulation

Abbreviations: ACV, acyclovir; d, day; GI gastrointestinal; HA, headache; HCl, hydrogen chloride; HIV, human immunodeficiency virus; IOP, intraocular pressure; IV, intravenous; mg, milligram; prn, as required; tid, three times a day.

age, if not exposed naturally to the virus, vaccination should occur. A single subcutaneous dose is given to children 12 months to 12 years of age, and two doses, administered 4 to 8 weeks apart, are given to those 13 years and older (Nightingale, 1995; Stover & Bratcher, 1998). A 10-year postvaccination study showed seroconversion in 97.9 or 93.5% (dose-dependent), with a modified chickenpox occurring in 2 to 3% (Johnson et al, 1997).

Pregnant women should not be vaccinated, and pregnancy should be deferred for 1 to 3 months after vaccination. Salicylates should be avoided for 6 weeks after vaccination. Adverse reactions to the vaccination include a mild generalized rash, pain, swelling, and induration at the injection site (Nightingale, 1995; Stover & Bratcher, 1998).

In patients vaccinated, there is little to no viremia, which contrasts the presence of viremia in those who acquire varicella naturally. Since there is usually no viremia associated with the vaccine, there is less chance that the vaccine virus will become latent in the ganglia, thereby decreasing the possibility of herpes zoster developing at a later date. If HZ does develop in those vaccinated, its clinical presentation is mild. When a large dose of the vaccine is given or in those who are immunocompromised, viremia and a rash may occur. Although questions have arisen as to waning immunity after vaccination, no evidence supports this (Liesegang, 1999).

Systemic

Varicella

Treatment and management of the primary infection of varicella or chickenpox is nonspecific, including palliative measures, compresses, and appropriate hygiene. Because varicella is highly contagious, measures should be taken to prevent spread to noninfected or immunocompromised individuals. This includes isolation of the infected patient or prophylactic use of varicella-zoster immune globulin (VZIG) within 96 hours of exposure, to modify or prevent the disease in susceptible individuals (such as the nonimmune, immunocompromised, or pregnant patient). In addition, aspirin should not be used because of its association with Reye syndrome. The exact pathogenesis of Reye syndrome is not known, but it has been associated with influenza or varicella and the use of salicylates, often leading to death. Oral acyclovir may be used in the treatment of chickenpox in healthy children. It simply hastens the healing time that would otherwise naturally occur (Dunkle et al, 1991).

Herpes Zoster

Management of HZ may include monitoring the patient or use of antiviral medications. As with varicella, appropriate hygiene and precautions should be taken. These include patient isolation from those never infected with the virus or from those immunocompromised, along with the use of gloves, until the lesions have crusted and the potential for spread has decreased.

The treatment of herpes zoster has been revolutionized with the antiviral agent acyclovir (ACV). ACV affects DNA synthesis through inhibition of DNA polymerase, resulting in decreased viral replication. ACV has replaced other antiviral medications as the drug of choice, with oral treatment generally safe for both the immunocompetent and immunosuppressed. Unlike ACV, other antiviral drugs such as idoxuridine are nonselective. Vidarabine has the same mechanism of action as ACV, but is not as specific.

> To be effective, antiviral medications should be given within 72 hours of the onset of the rash.

ACV affects viral cells as opposed to host cells. This specificity decreases its toxic side effects (see Table 47–6), making it a well-tolerated drug. ACV is most effective when used early in the course of the disease, within 3 days of the onset of the skin lesions, when it inhibits viral replication and dissemination. Although ACV's action is on the family of herpes viruses, a much higher concentration is needed for the varicella virus than the simplex virus. Consequently, high dosage is most effective in HZ.

ACV decreases acute pain (with no evidence of an affect on PHN), skin dissemination and duration, as well as providing a more expedient resolution of the signs and symptoms. Disseminated disease (eg, central nervous system involvement) or concurrent infection with HIV is usually treated with intravenous ACV.

Other antiviral drugs include valacyclovir and famciclovir. These drugs, along with acyclovir, are guanosine analogues. Valacyclovir is a prodrug of acyclovir, which once absorbed is cleaved to acyclovir. In comparison to acyclovir, it has an enhanced gastrointestinal absorption. Famciclovir is a prodrug of penciclovir. It has a prolonged half-life, with similar action to acyclovir. Both valacyclovir and famciclovir have a dosage of three times a day for 7 days. The choice of antiviral drug is individualized, with dosage and cost being potential factors.

Steroids used during the acute phase of HZ decrease inflammation, necrosis, and scarring. However, steroids have questionable effectivity, and can possibly cause numerous side effects. Oral ACV may be used in conjunction with steroids to decrease the potential of dissemination. In the immunosuppressed, steroids are generally contraindicated. However, if their use is needed, discontinuation with tapering should begin as soon as possible.

Skin Lesions

Specific lotions, ointments, or solutions may be used to sooth and soften the crusts of skin lesions. These include Burow solution (5% aluminum acetate), which provides a mildly antiseptic, drying effect; silver nitrate 0.25%, which provides a germicidal, astringent effect, but stains the skin brown; calamine lotion; and a cloth soaked with water to help remove exudates. In addition, oral antihistamines may be used to decrease itching, and antibiotic ointments may be used if bacterial infection is present.

Acute Pain and Postherpetic Neuralgia

Treatment for pain in HZ, both acute and postherpetic, remains a clinical challenge, often being ineffective or lacking supportive studies. Topical capsaicin (derived from the nightshade plant) cream (Zostrix) has been promising in decreasing acute and persistent pain. Its mechanism of action is related to substance P (a sensory or pain transmitter), which capsaicin depletes within several weeks of use (2 to 4 weeks), resulting in pain relief. The patient may continue to be pain free after discontinuation of capsaicin. However, some, particularly the elderly suffering from PHN, may need to continue with treatment indefinitely.

Other treatments for pain and PHN include analgesics, steroids, tricyclic antidepressants, and anticonvulsants. Gabapentin, an anticonvulsant, has shown promise as an effective treatment for the pain and sleep disturbances found with PHN (Rowbotham et al, 1998).

Local anesthetics, such as stellate ganglion blocks, appear to have good results in acute pain and should be reserved for use in certain cases not successfully treated by other means. The administration of local anesthetics, however, should be done by one experienced with the technique, such as an anesthesiologist. Neurosurgical techniques, as with sympathetic blocks, should only be considered as a final alternative in the most debilitating cases. Topical lidocaine (Xylocaine) patches may also reduce pain.

Disseminated Disease

For disseminated HZ disease, co-management with the respective specialist for the area involved is appropriate. In addition, a complete physical, with blood workup and chest x-ray should be done to rule out underlying disease, such as tuberculosis and malignancy. In patients younger than 45 years with no apparent cause for HZ, an evaluation should be done to rule out HIV infection.

Ocular

Varicella

The ocular treatment of varicella is as described in the systemic section. Iritis and keratitis may be treated with mydriatics. Cautious use of steroids may be efficacious for late interstitial keratitis.

Herpes Zoster

Ocular complications of HZ may be managed with systemic antivirals, steroids (topical or systemic), or specific treatment modalities dependent on the type of manifestation (see Table 47–6).

ACV has been noted to influence the incidence and severity of eye complications, including anterior uveitis, corneal disease, and lid scarring. Prompt ACV treatment is important for effectivity and is as discussed previously. Topical ACV 3% has shown inconsistent but favorable results in corneal disease. It is well tolerated, with few side effects including punctate keratopathy and burning. It is the antiviral drug of choice based on its ocular penetrance, where available.

Treatment with ACV is specific for the herpes virus; therefore, any inflammatory or immunologic process would need steroidal treatment. Steroids should be used cautiously, as noted previously, particularly in the immunosuppressed and in those with the potential for exacerbating a herpes simplex infection.

Pain

For control of pain (acute and persistent), stellate ganglion blocks have shown positive results in HZO. Ganglion blocks appear to decrease the course of the disease, relieve pain, and prevent PHN. Patients usually show relief of pain after 1 to 5 blocks (Currey & Dalsania, 1991). The mechanism of action is not known.

Lids and Skin

Lotions or ointment may be used for the periocular cutaneous lesions. If cicatricial lid retraction is present, skin graft or tarsorrhaphy may be needed.

Cornea

Punctate epithelial keratopathy and pseudodendrites are generally self-limited. However, because of viral presence, oral ACV may act prophylactically to decrease the progression of PEK to pseudodendrites.

Mucoid adherent plaques, sometimes associated with stromal inflammation and tear abnormalities, are also often self-limiting. Treatment ranges from monitoring only, to lubricants and mucolytics, or topical steroids.

Stromal involvement (anterior stromal infiltrates) may only need to be monitored. Topical steroids should only be used in cases of decreased vision, associated uveitis, secondary increased IOP from inflammation, and chronic stromal disease.

Various treatment modalities are recommended for neurotrophic keratopathy. Patients with decreased corneal sensation should be closely monitored and educated to the possible sequelae of neurotrophic complications (e.g., redness, decreased VA, change in corneal luster).

Penetrating keratoplasty was once not considered a treatment option for certain corneal manifestations because HZ patients were considered poor candidates because of affected corneal sensation and associated lid and tear disturbances. However, studies (Reed et al, 1989; Soong et al, 1989) have shown promising results in select patients, who receive careful postoperative management.

CONCLUSION

Almost every person is infected with the varicella-zoster virus in childhood, which usually follows a benign course. Reactivation of the latent virus, herpes zoster, occurs more commonly in the elderly and immunosuppressed population, and follows a more debilitating course, with the potential for long-standing sequelae. HZ has a number of clinical manifestations, including painful postherpetic neuralgia. Herpes zoster ophthalmicus occurs when reactivation affects the ophthalmic division of the trigeminal nerve, with the potential for sight-threatening complications.

Treatment of HZ, using the various antiviral drugs, has significantly improved the course of the disease. Prompt treatment can help to greatly minimize serious general and ocular sequelae. With widespread use of the varicella vaccine, elimination of this infection may occur, with the subsequent need to treat HZ becoming only a part of medical history.

REFERENCES

Amanat LA, Cant JS, Green FD. Acute phthisis bulbi and external ophthalmoplegia in herpes zoster ophthalmicus. *Ann Ophthalmol.* 1985;17:46–51.

Archambault P, Wise JS, Rosen J, et al. Herpes zoster ophthalmoplegia. Report of six cases. *J Clin Neuro-ophthalmol.* 1988;8:185–191.

Atmaca LS, Ozmert E. Optic neuropathy and central retinal artery occlusion in a patient with herpes zoster ophthalmicus. *Ann Ophthalmol.* 1992;24:50–53.

Benenson AB, ed. *Control of Communicable Diseases Manual.* An official report of the American Public Health Association. Washington, DC: American Public Health Association; 1995:87–91.

Borruat FX, Herbort CP. Herpes zoster ophthalmicus. Anterior ischemic optic neuropathy and acyclovir. *J Clin Neuro-ophthalmol.* 1992;12:37–40.

Browning DJ, Blumenkranz MS, Culbertson WW, et al. Association of varicella zoster dermatitis with acute retinal necrosis syndrome. *Ophthalmology.* 1987;94:602–606.

Bucci FA, Gabriels CF, Krohel GB. Successful treatment of postherpetic neuralgia with capsaicin. *Am J Ophthalmol.* 1988;106:758–759.

Büchi ER, Herbort CP, Ruffieux C. Oral acyclovir in the treatment of acute herpes zoster ophthalmicus. *Am J Ophthalmol.* 1986;102:531–532.

Burgoon CF, Burgoon JS, Baldridge GD. The natural history of herpes zoster. *JAMA.* 1957;164:265–269.

Chess J, Marcus DM. Zoster-related bilateral acute retinal necrosis syndrome as presenting sign in AIDS. *Ann Ophthalmol.* 1988;20:431–438.

Cobo LM. Corneal complications of herpes zoster ophthalmicus. Prevention and treatment. *Cornea.* 1988;7:50–56.

Cobo LM, Foulks GN, Liesegang T, et al. Observation on the natural history of herpes zoster ophthalmicus. *Curr Eye Res.* 1987;6:195–199.

Cobo LM, Foulks GN, Liesegang T, et al. Oral acyclovir in the therapy of acute herpes zoster ophthalmicus. *Ophthalmology.* 1986;93:763–770.

Cobo LM, Foulks GN, Liesegang T, et al. Oral acyclovir in the therapy of acute herpes zoster ophthalmicus. An interim report. *Ophthalmol.* 1985;92:1574–1583.

Cole EL, Meisler PM, Calabrese LH, et al. Herpes zoster ophthalmicus and acquired immune deficiency syndrome. *Arch Ophthalmol.* 1984;102:1027–1029.

Cooper M. The epidemiology of herpes zoster. *Eye.* 1987; 1:413–421.

Culbertson WW, Blumenkranz MS, Pepose JS. et al. Varicella zoster virus is a cause of the acute retinal necrosis syndrome. *Ophthalmology.* 1986;93:559–569.

Currey TA, Dalsania J. Treatment for herpes zoster ophthalmicus: Stellate ganglion block as a treatment for acute pain and prevention of postherpetic neuralgia. *Ann Ophthalmol.* 1991;23:188–189.

Dunkle LM, Arvin AM, Whitley RJ, et al. A controlled trial of acyclovir for chickenpox in normal children. *N Engl J Med.* 1991;325:1539–1544.

Edgerton AE. Herpes zoster ophthalmicus. *Arch Ophthalmol.* 1945;34:40–62, 114–153.

Harding SP, Lipton JR, Wells JCD. Natural history of herpes zoster ophthalmicus: Predictors of postherpetic neuralgia and ocular involvement. *Br J Ophthalmol.* 1987;71:353–358.

Harding SP, Porter SM. Oral acyclovir in herpes zoster ophthalmicus. *Curr Eye Res.* 1991;10(suppl):177–182.

Hoang-Xuan T, Bücchi ER, Herbort CP, et al. Oral acyclovir for herpes zoster ophthalmicus. *Ophthalmology.* 1992;99: 1062–1071.

Hope-Simpson RE. The nature of herpes zoster: A long-term study and a new hypothesis. *Proc Royal Soc Med.* 1965;58: 9–20.

Jessell TM, Iverson LL, Cuello AC. Capsaicin-induced depletion of substance P from primary sensory neurones. *Brain Res.* 1978;152:183–188.

Johnson CE, Stacin T, Fafflar D, et al. A long-term prospective study of varicella vaccine in healthy children. *Pediatrics.* 1997;100:761–766.

Karbassi M, Raizman MB, Schuman JS. Herpes zoster ophthalmicus. *Surv Ophthalmol.* 1992;36:395–410.

Karlin JD. Herpes zoster ophthalmicus: The virus strikes back. *Ann Ophthalmol.* 1993;25:208–215.

Karlin JD. Herpes zoster ophthalmicus and iris cysts. *Ann Ophthalmol.* 1990;22:414–415.

Kothe AC, Flanagan J, Trevino RC. True posterior ischemic optic neuropathy associated with herpes zoster ophthalmicus. *J Am Acad Optom.* 1990;67:845–849.

Liesegang TJ. Corneal complications from herpes zoster ophthalmicus. *Ophthalmology.* 1985;92:316–324.

Liesegang TJ. Diagnosis and therapy of herpes zoster ophthalmicus. *Ophthalmology.* 1991;98:1216–1229.

Liesegang TJ. Ophthalmic herpes zoster: Diagnosis and antiviral therapy. *Geriatrics.* 1991;46:64–71.

Liesegang TJ. The varicella-zoster virus: Systemic and ocular features. *J Am Acad Dermatol.* 1984;11:165–191.

Liesegang TJ. Varicella-zoster virus eye disease. *Cornea.* 1999; 18:511–531.

Lightman S, Marsh JR, Powell D. Herpes zoster ophthalmicus: A medical review. *Br J Ophthalmol.* 1981;65:539–541.

Lund J. Varicella zoster virus in the health care setting. *AAOHN J.* 1993;41:369–373.

Marsh RJ. Ophthalmic zoster. *Br J Ophthalmol.* 1992;76:244–245.

Marsh RJ, Cooper M. Double-masked trial of topical acyclovir and steroids in the treatment of herpes zoster ocular inflammation. *Br J Ophthalmol.* 1991;75:542–546.

Marsh RJ, Cooper M. Ophthalmic zoster: Mucous plaque keratitis. *Br J Ophthalmol.* 1987;71:725–728.

McGill J. The enigma of herpes stromal disease. *Br J Ophthalmol.* 1987;71:118–125.

Mondino BJ, Farley MK, Aizuss DH. Sectorial corneal infiltrates and pannus in herpes zoster ophthalmicus. *Clin Exp Ophthalmol.* 1986;224:313–316.

Nightingale SL. From the food and drug administration. *JAMA.* 1995;273:1564.

Ostler H, Thygeson P. The ocular manifestations of herpes zoster, varicella, infectious mononucleosis and cytomegalovirus disease. *Surv Ophthalmol.* 1976;21:148–159.

Pavan-Langston D. Varicella-zoster ophthalmicus. *Int Ophthalmol Clin.* 1975;15:171–185.

Ragozzino MW, Melton J, Kurland CT, et al. Risk of cancer after herpes zoster. A population-based study. *N Engl J Med.* 1982;307:393–397.

Reed JW, Joyner SJ, Knauer WJ. Penetrating keratoplasty for herpes zoster keratopathy. *Am J Ophthalmol.* 1989;107: 257–261.

Ross JVM. Herpes zoster ophthalmicus sine eruptione. *Arch Ophthalmol.* 1949;42:808–812.

Rowbotham M, Harden N, Stacey B, et al. Gabapentin for the treatment of postherpetic neuralgia. *JAMA.* 1998; 280:1837–1842.

Sandor EV, Millman A, Croxson S, Mildvan D. Herpes zoster ophthalmicus in patients at risk for the acquired immune deficiency syndrome (AIDS). *Am J Ophthalmol.* 1986; 101:153–155.

Schmader K, George LK, Burchett BM, et al. Racial differences in the occurrence of herpes zoster. *J Infect Dis.* 1995; 171:701–704.

Seiff SR, Margolis T, Graham SH, O'Donnell JJ. Use of intravenous acyclovir for treatment of herpes zoster ophthalmicus in patients at risk for AIDS. *Ann Ophthalmol.* 1988;20:480–482.

Soong HK, Schwartz AE, Meyer RF, Sugar A. Penetrating keratoplasty for corneal scarring due to herpes zoster ophthalmicus. *Br J Ophthalmol.* 1989;73:19–21.

Stankus SJ, Dlugopolski M, Packer D. Management of herpes zoster (shingles) and postherpetic neuralgia. *Am Fam Physician.* 2000;61:2437–2444.

Stover BH, Bratcher DF. Varicella-zoster virus: Infection, control, and prevention. *Am J Infect Control.* 1998;26: 369–384.

Straus SE. Clinical and biological differences between recurrent herpes simplex virus and varicella-zoster virus infections. *JAMA.* 1989;262:3455–3458.

Straus SE, Ostrove JM, Inchauspe G, et al. Varicella-zoster virus infections. Biology, natural history, treatment and prevention. *Ann Int Med.* 1988;108:221–237.

Strommen GL, Pucinol F, Tight RR, Beck CL. Human infection with herpes zoster: Etiology, pathophysiology, diagnosis, clinical course and treatment. *Pharmacotherapy.* 1988; 8:52–68.

Thibodeaux D. Herpes zoster ophthalmicus. In: Onofrey BE, ed. *Clinical Optometric Pharmacology and Therapeutics.* Philadelphia: Lippincott; 1991.

Tunis SW, Tapert MJ. Acute retrobulbar neuritis complicating herpes zoster ophthalmicus. *Ann Ophthalmol.* 1987; 19:453–460.

Verghese A, Sugar AM. Herpes zoster ophthalmicus and granulomatous angiitis. An ill-appreciated cause of stroke. *J Am Geriatr Soc.* 1986;34:309–312.

Watson PN, Evans RJ. Postherpetic neuralgia. *Arch Neurol.* 1986;43:836–840.

Weller TH. Varicella and herpes zoster. Changing concepts of the natural history, control, and importance of a not-so-benign virus (first of two parts). *N Engl J Med.* 1983a; 309:1362–1368.

Weller TH. Varicella and herpes zoster. Changing concepts of the natural history, control, and importance of a not-so-benign virus (second of two parts). *N Engl J Med.* 1983b; 309:1434–1440.

Wilson CA, Wander AH, Choromokos EA. Central retinal artery obstruction in herpes zoster ophthalmicus and cerebral vasculopathy. *Ann Ophthalmol.* 1990;22:347–351.

Womack LW, Liesegang TJ. Complications of herpes zoster ophthalmicus. *Arch Ophthalmol.* 1983;101:42–45.

Chapter 48

RUBELLA

Diane T. Adamczyk

Rubella, also known as German measles, was first recognized in the 1800s. Two hundred years later, with the use of the vaccination, the *potential* exists to eradicate the disease and its subsequent effect on the developing fetus.

Rubella is a relatively benign viral disease when it occurs postnatally, usually affecting children and young adults. However, when a pregnant woman is infected, its most damaging effects are to the developing fetus. The classic rubella triad of cataract, heart disease, and deafness in infants born during a rubella epidemic was first described in the 1940s. Congenital rubella syndrome encompasses a variety of systemic and ocular abnormalities that occur as a result of fetal infection.

EPIDEMIOLOGY

Systemic

- Rubella occurs worldwide, affecting all races and sexes equally.
- Reported rubella cases (1992–1996): annual average 183 cases; increase among Hispanics; (1994–1996): 12 infants with congenital rubella syndrome (MMWR, 1997)
- Specific patterns of infection are determined by population density, location, and climate, taking either an endemic or epidemic form.
    - In the United States, major epidemics have occurred in 1917, 1935, 1943, and 1964, with less severe epidemics in 1952 and 1958.
    - A typical annual incidence of 2000 cases of congenital rubella syndrome had been reported, but during the 1964 to 1965 epidemic, this increased 10 times to more than 20,000 cases (Cooper & Krugman, 1967).
    - An estimated 10,000 infants were born with moderate to severe rubella.
    - This worldwide epidemic is estimated to have affected 10% of pregnant females, with approximately 33% of the infants manifesting congenital disease (Diamond, 1994).
- Surviving patients from the prevaccination era of infection are still seen today.
- Rubella occurs more frequently in the winter and the spring.
- Approximately 90% of people are immune by adulthood, but more than 10% may still be susceptible.
- With consistent vaccination programs, the epidemiologic trends have shown a definite decline.
    - It was estimated that 5 years after vaccination programs were instituted, 10,000 to 20,000 cases of congenital rubella were avoided (Krugman & Katz, 1974).
    - Infrequent cases still occur because of vaccine failure and reinfection and because universal/worldwide immunization has not yet occurred.

- Infections occur, particularly in Latino communities, where unvaccinated individuals from Latin America come to the United States.
- Fetal exposure to rubella may result in stillbirth, spontaneous abortion, or early and/or late malformations, with the exact incidence difficult to determine.
  - Exposure, earlier in the pregnancy, has more likelihood of affecting the fetus, with the greatest detrimental effects occurring during this critical time of growth and development (the first 8 weeks of gestation). The fetuses are affected in the following percentages when infection occurs during the following time frames in pregnancy (below varies with study):
    - First month of pregnancy: up to 50% affected.
    - Second month of pregnancy: up to 25% affected.
    - Third month of pregnancy: approximately 10% affected.
    - Second trimester: up to 10% affected.
  - Fetal survival is as follows when infection occurs during the following time frames in pregnancy:
    - First month of pregnancy: approximately 20%.
    - Second month of pregnancy: 50%.
    - Third month: most survive.
- Postnatal complications:
  - Generally rare, with encephalitis occurring in 1 of 5000 cases.
  - The mortality rate for affected infants is higher than the average childhood population, with death in up to 20% within the first 18 months of life.
- Systemic manifestations of congenital rubella result in:
  - Heart disease in 52 to 61%, with patent ductus the most common manifestation.
  - Hearing loss in 29 to 66%.
  - Psychomotor retardation in up to 62%.
  - Mental retardation in 42%.
  - Low birth weight in 40%.
  - Thrombocytopenic purpura in up to 31%.
  - Transient bone changes in 40 to 50%.

Ocular

- Congenital rubella exposure results in ocular manifestations in 30 to 78% of infants.
  - Cataracts: 27 to 85%, bilateral involvement in 50 to 80%.
  - Retinopathy: 13 to 88% of cases.
  - Glaucoma: 2 to 29%.
  - Strabismus: 35% in the first 6 months, 60% by 18 months.
  - Nystagmus: 38%.
  - Iris hypoplasia: 33%.
  - Microphthalmia: 60 to 82%.
- Associated systemic findings with ocular manifestations of congenital rubella:
  - Heart defects in 96%.
  - Hearing loss in 50%.

PATHOPHYSIOLOGY/DISEASE PROCESS

Organism

- The rubella virus, identified in 1962, is a togavirus, which consists of an RNA core.
- Humans are the natural host, although animals may be artificially infected.
- Higher temperatures and extremes of pH affect infectivity.

Transmission

- Postnatally:
  - The virus is transmitted to the nonimmune through vaccination or is transmitted from an infected individual through airborne respiratory particles, such as from a cough or sneeze.
  - Once infected, incubation time is approximately 12 to 23 days.
  - The virus is communicable approximately 1 week before to 1 week after acute illness.
  - Once infected, life-long immunity usually results.
    - Reinfection may occur in those with low antibody levels (e.g., those vaccinated).
    - Reinfection in a pregnant woman has a significantly lower risk to the fetus than a primary infection.
- Prenatally:
  - The virus is transmitted to the embryo from the infected mother through the placenta.

Course of the Disease

Congenital rubella is considered a chronic infection, which may present with temporary, permanent, progressive, or late manifestations. The manifestations may be a result of the virus or immune responses.

> The classic congenital rubella clinical presentation includes cataract, heart disease, and deafness.

Systemic

- Postnatal rubella infection:
  - Generally follows a benign clinical course.
  - Children generally present with fewer symptoms than adults, particularly after inoculation with a vaccination.
    - Adults may experience arthralgic symptoms.
  - Clinical presentation (Table 48–1) includes:
  - Maculopapular rash, lymphadenopathy, headache, swollen joints, and more typically, a mild fever.
    - The rash follows the viral spread in the blood for 2 to 3 weeks postinfection.
  - Rubella may manifest subclinically or present with mild symptoms, without a rash.
- Viral antibodies occur at the same time as the rash.
  - Antibody titers peak at 7 to 10 days, initially consisting of IgM, which is present for about 1 month after the rash, and IgG, which is present for years.
  - Once infected, the individual usually maintains life-long immunity.
- Complications include:
  - Transient rheumatoid-like arthritis, thrombocytopenic purpura, and rarely encephalitis, necrotizing vasculitis, or neurologic deficit.

TABLE 48–1. SYSTEMIC MANIFESTATIONS OF RUBELLA

Postnatal Infection
• Upper respiratory tract inflammation
• Constitutional symptoms: fever, malaise, muscle ache, headache
• Lymphadenopathy
• Viremia
• Rash
Initially: transient blush
Maculopapular rash
• Antirubella virus antibodies
• Swollen joints
• Complications
Rheumatoid-like arthritis, thrombocytopenic purpura
Rare: encephalitis, necrotizing vasculitis, or neurologic deficit
Congenital Rubella Manifestations
• Cardiac
Patent ductus arteriosus (with or without stenosis of pulmonary artery or its branches)
Atrial and ventricular defects
Coarctation of the aorta, aortic stenosis
Congestive heart failure
Murmur
Necrotizing myocarditis
• Hearing loss
Mild or severe
Unilateral or bilateral
Sensory damage
Impaired vestibular function
• Psychomotor retardation
Spastic quadriparesis
Mental retardation
Focal neurologic deficits and seizures (uncommon)
• Miscellaneous
Thrombocytopenic purpura
Diabetes
Long bone lesions—evident on x-ray (transient)
Expanded rubella syndrome (usually transient): hepatosplenomegaly, hepatitis, hemolytic anemia, bulging anterior fontanelle, with or without pleocytosis
Bleeding tendencies
Low birthweight
CNS: microcephaly, mental disability, impaired motor development, neurosensory impairment, meningitis, encephalitis
Pneumonia
Dental defects
Cleft palate
Encephalomyelocele, meningocele
Esophageal atresia
Pancreatic insufficiency

- Congenital rubella:
  - Fetal infection may result in spontaneous abortion, stillbirth, malformations, and multiple organ involvement or may have no significant effect.
  - Time of maternal infection and fetal effect:
    - First trimester infection: greatest risk to fetal viability and malformation.
      - During this time cardiac, hearing, and psychomotor defects are most likely to occur.
    - Second and third trimester infections: less apparent manifestations.
    - End of the pregnancy: the infant may be born with rubella resembling a postnatal infection.
  - Persistent infection and viral isolation occurs in 60 to 80% of infants during the first month of life, and occasionally beyond 1 year, with the virus found in newborn excretions and secretions.
  - Systemic manifestations of congenital rubella:
    - Most common: cardiac involvement and loss of hearing.
      - Cardiac involvement may present without symptoms, or may develop into congestive heart failure within the first months of life, sometimes resulting in death.
      - Hearing loss is sensorineural, probably secondary to damage to the organ of Corti.
    - Central nervous system infection may result in psychomotor retardation.

- Development of diabetes later in life.
- Death in congenital rubella syndrome:
  - Usually within the first 3 to 6 months of life.
  - Results from pneumonia, congestive heart failure, encephalitis, or hepatitis, or sometimes following heart surgery.

Ocular

- Postnatal rubella ocular complications: rare.
- Congenital rubella ocular manifestations: common (Table 48–2).
  - Result from maternal infection during the first trimester of pregnancy.
    - Each eye may be affected differently because of a slower development or greater viral effect in one eye.
  - Cataract:
    - Results from viral encroachment in the lens.
    - Usually bilateral, but may be unilateral (Figure 48–1).
    - Central, pearly, white area, with a less dense cortical opacity surrounding the nuclear area.
      - May also present as a more uniformly dense opacity.
    - Usually present at birth, and may progress.
    - Decreased vision and nystagmus may result from the cataract.
    - Although rare, the lens may spontaneously absorb, either completely or partially (Boger & Peterson, 1981).

TABLE 48–2. OCULAR MANIFESTATIONS OF CONGENITAL RUBELLA SYNDROME

- Cataract
- Retinopathy
  - Pigment changes
  - Retinal folds
  - Subretinal neovascularization
  - Pallor of optic nerve
- Nystagmus (pendular or searching type)
  - Associated with cataracts or microphthalmia
- Iris
  - Pupil: miotic (thin sphincter), poor dilation (absent dilator), poor light reactions
  - Hypoplasia
  - Iridocyclitis
  - Transillumination defects
- Cornea
  - Clouding
  - Microcornea
- Microphthalmia
  - Often associated with cataracts
- Glaucoma

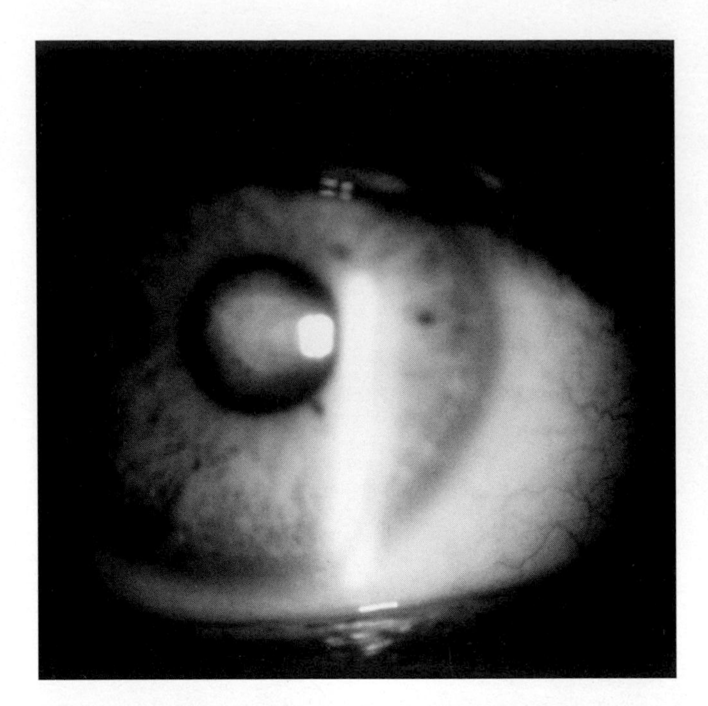

Figure 48–1. Central, white opacified area seen in rubella cataracts. *(Courtesy Dr. Scott Richter, SUNY, College of Optometry.)*

    - Frequently associated with microphthalmia.
    - The lens may be more oval, spherophakic, and smaller.
  - Retinal manifestations:
    - Common.
    - May be unilateral or bilateral, hyperpigmentation or hypopigmentation (Figure 48–2).
      - Characteristic appearance:
        - A fine, granular, mottled, pepper-like pigment clumping, of variable size.
        - Can affect any or all parts of the retina, a sector, the periphery, or more commonly involve the posterior pole and macula.
      - It appears that the classic rubella pigment retinopathy affects pigment distribution, rather than its function (Krill, 1972).
    - Generally not progressive.
    - Vision usually not affected, but may be.
    - In addition; retinal folds and subretinal neovascularization may occur.
    - Electrodiagnostic testing, including electroretinogram and electro-oculogram, is unaffected.
  - Glaucoma:
    - Present either at birth or during infancy.

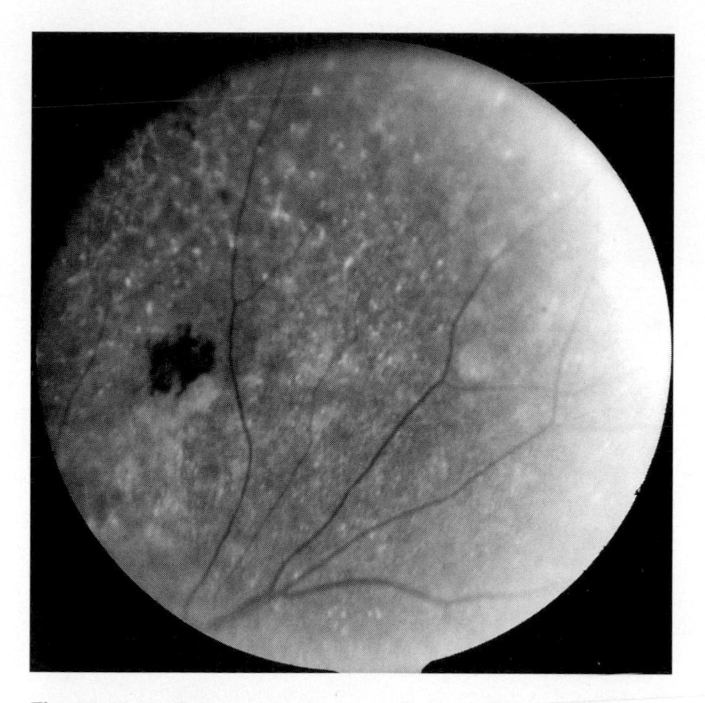

Figure 48–2. Retinal pigmentary variations. *(Courtesy Dr. Scott Richter, SUNY, College of Optometry.)*

- May result from abnormal angle development, secondary to inflammation, pupillary block, or cataract surgery.
- Strabismus:
  - A result of poor image as with cataract eye or CNS involvement as with brain damage.
  - Initially eso or convergent deviation, later becoming exo or divergent.
- Microphthalmia:
  - Results from abnormal development.
  - Vision is always poor, with an abnormal electroretinogram.
- Iris:
  - Hypoplasia.
  - Difficult to dilate pupil.

DIAGNOSIS

Table 48–3 lists the various diagnostic tests for rubella, and Table 48–4 provides the differential diagnosis.

Systemic

- Diagnosis of postnatal rubella infection (see Table 48–3):
  - Based on a history of exposure, clinical presentation or methods that detect either the virus or its antibodies.
  - Cultures.

TABLE 48–3. DIAGNOSTIC TESTS FOR RUBELLA

Postnatal Infection
- Cultures:
  - Pharyngeal secretions (1 week prior to, 2 weeks after rash)
  - Blood (1 week prior to, 2 days after rash)
- Serologic testing for rubella antibodies:
  - Complement fixing serum antibody (up to 1 to 2 years after infection)
  - ELISA
  - Radioimmunoassay
  - Inhibition of hemagglutination
  - Direct immunofluorescence technique
  - Immunoprecipitating reaction

Congenital Infection
- Tissue suspension
- Culture
- Complement fixation serum antibodies

- Serologic testing or assays that detect IgG and IgM.
  - Rubella antibodies may be found 2 to 4 days after the rash, and are present throughout life.
  - Complement-fixing antibody decreases with time; therefore testing is best done within 1 to 2 years of infection.
- Diagnosis of systemic manifestations of congenital rubella:
  - Based on clinical presentation or physical exam, or through viral isolation.

TABLE 48–4. DIFFERENTIAL DIAGNOSIS FOR RUBELLA

Systemic/Ocular
Herpes simplex
Cytomegalovirus
Scarlet fever
Drug rashes
Measles
Varicella/zoster virus
HIV
Secondary syphilis
Infectious mononucleosis
Rubeola

Ocular
Cataracts
- Associated with congenital cataracts
  - Various syndromes, Alport syndrome, Crouzon disease, Goldenhar syndrome, Usher syndrome, others
  - Infection related, varicella, herpes simplex
- Other causes of congenital leukocoria
  - Retinoblastoma, retrolental fibroplasia

Retinal changes
- Retinitis pigmentosa (RP)
- Syphilis
- Leber congenital amaurosis
- Radiation exposure

- The virus may be found beyond a year in the infant's throat, cerebral spinal fluid, stool, urine, conjunctiva, and lens.
- Also evaluate through tissue suspension, culture, and complement fixation serum antibodies.
- Observation of the child for unusual or abnormal behavior, for example, hearing loss.

Ocular

- Diagnosis of ocular manifestations of congenital rubella:
  - Based on clinical presentation, associated systemic findings, and ocular evaluation.
  - Electrodiagnostic testing.
  - Serologic testing.
  - Rubella is usually the underlying etiology when infantile glaucoma is associated with cerebral palsy and deafness.
  - Observing the child for unusual behavior:
    - Autostimulation, including the oculodigital phenomenon (pressing on the globe to produce pressure phosphenes) or the hand wagging phenomenon (hand waving over the eyes to change light intensity, while looking at a bright light), have been noted in infants with congenital cataracts who are trying to stimulate their retinas (Roy, 1967).

TREATMENT AND MANAGEMENT (Table 48–5)

Systemic

- Prevention of the infection:
  - Vaccination:
    - All nonimmune individuals, particularly children (older than 1 year of age) should be vaccinated.
      - Defer pregnancy at least 2 to 3 months after vaccination.
    - Avoid in those with depressed immune status.
    - Seroconversion is approximately >95%.
  - Isolate actively infected individuals from pregnant women, particularly during the first trimester.

> Worldwide vaccination can potentially lead to eradication of rubella.

TABLE 48–5. TREATMENT AND MANAGEMENT OF RUBELLA

Systemic
- MMR (measles/mumps/rubella) vaccination
  - First dose: 12–15 months
  - Second dose: 4–6 years
- Postnatal
  - Palliative measures
- Congenital
  - Gammaglobulin (injection during pregnancy)
  - Multidisciplinary care
  - Hearing aids
  - Special education/rehabilitation
  - Counseling

Ocular (Congenital)
- Cataract
  - Extraction
  - Appropriate refractive correction
- Strabismus
  - Remove cataract
  - Refractive correction
  - Vision therapy (e.g., occlusion)
  - Strabismic surgery (if necessary)
- Glaucoma
  - Medical (e.g., timolol, carbonic anhydrase inhibitor)
  - Surgical (e.g., goniotomy, filtering, cyclocryotherapy)

  - Injection of human gamma globulin may be considered if exposure during pregnancy occurs, in order to prevent infection.
    - Results vary as to its effectiveness.
- Postnatal infection: generally palliative.
- Congenital rubella syndrome:
  - Requires multispecialist care.
    - May include cardiologist, audiologist, special education, or rehabilitation programs.

Ocular

- Congenital rubella syndrome:
  - Aim: optimize and preserve visual function.
  - Cataract extraction.
  - Glaucoma: medical therapy; if uncontrolled, surgery.

CONCLUSION

Rubella is a viral infection that can follow a benign course in individuals affected postnatally, or follow a more devastating course in the developing fetus affected by maternal infection. Congenital rubella syndrome classically includes hearing loss and cardiac and ocular involvement. Optimal care includes comanagement of these patients with the appropriate specialists. Ultimately, the best treatment for the disease is its prevention. Since the discovery and use of a vaccine in the late 1960s, rubella epidemics are nonexistent and the potential for eradication exists. However, the threat of the disease to unborns will continue until everyone is effectively immunized.

REFERENCES

Arnold J. Ocular manifestations of congenital rubella. *Curr Opin Ophthalmol.* 1995;6:45–50.

Boger WP. Late ocular complications in congenital rubella syndrome. *Ophthalmology.* 1980;87:1244–1252.

Boger WP, Peterson RA, Robb RM. Spontaneous absorption of the lens in the congenital rubella syndrome. *Arch Ophthalmol.* 1981;99:433–434.

Boniuk M. Glaucoma in the congenital rubella syndrome. *Int Ophthalmol Clin.* 1972a;12:121–136.

Boniuk M, Zimmerman LE. Ocular pathology in the rubella syndrome. *Arch Ophthalmol.* 1967;77:455–473.

Boniuk V. Rubella. *Int Ophthalmol Clin.* 1975;15:229–241.

Boniuk V. Systemic and ocular manifestations of the rubella syndrome. *Int Ophthalmol Clin.* 1972b;12:67–76.

Bonomo PP. Involution without disciform scarring of subretinal neovascularization in presumed rubella retinopathy. *Acta Ophthalmol.* 1982;60:141–146.

Calvert DR. The rubella epidemic of 1964. *J Am Optom Assoc.* 1969;40:794–798.

Centers for Disease Control and Prevention. Rubella and congenital rubella syndrome: U.S., 1994–1997. *MMWR Weekly.* 1997;146:350–354.

Collis WJ, Cohen DN. Rubella retinopathy. A progressive disorder. *Arch Ophthalmol.* 1970;84:33–35.

Cooper LZ, Krugman S. Clinical manifestations of postnatal and congenital rubella. *Arch Ophthalmol.* 1967;77:434–439.

Diamond G. Ocular manifestations of genetic and developmental diseases. *Curr Opin Ophthalmol.* 1994;5:72–78.

Fleet WF, Benz EW, Karzon DT, et al. Fetal consequences of maternal rubella immunization. *JAMA.* 1974;227:621–627.

Geltzer AI, Guber D, Sears ML. Ocular manifestations of the 1964-65 rubella epidemic. *Am J Ophthalmol.* 1967; 63:221–229.

Givens KT, Lee DA, Jones T, Ilstrup DM. Congenital rubella syndrome: Ophthalmic manifestations and associated systemic disorders. *Br J Ophthalmol.* 1993;77:358–363.

Gregg NM. Congenital cataract following German measles in the mother. *Trans Ophthalmol Soc Aust.* 1941;3:35–46.

Gregg NM. Further observations on congenital defects in infants following maternal rubella. *Trans Ophthalmol Soc Aust.* 1944;4:119–130.

Hertzberg R. Congenital cataract following German measles in the mother. *Aust NZ J Ophthalmol.* 1985;13:303–309.

Hertzberg R. Twenty-five year follow-up of ocular defects in congenital rubella. *Am J Ophthalmol.* 1968;66:269–271.

Krill AE. Retinopathy secondary to rubella. *Int Ophthalmol Clin.* 1972;12:89–103.

Krugman S, Katz SL. Rubella immunization: A five year progress report. *N Engl J Med.* 1974;290:1375–1376.

Murphy AM, Reid RR, Pollard I, et al. Rubella cataracts. Further clinical and virologic observations. *Am J Ophthalmol.* 1967;64:1109–1119.

O'Neill JF. Strabismus in congenital rubella. *Arch Ophthalmol.* 1967;77:450–454.

O'Neill JF. Strabismus in rubella syndrome. *Int Ophthalmol Clin.* 1972;12:111–120.

O'Neill JF. The ocular manifestations of congenital infection: A study of the early effect and long-term outcome of maternally transmitted rubella and toxoplasmosis. *Trans Am Ophthalmol Soc.* 1998;96:813–879.

Orth DH, Fishman GA, Segall M, et al. Rubella maculopathy. *Br J Ophthalmol.* 1980;64:201–205.

Plotkin SA, Katz M, Cordero JF. The eradication of rubella. *JAMA.* 1999;281:561–562.

Rawls WE. Virology and epidemiology of rubella virus. *Int Ophthalmol Clin.* 1972;12:21–66.

Romano A, Weinberg M, Bar-Izhak R, et al. Rate and various aspects of eye infection resulting from congenital rubella. *J Pediatric Ophthalmol Strabismus.* 1979;16:26–30.

Roy FH. Microsurgery of congenital rubella cataract. *Am J Ophthalmol.* 1968;65:81–90.

Roy FH. Ocular autostimulation. *Am J Ophthalmol.* 1967; 63:1776–1777.

Roy FH, Deutsch AR. The congenital rubella syndrome. *Am J Ophthalmol.* 1966;62:236–238.

Roy FH, Fuste F, Hiatt RL, et al. The congenital rubella syndrome with virus recovery. *Am J Ophthalmol.* 1966; 62:222–232.

Roy FH, Hiatt RL, Korones SB, Roane J. Ocular manifestations of congenital rubella syndrome. *Arch Ophthalmol.* 1966;75:601–607.

Rudolph AJ, Desmond MM. Clinical manifestations of the congenital rubella syndrome. *Int Ophthalmol Clin.* 1972; 12:3–19.

Scheie HG, Schaeffer DB, Plotkin SA, Kertesz ED. Congenital rubella cataracts. Surgical results and virus recovery from intraocular tissue. *Arch Ophthalmol.* 1967;77: 440–444.

Sears ML. Congenital glaucoma in neonatal rubella. *Br J Ophthalmol.* 1967;51:744–748.

Slusher MM, Tyler ME. Rubella retinopathy and subretinal neovascularization. *Ann Ophthalmol.* 1982;14:292–294.

Tate HR. Congenital rubella syndrome. *Eye, Ear, Nose Throat Month.* 1969;48:33–41.

Weiss DI, Ziring PR, Cooper LZ. Surgery of the rubella cataract. *Am J Ophthalmol.* 1972;73:326–332.

Chapter 49

HISTOPLASMOSIS

Taryn Mathews

Histoplasmosis is a systemic disease caused by the fungus *Histoplasma capsulatum.* Although infection occurs throughout the world, it is endemic to the United States, particularly in the Ohio and Mississippi River valley regions. It is acquired by inhalation of fungal spores. The primary focus of infection is the lungs, but the fungus can also disseminate to other organs throughout the body, particularly the liver, spleen, and lymph nodes. Depending on the immune status of the patient, the disease manifests in a variety of ways, ranging from a benign, asymptomatic infection to a fatal disseminated disease.

The presumed ocular histoplasmosis syndrome (POHS) is a granulomatous choroiditis believed to result from dissemination of the fungus via the bloodstream during the primary systemic infection. It is characterized and diagnosed by the clinical presentation of peripapillary choroiditis, peripheral atrophic lesions, and exudative maculopathy. Although clinical and epidemiologic studies support *H. capsulatum* as the cause of the ocular syndrome, diagnosis remains presumptive until the organism is definitively isolated.

EPIDEMIOLOGY

Systemic

Systemic histoplasmosis occurs throughout the world, particularly in temperate and tropical areas. It is most frequently found in the river valleys of the central eastern United States. It is estimated that 50 million people in the United States have been infected. In highly endemic regions, over 80% of the population reacts positively to the histoplasmin skin test. However, the actual prevalence of infection is not known, because the skin test can become negative as a person ages.

Systemic histoplasmosis affects all age groups, but it is most prevalent at the extremes of life. Incidences of positive skin tests are the same for males and females, but the clinical disease is more common in adult men. Caucasians and African-Americans have equal rates of positive skin tests; however, the clinical disease is more common in Caucasians.

Ocular

The geographic distribution of POHS is consistent with the distribution of the systemic disease. This prevalence of POHS in endemic areas helps to substantiate the possible role of *H. capsulatum* in the syndrome.

POHS has been seen in patients ranging in age from 7 to 77 years, with most cases occurring from 20 to 50 years of age. Initial infection resulting in peripheral atrophic scars is believed to occur in childhood or early adulthood. About 70% of POHS patients have peripapillary changes. Macular manifestations normally occur 10 to 30 years after infection, with maculopathy most commonly seen in the fourth decade.

Macular involvement in POHS is more common in Caucasians than African-Americans by a ratio of 6 to 1. However, the frequency of peripheral histo spots is equal for the two races. Maculopathy, particularly bilateral, along with a greater sensitivity to histoplasmin, is more often found in men than women.

In endemic regions, up to 12% of adults have peripheral histo scars and 1 per 1000 adults is afflicted with maculopathy. Bilateral peripheral scars are present in 52% of patients with macular involvement. It is estimated that both maculas are involved in 10% of the patients. The average amount of time before the second macula becomes affected is 4.8 years. The incidence of pulmonary calcification on x-ray increases from 12.5 to 80% when patients have maculopathy as opposed to peripheral scars without macular involvement.

PATHOPHYSIOLOGY/DISEASE PROCESS

Systemic

The Organism

Histoplasma capsulatum is a dimorphic fungus, meaning that it exists as both a mold and yeast. At room temperature (23°C) and in its natural habitat, it exists as a mold. However, at 35° to 37°C and in vivo, it exists as the unicellular yeast. Its natural habitat is rich, moist, surface soil. Growth requirements, such as organic nitrogen, explain the high concentration of histoplasmosis in areas infested with the fecal material of birds and bats. Epidemics of histoplasmosis occur following the disturbance of areas where birds have roosted and in caves inhabited by bats.

Transmission

When contaminated soil is disturbed, the spores are released into the environment. Human infection only occurs when the tiny aerosolized spores are inhaled into the distal air spaces of the lung. In the alveoli, spores convert to the yeast form, the pathogenic form of *H. capsulatum*. Histoplasmosis is not contagious; transmission only occurs through inhalation of *H. capsulatum* spores.

Course of the Disease

The yeast cells proliferate in the lung parenchyma by budding or fission. The initial response by the lung tissue is the infiltration of polymorphonuclear leukocytes (PMNs). The PMNs are rapidly followed by the accumulation of macrophages, which phagocytize the yeasts. The yeasts then undergo an intense multiplication inside the macrophages, which results in the production of a pneumonitis. The yeast-laden macrophages are spread, via the lymphatics, to the regional hilar lymph nodes. From the lymph nodes, the fungus enters the circulation and is spread throughout the body, particularly to the liver and spleen.

Two to three weeks after the initial infection, a lymphocyte cellular immune response develops at the primary and metastatic infection sites. An intense inflammatory reaction occurs, followed by granuloma formation, caseation necrosis, and fibrotic encapsulation. Months to years later, the necrotic foci may undergo calcification. The healed encapsulated foci of infection are called histoplasmomas. Often, it is difficult to distinguish them from carcinoma, and in the past they were believed to be secondary to tuberculosis.

Prior to the histoplasmin skin test, histoplasmosis was considered to be a rare, fatal disease, and its detection occurred primarily at autopsies. The combination of positive histoplasmin skin test reactions, pulmonary calcifications, and negative tuberculin skin tests revealed histoplasmosis to be a common disease, particularly in an asymptomatic, benign form.

Benign Histoplasmosis

More than 90% of the infections in normal hosts caused by *H. capsulatum* are benign, asymptomatic, and resolve without treatment. Because these patients do not seek medical care, they are discovered inadvertently by a positive reaction to the histoplasmin skin test or by the presence of calcified lesions on a routine chest x-ray. However, when the lesions heal without the formation of fibrosis or calcification, the chest radiograph is normal. Asymptomatic reinfection may occur. It is believed that the POHS develops in people that have the benign form of the systemic disease. The remaining 5 to 10% of patients with symptomatic infection fall into three categories: primary acute histoplasmosis, disseminated histoplasmosis, and chronic pulmonary histoplasmosis (Table 49–1).

Primary Acute Histoplasmosis

Primary acute symptomatic histoplasmosis is uncommon and usually occurs in infants and children, possibly secondary to their immature immune systems. Three to 14 days after their initial exposure, these individuals present with a respiratory illness similar to the presentation of influenza, with varying severity. When the chest x-ray is abnormal, it shows one or more soft pulmonary infiltrates and enlargement of the hilar and mediastinal lymph nodes. In the acute form of histoplasmosis, it is common for the infection to spread without complication to extrapulmonary sites such as the liver, spleen, and lymph nodes.

A primary acute histoplasmosis infection usually resolves with no residual effects in 2 weeks to 3

TABLE 49–1. SYSTEMIC MANIFESTATIONS OF HISTOPLASMOSIS

Signs

- Benign systemic histoplasmosis
  - Chest x-ray may be (+) or (−) for pulmonary calcification
- Primary acute histoplasmosis
  - Pulmonary infiltration, calcification, cavitation
  - Enlargement and calcification of lymph nodes, liver, spleen
- Disseminated histoplasmosis
  - Pulmonary infiltration, calcification, cavitation
  - Enlargement and calcification of lymph nodes, liver, spleen
  - Adrenal gland insufficiency
  - Anemia, leukopenia, thrombocytopenia
  - Ulcerations of the mouth, tongue, nose, larynx, intestines
- Chronic pulmonary histoplasmosis
  - Cavitation, histoplasmomas, bronchiectasis

Symptoms

- Benign systemic histoplasmosis
  - None
- Primary acute histoplasmosis
  - Fever, chills, dry cough, malaise, myalgia, arthralgia, headache
- Disseminated histoplasmosis
  - Fever, cough, chills, malaise, headache, diarrhea, weight loss, dyspnea
- Chronic pulmonary histoplasmosis
  - Weight loss, fever, chronic cough, chest pain

months. Complete recovery without therapeutic intervention usually occurs, even when the patient appears to be very ill. During the illness, the histoplasmin skin test becomes positive. The lesions in the lungs, lymph nodes, and extrapulmonary organs can resolve completely, but they often calcify 6 months to several years after the symptomatic infection.

Although the acute form is usually benign, a severe pulmonary illness can occur in individuals who have inhaled a massive number of spores. These patients present with diffuse infiltrates, dyspnea, hypoxia, and acute respiratory distress. Early diagnosis and treatment are necessary to prevent death from respiratory insufficiency.

Disseminated Histoplasmosis

In disseminated histoplasmosis the T-cell immune response is weak or absent, and so the parasitic intracellular yeasts cannot be killed. The fungus undergoes extensive and uncontrolled multiplication inside the macrophages of the reticuloendothelial system. As the yeast continues to grow in multiple organs, additional macrophages are necessary to contain the organisms. The failure of the cell-mediated immune response results in a severe disseminated systemic illness.

Disseminated histoplasmosis can occur at any age, but usually affects young infants and the aged. In adults, disseminated histoplasmosis is a complication of immunosuppressive conditions such as underlying diseases, chemotherapy for hematologic malignancies, glucocorticoid therapy, therapy for organ transplant recipients, and acquired immunodeficiency syndrome. Some patients become ill when immunosuppressive therapy is initiated. This suggests that dormant *H. capsulatum* organisms within the body become active when the immune system falters.

Patients with disseminated histoplasmosis experience fever, cough, chills, malaise, headache, diarrhea, weight loss, and dyspnea. The widespread dissemination throughout the body has an effect on many organs. The uncontrolled growth of the fungus places extraordinary demands on the phagocyte system. The resulting suppression of the bone marrow causes anemia, leukopenia, and thrombocytopenia.

Pulmonary involvement is variable, but the most common presentation on the x-ray is diffuse interstitial infiltrates. Many of these patients have adrenal gland involvement; approximately 20% go on to develop Addison disease. Other findings include hepatosplenomegaly, lymphadenopathy, and ulcerations of the mouth, tongue, nose, larynx, and intestines. On rare occasions there is the presentation of chronic meningitis and endocarditis.

In addition to the disseminated form of histoplasmosis seen in infants and immunosuppressed patients, there is a chronic disseminated form that is found in healthy adults. These patients appear to have normal T-cell function. One explanation speculates that the development of this chronic form results from a temporary suppression of immunity secondary to an underlying viral infection. The clinical presentation of the two disseminated forms is similar. Both presentations of the disseminated disease can be devastating, but the chronic form tends to run a slower course.

If antifungal therapy is not instituted, up to 80% of patients suffering from disseminated histoplasmosis die. About 50% of the patients have negative skin tests. If left untreated, patients die within 4 to 10 months. Adrenal insufficiency is believed to be the most common cause of death in the disseminated form of the disease.

Chronic Pulmonary Histoplasmosis

Chronic pulmonary histoplasmosis results from the infection of lung tissue that has already been compromised by another disease process such as chronic obstructive pulmonary disease in older Caucasian males. Radiography shows the formation of histoplasmomas, cavitation (the formation of cavities), and bronchiectasis (dilation of the bronchial tubes). Symptoms associated with this form are weight loss, fever, chronic cough, and chest pain. The infection may resolve over a period of 1 to 3 months. Some patients suffer with progression of the disease, but it is difficult to separate the effects of histoplasmosis from the coexisting pulmonary disease.

Ocular

In 1959, Woods and Wahlen described POHS as the clinical triad of circumpapillary choroiditis, peripheral atrophic chorioretinal scars (histo spots), and exudative maculopathy. The syndrome is also characterized by clear media and linear streak lesions (Table 49–2). The typical patient is healthy, resides in an area endemic for histoplasmosis, and ranges in age from 20 to 50 years.

When *H. capsulatum* is disseminated throughout the body via the bloodstream, it is believed that the fungus enters the choroid through the choroidal vessels. The resulting POHS usually occurs after the benign form of the systemic disease. It is hypothesized that the fungus, after becoming entrapped in the choroid, replicates during a period of transient immunosuppression. The clinical picture of this process is focal areas of chorioretinitis resulting in the formation of a granulomatous mass. The presence or absence of symptoms will depend on whether these areas are located in the macula or the peripheral retina, respectively.

With the emergence of the lymphocytic immune response, the focal chorioretinitis begins to resolve as the fungal organisms are killed and healing takes place over a few weeks. During the inflammatory and healing processes, breaks may occur in the Bruch membrane, and there is atrophy and metaplasia of the surrounding retinal pigment epithelium (RPE), giving rise to the classic histo spots. The disruption of the Bruch membrane and RPE is a precursor for the development of a subretinal neovascular membrane, particularly in the macula.

TABLE 49–2. OCULAR MANIFESTATIONS OF HISTOPLASMOSIS

Signs
- Circumpapillary choroiditis
- Peripheral atrophic choroidal scars (histo spots)
- Exudative maculopathy
- No inflammatory reaction (no cells or flare)
- Linear streak lesions

Symptoms
- Decreased VA
- Metamorphopsia
- Photopsia

Stages of Maculopathy
- Stage 1: Macular yellow-white lesion of active choroiditis
- Stage 2: Neovascularization, macular pigment ring with overlying sensory retinal detachment
- Stage 3: Subretinal or subretinal pigment epithelial hemorrhage from the neovascular net
- Stage 4: White, edematous lipid exudates around area of serous detachment
- Stage 5: White elevated scar

Peripheral Atrophic Chorioretinal Scars

The peripheral atrophic histo spots are healed lesions most often found posterior to the equator, away from the macula (Figure 49–1). The number of scars per eye varies from 0 to 70. The spots are typically 0.2 to 0.7 DD in size, yellow-orange in color, bilateral, and depigmented. When pigment is present, it occurs in clumps at the borders of the histo spots. When the histo spots are outside of the disc and macular regions, visual loss does not occur. These lesions usually heal without neovascularization. The presence of inflammatory cells in the choroid and evidence of spots changing or disappearing suggest that these histo spots may be active. The random distribution of the histo spots in both eyes in areas of the fundus with greater blood supply supports the hypothesis of the fungus reaching the choroid through the bloodstream.

Peripapillary Choroiditis

The choroiditis surrounding the disc is important for making the diagnosis of POHS. These scars are in the choroid and RPE, and the degree of involvement of these two areas is variable. The area involved can have a diffuse and/or nodular appearance extending from 0.125 to 0.5 DD from the disc. At the level of the RPE there is a pigment line located at the inside border of the area of peripapillary depigmentation. The outer margin has an irregular and indistinct appearance (Figure 49–2).

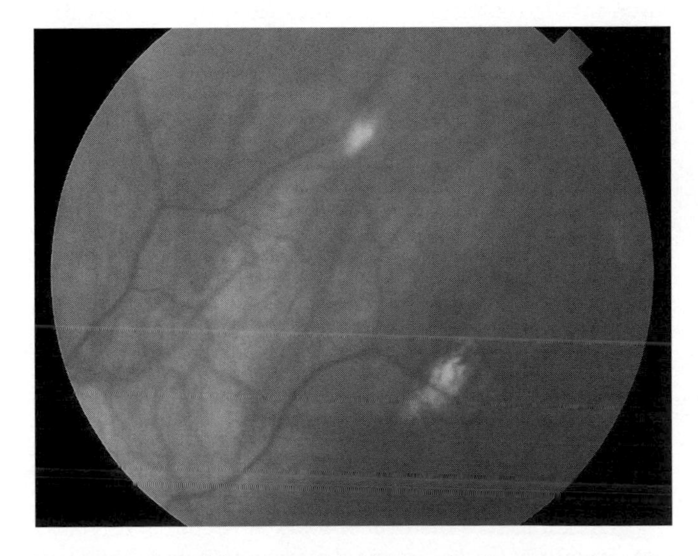

Figure 49–1. Peripheral atrophic histo spots. *(Courtesy of the Optometry Service, FDR VA Hospital, Montrose, NY.)*

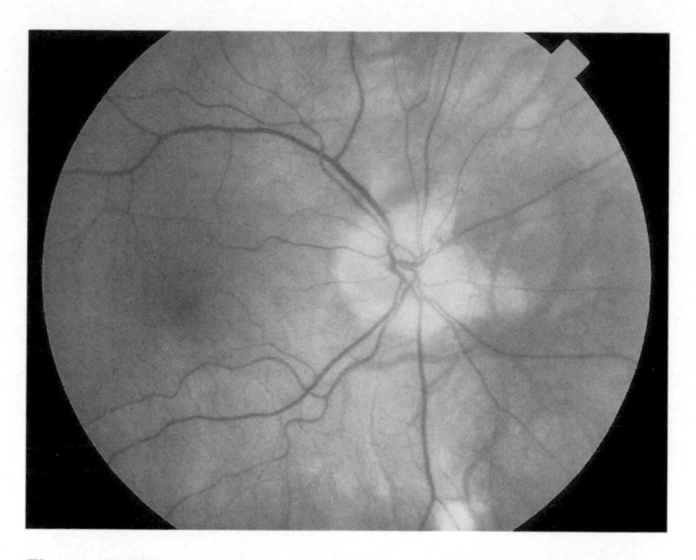

Figure 49–2. Peripapillary RPE changes secondary to histoplasmosis. *(Courtesy of the Optometry Service, FDR VA Hospital, Montrose, NY.)*

In most cases, the peripapillary changes are inactive and the patient is usually asymptomatic. However, these changes will always cause an increase in the blind spot on visual field testing. Ten percent of POHS patients become symptomatic when the scars around the disc become activated. Activation involves disruption of the RPE and Bruch membrane with subsequent neovascularization and possible hemorrhage.

Hemorrhage leads to detachment of the sensory retina and/or the RPE, which can extend from the disc out to the macula. Visual prognosis is poor in patients that develop a hemorrhage. If left untreated, about half of these patients will become legally blind.

Maculopathy

The development of maculopathy (Figure 49–2) occurs 10 to 30 years after the peripheral histo spots have formed and healed. There have been a number of speculations to explain this reactivation process. Because macular lesions usually originate from areas of previous scarring, vascular decompensation may be the mechanism of reactivation. Another possibility is that the unique structure of the macular region predisposes the area to neovascularization. An immunologic mechanism is a more likely etiology, because lymphocytes have been found to persist in the choroid many years after the primary active disease. It is hypothesized that these T lymphocytes remain sensitized from the primary infection. When the antigen or part of the antigen is reintroduced to the choroid, either from active foci in the body or from an outside source, the sensitized T cells react and an inflammatory reaction results.

The problem with the immunologic explanation is that no organism has ever been found in the choroid or retina of patients with the POHS. Yet patients with the benign form of systemic histoplasmosis are found to have old dead organisms in the granulomatous lesions in their lungs. The reason for the difference is not known. One hypothesis is the pathogenesis of the ocular lesions is different from that of the lung lesions. When granulomas form in the lung, the fibrotic scar tissue encapsulates the dead fungal organisms. In the eye, the scarring process in POHS does not result in the *Histoplasma* organisms being walled off in the lesions. Researchers continue to search for the fungus in the ocular lesions.

It is involvement of the macula, particularly the fovea, that causes ocular symptoms. The patient is usually not aware of the histo spots in the periphery. It is believed that the maculopathy does not occur until after the peripheral histo lesions have become atrophic. The patient presents with symptoms of decreased visual acuity, metamorphopsia, and photopsia. Often, the symptoms of a developing lesion precede the ophthalmoscopic signs.

> Patients with POHS are asymptomatic until the macula is involved.

The maculopathy of POHS passes through a number of stages. In the first stage, there is a yellow-white spot, which represents an area of active choroiditis. The lesion may stabilize, but usually progresses to the later stages, eventually resulting in exudative macular disease.

In this early, mild stage, the choroiditis is most often caused by the activation of an old histo scar. A granulomatous mass forms in the choroid with overlying disruption of the Bruch membrane and depigmentation of the RPE. These early lesions often have the following characteristics: locations near the macular periphery; completely flat, fuzzy white borders, less than 1 DD in size; and a window defect without leakage or late staining on fluorescein angiography. On rare occasions, these histo spots may become elevated with an underlying neovascular net and/or enlarge laterally.

The main feature in the second stage of maculopathy is a pigment ring in the macula with an overlying sensory retina detachment. The inflammatory process in the choroid causes a hole in the Bruch membrane and the pigment epithelium. This hole allows the ingrowth of neovascularization from the choroid. The pigment ring represents hyperpigmentation of the RPE in its attempt to stop the growth of the neovascular net.

When the choroiditis does not produce a hole, a gray nodule may form. This nodule is believed to be a localized area of RPE detachment that later converts to a pigment ring.

Blood vessel growth starts inside the pigment ring and then radiates outward in a sea fan fashion under the sensory retina or in the subpigment epithelial space. It is difficult to determine if the vessels lie under the sensory retina or RPE, because the RPE is usually depigmented from the choroiditis.

The combination of blood vessel growth and leakage causes the sensory retina to elevate and detach. Because the bond between the sensory retina and RPE is weak, the area of sensory retina detachment is usually much greater than the original area of choroiditis and RPE detachment. The size of the detachment corresponds to the size of the scotoma. This stage is similar to stage 1 in that it can stop or undergo regression.

Stage 3 of POHS maculopathy consists of subretinal or subretinal pigment epithelial hemorrhage from the choroidal neovascularization (CNV). When the sensory retinal detachment is extensive, the underlying hemorrhage is difficult to view even on fluorescein angiography.

Stage 3 progresses to stage 4 maculopathy with the addition of white edematous residues such as lipid exudates around the area of serous detachment. The hemorrhaging and accumulation of exudates recur and persist for 2 years or longer. Finally, in stage 5, there is a white elevated scar. The size of the scar ranges from 0.33 to 1 DD. The scar can be atrophic, fibrous, or microcystic (Figure 49–3). Microcystic degeneration occurs when there is chronic sensory retina detachment with minimal hemorrhage. Fibrosis of the scar develops when there has been a great deal of blood under the retina.

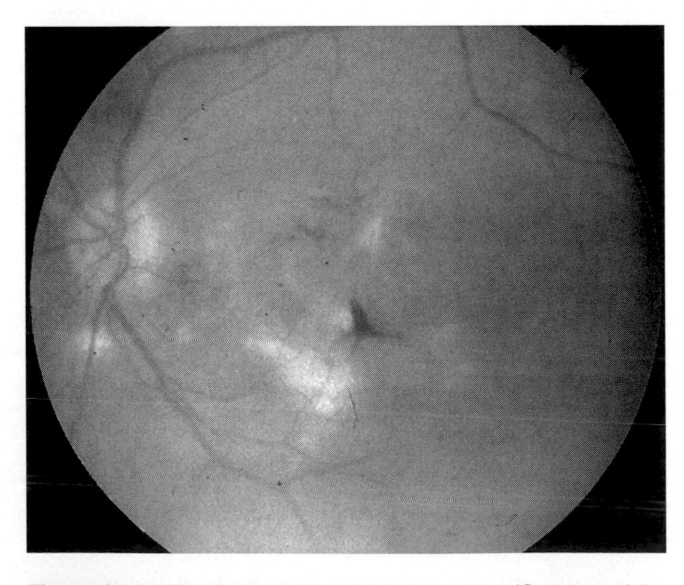

Figure 49–3. Macular scarring in histoplasmosis. *(Courtesy of the Optometry Service, FDR VA Hospital, Montrose, NY.)*

Other Manifestations

An important part of the clinical presentation of POHS is lack of an inflammatory reaction in the aqueous or vitreous. If cells are seen in the anterior chamber or the vitreous, then the diagnosis is not POHS and another cause should be considered, such as inflammatory pseudohistoplasmosis syndrome. Here, patients present with the triad of signs classic for POHS along with inflammatory cells in the ocular media. Although the cause of this syndrome is not known, it is believed to be the manifestation of inflammatory ocular diseases caused by sarcoidosis, tuberculosis, or syphilis.

Another sign that occurs in approximately 5% of POHS patients is linear streak lesions. They usually run parallel to the ora serrata at the equator in both eyes. All four quadrants can be affected. Their length varies from half a clock hour to 11 clock hours. The degree of pigmentation is variable, but most are completely depigmented. Often, large choroidal vessels can be seen running perpendicular to these streaks. These streaks seem to be the result of loss of choriocapillaris and RPE. Many believe that they are simply a linear aggregation of peripheral histo spots. The differential diagnosis includes lattice degeneration.

Prognosis

Visual prognosis depends on the degree of macular involvement, frequency of recurrent macular detachment, and duration of detachment. The most important factor is the distance of the neovascular membrane from the fovea. The prognosis is good when the CNV membrane is located greater than 1 DD from the foveal center, even with a macular detachment. On rare occasions, a patient with foveal involvement will spontaneously recover with good acuity. Patients with sensory retina detachments and CNV membranes outside the foveal avascular zone have a 60 to 70% chance of retaining 20/40 acuity or better. If the neovascularization is inside the foveal avascular zone (FAZ), the chance of good vision is 15% or less. Without treatment, approximately 59% of patients become legally blind.

Studies have shown that histo spots are not static; they change in size, shape, and density. A patient with scars in the macula has a 1 in 4 chance of developing problems over the next 3 years. If the macula is unaffected, the chance of developing visual symptoms is reduced to 1 in 50.

If a patient has symptomatic macular involvement in one eye, the fellow eye has a 20 to 30% chance of developing symptoms. The risk of developing symptoms in the second eye increases if the patient has circumpapillary and macular scars. Some patients report an improvement in acuity in the first eye when the second eye becomes symptomatic.

In the early 1980s, the Macular Photocoagulation Study (MPS) was conducted to determine the long-term benefits of laser photocoagulation of CNV membranes secondary to age-related macular degeneration, ocular histoplasmosis, or idiopathic causes. The MPS was a multicenter randomized controlled clinical trial conducted to determine whether laser photocoagulation is useful in preventing or delaying loss of visual acuity in eyes that have CNV 1 to 199 microns from the center of the FAZ or CNV 200 microns or farther from the FAZ. The MPS has shown that the loss of vision in POHS can be prevented or delayed by lasering extrafoveal and juxtafoveal CNV. The 5-year follow-up of the laser-treated eyes showed almost half of the treated study eyes had visual acuity of worse than 20/40, but 81% of their histo patients had 20/20 acuity in at least one eye and 20% had 20/20 in both eyes. Since the MPS group and other investigators have found an incidence rate of neovascular maculopathy in fellow eyes to be about 2% per year, it is important to monitor the condition of both eyes.

Past studies have shown that patients with the typical atrophic histo spots in the macula are at a greater risk of developing CNV. New findings by the MPS group suggest that macular CNV develops at sites that do not have the typical appearance of histo spots. These scars, referred to as "atypical" histo spots, are thick with irregular margins. Close observation of these new histo spots is recommended. If CNV develops in these areas, early detection may allow for better results with laser treatment.

The relationship between the systemic and ocular forms of histoplasmosis is uncertain. Exposure to the fungus rarely results in visual loss. The classic ocular syndrome only seems to occur in the benign form of the disease. It is hypothesized that certain individuals are predisposed or genetically susceptible to the visual syndrome. Support can be found in studies that have shown that patients with the POHS are more likely to have the HLA-B7 and HLA-DRw2 antigens.

DIAGNOSIS

Systemic

Making the diagnosis of systemic histoplasmosis begins with a careful and thorough history. If the patient presents with a respiratory infection, histoplasmosis should be considered as a cause, particularly in patients who live or have lived in an endemic region. If histoplasmosis is suspected, questions should be directed at determining if the patient has been exposed to the fungus, particularly at potential exposure sites such as chicken coops, caves inhabited by bats, storm cellars, gardens, and construction sites. Often diagnosis is difficult because histoplasmosis can mimic tuberculosis, influenza, sarcoidosis, and other fungal infections (Table 49–3). In addition, it is important to consider that histoplasmosis can coexist with other infections.

A definitive diagnosis (Table 49–4) of histoplasmosis is made when the fungus is isolated by culture or histology. Culturing is the preferred method, because direct examination of the fungus is difficult as a result of its small size and intracellular location. Smears of bone marrow and blood also may be useful for diagnosing patients with disseminated disease. If body secretions do not reveal the fungus, then the visceral organs involved should be biopsied.

Obtaining the results of a culture can take from 5 days to 6 weeks because *H. capsulatum* is a slow-growing organism. The culture time lessens as the number of organisms in the specimen increases.

The histoplasmin skin test cannot be used to diagnose histoplasmosis, with two exceptions. The first is in a young infant with active infection, and the second is in a previously known negative skin reactor who tests positive after a recent exposure to the fungus. In all other cases, a positive skin test simply indicates that at some time in the patient's life, infection with the fungus occurred. It provides no information concerning age or activity of the disease. In endemic

TABLE 49–3. DIFFERENTIAL DIAGNOSIS OF HISTOPLASMOSIS

Systemic
- Influenza
- Lymphoma
- Tuberculosis
- Sarcoidosis
- Other fungal infections

Ocular
- Pseudohistoplasmosis syndrome
- Lattice degeneration
- Toxoplasmosis
- Syphilis
- Sarcoidosis
- Toxocariasis
- Multifocal choroiditis
- Vitiliginous chorioretinitis
- Myopic degeneration
- Drusen of the optic disc
- Angioid streaks
- Age-related macular degeneration

TABLE 49–4. DIAGNOSTIC TESTS FOR HISTOPLASMOSIS

Systemic
- Culture
- Complement-fixation test
- Immunodiffusion
- Radioimmunoassay
- Chest x-ray

Ocular
- None—diagnosis based on classic clinical presentation

areas, up to 90% of the population tests positive to histoplasmin. In addition, a negative skin test occurs in many patients with disseminated histoplasmosis as a result of their weakened immune systems. Despite its limitations in diagnosing histoplasmosis, the histoplasmin skin test has been and continues to be invaluable in epidemiologic studies of the disease.

Serologic tests are helpful in making a presumptive diagnosis because isolation of the fungus by culture is slow and a positive skin test is not diagnostic. The serologic tests most commonly used for histoplasmosis are the complement-fixation test, immunodiffusion, and radioimmunoassay. The complement-fixation test is considered to be more specific than the others, and some consider it to be the best serologic test. However, it is negative in 30% of patients with acute histoplasmosis and in approximately 50% of patients with disseminated disease. In addition, a previously performed histoplasmin skin test can induce antibody production, resulting in a false-positive result on the complement-fixation test. The immunodiffusion test is not as sensitive as the complement-fixation test and is negative in up to 50% of patients with acute histoplasmosis. Radioimmunoassay is the most sensitive test, which makes it very useful in screening for histoplasmosis.

Unfortunately, all of the serologic tests have limited usefulness in diagnosing histoplasmosis because of the large number of false-negatives and false-positives. Another disadvantage is the 2- to 3-week wait for test results. Patients with the acute form of the disease often show signs of recovery before the test results are known, and severely ill patients require immediate therapy.

Another important diagnostic tool is x-ray examination. The classic x-ray picture of healed histoplasmosis is multiple calcified foci in both lungs. These lesions can be distinguished from those caused by tuberculosis because they are larger in size. These pulmonary foci are often found during routine examination in patients who are totally asymptomatic. Patients who are under 30 years of age and nonsmokers should be monitored with repeat chest films every 3 to 6 months. Histoplasmomas and cavitations may require more invasive procedures to confirm the diagnosis and to rule out carcinoma and tuberculosis.

Ocular

The diagnosis of ocular histoplasmosis is presumptive, because *H. capsulatum* has never been definitively identified in the eye of a patient with the POHS. There have been a handful of cases in which the investigators claim to have isolated the organism, but none of these cases have been substantiated. The diagnosis is made by finding the classic clinical presentation of the syndrome (Table 49–4).

When Woods and Wahlen (1959) described the clinical syndrome, they established criteria for a diagnosis of POHS. Their findings were categorized based on those patients who were most likely to have a choroiditis as a result of histoplasmosis, to those least likely to be associated with the disease. In addition to the classic funduscopic findings, the diagnostic criteria include clear media, a positive histoplasmin skin test, pulmonary calcifications on the x-ray, and a negative tuberculin reaction.

Because the clinical picture of POHS is so typical, the other tests are more useful in establishing past exposure to the fungus rather than in making a diagnosis. As with systemic histoplasmosis, the histoplasmin skin test is not very useful because the majority of the endemic population tests positive. Negative reactions do occur in patients with the syndrome, and no relationship between skin sensitivity and chorioretinitis has actually been established. Also, the test causes 7% of the patients to suffer a recurrence of their maculopathy.

The differential diagnosis (Table 49–3) includes other causes of inflammatory disease of the fundus such as toxoplasmosis, syphilis, sarcoidosis, toxocariasis, multifocal choroiditis, and vitiliginous chorioretinitis. Noninflammatory conditions such as myopic degeneration, drusen of the optic disc, and angioid streaks can also mimic ocular histoplasmosis. When the syndrome is found in patients who reside in nonendemic regions and have negative skin tests, other causative organisms should be considered.

TREATMENT AND MANAGEMENT

Systemic

The treatment regimen for systemic histoplasmosis (Table 49–5) depends on the form of the disease and the status of the patient's immune system. When antifungal therapy is required, amphotericin B is the primary antifungal drug. Amphotericin B is a polyene antibiotic

TABLE 49–5. TREATMENT AND MANAGEMENT OF HISTOPLASMOSIS

Systemic
- Antifungal drugs: amphotericin B, ketoconazole, itraconazole
- Corticosteroids
- Pulmonary surgery (rare)

Ocular
- Patient monitoring: home Amsler grid
- Avoidance of stress, aspirin, and the Valsalva maneuver
- Corticosteroids when indicated: 200 mg/day for 2–3 weeks in divided dosages, then in single dose every other day at breakfast; taper gradually
- Fluorescein angiogram performed (when neovascular net is suspected) less than 72 hours prior to laser treatment and within 2 weeks after treatment
- Laser photocoagulation of neovascular membranes 200 μm or more from foveal center
- Surgical removal of subfoveal neovascular nets (Submacular Surgery Trial in progress)

that binds to the cell membrane and disrupts the cell's metabolic activity. It is administered intravenously and is very toxic. Because human and fungal cytoplasmic membranes are similar, antifungal drugs that act on these membranes can cause toxicity in humans. Side effects include hypotension, thrombophlebitis, chills, fever, nausea, anemia, and nephrotoxicity.

Two oral fungal drugs recommended for treatment are ketoconazole and itraconazole. Both are effective with less toxicity than amphotericin B. Ketoconazole is an oral imidazole that can cause nausea, vomiting, liver dysfunction, and abnormal synthesis of steroids. Patients tolerate itraconazole better, but ketoconazole is less expensive. To reduce inflammation, corticosteroids may be administered in conjunction with the antifungal drugs.

The vast majority of acute pulmonary histoplasmosis infections are benign and resolve without complications; therefore, treatment is usually not indicated. Patients with the severe life-threatening form of acute histoplasmosis require antifungal therapy with amphotericin B. Disseminated histoplasmosis also requires aggressive antifungal therapy, because without medication, this form of the disease is fatal. With treatment, mortality is reduced from 85% to 15%. Chronic pulmonary histoplasmosis responds well to amphotericin B, ketoconazole, and itraconazole. On rare occasions, surgery is required for cavitations and lesions indistinguishable from pulmonary carcinoma.

About half of the patients with AIDS relapse after treatment. Over the past 10 years, AIDS patients with disseminated histoplasmosis have required aggressive treatment to prevent relapse. Severely ill patients such as those with AIDS are treated with amphotericin B until they show improvement. Then, therapy is continued with itraconazole. Investigators have found that immunosuppressed patients respond well to a lifelong maintenance dose of itraconazole. For patients intolerant of itraconazole, fluconazole is an effective alternative.

Ocular

It is essential that ocular management (Table 49–5) includes daily monitoring with an Amsler grid, because the patient often notices changes in vision prior to the appearance of ophthalmoscopic signs. Emotional or physical stress, aspirin, and the Valsalva maneuver should be avoided because they may reactivate or aggravate maculopathy.

Medical therapy, particularly the antifungal agents discussed in the treatment of symptomatic systemic histoplasmosis, has been found to be ineffective in the treatment of POHS. The use of oral and periocular corticosteroids is controversial, but patients often report improved vision after being treated with them. The main concern is determining if the benefits from steroid treatment outweigh the potential risks and side effects.

The infiltration of T lymphocytes to combat the choroiditis of POHS has been hypothesized. Steroids indirectly interfere with the T-lymphocyte immune reaction by adversely affecting the ability of macrophages to phagocytize and process antigens. In addition, by reducing the permeability of capillaries, steroids decrease leakage from the choroidal neovascular net. In suppressing the inflammatory reaction, corticosteroids possibly prevent the progression to the destructive later stages of maculopathy.

Because steroid therapy suppresses the inflammatory reaction before the macula is severely damaged, patients are instructed to take prednisone immediately after noticing a change in vision. Once patients learn to properly assess their symptoms, they are quite reliable in determining a recurrence of macular involvement and usually can be trusted to initiate their own therapy.

Oral and periocular steroids can be given separately or simultaneously. Because patient reaction to steroids varies, it is advantageous to administer tablets and injections at the same time. This allows the determination of the best route according to the patient's experience. If the patient is compliant, tablets are the preferred route, because they are easy to take and less costly. Advantages of steroid injection include placing the drug directly at the site of inflammation, uniocular treatment, and avoidance of most systemic effects.

The clinical presentation of each individual patient will determine the recommended dosage, tapering regimen, and duration of treatment. An initial

choroiditis is believed to be active for 8 weeks. If CNV has developed, treatment may be required for 2 years. The patient will require close monitoring for the potential development of increased intraocular pressure and posterior subcapsular cataracts from long-term corticosteroid use.

If the patient does not improve or worsens on corticosteroid therapy after 2 to 3 weeks of treatment, then photocoagulation should be considered. Laser treatment is used to prevent further visual loss and to maintain and prolong the vision that remains. Vision may be worse after treatment, and even when treatment is successful, the visual field defect will be larger. Because the underlying disease process still exists, CNV can recur after laser therapy.

A thorough examination should be performed to aid in the preparation and planning of the laser treatment. Tests of particular importance are the Amsler grid, visual field, and fluorescein angiography. Because a neovascular net can change and grow rapidly, the fluorescein must be performed less than 72 hours before treatment. In fact, it is best to do the fluorescein angiogram on the day of treatment, using it as a guide to make certain that the entire choroidal neovascular net is localized and destroyed.

Inactive histo lesions are not prophylactically treated, because treatment can result in activation and histo spots can disappear on their own. In some cases, a laser is used in conjunction with corticosteroids. Studies have shown that when active maculopathy is left untreated, 59% of the eyes have 20/200 vision or worse result. The effectiveness of argon laser photocoagulation of CNV membranes 200 μm or more from the foveal center has been proven by the MPS. Lasering of neovascularization inside the foveal avascular zone is not recommended, because the resulting visual acuity is poor with or without therapy.

Both the blue-green argon laser and the red krypton laser have been shown to be effective in destroying the choroidal neovascular net in the POHS. It has been determined that the argon laser should be used on neovascularization that is greater than 0.25 DD away from the fovea. The blue-green laser is more damaging because it is absorbed by macular pigment and blood; therefore, the krypton laser is preferred for treating areas less than 0.25 DD from the fovea. The red wavelength penetrates deeper to destroy the underlying neovascular membrane, causing less damage to the inner macular layers.

After treatment, careful follow-up examinations are performed. The patient uses the Amsler grid daily to detect visual change due to a persistent or recurrent net. Within 2 weeks after the treatment, a fluorescein angiogram is performed. If leakage is detected, the patient is retreated. These patients must be monitored carefully for the rest of their lives, because recurrent neovascular nets can occur years after laser treatment.

Visual prognosis following corticosteroid and/or laser therapy depends on both the condition of the patient before treatment and the possible side effects of the treatment. If the patient has symptoms of maculopathy for more than 6 months, a large neovascular membrane, or a neovascular membrane close to the fovea, then the visual prognosis after treatment is poor. If the CNV does not recur 1 year after treatment, then the likelihood of recurrence is extremely low. Adverse effects of laser treatment include choroidal bleeding, thermal vasculitis, retinal edema, and internal limiting membrane wrinkling.

Despite the adverse effects of laser treatment and the high rate of CNV recurrence, 1-, 3-, and 5-year follow-ups of the MPS show a reduction or delay in visual acuity loss in laser-treated eyes. In some cases, there was even a gain in visual acuity. Laser treatment is recommended for extrafoveal and juxtafoveal CNV secondary to ocular histoplasmosis. Also, patients with peripapillary CNV or CNV nasal to the fovea have less visual loss if the CNV is treated with a laser. However, there is a reduction in the treatment benefit for both extrafoveal and juxtafoveal CNV in patients with hypertension.

> Laser treatment of extrafoveal and juxtafoveal CNV in POHS is recommended to prevent or delay the loss of visual acuity.

The goal of photocoagulation is to aggressively and completely ablate the entire neovascular net without damaging the fovea. The use of partial photocoagulation is controversial. However, the overriding consensus is that it is contraindicated, because it may stimulate the remaining net to grow. To ensure that the entire area is obliterated, the laser burns are applied 100 to 150 μm beyond the border of the choroidal neovascularization. The MPS results show a decrease in visual acuity loss when the CNV is completely treated. However, complete treatment to prevent persistence or recurrence of CNV requires lasering CNV close to the fovea (less than 200 μm from the FAZ). Retinal specialists are reluctant to perform complete lasering of CNV because they fear inaccuracy will result in damaging healthy retina.

The likelihood of having a subfoveal lesion 5 years after treatment is the same in laser-treated eyes versus untreated eyes. However, the nature of the scarring is different. Treated eyes have less CNV and better visual acuity, and the scarring is secondary to the laser. Untreated eyes have subfoveal disciform scars and more active CNV.

Another form of treatment involves the surgical removal of the subfoveal neovascular membranes. It began in 1991 when Thomas and Kaplan successfully performed this surgery on two patients with resulting improved visual acuity and no recurrence. To better define the role of submacular surgery in POHS, the Submacular Surgery Trial (SST) is currently underway. This multicenter research group was formed to determine whether submacular surgery improves visual acuity in patients with CNV from age-related macular degeneration, POHS, and idiopathic causes. The patients in this study are being randomly assigned to surgery or observation.

Patients with POHS who present with choroidal neovascularization beneath the fovea do not benefit from laser photocoagulation. The laser causes significant damage to the overlying neurosensory retina, resulting in permanent loss of central vision. Surgical excision of subfoveal CNV is being investigated because it has the potential to allow for eradication without damaging the function of the retina. Clinical studies of surgery for subfoveal CNV suggest an improvement in visual function compared with the natural history of POHS or with laser photocoagulation.

In recent years, studies of the surgical removal of subfoveal neovascular membranes in POHS patients show an improvement in visual acuity. The findings indicate that 40% of patients have a marked improvement in central vision. It is believed that this favorable visual prognosis is dependent upon the location of the neovascular membrane. In POHS, the CNV arises from focal defects in the Bruch membrane and proliferates anterior to the RPE. Membranes anterior to the RPE can be removed without damaging the underlying RPE and choriocapillaries. Since the ability of the neurosensory retina to function is dependent upon the integrity of the underlying RPE and choriocapillaries, POHS patients have a better chance of visual recovery after surgery.

Preliminary review of postoperative results shows that 35% of eyes have a final visual acuity of 20/40 or better. Follow-up of these patients over a 1-year interval shows the visual improvement is relatively stable. Postoperative visual results are better in patients with moderate preoperative visual loss (20/100 or better). Postoperative recurrent neovascularization is common (50%) and responds best to laser photocoagulation as opposed to repeat surgery or observation. The continued research of the SST will hopefully provide more information on the risks and benefits of submacular surgery.

CONCLUSION

The presumed ocular histoplasmosis syndrome is a common cause of visual loss in endemic areas. Despite the understanding of the systemic disease from its benign to fatal presentations, the relationship between the ocular and nonocular forms remains uncertain. Epidemiologic and experimental studies have provided some answers, but they have not substantiated *H. capsulatum* as the cause of the ocular syndrome. However, both forms of the disease can be devastating. As researchers continue to look for a correlation, the focus should be on proper diagnosis, management, and treatment.

REFERENCES

Akduman L, Del Priore LV, Desai VN, et al. Perfusion of the subfoveal choriocapillaris affects visual recovery after submacular surgery in presumed ocular histoplasmosis syndrome. *Am J Ophthalmol.* 1997;123910:90–96.

Atebara NH, Thomas MA, Holekamp NM, et al. Surgical removal of extensive peripapillary choroidal neovascularization associated with presumed ocular histoplasmosis syndrome. *Ophthalmology.* 1998;105:1598–1605.

Beck RW, Sergott RC, Barr CC, Annesley H. Optic disc edema in the presumed ocular histoplasmosis syndrome. *Ophthalmology.* 1984;91:183–185.

Berger AS, Conway M, Del Priore LV, et al. Submacular surgery for subfoveal choroidal neovascular membranes in patients with presumed ocular histoplasmosis. *Arch Ophthalmol.* 1997;115:991–996.

Berger AS, Kaplan HJ. Clinical experience with the surgical removal of subfoveal neovascular membranes. *Ophthalmology.* 1992;99:969–975.

Bindschadler D. Fungal diseases. In: Mitchell R, Petty T, Schwarz M, eds. *Synopsis of Clinical Pulmonary Disease.* 4th ed. St. Louis: Mosby; 1989:106–117.

Bottoni FG, Deutman AF, Aandekerk AL. Presumed ocular histoplasmosis syndrome and linear streak lesions. *Br J Ophthalmol.* 1989;73:528–535.

Braley RE, Meredith TA, Aaberg TM, et al. The prevalence of HLA-B7 in presumed ocular histoplasmosis. *Am J Ophthalmol.* 1978;85:859–861.

Campochiaro PA, Morgn KM, Conway BP, Stathos J. Spontaneous involution of subfoveal neovascularization. *Am J Ophthalmol.* 1990;109:668–675.

Canadian Ophthalmology Study Group. Argon green vs krypton red laser photocoagulation for extrafoveal choroidal neovascularization. One-year results in ocular histoplasmosis. *Arch Ophthalmol.* 1994;112:1166–1173.

Chandler FW, Watts JC. Fungal infections. In: Dail DH, Hammar SP, eds. *Pulmonary Pathology.* New York: Springer-Verlag; 1988:189–201.

Check IJ, Diddie KR, Jay WM, et al. Lymphocyte stimulation by yeast phase *Histoplasma capsulatum* in presumed ocular histoplasmosis syndrome. *Am J Ophthalmol.* 1979; 87:311–316.

Cummings HL, Rehmar AJ, Wood WJ, Isernhagen RD. Long-term results of laser treatment in the ocular histoplasmosis syndrome. *Arch Ophthalmol.* 1995;113:465–468.

Deutsch TA, Tessler HH. Inflammatory pseudohistoplasmosis. *Ann Ophthalmol.* 1985;17:461–465.

Dismukes WE. Histoplasmosis. In: Bennett JC, Plum F, eds. *Cecil Textbook of Medicine.* Philadelphia: WB Saunders; 1996:20.

Dreyer RF, Gass DM. Multifocal choroiditis and panuveitis. *Arch Ophthalmol.* 1984;102:1776–1784.

Feman SS, Tilford RH. Ocular findings in patients with histoplasmosis. *JAMA.* 1985;253:2534–2537.

Fountain JA, Schlaegel TF. Linear streaks of the equator in the presumed ocular histoplasmosis syndrome. *Arch Ophthalmol.* 1981;99:246–248.

Gass JD. Biomicroscopic and histopathologic considerations regarding the feasibility of surgical excision of subfoveal neovascular membranes. *Am J Ophthalmol.* 1994;118: 285–298.

Gass JD. *Stereoscopic Atlas of Macular Diseases.* 3rd ed. St. Louis: Mosby;1987:112–128.

Graybill JR. Infections caused by fungi and the higher bacteria *(Actinomyces* and *Nocardia).* In: Stein JH, ed. *Internal Medicine.* Boston: Little, Brown;1990:1556–1562.

Grossniklaus HE, Green WR. Histopathologic and ultrastructural findings of surgically excised choroidal neovascularization. Submacular Surgery Trials Research Group. *Arch Ophthalmol.* 1998;116:745–749.

Han DP, Folk JC. Internal limiting membrane wrinkling after argon and krypton laser photocoagulation of choroidal neovascularization. *Retina.* 1986;6:215–219.

Han DP, Folk JC, Bratton AR. Visual loss after successful photocoagulation of choroidal neovascularization. *Ophthalmology.* 1988;95:1380–1384.

Holekamp NM, Thomas MA, Dickinson JD, Valluri S. Surgical removal of subfoveal choroidal neovascularization in presumed ocular histoplasmosis: Stability of early visual results. *Ophthalmology.* 1997;104:22–26.

Holland GN. Endogenous fungal infections of the retina and choroid. In: Ryan SJ, ed. *Retina.* vol.2. St. Louis: Mosby; 1989;2:625–635.

Johnston RL, Mitchell PC, Berman AM. Presumed ocular histoplasmosis syndrome. *J Am Optom Assoc.* 1988;59:401–405.

Joondeph BC, Tessler HH. Clinical course of multifocal choroiditis: Photographic and angiographic evidence of disease recurrence. *Ann Ophthalmol.* 1991;23:424–429.

Kleiner RC, Ratner CM, Enger C, Fine SL. Subfoveal neovascularization in the ocular histoplasmosis syndrome. *Retina.* 1988;6:225–229.

Klintworth GK, Hollingsworth AS, Lusman PA, Bradford WD. Granulomatous choroiditis in a case of disseminated histoplasmosis. *Arch Ophthalmol.* 1973;90:45–48.

Lewis ML, Van Newkirk MR, Gass JD. Follow-up study of presumed ocular histoplasmosis syndrome. *Ophthalmology.* 1980;87:390–399.

Loewenstein A, Sunness JS, Bressler NM, et al. Scanning laser ophthalmoscope fundus perimetry after surgery for choroidal neovascularization. *Am J Ophthalmol.* 1998; 125:657–665.

Louria DB. Fungus, *Actinomyces,* and *Nocardia* infections of the lungs. In: Baun GL, Wolinsky E, eds. *Textbook of Pulmonary Diseases.* Boston: Little, Brown; 1983;459–467.

Macular Photocoagulation Study Group. Argon laser photocoagulation for neovascular maculopathy. Five-year results from randomized clinical trials. *Arch Ophthalmol.* 1991;109:1109–1114.

Macular Photocoagulation Study Group. Argon laser photocoagulation for ocular histoplasmosis. *Arch Ophthalmol.* 1983;101:1347–1357.

Macular Photocoagulation Study Group. Five-year follow-up of fellow eyes of individuals with ocular histoplasmosis and unilateral extrafoveal or juxtafoveal choroidal neovascularization. *Arch Ophthalmol.* 1996;114:677–688.

Macular Photocoagulation Study Group. Laser photocoagulation for juxtafoveal choroidal neovascularization Five-year results from randomized clinical trials. *Arch Ophthalmol.* 1994;112:500–509.

Macular Photocoagulation Study Group. Laser photocoagulation for neovascular lesions nasal to the fovea. Results from clinical trials for lesions secondary to ocular histoplasmosis or idiopathic causes. *Arch Ophthalmol.* 1995; 113:56–61.

Macular Photocoagulation Study Group. *MPS Manual of Procedures.* Springfield, VA: National Technical Information Service; 1991. Accession No. PB91159368.

Macular Photocoagulation Study Group. The influence of treatment extent on the visual acuity of eyes treated with krypton laser for juxtafoveal choroidal neovascularization. *Arch Ophthalmol.* 1995;113:190–194.

McMillan TA, Lashkari K. Ocular histoplasmosis. *Int Ophthalmol Clin.* 1996;36:179–186.

Melberg NS, Thomas MA, Dickinson JD, Valluri S. Managing recurrent neovascularization after subfoveal surgery in presumed ocular histoplasmosis syndrome. *Ophthalmology.* 1996;103:1064–1067.

Meredith TA, Smith RE, Duquesnoy RJ. Association of HLA-DRw2 antigen with presumed ocular histoplasmosis. *Am J Ophthalmol.* 1980;89:70–76.

Negroni P. *Histoplasmosis.* Springfield, IL: Thomas; 1965.

Olk RJ, Burgess DB. Treatment of recurrent juxtafoveal subretinal neovascular membranes with krypton red laser photocoagulation. *Ophthalmology.* 1985;92:1035–1046.

Olk RJ, Burgess DB, McCormick PA. Subfoveal and juxtafoveal subretinal neovascularization in the presumed ocular histoplasmosis syndrome. *Ophthalmology.* 1984; 91:1592–1602.

Patterson TF, Graybill JR. Infections caused by common fungi. In: Stein JH, ed. *Internal Medicine.* St. Louis: Mosby; 1998:5.

Roth AM. *Histoplasma capsulatum* in the presumed ocular histoplasmosis syndrome. *Am J Ophthalmol.* 1977;84: 293–298.

Sabates FN, Lee KY, Ziemianski MC. A comparative study of argon and krypton laser photocoagulation in the treatment of presumed ocular histoplasmosis syndrome. *Ophthalmology.* 1982;89:729–734.

Sarosi GA, Davies SF, eds. *Fungal Diseases of the Lung.* Orlando, FL: Grune & Stratton; 1986.

Sarosi GA, Davies SF. Histoplasmosis. In: Fishman A, ed. *Pulmonary Diseases and Disorders.* 2nd ed. New York: McGraw-Hill; 1988;1775–1781.

Sawelson H, Goldberg RE, Annesley WH, Tomer TL. Presumed ocular histoplasmosis syndrome: The fellow eye. *Arch Ophthalmol.* 1976;94:221–224.

Saxe SJ, Grossniklaus HE, Lopez PF, et al. Ultrastructural features of surgically excised subretinal neovascular membranes in the ocular histoplasmosis syndrome. *Arch Ophthalmol.* 1993;111:88–95.

Schlaegel TF. *Ocular Histoplasmosis.* New York: Grune & Stratton; 1977.

Schlaegel TF. Presumed ocular histoplasmosis. In: Tasman W, Jaeger EA, eds. *Duane's Clinical Ophthalmology.* Philadelphia: Lippincott; 1991;4.

Schlaegel TF. *Update on Ocular Histoplasmosis.* Boston: Little, Brown; 1983.

Scholz R, Green WR, Kutys R, et al. *Histoplasma capsulatum* in the eye. *Ophthalmology.* 1984;91:110–1104.

Schwarz J. *Histoplasmosis.* New York: Praeger; 1981.

Sheffer A, Green R, Fine SL, Kincaid M. Presumed ocular histoplasmosis syndrome—A clinicopathologic correlation of a treated case. *Arch Ophthalmol.* 1980;98:335–340.

Singerman LJ. Important points in management of patients with choroidal neovascularization. *Ophthalmology.* 1985; 92:610–614.

Singerman LJ, Wong B, Ai E, Smith S. Spontaneous visual improvement in the first affected eye of patients with bilateral disciform scars. *Retina.* 1985;5:135–143.

Thomas MA, Dickinson JD, Melberg NS, et al. Visual results after surgical removal of subfoveal choroidal neovascular membranes. *Ophthalmology.* 1994;101:1384–1396.

Thomas MA, Kaplan HJ. Surgical removal of subfoveal neovascularization in the presumed ocular histoplasmosis syndrome. *Am J Ophthalmol.* 1991;111:1–7.

Watzke RC. Histoplasmosis. In: Gold DH, Weingeist TA, eds. *The Eye in Systemic Disease.* Philadelphia: Lippincott; 1990:200–202.

Wilkinson CP. Presumed ocular histoplasmosis. *Am J Ophthalmol.* 1976;82:140–142.

Woods AC, Wahlen HE. The probable role of benign histoplasmosis in the etiology of granulomatosis uveitis. *Trans Am Ophthalmol Soc.* 1959;57:318.

Yassur Y, Gilad E, Ben-Sira I. Treatment of macular subretinal neovascularization with the red-light krypton laser in presumed ocular histoplasmosis syndrome. *Am J Ophthalmol.* 1981;91:172–176.

Chapter 50

CHLAMYDIA

Taryn Mathews

For thousands of years, humans have suffered from systemic and ocular infections caused by the intracellular parasite chlamydia. The genus *Chlamydia* has three species, *C. trachomatis, C. psittaci,* and *C. pneumoniae,* and each species has a number of serotypes responsible for various chlamydial diseases. This chapter will be restricted to diseases caused by *C. trachomatis.*

In the developing world, the severest form of chlamydia, called trachoma, is the greatest cause of preventable vision loss despite improvements in living conditions. In the industrialized world, chlamydia causes the most common sexually transmitted disease. Genital chlamydial infections are transmitted to the eye, causing adult inclusion conjunctivitis and neonatal conjunctivitis. Oculogenital chlamydial infections can be difficult to diagnose, because many of those afflicted are asymptomatic and clinical features are shared with other common infections.

The acronym TRIC, which stands for trachoma-inclusion conjunctivitis, is given to all the serotypes that cause trachoma, inclusion conjunctivitis, and the associated systemic complications. Recognizing the clinical presentation, in combination with appropriate testing, allows for the correct diagnosis and choice of treatment. Reinfection and further spread of the disease can be prevented by examining the patient and the sexual partners.

EPIDEMIOLOGY

Systemic

Each year, there are 3 to 4 million new cases of genital infection caused by *C. trachomatis.* In fact, it is the most common sexually transmitted disease in the United States. A significant number of patients infected with *Neisseria gonorrhoeae* have a concurrent chlamydial infection. However, in the comparison of chlamydial and gonococcal infections, chlamydial infections producc fewer symptoms and signs. In many cases, particularly in chlamydial infections of female genital tracts, there are no symptoms. Approximately 25% of heterosexual men suffer with concurrent infection. In women, 30 to 50% with gonorrhea also have a chlamydial infection.

Combined infections are more prevalent in single, non-Caucasian or Asian females in their late teens and early twenties. In industrialized countries, chlamydial infections are more prevalent than gonorrhea because routine diagnostic testing and treatment of gonorrhea (in both sexual partners) has been more effectively instituted. However, in areas where programs have been implemented to control chlamydial infections, there has been a decrease in the number of cases.

Chlamydial cervicitis develops in 60% of women who engage in sexual activity with infected men. In sexually transmitted disease (STD) clinics, over 20% of women have cervical infection from chlamydia. In family planning clinics, the prevalence of cervicitis is over 10%. In the United States, chlamydial cervicitis in pregnant women is 5 to 10 times more prevalent than gonorrhea. Infants exposed during birth have a 60% chance of developing a chlamydial infection. Approximately 10 to 20% of these newborns develop pneumonia.

Thirty-five to fifty percent of patients with nongonococcal urethritis (NGU) test positive for *C. trachomatis,* making it the leading cause of NGU and of postgonococcal urethritis (PGU). In the United States, the number of new NGU cases increases by half a million each year. Chlamydia causes two thirds of epididymitis cases. Chlamydial urethral infections are found in 15 to 20% of young heterosexual men examined in STD clinics. Homosexual males have rectal infections more often than urethral infections due to anorectal intercourse. Although chlamydia has not been established as the cause of Reiter syndrome, 40 to 70% of male patients with this syndrome have *C. trachomatis* in their urethras.

Ocular

Trachoma

Trachoma is one of the major causes of blindness throughout the world. Although the blindness is preventable, approximately 200 million of the estimated 700 million cases of trachoma involve blindness or severe visual loss. The blinding form, known as endemic trachoma, is most prevalent in countries of low socioeconomic status with a dry, sandy climate. Trachoma is associated with impoverished rural communities of underdeveloped countries plagued with poor sanitation, overcrowding, and unhealthy living conditions. Today, the regions most affected by trachoma include North Africa, sub-Saharan Africa, the Middle East, and parts of the Indian subcontinent, Asia, Latin America, Australia, and the Pacific Islands. In the United States, trachoma is prevalent in southwestern American Indians and Mexicans, and in the states of Arkansas, Missouri, Oklahoma, West Virginia, and Kentucky.

Adult Inclusion Conjunctivitis

The typical patient with inclusion conjunctivitis is a young, sexually active adult ranging in age from 18 to 35 years. In many cases, the patient reports having a new sexual partner. It is more frequently seen in industrialized countries, and all social classes are known to be affected by the disease. But like trachoma, it is more prevalent in people with poor hygiene. In about 70% the condition affects only one eye. Recurrences occur when both sexual partners are not treated. The incidence of inclusion conjunctivitis has increased dramatically with the rise in chlamydial genital infections and other venereal diseases. Each year, over 4 million Americans contract genital chlamydial disease. Approximately 1 in 300 of these patients develops inclusion conjunctivitis.

Neonatal Inclusion Conjunctivitis

Neonatal inclusion conjunctivitis or blennorrhea is the most common form of eye disease caused by chlamydia. The number of cases in industrialized countries is on the rise. Two to six percent of all newborns in the United States contract chlamydia as a result of exposure to infected birth canals. Children born to infected mothers have a 50% chance of developing inclusion conjunctivitis.

PATHOPHYSIOLOGY/DISEASE PROCESS

Systemic

The Organism

Chlamydia is an obligate, intracellular parasite that possesses characteristics of bacteria and viruses. For many years, this parasite was considered to be a virus, but is now classified as a bacterium with a separate order, genus, and species. Similar to a bacterium, chlamydia possesses deoxyribonucleic acid (DNA) and ribonucleic acid (RNA), divides by binary fission, and is sensitive to antibiotics. However, like a virus, chlamydia is unable to produce ATP, and is therefore dependent on the host epithelial cell for energy. *C. trachomatis* is subdivided into several serotypes. Sexually transmitted diseases and neonatal infections are caused by serotypes D through K, whereas trachoma is caused by serotypes A through C.

Transmission

Chlamydia has a unique life cycle that involves two forms, the elementary body (EB) and the reticulate or initial body (RB). A brief description of the life cycle provides an explanation for the basis of diagnostic testing. The EB is the infectious form, which is phagocytized by its target, the epithelial cell (genital or ocular). After it enters the cell, it changes into the larger RB. The RB then multiplies into aggregates of EBs near or attached to the nucleus. An aggregate of EBs is called an inclusion body. When the cell ruptures, the EBs are released to infect other epithelial cells. The life cycle requires about 48 hours.

Chlamydia, transmitted via sexual contact, results in genital infection. Newborns of infected mothers acquire the parasite through exposure to the infected birth canal. Transmission of the oculogenital disease is primarily through sexual contact, either from the genital tract to the fingers and then to the eye, or directly from the genitals to the eye. It is very rare for transmission of inclusion conjunctivitis to occur through eye to eye contact. Before chlorination, adult inclusion conjunctivitis was transmitted from genital secretions in swimming pools. Today, swimming pool conjunctivitis is rare and is caused by adenovirus.

The transmission of trachoma occurs by eye-to-eye or hand-to-eye contact via flies, fomites, contaminated towels, and water. It is believed that trachoma develops after repeated, prolonged exposure to the organism over months or years.

Course of the Disease

C. trachomatis is a major cause of a number of genital infections in men and women (Table 50–1). In men, it has been associated with a large percentage of the NGU and PGU cases. Nongonococcal urethritis, as the name implies, is urethritis not caused by gonorrhea but with the clinical presentation of gonorrhea. PGU is a type of NGU that develops 2 to 3 weeks after successful gonorrhea treatment.

One to three weeks after exposure, NGU patients present with a mucopurulent discharge. The presentation is similar to gonorrhea, but chlamydial urethritis is not as severe. Other symptoms include dysuria and urethral pruritus. Meatal erythema and tenderness are found upon examination. However, in about one third of men diagnosed with chlamydial urethritis, there are no signs or symptoms.

PGU patients complain of a persistent urethral discharge after being treated with penicillin for gonorrhea. These patients had concurrent infection that was unknown until the gonorrhea was treated. However, the incidence of PGU caused by chlamydia has decreased in recent years because patients with gonorrhea are concurrently prescribed medication for chlamydia.

Epididymitis is a complication that often occurs secondary to chlamydial urethritis. Patients with Reiter syndrome have urethritis, arthritis, conjunctivitis, and a rash. The relationship of chlamydia to Reiter syndrome is unknown, but a genital infection caused by *C. trachomatis* often precedes the syndrome.

Proctitis caused by chlamydia occurs in men or women who have anorectal intercourse. It is an inflammatory condition that is often asymptomatic or mild. Examination reveals rectal mucosa erythema and a mucopurulent discharge. Patients complain of anorectal discharge, constipation, tenesmus (the unsuccessful urge to void), and pruritus.

In women, the most common complication of chlamydial infection is a mucopurulent cervicitis.

TABLE 50–1. SYSTEMIC MANIFESTATIONS OF CHLAMYDIA

Nongonococcal Urethritis (NGU)
- May or may not be asymptomatic
- Mucopurulent discharge
- Dysuria and urethral pruritis
- Meatal erythema and tenderness
- Possible association with Reiter syndrome: urethritis, uveitis, conjunctivitis, arthritis

Postgonococcal Urethritis (PGU)
- Persistent urethral discharge despite penicillin (PCN) treatment for gonorrhea
- Epididymitis
- Proctitis

Rectal mucopurulent discharge
Rectal mucosa erythema
Constipation
Tenesmus
Pruritis

Complications in Women
- Cervicitis
  - Often concurrently infected with *Neisseria gonorrhoeae*
  - Yellow, mucopurulent discharge
  - Erythematous, edematous cervix
  - Bleeds easily with minor trauma
- Salpingitis
  - Subsequent fallopian tube scarring and sterility may result
- Pelvic inflammatory disease
  - Multiple infecting organisms
  - Cervicitis
  - Endometritis (vaginal bleeding, abdominal pain, uterine tenderness)
  - Endosalpingitis (subsequent scarring and sterility may result)
  - Pelvic peritonitis
  - Perihepatitis (also known as Fitz-Hugh–Curtis syndrome, characterized by inflammation of the liver capsule with fibrinous adhesions and pleuritic upper abdominal pain and tenderness)

Complications in Pregnant Women
- Increased risk of ectopic pregnancy
- Premature delivery
- Postpartum endometritis

Complications in Newborns
- Pneumonia: afebrile, coughing, tachypneic
- Otitis with potential hearing loss
- Vaginitis

Some patients have mild symptoms, whereas many others have no symptoms. The cervix becomes red and edematous, bleeds easily from minor trauma, and produces a yellow mucopurulent discharge. As with urethritis in men, many patients have simultaneous infections from *C. trachomatis* and *N. gonorrhoeae*.

Further complications of chlamydial infection in women include urethritis, salpingitis (inflammation of the fallopian tubes), pelvic inflammatory disease, secondary peritonitis, and fallopian tube scarring with subsequent sterility. Tubal scarring from chlamydia may be a contributing factor in the increase of ectopic pregnancies. Chlamydial infection during pregnancy may lead to premature delivery and postpartum endometritis.

Pelvic inflammatory disease is caused by multiple organisms, particularly *N. gonorrhoeae* and *C. trachomatis*. Microorganisms travel from the lower genital tract to the fallopian tubes and endometrium. The disease is characterized by cervicitis, endometritis, endosalpingitis, and pelvic peritonitis. In endometritis, patients suffer with vaginal bleeding, abdominal pain, and uterine tenderness. Perihepatitis (inflammation of the liver capsule) may also occur.

Systemic complications in newborns infected during delivery include pneumonia, otitis, vaginitis, and hearing loss. The development of pneumonia occurs from 2 to 12 weeks of age. Clinical examination reveals afebrile, coughing, and tachypneic (breathing very rapidly) newborns.

Lymphogranuloma venereum (LGV) is a systemic sexually transmitted disease caused by *C. trachomatis* serotypes L1, L2, and L3. Although still endemic in tropical countries, LGU is rare in the United States, and rarely causes ocular manifestations. Therefore, this chlamydial disease will not be discussed.

Ocular

Table 50–2 summarizes the ocular manifestations of chlamydia.

Trachoma

The clinical presentation of trachoma is variable due to differences in the various strains, the occurrence of concurrent bacterial infections, and the climate. In endemic regions, trachoma primarily affects young children. In fact, almost all the children acquire the infection by the age of 1 or 2 years, and then the disease slowly runs its course through the adult years. It is uncommon for the infection to start during adulthood. Relapses or recurrences of disease may occur because of latency or the failure to develop immunity. It is common to see recurrent disease in children, even after they have been treated. The severe blinding complications of trachoma are more common in adults.

Endemic trachoma is a chronic, bilateral follicular keratoconjunctivitis. The layer most involved in trachoma infections is the epithelium of the conjunctiva and cornea. The pathologic changes of the conjunctival epithelium include weakened cell-to-cell adhesions, hyperplasia, irregularity of cell size, and the infiltration of lymphocytes and polymorphonuclear leukocytes. The area of the conjunctiva most affected is the upper tarsal plate.

Following the epithelial change is a chronic inflammatory reaction in the subepithelial tissues. The infiltration of inflammatory cells results in edema, hy-

TABLE 50–2. OCULAR MANIFESTATIONS OF CHLAMYDIA

Trachoma
- MacCallan trachoma grading
  - Stage I: Soft, immature follicles in the upper palpebral conjunctiva without scarring
    - Serous exudation of variable degree is usually present
    - Follicles may be present at limbus (especially superior) and caruncle
  - Stage IIA: Mature upper tarsal plate follicles and moderate papillary hypertrophy
  - Stage IIB: Papillary hypertrophy predominates, resulting in obscuration of follicles
  - Stage III: Cicatricial or conjunctival scarring
  - Stage IV: Healed trachoma (the inflammatory reaction, follicles, and papillae have subsided and are replaced by scar tissue)
- The WHO trachoma grading
  - Based on number of follicles and the degree of papillary hypertrophy
- Symptoms
  - Erythema, tearing, mucopurulent discharge
  - Photophobia, pain
  - Edematous lids and conjunctiva
  - Tender preauricular lymph node
- Complications
  - Vision loss secondary to conjunctival (Arlt lines) and corneal scarring
  - Dry eye syndrome secondary to lacrimal gland and goblet cell damage
  - Dacryocystitis secondary to lacrimal sac damage
  - Lid deformities (entropion, ectropion, trichiasis)
  - Corneal ulceration and scarring secondary to trichiasis
  - Secondary bacterial infections

Adult Inclusion Conjunctivitis
- Symptoms
  - Mild irritation, foreign-body sensation, tearing, photophobia
  - Conjunctival erythema, mild mucopurulent discharge
  - Lid edema, lids sealed shut in morning
  - (+) or (−) genital symptoms
- Signs
  - Ipsilateral tender palpable preauricular node
  - (−) fever, (−) upper respiratory infection
  - Hyperemic, edematous conjunctiva
  - Follicular/papillary palpebral conjunctiva hypertrophy (especially lower tarsal conjunctiva and fornix)
  - Superiorly located keratitis with yellow subepithelial infiltrates (peripheral > central cornea)
  - Corneal vascularization, limbal swelling, and micropannus formation (resolves with treatment)
- Less common findings
  - Pseudoptosis
  - Mild anterior uveitis
  - Association with Reiter syndrome
  - Ipsilateral otitis media

Neonatal Inclusion Conjunctivitis
- Usually presents bilaterally 5 days after birth
- Signs
  - Profuse mucopurulent discharge
  - Edematous lids
  - Hyperemic conjunctiva
  - Papillary hypertrophy
  - Inflammatory pseudomembrane
  - Corneal infiltration and pannus formation

peremia, papillary hypertrophy, and the formation of follicles. Follicles do not form during the first year of life. A unique feature of trachomatous follicles is their softness, allowing their contents of lymphocytic cells to be easily expressed onto the conjunctiva, resulting in necrosis and scarring. Scarred follicles at the limbus form depressions called Herbert pits. These pits have a serrated appearance and are pathognomonic of trachoma. The follicular response is sometimes masked by the papillary hypertrophy and inflammation.

MacCallan (1931) was the first to classify the clinical features of the conjunctiva in trachoma into four stages (see Table 50–2). The first three stages, lasting months to years, are characterized by follicles in the superior palpebral conjunctiva, superior limbus, and caruncle. Serous exudation is usually present. Papillary hypertrophy eventually obscures the follicles. Cicatricial or conjunctival scarring eventually occurs. The inflammatory reaction, follicles, and papillae subside and are replaced by scar tissue in the final stage.

The amount of scarring varies depending on the severity of the inflammatory reaction in the earlier stages. The MacCallan system is limited as it only addresses the conjunctival involvement. The World Health Organization (WHO) developed a grading system to enable personnel (other than eyecare providers) to assess the degree of severity of trachoma within a community. The system is based on the number of upper tarsal follicles and the degree of upper tarsal papillary hypertrophy (see Table 50–2).

Endemic trachoma has a gradual onset. The typical patient is less than 2 years of age. The presenting symptoms are redness, tearing, photophobia, pain, mucopurulent discharge, swollen lids and conjunctiva, and a tender preauricular lymph node. The degree of pain and photophobia depends on the extent of corneal involvement. The amount of discharge will vary depending on the development of secondary bacterial infection.

Visual impairment in trachoma results from complications of the active disease. As the inflammation subsides, the conjunctiva becomes severely scarred and fibrotic. Damage to the goblet cells and the ductules of the lacrimal gland leads to dry eye syndromes. Dacryocystitis often occurs from scarring of the lacrimal sac. The scarred conjunctiva shrinks and contracts, forming a white horizontal scar across the upper tarsal plate approximately one third of the distance from the lid margin. These linear scars, called Arlt lines, contract to produce entropion. Scarring at the lid margin results in further distortion and deformity of the lids and trichiasis.

Blindness in trachoma ultimately is due to the effects of the secondary complications on the cornea

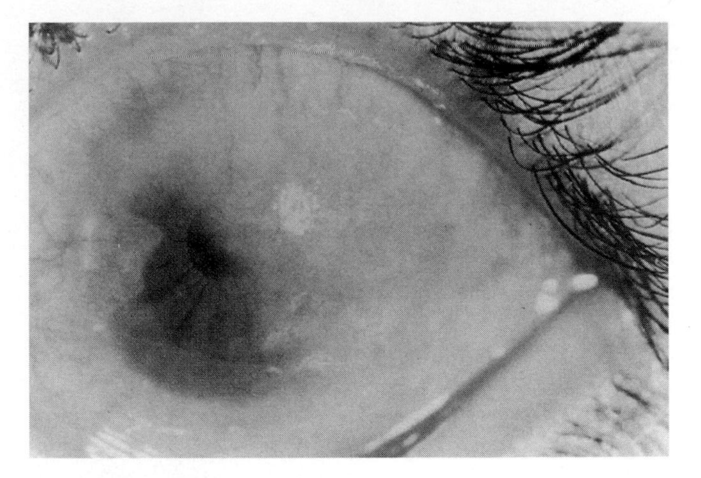

Figure 50–1. Severe corneal pannus and scarring in endstage trachoma. *(Reprinted with permission from Mandel ER, Wagoner MD.* Atlas of Corneal Disease. *Philadelphia: WB Saunders Co, 1989.)*

(Figure 50–1). In fact, entropion and trichiasis are the most common causes of severe visual loss. Recurrent abrasion of the cornea by the lashes, combined with keratitis sicca and abnormal lid closure, results in corneal ulceration and scarring. In addition, the compromised cornea is more susceptible to secondary bacterial infections. A concurrent bacterial infection increases the severity of the disease. The presentation of disease can range from very mild with few or no complications to complete degeneration of the cornea and conjunctiva.

Adult Inclusion Conjunctivitis

Adult inclusion conjunctivitis is an oculogenital disease, affecting the conjunctiva and the genital or urinary tract. It is caused by *C. trachomatis* serotypes D through K. The ocular clinical presentation has a similar appearance to the early stages of trachoma, but the condition is benign and self-limiting without the scarring and other severe complications. To differentiate the condition from endemic trachoma, it is sometimes referred to as paratrachoma.

One to two weeks after exposure, adults present with an acute follicular conjunctivitis. Symptoms include mild irritation, foreign-body sensation, tearing, photophobia, redness, lid swelling, and mild mucopurulent discharge. Patients report sticky eyelids sealed shut upon awakening. Upper respiratory symptoms and fever are absent, helping to differentiate inclusion conjunctivitis from conjunctivitis caused by viruses, especially adenovirus. However, a small, mildly tender preauricular node does occur on the affected side. Symptoms of systemic or genital manifestations consistent with chlamydia may or may not be present.

> Adult inclusion conjunctivitis can mimic bacterial and/or viral keratoconjunctivitides. Chlamydia should be suspected in cases with prolonged bacterial signs and symptoms, unresponsive to standard topical antibiotic treatment. Patients and sexual partners should be counseled and tested for venereal disease.

The conjunctiva is injected, hyperemic, and edematous with a combination of follicular and papillary hypertrophy in the upper and lower conjunctiva (Figure 50–2). In contrast to endemic trachoma, the conjunctival response is greatest in the lower tarsal conjunctiva and fornix, and the follicles may take up to 3 weeks to appear.

Corneal involvement usually occurs during the second week of the disease. The keratitis occurs in the superficial epithelium and is usually localized to the superior cornea. Subepithelial infiltration and opacification occur in the peripheral and central cornea, although the marginal infiltrates are more common. The infiltrates have a yellow appearance and stain with fluorescein. Superior superficial corneal vascularization and limbal swelling occur, followed by the formation of a micropannus of 1 to 3 mm. Most of the corneal changes resolve with treatment.

Additional less common clinical findings include a pseudoptosis, persistent superficial punctate keratitis, mild anterior uveitis, Reiter syndrome, and (in 14% of cases) otitis media on the involved side. There have been reports of patients with genital chlamydia having inclusion conjunctivitis without symptoms. On occasion, inclusion conjunctivitis can become a chronic condition.

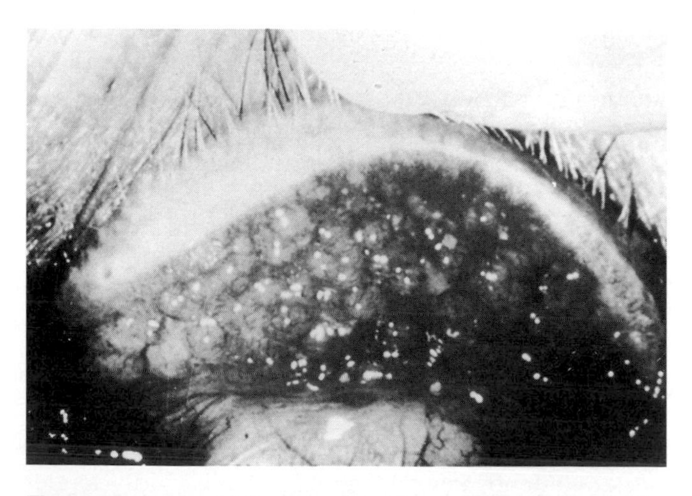

Figure 50–2. Mixed follicular and papillary hypertrophy in adult inclusion conjunctivitis. *(Reprinted with permission from Wallace W. Diseases of the conjunctiva. In: Bartlett JD, Jaanus SD, eds.* Clinical Ocular Pharmacology. *Boston: Butterworths 1989:546.)*

Untreated, inclusion conjunctivitis has a natural course of 6 to 18 months. The disease resolves without complications, although a few cases of conjunctival scarring have been reported. With topical and systemic treatment, the disease resolves over a 3-week period. Patients report feeling better after 1 week of treatment.

Neonatal Inclusion Conjunctivitis

Neonatal inclusion conjunctivitis usually presents bilaterally on the fifth day after birth. However, the duration of incubation is variable, a range of 3 to 21 days. The clinical presentation is indistinguishable from other forms of acute neonatal conjunctivitis without diagnostic testing. The signs include edematous lids, conjunctival hyperemia, papillary hypertrophy, and a profuse mucopurulent discharge. Corneal pannus and infiltration are also seen.

The clinical presentation of the neonatal form is similar to the adult form of inclusion conjunctivitis. However, there are a number of distinguishable differences. Because newborns lack mature conjunctival lymphoid tissue, follicles cannot develop until 4 or 5 months of age. Therefore, the conjunctival reaction is primarily one of papillary hypertrophy rather than follicular. Newborns have more mucopurulent discharge than adults. In severe cases, infants can develop an inflammatory pseudomembrane in the palpebral conjunctiva. Membranes are not seen in the adult form. Newborns have more intracytoplasmic inclusion bodies. Lastly, the infant form responds better to topical medication than the adult variety.

When infected infants are not treated both orally and topically, they are more likely to develop conjunctival scarring and pannus. Untreated neonates are also more likely to develop chlamydial pneumonia.

DIAGNOSIS

Systemic

Despite the availability of many diagnostic techniques, chlamydial infections are often difficult to diagnose (Table 50–3). Many cases go unnoticed because of their mild or asymptomatic nature. Furthermore, chlamydial infections are often masked by a concurrent infection, especially gonorrhea. The variability and limitations of the various tests also hinder the diagnostic process. Therefore, the clinical presentation plays a crucial part in chlamydial diagnosis. Patient history, genital examination, cultures, smears, routine blood work, urinalysis, serologic tests, and in the case of sus-

TABLE 50–3. DIFFERENTIAL DIAGNOSIS OF CHLAMYDIA

Systemic
- *Neisseria gonorrhoeae*
- *Ureaplasma urealyticum*
- *Trichomonas vaginalis*
- Herpes simplex virus

Ocular
Trachoma
- Atopic keratoconjunctivitis
- Bacterial keratoconjunctivitis
- Adult inclusion conjunctivitis
- Cicatricial
- Giant papillary conjunctivitis
- Superior limbic keratoconjunctivitis
- Vernal keratoconjunctivitis

Adult inclusion conjunctivitis
- Bacterial keratoconjunctivitis
- Viral keratoconjunctivitis
- Epidemic keratoconjunctivitis
- Episcleritis
- Scleritis
- Trachoma
- Superficial keratitis
- Reiter syndrome
- Pharyngoconjunctival fever

Neonatal inclusion conjunctivitis
- Chemical (eg, silver nitrate)
- *Neisseria gonorrhoeae*
- Bacteria
- Herpes simplex virus
- Dacryocystitis
- Nasolacrimal duct obstruction
- Trachoma

pected pneumonia, chest x-rays, are all employed in the diagnosis (Table 50–4).

Before present-day diagnostic tests were available, chlamydia was cultured by inoculating the yolk sac of embryonated chicken eggs. Today, the standard diagnostic test is the McCoy cell tissue culture. In this test, irradiated tissue culture cells, called McCoy cells, are inoculated with the presumed infected specimens. After a 3-day incubation, iodine or Giemsa stain is applied to identify inclusion bodies. Although the McCoy cell tissue culture is the definitive test for the diagnosis of chlamydia, there are a number of disadvantages associated with it. It is expensive, not readily available, and can be negative in half the cases.

TABLE 50–4. DIAGNOSTIC TESTS FOR CHLAMYDIA

Systemic
- McCoy cell tissue culture
- Fluorescein-conjugated monoclonal antibody test
- ELISA (enzyme-linked immunosorbent assay)
- Polymerase chain reaction (PCR) test
- Chest x-ray if pneumonia suspected

Ocular
- Conjunctival culture
- Giemsa stain
- Fluorescein-conjugated monoclonal antibody test
- Polymerase chain reaction (PCR) test

Because of the problems associated with culturing, antigen detection tests for diagnosing chlamydial infections were developed. One of the most sensitive tests for diagnosis is the fluorescein-conjugated monoclonal antibody test. The technique entails fixing the genital or ocular specimen on a slide and then incubating it with the fluorescein-conjugated monoclonal antibody. When the antibodies bind to the chlamydial inclusions, they become bright fluorescent green in the cytoplasm. This test is highly sensitive and specific for diagnosing urethral, cervical, and ocular infections. A main advantage of this technique, in addition to reliability, is that results are obtained in as little as 30 minutes.

In urethritis, the specimen should be obtained by inserting the swab at least 2 cm into the urethra. To diagnose cervicitis, a Pap smear should be performed. The cervix should be cleaned first and the swab should be rotated inside the cervix. An increase in neutrophils and inflammatory cells will also be found on Pap smears.

The other antigen test is the serologic technique called enzyme-linked immunosorbent assay (ELISA). It is rapid, inexpensive, relatively sensitive and specific, and especially useful in screening large numbers of specimens. Other serologic tests can also be used to diagnose chlamydia, but are only useful for certain conditions. The microimmunofluorescence test, which allows the differentiation of the various serotypes of chlamydia, is useful for infant pneumonia and salpingitis.

Newborns suspected to have systemic complications from chlamydia should be examined for pneumonia, genital infection, and ear involvement. Chest x-ray will demonstrate mild interstitial infiltrates and hyperexpansion of the lungs. Also, there is an increase in immunoglobulins and eosinophilia.

In recent years, a new nonculture laboratory technique has been developed for the diagnosis of chlamydia. It is called the polymerase chain reaction (PCR) test (Amplicor). The PCR allows for the detection of chlamydial DNA in clinical specimens. In this three-step test, the chlamydial DNA is amplified into millions of copies using nucleic acid probes in the PCR. The amplified product is detected using a modified ELISA.

In several recent studies, the PCR test has been shown to be more sensitive than the fluorescent monoclonal antibody assay and cell culture techniques. In fact, the PCR test has become the most sensitive diagnostic test available.

In addition to being sensitive, the PCR test has a number of advantages over other diagnostic tests. Unlike cultures, it is a rapid procedure, reaching completion within 6 hours. Since the PCR test only requires the presence of chlamydial DNA in the specimens, the problems associated with maintaining viable organisms for culture are avoided. The PCR test can detect chlamydial DNA in first-void urine. Therefore, patients are spared the invasive and painful urethral and cervical probing and swabbing. The use of urine specimens also allows for a noninvasive screening of the population for chlamydia and for chlamydia control programs.

Ocular

The diagnosis of ocular chlamydial infections (trachoma or inclusion conjunctivitis) relies on patient history and ocular examination with thorough slit-lamp evaluation of the anterior segment (Table 50–3). If a chlamydial infection is suspected, a conjunctival scraping should be obtained. The purpose of scraping is to collect epithelial cells, not the mucopurulent discharge. If this is not possible, diagnosis may be made by clinical presentation. For example, endemic trachoma has a number of distinguishing signs that are useful for clinical diagnosis. The signs are lymphoid follicles on the superior tarsal conjunctiva, conjunctival scarring, vascular pannus, and limbal follicles or Herbert pits. The presence of two of the four signs is sufficient for diagnosis of trachoma. The patient should be questioned concerning the presence of eye disease in family members or friends. In suspected inclusion conjunctivitis the patient, or in the case of a newborn, the mother, should be questioned concerning the presence of genital infection.

The main method for diagnosing chlamydial ocular infections is by Giemsa staining of the typical inclusion bodies. When Giemsa stain is applied to a smear of conjunctival scrapings, the cytoplasmic inclusions of the epithelial cells appear reddish blue. The singular or multiple inclusions are seen next to the nucleus. Occasionally, elementary bodies can be seen from ruptured epithelial cells. The cytology of the smear becomes important in old cases of trachoma or inclusion conjunctivitis that lack the classic inclusion bodies. Diagnosis in these cases depends on the presence of PMNs, plasma cells, Leber cells (giant macrophages with phagocytized debris), and lymphocytes.

Giemsa staining is especially useful for the diagnosis of ocular conjunctivitis in newborns because they have large numbers of inclusions. Giemsa staining is not as useful a diagnostic test in adult inclusion conjunctivitis and systemic chlamydial disease because the sensitivity is low and false-positives are high. Furthermore, in trachoma and inclusion conjunctivitis, the inclusions appear the same on Giemsa staining. Therefore, the test cannot be used to differentiate the two conditions.

The fluorescein-conjugated monoclonal antibody test (MicroTrak, Syva) is the preferred test over the Giemsa stain for evaluating adult inclusion conjunctivitis and trachoma. The test results are reliable and are obtained quickly, which is especially important in cases such as newborn conjunctivitis in which treatment should be administered rapidly.

Several studies have shown the newer PCR test to be more sensitive than the other diagnostic options for ocular chlamydial infections. Detection of chlamydial DNA with the PCR technique in trachoma patients with negative cultures suggests that they have persistent or latent infections. If persistent infection is prevalent, then it may play a role in the scarring process. Positive PCR results in patients with no clinical signs of trachoma suggest a natural immunity to the disease. Although efforts to develop a trachoma vaccine have been unsuccessful, studies of these patients with immunity may help to develop a vaccine.

The PCR test has been shown to be especially useful in the early diagnosis of neonatal chlamydial conjunctivitis. Cultures of specimens collected at birth are often false because the number of organisms present is insufficient. Early detection with the PCR in the newborn allows for earlier treatment with a subsequent decrease in ocular and systemic complications.

If diagnostic testing is not readily available or affordable, the Centers for Disease Control and Prevention (CDC) recommend instituting treatment without confirmation through diagnostic techniques. This approach (for both systemic and ocular infections) involves oral treatment for 6 days. If there is significant improvement within 3 to 4 days, then the clinician may assume that the suspicion of chlamydial infection was correct and therapy should be continued. However, it is better to confirm the diagnosis with testing rather than relying on the clinical presentation (Table 50–4).

TREATMENT AND MANAGEMENT

Systemic

The treatment of choice for adult chlamydial genital infections, as well as all other chlamydial infections, is oral tetracyclines (Table 50–5). Chlamydial infections require a minimum of 7 days of treatment and often need 2 to 3 weeks of therapy. *C. trachomatis* infections

TABLE 50–5. TREATMENT AND MANAGEMENT OF CHLAMYDIA

Genital Chlamydial Infections

- Adults
  - Tetracycline hydrochloride 500-mg tabs PO qid × minimum 1 week (max 3 weeks), *OR*
  - Doxycycline 100-mg tabs PO bid × minimum 1 week *OR*
  - Erythromycin 500-mg tabs PO qid × minimum 1 week *OR*
  - Ofloxacin 300-mg po bid × week *OR*
  - Azithromycin single 1-g dose
  - *Sexual partners must be tested and treated if indicated*
- Pregnant women
  - Erythromycin 500-mg tabs PO qid × 10–14 days *OR*
  - Amoxicillin 500-mg tabs PO tid × 10 days
  - *Sexual partners must be tested and treated if indicated*
- Neonates (all chlamydial infections)
  - Erythromycin ethylsuccinate or estolate 50 mg/kg/day × 14 days
  - *Parents and their sexual partners must be tested and treated if indicated*

Ocular Chlamydial Infections

- **Trachoma**
  - Medical Therapy
    - Adults
      - Tetracycline 250-mg tabs PO qid × 3 weeks
    - Pregnant women
      - Erythromycin 500-mg tabs PO qid × 3 weeks
    - Children
      - Tetracycline or erythromycin ung bid to tid × 21–60 days *PLUS*
      - Tetracycline 250-mg tabs PO qid × 3 weeks (if child $>$ 8 years old) *OR*
      - Erythromycin 500-mg tabs PO qid × 3 weeks (if child $<$ 8 years old)
  - Surgical therapy
    - Corrective lid surgery may be indicated
    - Penetrating keratoplasty
    - Phototherapeutic keratectomy
- **Adult inclusion conjunctivitis**
  - Adults
    - Tetracycline 250-mg tabs PO qid × 3 weeks or 500-mg qid × 2 weeks *OR*
    - Doxycycline 100-mg tabs PO qd × 2 weeks *PLUS*
    - Tetracycline, erythromycin, or sulfacetamide ung bid to tid × 2–3 weeks
    - *Patients and their sexual partners must be tested for genital infection and treated if indicated*
  - Pregnant women
    - Erythromycin 500-mg tabs PO qid × 2 weeks *PLUS*
    - Erythromycin (preferably) or sulfacetamide ung bid to tid × 2–3 weeks
    - *Patients and their sexual partners must be tested for genital infection and treated if indicated*
- **Neonatal inclusion conjunctivitis**
  - Erythromycin ethylsuccinate 50 mg/kg/day × 2 weeks *PLUS*
  - Erythromycin or sulfacetamide ung qid × 2 weeks
  - *Parents and their sexual partners must be tested for genital infection and treated if indicated*

Abbreviations: bid, twice a day; g, gram; kg, kilogram; mg, millogram; PO, orally; qid, four times a day.

may also be treated with oral doxycycline or erythromycin. The treatment for infected pregnant women is erythromycin or amoxicillin.

In recent years, two other antibiotics have become available for the treatment of chlamydial genital infections. The first is a 7-day course of ofloxacin. This antibiotic is safe, well tolerated, and as effective a treatment as doxycycline. The second antibiotic treatment is a single 1-g dose of the macrolide azithromycin. It is safe, unlikely to cause gastrointestinal upset, assures compliance, and is also as effective as a 7-day course of doxycycline. These two antibiotics are not recommended for treating pregnant women. Azithromycin has been shown to be safe and effective in the treatment of pregnant women, but the FDA has not approved it.

A crucial part of the treatment of genital chlamydial infections is the education and treatment of the patient's sexual partners. When treatment is unsuccessful, it is often due to reinfection by the untreated partner. Even if the sexual partner of an infected patient is asymptomatic, treatment should still be instituted.

Tetracyclines cause skeletal and dental defects in the fetus and in children less than 8 years old; therefore, neonates with chlamydial infections (ocular and/or systemic) should be treated with erythromycin ethylsuccinate or estolate. Absorption of this antibiotic is enhanced by milk. Both parents of the infected infant should also be tested and treated if necessary.

Ocular

Trachoma

Mass treatment programs with topical tetracycline or erythromycin have been instituted for endemic trachoma. The ointment is applied to the eyes of all the infected children. Topical therapy alone does not eradicate trachoma, but does prevent the blinding complications. Ideally, topical treatment should be combined with systemic antibiotics. Unfortunately, it is difficult and potentially dangerous to administer mass treatment with systemic antibiotics. However, with the advent of single-dose azithromycin therapy, mass antibiotic treatment may be possible. Azithromycin, like the ointment, does not cure the patient systemically, but it may prove to be the preferred method for preventing the blinding complications when considering the administration of a single-dose therapy to masses of people versus 2 months of topical therapy.

The treatment for adult trachoma is oral tetracycline. For pregnant women and children under 8 years old, the treatment of choice is oral erythromycin. Sulfonamides may also be used, but the toxic and allergic side effects make them a secondary choice. In addition to medical therapy for trachoma, surgery may be necessary to correct entropion and trichiasis. Corneal scarring can be treated with penetrating keratoplasty and phototherapeutic keratectomy.

The rise of industrialization with improved living conditions has also contributed to the decline of the incidence and severity of trachoma in many parts of the world. Basic improvements in living standards, personal hygiene (particularly face washing), and the reduction of household flies are helping to decrease the prevalence of trachoma. Research is ongoing to develop a vaccine for trachoma.

Adult Inclusion Conjunctivitis

The treatment of choice for adult inclusion conjunctivitis is oral tetracycline. In patients that are not compliant, it may be better to prescribe doxycycline, as it only requires single daily doses. Pregnant women should be given erythromycin. Topical medications (erythromycin, tetracycline, or sulfacetamide ointment) do not cure inclusion conjunctivitis, but their use may reduce the duration of the infection. It is important to emphasize to the patient that sexual partners must be evaluated and treated if necessary.

> The clinical signs of adult inclusion conjunctivitis may take 2 to 3 months to resolve and there is a risk of recurrence.

Neonatal Inclusion Conjunctivitis

Neonatal inclusion conjunctivitis is treated with topical erythromycin or sulfacetamide ointment as well as oral erythromycin ethylsuccinate. Inadequate treatment of neonatal conjunctivitis can lead to the development of pneumonia. The infant's parents (and their sexual partners) must be evaluated for infection and treated if necessary.

CONCLUSION

Chlamydial infections in humans are common throughout the world. The clinical presentation is quite variable, ranging from trachoma, which causes severe visual loss in millions of people, to oculogenital infections, which usually resolve with treatment, leaving few or no complications. The clinical presentation, diagnostic testing, and evaluation of both the patient and the source of infection are important in the treatment and management of chlamydial disease.

REFERENCES

An BB, Adamis AP. Chlamydial ocular diseases. *Int Ophthalmol Clin.* 1998;38:221–230.

Arffa RC. Chlamydial infections. In: Kist K, ed. *Grayson's Diseases of the Cornea.* St. Louis: Mosby–Year Book; 1991: 151–162.

Bailey RL, Hampton TJ, Hayes LJ, et al. Polymerase chain reaction for the detection of ocular chlamydial infection in trachoma-endemic communities. *J Infect Dis.* 1994;170: 709–712.

Bialasiewicz AA, Jahn GJ. Evaluation of diagnostic tools for adult chlamydial keratoconjunctivitis. *Ophthalmology.* 1987;94:532–537.

Carta F, Zanetti S, Pinna A, et al. The treatment and follow up of adult chlamydial ophthalmia. *Br J Ophthalmol.* 1994; 78:206–208.

Cotran RS, Kumar V, Robbins SL. Chlamydia diseases. In: Cotran RS, Kumar V, Robbins SL, eds. *Robbins Pathologic Basis of Disease.* 4th ed. Philadelphia: Saunders; 1989: 326–328.

Dawson CR. Pathogenesis and control of blinding trachoma. In: Tasman W, Jaeger EA, eds. *Duane's Clinical Ophthalmology. Philadelphia*: Lippincott; 1991:5.

Dawson CR, Sheppard JD. Follicular conjunctivitis. In: Tasman W, Jaeger EA, eds. *Duane's Clinical Ophthalmology.* Philadelphia: Lippincott; 1991:4.

Elnifro EM, Storey CC, Morris DJ, Tullo AB. Polymerase chain reaction for detection of *Chlamydia trachomatis* in conjunctival swabs. *Br J Ophthalmol.* 1997;81:497–500.

Forster RK, Dawson CR, Schachter J. Late follow-up of patients with neonatal inclusion conjunctivitis. *Am J Ophthalmol.* 1970;69:467–472.

Hammerschlag MR, Roblin PM, Gelling M, et al. Use of polymerase chain reaction for the detection of *Chlamydia trachomatis* in ocular and nasopharyngeal specimens from infants with conjunctivitis. *Pediatr Infect Dis J.* 1997;16: 293–297.

Harrison HR, Phil D, English MG, et al. *Chlamydia trachomatis* infant pneumonitis. *N Engl J Med.* 1978;298:702–708.

Hawkins DA, Wilson RS, Thomas BJ, Evans RT. Rapid, reliable diagnosis of chlamydial ophthalmitis by means of monoclonal antibodies. *Br J Ophthalmol.* 1985;69:640–644.

Holmes KK. Pelvic inflammatory disease. In: Wilson JD, et al, eds. *Harrison's Principles of Internal Medicine.* New York: McGraw-Hill; 1991:533–537.

Holmes KK. The chlamydia epidemic. *JAMA.* 1981;245:1718–1723.

Kowalski RP, Uhrin M, Karenchak LM, et al. Evaluation of the polymerase chain reaction test for detecting chlamydial DNA in adult chlamydial conjunctivitis. *Ophthalmology.* 1995;102:1016–1019.

Milano M, Gorini G, Olliaro P, et al. Evaluation of diagnostic procedures in chlamydial eye infection. *Ophthalmologica.* 1991;203:114–117.

Peterson HB, Walker CK, Kahn JG, et al. Pelvic inflammatory disease. *JAMA.* 1991;266:2605–2611.

Polack FM. *External Diseases of the Eye.* Barcelona: Ediciones Scriba; 1991:49–56.

Quinn TC, Bender B. Sexually transmitted diseases. In: Harvey AM, Johns RJ, McKusick VA, et al, eds. *The Principles and Practice of Medicine.* Norwalk, CT: Appleton & Lange; 1988:657–659.

Sanders LL, Harrison HR, Washington AE. Treatment of sexually transmitted chlamydial infections. *JAMA.* 1986; 255:1750–1756.

Schachter J. Chlamydial infection (first of three parts). *N Engl J Med.* 1978;298:428–435.

Sheppard JD, Dawson CR. Chlamydial infections. In: Gold DH, Weingeist TA, eds. *The Eye in Systemic Disease.* Philadelphia: Lippincott; 1990:169–174.

Stamm WE. Chlamydial infections. In: Fauci et al, eds. *Harrison's Principles of Internal Medicine.* New York: McGraw-Hill; 1998:1055–1064.

Stamm WE, Holmes KK. Chlamydial infections. In: Wilson JD, et al, eds. *Harrison's Principles of Internal Medicine.* New York: McGraw-Hill; 1991:764–772.

Stenberg K, Mardh PA. Chlamydial conjunctivitis in neonates and adults. *Ophthalmologica.* 1990;68:651–657.

Talley AR, Garcia-Ferrer F, Laycock KA, et al. The use of polymerase chain reaction for the detection of chlamydial keratoconjunctivitis. *Am J Ophthalmol.* 1992;114:685–692.

Talley AR, Garcia-Ferrer F, Laycock KA, et al. *Am J Ophthalmol.* 1994;117:50–57.

Terry JE. Diseases of the cornea. In: Bartlett JD, Jaanus SD, eds. *Clinical Ocular Pharmacology.* Boston: Butterworths; 1989:570–572.

Wallace W. Diseases of the conjunctiva. In: Bartlett JD, Jannus SD, eds. *Clinical Ocular Pharmacology.* Boston: Butterworths; 1989:544–547.

Whitcher JP. Chlamydial diseases. In: Smolin G, Thoft RA, eds. *The Cornea.* Boston: Little, Brown; 1983:210–220.

Yanoff M, Fine BS. Specific inflammations. In: Cooke DB, Patterson D, Anderson W, eds. *Ocular Pathology.* Philadelphia: Lippincott; 1989:221–224.

Chapter 51

TOXOPLASMOSIS

Brad M. Sutton, Julie K. Torbit

Toxoplasma gondii is an intracellular parasite requiring a host to maintain its existence. Felines are the definitive host. The organism also infects humans and domesticated animals. Toxoplasmosis is the most common etiology of human retinochoroiditis (Pearson et al, 1999). The brain, skeletal muscles, heart, and other internal organs may also be affected. The disease can be contracted as a maternally transmitted congenital infection or acquired later in life, occurring most commonly in immunocompromised individuals.

EPIDEMIOLOGY

Systemic

Toxoplasmosis is a common infection throughout the world, affecting an estimated 500 million people (Pavesio & Lightman, 1996). The infection is most prevalent in warm, moist climates. Arid areas, cold regions, and high elevations are less conducive to survival of the organism (Beaman et al, 1995). Antibodies to *Toxoplasma gondii* will increase with age and in the United States approximately 50% of the population shows seropositivity by the fourth decade (McCabe & Remington, 1990).

Congenital toxoplasmosis occurs when a pregnant woman becomes infected. The reported rates of congenital infection in the United States vary from as low as 1 in 10,000 (Hunter et al, 1983) to as high as 13 in 10,000 (Kimball et al, 1971). Prevalence rates will vary depending upon geographic locale and the population base. Factors that influence these rates include climate, cat population, hygiene, cultural habits of food preparation, and the type of testing utilized to determine infection.

Ocular

Retinochoroiditis will develop in fewer than 1% of patients with acquired *Toxoplasma* infection as compared to greater than 80% of patients with congenital toxoplasmosis (Alexander, 1994). The estimates of the percentage of all cases of posterior uveitis that are caused by toxoplasmosis infection range from a low of 16% (Schlaegel, 1978) to a high of 70% (Cassady, 1960). A conclusive diagnosis of ocular toxoplasmosis in the adult is difficult because it requires isolation of the *Toxoplasma* organism from ocular tissue in the patient suffering from active disease.

PATHOPHYSIOLOGY/DISEASE PROCESS

The Organism

As an obligate intracellular parasite, *Toxoplasma gondii* requires a host to maintain its existence. Feline species are the definitive hosts while intermediate hosts include humans, other mammals, rodents, and birds. The organism's life cycle consists of three distinct stages:

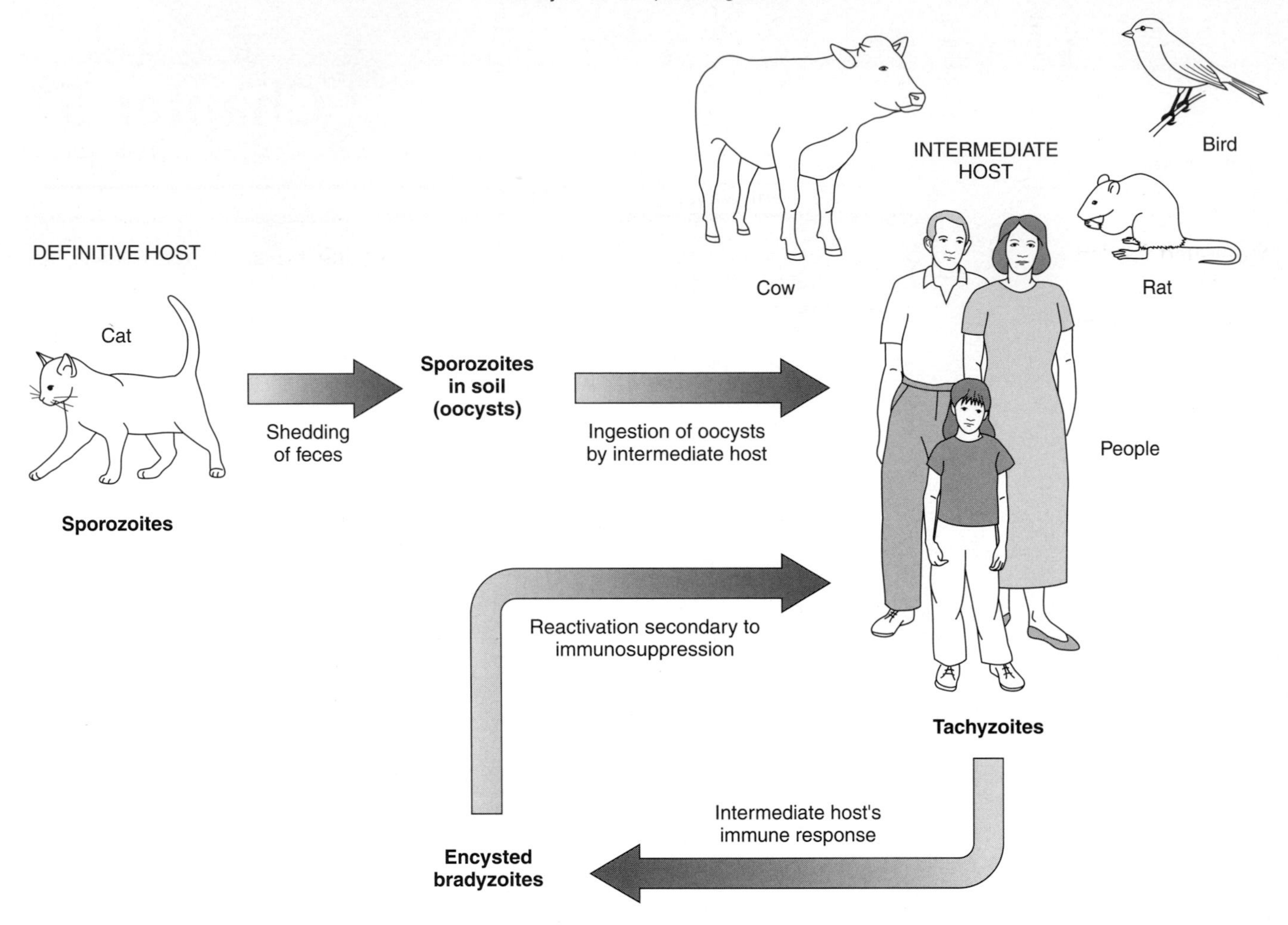

Figure 51–1. Life cycle of *Toxoplasma gondii. (Reprinted with permission from* Am J Dis Child. *1975;129:777–779. Copyright 1975 American Medical Association.)* *Adapted from Life cycle of *Toxoplasma gondii.* Am J Dis Child, *1975;129:777–779.* Copyright 1975. American Medical Association.

> Toxoplasmosis is the most common cause of human retinochoroiditis.

sporozoite, tachyzoite, and bradyzoite (Figure 51–1). The sporozoite is found only in the intestine of infected cats. The afflicted animal will shed millions of these organisms per day contained within hardy oocysts. The sporozoites within these cysts can remain viable in the soil in warm, moist climates for up to 1 to 2 years (Pavesio & Lightman, 1996). As intermediate hosts ingest these oocysts, the gastric enzymes cause the cyst wall to rupture, releasing the sporozoites. They then transform into the mobile, active tachyzoite form of the parasite. It is this form that invades and lyses host cells.

> Reactivation of congenital infection typically occurs at the border of an old chorioretinal scar and results in an inflammatory lesion with an overlying vitritis (described as a "headlight in the fog").

When the organisms reproduce and infect surrounding cells, they are eventually disseminated throughout the body via the bloodstream. As the host's immune response battles the infection, the tachyzoites become encysted and revert into inactive bradyzoites. The bradyzoites then lie dormant for many years until the cysts rupture, at which time they transform back into tachyzoites.

> Toxoplasmosis infection is most common in warm, moist climates.

Transmission

Humans can acquire *T. gondii* in many different ways. Major modes of transmission include ingestion of contaminated foodstuffs, handling or disposing of cat feces, and transplacental transmission from mother to fetus during pregnancy (Jabs & Quinlan, 1994). Ingestion of undercooked meat (usually pork or lamb), unwashed vegetables, or raw milk can lead to infection. Contraction of the organism can also occur from direct contact with infected cats, contaminated litter boxes and sandboxes, or soil (Jabs & Quinlan, 1994). Other forms of transmission include blood transfusions, organ transplants, and accidental laboratory inoculations (Rutzen et al, 1994). Contaminated drinking water has also been linked to a widespread outbreak of toxoplasmosis (Bowie et al, 1997; Burnett et al, 1998).

> Transmission of the organism to humans may occur through the ingestion of undercooked meats or raw vegetables and through the handling of cat feces.

> Eighty percent of congenitally infected individuals will develop ocular complications as opposed to only 1% of those with acquired disease.

Course of the Disease

Clinically, toxoplasmosis infection in humans may be divided into the following types: acquired toxoplasmosis, congenital toxoplasmosis, and toxoplasmosis in the immunosuppressed individual (Table 51–1).

Acquired Toxoplasmosis

Systemic

Typically, an acute, acquired infection goes undetected because most individuals are asymptomatic. However, 10 to 20% will experience flu-like symptoms (Jabs & Quinlan, 1994) that can mimic influenza, infectious mononucleosis, and a host of other conditions (Tables 51–1 and 51–2). Cervical lymphadenopathy is the most common systemic manifestation of acquired toxoplasmosis (Primo, 1994). Seven to twenty-one days after exposure to the parasite, enlargement of one or more cervical nodes (usually nontender) can occur in the symptomatic patient. Other symptoms include fever, malaise, myalgia, fatigue, headache, sore throat, and a maculopapillar rash that spares the palms of the hands and soles of the feet (Jabs & Quinlan, 1994). In severe cases, central nervous system involvement may lead to potentially fatal encephalitis.

TABLE 51–1. SYSTEMIC MANIFESTATIONS OF TOXOPLASMOSIS

Type of Toxoplasmosis	Symptoms	Signs
• Acquired systemic toxoplasmosis	• Fever • Malaise • Sore throat • Myalgia	• Cervical lymphadenopathy • Maculopapillar rash • Liver and spleen enlargement • Rising *Toxoplasma* antibody titers
• Congenital toxoplasmosis	• Rash • Fever • Psychomotor retardation • Jaundice	• Hydrocephaly or microcephaly • CSF abnormalities • Cerebral calcifications • Lymphadenopathy • Enlarged spleen • Endocrinological disease
• Toxoplasmosis in the immunocompromised	• Same as in acquired toxoplasmosis PLUS • Confusion • Headache	• Same as in acquired toxoplasmosis EXCEPT serologic tests may give false-negative results PLUS • Encephalitis • Coma • Myositis • Myocarditis • Pneumonitis

TABLE 51–2. DIFFERENTIAL DIAGNOSIS OF TOXOPLASMOSIS

Systemic	Ocular
• Hodgkin lymphoma	• Histoplasmosis
• Mononucleosis	• Toxocariasis
• Influenza	• Sarcoidosis
• Metastatic cancer	• Tuberculosis
• Cat scratch disease	• Syphilis
• AIDS	• CMV
• Sarcoidosis	• Fungal infections
• Tuberculosis	• DUSN
• CMV	• CHRPE

Ocular

Once the mobile tachyzoite reaches the eye, it enters the retinal cells, causing a retinitis. Infection of the retinal tissue in turn leads to inflammation of the choroid and sclera. Therefore, this process is termed "retinochoroiditis" as opposed to the chorioretinitis typically seen in other inflammatory conditions. The retinochoroiditis often results in a vitreitis caused by the release of inflammatory cells and *Toxoplasma* antigens into the vitreous. This vitreitis may be associated with an anterior uveitis that can be granulomatous or nongranulomatous. Retinal scars consistent with ocular toxoplasmosis have been seen in patients with Fuchs heterochromic cyclitis. It has been suggested that toxoplasmosis causes anterior segment inflammation that leads to heterochromia, posterior cataract, and iridocyclitis that mimics Fuchs heterochromic disease (Pavesio & Lightman, 1996). However, a study by La Hey and associates (1992) found no statistical association between Fuchs and toxoplasmic scars.

The host's immune response typically results in the conversion of the active tachyzoite into the inactive bradyzoite. These inactive organisms become encysted in the retinal tissue with a single cyst containing up to 3000 bradyzoites (Tabbara, 1990). These cysts then lie dormant in the tissue, often for many years. For unknown reasons, the cysts can burst and release organisms into the surrounding tissue. It has been postulated that the cysts may rupture because of slow reproduction of the bradyzoites within the cyst walls or enzymes released from degenerating organisms (Morhun et al, 1996; Pavesio & Lightman, 1996). A compromise in the immune status of the host may also play a role (Morhun et al, 1996). Rupture of the cyst leads to a focal retinochoroiditis consisting of one or more white, fluffy lesions affecting the inner retinal layers (Figure 51–2). These lesions are often surrounded by edema and may vary in size and location. Large lesions may lead to granuloma formation and can often be associated with a significant vitreitis. Lesions affecting the outer retinal layers are grayer in appearance and do not lead to severe vitreitis. Indocyanine green angiography may reveal multiple, hypofluorescent spots surrounding active lesions. These spots are not visible with ophthalmoscopy or fluorescein angiography and are believed to be a result of inflammation of the choriocapillaris (Auer et al, 1997; Guex-Crosier et al, 1998).

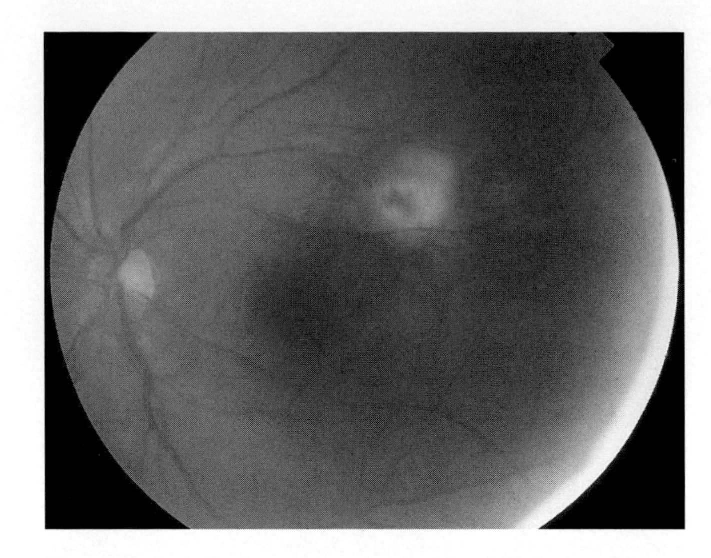

Figure 51–2. Active toxoplasmosis retinochoroiditis lesion with hazy borders.

Floaters and photophobia are common presenting complaints (Table 51–3). Loss of visual acuity will depend upon the degree of vitreitis and location of the lesion. If the organism affects the papillomacular bundle, macula, or optic nerve, there will be significant loss of visual acuity. In addition, active infection can lead to a papillitis in the absence of any retinal complications. Patients with active retinal infection must also be monitored closely for the development of tractional retinal tears and subsequent detachment. Healing of the inflammatory area results in a chorioretinal scar, usually with pigmented borders (Figures 51–3, 51–4, and 51–5). These scars can, on occasion, be associated with the formation of subretinal neovascularization (Chalam & Tripathi, 1997). When the inflammatory reaction has subsided, the visual acuity will improve unless the macula or optic nerve has been affected.

Congenital Toxoplasmosis

Systemic

Congenital toxoplasmosis is believed to result from an acute infection acquired during pregnancy (Pavesio & Lightman, 1996). Transmission of the organism to the fetus has been reported to be as high as 60% (Tabbara,

TABLE 51–3. OCULAR MANIFESTATIONS OF TOXOPLASMOSIS

Type of Toxoplasmosis	Symptoms	Signs
• Acquired systemic toxoplasmosis	• Reduced visual acuity • Photophobia • Floaters	• Retinochoroiditis • Vitritis • Anterior uveitis • Optic neuritis or papillitis • Retinal tears • Retinal detachments • Well-pigmented chorioretinal scars • New lesions originating near old scars
• Congenital toxoplasmosis	• Reduced vision from birth or shortly after birth	• Retinochoroiditis (often bilateral macular lesions) • Microphthalmia • Enophthalmos • Ptosis • Nystagmus • Strabismus
• Toxoplasmosis in the immunocompromised	• Reduced vision if lesions affect macula, optic nerve, or papillomacular bundle	• Retinochoroiditis • Poorly pigmented scars • Minimal vitreitis • New lesions unassociated with previous scars

1990). The incidence of transmission varies depending upon the trimester in which the mother becomes infected. The incidence is lowest during the first trimester and highest in the third trimester (Tabbara, 1990). However, the earlier in pregnancy the disease is acquired, the more severe the systemic manifestations. Future offspring from a previously infected mother will not be affected because of the maternal immunity that develops subsequent to the initial infection.

Infection during pregnancy can lead to stillbirth, spontaneous abortion, or live births with offspring who have significant systemic sequelae. The majority of infants are not born with overt manifestations of the disease; however, 80% of subclinically infected children develop ocular complications later in life (Meeken et al, 1995). Signs of clinical systemic congenital toxoplasmosis in the newborn can vary (Table 51–1) and may include hydrocephaly or microcephaly, endocrine disease, cerebral calcifications, rash, fever, psychomotor retardation, jaundice, lymphadenopathy, enlarged spleen, and cerebrospinal fluid abnormalities (Meeken et al, 1995).

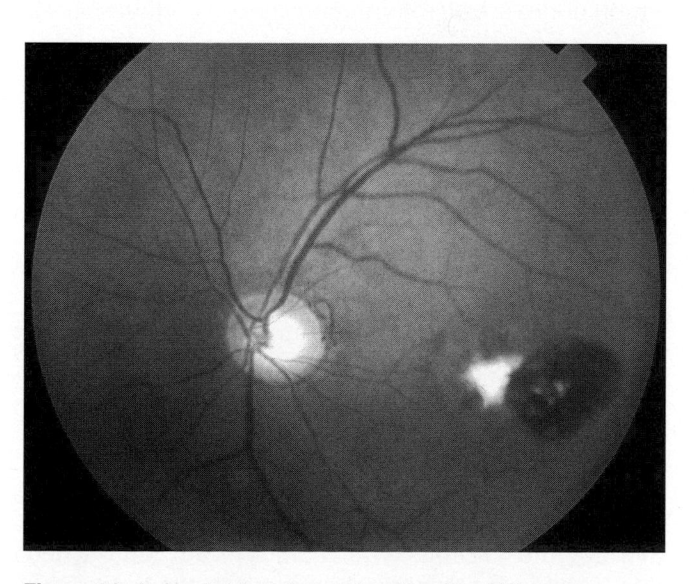

Figure 51–3. Healed toxoplasmosis retinochoroiditis lesion.

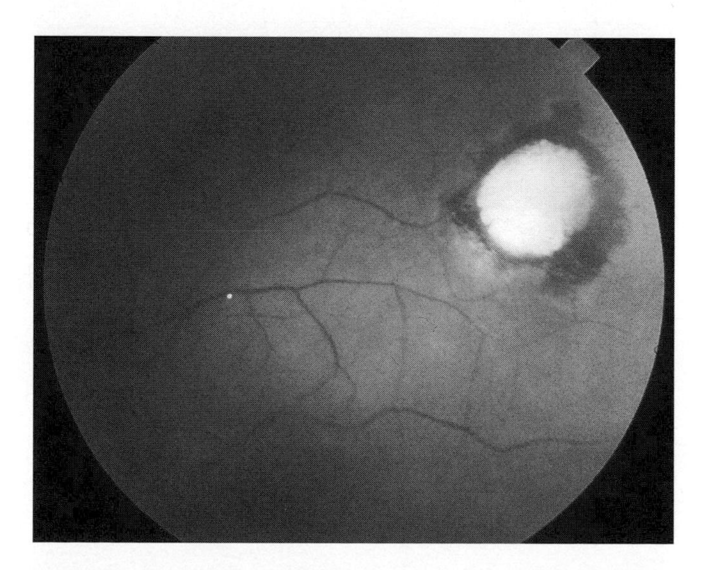

Figure 51–4. Healed toxoplasmosis lesion with visible sclera and pigmented borders.

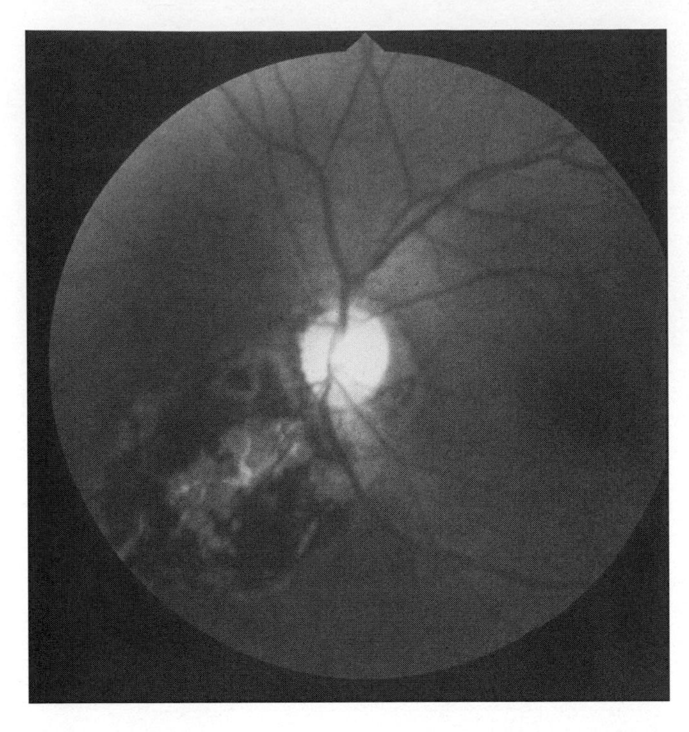

Figure 51–5. Juxtapapillary scar secondary to toxoplasmosis retinochoroiditis.

Ocular

The most common ocular manifestation of congenital toxoplasmosis is a retinochoroiditis with a predilection for the macula (Table 51–3). Tabbara (1990) has theorized that this predilection may be due to tachyzoites being trapped in the small perifoveal capillaries. The resultant macular scar (Figure 51–6) often mimics a coloboma and leads to severe visual acuity loss (Meeken et al, 1995). Other ocular signs of congenital infection include optic nerve head atrophy, nystagmus, strabismus, micropthalmos, enophthalmos, cataracts, and iris abnormalities. In congenitally infected individuals, reactivation of retinochoroiditis typically occurs at the edge of an old scar. This is due to the predilection for tissue cysts to be located at the borders of healed lesions.

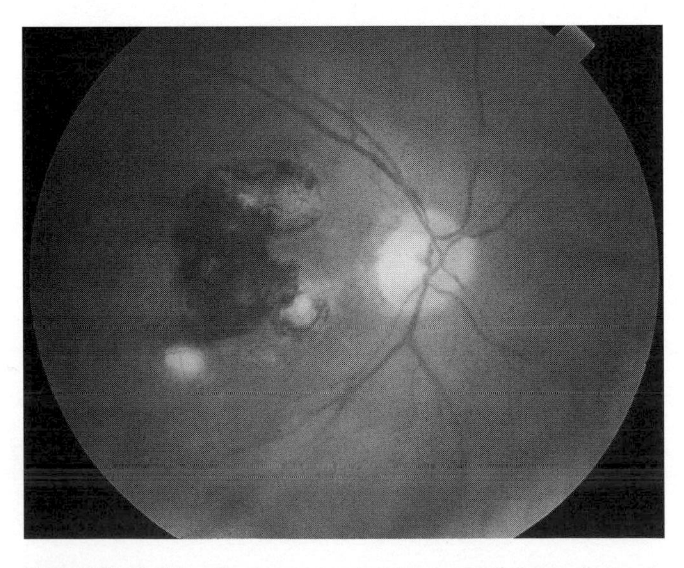

Figure 51–6. Macular scar secondary to congenital toxoplasmosis infection.

> Congenital infection often leads to a bilateral retinochoroiditis with a predilection for affecting the macula.

Toxoplasmosis in the Immunosuppressed Patient

Systemic

Individuals who have a compromised immune system are at great risk for multiorgan infection. Immunosuppression may result from malignancies, chronic immunosuppressive therapies, AIDS, organ transplantation, or connective tissue disorders (Johnson et al, 1997; Pavesio & Lightman, 1996). *Toxoplasma gondii* is one of the most common causes of focal lesions and nonviral infections of the CNS. Encephalitis, pneumonitis, myocarditis, and retinochoroiditis can be associated findings in the immunocompromised host (Beaman et al, 1995). Ten to twenty percent of patients with encephalitis have a concomitant retinochoroiditis. However, it is much more common for those patients presenting with a retinochoroiditis to have a concurrent encephalitis (Mansour, 1997). The liver, spleen, and lymph nodes are also commonly involved (Table 51–1).

Ocular

Ocular manifestations in the immunocompromised host include lesions that tend to be bilateral and multifocal rather than unilateral and discrete as seen in healthy individuals (Table 51–3). There may be no preexisting retinal scars in the immunosuppressed patient, which suggests an acquired infection or dissemination of the organism from other parts of the body. These patients may have a diffuse retinochoroiditis that can mimic acute retinal necrosis (ARN) (Johnson et al, 1997; Mansour, 1997). As a result of their immunocompromised state, there is only a moderate associated vitritis and uveitis. The lesions also do not pigment as well as those found in immunocompromised patients. In addition, *T. gondii* may infect the iris, choroid, and vitreous, which are typically untouched areas in those with normal immune systems.

TABLE 51–4. SEROLOGIC TESTING

Tests	Key Points	Reference Ranges
• Sabin–Feldman	• Reference test • Very sensitive and specific • Limited by need to maintain a live *Toxoplasma* supply	• Titer >1:4 considered positive • May reach 1:1000 in acute infection • Titer level does not correlate with severity of disease
• Indirect fluorescent antibody	• Most widely utilized test • Does not require live organisms • ANA, RA factors lead to false-positives • Excellent for detection of congenital infection in newborns	• Titer >1:8 considered positive • IgG may reach level 1:1000 • IgM may reach level 1:64
• Indirect hemagglutination	• High rate of false-negatives • Will not become positive until 2–4 weeks after infection	• Titer >1:16 is considered positive • May be >1:1000 in acute infection
• ELISA	• Can detect *Toxoplasma* organism • IgG antibody levels not useful in determining congenital infection • IgM and IgA antibody levels excellent for determining congenital infection • IgG and IgE antibody levels utilized to detect acquired infection	• IgG titer >1:4 is considered positive • IgG titer >1:1024 denotes acute infection • IgM titer >1:4 in infants is considered positive • IgM titer >1:64 in adults is considered positive • IgM titer >1:256 denotes acute infection

DIAGNOSIS

Systemic

Serologic testing is often utilized in the differential diagnosis of systemic *Toxoplasma* infection (Table 51–4). These tests are limited, however, because of the high incidence of seropositivity in healthy individuals and potentially significant problems with false-positive results. Immunocompromised patients can exhibit false-negative responses secondary to their immune system's poor response to infection and subsequent low antibody production (Montoya & Remington, 1996). In spite of these limitations, serologic testing plays a key role in diagnosing toxoplasmosis. The most frequently used serologic tests include the Sabin–Feldman (methylene blue) dye test, indirect fluorescent antibody (IFA) test, indirect hemagglutination test, and enzyme-linked immunosorbent assay (ELISA) tests. Other less frequently utilized procedures include complement-fixation techniques and IgG avidity testing.

> ELISA testing is the most commonly employed method utilized for serologic confirmation of systemic toxoplasmosis.

The Sabin–Feldman or methylene blue dye test is the reference against which all others are judged (Beaman et al, 1995). It is highly sensitive and specific, but its use is severely limited by the need to maintain a live supply of *Toxoplasma* parasites for performing the procedure. Live organisms are combined with serum to be tested. If antibodies are present, the cell membrane will lyse and it will fail to stain with methylene blue dye. The antibody titer is reported as the serum dilution at which greater than 50% of the organisms remain unstained. Tests are considered to be positive when a level greater than 1:4 is reached, and acute infection may result in levels upward of 1:1000 (Jabs & Quinlan, 1994).

The indirect fluorescent antibody test is the most widely employed serologic test for the detection of toxoplasmosis because it utilizes dead rather than live organisms and has excellent sensitivity, specificity, and reliability. A slide preparation of dead tachyzoites is tested with the patient's serum to detect IgG and IgM antibodies. Unfortunately, antinuclear antibodies and rheumatoid factors will often lead to false-positive results, and false-negative findings will occur in immunocompromised individuals. Artificially elevated levels of anti-*Toxoplasma* serum antibodies have also been reported in patients suffering from a thymoma (Shaikh et al, 1997).

The indirect hemagglutination test is very simple to perform but has significant drawbacks. It is based upon the fact that red blood cells that have been exposed to an antigen will agglutinate when confronted with the appropriate antibodies (Remington et al, 1995). Different antibodies are detected in this process than those measured with the IFA or Sabin–Feldman tests (Tabbara, 1990). Unfortunately, false-negative results are quite frequent, and the antibody titer will not become positive until 2 to 4 weeks have elapsed after infection (Beaman et al, 1995).

ELISA testing can be utilized to detect both IgG and IgM antibodies as well as the presence of the antigen itself. IgG antibodies can be passed from the mother to the developing fetus, so they are of limited value in confirming congenital infections. IgM antibodies are an excellent indicator of congenital infection because they are produced strictly by the fetus and are not transferred from the mother. Their levels rise faster and drop sooner than do those of serum IgG. Therefore, IgM antibodies can be detected very shortly after contracting the disease. Testing for them several weeks after suspected infection, however, is of limited value because their levels may return rapidly to a near normal state.

ELISA testing can also be modified to detect IgA antibodies that are an even more accurate predictor of congenital infection than IgM levels. IgE antibody detection is very useful to indicate acute infection in acquired cases but is limited in its ability to predict infection in the fetus or the newborn. Advanced ELISA techniques known as "double-sandwiching" methods have eliminated false-positives from antinuclear antibody (ANA) and rheumatoid factors (Beaman et al, 1995). This process can be employed when testing for any of the various immunoglobulin antibodies.

Neuroimaging is not routinely utilized in the diagnosis of toxoplasmosis. It may be of value, however, in those cases involving symptomatic newborns and immunocompromised individuals. In these instances, encephalitis can lead to calcific plaque formation and multiple, diffuse lesions that appear with contrast-enhanced CT scan or MRI (Alexander, 1994).

Ocular

The diagnosis of ocular toxoplasmosis is based mostly upon ocular signs and symptoms. Serologic testing can be helpful as an adjunct or confirmatory measure. Tests for specific ocular antibodies utilizing a sample of aqueous humor have also been advocated (Bloch-Michel et al, 1998; Boer & et al, 1995; Bornand & Gottrau, 1997). Techniques exist as well that are capable of identifying the presence of *Toxoplasma* enzymes in the intraocular fluids (Klaren et al, 1998). These measures are rarely employed clinically, however, because of the necessity of performing a paracentesis or vitrectomy to obtain fluid samples.

TREATMENT AND MANAGEMENT

Traditionally, a small core group of medications has been employed to fight toxoplasmosis infection. Many of these drugs have significant side effects associated with their use; therefore, prevention of infection is critical. All meat that is prepared for human consumption should be thoroughly cooked. Hands must be washed after contact with cats, litter boxes, raw vegetables, and soil. Pregnant women should be advised to refrain from handling litter boxes when possible.

The decision to treat an infected patient depends upon the activity of the disease. Newborns with congenital toxoplasmosis are invariably treated. Adults with ocular toxoplasmosis are treated during recurrences of retinochoroiditis when lesions threaten the macula, papillomacular bundle, or optic nerve. Treatment is particularly important in immunocompromised individuals suffering from CNS and ocular complications. In these patients, maintenance therapy often must continue indefinitely to prevent recurrences (Beaman et al, 1995).

Systemic

Classic triple therapy consists of pyrimethamine (Daraprim) and sulfadiazine in conjunction with corticosteroids. Pyrimethamine and sulfadiazine both inhibit the formation of nucleic acid but work at different steps in the pathway of its synthesis. For this reason, they work synergistically and are particularly effective in combination. Treatment should begin with a loading dose and continue for 3 to 4 weeks (Table 51–5). Folinic acid must be given in conjunction with the use of pyrimethamine to counteract possible folate deficiency induced by the medication. In addition, patients taking pyrimethamine require weekly blood counts to detect potentially harmful thrombocytopenia and leukopenia. Individuals using sulfadiazine must increase their fluid intake to decrease the likelihood of renal stone formation (Jabs & Quinlan, 1994).

> Commonly utilized pharmaceutical agents include pyrimethamine, sulfadiazine, clindamycin, and corticosteroids.

Clindamycin has been advocated as an adjunct therapy for toxoplasmosis and as a stand-alone treatment (Auer et al, 1997; Guex-Crosier et al, 1998). It may be used as an alternative to pyrimethamine when the latter drug's side effects are intolerable. Likewise, trisulfapyrimidine (triple sulfa) can be substituted for

> Folinic acid must be given to patients taking pyrimethamine.

TABLE 51–5. TREATMENT AND MANAGEMENT OF TOXOPLASMOSIS (SYSTEMIC AND OCULAR)

Adult Patient

1. Pyrimethamine
   Loading dose 75–100mg PO × 2 days, then
   25 mg/day × 3–6 weeks
   A. Can be combined with sulfadiazine or trisulfapyrimidine
      Loading dose 2 g PO followed by 1 g qid × 3–6 weeks
   Monitor blood counts for leukopenia and thrombocytopenia
   Adjunct: folinic acid 3–5 mg IM or PO 2 × /week

OR

2. Clindamycin
   300 mg PO qid × 3–6 weeks
   Does not cross blood–brain barrier; do not use in toxoplasmosis encephalitis
   May cause colitis
   A. Can be combined with sulfadiazine or trisulfapyrimidine
      Loading dose 2 g PO followed by 1 g qid × 3–6 weeks

plus

   Prednisone when indicated
   20–80 mg PO daily with 3- to 6-week taper

OR

3. Trimethoprim-sulfamethoxazole (Bactrim)
   160 mg (trimethoprim) plus 800 mg (sulfamethoxazole) PO bid 4–6 weeks
   May cause skin rash and/or mild diarrhea
   A. Can be combined with clindamycin 300 mg qid × 2 weeks

plus

   Prednisone
   80 mg qd × 2 days, tapered 20 mg qid to 20 mg qd × 4 weeks

OR

4. Atovaquone
   750 mg (5 mL of suspension) PO bid × 3 months
   Take with food at least moderately high in fat to enhance absorption

OR

5. Ocular topical agents used in cases of anterior uveitis.
   Prednisolone acetate 0.5–1.0% variable frequency and/or homatropine 2–5% bid–qid

Immunocompromised Patient

1. Same regimen as adult patient (doses may be increased)
2. *Exception:* Prednisone is contraindicated

Infant Patient

1. Pyrimethamine 1 mg/kg/PO once every 3 days × 2–6 months
   Monitor blood counts for leukopenia and thrombocytopenia
   Combined with sulfadiazine 50–100 mg/kg/day PO in 2 divided doses × 3 weeks

Pregnant Patient

1. Pyrimethamine not advised because it is teratogenic during the first trimester
2. Sulfadiazine
   Loading dose 2 g PO followed by 1 g qid × 4 weeks
3. Counseling/therapeutic abortion may be considered

Abbreviations: bid, twice a day; g, gram; mg, milligram; PO, by mouth, orally; qd, every day; qid, four times daily.

sulfadiazine in the standard treatment protocol. Clindamycin does not cross the blood–brain barrier and is therefore ineffective against *Toxoplasma* encephalitis. Its use has also been associated with pseudomembranous colitis (Jabs & Quinlan, 1994). Spiramycin, minocycline, and trimethoprim-sulfamethoxazole (Bactrim) have also been shown to be somewhat effective as adjunct or alternative agents.

> Corticosteroids should not be used in the absence of concomitant antimicrobial therapy or in immunocompromised patients.

Atovaquone (Mepron), an antimalarial agent also utilized in the treatment of *Pneumocystis carinii* pneumonia, has been shown to be effective against the *Toxoplasma* organism. Beginning in the early 1990s, its use was advocated in cases resistant to other treatment modalities. It also appears to have promise as a monotherapy (Pearson et al, 1999). All of the traditionally employed anti-*Toxoplasma* medications work by killing active tachyzoites and have no effect on encysted bradyzoites. Atovaquone, however, has been shown to destroy bradyzoites in both retinal and cerebral cysts as well as tachyzoites (Gormley et al, 1998). Although further trials are needed, it has tremendous potential because of its ability to prevent or decrease future recurrences.

Immunocompromised individuals are treated with the same drugs as immunocompetent patients, with the exception of corticosteroids, which are contraindicated (Boch-Driessen & Rothova, 1998). In this patient population, pyrimethamine is often used as a chronic maintenance therapy to prevent relapses. During acute infections, higher doses of medication are required in the immunosuppressed.

Drug therapy during pregnancy is complicated by the teratogenic effects of pyrimethamine. It cannot be used during the first trimester; therefore, sulfadiazine or trisulfapyrimidine must be employed. In Europe, spiramycin has been prescribed but it is not commercially available in the United States (Remington et al, 1995). Because of the potentially severe effects of early term maternal infection on the developing fetus, therapeutic abortion may need to be considered in high-risk cases. Infants and newborns with congenital toxoplasmosis are treated with reduced doses of the same medication utilized in infected adults (Table 51–5).

Ocular

Systemic drug therapy is also the mainstay of treatment for ocular toxoplasmosis. Topical corticosteroids and cycloplegics are employed only in those cases involving an anterior uveitis. Treatment with oral corticosteroids in the absence of concomitant antiparasitic agents may lead to significant progression of the disease and should be avoided. Corticosteroids are necessary only when inflammatory lesions affect the optic nerve, macula, or papillomacular bundle, or when a significant vitreitis is present. Active peripheral lesions that do not result in vision loss from vitreitis may be safely monitored without therapy.

In severe, recalcitrant cases vitrectomy may be necessary. Photocoagulation and cryotherapy of active lesions have been attempted in hopes of destroying the parasite and/or denaturing protein to shorten the inflammatory process. Unfortunately, this can be associated with vitreal hemorrhage and retinal detachment (Demestre et al, 1996). Laser treatment decreases the rate of recurrence around active lesions but is ineffective for preventing inactive chorioretinitis from progressing in the future (Demestre et al, 1996). In addition to these drawbacks, tissue cysts are often scattered throughout the retina in uninvolved areas. This makes it impossible to destroy potential sites of future recurrence using this technique.

Follow-up visits should occur at least weekly during active infections. Visual acuity, IOP, anterior segment status, and fundus appearance must be monitored closely. Inactive lesions require only yearly examinations, but patients must be thoroughly educated regarding the need to return promptly for evaluation if symptoms recur.

CONCLUSION

Toxoplasma infection remains a significant cause of morbidity worldwide. Despite an excellent understanding of the transmission of the organism to humans, the number of afflicted individuals continues to grow. Development of a vaccine is critical to future prevention of the disease. New nonteratogenic medications that can safely be utilized during the first trimester of pregnancy are needed. An effective, reliable pharmaceutical agent that is capable of destroying encysted organisms would greatly enhance our current ability to manage afflicted individuals. Improved methods of detecting the presence of fetal infection in utero must be developed, and further understanding of the cause of tissue cyst reactivation is essential.

REFERENCES

Alexander L. *Primary Care of the Posterior Segment.* 2nd ed. Norwalk, CT: Appleton & Lange; 1994:315–319, 324.

Auer C, Bernasconi O, Herbort CD. Toxoplasmic retinochoroiditis: New insights provided by indocyanine green angiography. *Am J Ophthalmol.* 1997;123:131–133.

Beaman MH, McCabe RE, Wong SY, Remington JS. *Toxoplasma gondii.* In: Mandell GL, Bennett JE, Dolin R, eds. *Principles and Practice of Infectious Diseases.* 4th ed. New York: Churchill Livingstone; 1995:2455–2475.

Bloch-Michel E, Lambin P, Debbia M, et al. Local production of IgG and IgG subclasses in the aqueous humor of patients with Fuchs heterochromic cyclitis, herpetic uveitis and toxoplasmic chorioretinitis. *Int Ophthalmol.* 1998; 21:187–194.

Boch-Driessen EH, Rothova A. Sense and nonsense of corticosteroid administration in the treatment of ocular toxoplasmosis. *Br J Ophthalmol.* 1998;82:858–860.

Boer JH, Luyendijk L, Rothova A, Kijlstra A. Analysis of ocular fluids for local antibody production in uveitis. *Br J Ophthalmol.* 1995;79:610–616.

Bornand JE, deGrottrau. Uveitis: Is ocular toxoplasmosis only a clinical diagnosis? *Ophthalmologica.* 1997;211:87–89.

Bowie WR, King AS, Werker DH, et al. Outbreak of toxoplasmosis associated with municipal drinking water. *Lancet.* 1997;350:173–177.

Burnett AJ, Shortt SG, Isaac-Renton J, et al. Multiple cases of acquired toxoplasmosis retinitis presenting in an outbreak. *Ophthalmology.* 1998;105:1032–1037.

Cassady JV. Toxoplasmic retinochoroiditis. *Trans Am Ophthalmol Soc.* 1960;58:392.

Chalam KV, Tripathi RC. Toxoplasmic chorioretinal scar as a cause of unusual neovascularization. *Ann Ophthalmol.* 1997;29:306–308.

Demestre T, Labalette P, Fortier B, et al. Laser photocoagulation around the foci of toxoplasma retinochoroiditis: A descriptive statistical analysis of 35 patients with long term follow-up. *Ophthalmologica.* 1996;210:90–94.

Gormley PD, Pavesio CE, Minnasian D, Lightman S. Effects of drug therapy on toxoplasma cysts in an animal model of acute and chronic disease. *Invest Ophthalmol Vis Sci.* 1998;39:1171–1175.

Guex-Crosier Y, Auer C, Bernasconi O, Herbort CP. Toxoplasmic retinochoroiditis: Resolution without treatment of the perilesional satellite dark dots seen by indocyanine green angiography. *Graefes Arch Clin Exp Ophthalmol.* 1998; 236:476–478.

Hunter D, Stagno S, Capps E, et al. Prenatal screening of pregnant women for infections caused by cytomegalovirus, Epstein–Barr virus, herpesvirus, rubella, and *Toxoplasma gondii. Am J Obstet Gynecol.* 1983;145:269–273.

Jabs DA, Quinlan P. Ocular toxoplasmosis. In: Ryan SJ, Schachat AP, Murphy RP, eds. *Retina.* 2nd ed. St. Louis: Mosby–Year Book; 1994:1531–1543.

Johnson MW, Greven CM, Jaffe GJ, et al. Atypical, severe toxoplasmic retinochoroiditis in elderly patients. *Ophthalmology.* 1997;104;48–57.

Kimball AC, Kean BH, Fuchs F. Congenital toxoplasmosis. A prospective study of 4,048 obstetric patients. *Am J Obstet Gynecol.* 1971;111:211–218.

Klaren V, Van Doornik C, Ongkosuwito JV, et al. Differences between intraocular and serum antibody responses in patients with ocular toxoplasmosis. *Am J Ophthalmol.* 1998; 126:698–706.

La Hey E, Rothova A, Baarsma GS, et al. Fuchs heterochromic iridocyclitis is not associated with ocular toxoplasmosis. *Arch Ophthalmol.* 1992;110:806–811.

Mansour SE. Non-cytomegalovirus posterior segment opportunistic infections in AIDS patients. *Ophthalmol Clin North Am.* 1997;10:45–60.

McCabe RE, Remington JS. Toxoplasmosis. In: Warren KS, Maltound AAF, eds. *Tropical and Geographical Medicine.* New York: McGraw-Hill; 1984:281.

Meeken C, Assies J, van Nieuwenhuizen O, et al. Long term ocular and neurological involvement in severe congenital toxoplasmosis. *Br J Ophthalmol.* 1995;79:581–554.

Montoya JG, Remington JS. Toxoplasmic chorioretinitis in the setting of acute acquired toxoplasmosis. *Clin Infect Dis.* 1996;23:277–282.

Morhun PJ, Weisz JM, Elias SJ, Holland GN. Recurrent ocular toxoplasmosis in patients treated with systemic corticosteroids. *Retina.* 1996;16:383–387.

Pavesio CE, Lightman S. *Toxoplasma gondii* and ocular toxoplasmosis pathogenesis. *Br J Ophthalmol.* 1996;80:1099–1107.

Pearson PA, Piracha AR, Sen HA, Jaffe GJ. Atovaquone for the treatment of toxoplasma retinochoroiditis in immunocompetent patients. *Ophthalmology.* 1999;106:148–153.

Primo SA. Infectious/inflammatory diseases. In: Paorgis CJ, Classe JG, eds. *Optometry Clinics, Systemic Disease and the Eye.* Norwalk, CT: Appleton & Lange; 1994:112–126.

Remington JS, McLeod R, Desmonts G. Toxoplasmosis. In: Remington JS, Klein JO, eds. *Infectious Diseases of the Fetus and Newborn.* 4th ed. Philadelphia: WB Saunders; 1995: 140–267.

Rutzen AR, Smith RE, Roa NA. Recent advances in the understanding of ocular toxoplasmosis. *Curr Opin Ophthalmol.* 1994;5:3–9.

Schlaegel TF. *Ocular Toxoplasmosis and Pars Planitis.* New York: Grune & Stratton; 1978:8.

Shaikh S, Schwab IR, Morse LS. Association of ocular toxoplasmosis and thymoma. *Retina.* 1997;17:354–356.

Tabbara KF. Toxoplasmosis. In: Tasman W, Jaeger EA, eds. *Clinical Ophthalmology.* Philadelphia: Harper & Row; 1990; 1,14.

Chapter 52

TOXOCARIASIS

Diane T. Adamczyk

Toxocariasis, currently also known as toxocarosis, is caused by the parasite *Toxocara canis*, a roundworm commonly found in dogs, or *T. cati*, found in cats. Human infection occurs most frequently in children, who often have a history of eating dirt that is contaminated with parasite eggs, from dog or cat excrement. Once infected, *Toxocara* in humans manifests as either the systemic disease, visceral larva migrans (VLM), or the ocular disease, ocular larva migrans. VLM may involve multiple organs (eg, the liver, lungs, and heart) along with the central nervous system. Ocular manifestations vary from minimal or no symptoms to marked symptomatology. Correct diagnosis is important, particularly with ocular involvement, because appropriate management can preserve both vision and the eye.

EPIDEMIOLOGY

Systemic

Toxocara is a common, global parasitic infection that occurs in domestic animals, particularly dogs and cats. Although *T. cati* may be involved more than previously thought, most reports on *Toxocara* center around its relationship with dogs and its subsequent infection in humans.

Reports worldwide indicate that 13.5 to 93% of dogs may be infected. Puppies in particular are at greatest risk of infection, with more than 80% found to be infected between 2 and 6 months of age, decreasing to less than 20% in those older than 1 year. Transmission of *Toxocara* eggs may occur through dog excretion, with the eggs often found in dirt. Soil contaminated with *Toxocara* may be found in 10 to 30% of public areas (parks and playgrounds), while 11% of private areas (backyards and gardens) are contaminated (Childs, 1985). VLM is found more commonly in the south central and southeastern part of the United States, possibly because soil and climatic conditions harbor *Toxocara* eggs better.

The risks of infection, particularly for children, are high, especially in those with a history of pica or geophagia (eating dirt) or owning a puppy. Although any age may be affected, VLM occurs most commonly in children between 1 and 4 years, with an average age of 2 years. Although both sexes and all races are affected, boys, African-American children, and children of parents with an education below high school level are more commonly infected. Although studies are inconsistent, those individuals having greater contact with dogs through occupations such as dog breeding may have increased exposure to *Toxocara*.

The exact incidence of *Toxocara* infection in humans is not known, because many cases go undiagnosed or unrecognized. In the United States, it is estimated that 10,000 cases of human *Toxocara* infection occur. Serologic evidence of infection may be found in up to 6.5% of the general population, with up to 30%

in children. Systemic involvement commonly includes hepatomegaly in 87% and pulmonary manifestations in approximately 50%, with *Toxocara* reported in 13.6% of patients with poliomyelitis and 7.5% of patients with epilepsy (Mok, 1968).

Ocular

As with VLM, ocular involvement from *Toxocara* occurs most commonly in children, but at a slightly older age. Although any age may be affected, ocular manifestations are seen in 4 to 8 year olds, with an average age of 7.5 years. Central lesions occur more commonly in children 6 to 14 years of age, with peripheral lesions more common in adolescents and adults (Wan et al, 1991).

Usually one eye is affected, with 2.4% having bilateral involvement (Brown, 1970). Ten percent of uveitis in children may be secondary to *Toxocara* (Perkins, 1966). Ocular and systemic disease rarely occur together.

PATHOPHYSIOLOGY/DISEASE PROCESS

The Organism

Toxocara is a roundworm that infects domestic animals, with *T. canis* commonly infecting the dog and *T. cati* infecting cats. Because of the fastidious "toilet behavior" of cats, human infection is believed to be much less likely due to *T. cati* than *T. canis*. Therefore most of the literature centers around *T. canis*. In order to more definitively understand *T. cati's* role in toxocariasis, determination of antibodies that differentiate it from *T. canis* are necessary. The following discussion uses *T. canis* and dogs as the prototype.

The complete life cycle of *T. canis* occurs in the dog, its natural host. Infection in the dog may occur through reactivation of larvae from hormonal changes in a pregnant bitch, with transplacental transfer to the puppy; from a nursing bitch's milk; from a nursing bitch licking her young; from ingesting feces; or from eating an infected mouse or rabbit. In the prenatally infected puppy, at birth, a third-stage larva is formed in the lungs, which the puppy coughs up and swallows. This then goes to the small intestine, maturing to adult worms in approximately 3 weeks. The adult worm sheds 200,000 eggs per day through the puppy's feces, until 4 to 6 months of age, when the infection decreases. Eggs are also shed through a lactating bitch's feces. These eggs become infectious in 2 to 7 weeks, and may remain viable, dependent on soil type and climate, for months to years. The adult dog may ingest the eggs, which hatch in the small intestine, with second-stage larvae passing through the intestinal wall. These travel to various organs and tissues (liver, lungs, brain, eye), usually remaining in these tissues, instead of completing the cycle as in a puppy.

Transmission

Humans are infected through pica or geophagia, poor hygiene (particularly after playing or working in dirt or around infected puppies), or sometimes by ingesting food contaminated with eggs from infected soil, such as lettuce. In the small intestine the ova hatch, with the larvae going through the intestinal wall, traveling to various tissues and organs, via the blood or lymphatic system. When the larvae cannot pass through the blood vessel because of its size, they travel through the blood vessel wall into the surrounding tissue. Larvae may remain viable in these tissues for weeks, months, or even years, eventually dying. The larvae may become dormant, later to reactivate. In humans, a complete life cycle to mature adult worms does not occur, which explains why human feces lack ova. Inflammation, hemorrhage, necrosis, or an eosinophilic granulomatous response may occur with infection in either systemic or ocular disease.

Course of the Disease

Systemic

As the life cycle of *Toxocara* evolves in humans, various organs and tissues may be affected, with numerous systemic manifestations resulting (Table 52–1) in VLM. These manifestations are related to larval mi-

TABLE 52–1. SYSTEMIC MANIFESTATIONS OF TOXOCARIASIS (VISCERAL LARVA MIGRANS)

Signs/Symptoms
- Fever, abdominal pain, fatigue/malaise, headache, pallor, anemia, anorexia/weight loss, irritability, sleep/behavioral disturbances, nausea, vomiting, pharyngitis, limb pains, dizziness, constipation, poliomyelitis
- Eosinophilia, leukocytosis, elevated isohemagglutinations, increased serum gammaglobulin (IgG, IgM)
- Lymphadenopathy
- Covert disease: headache, abdominal pain, cough (nonspecific signs/symptoms)

Visceral Involvement
- Splenomegaly
- Hepatomegaly
- Pulmonary involvement
  Pneumonia, cough, wheeze, bronchitis, asthma, transient pulmonary infiltrates on chest films
- Neurologic involvement
  Seizures or epilepsy, behavior disorders, increased eosinophils in cerebrospinal fluid
- Dermatologic involvement
  Urticarial, pruritic, or nodular skin rash
- Cardiac involvement
  Myocarditis

gration and its sequelae, along with larval death, which may produce more severe reactions than the live larva. Eosinophils surround the larva, with the development of an inflammatory, granulomatous reaction along with fibrous tissue. Clinical manifestations most commonly include fever, fatigue, lymphadenopathy, and eosinophilia. Toxocariasis generally follows an unremarkable course, resolving in weeks, with an incubation time of days to months. Eosinophilia may last for years, with the antibody titer often decreasing over time. Rarely, the course of the disease results in death, which is usually from complications of myocarditis or encephalitis.

In addition to VLM, a covert form of the disease may occur. Here distinct signs and symptoms described are not present. Instead, nonspecific symptoms, such as headache, abdominal pain, or cough, may occur.

Ocular

The effect of *Toxocara* in the eye (Table 52–2) differs in a number of respects from systemic involvement. Ocular symptoms may result from just one or two larvae, whereas many larvae are needed to elicit symptoms from larger organs, such as the liver. Ocular manifestations occur at a later age than VLM. This may be due to a latent period that follows the initial infection. Reactivation occurs years later, resulting in ocular manifestations.

TABLE 52–2. OCULAR MANIFESTATIONS OF *TOXOCARA*

Vitreoretinal Involvement
- Retinochoroiditis
- Vitritis
- White mass/granuloma (1/2 to 4 disc diameters)
- Retinal traction
- Vitreous bands
- Traction bands (extend from lesion to disc or macula)
- Retinal folds
- Heterotropic macula
- Tortuous/deviated vessels
- Distorted optic nerve head
- Macular granuloma, associated with hemorrhages or serous detachment
- Peripheral-falciform fold, unilateral pars planitis, retinal fold from peripheral mass to optic nerve head
- Other: retinal hemorrhage, retinal edema, papillitis (rare), secondary retinal artery occlusion

Endophthalmitis
- Minimal pain or photophobia
- Leukocoria
- Cyclitic membrane
- Eosinophils in vitreous
- Vitritis
- Keratic precipitates
- Hypopyon (rare)
- Anterior chamber reaction (less common)
- Secondary cataract and glaucoma, synechiae, iris bombe, phthisis bulbi

Miscellaneous
- Strabismus, keratitis (rare), conjunctivitis, larva in lens (rare), iris nodules (rare), diffuse unilateral subacute neuroretinitis, choroidal neovascular membrane

The larva enters the eye through the choroidal (posterior ciliary) and retinal circulation, migrating to the subretinal area or vitreous. The incubation period may take months to years, with death of the larva eventually occurring. *Toxocara* causes damage to the eye by direct affect of the larva to the eye and/or from the inflammatory response. Larval death results in a more marked inflammatory response than that of the live larva.

Toxocara usually affects only one eye, manifesting as a focal retinal granuloma, peripheral inflammatory mass, and/or endophthalmitis. As the larva migrates through the choroid and retina, a retinochoroiditis with an overlying vitreous reaction may occur, either centrally or peripherally. A granulomatous reaction and a white fibrous mass may result. The granuloma most commonly is found in the macular or peripapillary area, but may also occur in the periphery. Eventually this lesion takes on a more glistening white or gray appearance, with the inflammation subsiding. Vitreous bands, retinal dragging, strabismus, heterotropia of the macula, and vision loss may subsequently occur (Figures 52–1 and 52–2). Vision may be preserved in cases of peripheral lesions.

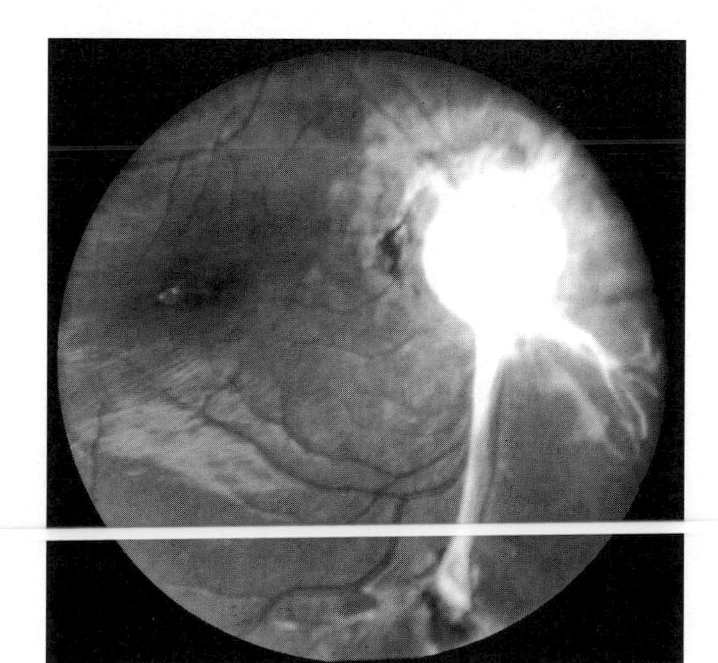

Figure 52–1. Vitreoretinal band to the optic nerve head in toxocariasis. *(Photo courtesy of Dr. Jerome Sherman, SUNY, College of Optometry.)*

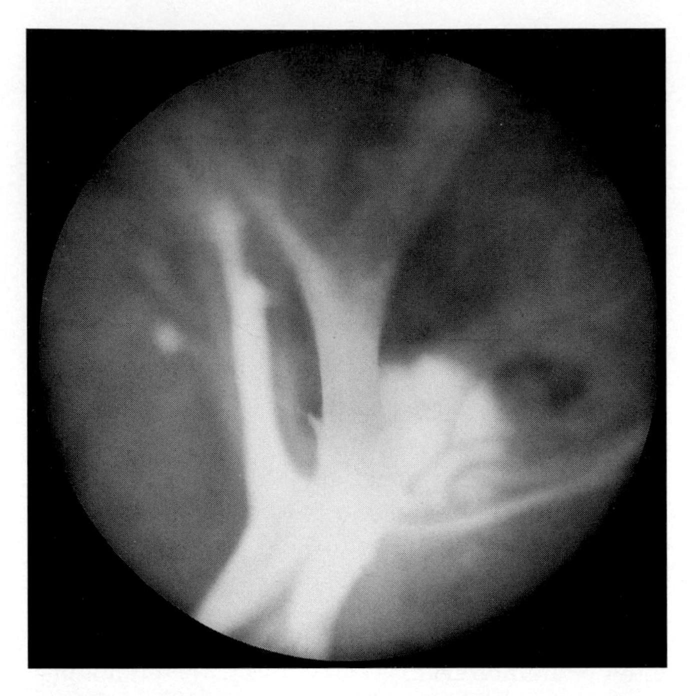

Figure 52–2. Marked vitreous band in suspected *T. canis. (Photo courtesy of Dr. Scott Richter, SUNY, College of Optometry.)*

Endophthalmitis is usually associated with minimal pain and photophobia, possibly resulting in leukocoria, retinal detachment, retrolental mass, or cyclitic membrane. Visual prognosis with cyclitic membranes is generally poor, requiring prompt surgical intervention.

DIAGNOSIS

Table 52–3 lists diagnostic laboratory tests, and Table 52–4 lists differential considerations.

Systemic

Many cases of VLM may be misdiagnosed or go undetected. The definitive diagnosis of *Toxocara* is made based on tissue biopsy; however, this is often not possible. A history of geophagia, exposure to dogs, suggestive clinical manifestations, and other testing procedures will support the diagnosis. *Toxocara* infection should be ruled out in children with seizures or epilepsy.

Enzyme-linked immunosorbent assay (ELISA) has proven to be one of the most reliable and sensitive tests for *Toxocara*. ELISA may indicate past or present infection. The recommended titer for diagnosis of VLM is 1 in 32, which has a sensitivity of 78% and specificity of 92%.

> *Toxocara* should be considered in the differential diagnosis of children with seizures or epilepsy.

Eosinophilia is frequently present in *Toxocara*. However, its absence does not preclude the diagnosis. When eosinophilia is present, it may remain for months, possibly years after the initial infection. Leukocytosis, elevated serum gamma globulin (IgG and IgM), and isohemaglutinin titers against A and B blood may be found.

Other tests must be interpreted with caution because of cross-reactions with other parasites, and lack of sensitivity and specificity (e.g., fluorescent antibody and hemagglutinin tests). Stool and urine testing does not assist in the diagnosis, since *Toxocara* is not excreted in humans.

> A unilateral inflammation, pars planitis, or leukocoria in a child should make the practitioner suspicious of *Toxocara.*

TABLE 52–3. DIAGNOSTIC TESTING FOR TOXOCARA INFECTION

ELISA
VLM: 1 in 32
OLM: 1 in 8
Biopsy
Workup for eosinophilia

TABLE 52–4. DIFFERENTIAL DIAGNOSIS OF *TOXOCARA* INFECTION (SYSTEMIC/OCULAR)

Visceral Toxocariasis
Toxoplasmosis
Infectious diseases
Consider parasites, protozoa, virus
Seizure-related
Consider idiopathic, tuberous sclerosis, encephalitis, neurofibromatosis, febrile-related
Ocular Toxocariasis
Toxoplasmosis
Intraocular neoplasms
Consider retinoblastoma, amelanotic melanoma, glioma
Persistent hyperplastic primary vitreous
Retinochoroidal coloboma
Coat disease
Tuberous sclerosis
Retinopathy of prematurity

Ocular

Ocular diagnosis of *Toxocara* is based on clinical presentation, history, and a complete eye evaluation. A unilateral inflammation, pars planitis, or leukocoria in a child should make the practitioner suspicious of *Toxocara*. Definitive diagnosis, although not always determined, is made through histologic evidence of the organism in an enucleated eye.

Diagnosis may be relatively easy, based on the classic clinical presentation of a granuloma, with associated retinal manifestations. However, the use of specific tests (e.g., for eosinophilia or ELISA), which are often helpful in VLM, may be equivocal in ocular disease. Antibody levels in ocular *Toxocara* are weaker than in VLM. An ELISA of 1 in 8 is the criterion for ocular diagnosis. With this criteria, ELISA has a 90% sensitivity and 91% specificity for ocular *Toxocara* (Pollard, 1979). However, the presence of an elevated titer does not provide a definitive diagnosis, but in the presence of clinical signs may be supportive of one. When the diagnosis is questionable, aqueous or vitreous samples should be taken, which may demonstrate eosinophils and positive ELISA findings, along with absence of tumor cells that may be present in retinoblastoma.

History, associated findings, computed tomography (CT), and ultrasound may assist in the differential diagnosis of *Toxocara* from other ocular diseases. For example, the CT and ultrasound may show calcification in retinoblastoma, but this is rarely found in *Toxocara*. Microphthalmia is an associated finding in persistent primary hyperplastic vitreous, but not in *Toxocara*. Correct diagnosis is essential, because many cases of *Toxocara* are misdiagnosed, resulting in inappropriate management, as evidenced by cases of enucleation when a misdiagnosis of retinoblastoma is made.

TREATMENT AND MANAGEMENT

Systemic

The optimal management of *Toxocara* is prevention. This may include deworming puppies and appropriate hygiene when dealing with soil and dogs (Table 52–5).

When VLM does occur, mild disease may simply be monitored, with referral to a pediatrician who is trained to deal with any potential complications, such as pulmonary, hepatic, neurologic, or cardiac involvement. Specific treatment is determined by patient symptomatology, disease severity and organ involvement. Steroids may be used for severe respiratory and myocardial involvement. Anthelmintic drugs, such as diethylcarbamazine and thiabendazole, may relieve symptoms and duration by killing the larvae. However, these drugs should be used sparingly and in those who are very sick, because severe side effects may result. Often the organism is best left untreated.

> The best treatment for *Toxocara* infection in humans is prevention through deworming and appropriate hygiene of dogs and cats.

TABLE 52–5. TREATMENT AND MANAGEMENT OF *TOXOCARA*

Systemic

Prevention
- Deworm dogs
- Hygiene (when dealing with soil, dogs)
- Educate dog owners
- Enforce pooper scooper/leash laws
- Keep children from contaminated areas

Visceral larva migrans
- Monitor
- Referral to physician or pediatrician with appropriate training to deal with potential complications (pulmonary, hepatic, neurologic, or cardiac)
- Severe respiratory and myocardial involvement: steroids
- Anthelmintic drugs (eg, diethylcarbamazine, thiabendazole)

Ocular
- Inflammation
  Steroids (topical, subconjunctival, subtenon, oral), cycloplegic agents
- Anthelminthics
  (variable success), used with steroids
- Surgical
  Vitrectomy, laser photocoagulation/cryotherapy, pars plana vitrectomy, secondary cataract removal
- Secondary glaucoma
  Medication, surgery (eg, trabeculectomy)

Ocular

Treatment of ocular involvement of *Toxocara* is dependent on the severity and potential threat to the eye and vision. For example, monitoring the patient with a nonthreatening peripheral granuloma may be the best treatment option. Steroid treatment may be necessary for some cases of inflammation. Although the use of anthelminthics in ocular disease is of questionable value, they may be used in conjunction with steroids. Surgical intervention may ultimately be necessary. Pars plana vitrectomy may be needed in cases of chronic endophthalmitis, to remove vitreous bands and to prevent the possible sequelae of retinal detachment, phthisis bulbi, or amblyopia. Photocoagulation or cryotherapy may be used to kill the larvae; however, this treatment is reserved for those cases where the resultant inflammatory response to the dead larvae outweighs the risk of no treatment.

CONCLUSION

Toxocara is a parasitic infection that occurs commonly in its natural host, the domestic dog, with infection and an incomplete life cycle occurring in humans. The disease in humans affects children most commonly, resulting in systemic (visceral larva migrans) or ocular manifestations (ocular larva migrans), with each rarely occurring concurrently. *Toxocara* usually follows a benign course, or may manifest in ways such that the underlying cause may go undiagnosed. Correct diagnosis may therefore prevent inappropriate treatment and allow prompt management when indicated.

REFERENCES

Arpino C, Curatolo P. Toxocariasis in children. *Lancet.* 1988; 1:1172.

Arpino C, Gattinara GC, Piergili D, Curatolo P. *Toxocara* infection and epilepsy in children: A case-control study. *Epilepsia.* 1990;31:33–36.

Belmont JB, Irvine A, Benson W. O'Connor R. Vitrectomy in ocular toxocariasis. *Arch Ophthalmol.* 1982;100:1912–1915.

Berrocal J. Prevalence of *Toxocara canis* in babies and in adults as determined by the ELISA test. *Trans Am Ophthalmol Soc.* 1980;78:376–413.

Biglan AW, Glickman LT, Lobes LA. Serum and vitreous toxocara antibody in nematode endophthalmitis. *Am J Ophthalmol.* 1979;88:898–901.

Brown DH. Ocular *Toxocara canis. J Pediatr Ophthalmol.* 1970; 7:182–191.

Brown GC, Tasman WS. Retinal arterial obstruction in association with presumed *Toxocara canis* neuroretinitis. *Ann Ophthalmol.* 1981;13:1385–1387.

Byers B, Kimura SJ. Uveitis after death of a larva in the vitreous cavity. *Am J Ophthalmol.* 1974;77:63–66.

Caucanas JP, Magnaval JF, Pascal JP. Prevalence of toxocaral disease. *Lancet.* 1988;1:1049.

Centers for Disease Control and Prevention. Division of Parasitic Diseases. Fact sheet: Toxocariasis. Updated June 13, 2000. http:\\www.cdc.gov\ncidod\dpd\parasites\toxocara\factsheet.

Childs JE. The prevalence of *Toxocara* species ova in backyards and gardens of Baltimore, Maryland. *AJPH.* 1985; 75:1092–1094.

Clemett RS, Allardyce RA, Williamson HJE, et al. Ocular *Toxocara canis* infections: Diagnosis by enzyme immunoassay. *Aust NZ J Ophthalmol.* 1987;15:145–150.

Cox TA, Haskins GE, Gangitano JL, Antonson DL. Bilateral *Toxocara* optic neuropathy. *J Clin Neuro-ophthalmol.* 1983; 3:267–274.

Dernouchamps JP, Verougstraete C, Demolder E. Ocular toxocariasis: A presumed case of peripheral granuloma. *Int Ophthalmol.* 1990;14:383–388.

Dinning WJ, Gillespie GH, Cooling RJ, Maizels RM. Toxocariasis: A practical approach to management of ocular disease. *Eye.* 1988;2:580–582.

Duguid IM. Features of ocular infestation by *Toxocara. Br J Ophthalmol.* 1961;45:789–796.

Eberhard ML, Alfano E. Adult *Toxocara cati* infections in U.S. children: Report of four cases. *Am J Trop Med Hyg.* 1998; 59:404–406.

Ellis GS, Pakalnis VA, Worley G. *Toxocara canis* infection. Clinical and epidemiological associations with seropositivity in kindergarten children. *Ophthalmology.* 1986;93:1032–1037.

Ferguson EC, Olson LJ. *Toxocara* ocular nematodiasis. *Int Ophthalmol Clin.* 1967;7:583–603.

Gill D, Dunne K, Kenny V. Toxocariasis in children. *Lancet.* 1988;1:1172.

Jones WL. *Toxocara canis. J Am Optom Assoc.* 1979;4:450–454.

Kennedy JJ, Defeo E. Ocular toxocariasis demonstrated by ultrasound. *Ann Ophthalmol.* 1981;13:1357–1358.

Kielar RA. *Toxocara canis* endophthalmitis with low ELISA titer. *Ann Ophthalmol.* 1983;15:447–449.

Kirber WM, Nichols CW, Braunstein SN. Unusual presentation of ocular toxocariasis in friends. *Ann Ophthalmol.* 1979;11:573–576.

Lampariello DA, Primo SA. Ocular toxocariasis: A rare presentation of a posterior pole granuloma with an associated choroidal neovascular membrane. *J Am Optom Assoc.* 1999;70:245–252.

Liesegang TJ. Atypical ocular toxocariasis. *J Pediatr Ophthalmol.* 1977:14:349–353.

Maguire AM, Green WR, Michels RG, Erozan YS. Recovery of intraocular *Toxocara canis* by pars plana vitrectomy. *Ophthalmology.* 1990;97:675–680.

Maguire AM, Zarbin MA, Connor TB, Justin J. Ocular penetration of thiabendazole. *Arch Ophthalmol.* 1990;108: 1675.

Marmor M, Glickman L, Shofer F, et al. *Toxocara canis* infection of children: Epidemiologic and neuropsychologic findings. *Am J Public Health.* 1987;77:554–559.

Mok CH. Visceral larva migrans. A discussion based on review of the literature. *Clin Pediatr.* 1968;7:565–573.

Molk R. Ocular toxocariasis: A review of the literature. *Ann Ophthalmol.* 1983;15:216–231.

Molk R. Treatment of toxocaral optic neuritis. *J Clin Neuro-ophthalmol.* 1982;2:109–112.

O'Connor PR. Visceral larva migrans of the eye. *Arch Ophthalmol.* 1972;88:526–529.

Overgaauw PAM. Aspects of *Toxocara* epidemiology: Human toxocarosis. *Crit Rev Microbiol.* 1997;23:215–231.

Perkins ES. Pattern of uveitis in children. *Br J Ophthalmol.* 1966;50:169–185.

Pollard ZF. Long-term follow-up in patients with ocular toxocariasis as measured by ELISA titers. *Ann Ophthalmol.* 1987;19:167–169.

Pollard ZF. Ocular *Toxocara* in siblings of two families. *Arch Ophthalmol.* 1979;97:2319–2320.

Pollard ZF, Jarrett WH, Hagler WS, et al. ELISA for diagnosis of ocular toxocariasis. *Ophthalmology.* 1979;86:743–752.

Richer SP, Stiles WR. Presumed *Toxocara canis* with peripheral retinal granuloma and secondary macular hole. *J Am Optom Assoc.* 1987;58:404–407.

Rodriguez A. Early pars plana vitrectomy in chronic endophthalmitis of toxocariasis. *Graefe's Arch Clin Exp Ophthalmol.* 1986;224:218–220.

Schantz PM, Glickman LT. Toxocaral visceral larva migrans. *N Engl J Med.* 1978;298:436–439.

Schantz PM, Weis PE, Pollard ZF, White MC. Risk factors for toxocaral ocular larva migrans: A case control study. *Am J Public Health.* 1980;70:1269–1272.

Schimek RA, Perez WA, Carrera GM. Ophthalmic manifestations of visceral larva migrans. *Ann Ophthalmol.* 1979; 11:1387–1390.

Searl SS, Moazed K, Albert DM, Marcus LC. Ocular toxocariasis presenting as leukocoria in a patient with low ELISA titer to *Toxocara canis. Ophthalmology.* 1981;88:1302–1306.

Sharkey JA, McKay PS. Ocular toxocariasis in a patient with repeatedly negative ELISA titre to *Toxocara canis. Br J Ophthalmol.* 1993;77:253–254.

Shields JA. Ocular toxocariasis. A review. *Surv Ophthalmol.* 1984;28:361–381.

Shields JA, Felberg NT, Federman JL. Discussion of presentation by Dr Zane F. Pollard, et al. *Ophthalmology.* 1979; 86:750–752.

Taylor MRH, Keane CT, O'Connor P, et al. The expanded spectrum of toxocaral disease. *Lancet.* 1988:692–694.

Wan WL, Cano MR, Pince KJ, Green RL. Echographic characteristics of ocular toxocariasis. *Ophthalmology.* 1991; 98:28–32.

Zinkham WH. Visceral larva migrans. A review and reassessment indicating two forms of clinical expression: Visceral and ocular. *Am J Dis Child.* 1978;132:627–633.

Section XI

HEMATOLOGIC DISORDERS

Chapter 53

ANEMIAS

Lori R. Reminick

Anemia is defined as a decrease in the circulating red blood cell mass. Anemia may be classified according to cell morphology (microcytic, normocytic, and macrocytic) or etiology (impaired production, hemolytic, and acute blood loss). Systemic signs and symptoms shared by most anemias are pallor, weakness, lethargy, dyspnea, palpitations, bruising, lymphadenopathy, bone tenderness, hepatosplenomegaly, and epithelial abnormalities. Ocular signs and symptoms are numerous as well, affecting the conjunctiva, retina, optic nerve, and extraocular muscles. Iron-deficiency, pernicious, and aplastic anemias will be discussed with emphasis on their ocular manifestations.

EPIDEMIOLOGY

Systemic

Iron-deficiency anemia is the most common anemia in the United States. Iron deficiency is more common in infants, childhood, pregnancy, and women during childbearing years. The adult male has no increased demands for iron, and therefore can live without dietary iron for approximately 3 to 4 years before iron-deficiency anemia results (Brown, 1993). Results from the third National Health and Nutrition Examination Survey (NHANES III, 1988–1994) revealed the prevalence of iron-deficiency anemia to be highest in females ages 20 to 49 (5%), ages 16 to 19 (3%), and infants between the ages of 1 and 2 (3%). The lowest prevalence is in males ages 12 to 49 (<1%). This translates into 3.3 million adolescent girls and women of childbearing age affected and 240,000 toddlers in the United States.

Pernicious anemia is most often found in patients above 60 and rarely below 40 years of age (Brown, 1993). There is strong evidence that this disorder may be an inherited autoimmune disease. Frequency of diagnosed cases has been variously estimated from as low as 0.1% of the population and rising to 1% in northern European elderly. The frequency of undiagnosed cases has been estimated to be 1.9% (Carmel, 1996). The highest frequencies were in African-American women.

Aplastic anemia is idiopathic in about 50% of cases with the remaining cases secondary to chemical agents and infections, and to metabolic, immunologic, and neoplastic etiologies (Erslev & Gabuzda, 1985). The incidence of aplastic anemia in the United States has been reported in different studies. One study took place in South Carolina, comparing the incidence rates with a study in Baltimore. The same general age-specific incidence pattern was found in the two areas. Nonwhite average annual age-adjusted rates in South Carolina were 6.8 and 13.7 per 1,000,000 per year for males and females, respectively, and 4.7 and 7.3 per 1,000,000 per year for males and females, respectively, in Baltimore. For whites, the rates in South Carolina were 11.7 and 5.4 per 1,000,000 per year for males and females, respectively, and 7.1 and 5.4 in Baltimore (Linet et al, 1986).

Ocular

Retinal manifestations are the most common ocular finding. Rubenstein et al (1968) found that only 10% of persons with anemia alone had retinopathy, whereas 70% developed retinopathy when both anemia and thrombocytopenia were present.

PATHOPHYSIOLOGY/DISEASE PROCESS

Systemic

Table 53–1 lists the classification of the anemias.

Iron-Deficiency Anemia

Iron is necessary for hemoglobin and myoglobin synthesis. The body has roughly 4000 mg of iron. Approximately 60% or more circulates in the peripheral blood as red blood cell hemoglobin (RBCHb), and 40% is stored as ferritin in the reticuloendothelial cells of the bone marrow. Normal iron balance is maintained by adequate iron absorption. The usual Western diet contains 10 to 20 mg of iron. The normal gastrointestinal (GI) tract can absorb 10% of its intake. This results in absorption of 1 to 2 mg daily, which adequately replaces daily loss due to red blood cell (RBC) turnover (Rubin & Leopold, 1998). Therefore, unless there is an increased need for iron (infancy, pregnancy, menstruation, GI bleeding), deficiency will not develop. Normal red blood cell and iron values are given in Table 53–2.

Iron-deficiency anemia (IDA) occurs in three stages. First, there is a depletion of iron stores in which iron is being utilized by the red blood cells at an increased rate and the dietary intake is not enough to keep up with the demand. At this stage the cells are normochromic and normocytic. Next, iron-deficient erythropoiesis takes place in which the stores become exhausted and the erythrocytes become microcytic. In the final stage, the stores are depleted and the cells become characteristically microcytic and hypochromic. IDA presents at this stage (Brown, 1993).

In addition to the generalized symptoms common to most anemias, such as palpitations, weakness, fatigue, and dyspnea on exertion, there are signs specific to iron deficiency (Table 53–3). Pica (cravings for strange food and things such as starch, clay, and ice) is a symptom of IDA. Additionally, brittle, spooned nails (koilonychia), atrophic tongue, gastritis with atrophy, and dysphagia secondary to esophageal webs are specific signs and symptoms of IDA (Rubin & Leopold, 1998). Iron-deficiency anemia is usually mild;

TABLE 53–1. CLASSIFICATION OF ANEMIAS

Etiologic

Inadequate erythropoiesis
Aplastic anemia
Myelophthisic anemia
Bone marrow carcinoma
Iron-deficiency anemia
Thalassemia
Anemia of chronic disease

Excessive blood loss
Hemorrhagic anemia

Excessive blood destruction
Congenital hemolytic and acquired anemias
Sickle cell anemia

Morphologic

Microcytic
Iron-deficient anemia
Thalassemia
Anemia of chronic disease

Normocytic
Aplastic anemia
Infectious anemia
Pure red cell aplasia
Inflammation
Renal disease
Neoplasms
Pituitary/thyroid failure
Starvation

Macrocytic
Megaloblastic
- Vitamin B_{12} deficiency
- Folate deficiency

Nonmegaloblastic
- Myelodysplasia
- Chemotherapy
- Myxedema

TABLE 53–2. NORMAL RED CELL BLOOD AND IRON VALUES FOR ADULTS

	Males	Females
Normal Red Blood Cell Values		
Hematocrit (Hct)	47%±7	42%±5
Hemoglobin (Hgb)	16 g/dL±2	14 g/dL±2
Red blood cell count (RBC)	$5.4 \times 10^6/\mu L \pm 0.8$	$4.8 \times 10^6/\mu L \pm 0.6$
Mean cell volume (MCV)	90 fL±8	90 fL±8
Mean cell hemoglobin (MCH)	29 pg/cell±2	29 pg/cell±2
MCH concentration (MCHC)	33.5 g/dl±2	33.5 g/dl±2
Normal Iron Balance		
Normal Hgb	16 g/dL	14 g/dL
Hgb iron	2500 mg	1900 mg
Iron intake per day	10–15 mg	10–15 mg
Storage iron	1000 mg	500 mg
Iron absorbed per day	1.0 mg	1.0–2.5 mg
Iron loss per day	1.0 mg	1.0–2.5 mg

Adapted from Spivak JL, The anemic patient. In: Harvey AM, et al, eds. The Principles and Practice of Medicine. *2nd ed. Norwalk, CT: Appleton & Lange; 1988:310–322.*

TABLE 53–3. SYSTEMIC MANIFESTATIONS OF ANEMIAS

General Systemic Signs and Symptoms of Anemia
- Pallor
- Weakness
- Lethargy
- Dyspnea
- Tachycardia
- Palpitations
- Tachypnea (very rapid breathing) on exertion
- Cutaneous hemorrhage (bruise)
- Lymphadenopathy
- Bone tenderness
- Hepatosplenomegaly
- Epithelial abnormalities

Systemic Signs and Symptoms of Specific Anemias
- **Iron-deficiency anemia**
  - Headache
  - Light-headedness
  - Pica
  - Glossitis
  - Koilonychia
  - Dysphagia
- **Aplastic anemia**
  - Easy bruisability
  - Epistaxis
  - Increased menstrual flow
  - Bacterial infections of mouth and perirectal area
- **Pernicious anemia**
  - Glossitis
  - GI disturbances
    - Atrophic gastritis
    - Anorexia
    - Diarrhea
  - Neurogenic disturbances
    - Subacute combined degeneration
  - Autoimmune diseases

however, it may become severe enough to be life-threatening.

Pernicious Anemia

Pernicious anemia is a megaloblastic anemia caused by a deficiency in vitamin B_{12} (cobalamin) resulting from an inability of the gastric mucosa to secrete intrinsic factor necessary for B_{12} absorption. There is strong evidence at present that this disorder may be an inherited autoimmune disease. Antibodies to intrinsic factor have been found in over half of the cases, and antibodies to the parietal cells of the stomach (which secrete intrinsic factor) have been found to be present in over 85% of patients with pernicious anemia (Brown, 1993). The major abnormality is the decreased synthesis of DNA caused by depleted stores of thymidine triphosphate. The cells become larger than normal because maturation of the cell nuclei is slowed relative to maturation of the cytoplasm. This results in enlarged (macrocytic), normochromic red blood cells.

The clinical symptoms are weakness, shortness of breath, and a lemon yellow pallor (see Table 53–3). Additionally, patients may have glossitis, GI symptoms, and neurologic symptoms. Patients may experience numbness, tingling of the extremities, loss of position sense, muscle weakness, and decreased tendon reflexes. In advanced stages the patient may become emotionally unstable and show personality changes referred to as "megaloblastic madness" (Brown, 1993). The clinical symptoms evolve slowly over a period of several months. Other causes of megaloblastic anemia are nutritional deficiencies of vitamin B_{12} and folate resulting from inadequate diet and/or alcohol abuse (Lam & Lam, 1992).

Aplastic Anemia

Aplastic anemia is characterized by pancytopenia (failure to produce red blood cells, white blood cells, and platelets). Most evidence suggests this is due to damage to the hematopoietic stem cells. In aplastic anemia the red blood cells are usually normocytic and normochromic. Aplastic anemia may be acquired (secondary), from exposure to chemicals, drugs, radiation, infections, or autoimmune diseases, or idiopathic (primary) in about 50% of cases. The clinical course varies with disease severity and may show rapid onset and progression to death, or may have a slow onset and chronic course (Brown, 1993). Clinical manifestations are all directly related to the pancytopenia. Patients may experience weakness, fatigue, pallor, fever, infections, and hemorrhages. Severe aplastic anemia is dominated by skin and mucosal bleeding, fatigue, and infection (see Table 53–3). Death is usually due to infections with bacterial and fungal pathogens (Rubin & Leopold, 1998).

Ocular

Ocular manifestations are not usually present unless anemia is severe. Numerous ocular findings have been reported such as conjunctival pallor or hemorrhage, hyphema, optic neuropathy, papilledema, cranial nerve palsies, and retinopathy (Table 53–4). Anemic retinopathy consists of any combination of superficial streak hemorrhages, dot and blot hemorrhages, flame-shaped hemorrhages with pale centers (Roth spots), boat-shaped subhyaloid hemorrhages, vitreous hemorrhages, cotton-wool spots, and hard exudates (Figure 53–1) (Koh & Yeo, 1998). Dilated and tortuous retinal veins may be present, and in extreme cases they lead to central retinal vein occlusion.

> Anemic retinopathy is the most common ocular manifestation of anemia.

TABLE 53–4. OCULAR MANIFESTATIONS OF ANEMIAS

Generalized Ocular Signs of Anemia
- Conjunctival findings
  - Pallor/hemorrhage
- Retinal findings
  - Retinal and preretinal hemorrhages
  - Roth spots
  - Breakthrough vitreous hemorrhages
  - Cotton-wool spots
  - Dilated tortuous veins
  - Exacerbation of diabetic retinopathy
  - Hard exudates

Ocular Signs of Specific Anemias

Iron-deficiency anemia
- Central retinal vein occlusion with or without macular edema
- Incomplete central retinal artery occlusion
- Blue sclera

Pernicious anemia
- Optic neuropathy
- Optic disc edema
- Ophthalmoplegia
- Anterior ischemic optic neuropathy

Aplastic anemia
- Hyphema
- Papilledema

There seems to be a relationship between the severity of anemia and the presence of anemic retinopathy (Koh & Yeo, 1998). Retinopathy caused by anemia probably does not occur unless the hemoglobin titer is less than 8 g/100 mL. Additionally, severe anemia (hemoglobin <8 g/100 mL) or thrombocytopenia (<50,000/mm^3) alone is less likely to cause retinopathy than both occurring simultaneously. Anoxia alone is not sufficient to cause hemorrhage, as long as sufficient numbers of platelets are present to protect the integrity of the capillary endothelium. The pathogenesis of retinopathy of anemia is uncertain. Little has been published regarding the pathophysiology of anemic retinopathy; however, several factors have been implicated. Retinal vascular endothelial incompetence caused by hypoxia is believed to be one etiology (Kirkham et al, 1971). Anemia results in diminished capillary oxygenation, producing increased permeability and extravasation of blood. In a study by Merin and Freund (1968), children appeared to be more resistant to the development of anemic retinopathy than adults, which may indicate that aging of the retinal vessels could play a role in the retinopathy.

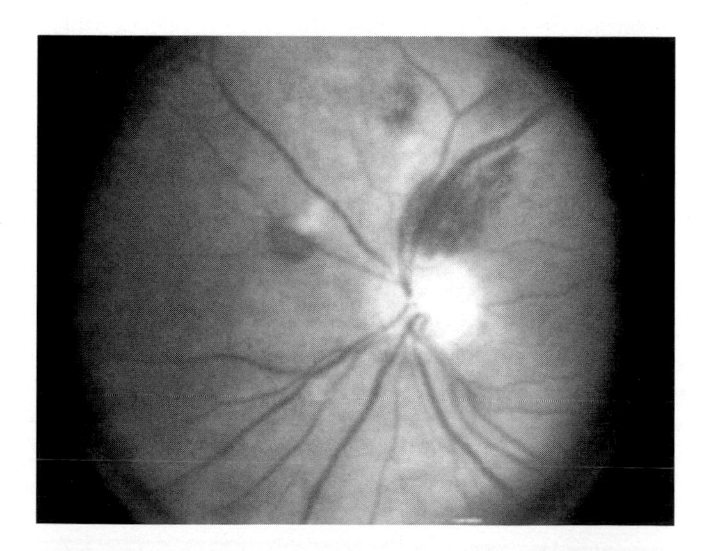

Figure 53–1. Fundus of a patient with severe anemia. Note intraretinal hemorrhages and cotton-wool spots. *(Reprinted with permission from Lowenstein JI. Retinopathy associated with blood anomalies. In: Albert DM, Jakobiec FA, eds.* Principles and Practices of Ophthalmology. *Vol 2, Clinical Practice. Philadelphia: Saunders; 1994:399–408.)*

Severe IDA may exacerbate diabetic retinopathy. Shorb (1985) reported three patients with mild to moderate background diabetic retinopathy that developed marked IDA and then rapidly progressed to severe proliferative retinopathy. It was suggested that hypoxia, resulting from anemia, can cause the release of a vasoproliferative factor, and thus increase the tendency for the development of proliferative disease. Qiao et al (1997) found that subjects with normocytic anemia tended to have an increased risk for severe diabetic retinopathy.

There are a few ocular signs reported in association with specific types of anemia (see Table 53–4).

> Hypoxia caused by severe anemia may cause the release of a vasoproliferative factor, thus increasing the tendency for the development of proliferative diabetic retinopathy.

Iron-Deficiency Anemia

IDA associated with an incomplete central retinal artery occlusion has been reported (Matsuoka et al, 1996). There also is an association reported between blue sclera and IDA in adults (Kalra, 1986). The blue color of the sclera results from thinning of the underlying uveal tissue. Since iron is a cofactor in the synthesis of collagen, iron deficiency may lead to an abnormally thin sclera (Beghetti et al, 1993). Papilledema is an uncommon complication of severe anemia. Among patients with this association, the anemia usually is related to iron deficiency (Lilley et al, 1990).

Pernicious Anemia

Optic neuropathy is present in 5% of cases (Vaughan et al, 1989). The optic neuropathy is usually bilateral and may precede other clinical signs. Visual loss is usually slow and progressive with vision ranging from 20/40 to 20/200. Advanced cases are marked by eventual optic nerve atrophy. Visual field defects are usually central or cecocentral. If vitamin B_{12} therapy is administered before optic atrophy occurs, visual recovery is good (Foulds, 1969). Ophthalmoplegia occurs rarely although Sandyk (1984) reported a case of paralysis of upward gaze as a presenting sign of vitamin B_{12} deficiency. Golnik & Newman (1990) reported a case of anterior ischemic optic neuropathy (AION) associated with a severe macrocytic anemia secondary to folate-deficiency anemia. Decreased oxygen delivery to the prelaminar optic nerve caused by a low hemoglobin concentration was postulated as the most plausible mechanism for this AION. Lam and Lam (1992) reported a case of bilateral retinal hemorrhages with optic disc edema in a patient with megaloblastic anemia and thrombocytopenia secondary to vitamin B_{12} and folate deficiencies from inadequate diet and alcohol abuse. In Africa, retinal hemorrhages were reported more frequently in megaloblastic anemia than in iron-deficiency anemia (Holt & Gordon-Smith, 1969). Since thrombocytopenia is a common feature in megaloblastic anemia, whereas platelet counts tend to be elevated in iron-deficiency anemia, this lends further support to thrombocytopenia playing an important factor in the development of anemic retinopathy.

Aplastic Anemia

Papilledema is an uncommon complication that has been reported in a child with idiopathic aplastic anemia (Lilley et al, 1990) (Figure 53–2).

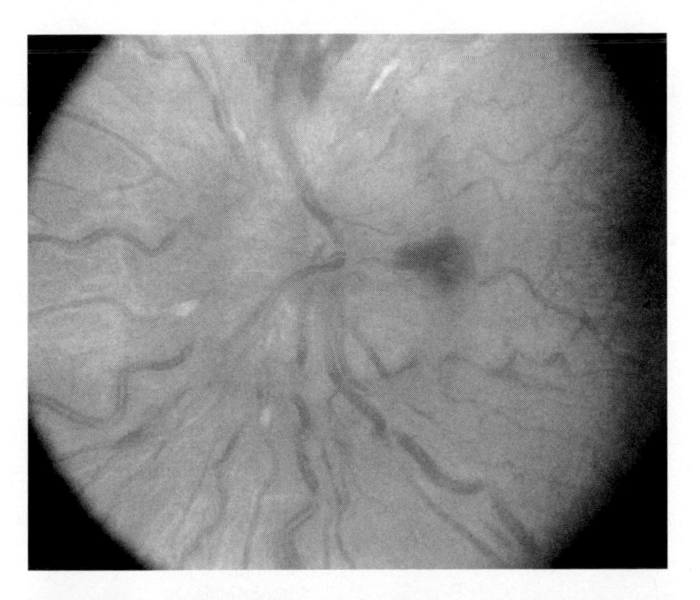

Figure 53–2. Disc swelling and flame-shaped hemorrhages in a patient with aplastic anemia. *(Reprinted with permission from Lilley ER, Bruggers CS, Pollock SC. Papilledema in a patient with aplastic anemia. Case report.* Arch Ophthalmol. *1990;108:1674.)*

DIAGNOSIS

Systemic

Iron-Deficiency Anemia

The laboratory tests performed to diagnose IDA are a complete blood count (CBC) with differential, peripheral blood smears, reticulocyte count, bone marrow iron stain, plasma ferritin studies, and iron-binding capacity studies. The laboratory findings are summarized in Table 53–5. The red blood cells are usually microcytic and hypochromic, characterized by a low mean corpuscular volume (MCV), mean corpuscular hemoglobin (MCH), and mean corpuscular hemoglobin concentration (MCHC). Increased platelet counts (thrombocytosis) are quite common. Reticulocyte counts are low. Bone marrow studies are characterized by lack of stainable iron. Serum iron studies demonstrate low serum iron and ferritin with elevated total iron-binding capacity (TIBC) (Rubin & Leopold, 1998). The most reliable test in detecting iron deficiency is a bone marrow iron stain. The most conclusive evidence for iron deficiency is a therapeutic trial of iron. This should be followed by further exploration to determine the underlying etiology of the deficiency as

TABLE 53–5. DIAGNOSTIC FINDINGS IN ANEMIAS

Iron-Deficiency Anemia

	Normal	Iron deficient
MCV(fL)	80–99	<80
Plasma iron (μg/dL)	65–175	<30
Iron-binding capacity (μg/dL)	300–360	400
Transferrin saturation(%)	25–50	<16
Plasma ferritin (μg/L)	20–250	<12
Erythrocyte-free protoporphyrin (μg/dL)	27–61	180
Basophilic stippling	Absent	Absent
Marrow iron stores	Present	Absent

Aplastic Anemia

Severe

Platelet count <20,000/μL
Reticulocyte count <60,000/μL
Granulocyte count <500/μL
Bone marrow biopsy: hypocellular or aplastic

Mild

Platelet count <1800/μL
Hematocrit <38%
Granulocyte count <1800/μL
Bone marrow biopsy: at least one hypocellular biopsy

Pernicious Anemia

Peripheral blood	Bone marrow
Oval macrocytes	Hypercellularity
Anisocytosis	Erythroid hyperplasia
Poikilocytosis	Giant metamyelocytes
Howell–Jolly bodies	Neutrophil hypersegmentation
Neutrophil hypersegmentation	

nutritional, physiologic, hemorrhagic, or secondary to another disease process (Table 53–6).

Pernicious Anemia

The laboratory findings for diagnosis of pernicious anemia are summarized in Table 53–5. A CBC with differential shows macrocytic red blood cells, or an elevated MCV. The most important variants of macrocytic anemias are the megaloblastic anemias characterized by enlarged red blood cells resulting from impaired DNA synthesis. Reticulocyte counts are low. Blood smear reveals large, oval macrocytes with hypersegmented polymorphonuclear cells. Vitamin B_{12} and folate levels are measured in order to differentiate the two. The Schilling test is not as commonly performed as in the past, but can be used to investigate vitamin B_{12} absorption. This is done by administering radioactive vitamin B_{12} and comparing the ratio of isotopes in the urine and peripheral blood. This test differentiates whether the defect is a deficiency of intrinsic factor or caused by small bowel malabsorption (Isbister, 1988).

Aplastic Anemia

The diagnosis of aplastic anemia is defined as pancytopenia of the peripheral blood (failure to produce red blood cells, white blood cells, and platelets) with bone marrow hypocellularity (see Table 53–5). The red blood cells are usually normocytic and normochromic (Brown, 1993). Severe aplastic anemia is defined when two of the following three conditions are met: (1) absolute neutrophil count less than 500/μL; (2) reticulocytes under 1%; and (3) platelet count less than 20,000/μL without excess marrow fibrosis, granulomas, or tumor cells (Rubin & Leopold, 1998).

Ocular

The ocular manifestations of anemia may be suggestive of the underlying disease process, but diagnosis is based on the associated laboratory and systemic findings. The differential diagnoses of the ocular manifestations of anemias are summarized in Table 53–6.

TABLE 53–6. DIFFERENTIAL DIAGNOSIS OF ANEMIAS

Systemic	
Dyspnea	Pulmonary/embolus Congestive heart failure Emphysema Asthma Myasthenia gravis Polyneuritis
Dysphagia	Myasthenia gravis Structural abnormalities
Fatigue	Emotional/psychological Malignant disease Chronic infection Postviral fatigue Connective tissue disease Hypothyroidism Malnutrition Chronic pain Multiple sclerosis Myasthenia gravis Chronic drug intoxication
Pallor	Hypotension Acromegaly Myxedema
Pica	Emotionally deprived children
Ocular	
Subconjunctival hemorrhage	Coumadin therapy Valsalva maneuver Bleeding disorder Idiopathic
Roth spots	Leukemia Septic chorioretinitis Diabetes mellitus
Retinal hemorrhages/ hard exudates/ cotton-wool spots	Diabetes mellitus Hypertension
Cranial nerve palsies	Microvascular disease Aneurysm Cavernous sinus syndrome Trauma Orbital disease Leukemia Giant cell arteritis Multiple sclerosis Stroke Idiopathic Congenital
Optic neuropathy	Ischemic Toxic/metabolic Infectious Compressive
Papilledema	Intracranial tumor Aqueductal stenosis Pseudotumor cerebri Subdural hematoma Subarachnoid hemorrhage Arteriovenous malformation Meningitis Encephalitis Sagittal sinus thrombosis

TREATMENT AND MANAGEMENT

Systemic

Iron-Deficiency Anemia

IDA is treated with iron replacement therapy (Table 53–7). The ferrous form is given as a daily supplement on an empty stomach to enhance absorption. Side effects are dark stool and constipation. Anemia usually corrects rapidly with 50% correction by 3 to 4 weeks of therapy, and normalization within 2 to 3 months.

TABLE 53–7. TREATMENT AND MANAGEMENT OF ANEMIAS

Iron-Deficiency Anemia
- 200 mg ferrous sulfate daily

Pernicious Anemia
- Intramuscular (IM) injections of vitamin B_{12}
  - 1000 μg for 1 week
  - Then weekly for a month
  - Then every 2–3 months for life

Aplastic Anemia
- Bone marrow transplant
- Remove causative agent
- Platelet and red blood cell (RBC) transfusions
- Antibiotics
- Immunosuppressive therapy

An additional 3 months of therapy will replete iron stores. In unusual circumstances, cautious intravenous therapy can be administered (Rubin & Leopold, 1998).

Pernicious Anemia

Therapy for pernicious anemia is easy and efficacious. Treatment is performed with daily intramuscular injections of vitamin B_{12}, 1000 μg for 1 week, then weekly for 1 month, and then every 2 to 3 months for life (see Table 53–7). Neurologic response to vitamin B_{12} and prognosis for recovery are more problematic. As a rule, neurologic changes present for less than 3 months are fully reversible, for 3 to 6 months variable, and for longer than 6 months irreversible (Rubin & Leopold, 1998).

Aplastic Anemia

Treatment for aplastic anemia is bone marrow transplantation (in patients under 50), with removal of the offending agent when identified (see Table 53–7). Platelet and red blood cell transfusions should be given as indicated for each individual patient, as well as antibiotics to prevent infection. Immunosuppressive therapies employing antithymocyte globulin (ATG) and cyclosporin result in disease remission rates similar to those of bone marrow transplantation.

Ocular

There is no specific treatment for the ocular signs of anemia. Ocular findings related to most forms of anemia tend to resolve when the systemic manifestations are treated, with the exception of optic nerve damage severe enough to be permanent.

> Most ocular manifestations of anemia will resolve when the systemic manifestations are treated.

CONCLUSION

The anemias include a wide variety of disorders, all resulting in a decrease in the number or size of circulating red blood cells. Systemic manifestations associated with anemia vary depending on type and severity of the disease. Common features to most anemias are fatigue, pallor, palpitations, bruising, lymphadenopathy, bone tenderness, hepatosplenomegaly, and epithelial abnormalities. Laboratory testing is used to identify the specific type of underlying anemia.

Ocular abnormalities may be accompanying or initial signs of anemia, and the eyecare practitioner should therefore be aware of associated clinical manifestations. The most common ocular finding is anemic retinopathy consisting of retinal hemorrhages, cotton-wool spots, and venous tortuosity. Additionally, signs such as conjunctival pallor and hemorrhage should be routinely observed since this is an easy screening tool that may aid in diagnosis, along with clinical and laboratory findings. Patients presenting with the above ocular findings along with vague systemic complaints should have anemia considered in the differential diagnosis.

REFERENCES

Baumelou MJ, Guignet M, et al. Epidemiology of aplastic anemia in France: A prospective multicentric study. *Blood.* 1990;75:1646–1653.

Beghetti M, Mermillod B, Halperin DS. Blue sclerae: A sign of iron deficiency anemia in children? *Pediatrics.* 1993;91: 1195–1196.

Brown BA. *Hematology: Principles and Procedures.* 6th ed. Philadelphia: Lea & Febiger; 1993:279–292.

Carmel R. Prevalence of undiagnosed pernicious anemia in the elderly. *Arch Intern Med.* 1996;156:1097–1000.

Duke-Elder S, Dobree JH. The blood diseases. In: *System of Ophthalmology.* Duke-Elder S, ed. St. Louis: CV Mosby; 1967:373–407.

Erslev AJ, Gabuzda TG. *Pathophysiology of Blood.* Philadelphia: WB Saunders; 1985:54–58.

Foulds WS, Chisholm IA, Stewart JB, et al. The optic neuropathy of pernicious anemia. *Arch Ophthalmol.* 1969;82:427.

Golnik KC, Newman SA. Anterior ischemic optic neuropathy associated with macrocytic anemia. *J Clin Neuro-ophthalmol.* 1990;104:244–247.

Holt JM, Gordon-Smith EC. Retinal abnormalities in disease of the blood. *Br J Ophthalmol.* 1969;53:145–160.

Hurst JW. Medicine for the practicing physician. Boston: Butterworth; 1983:799–801.

Isbister JP, Pittiglio DH. *Clinical Hematology: A Problem-Oriented Approach.* Baltimore: Williams & Wilkins; 1988:58.

Kalra L, Hamlyn AN, Jones BJM. Blue sclerae: A common sign of iron deficiency? *Lancet.* 1986;2:1267–1268.

Kirkham TH, Wrigley PFM, Holt JM. Central retinal vein occlusion complicating iron deficiency anemia. *Br J Ophthalmol.* 1971;55:777–780.

Koh AHC, Yeo KT. Anaemia—more than meets the eye. *Singapore Med J.* 1998;39:222–225.

Lam S, Lam BL. Bilateral retinal hemorrhages from megaloblastic anemia: Case report and review of literature. *Ann Ophthalmol.* 1992;24:86–90.

Lilley ER, Bruggers CS, Pollock SC. Papilledema in a patient with aplastic anemia. *Arch Ophthalmol.* 1990;108:1674–1675.

Linet MS, McCaffrey LD, Morgan WF, et al. Incidence of aplastic anemia in a three county area in South Carolina. *Cancer Res.* 1986;46:426–429.

Looker AC, Dallman PR, Carroll MD, et al. Prevalence of iron deficiency in the United States. *JAMA.* 1997;277:973–976.

Matsuoka Y, Hayasaka S, Yamada K. Incomplete occlusion of central retinal artery in a girl with iron deficiency anemia. *Ophthalmologica.* 1996;210:358–360.

Merin S, Freund M. Retinopathy in severe anemia. *Am J Ophthalmol.* 1968;66:1102–1106.

Qiao Q, Keinanen-Kiukaanniemi S, Laara E. The relationship between hemoglobin levels and diabetic retinopathy. *J Clin Epidemiol.* 1997;50:153–158.

Rubenstein RA, Yanoff M, Albert DM. Thrombocytopenia, anemia and retinal hemorrhage. *Am J Ophthalmol.* 1968;65:435–439.

Rubin RN, Leopold LH. *Hematologic Pathophysiology.* Madison, CT: Fence Creek; 1998:21–22.

Sandyk R. Paralysis of upward gaze as a presenting symptom of vitamin B_{12} deficiency. *Eur Neurol.* 1984;23:198–200.

Shorb SR. Anemia and diabetic retinopathy. *Am J Ophthalmol.* 1985;100:434–436.

Vaughan D, Asbury T, Tabbara KF. *General Ophthalmology.* Norwalk, CT: Appleton & Lange; 1989:288.

Chapter 54

SICKLE HEMOGLOBINOPATHIES

Felicia Fodera

Sickle-cell anemia was first described clinically by James B. Herrick in 1910. He presented a case of a black patient from the West Indies suffering from anemia with elongated sickle-shaped red blood cells.

A point mutation in the hemoglobin gene is responsible for the inherited abnormality that causes the sickle-cell hemoglobinopathies. Erythrocytes with normal adult hemoglobin (hemoglobin A) have a biconcave disk configuration. They are flexible, pliable, and flow easily through capillaries delivering oxygen to surrounding tissues. Erythrocytes with sickle-cell hemoglobin (hemoglobin S) are more rigid and elongated, which is referred to as "sickled" or a "sickle cell." These red blood cells cannot pass through capillaries, which results in ischemia, hypoxia, and necrosis of surrounding tissues. With increasing levels of hypoxia, the sickling of red blood cells tends to increase. This causes the blood viscosity to increase and leads to vascular occlusion.

Vaso-occlusion and tissue ischemia in sickle-cell disease can result in acute and chronic injury to virtually every organ of the body (Lane, 1996). Sickle-cell retinopathy, the most significant ocular manifestation, can be divided into proliferative and nonproliferative types. The conjunctiva, iris, and anterior chamber can also be affected.

EPIDEMIOLOGY

Systemic

Epidemiologic studies have shown that sickle-cell disease occurs with high frequency among various ethnic groups in which malaria is endemic. Protection against the lethal effects of malaria is provided by sickle-cell disease. Individuals of African, Mediterranean, Middle Eastern, and Indian ancestry are at highest risk.

Sickle-cell syndromes are present in approximately 10% of African-Americans. Of this group, approximately 8 to 9% have sickle-cell trait (SA), 0.4% have sickle-cell anemia (SS), 0.1 to 0.3% have sickle-cell hemoglobin C disease (SC), and 0.5 to 1% have sickle-cell thalassemia (SThal) (Goldberg, 1992). Only in rare instances do whites have sickle-cell hemoglobin.

Ocular

Nonproliferative retinal changes can be seen in about 30% of children with sickle-cell disease but are less prevalent in children with hemoglobin SC disease. In contrast, adults show a higher prevalence of proliferative retinopathy, and those with hemoglobin SC disease appear to have more retinopathy than those with sickle-cell anemia. Proliferative sickle-cell retinopathy (PSR) is primarily seen in those between 40 and 50 years of age and is rare in patients under 20 years of age. Vision loss occurs in 34% of patients with PSR and in 2% of patients without PSR (Moriarity et al, 1988).

PATHOPHYSIOLOGY/DISEASE PROCESS

Systemic

Specific hemoglobin inheritance patterns form five major sickle-cell syndromes (Table 54–1), each with a wide range of systemic and ocular complications (Table 54–2). They are sickle-cell anemia (SS), sickle-cell trait (SA), sickle-cell C disease (SC), sickle-cell thalassemia (SThal), and hemoglobin C trait (AC).

Of these syndromes, SS has the most acute, life-threatening systemic manifestations. SA patients normally do not have any systemic findings. SC and SThal patients have relatively fewer systemic complications compared to SS. Systemic findings are rare in AC.

SS is homozygous for hemoglobin S and causes an unrelenting hemolytic anemia. Most manifestations of the disease are related to the vaso-occlusive phenomena that result from the elongated or sickling characteristics of the abnormal hemoglobin in the presence of decreased oxygen.

> Sickle-cell anemia has the most acute, life-threatening systemic manifestations and fewer ocular complications, whereas sickle-cell C disease and sickle-cell thalassemia demonstrate a high incidence of proliferative retinopathy but have fewer systemic complications.

Vascular occlusion, of both the microcirculation and macrocirculation, is responsible for the clinical course of sickle-cell anemia. Occlusion within the microcirculation results in acute painful crisis, whereas occlusion of the macrocirculation is associated with organ failure.

Microcirculation occlusion begins with hemoglobin S polymerization, which leads to decreased red cell deformability. These more rigid red blood cells occlude small blood vessels, creating ischemia, hypoxia, and necrosis of the surrounding tissues. This tissue damage triggers the painful response and a vicious cycle is created with increased hypoxia resulting in increased sickling of the red blood cells.

Vascular intimal hyperplasia of the large vessels within the lungs, kidneys, and cerebrum results in macrovascular occlusion. These occlusions clinically present themselves as cerebral infarctions, acute renal infarctions, and acute chest syndrome.

Acute sickle cell crises are periodic occurrences of acute pain and fever caused by recurrent occlusive events in various parts of the body (back, chest, and extremities). The episode can last from hours to days and can be precipitated by influenza, trauma, surgery, dehydration, stress, and exposure to heat or cold. Chronic damage can occur as a result of these episodes. Skin ulcers, bone infarcts, papillary infarcts, and autosplenectomy may occur. These patients also have increased susceptibility to infection and gallstone formation and have abnormal growth and development.

TABLE 54–1. SICKLE-CELL HEMOGLOBINOPATHIES

Normal Hemoglobin
Hemoglobin F (HbF): fetal hemoglobin
Hemoglobin A (HbA): normal adult hemoglobin

Abnormal Hemoglobin
Hemoglobin S (HbS): valine is substituted for glutamic acid
Hemoglobin C (HbC): lysine is substituted for glutamic acid
Thalassemia (Thal): disorder of the rate of globin chain synthesis

Inheritance/Severity

HbS + HbS = SS	Sickle-cell anemia	Clinically severe
HbS + HbA = SA	Sickle-cell trait	Asymptomatic without anemia
HbS + HbC = SC	Sickle-cell C disease	Moderate severity
HbS + Thal = SThal	Sickle-cell thalassemia	Moderate severity
HbA + HbC = AC	Hemoglobin C trait	Systemic findings are rare

TABLE 54–2. SYSTEMIC MANIFESTATIONS OF SICKLE-CELL SYNDROMES

Acute Sickle-Cell Crisis
- Extreme pain
  - Back
  - Chest
  - Extremities
- Complications
  - Cerebral vascular accident
  - Acute chest syndrome from pulmonary vessel involvement
  - Hepatic crisis
  - Acute renal failure

Chronic Organ Damage
- Skin ulcers
  - Particularly legs
- Bone infarcts
  - Associated with bone pain
- Renal medulla microinfarct
  - Inability to concentrate urine
- Papillary infarcts
  - Prolonged painless hematuria
- Autosplenectomy
  - Common in patients with SS

Additional Manifestations Not Related to Vaso-occlusion
- Increased susceptibility to infections
- Gallstone formation
- Abnormal growth and development

SC and SThal are associated with mild anemia, and patients may be asymptomatic. Splenomegaly is common, and infarction may occur in some cases.

Ocular

In contrast to what might be expected, the degree of ocular involvement cannot be based on the severity of the systemic disease. Patients with SS have the most acute life-threatening systemic manifestations but have fewer ocular complications than patients with SC and SThal disease. Although SC and SThal patients have fewer systemic complications, they demonstrate a much higher incidence of proliferative retinopathy.

The many ocular manifestations of the sickle-cell syndromes affect virtually every tissue and are caused by microvascular occlusion (Table 54–3). Retinal changes are of primary concern because proliferative retinopathy causes profound and permanent visual loss. The anterior segment, however, may be the initial site of the sickling process. The conjunctival capillaries, particularly in the inferior quadrant, appear comma-shaped and may appear isolated. This can be observed with the naked eye and may actually be hidden under the slit lamp since heat may dilate the vessels. Phenylephrine will enhance this sign by causing vasoconstriction. It is seen in 97% of SS patients, 80% of SC patients, and 64% of SThal patients and is considered to be a very reliable indicator of sickle-cell disease (Paton, 1961).

Microhyphemas from trauma, normally benign, can cause a severe secondary glaucoma in sickle-cell patients. Sickling increases in the anterior chamber, obstructs outflow, and increases intraocular pressure (IOP).

The well-vascularized uveal tract can be affected by the blood sludging from the sickled cells. Focal iris atrophy, rubeosis irides, and choroidal vessel occlusion have all been observed. Transient plugs of deoxygenated erythrocytes can be seen in small vessels on the surface of the optic nerve head. No functional visual impairment occurs.

Various retinal findings may occur in many combinations. Nonproliferative changes include venous tortuosity, black sunbursts, dark without pressure, refractile deposits, salmon patch hemorrhages, and retinal holes and tears.

Tortuosity of the venous system is seen in 47% of patients with SS and 32% of patients with SC. It is not common in SA or SThal (Goldberg, 1992).

Sunbursts are black fundus lesions with stellate borders usually 0.5 to 2.0 disc diameters in size. They appear as focal areas of retinal pigment epithelium (RPE) migration, hyperplasia, and hypertrophy, and are thought to be the result of acute vascular occlusion of the retina that leads to deep retinal hemorrhages near the RPE (Figure 54–1).

TABLE 54–3. OCULAR MANIFESTATIONS IN SICKLE-CELL SYNDROMES

General
- Conjunctival sickling sign
- Focal iris atrophy
- Refractory increase in intraocular pressure (IOP) with microhyphemias
- Rubeosis irides
- Optic disc sign
- Choroidal vascular occlusion

Retinopathy
- Nonproliferative
  - Venous tortuosity
  - Black sunbursts
  - Refractile deposits
  - Silver-wire arterioles
  - Salmon patch hemorrhages
  - Retinal holes/tears
  - Central retinal artery occlusion (CRAO)
  - Macular arteriole occlusions
  - Retinal venous occlusions
  - Angioid streaks
  - Macular holes
  - Dark without pressure
- Proliferative
  - Stage I: Peripheral arteriolar occlusions
    - Capillary bed and vernule fail to fill
    - Grayish-brown coloration of retina
    - Silver-wire or chalky white arterioles
    - Interface of perfused to nonperfused retina visible with FA
  - Stage II: Peripheral arteriolar–venule anastomoses
    - Anastomoses at interface of nonperfused retina, blood shunted from occluded arterioles to nearest venule
    - Enlargement of preexisting capillaries
    - Resemble telangiectases and microaneurysms
  - Stage III: Neovascular proliferation
    - Neovascular capillary buds from perfused to nonperfused retina
    - Attempt to revascularize ischemic retina
    - Fan-shaped neovascularization
    - FA: vitreous leakage
  - Stage IV: Vitreous hemorrhage
    - Due to minor ocular trauma, vitreous collapse, or traction on adherent neovascular tissue
    - Small and localized or massive
    - Clotted hemorrhage becomes organized to form white fibrous tissue
    - Intermittent bleed in fibrovascular area
  - Stage V: Retinal detachment
    - Associated retinal holes
    - Vitreous hemorrhage

A granular, refractile substance is often seen in the retinal periphery and can be associated with arteriolar occlusions. In addition, when hemoglobin degrades, small schisis cavities are formed intraretinally and hemosiderin is trapped within these spaces. These rarely involve the macular area and are a prognostic sign for the subsequent development of neovascularization.

Geographic brown mottled areas in the retina, which have been called "dark without pressure," have

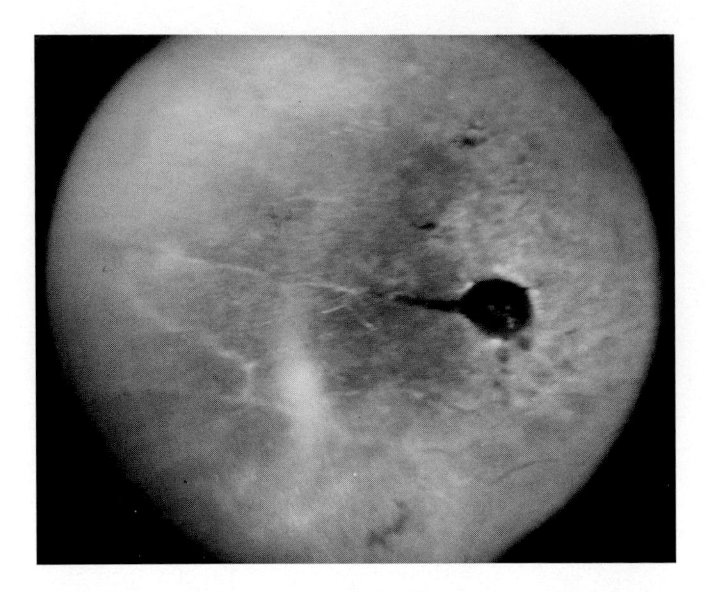

Figure 54–1. Patient with SS disease. Note vascular nonperfusion, pigment clumping, and large "black sunburst." *(Courtesy of Jane Stein, The Eye Institute, Pennsylvania College of Optometry.)*

been reported in patients with SS, SC, and SThal. They were originally reported to be the sequel to vascular occlusive events in the area. However, these transient areas, which leave no trace of their presence after their disappearance, have not been shown to be related to any retinal or choroidal vascular changes.

Salmon patch hemorrhages are located in the midperipheral sensory retina but can break through into the subretinal space. They appear oval or round with defined borders. They are bright red early on in their course, then change to orange, and then to a yellow or white nodule. They measure between 0.25 and 2.0 disc diameters and are usually caused by occlusion of an adjacent arteriole. The hemorrhage may last days to weeks and will result in a schisis cavity with refractile bodies within it.

Retinal holes or tears may be found in the equatorial region or slightly posterior to it. Small to moderate in size, they are usually oval or horseshoe-shaped. There may be adjacent or overlying vitreous bands.

Various retinal vascular occlusions can occur in sickle-cell disease. Central retinal artery occlusion, although rare, has been reported in SS, SA, and SC. Macular arteriole occlusions have been reported in SS and SThal. Discrete occlusions of the capillary network result in avascular zones and subsequent visual field defects. Venous occlusions have been reported rarely. Extensive choroidal or posterior ciliary vessel occlusion has been reported in SC, SA, and SThal.

Angioid streaks, although rare, have been reported most frequently in SS. When present, they rarely cause visual disability.

Proliferative sickle-cell retinopathy (PSR) occurs primarily between 40 and 50 years of age and rarely occurs in patients under 20 years of age. Vision loss occurs in 34% of patients with PSR and in only 2% of patients without PSR. Proliferative disease is classically characterized by seafan neovascularization (Figures 54–2 and 54–3). Seafans may regress spontaneously with resulting fibrous tissue or may progress and ultimately result in a retinal detachment. Vitreous hemorrhage and retinal detachment are common in SC and occur rarely in SS or SA.

PSR may be divided into five stages that mark its progression. Stage I is peripheral arteriolar occlusion, stage II is peripheral arteriolar–venule anastomoses, stage III is neovascular proliferation, stage IV is vitreous hemorrhage, and stage V is retinal detachment (Table 54–3).

DIAGNOSIS

Systemic

The sickle-cell hemoglobinopathies are characterized by the presence of hemoglobin S in the absence of, or in greater amounts than, normal hemoglobin A. Sickle-cell disease is an exception in that the level of hemoglobin S is always lower than that of hemoglobin A. A blood cell count will typically show moderately severe anemia. Solubility testing (Sickledex, Sickleprep, or Sicklequik) can be used as a screening mechanism for the presence of hemoglobin S. Hemoglobin electrophoresis is used to identify a particular sickle syndrome (Table 54–4).

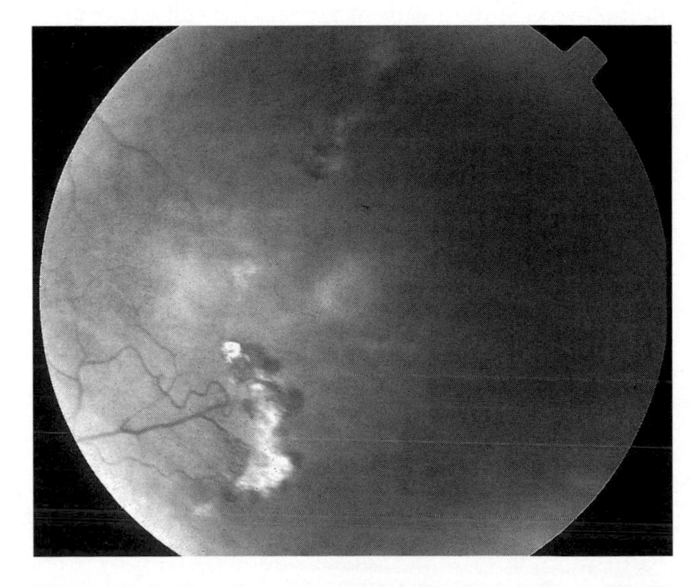

Figure 54–2. Sea fan neovascularization in a patient with SC disease.

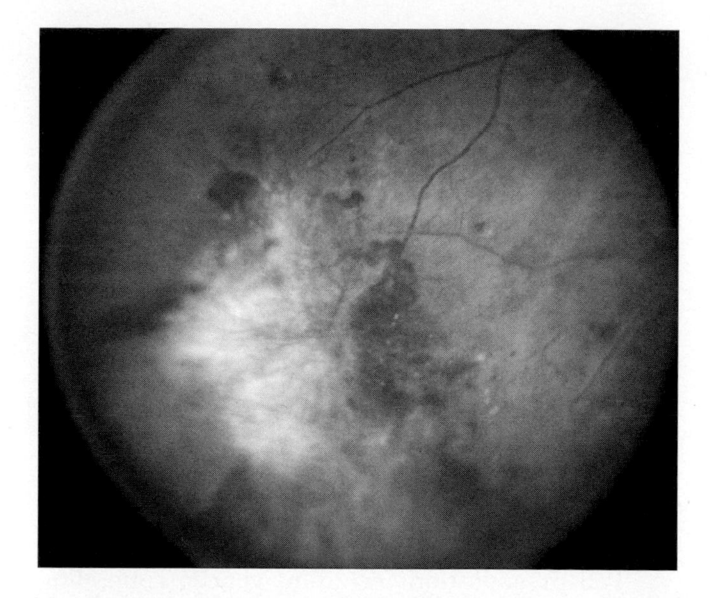

Figure 54–3. Another patient with SC disease and seafan neovascularization, hemorrhage, and fibrosis. *(Courtesy of Jane Stein, The Eye Institute, Pennsylvania College of Optometry.)*

The hemolysis and vascular occlusive events that cause tissue ischemia and organ dysfunction present with varying degrees of severity. They can manifest as chronic anemia, recurrent acute pain, stroke, chronic nephropathy, and retinopathy.

Ocular

Diagnosing a sickle-cell syndrome can begin with observation during ocular examination. A significant anterior segment finding, comma-shaped blood vessels, can be seen in the conjunctiva of patients with clinically significant sickling disorders. These blood vessels appear disconnected from other vasculature but pose no clinical disability. Although this is a reliable indicator for sickle cell, the differential diagnosis should include other etiologies associated with conjunctival vascular changes and blood sludging such as polycythemia (Table 54–5).

TABLE 54–4. DIAGNOSTIC TESTS IN SICKLE HEMOGLOBINOPATHIES

First-line: solubility testing: screens for the presence of hemoglobin S
- Sicklequik
- Sickledex
- Sickleprep

Follow-up: hemoglobin electrophoresis: identifies the particular sickle syndrome

		Findings (%)			
Genotype	**Clinical Condition**	**HbS**	**HbA**	**HbF**	**HbC**
SS	Sickle-cell anemia	85–95	2–3	5–15	—
SA	Sickle-cell trait	55–60	40–45	2–3	1
SC	Sickle-cell C disease	45–50	2–3	1	45–50
SThal	Sickle-cell thalassemia	70–80	3–5	10–20	—

TABLE 54–5. DIFFERENTIAL DIAGNOSIS OF SICKLE-CELL DISEASE

Systemic
Polycythemia

Ocular
Sickle-cell retinopathy
- Sarcoidosis
- Diabetic retinopathy
- Polycythemia
- Branch retinal vein occlusion
- Takayasu pulseless disease
- Retinopathy of prematurity
- Eales disease
- Chronic myelogenous leukemia

> Proliferative retinopathy requires treatment only after neovascularization appears (stage III).

Hyphema poses a significant problem in sickle-cell patients. Red blood cells containing hemoglobin S can sickle in the aqueous and occlude aqueous outflow channels, leading to increased intraocular pressure. An African-American who presents with hyphema of unknown etiology warrants sickle-cell testing. Iris atrophy from the pupillary border to the collarette can also be seen with sickle-cell syndromes.

> Hyphema poses a significant problem in sickle-cell patients. African-Americans who present with hyphema warrant sickle-cell testing.

Posterior segment findings can be divided into nonproliferative and proliferative retinopathies. Asymptomatic nonproliferative sickle retinopathies include venous tortuosity, black sunbursts, salmon patch hemorrhages, refractile deposits, silver wire arterioles, and retinal holes. Symptomatic nonproliferative retinopathies associated with sickle-cell syndromes include central retinal artery occlusion, macular arteriole occlusion, retinal venous occlusions, choroidal vascular occlusions, and angioid streaks.

Proliferative sickle retinopathies are located in the peripheral retina and can be classified from stages I through V as follows: arterial obstruction, arteriolar–

venular anastomosis, neovascular proliferations, vitreous hemorrhage, and retinal detachment, respectively. Fluorescein angiography can aid in the diagnosis and treatment of proliferative disease.

Other retinopathies, characterized by retinal vascular closure, may have similar appearances to sickle-cell retinopathies. These include sarcoidosis, chronic myelogenous leukemia, Takayasu pulseless disease, retinopathy of prematurity, branch retinal vein occlusion, Eales disease, and diabetes (Table 54–5).

TREATMENT AND MANAGEMENT

Systemic

Although the cause of sickle-cell disease has been known for some time, there is still no specific therapy to successfully treat it. Supportive therapy, bed rest, analgesics, and hydration help manage the events. Currently, three therapeutic approaches offer hope to prevent manifestations of the disease (Table 54–6).

Blood transfusions are indicated in acute exacerbations of anemia, severe vasoocclusive events, acute organ dysfunction, chronic organ failure, and high-risk procedures. The objective is to replace the sickle cells with normal red blood cells in an attempt to stop the vaso-occlusive process and increase perfusion to ischemic areas. Unfortunately, transfusions are met with significant complications, including hyperviscosity and viral infection transmission; however, transfusions remain the mainstay of treatment at this time.

Two not-yet-conventional therapies include bone marrow transplantation and hydroxyurea. Although bone marrow transplant provides a hematologic cure for sickle-cell disease, significant complications, including intracranial hemorrhage, have limited its application. Hydroxyurea shows promise of reducing episodes of painful crisis and blood transfusions; however, approximately 25% of patients do not respond to it (Rodgers, 1997).

TABLE 54–6. SYSTEMIC TREATMENT AND MANAGEMENT OF SICKLE-CELL SYNDROMES

- Acute pain crisis
  - Variable depending on severity; vigorous hydration, analgesics, bed rest
- Hypoxia
  - Oxygen
- Supportive management
  - Nutrition, education on genetic counseling and prompt medical care
- Transfusions
- Bone marrow transplant
- Hydroxyurea

TABLE 54–7. OCULAR TREATMENT AND MANAGEMENT OF SICKLE-CELL SYNDROMES

- Retinal preneovascularization (stages I and II)
  - No treatment to prevent retinal neovascularization
- Retinal neovascularization (stages III to V)
  - Treatment includes direct focal ablation, feeder vessel treatment, panretinal scatter
- Nonresolving vitreous hemorrhage
  - Vitrectomy
- Retinal detachment
  - Standard techniques while preventing anterior ischemia
- Hyphema/secondary glaucoma
  - Topical agents
  - Carbonic anhydrase inhibitors and oral osmotics are contraindicated
  - Paracentesis for secondary glaucoma with hyphema

Patient education including genetic counseling and the understanding to seek prompt medical attention for symptoms of pain, fever, and infection is key to managing the disease.

Ocular

Treatment is indicated in cases of retinal neovascularization, nonresolving vitreal hemorrhage, retinal detachment, and secondary glaucoma (Table 54–7). Proliferative sickle retinopathy need not be treated until stage III is reached. Treating stage I and II lesions has no benefit. Panretinal photocoagulation and direct focal ablation techniques can be used to treat stage III lesions. Fluorescein angiography is useful in determining the effectiveness of the therapy.

Nonresolving vitreous hemorrhage may require vitrectomy. In cases of retinal detachment, standard corrective techniques should be employed.

Treating glaucoma in sickle-cell patients requires specific considerations. Carbonic anhydrase inhibitors and oral osmotic agents are contraindicated. Carbonic anhydrase inhibitors increase hemoconcentration and blood viscosity, causing systemic acidosis, which potentiates sickling. Oral osmotic agents may also increase blood viscosity. In sickle-cell patients with hyphema and an acute intraocular pressure rise, ocular paracentesis appears to be the most effective treatment.

CONCLUSION

Sickle-cell syndromes are relatively common in African-Americans. Depending on the type, sickle-cell syndromes have the potential for severe systemic and ocular complications. Patients with sickle-cell anemia are at greatest risk for developing life-threatening systemic manifestations. Patients with sickle-cell hemoglobin C disease and sickle-cell thalassemia need to be monitored closely for evidence of proliferative retinopathy. Appropriate and timely treatment should be initiated to prevent further complications such as retinal detachment.

REFERENCES

Ballas SK, Mohandas N. Pathophysiology of vaso-occlusion. *Hematol Oncol Clin North Am.* 1996;10:1221–1235.

Bookchin RM, Lew VL. Pathophysiology of sickle cell anemia. *Hematol Oncol Clin North Am.* 1996;10:1241–1251.

Browne P, Shalev O, Hebbel RP. The molecular pathobiology of cell membrane iron: The sickle red cell as a model. *Free Radic Biol Med.* 1998;24:1040–1048.

Charache S. Experimental therapy. *Hematol Oncol Clin North Am.* 1996;10:1373–1382.

Charache S. Eye disease in sickling disorders. *Hematol Oncol Clin North Am.* 1996;10:1357–1362.

Charache S. Mechanism of action of hydroxyurea in the management of sickle cell anemia in adults. *Semin Hematol.* 1997;34:15–21.

Curran EL, Fleming JC, Rice K, Wang WC. Orbital compression syndrome in sickle cell disease. *Ophthalmology.* 1997; 104:1610–1615.

Dale GL. Is there a correlation between raised erythropoietin and thrombotic events in sickle-cell anaemia? *Lancet.* 1998; 352:566–567.

Fekrat S, Lutty G, Goldberg MF. Hemoglobinopathies. In: Guyer DR, Yannuzzi LA, Chang S, et al, eds. *Retina, Vitreous, Macula.* Philadelphia: WB Saunders; 1999:438–458.

Feldman SD, Tauber AI. Sickle cell anemia: Reexamining the first molecular disease. *Bull Hist Med.* 1997;71:623–650.

Goldberg MF. Sickle cell retinopathy. In: Tasman W, Jaeger EA, eds. *Duane's Clinical Ophthalmology.* Philadelphia: Lippincott; 1992:3.

Hillery CA. Potential therapeutic approaches for the treatment of vaso-occlusion in sickle cell disease. *Curr Opin Hematol.* 1998;5:151–155.

Howlett DC, Hatrick AG, Jarosz JM, et al. Pictorial review: The role of CT and MR in imaging the complications of sickle cell disease. *Clin Radiol.* 1997;52:821–829.

Jackson H, Bentley CR, Hingorani M, et al. Sickle retinopathy in patients with sickle trait. *Eye.* 1995;9:589–593.

Kachmaryk MM, Trimble SN, Gieser RG. Cilioretinal artery occlusion in sickle cell trait and rheumatoid arthritis. *Retina.* 1995;15:501–504.

King KE, Ness PM. Treating anemia. *Hematol Oncol Clin North Am.* 1996;10:1305–1317.

Lane PA. Sickle cell disease. *Hematol Oncol Clin North Am.* 1996;10:639–664.

Mcleod DS, Merges C, Fukushima A, et al. Histopathologic features of neovascularization in sickle cell retinopathy. *Am J Ophthalmol.* 1997;124:455–472.

Moriarty BJ, Acheson RW, Condon PI, Sergeant GR. Patterns of visual loss in untreated sickle cell retinopathy. *Eye.* 1988; 2:330–335.

Oh SO, Ibe BO, Johnson C, et al. Platelet-activating factor in plasma of patients with sickle cell disease in steady state. *J Lab Clin Med.* 1997;130:191–196.

Ohene-Frempong K, Weiner SJ, Sleeper LA, et al. Cerebrovascular accidents in sickle cell disease: Rates and risk factors. *Blood.* 1998;91:288–294.

Paton D. The conjunctival sign of sickle cell disease. *Arch Ophthalmol.* 1961;66:90–94.

Rodgers GP. Overview of pathophysiology and rationale for treatment of sickle cell anemia. *Semin Hematol.* 1997;34:2–7.

Roy MS, Gascon P, Giuliani D. Macular blood flow velocity in sickle cell disease: Relation to red cell density. *Br J Ophthalmol.* 1995;79:742–745.

Schnog JJ, Lard LR, Rojer RA, et al. New concepts in assessing sickle cell disease severity. *Am J Hematol.* 1998; 58:61–66.

Solovey A, Lin Y, Browne P, et al. Circulating activated endothelial cells in sickle cell anemia. *N Engl J Med.* 1997; 337:1584–1590.

Thomas PW, Higgs DR, Sergeant GR. Benign clinical course in homozygous sickle cell disease: A search for predictors. *J Clin Epidemiol.* 1997;50:121–126.

van Meurs JC. Evolution of a retinal hemorrhage in a patient with sickle cell-hemoglobin C disease. *Arch Ophthalmol.* 1995;113:1074–1075.

Wun T, Paglieroni T, Tablin F, et al. Platelet activation and platelet-erythrocyte aggregates in patients with sickle cell anemia. *J Lab Clin Med.* 1997;5:507–516.

Chapter 55

LEUKEMIAS

Lori R. Reminick

Leukemia is a hematologic malignancy of the bone marrow, with the neoplasm consisting of abnormal, uncontrolled proliferation of one or more hematopoietic or lymphoid cells. Leukemias are classified broadly into acute and chronic according to the time span of their clinical course. In general, acute leukemia behaves in an acute and rapidly fatal manner, and is characterized by immature cells called blasts. Chronic leukemias involve more differentiated, mature cells and have a more prolonged clinical course (Isbister, 1998). Leukemias are further classified on the basis of their cell of origin and referred to as acute lymphocytic leukemia (ALL), acute myelogenous or myeloblastic leukemia (AML), chronic lymphocytic leukemia (CLL), and chronic myelogenous leukemia (CML). Ocular involvement in leukemia may be an initial feature of the disease (Bhadresa, 1971), or the first manifestation of relapse after remission-inducing chemotherapy (Rosenthal, 1983).

EPIDEMIOLOGY

Systemic

ALL comprises 90% of childhood leukemias but only 20% of adult acute leukemias (Cook & Bartley, 1997). The disease occurs more commonly in males. AML constitutes 25% of all leukemias and is most common in the middle-aged and elderly. CLL has recently been reported as the most frequent form of leukemia in the Western hemisphere, with an incidence of 40 per 100,000 by the eighth decade of life. This represents approximately one third of all leukemias. It usually affects the middle-aged or elderly with males more frequently affected 2.5:1. CML accounts for 20% of all cases of leukemia and carries a death rate of 1.5 per 100,000 (Rubin & Leopold, 1998).

Ocular

Some studies have found that the eye is involved more often in the acute than chronic leukemias, 82% and 75%, respectively (Kincaid & Green, 1983). Other studies have detected no significant difference (Leonardy et al, 1990). Most of the ocular involvement in leukemia can be related to direct invasion by neoplastic cells. Almost every ocular structure has been found to be involved in this group of diseases (Karesh et al, 1989).

Involvement of the anterior segment is detected clinically and pathologically in about only 1.5% of patients with leukemia and is seen most commonly with ALL (Kincaid & Green, 1983). Anterior segment relapse accounts for 0.2 to 2% of all cases. Fundus abnormalities are the most common ocular findings found in 53% of patients by Karesh and associates (1989).

PATHOPHYSIOLOGY/DISEASE PROCESS

Systemic

Although the etiologies of the leukemias still remain unclear, ionizing radiation and exposure to certain toxins can induce some types of leukemia. The human T-cell leukemia has been associated with a retrovirus in some patients, and several chromosomal abnormalities have been isolated such as the Philadelphia chromosome in CML.

Signs and symptoms of acute leukemia include bleeding, petechial hemorrhages, pallor, fever, easy bruisability, infection, CNS involvement, and joint pain (Table 55–1). Signs and symptoms of chronic leukemia include fatigue, night sweats, anorexia, weight loss, lymphadenopathy, and sense of abdominal fullness (Rubin & Leopold, 1998). Patients with chronic leukemia may be asymptomatic in early stages (Table 55–1).

Acute Myelogenous Leukemia

AML, which has been classified into seven subtypes, presents clinically with anemia, infections, bruising, or bleeding. Leukemic cells may infiltrate the CNS, lymph nodes, and skin. AML is rapidly fatal without treatment, and commonly cured with conventional chemotherapy or bone marrow transplantation (BMT) (Rubin & Leopold, 1998).

TABLE 55–1. SYSTEMIC MANIFESTATIONS OF LEUKEMIA

Acute Leukemia
• Failure of normal hematopoiesis
Bleeding
Petechiae
Pallor
Fever
Easy bruisability
Mucous membrane hemorrhage
• Infection
• CNS involvement
Headaches
Vomiting
Irritability
• Joint and bone pain
Chronic Leukemia
• Possibly asymptomatic in early stages
• Insidious onset of nonspecific symptoms
Fatigue
Weakness
Fever
Night sweats
Anorexia
Weight loss
Sense of abdominal fullness
• With disease progression
Pallor
Fever
Marked splenomegaly
Marked lymphadenopathy
Bleeding
Easy bruisability

> Untreated, acute leukemia results in death, usually a few months after diagnosis.

Acute Lymphocytic Leukemia

ALL presents with findings similar to AML, with an increased chance of mediastinal and CNS involvement. ALL is histologically classified into subtypes L1, L2, and L3. L1 is the subtype most common in childhood and is composed of small and homogenous cells. Treatment of ALL results in remission in approximately 50% of cases (Kincaid & Green, 1983).

Chronic Myelogenous Leukemia

CML is a clonal myeloproliferative disorder that involves the stem cells and affects the myeloid, erythroid, megakaryocytic, and lymphoid elements. Virtually all cases of CML involve a chromosomal translocation in which a small portion of the long arm of chromosome 9 is translocated to the long arm of chromosome 22, called the Philadelphia chromosome. CML presents with an elevated white blood cell (WBC) count and an enlarged spleen. CML usually presents in an indolent chronic phase, which lasts 4 to 6 years. Although typically asymptomatic, patients may have symptoms of anemia, leukostasis, or splenomegaly, or develop thrombotic/hemorrhagic complications (Rubin & Leopold, 1998).

Chronic Lymphocytic Leukemia

Nearly half of newly diagnosed cases of CLL are asymptomatic patients who had phlebotomy for other reasons. When present, symptoms include fatigue, weight loss, and lymphadenopathy. Hepatosplenomegaly, anemia, and thrombocytopenia develop. CLL may evolve into a more aggressive large cell lymphoma in up to 10% of patients (Richter syndrome).

Ocular

Ocular manifestations of leukemia are summarized in Table 55–2.

Anterior Segment

Anterior segment manifestations of leukemia are uncommon, generally occurring in patients with bone marrow or central nervous system (CNS) relapse (Katz et al, 1997). The cornea is normally avascular; therefore, direct invasion by leukemic cells would not be expected. However, leukemia can induce formation of a sterile ring ulcer with iritis and pannus. Conjunctival

TABLE 55–2. OCULAR MANIFESTATIONS OF LEUKEMIA

- **Ocular adnexa**
  - Lacrimal gland infiltration (dry eye)
  - Dacryocystitis secondary to infiltration (epiphora)
  - Extraocular muscle infiltration (paresis)
  - Infiltration of skin of lid (lid swelling)
- **Orbit**
  - Infiltration with associated exophthalmos, lid edema, chemosis, pain
- **Conjunctiva**
  - Infiltrates in perivascular regions
  - Conjunctival swellings
  - Subconjunctival hemorrhage
  - Necrosis secondary to ischemia
- **Cornea**
  - Sterile peripheral corneal ulcers with pannus
- **Episcleral sclera**
  - Episcleritis
  - Infiltrates in perivascular regions (rare)
- **Iris and ciliary body**
  - Infiltration
  - Iris color change
  - Associated pseudohypopyon (gray-yellow in color)
- **Retina**
  - Dilated and tortuous venules
  - Yellowing of vascular reflex
  - Hemorrhages (flame, dot, blot, white-centered)
  - Retinal leukemia infiltrates (perivascular gray-white sheathing)
  - Retinal infiltration tumors
  - Vitreal infiltrates
  - Cotton-wool spots
  - Microaneurysm
  - Peripheral retinal neovascularization
- **Choroid**
  - Serous sensory retinal detachment
  - RPE hypertrophy hyperplasia atrophy
  - Photoreceptor disruption
  - Cystoid retinal edema
  - Drusen
- **Optic nerve**
  - Direct infiltration of optic nerve (vision loss, field loss)
  - Papilledema secondary to CNS infiltration
- **Opportunistic infections**
  - Cytomegalovirus
  - Herpes simplex
  - Herpes zoster ophthalmicus
  - Mumps
  - Toxoplasmosis
  - Bacterial infection
  - Fungal infection (e.g., *Candida, Aspergillus*)

involvement occurs most often in patients with lymphocytic leukemia. This can present as infiltration with conjunctival nodules and localized injection resembling an episcleritis, often with subconjunctival hemorrhage (Kincaid & Green, 1983) (Figure 55–1).

A clear pattern has emerged of a high-risk period for anterior chamber leukemic relapse in the first few months following maintenance therapy withdrawal in patients with ALL (Maclean et al, 1996). Anterior segment, orbital, and periocular findings are rarely described in the myeloid leukemias (Karesh et al, 1989). Manifestations include infiltration of the iris, ciliary body, and anterior chamber structures. The first presenting sign may be a change in iris color. Iris involvement may be diffuse or nodular. Iritis with accompanying pseudohypopyon that is grey-yellow in color may occur, as well as elevated intraocular pressure and spontaneous hyphema in children (Kincaid & Green, 1983). The diagnosis can be confirmed by paracentesis. The anterior segment of the eye has been reported as a "pharmacologic sanctuary" because it is only marginally affected by systemic chemotherapy. This implies that leukemic cells present in the iris at the onset of the disease are suppressed but not eradicated during systemic chemotherapy (Rosenthal, 1983).

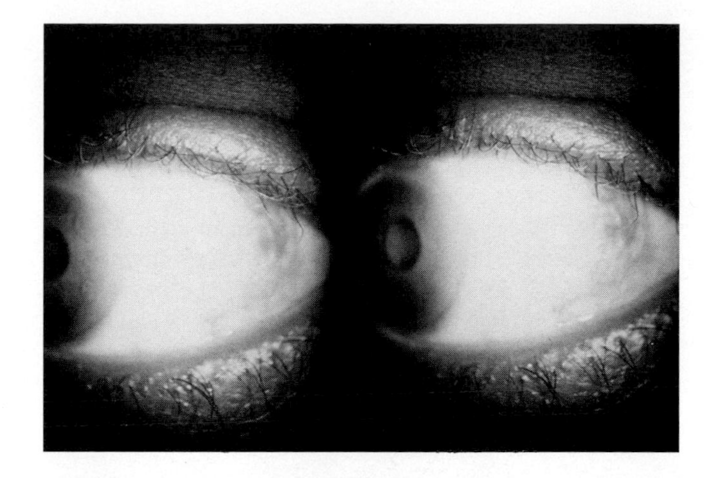

Figure 55–1. Stereophotograph of subconjunctival hemorrhage that can occur in patients with leukemia. *(Courtesy of Jane Stein, The Eye Institute, Pennsylvania College of Optometry.)*

> Almost every ocular structure may be affected by leukemia.

Posterior Segment

Most of the retinal findings in leukemia (Figure 55–2) are not caused by neoplastic cells but rather associated hematologic abnormalities (Char, 1997). Hematologic abnormalities associated with ocular complications are anemia (leukemic retinopathy) and hyperviscosity (microaneurysm formation, capillary closure, and retinal neovascularization) (Rosenthal, 1983). The term "leukemic retinopathy" typically refers to the intraretinal hemorrhages, white-centered hemorrhages,

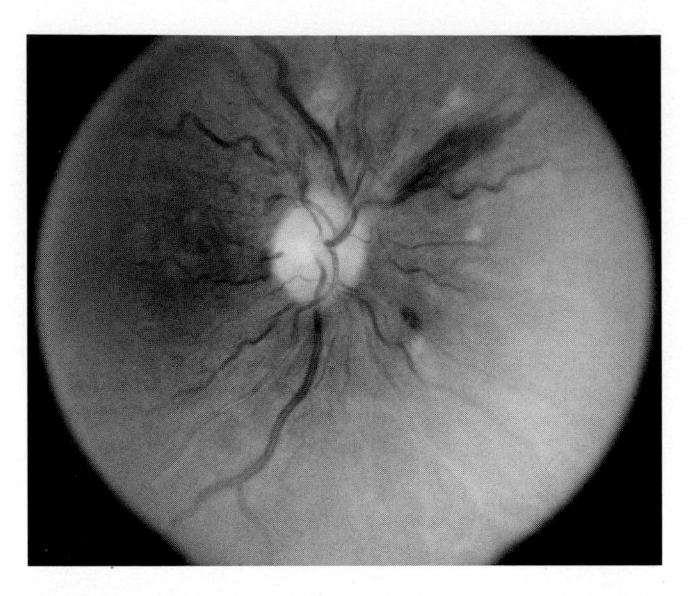

Figure 55–2. Fundus photograph of retinal hemorrhages and cotton-wool spots commonly seen in leukemic retinopathy. *(Courtesy of Jane Stein, The Eye Institute, Pennsylvania College of Optometry.)*

and cotton-wool spots seen in patients with leukemia (Schachat, 1989) (Figure 55–3).

Leukemic retinopathy is observed in both the acute and chronic forms of leukemia, though it is more common in the acute forms (Holt & Gordon-Smith, 1969). Tortuous, dilated retinal veins are one of the classic features of the retinopathy. The dilation may be irregular in caliber and gives a sausage-like appearance to the retinal vessels. Retinal vascular sheathing is often present, and is felt to be caused by actual perivascular infiltration by leukemic cells (Rosenthal, 1983).

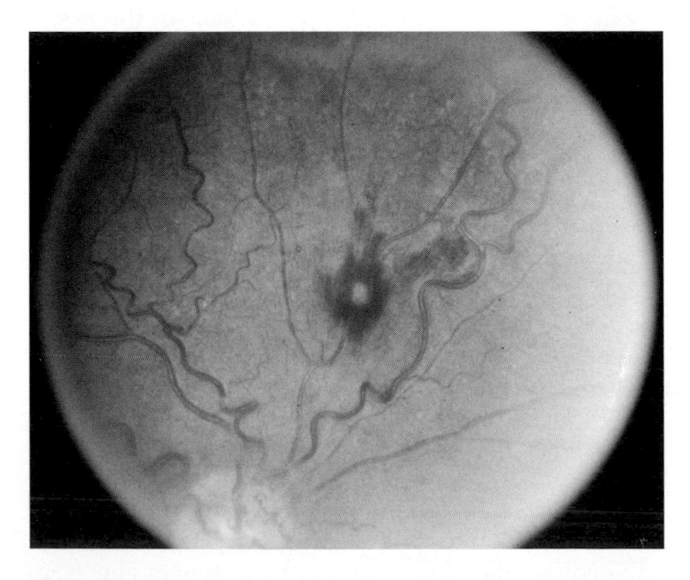

Figure 55–3. Fundus photography of a white-centered hemorrhage. The white center usually consists of leukemic cells. *(Courtesy of Jane Stein, The Eye Institute, Pennsylvania College of Optometry.)*

Retinal hemorrhages are most commonly located in the posterior pole. The hemorrhages are usually intraretinal and either round or flame-shaped, but may also appear boat-shaped (Rosenthal, 1983). The intraretinal hemorrhage may contain a white center (Roth spot), which is thought to represent cellular debris, platelet–fibrin aggregates, capillary emboli, or accumulation of leukemic cells.

> The retina and the choroid represent the most frequent sites of ocular involvement and may be the initial sign of the disease or its relapse.

Retinal infiltrates are large grayish-white nodules of varying sizes associated with local destruction, necrosis, and hemorrhage. They occur in association with elevated leukocyte counts and a high proportion of blast cells (Robb et al, 1978). Leukemic retinal infiltration combined with a high leukocyte count is an ominous prognostic sign (Rosenthal, 1983).

Retinal microaneurysms, capillary closure, and neovascularization are retinal changes observed in chronic leukemia and found more commonly in CML than CLL (Duke et al, 1968). Prolonged leukocytosis (increased white blood cell count) has been reported to be a necessary factor in the development of peripheral microaneurysms (Jampol & Goldberg, 1975), as well as for the development of seafan-like neovascularization, similar to that seen in sickle-cell hemoglobinopathies (Morse & McCready, 1971). The pathogenesis of retinal vascular disease is thought to be the result of hyperviscosity caused by the increased number of circulating leukocytes or platelets. This increased viscosity leads to reduced blood flow, producing capillary dropout, microaneurysm formation, and proliferative retinopathy (Rosenthal, 1983).

The relationship between fundus findings in leukemic retinopathy and hematologic parameters varies depending on the study. Retrospective studies are influenced by treatment. However, prospective studies on patients with acute leukemia allow collection of data prior to any therapeutic intervention. Karesh and colleagues (1989) and Guyer and co-workers (1989) found that patients with lower levels of circulating platelets (thrombocytopenia) and marked anemia demonstrated retinopathy more frequently. It is possible that the absence of an adequate number of platelets to form the microclots that plug tiny areas of ischemic or mechanical capillary damage is particularly critical in patients with leukemia.

Jackson and associates (1996) found no such relation with thrombocytopenia, but rather a significant association with leukocytosis. They postulated four mechanisms whereby a high WBC count could have a pathogenic role in leukemic retinopathy: (1) hyperviscosity causing raised intracapillary pressure; (2) vaso-occlusion leading to ischemia; (3) intra-/periendothelial infiltration by WBCs; and (4) formation of microaneurysms.

Optic nerve infiltration occurs mainly in children with ALL. Two distinct clinical patterns of optic nerve head infiltration have been observed: those in which there is prelaminar invasion of the optic nerve head and those in which there is a retrolaminar invasion. In prelaminar infiltration, a fluffy infiltrate with or without edema and hemorrhage is observed. The visual acuity may be altered minimally or significantly depending on associated edema and hemorrhage extending into the macular area. In retrolaminar invasion, visual acuity will be significantly impaired. Moderate to pronounced disc elevation and edema, as well as hemorrhage, may also be present.

In either type of infiltration the response to radiation is dramatic. It is essential that optic nerve head infiltration with leukemic cells be differentiated from papilledema from increased intracranial pressure. A lumbar puncture must be performed in every case to aid this differentiation since radiation therapy would be of no benefit in papilledema whereas it is the treatment of choice for direct optic nerve infiltration. It is not unusual for optic nerve infiltration to occur simultaneously with papilledema caused by meningeal infiltration (Rosenthal, 1983).

The choroid is commonly infiltrated with leukemic cells histopathologically, although ophthalmoscopic changes are difficult to detect clinically. Although the retina may be the ocular tissue most often involved clinically, on histopathologic examination the choroid shows leukemic infiltration most consistently. However it is almost never clinically apparent (Kincaid & Green, 1983). There have been reports of bilateral serous detachments of the retina as well as retinal pigment epithelial disturbances in a leopard-spot pattern (Kincaid et al, 1979).

Leukemia patients are susceptible to opportunistic infections due to immunosuppression. One of the most common viral infections is cytomegalovirus. Herpes simplex, herpes zoster, and measles may cause a necrotizing retinitis. Fungal infections include *Candida* retinitis, uveitis, and vitreitis, as well as *Aspergillus* choroiditis and vitreitis (Kincaid & Green, 1983).

Orbital involvement in leukemia may be due either to soft tissue infiltration by leukemic cells or to hemorrhage. Infiltration of the lid, orbit, lacrimal gland, or rarely the lacrimal sac may be observed (Rosenthal, 1983). Munro and colleagues (1994) reported two patients with CLL who had nasolacrimal obstruction secondary to neoplastic lymphocytic infiltrates in the region of the lacrimal sac. Orbital granulocytic sarcoma is a rare tumor composed of immature granulocytes and is usually diagnosed in children with a history of AML, although rare cases have been reported in adults with AML (Watkins et al, 1997). The cells elicit an enzyme, myeloperoxidase, that is responsible for the tumor's greenish color; the tumor is also called a chloroma. It may appear at any time in the course of myelogenous leukemia and often before systemic involvement is noted. The patient may present with proptosis secondary to a discrete orbital mass or diffuse orbital involvement simulating inflammatory pseudotumor. The prognosis of a patient with granulocytic sarcoma is usully poor despite aggressive therapy (Kincaid & Green, 1983).

DIAGNOSIS

Systemic

See Table 55–3 for an overview of leukemia diagnosis, and Table 55–4 for differential diagnoses.

Acute Leukemias

In acute leukemia, patients present because of symptoms related directly to the leukemic process. Diagnosis is based on patient history, clinical presentation, and laboratory testing for anemia, thrombocytopenia, and leukemic blast cells in a bone marrow smear. A bone marrow biopsy confirms the diagnosis and differentiates ALL from AML. CNS involvement may be diagnosed by examination of the CSF for leukemic cells.

TABLE 55–3. DIAGNOSIS OF LEUKEMIA

Acute Leukemia
Anemia
Thrombocytopenia
Leukemic blast cells usually found in blood smear
Bone marrow biopsy differentiates types of acute leukemias
Chronic Leukemia
White blood cell (WBC) count
Asymptomatic patient: <50,000 μL
Symptomatic patient: 200,000–1,000,000 μL
Platelet count normal to slightly elevated
Hemoglobin greater than 10 gm/dL
Blood smears
Increase in absolute eosinophil and basophils
Bone marrow biopsy and aspirate hypercellular

TABLE 55–4. DIFFERENTIAL DIAGNOSIS OF LEUKEMIA

Systemic	
Bleeding	Peptic ulcer Hemophilia Coumadin therapy Thrombocytopenia
Fever	Infectious mononucleosis Bacteremia Localized infection (e.g., abscess) Inflammatory disease (e.g., sarcoid) Hepatic infections Connective tissue disorders Diseases of the tropics (e.g., malaria) Meningeal hemorrhage Malignancy Drug reactions
Weight loss	Malnutrition Malignant disease Chronic infection Hyperthyroidism Diabetes mellitus Anorexia nervosa
Joint pain	Arthropathies
Pallor	Hypotension Acromegaly Myxedema
Ocular	
Subconjunctival hemorrhage	Coumadin therapy Valsalva maneuver Bleeding disorder Idiopathic
Episcleritis	Idiopathic Collagen vascular disease Gout Herpes zoster virus Syphilis
Pseudo- versus true hypopyon	Infectious corneal ulcer Endophthalmitis Severe uveitis Reaction to IOL Intraocular tumor
Retinal hemorrhages and cotton-wool spots	Diabetes mellitus Hypertension Anemia
Roth spots	Anemia Septic chorioretinitis Diabetes mellitus
Peripheral neovascularization	Sickle hemoglobinopathies
Opportunistic retinal necrosis	Other causes of immunosuppression

Chronic Leukemias

In contrast, chronic leukemia is usually diagnosed as an incidental finding during elective surgery, or medical workups for unrelated problems. The diagnosis of chronic leukemia is based on patient history; clinical presentation, particularly the delay of pallor, bleeding, and bruisability at the early stages of the disease; and a blood workup. Laboratory testing includes complete blood cell count (CBC) and blood smear. Bone marrow is hypercellular on both aspirate and biopsy.

Ocular

Diagnosis of ocular involvement is made by funduscopic examination. Fluorescein angiography may assist with diagnosis of microaneurysms and serous detachment. Aspiration of the anterior chamber may reveal leukemic cells.

TREATMENT AND MANAGEMENT

Systemic

Table 55–5 describes systemic leukemia treatment and management. Chemotherapy is the primary treatment modality for leukemia patients. Adjuvant radiotherapy is also useful particularly for enlarged nodes and the CNS. Transfusions may be necessary to control the secondary cytopenias, and antibiotics may be needed for superinfections. BMT is useful in patients with nonlymphocytic leukemia. Patients' own marrow is destroyed during chemotherapy and radiotherapy, at which time marrow may be received from an HLA-tissue-matched sibling. Graft-versus-host disease occurs when the immunocompetent transfused lymphocytes attack the graft recipient. There is considerable debate regarding the timing of BMT.

The acute leukemias are treated in three phases: induction, consolidation, and maintenance therapy. Currently, cytarabine, administered by continuous infusion over 7 days at doses of 100 to 200 mg/m^2, with anthracycline (idarubicin or daunorubicin), administered for 3 days, is the most common induction regimen for AML. ALL is also treated with aggressive anthracycline-based chemotherapy plus additional CNS prophylaxis in patients with a high likelihood of CNS relapse (Rubin & Leopold, 1998).

There are no conventional therapies that have resulted in cures for CML. Hydroxyurea and alkylating agents are used to control leukocytosis and splenomegaly. It has been recently shown that alpha interferon may suppress the expression of the Philadelphia chromosome–positive clone in up to 25% of CML patients. Allogenic BMT following high-dose myeloablative chemoradiotherapy has been curative in up to 85% of cases. Conventional therapy is not curative for CLL either. Patients with indolent CLL may do well without therapy for over a decade. Conventional therapy includes alkylating agents and new nucleotide ana-

TABLE 55–5. TREATMENT AND MANAGEMENT OF LEUKEMIA

Systemic
- Chemotherapy
- Radiation
- Bone marrow transplantation

AML
- Three phases of chemotherapy: induction, consolidation, and maintenance
- Chemotherapy (cytarabine with doxorubicin or daunorubicin)
- Bone marrow transplant
- Chemotherapy and/or radiation followed by bone marrow transplantation
- Monitor for infection and potential antibiotic treatment
- Monitor for potential of increased bleeding (e.g., care with brushing teeth, stool softener, hormonally suppressed menstruation

ALL
- Three phases of chemotherapy: induction, consolidation, and maintenance
- Prednisone; vincristine; doxorubicin; L-asparaginase
- Prophylaxis for potential meningeal involvement (radiation, intrathecal methotrexate, or cytarabine)
- Monitor for infection and bleeding as above

CLL
- Monitor
- Alkylating agent
- Chemotherapy
- Steroid

CML
- Cytotoxic agent (Busulfan)
- Bone marrow transplantation

Ocular
- Systemic chemotherapy (for ocular leukemic infiltration)
- Irradiation and intrathecal chemotherapy (for retrolaminar infiltration)
- Bone marrow transplantation

Ocular side effects of treatment
- Cytotoxic drugs
  Cataracts, cranial nerve palsy, optic atrophy, intraocular inflammation
- Bone marrow transplantation with chemotherapy
  Graft-versus-host disease (Sjögren- or scleroderma-like illness: dry eye, conjunctival keratinization, ectropion, uveitis)

logue drugs. Allogenic and autologous BMTs are being investigated in younger patients with CLL (Rubin & Leopold, 1998).

Ocular

Table 55–5 describes ocular leukemia treatment and management. Conjunctival infiltration responds well to systemic chemotherapy. Prophylaxis for CNS leukemia with intrathecal methotrexate and radiation to the head and spine is given routinely for ALL; however, the eye is beyond the reach of these agents (Ellis & Little, 1973). Some have suggested prophylactic irradiation to the eyes (Ridgway et al, 1976).

Anterior chamber disease affected by iris infiltration and pseudohypopyon has been treated with varying doses of local irradiation (Kincaid & Green, 1983). Subconjunctival steroid injection and intrathecal methotrexate have also been reportedly helpful in iris infiltration and secondary glaucoma. Iris infiltration and hypopyon uveitis may respond to topical and periocular steroids; however, recurrence is frequent, and therefore local anterior segment irradiation should be used as primary therapy because it leads to complete resolution.

Leukemic infiltration of the optic nerve has been treated with higher doses of irradiation ranging from 700 to 2000 rads over a 1- to 2-week period and often results in complete resolution and return of visual acuity to normal. Granulocytic sarcoma is managed by removal with lateral orbitotomy and subsequent orbital irradiation. It carries a poor prognosis despite treatment.

Ocular Toxicity

Many ocular side effect exist from the treatment of leukemia (Table 55–5). Cytotoxic drugs have caused posterior subcapsular cataracts (Podos & Canellos, 1969). Cranial nerves palsies of III, IV, VI, and VII as well as corneal hypesthesia of V have been reported from treatment with vincristine and vinblastine (Albert et al, 1967). Vincristine has also been shown to disrupt neurotubules and cause optic atrophy (Green, 1975). Cytosine Arabinoside has been shown to be toxic to the corneal epithelium, causing symptoms of blurred vision and foreign-body sensation (Hopen et al, 1981). The side effects of BMT with associated chemotherapy can cause acute graft-versus-host disease with a Sjögren-like or scleroderma-like dry eye, conjunctival keratinization, ectropion of the eyelid, and uveitis (Jabs et al, 1983).

CONCLUSION

The leukemias are a group of neoplastic bone marrow diseases in which there is abnormal proliferation of hematopoietic or lymphoid cells affecting the entire body. The leukemias may affect all of the ocular tissues, with the well-vascularized retina and uveal tract most commonly affected. Although some of the ocular manifestations are rare, the prompt diagnosis and treatment of leukemia patients is critical, particularly when the ocular manifestation is the initial sign of disease or relapse. Therefore, eyecare practitioners need to be aware of the systemic as well as ocular manifestations of leukemia in order to properly diagnose and manage these patients.

REFERENCES

Albert DW, Wond VG, Henderson ES. Ocular complication of vincristine therapy. *Arch Ophthalmol.* 1967;78:709–713.

Bhadresa GN. Changes in the anterior segment as a presenting feature in leukaemia. *Br J Ophthalmol.* 1971;55:133–135.

Char DH. *Clinical Ocular Oncology.* Philadelphia: Lippincott-Raven; 1997:192–194.

Cook BE, Bartley GB. Acute lymphoblastic leukemia manifesting in an adult as a conjunctival mass. *Am J Ophthalmol.* 1997;124:104–105.

Duane TD, Osher RH, Green WR. White centered hemorrhages: Their significance. *Ophthalmology.* 1980;87:66–69.

Duke JR, Wilkinson CP, Sigelman S. Retinal microaneurysms in leukaemia. *Br J Ophthalmol.* 1968;52:368–374.

Ellis W, Little HL. Leukemic infiltration of the optic nerve head. *Am J Ophthalmol.* 1973;75:867–871.

Green WR. Retinal and optic nerve atrophy *induced* by intravitreous vincristine in the primate. *Trans Am Ophthalmol Soc.* 1975;73:389–416.

Guyer DR, Schchat AP, Vitale S, et al. Leukemic retinopathy. Relationship between fundus lesions and hematologic parameters at diagnosis. *Ophthalmology.* 1989;96:860–864.

Holt JM, Gordon-Smith EC. Retinal abnormalities in diseases of the blood. *Br J Ophthalmol.* 1969;53:145–160.

Hopen G, Mondino BJ, Johnson BL, et al. Corneal toxicity with systemic cytarabine. *Am J Ophthalmol.* 1981;91:500–504.

Isbister JP, Pittiglio DH. *Clinical Hematology: A Problem-Oriented Approach.* Baltimore: Williams & Wilkins; 1988:181.

Jabs DA, Hirst W, Green WR, et al. The eye in bone marrow transplantation. *Am J Ophthalmol.* 1983;101:585–590.

Jackson N, Reddy SC, Hishamuddin MD, et al. Retinal findings in adult leukaemia: Correlation with leukocytosis. *Clin Lab Haematol.* 1996;18:105–109.

Jampol LM, Goldberg MF, Busse B. Peripheral retinal microaneurysms in chronic leukemia. *Am J Ophthalmol.* 1975; 80(2):292–298.

Karesh JW, Goldman EJ, Reck K, et al. A prospective ophthalmic evaluation of patients with acute myeloid leukemia: Correlation of ocular and hematologic findings. *J Clin Oncol.* 1989;7:1528–1532.

Katz SE, Wade NK, Anderson DP, et al. Anterior segment recurrence of acute myelogenous leukemia: Treatment with subconjunctival injections of methotrexate and triamcinolone acetonide. *Can J Ophthalmol.* 1997;32:265–267.

Kincaid MC, Green WR. Ocular and orbital involvement in leukemia. *Surv Ophthalmol.* 1983;27:211–232.

Kincaid MC, Green WR, Kelley JS. Acute ocular leukemia. *Am J Ophthalmol.* 1979;87:698–702.

Leonardy NJ, Rupani M, Dent G, et al. Analysis of 135 autopsy eyes for ocular involvement in leukemia. *Am J Ophthalmol.* 1990;109:436–444.

Maclean H, Clarke MP, Strong NP, et al. Primary ocular relapse in acute lymphoblastic leukaemia. *Eye.* 1996;10: 719–722.

Morse PH, McCready JL. Peripheral retinal neovascularization in chronic myelocytic leukemia. *Am J Ophthalmol.* 1971;72:975–978.

Munro S, Brownstein S, Jordan DR, et al. Nasolacrimal obstruction in two patients with chronic lymphocytic leukemia. *Can J Ophthalmol.* 1994;29:137–140.

Podos SM, Canellos GO. Lens changes in chronic granulocytic leukemia: Possible relationship to chemotherapy. *Am J Ophthalmol.* 1969;68:500–504.

Ridgway EW, Jaffe N, Walton DS. Leukemic ophthalmopathy in children. *Cancer.* 1976;38:1744–1749.

Robb RM, Ervin LD, Sallan SE. A pathological study of eye involvement in acute leukemia of childhood. *Tr Am Ophthalmol Soc.* 1978;76:90–101.

Rosenthal AR. Ocular manifestations of leukemia. *Ophthalmology.* 1983;90:899–905.

Rubin RN, Leopold LH. *Hematologic Pathophysiology.* Madison, CT: Fence Creek; 1998:56–74.

Schachat AP. The leukemias and lymphomas. In: Ryan SJ, ed. *Retina.* Vol. 2. St. Louis: CV Mosby; 1989:873–890.

Watkins LM, Remulla HD, Rubin PA. Orbital granulocytic sarcoma in an elderly patient. *Am J Ophthalmol.* 1997; 123:854–857.

Section XII

ONCOLOGIC DISORDERS

Chapter 56

METASTASIS OF SYSTEMIC MALIGNANCIES TO THE EYE AND ORBIT

Leonard J. Oshinskie

Cancer is a leading cause of morbidity and mortality in the United States. Metastasis to the eye or orbit occurs in 1 to 10% of those with systemic cancer. Since eyecare providers routinely see patients with a history of systemic malignancies, an awareness of the signs and symptoms of metastasis of these malignancies to the ocular structures is important to providing good care.

Metastasis occurs when malignant cells separate from a primary site and establish a new colony of cells through adherence and invasion at a secondary site. This dissemination occurs through interstitial spread of tumor cells at the primary site into the bloodstream or lymphatic channels. Metastasis of systemic cancers may involve several ophthalmic structures including most commonly the choroid and orbit. It is uncommon for patients to present with metastasis of systemic cancer to the retina, optic nerve, iris, ciliary body, and sclera. Most patients who present with ocular metastasis are aware of their cancer diagnosis; however, it is not uncommon for ocular metastasis to be the presenting sign of systemic cancer.

EPIDEMIOLOGY

Systemic

- Carcinoma is by far the most common general form of malignancy metastatic to the uvea. Sarcomas, melanomas, and carcinoid tumors together account for less than 5% of primary tumor types metastatic to the uvea.
- The most common primary sites for systemic cancers metastatic to eye are the breast, followed by the lung. Less common primary sites are the skin, gastrointestinal and genitourinary (kidney) systems.
- Metastasis to the eye from the thyroid, skin, or uterus is rare.
- One-third to one-half of patients with ocular metastasis have no known primary site at the time of diagnosis of the ocular disease.
- Orbital metastasis is less common than intraocular metastasis (an estimated 1:8 ratio of orbital to intraocular).

> Most common systemic malignancies metastatic to the eye are breast cancer and lung cancer.

Ocular

- There is no gender predilection in the overall population with cancer, but lung cancer is the most common primary site in males with ocular metastasis and breast cancer is the most likely in females.
- The vast majority of cases of metastatic ocular and adnexal disease occur in patients ages 40 to 70.
- The cases are bilateral in 10 to 25% of patients, with the right eye affected equally as often as the left.
- The uveal tract is the most commonly involved structure, especially the choroid in the posterior pole region because of high blood flow in this area. Orbital metastasis is less common; only rarely are the iris, ciliary body, retina, or sclera affected.
- Prevalence of ocular metastasis in those with systemic cancer ranges from approximately 1 to 10%.

PATHOPHYSIOLOGY/DISEASE PROCESS

Systemic

- Metastasis requires spread through the hematologic system or lymphatics.
- Systemic manifestations of cancer are many, but some common signs and symptoms are listed in Table 56–1.
- Once ocular metastasis is noted , there is a poor prognosis for survival with mean survival of generally 6 to 12 months, although there are exceptions depending on cancer type and patient age.
- There is longer survival for those with metastatic breast cancer compared to metastatic lung cancer.

TABLE 56–1. MANIFESTATIONS SUGGESTIVE OF VARIOUS TYPES OF SYSTEMIC CANCER

- Unexplained weight loss
- Persistent cough
- Dysphagia
- Irregular bowel or bladder habits
- Loss of appetite
- Lump in breast
- Blood in feces or urine

- Patients with carcinoid tumors have a better prognosis than those with other malignancies.
- In general, lung, renal cell, and prostate cancer metastasizes to the eye earlier than breast cancer or cutaneous melanoma.

Ocular

Ocular manifestations of metastasis are outlined in Table 56–2.

- Metastasis occurs most commonly from the primary site via blood vessels to the highly vascularized choroid.
- Intraocular metastasis is often associated with subretinal fluid and decreased vision.
- Consider metastatic disease in any patient with a nonrhegmatogenous retinal detachment (Figure 56–1), especially one with an established history of systemic cancer or other systemic signs of cancer.
- Orbital metastasis can lead to exophthalmos, exposure keratitis, or diplopia.
- Ocular signs that indicate metastasis to nonocular structures include papilledema, Horner's syndrome, or palsies of cranial nerves 3, 4, 5, 6 or 7.

> The most common symptom of metastasis to the eye is blurred vision.

TABLE 56–2. MANIFESTATIONS OF METASTATIC DISEASE TO INTRAOCULAR AND ORBITAL STRUCTURES

Intraocular
- Decreased visual acuity
- Visual field defect
- Floaters
- Headache/pain
- Conjunctival erythema
- Uveitis (anterior or posterior)
- Disc edema
- Vitritis
- Nonrhegmatogenous retinal detachment
- Secondary glaucoma
- Iris mass

Orbital
- Ptosis
- Proptosis
- Headache/pain
- Diplopia
- Decreased visual acuity
- Conjunctival erythema

Adapted from Freedman MI, Folk JC. Metastatic tumors to the eye and orbit. Arch Ophthalmol. *1987;105:1215–1219.*

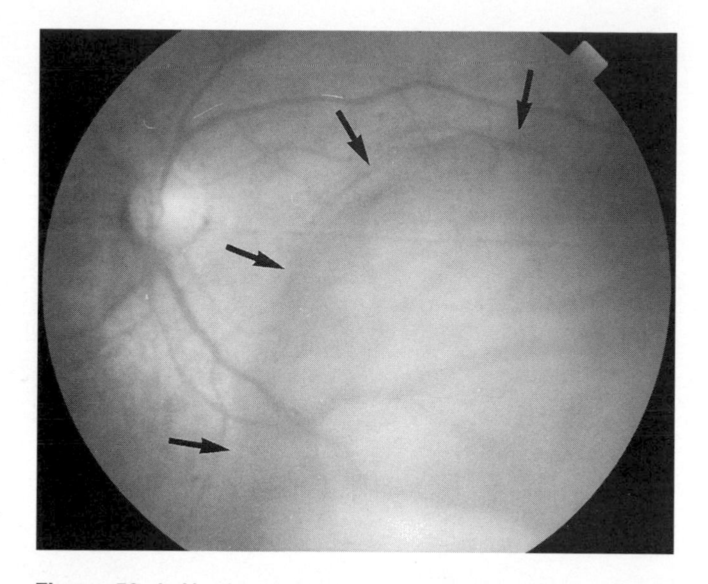

Figure 56–1. Nonrhegmatogenous retinal detachment overlying choroidal metastasis from lung carcinoma. Patient had no previous history of cancer at time of presentation. *(Reprinted with permission from Teague BL, Oshinskie LJ, Stoj MJ. Ocular metastasis of pulmonary oat cell carcinoma.* J Am Optom Assoc. *1991;61:124–130.)*

- For uveal metastasis:
  - The choroid is much more commonly involved than the iris or ciliary body.
  - Choroidal lesions have been described as creamy, yellow, yellow-gray, brown-gray, orange, or pinkish-white in color; they are typically flat and diffuse with average sizes of 8 to 10 mm wide and 1 to 4 mm thick (Figure 56–2).
  - Metastasis is most commonly found in the posterior pole between the macula and equator because of the rich blood supply to short posterior ciliary arteries, and more commonly seen in the temporal or superior regions compared to inferior or nasal regions.
- Metastasis may be bilateral or multifocal.
- Common signs/symptoms include decreased visual acuity, pain, or serous/nonrhegmatogenous retinal detachment.
- Metastasis may cause hyperopic shift in refractive error.

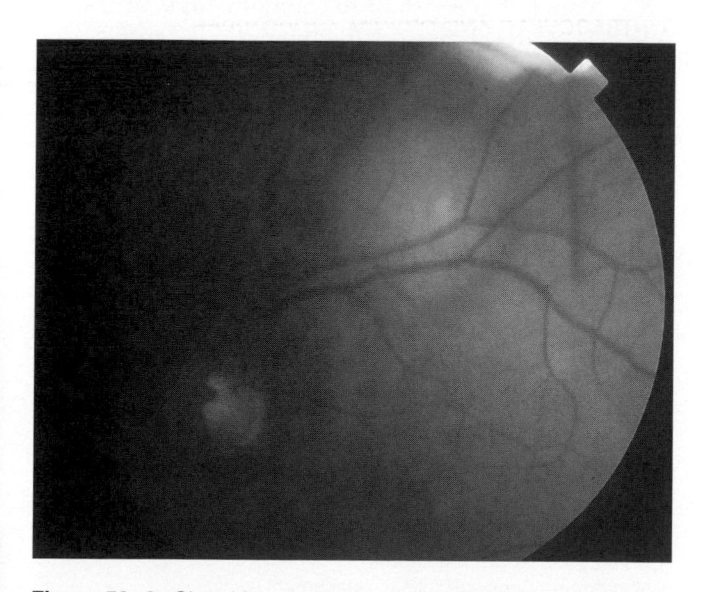

Figure 56–2. Choroidal metastatic disease in a patient with a history of lung cancer.

> Metastasis to the eye is commonly associated with short life expectancy.

- For iris metastasis (Figure 56–3):
  - Although uncommon, metastasis to the iris usually appears as a solitary lesion that is yellow, white, or orange-pink.
  - It is seen almost exclusively in adults.
  - It is often associated with secondary glaucoma, misshapen pupil, and a red eye.
  - Common symptoms are blurred vision or ocular pain.
- For orbital metastasis:
  - Signs/symptoms of orbital metastasis include classic "orbital signs" (i.e., diplopia, proptosis, decreased vision, ptosis, pain, and erythema).
- For metastasis to other ocular sites:
  - Isolated metastases to the retina, optic nerve, eyelid, sclera, conjunctiva, and vitreous are rare.

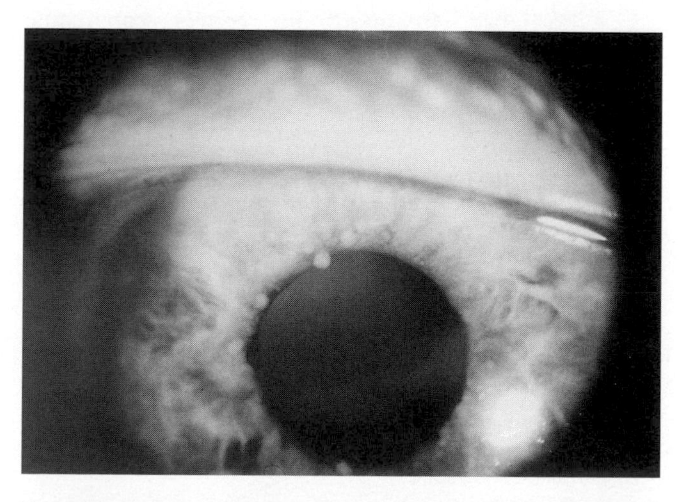

Figure 56–3. Metastatic iris nodules in patient with lung carcinoma. *(Reprinted with permission from Teague BL, Oshinskie LJ, Stoj MJ. Ocular metastasis of pulmonary oat cell carcinoma.* J Am Optom Assoc. *1991;61:124–130.)*

DIAGNOSIS

Systemic

Commonly used tests for systemic and ocular cancer diagnosis/metastatic workup are listed in Table 56–3.

Ocular

- For uveal metastasis:
  - Fluorescein angiography shows blockage early with late staining.
  - B-scan ultrasonography (Figure 56–4), fine needle biopsy, vitreous aspiration, magnetic resonance imaging (MRI), and computed tomography (CT) are also employed in diagnosis.
  - The differential diagnosis is listed in Table 56–4.
- For orbital metastasis:
  - MRI/CT and fine needle biopsy are helpful in diagnosis.

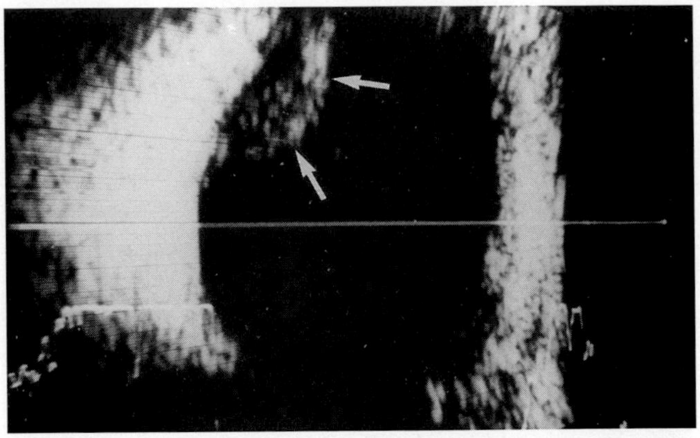

Figure 56–4. B-scan ultrasonography of retinal detachment and thickened choroid of patient in Figure 71–2. *(Reprinted with permission from Teague BL, Oshinskie LJ, Stoj MJ. Ocular metastasis of pulmonary oat cell carcinoma.* J Am Optom Assoc. *1991;61:124–130.)*

TREATMENT AND MANAGEMENT

Treatment and management of ocular metastasis are outlined in Table 56–5.

Systemic

- A variety of chemotherapeutic or hormonal agents, irradiation, or surgery are used.
- Many of the agents used have ocular side effects including keratopathy, conjunctivitis, blepharitis, dry eye, uveitis, cataract, retinopathy, optic neuropathy, ocular pain, diplopia, and others (Imperia et al, 1989; Young & Koda-Kimble, 1992).
- Radiation treatment for cancer can cause retinopathy similar in appearance to diabetic retinopathy, as well as optic atrophy, dry eyes, and cataracts.

> Chemotherapy and radiotherapy can cause a number of ocular complications including dry eye, cataract, retinopathy, and optic neuropathy.

Ocular

- Chemotherapy is generally used for choroidal disease that is localized and relatively nonprogressive.
- External beam radiotherapy is used if the tumor is large, there is vision loss or secondary glaucoma, it is resistant to chemotherapy, or if there is bilateral disease. Plaque radiotherapy is used if it is not responsive to external beam or there is no evidence of systemic disease.
- Radiation is often used in cases of orbital metastasis.

TABLE 56–3. DIAGNOSTIC TESTING FOR METASTATIC DISEASE TO THE EYE

Systemic
- Magnetic resonance imaging and computed tomography
- Bone scans
- Chest x-rays
- Lumbar puncture
- Laboratory testing with tumor markers such as carcinoembryonic antigen (CEA) or prostate-specific antigen (PSA)

Ocular
- Fluorescein angiography
- B-scan ultrasonography
- Fine needle biopsy
- Vitreous aspiration
- Magnetic resonance imaging
- Computed tomography

TABLE 56–4. DIFFERENTIAL DIAGNOSIS OF SYSTEMIC METASTASIS TO THE UVEA

- Rhegmatogenous retinal detachment
- Amelanotic melanoma
- Serous or retinal pigment epithelial detachment or disciform scar due to choroidal neovascularization
- Choroidal osteoma
- Localized choroidal hemangioma
- Choroiditis
- Choroidal granuloma
- CMV retinitis
- Primary malignant melanoma
- Nonrhegmatogenous retinal detachment
- Posterior scleritis

TABLE 56–5. TREATMENT AND MANAGEMENT OF OCULAR METASTASIS

- Referral to oncologist or internist for diagnosis of primary site if unknown
- Chemotherapy (agent varies by cancer type)
- Radiation
- Hormonal therapy
- Debulking of tumor in orbital cases causing proptosis and exposure
- Enucleation for patient in intractable pain
- Fundus/biomicroscopic photography
- Visual fields
- Ultrasonography
- Fluorescein angiography
- Lubrication for exposure secondary to proptosis
- Fresnal prism or patching for diplopia

- Hormonal therapy is used in cases of prostate or breast cancer.
- Enucleation is used for intractable pain.
- In cases of proptosis, lubrication or orbital surgery is helpful.
- In cases of diplopia, prisms (ground-in or press-on type) or patching may be necessary.
- Fundus photography may be needed for monitoring size and extent of the lesion.
- Patient's internist, oncologist, retina specialist, or ocular oncologist is usually involved in the care of a patient with ocular/orbital metastatic disease.

REFERENCES

Char DH, Miller T, Kroll S. Orbital metastases: Diagnosis and course. *Br J Ophthalmol.* 1997;81:386–390.

Eliassi-Rad B, Albert DA, Green WR. Frequency of ocular metastasis in patients dying of cancer in eye bank populations. *Br J Ophthalmol.* 1996;80:125–128.

Ferry AP, Font RL. Carcinoma metastatic to the eye and orbit: A clinicopathologic study of 227 cases. *Arch Ophthalmol.* 1974;92:276–286.

Freedman MI, Folk JC. Metastatic tumors to the eye and orbit. *Arch Ophthalmol.* 1987;105:1215–1219.

Goldberg RA, Rootman J, Cline RA. Tumors metastatic to the orbit: A changing picture. *Surv Ophthalmol.* 1990;35:1–24.

Imperia PS, Lazarus HM, Lass JH. Ocular complications of systemic cancer chemotherapy. *Surv Ophthalmol.* 1989; 34:209–230.

Mack HG, Jakobiec FA. Isolated metastases to the retina or optic nerve. *Int Ophthalmol Clin.* 1997;37:251–260.

Merrill CF, Kaufman DI, Dimitrov NV. Breast cancer metastatic to the eye is a common entity. *Cancer.* 1991;68:623–627.

Purtilo DT, Purtilo RB. A survey of human diseases. Boston: Little, Brown; 1989.

Ratanatharathorn V, Powers WE, Grimm J, et al. Eye metastasis from carcinoma of the breast: Diagnosis, radiation treatment and results. *Cancer Treat Rev.* 1991;18:261–276.

Ruddon RW, Norton SE. Use of biological markers in diagnosis of cancers of unknown primary tumor. *Semin Oncol.* 1993;20:251–260.

Shields JA. Metastatic tumors of the uvea. *Int Ophthalmol Clin.* 1993;33:155–161.

Shields CL, Shields JA, De Potter P, et al. Plaque radiotherapy for the management of uveal metastasis. *Arch Ophthalmol.* 1997;115:203–209.

Shields CL, Shields JA, Gross NE, et al. Survey of 520 eyes with uveal metastasis. *Ophthalmology.* 1997;104:1265–1276.

Shields JA, Shields CL, Kiratli H, De Potter P. Metastatic tumors of the iris in 40 patients. *Am J Ophthalmol.* 1995; 119:422–430.

Smith JA, Gragoudas ES, Dreyer EB. Uveal metastasis. *Int Ophthalmol Clin.* 1997;37:183–199.

Watkins LM, Rubin PAD. Metastatic tumors of the eye and orbit. *Int Ophthalmol Clin.* 1997;37:117–128.

Young LY, Koda-Kimble MA, eds. *Applied Therapeutics: The Clinical Uses of Drugs.* Vancouver: Applied Therapeutics; 1992.

Chapter 57

NON-HODGKIN LYMPHOMA AND INTRAOCULAR LYMPHOMA

Leonard J. Oshinskie

Lymphomas represent a group of diseases that are the result of abnormal arrest and clonal proliferation of T or B lymphocytes. These malignant cells infiltrate tissues throughout the body with morbid consequences such as lymphadenopathy, splenomegaly, and hematologic or immunologic abnormalities. Lymphomas are generally classified as Hodgkin or non-Hodgkin (NHL). When these malignant lymphoid cells infiltrate the uvea, retina, vitreous, or optic nerve, the condition is referred to as intraocular lymphoma. Intraocular lymphoma may present as a primary ocular form or be associated with a systemic form of NHL or a central nervous system lymphoma. Ocular manifestations typically include a chronic uveitis or vitritis.

EPIDEMIOLOGY

Systemic

- NHL comprises 5% of newly diagnosed cases of cancer.
- It is a leading cause of cancer death in males less than 55 years old.
- Annual incidence is 7 per 100,000 in the United States.
- It typically affects patients ages 50 to 60.
- The incidence of primary CNS lymphoma was recently noted to be increasing in both the immunocompetent and immunocompromised patient population.

Ocular

- The intraocular form is often found in association with CNS lymphoma (56%), in isolation (22%), with systemic lymphoma (16%), or with both CNS and systemic disease (6%) (Freeman et al, 1987).
- Patient average age is 60 although it can occur in much younger patients.
- It is often bilateral (44 to 80%).
- Despite an increased incidence of CNS lymphoma in HIV-infected patients, intraocular lymphoma is still relatively uncommon in this population.

PATHOPHYSIOLOGY/DISEASE PROCESS

Systemic

- Lymphocytes typically invade lymph glands, spleen, and hematologic systems with morbid consequences.

> The patient with non-Hodgkin lymphoma is typically aged 50 to 60.

- Signs and symptoms vary but may include those listed in Table 57–1.
- Signs of intraocular lymphoma often precede systemic involvement.
- Survival rates vary widely depending on stage, organ systems involved, and chemotherapy regimen.
- If CNS is involved, then mean life expectancy is about 3 years although some survive for longer periods.
- Survival for AIDS patients with primary CNS lymphoma is short (2.6 months).

Ocular

- Abnormal lymphocytes infiltrate uvea, retina, vitreous, or optic nerve (Table 57–2).
- Ocular manifestations are often the first sign of CNS or systemic involvement.
- Complications include exudative retinal detachment, secondary glaucoma, vitreous hemorrhage, proptosis, and pain.
- The survival rate for those with primary intraocular lymphoma is often short (3 months).

> The intraocular form may be the first sign of CNS lymphoma.

DIAGNOSIS

Systemic

- Workup (Table 57–3) includes CT/MRI to rule out involvement of CNS or internal organs, and lumbar puncture or biopsy of lymph nodes.
- If CNS lymphoma is present, then CT may show isodense or hyperdense cortical lesions with relatively little associated edema. These lesions commonly show enhancement in contrast-enhanced studies.

Ocular

- Intraocular lymphoma should be suspected in cases of chronic uveitis or vitreitis, especially in an older patient whose inflammation is unresponsive to corticosteroids.
- Vitreous or retinal biopsy is used together with biopsies from other systemically involved sites.
- A repeat biopsy may be necessary.
- The polymerase chain reaction of vitreous washings was recently reported to be helpful in diagnosis.
- Table 57–4 includes the differential diagnosis.
- Fundus photography is helpful to monitor progression/regression.

> Intraocular lymphoma commonly presents as uveitis or vitreitis unresponsive to steroids.

TABLE 57–1. SYSTEMIC MANIFESTATIONS OF NON-HODGKIN LYMPHOMA

- Weight loss
- Malaise
- Fever
- Night sweats
- Enlargement of lymph nodes or other internal organs
- Hematologic abnormalities

TABLE 57–2. MANIFESTATIONS OF INTRAOCULAR AND ORBITAL LYMPHOMA

Intraocular
- Blurred vision/floaters
- Posterior uveitis
- Vitreitis
- Keratic precipitates
- Anterior uveitis
- Hypopyon
- Exudative retinal detachment
- Neovascular glaucoma
- Optic nerve head edema
- Subretinal infiltrates
- Cranial nerve palsies (with CNS involvement)

Orbital
- Proptosis
- Orbital mass
- Eyelid edema
- Pain

TABLE 57–3. DIAGNOSTIC WORKUP OF LYMPHOMA

Systemic
CT/MRI
Lumbar puncture
Lymph node biopsy

Ocular
Vitreous/retinal biopsy
Polymerase chain reaction

TABLE 57–4. DIFFERENTIAL DIAGNOSIS OF OCULAR LYMPHOMA

- CMV retinitis
- Multifocal chorioretinopathy
  Acute posterior multifocal placoid pigment epitheliopathy or birdshot chorioretinitis

TREATMENT AND MANAGEMENT

Systemic

The treatment regimen (Table 57–5) considers factors such as cell type, tumor staging, tumor site, age, and general systemic condition.

- Irradiation and combination chemotherapy are commonly used.
- Chemotherapy includes agents such as methotrexate, cytarabine(ARA-C), dexamethasone, vincristine, and leucovorin.
- If CNS involvement is minimal, then therapy can extend life considerably.
- If significant CNS involvement and concurrent intraocular lymphoma exist, then the prognosis is poor.

Ocular

- Local irradiation is delivered in fractionated doses of approximately 35 to 40 Gy.

TABLE 57–5. TREATMENT AND MANAGEMENT OF INTRAOCULAR AND ORBITAL LYMPHOMA

- Local radiation treatment to eye
- Radiation treatment to local CNS sites
- Chemotherapy of systemic cases with CHOP therapy (cyclophosphamide, hydroxyldaunomycin, Oncovin, prednisone) and bleomycin
- Refer for vitreous biopsy for definitive diagnosis
- Fundus photography
- Referral to oncologist for radiation and/or chemotherapy

- If concurrent CNS disease exists, then chemotherapy and irradiation of CNS are also performed.

REFERENCES

Armitage JO. Treatment of non-Hodgkin's lymphoma. *N Engl J Med*. 1993;328:1023–1030.

Buettner H, Bollin JP. Intravitreal large-cell lymphoma. *Mayo Clin Proc*. 1993;1011–1015.

Char DH. *Clinical Ocular Oncology*. New York: Churchill Livingstone; 1989.

Char DH, Ljung BM, Miller T, Phillips T. Primary intraocular lymphoma (ocular reticulum cell sarcoma) diagnosis and management. *Ophthalmology*. 1988;95:625–630.

Fine HA, Mayer RJ. Primary central nervous system lymphoma. *Ann Intern Med*. 1993;119:1093–1104.

Freeman LN, Schachat AP, Knox DL, Michels DG. Clinical features, laboratory investigations and survival in ocular reticulum cells sarcoma. *Ophthalmology*. 1987;94:1631–1639.

Margolis L, Fraser R, Lichter A, Cahr DH. The role of radiation therapy in the management of ocular reticulum cells sarcoma. *Cancer*. 1980;45:688–692.

Non-Hodgkin's Lymphoma Pathologic Classification Project. National Cancer Institute sponsored study of classifications of non-Hodgkin's lymphomas: Summary and description of a working formulation for clinical usage. *Cancer*. 1982;49:2112–2135.

Rivero ME, Kupperman BD, Wiley CA, et al. Acquired immunodeficiency syndrome-related intraocular B-cell lymphoma. *Arch Ophthalmol*. 1999;117:616–622.

Sandor V, Stark-Vancs V, Pearson D, et al. Phase II trial of chemotherapy alone for primary CNS and intraocular lymphoma. *J Clin Oncol*. 1998;16:3000–3006.

Valluri S, Moorthy RS, Khan A, Rao NA. Combination treatment of intraocular lymphoma. *Retina*. 1995;15:125–129.

Whitcup SM, de Smet MD, Rubin BI, et al. Intraocular lymphoma: Clinical and histopathologic diagnosis. *Ophthalmology*. 1993;100:1399–1406.

White VA, Gascoyne RD, Paton KE. Use of polymerase chain reaction to detect B- and T-cell gene rearrangements in vitreous specimens from patients with intraocular lymphoma. *Arch Ophthalmol*. 1999;117:761–765.

Section XIII

METABOLIC DISORDERS

Chapter 58

HYPERLIPIDEMIA

Esther S. Marks

Hyperlipidemia refers to an elevation in one or both of the major classes of circulating lipids: cholesterol and triglycerides. Primary (genetic) lipid disorders are due to inherited or sporadic inborn errors of lipid metabolism. Secondary (acquired) lipid disorders are due to an underlying disease, such as diabetes mellitus or dietary excess, or to medications such as diuretics, beta-blockers, and steroids.

The potential consequences of hyperlipidemia, whether primary or secondary, are similar: most importantly, an increased risk for atherosclerosis and its vascular complications [mainly coronary artery disease (CAD)], the cutaneous manifestation of xanthomas, and pancreatitis. The number 1 cause of death in the United States for both men and women is coronary heart disease (CHD); therefore, much research has been devoted to the association between lipid disorders and atherosclerotic cardiovascular disease. Coronary heart disease morbidity and mortality are a heavy economic burden, costing billions of dollars each year in hospitalizations, medical procedures, and lost productivity.

Lipid disorders have well-documented ocular manifestations. Corneal arcus has been studied extensively as a potential identifiable risk factor in coronary heart disease and cardiovascular disease mortality. Other ocular manifestations include xanthelasmas and lipemia retinalis.

EPIDEMIOLOGY

Systemic

The incidence and prevalence of hyperlipidemia are difficult to extract from the literature. This is due to the enormous variety of hyperlipidemias, the varying laboratory and clinical guidelines for the definition of hyperlipidemia, and the tendency to discuss these conditions in terms of their relationship (especially hypercholesterolemia) to coronary artery disease.

However, using the criteria established by the National Cholesterol Education Program (NCEP), it is believed that 36% of the U.S. population (between the ages of 20 and 74 years) suffers from hypercholesterolemia. In terms of gender, 41% of males and 32% of females are hypercholesterolemic. The incidence increases with age from 20% in ages 20 to 39 years, to 47% in ages 40 to 59 years, and to 58% in ages 60 to 74 years (Sempos et al, 1989). African-Americans and Caucasians appear to have similar cholesterol levels. Increased cholesterol levels (both primary and secondary forms) are strongly associated with an increased risk for atherosclerotic vascular disease and its complications. Xanthomas are usually associated with only the primary forms of elevated cholesterol.

The heterozygous form of familial hypercholesterolemia affects 1 per 500 persons with anywhere from

40 to 90% developing xanthomas. Premature CHD often occurs by the fourth decade. The homozygous form affects only 1 per million persons with profound premature CHD and aortic stenosis by age 20 years. Nonfamilial hypercholesterolemia is a common form of primary hyperlipidemia with both genetic and environmental components. Although not associated with xanthoma formation, it is associated with an increased risk for premature CHD.

Hypertriglyceridemia is usually more common in males than females, and generally more common in Caucasians than African-Americans. Acute pancreatitis and eruptive xanthomas along with lipemia retinalis (known as the chylomicronemia syndrome) most commonly result from the coexistence of a primary and secondary form of hypertriglyceridemia. Familial hypertriglyceridemia affects approximately 1 per 200 persons.

Combined hyperlipidemia, in which both cholesterol and triglyceride levels are elevated, may be familial or acquired. The familial form affects about 1 per 100 persons. More than 15% of patients with premature CHD have familial combined hyperlipidemia. Dysbetalipoproteinemia (Type III hyperlipidemia), although phenotypically distinct from familial combined hyperlipidemia, also is characterized by elevated cholesterol and triglyceride levels, and affects 1 per 10,000 persons. Approximately 25% of these patients develop tendon xanthomas, 64% have palmar xanthomas, and 80% develop tuberous xanthomas. Combined hyperlipidemia is frequently observed in patients with type II diabetes mellitus.

Ocular

Corneal arcus exists in 20 to 30% of the population. Its incidence increases with age. It is more common in males than females, and appears at a younger age in African-Americans than Caucasians. Although more than 50% of patients with corneal arcus are normolipidemic, the presence of arcus in patients under 50 years may suggest hyperlipidemia and a risk for CHD. Fifty percent of patients with heterozygous familial hypercholesterolemia will demonstrate arcus after 30 years of age.

Xanthelasmas are associated with elevated blood lipid levels in only 30 to 50% of patients. They are more common in females, increase in prevalence with age, and are highly associated with corneal arcus. The younger the patient with xanthelasmas, the more likely a lipid disorder exists. Xanthelasmas occur in 23% of patients with familial hypercholesterolemia.

The incidence of lipemia retinalis, a rare phenomenon, is not available in the literature. However, it only occurs in patients with extremely high triglyceride levels.

PATHOPHYSIOLOGY/DISEASE PROCESS

Lipoproteins are complex macromolecules composed of a core of cholesterol and triglycerides, surrounded by phospholipids and apolipoproteins. Lipoproteins may be categorized by several different methods: ultracentrifugation, electrophoresis, or immunological techniques. Ultracentrifugation divides the lipoproteins by density into their familiar classes of chylomicrons, very-low-density lipoproteins (VLDLs), intermediate-density lipoproteins (IDLs), low-density lipoproteins (LDLs), and high-density lipoproteins (HDLs). Electrophoresis separates the lipoproteins by electrical charge and size into beta, prebeta, and alpha lipoproteins. Immunological techniques separate the lipoproteins by their apolipoprotein categories. The 11 major apolipoproteins are: apo A-I, -II, and -IV, apo (a), apo B-48 and -100, apo C-I, -II, and -III, apo D, and apo E.

Triglycerides are the major lipid in chylomicrons and VLDLs. Synthesized from carbohydrates, triglycerides are stored in adipose and muscle tissue to serve as an energy source. Cholesterol, the major lipid in LDL and HDL, is a structural component of all cell membranes, and is a precursor for liver bile acids as well as steroid hormones. Cholesterol and triglycerides are obtained by diet, and by synthesis in the liver.

Chylomicrons transport the exogenous lipids from the small intestine into the circulation. Triglycerides are released into the peripheral tissues when the chylomicrons are exposed to the enzyme lipoprotein lipase. Special receptors on the liver take up the chylomicron remnants. These remnants may then be excreted into the bile, or used to form VLDL. VLDL may then be degraded into IDL for hepatic removal, or converted into LDL. LDL, a cholesterol-rich lipoprotein, is then delivered to receptors on peripheral tissues and organs. HDL, synthesized both by the liver and intestine, facilitates the removal of peripheral cholesterol to the liver, and has therefore always been viewed as cardioprotective. This occurs via the enzyme lethicin–cholesterol acyltransferase (LCAT), which allows the transfer of cholesterol to IDL. IDL is then converted to LDL, which is excreted by the liver via bile into the intestine. The apolipoproteins are largely responsible for the rate of lipoprotein biosynthesis and breakdown.

Systemic

Hyperlipidemia, an elevation in cholesterol and/or triglycerides, may be primary or secondary (Table 58–1). The primary forms are due to an inborn error of lipid metabolism as a result of structural defects or deficiencies in apolipoproteins, enzymes, lipid transfer proteins, or receptors. The secondary forms are due to underlying conditions or diseases that alter lipid

TABLE 58–1. TYPES OF HYPERLIPIDEMIAS (ABBREVIATED LIST)

Primary *(due to inherited or sporadic inborn error of lipid metabolism)*
- Familial hypercholesterolemia—heterozygous and homozygous
- Nonfamilial hypercholesterolemia
- Familial hypertriglyceridemia
- Familial combined hyperlipidemia
- Familial dysbetalipoproteinemia

Secondary *(due to underlying conditions or drugs)*
- Diet
  - Excessive intake of saturated fats
  - Excessive intake of cholesterol
  - Excessive caloric intake
- Conditions
  - Diabetes mellitus
  - Obesity
  - Pregnancy
  - Hypothyroidism
  - Systemic lupus erythematosus
  - Renal failure
  - Nephrotic syndrome
  - Obstructive liver disease
  - Cushing syndrome
  - Acromegaly
  - Anorexia nervosa
  - Porphyria
- Drugs
  - Alcohol
  - Estrogen
  - Beta-blockers
  - Diuretics
  - Glucocorticoids
  - Progestogens
  - Anabolic steroids
  - Retinoids
  - Phenytoin

metabolism, such as diabetes mellitus, obesity, hypothyroidism, renal failure, nephrotic syndrome, and obstructive liver disease. Drugs such as alcohol, beta-blockers, diuretics, glucocorticoids, estrogen, and progestogens may also alter lipid profiles resulting in secondary hyperlipidemias.

The manifestations of hyperlipidemia (Table 58–2) may be due directly to the elevated lipid levels themselves. Systemically, this may present as xanthomas and pancreatitis and ocularly, as corneal arcus, xanthalasmas, and lipemia retinalis. Often, the manifestations are due to a condition to which hyperlipidemia contributes—atherosclerosis and its complications. The manifestations may vary with each type of lipid disorder (Table 58–3). Finally, the hyperlipidemia may manifest secondary to or as a sign of an underlying condition such as diabetes mellitus.

Xanthomas are deposits of lipids that occur most commonly in the skin and tendons, although they may

TABLE 58–2. GENERAL SYSTEMIC AND OCULAR MANIFESTATIONS OF HYPERLIPIDEMIAS

Systemic
- Elevated lipid levels
- Atherosclerosis and its thromboembolic vascular complications
  - Cardiovascular
  - Peripheral vascular
  - Cerebrovascular
  - Angina
  - Myocardial infarction
  - Intermittent claudication
  - Transient ischemic attacks
  - Cerebrovascular accidents
- Xanthomas
  - Planar, palmar, tendon, subperiosteal, eruptive, tuberous, mediastinum, retroperitoneum
- Abdominal pain
- Chylomicronemia syndrome
  - Pancreatitis, hepatomegaly, eruptive xanthomas, lipemia retinalis, and neurologic involvement

Ocular
- Corneal arcus
- Xanthelasma
- Lipemia retinalis

also develop in the mediastinum, retroperitoneum, and bone. Although the presence of such lesions suggests a lipid disorder (primary or secondary), patients with normal lipid profiles may also demonstrate these findings. More importantly, the absence of xanthomas does not eliminate the presence of a lipid disorder.

Planar xanthomas are flat or slightly raised cutaneous yellowish to yellowish-orange lesions associated with the homozygous form of familial hypercholesterolemia. They may occur throughout the body, especially on the knees, ankles, upper trunk, neck, face, and dorsal aspects of the hands. Palmar xanthomas are flat yellowish-orange cutaneous lesions occurring in the creases of the palms and on the palmar surface of the fingers, and are usually associated with familial dysbetalipoproteinemia.

Tendon xanthomas are nontender, firm, smooth, elevated nodular lesions within the tendon. They may occur in any tendon, although the Achilles and the extensor tendons of the fingers appear to be the most common. If particularly large, the overlying skin may break down due to mechanical irritation. Tendon xanthomas are of particular importance as their size often parallels that of underlying coexistent atherosclerotic plaques.

Eruptive xanthomas (Figure 58–1) are multiple, small, yellowish-orange lesions usually associated with profound hypertriglyceridemia (a condition that may occur in uncontrolled diabetes mellitus). They usually develop on extensor surfaces, the buttocks, and

TABLE 58–3. SYSTEMIC AND OCULAR MANIFESTATIONS SPECIFIC TO TYPE OF HYPERLIPIDEMIA

PRIMARY HYPERLIPIDEMIAS

Familial Hypercholesterolemia

Systemic
- Elevated plasma LDL cholesterol
- Premature coronary artery disease
- Myocardial infarction especially in males in early forties
- Tendon xanthomas usually on extensor surfaces

Ocular
- Premature corneal arcus
- Xanthelasma common in heterozygotes only

Nonfamilial Hypercholesterolemia

Systemic
- Plasma LDL cholesterol 160–220 mg/dL
- Increased risk of premature coronary artery disease

Ocular
- Corneal arcus
- Xanthelasma possible

Familial Hypertriglyceridemia

Systemic
- Elevated triglyceride levels
- Usually asymptomatic
- May develop chylomicronemia syndrome especially if diabetes is present

Ocular
- Lipemia retinalis possible

Familial Combined Hyperlipidemia

Systemic
- Elevated triglyceride and cholesterol levels
- Premature coronary artery disease
- Myocardial infarction around age 40 years
- May develop chylomicronemia syndrome especially if diabetes is present

Ocular
- Corneal arcus and xanthelasma possible
- Lipemia retinalis possible

Familial Dysbetalipoproteinemia

Systemic
- Elevated triglyceride and cholesterol levels
- Atherosclerosis: in men prematurely, in women after menopause
- Xanthomas: tendon, tuberous, or palmar
- Peripheral vascular disease predominates
- Coronary artery disease may also occur

Ocular
- Premature corneal arcus
- Xanthelasma and lipemia retinalis possible

SECONDARY HYPERLIPIDEMIAS

Acquired Hypercholesterolemia

Systemic
- Elevated plasma cholesterol levels
- May be due to dietary excess, anorexia nervosa, porphyria, or diuretic drugs

Ocular
- Corneal arcus and xanthelasma possible

Acquired Hypertriglyceridemia

Systemic
- Elevated plasma triglyceride levels
- May be due to uncontrolled diabetes mellitus, obesity, estrogen use, alcohol, retinoids, or beta-blockers
- In severe cases may develop chylomicronemia syndrome especially if diabetes and a primary form of hypertriglyceridemia are present

Ocular
- Lipemia retinalis possible

Acquired Combined Hyperlipidemia

Systemic
- Elevated plasma cholesterol and triglyceride levels
- May be due to hypothyroidism, nephrotic syndrome, and excess glucocorticoid

Ocular
- Corneal arcus and xanthelasma possible

the trunk. Tuberous xanthomas are believed to arise when eruptive xanthomas coalesce into soft elevated papules. They are found on extensor surfaces, knees, elbows, buttocks, and palmar surfaces of the hands. These usually occur in primary hypertriglyceridemias.

The chylomicronemia syndrome, most commonly caused by the simultaneous presence of both a primary and secondary form of hypertriglyceridemia, results in a constellation of clinical signs and symptoms. These include acute pancreatitis, abdominal pain, hepatomegaly, eruptive xanthomas, lipemia retinalis, memory loss, dementia, peripheral neuropathy, and paresthesias. Either the inflamed pancreas (irritated by chemicals released by chylomicrons) and/or the enlarged liver (due to fatty infiltration) result in the abdominal pain. It may be mild to severe, and may extend into the chest area. Xanthomas erupt over the extensor surfaces and the buttocks. Lipemia retinalis may be observed. Dementia in the form of memory loss occurs. The peripheral neuropathy and paresthesias may present like a carpal tunnel syndrome. All of these manifestations are reversible with treatment.

It is not hyperlipidemia per se that leads to increased morbidity and mortality, but rather the interaction of hyperlipidemia (especially increased LDL) with multiple other risk factors (e.g., males 45 years of age, females 55 years, family history of premature CHD, hypertension, low HDL levels, diabetes mellitus, cigarette smoking, obesity, lack of physical exercise, alcohol, certain medications, and other diseases). Hyperlipidemic states will aggravate and accelerate the atherosclerotic process, thereby increasing the risk for vascular disease and its complications. The combination of elevated total cholesterol, elevated LDL, elevated triglycerides, and lowered HDL clearly contributes to vascular disease, but the individual contribution of each class of lipids is less clear. There is currently widely accepted evidence that elevated total cholesterol levels as well as elevated LDL cholesterol levels play significant roles in the development

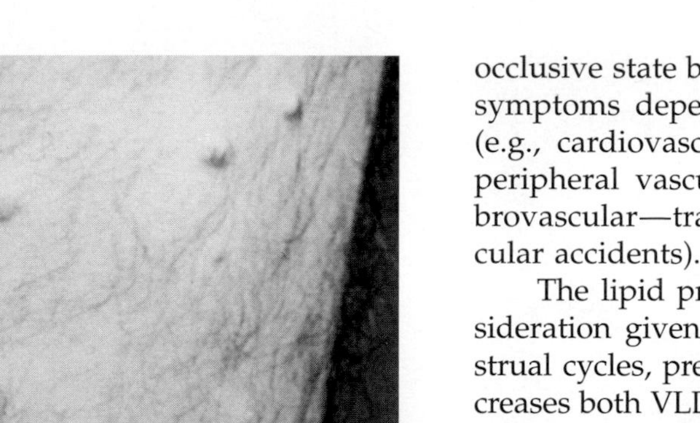

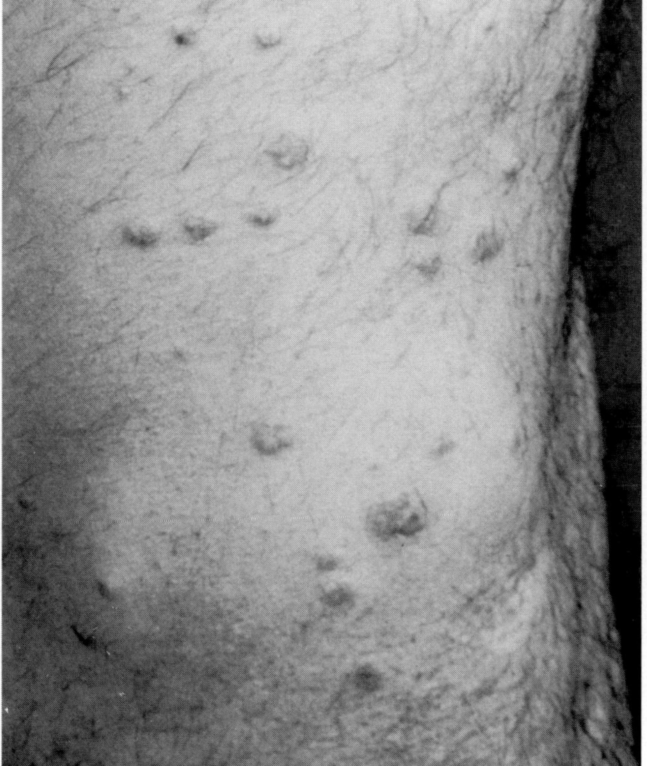

Figure 58–1. Eruptive xanthomas on the leg of a diabetic patient with uncontrolled diabetes and hypertriglyceridemia. *(Reprinted with permission from Steiner G, Shafrir E.* Primary Hyperlipoproteinemias. *New York: Mc Graw-Hill; 1991.)*

of coronary heart disease (Gotto, 1999), and established guidelines exist for managing these conditions. Although low HDL cholesterol levels (even in isolation) have been shown to increase the risk for cardiac complications due to atherosclerosis, the clinical management is less clear (Harper & Jacobson, 1999). The same holds true for elevated triglyceride levels, which have been recognized as playing a role in the atherogenic process (Kraus, 1998). It is well known that the process of atherosclerosis is life-long, commencing in childhood and progressing into adulthood until it becomes clinically apparent. Fatty streaks appear initially in the aorta of children and then spread to the coronary arteries, with eventual potential involvement of the peripheral and cerebrovascular systems. The progression of these streaks to fibrous plaques usually occurs in adulthood (20 years or older).

If the atherosclerotic lesions develop sufficiently, the clinical signs and symptoms of a thromboembolic occlusive state become evident. The type of signs and symptoms depend on the vascular system involved (e.g., cardiovascular—angina, myocardial infarction; peripheral vascular—intermittent claudication; cerebrovascular—transient ischemic attacks, cerebrovascular accidents).

The lipid profile in females deserves special consideration given the changes that occur during menstrual cycles, pregnancy, and menopause. Estrogen increases both VLDL and HDL levels and decreases LDL levels, whereas progestogens decrease the cardioprotective HDL levels. Women have significant increases in cholesterol and triglyceride levels during pregnancy, yet there is considerable disagreement concerning whether or not this increases their risk for coronary artery disease. Oral contraceptives as well as menopause appear to alter the lipid profile to a more atherogenic state. However, postmenopausal estrogen replacement dramatically reduces mortality (30 to 60%) from coronary artery disease.

Ocular

The ocular manifestations of hyperlipidemia include corneal arcus, xanthelasmas, and lipemia retinalis. Corneal arcus is a greyish-white ring of lipid deposition in the corneal stroma (Figure 58–2). It occurs at the limbus with a clear interval (0.3 to 1.0 mm) between the limbus and the lesion, never involves the central cornea, and therefore never affects visual acuity. Arcus usually starts superiorly, followed by inferiorly, slowly progressing completely around the corneal circumference. It is almost always a bilateral phenomenon. Although more common with increasing age in all populations, arcus may occur prematurely in lipid disorders, particularly the genetic forms. It is felt to be primarily due to elevated cholesterol levels. A study by Varnek and associates (1979) suggested that marked nasal arcus in particular is linked to high cholesterol levels. Below the age of 50 years (in men) the presence of corneal arcus has been shown to be a risk factor for coronary heart disease mortality, especially in the presence of a hyperlipidemic state (Chambless et al, 1990).

Xanthelasmas are a form of xanthoma (Figure 58–3). Located on the eyelids, they are yellowish, slightly elevated soft lesions of lipid deposition. As with corneal arcus, they are seen more commonly with increasing age. Fifty percent of patients with xanthelasmas have coexisting hyperlipidemia (especially elevated cholesterol and triglyceride levels), which is responsible for an increased risk for atherosclerosis and its complications. However, the other 50% of patients with xanthelasmas are normolipidemic. The risk for atherosclerosis in this population is unclear. However, the younger the patient with xanthelasma, the more

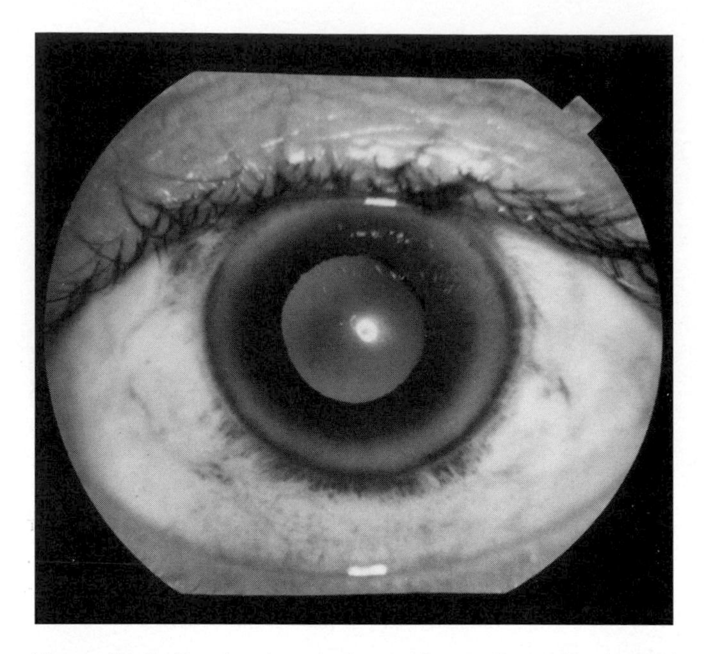

Figure 58–2. Prominent corneal arcus in a patient with elevated cholesterol levels.

likely it is due to a lipid disorder, particularly elevated cholesterol levels.

Lipemia retinalis occurs in the presence of extremely elevated triglyceride levels (exceeding 1000 mg/dL). It tends to occur in the retinal periphery first; then as triglyceride levels continue to rise, it extends back to involve the posterior pole and the optic disc.

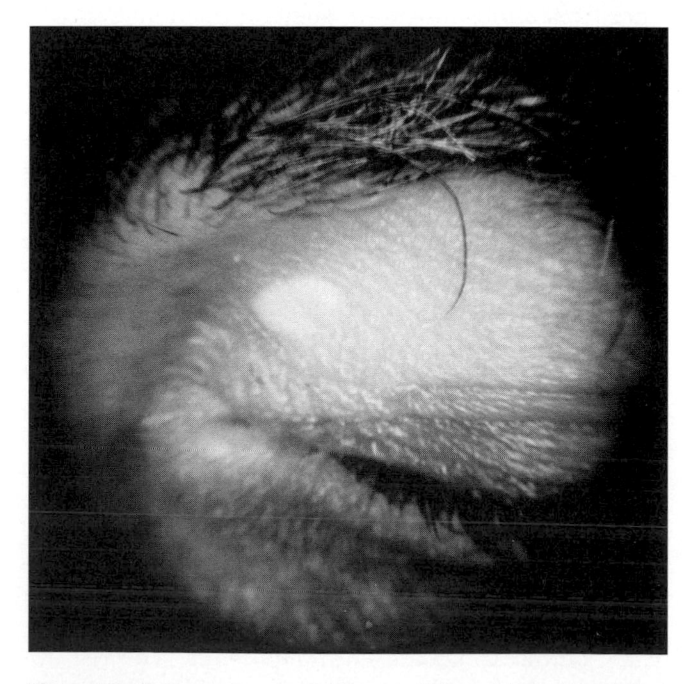

Figure 58–3. Xanthelasma of the upper lid in a 44-year-old patient with hypercholesterolemia.

> Whereas the presence of corneal arcus and/or xanthelasma, particularly in the younger patient, is suggestive of hyperlipidemia, lipemia retinalis is pathognomonic specifically for severe hypertriglyceridemia.

The retinal vessels become salmon or creamy, milky white in color. As the triglyceride levels are brought under control, the color recedes first from the disc and posterior pole, and then from the peripheral fundus. Visual impairment or complications, either transient or permanent, have rarely been noted.

DIAGNOSIS

Systemic

The diagnosis of hyperlipidemia (and its differential; Table 58–4) should include a full history (including family), a physical examination, and laboratory evaluation. The history should inquire about diet, underlying diseases (e.g., diabetes or hypothyroidism), drugs, hyperlipidemia in the family, as well as any premature CHD or deaths. A routine physical examination should be performed noting body weight and the presence of any xanthomas. Laboratory lipid diagnosis (Table 58–5) is usually limited to routine tests of total cholesterol, triglycerides, and HDL and LDL cholesterol levels. Other laboratory tests, such as blood glucose, urinalysis, serum chemistry, serum protein electrophoresis, thyroid profile, and liver function tests, may be warranted in patients suspected to have an underlying disease giving rise to a secondary hyperlipidemia.

A fasting lipid profile (including no alcohol intake 24 to 48 hours prior to testing) should include total

TABLE 58–4. DIFFERENTIAL DIAGNOSIS OF HYPERLIPIDEMIAS

Systemic
- See Table 58–1

Ocular
- Corneal arcus
  - Kaiser-Fleischer ring
- Xanthelasma
  - Cysts
  - Nevus
  - Neurofibroma
  - Necrobiotic xanthogranuloma nodules of multiple myeloma
- Lipemia retinalis
  - None

TABLE 58–5. ROUTINE DIAGNOSTIC TESTS FOR HYPERLIPIDEMIA AND THE RISK FOR CORONARY HEART DISEASE

Total cholesterol	
Desirable	<200 mg/dL
Borderline-high	200–239 mg/dL
High	>239 mg/dL
LDL cholesterol	
Desirable	<130 mg/dL
Borderline-high	130–159 mg/dL
High	>159 mg/dL
HDL cholesterol	
Recommended	≥35 mg/dL
Atherosclerotic Coronary Heart Disease Risk Ratios	
LDL/HDL	
Desirable	<4
High	≥4
Total cholesterol/HDL	
Desirable	<5
High	≥5
Triglycerides	
Normal	<200 mg/dL
Borderline-high	200–399 mg/dL
High	400–1000 mg/dL
Very high	>1000 mg/dL

cholesterol, triglycerides, HDL cholesterol, and LDL cholesterol. Although there is variation in suggested laboratory values and clinical application, the second Adult Treatment Panel of the U.S. National Cholesterol Education Program (NCEP), updated its 1988 guidelines in 1993 for the classification of cholesterol levels in adults aged 20 years and older (see Table 58–5). As a general rule total cholesterol levels more than 240 mg/dL and LDL cholesterol levels more than 160 mg/dL are considered high and place the patient at increased risk for coronary artery disease. These values will be lower with children, and higher with older adults. HDL cholesterol levels less than 35 mg/dL are considered risky for coronary heart disease. Atherosclerosis risk ratios were also developed using LDL, HDL, and total cholesterol. The higher the LDL/HDL and total cholesterol/HDL ratios are, the higher the risk for developing coronary heart disease.

The role triglyceride levels play in atherosclerotic disease is still controversial; therefore, fewer guidelines exist for identifying different levels of risk. Many laboratories consider approximately 30 to 150 mg/dL desirable. Levels are slightly lower for women and children. However, the second Adult Panel of the NCEP developed a classification for triglyceride levels in which levels under 200 mg/dL may be considered normal because little evidence exists predicting an increased risk for coronary heart disease. Triglyceride levels are considered borderline-high at 200 to 400 mg/dL, high at 400 to 1000 mg/dL, and very high at over 1000 mg/dL. Levels higher than 500 mg/dL run increasingly higher risks for pancreatitis.

Additional testing, such as lipoprotein electrophoresis, beta-quantification, lipoprotein lipase assay, lipoprotein-a, and apo-E genotyping, is usually limited to patients with certain genetic lipid disorders. Future tests may include levels of fibrinogen, homocysteine, antiphospholipid antibodies, antioxidants, LDL oxidizability, and subclasses of HDL and LDL (Jialal, 1996).

Ocular

External and biomicroscopic examination will easily reveal palpebral xanthelasmas and corneal arcus. Lipemia retinalis may be observed as salmon to milky colored retinal blood vessels on dilated fundus examination.

TREATMENT AND MANAGEMENT

Systemic

The treatment of hyperlipidemia is essentially similar whether primary or secondary in nature (Table 58–6). Any existing CHD risk factors should be evaluated and treated if possible. Any underlying systemic condition that contributes to the lipid disorder must be controlled. Any medications that adversely affect lipid levels should be changed if possible. Smoking should cease. Diet and body weight management are crucial to lipid level control, and are strongly recommended as the initial treatment (Expert Panel, 1993), and the foundation for any further treatment. Modifying the diet by limiting animal products, saturated fats, and processed foods and increasing fresh fruits, vegetables, and whole grain starches may not only improve serum lipid levels, but provide other health benefits (eg, reduced risk for cardiovascular disease) (Hensrud, 2000). Physical activity, the cessation of smoking, and limited alcohol intake should be encouraged. When these measures fail to lower lipid levels sufficiently, pharmacologic intervention may be required.

Caloric intake should be adjusted to achieve appropriate body weight. Daily cholesterol intake should be restricted to under to 200 to 300 mg. Total fat intake

> Diet modification, weight reduction, and physical activity are the foundation of hyperlipidemia treatment. The addition of drug therapy may be necessary, but *cannot replace* lifestyle modification.

TABLE 58–6. TREATMENT AND MANAGEMENT OF HYPERLIPIDEMIA

Systemic
- **Nonpharmacologic modalities—all of the following:**
  - Physical activity recommended
  - Cessation of cigarette smoking
  - Dietary regimen:
    - Limitation or elimination of alcohol
    - Adjust caloric intake to achieve appropriate body weight
    - Daily cholesterol intake <200–300 mg
    - Total fat intake <30% of total caloric intake
      - Polyunsaturated fat ≤ 10%
      - Monounsaturated fat 10–15%
      - Saturated fat <7–10%
    - Carbohydrates 50–60% of total caloric intake
    - Protein 10–20% of total caloric intake
    - 25–35 g daily fiber (psyllium)

If insufficient, add:

- **Pharmacologic modalities**
  - Control any underlying disease
  - Change any medication that adversely affects lipid levels if possible
  - **Plus one or more of the following:**
    - HMG-CoA reductase inhibitors
      - Atorvastatin: 10–80 mg qd
      - Cerivastatin: 0.3 mg qhs
      - Fluvastatin: 20–40 mg qhs
      - Lovastatin: 20–80 mg qd
      - Pravastatin: 10–40 mg qhs
      - Simvastatin: 5–40 mg qhs
    - Bile-acid resins
      - Cholestyramine: 4–16 g bid
      - Colestipol: 10–30 g/day
    - Nicotinic acid
      - 1.5–6 g/day
    - Fibric acids
      - Gemfibrozil: 600 mg bid
      - Clofibrate: 500 mg qid
- **Other therapeutic modalities**
  - Multivitamins/antioxidants
  - Estrogen replacement therapy
  - New lipid-lowering agents—lifibrol
  - Gene therapy
  - Plasmapheresis
  - Surgery

Ocular

Treatment of underlying lipid disorder if present

Corneal arcus
- No direct treatment

Xanthelasma
- No direct treatment necessary
- May be surgically removed for cosmesis

Lipemia retinalis
- No direct treatment

Abbreviations: bid, twice a day; qd, every day; qhs, every hour of sleep; qid, four times daily.

should be limited to 30% or less of total calories, with polyunsaturated fat 10% or less, monounsaturated fat 15% or less, and saturated fat less than 7 to 10% of total fat. Carbohydrates should be 55% or less, and protein should be approximately 15% of total calories (Expert Panel, 1993). Studies have found that the daily addition of 25 to 35 g of fiber (psyllium—Metamucil) to a low-fat, low-cholesterol diet is efficacious in further lowering cholesterol levels (Lipsky et al, 1990).

Antioxidants may provide some protection by preventing the oxidation and glycosylation of LDL cholesterol, which is atherogenic. Antioxidant vitamins, including C and E, and beta carotene may be taken in pill form or in the form of fruits and vegetables (dark-green and deep-yellow) (Ahmed et al, 1998). Compliance is the most difficult aspect of any dietary regimen, requiring the combined efforts of the patient, physician, and often a nutritionist or dietician.

If a patient has desirable cholesterol levels (less than 200 mg/dL), general dietary and risk reduction information should be provided. Remeasurement is advised in 5 years. Borderline-high cholesterol levels (200 to 239 mg/dL) in the absence of coronary heart disease and risk factors require slightly stricter dietary and risk reduction information, along with remeasurement in 1 year. Risk factors include male sex, family history of premature coronary heart disease, cigarette smoking, hypertension, low HDL cholesterol (less than 35 mg/dL), diabetes mellitus, history of cerebrovascular or peripheral vascular disease, and severe obesity (defined as more than 30% overweight). Borderline-high cholesterol levels in the presence of coronary heart disease or two risk factors require lipoprotein analysis. High cholesterol levels (more than 240 mg/dL) also require lipoprotein analysis.

Upon analysis, if LDL cholesterol levels are desirable (less than 130 mg/dL), once again simple dietary and risk reduction information should be provided, with remeasurement within 5 years. Borderline-high LDL cholesterol levels (130 to 159 mg/dL) in the absence of coronary heart disease and risk factors require slightly stricter dietary and risk reduction information, along with remeasurement in 1 year. Borderline-high LDL cholesterol levels in the presence of coronary heart disease or two risk factors and high LDL cholesterol levels (more than 160 mg/dL) both require a full clinical evaluation. Special care should be taken to rule out the presence of underlying diseases or primary lipid disorders.

In the absence of coronary heart disease and risk factors, the goal is LDL cholesterol less than 160 mg/dL and total cholesterol less than 240 mg/dL. In the presence of coronary heart disease or two risk factors, the goal is LDL cholesterol under 130 mg/dL, and total cholesterol under 200 mg/dL. The first step is strict dietary management. If the cholesterol goals are met within 3 months, long-term monitoring is suggested by remeasurement of lipid levels four times the first year, and two times per year thereafter. If the cholesterol goals are not met within the first 3 months, then even stricter dietary management is required under supervision. If the cholesterol goals are met within 6 months, long-term monitoring again is suggested. If the goal is not met, medication must be considered.

Treatment modalities for hypertriglyceridemia are less clear because of controversy concerning the role triglycerides play in cardiovascular disease. If nonpharmacological modalities fail (e.g., diet, exercise, weight reduction), drug therapy should be considered. Patients with severe hypertriglyceridemia must follow an extremely restrictive diet, limiting fat intake to less than 20% of total calories. Should chylomicronemia syndrome occur, strict elimination of all oral intake and alcohol will quickly decrease triglyceride levels. Refeeding may be initiated with severe fat intake reduction. Drug therapy may be required.

The type of lipid disorder determines the appropriate medication(s) because some of the drugs affect cholesterol only, triglycerides only, or both. Hypercholesterolemia is treated with HMG-CoA (3-hydroxy-3-methylglutaryl coenzyme A) reductase inhibitors, bile acid resins, or nicotinic acid. Combined hyperlipidemia is treated with nicotinic acid, HMG-CoA reductase inhibitors, or fibric acid derivatives. Hypertriglyceridemia is treated with nicotinic acid or fibric acid derivatives.

HMG-CoA reductase inhibitors (e.g., lovastatin, pravastatin, simvastatin, fluvastatin, cerivastatin, or atorvastatin) inhibit the synthesis of cholesterol in the liver, stimulating the synthesis of LDL receptors. Circulating LDL and VLDL levels drop, as do triglyceride levels. Although generally well tolerated, diarrhea, insomnia, liver toxicity, and muscle pain may occur. Liver function and creatinine kinase levels should be monitored. Lovastatin has produced cataracts in studies using dogs (Fraunfelder, 1988). The evidence in humans is inconclusive; therefore, prior to initiating lovastatin therapy an examination of the crystalline lens is recommended, with routine annual examinations thereafter.

Bile acid resins (cholestyramine and colestipol) reduce total and LDL cholesterol levels by removing bile acids from the intestine. This prevents reabsorption by the liver, dropping cholesterol levels and increasing LDL receptor synthesis. Circulating LDL cholesterol levels drop. Its major side effect is constipation. These drugs may also interfere with the absorption of other drugs (e.g., warfarin, thyroxine, thiazide diuretics, betablockers, penicillin G, phenobarbitol, acetaminophen, and nonsteroidal anti-inflammatory drugs).

Nicotinic acid (niacin) inhibits the production of VLDL and triglycerides, which also lowers the level of LDL. Frequent side effects occur, including skin rashes, flushing, gastrointestinal symptoms, hyperglycemia, hyperuricemia, fatigue, and liver toxicity. Therefore, nicotinic acid is contraindicated in peptic ulcer disease, gouty arthritis, hyperuricemia, liver disease, and diabetes mellitus. Patients on nicotinic acid should have uric acid, liver function, and glucose levels monitored.

Fibric acids (gemfibrozil and clofibrate) lower triglyceride levels by increasing the activity of lipoprotein lipase. Cholesterol gallstones, gastrointestinal symptoms, skin rashes, leukopenia, muscle pain, and hepatic malignancy may occur. Care should be taken with patients on oral anticoagulants because gemfibrozil potentiates their effects.

Multiple drug therapy may be necessary in a high-risk patient with coronary artery disease who is unable to reach treatment goals with lifestyle modification and one medication. In postmenopausal women, estrogen replacement therapy should be considered since it lowers LDL and increases HDL cholesterol levels. Other therapeutic modalities such as new lipid-lowering drugs and gene therapy are under investigation. Plasmapheresis is used commonly for the treatment of severe hypercholesterolemia in order to drastically lower triglyceride levels and reduce the risk of pancreatitis. Surgical treatments (GI and liver) may be effective in severe refractory cases of hyperlipidemia (Ahmed et al, 1998).

Ocular

There is no treatment for corneal arcus. Although it has no adverse effect on ocular structures, arcus noted in patients under 50 years old is a strong risk factor for coronary heart disease mortality. Therefore, arcus noted in any patients under 50 years, particularly if unaware of their lipid levels, warrants blood cholesterol testing.

Xanthelasmas, although cosmetically unappealing, also have no adverse effect on the ocular adnexa. However, these patients also warrant blood cholesterol testing, particularly if arcus and xanthelasmas coexist. With antilipidemic medications, the xanthelasmas may slowly regress. Surgical removal of these lid lesions is feasible; however, approximately 40% recur.

Lipemia retinalis itself requires no treatment as it rarely adversely affects the eye. However, its presence occurs only with triglyceride levels well over 1000 mg/dL. Lipemia retinalis in a patient with a known lipid disorder warrants referral back to the physician for immediate control. Clearly, if the patient presents with lipemia retinalis and is unaware of an existing lipid disorder, urgent referral to a lipid metabolism specialist is warranted, considering the risk of developing pancreatitis.

CONCLUSION

Hyperlipidemia is often labeled a disease of modern civilization with its high-cholesterol, high-fat diet. Both primary and secondary forms of hyperlipidemia demonstrate clear associations with atherosclerotic cardiovascular disease, particularly coronary heart disease. Due to the significant morbidity and mortality associated with such thromboembolic heart disease, patients suspected of hyperlipidemia warrant, at minimum, a test of cholesterol levels, if not an entire lipid profile. The ocular manifestations of hyperlipidemia, in particular corneal arcus, are potential prognostic factors for coronary heart disease. Thus, the eyecare practitioner plays an integral role in the potential diagnosis, treatment, and management of lipid disorders.

REFERENCES

Ahmed SM, Clasen ME, Donnelly JF. Management of dyslipidemia in adults. *Am Fam Physician.* 1998;57:2192–2204.

Alexander LJ. Ocular signs and symptoms of altered blood lipids. *J Am Optom Assoc.* 1983;54:123–126.

Alexander LJ. The prevalence of corneal arcus senilis in known insulin-dependent diabetic patients. *J Am Optom Assoc.* 1985;56:556–559.

Assman G, et al. Management of hypertriglyceridemic patients: A. Treatment classifications and goals. *Am J Cardiol.* 1991;68:30A–34A.

Assman G, Brewer HB. Genetic (primary) forms of hypertriglyceridemia. *Am J Cardiol.* 1991;68:13A–16A.

Barchiesi BJ, Eckel RH, Ellis PP. The cornea and disorders of lipid metabolism. *Surv Ophthalmol.* 1991;36:1–22.

Bergman R. The pathogenesis and clinical significance of xanthelasma palpebrarum. *J Am Acad Dermatol.* 1994; 30:236–242.

Berman EL. Clues in the eye: Ocular signs of metabolic and nutritional disorders. *Geriatrics.* 1995;50:34–37.

Breslow JL. Genetics of lipoprotein disorders. *Circulation.* 1993;87:III-16–III-21.

Brunzell JD. The hyperlipoproteinemias. In: Wyngaarden JB, Smith LH, eds. *Cecil Textbook of Medicine.* Philadelphia: WB Saunders; 1988:1137–1144.

Carmena R, Grundy SM. Management of hypertriglyceridemic patients: B. Dietary management of hypertriglyceridemic patients. *Am J Cardiol.* 1991;68:35A–42A.

Castelli WP, et al. Incidence of coronary heart disease and lipoprotein cholesterol levels: The Framingham Study. *JAMA.* 1986;256:2835–2838.

Chait A, Brunzell JD. Acquired hyperlipidemia (secondary hyperlipoproteinemias). *Endocrinol Metab Clin North Am.* 1990;19:259–278.

Chambless LE, et al. The association of corneal arcus with coronary heart disease and cardiovascular disease mortality in the Lipid Research Clinics Mortality Follow-up Study. *Am J Public Health.* 1990;80:1200–1204.

Davidson MH. Implications for the present and direction for the future. *Am J Cardiol.* 1993;71:32B–36B.

Drood JM, et al. Nicotinic acid for the treatment of hyperlipoproteinemia. *J Clin Pharmacol.* 1991;31:641–650.

Dunn FL. Management of hyperlipidemia in diabetes mellitus. *Endocrinol Metab Clin North Am.* 1992;21:395–414.

Expert Panel. Report of the National Cholesterol Education Program Expert Panel on Detection, Evaluation, and Treatment of High Blood Cholesterol in Adults. *Arch Intern Med.* 1988;148:36–69.

Expert Panel. Summary of the second report of the National Cholesterol Education Program (NCEP) Expert Panel on Detection, Evaluation, and Treatment of High Blood Cholesterol in Adults (Adult Treatment Panel II). *JAMA.* 1993;269:3015–3023.

Franklin FA, Brown RF, Franklin CC. Screening, diagnosis, and management of dyslipoproteinemia in children. *Endocrinol Metab Clin North Am.* 1990;19:399–449.

Fraunfelder FT. Ocular examination before initiation of lovastatin (Mevacor) therapy. *Am J Ophthalmol.* 1988;105:91–92.

Ginsberg HN. Lipoprotein physiology and its relationship to atherogenesis. *Endocrinol Metab Clin North Am.* 1990; 19:211–228.

Ginsberg HN. Lipoprotein physiology in nondiabetic and diabetic states: Relationship to atherogenesis. *Diabetes Care.* 1991;14:839–855.

Goodman DS. New guidelines for lowering blood cholesterol. *Clin Lab Med.* 1989;9:17–27.

Gordon DJ. Role of circulating high-density lipoprotein and triglycerides in coronary artery disease: Risk and prevention. *Endocrinol Metab Clin North Am.* 1990;19:299–309.

Gotto AM: Dyslipidemia and atherosclerosis: A forecast of pharmaceutical approaches. *Circulation.* 1993;87:III-56–III-59.

Gotto AM. Hypertriglyceridemia: Risks and perspectives. *Am J Cardiol.* 1992;70:19H–25H.

Gotto AM. Overview of current issues in management of dyslipidemia. *Am J Cardiol.* 1993;71:3B–8B.

Gotto AM. Prognostic and therapeutic significance of low levels of high-density lipoprotein cholesterol. *Arch Intern Med.* 1999;159:1038–1040.

Gotto AM. Rationale for treatment. *Am J Med.* 1991;91(suppl 1B):31S–36S.

Grundy SM. Cholesterol and coronary heart disease: A new era. *JAMA.* 1986;256(20):2849–2858.

Grundy SM. Cholesterol lowering drugs as cardioprotective agents. *Am J Cardiol.* 1992;70:271–321.

Haffner SM. Diabetes, hyperlipidemia, and coronary artery disease. *Am J Cardiol.* 1999;83:17F–21F.

Harper CR, Jacobson TA. New perspectives on the management of low levels of high-density lipoprotein cholesterol. *Arch Intern Med.* 1999;159:1049–1057.

Hensrud DD. Clinical preventive medicine in primary care: Background and practice: 3. Delivering preventive screening services. *Mayo Clin Proc.* 2000;75:381–385.

Hunningshake DB: Drug treatment of dyslipoproteinemia. *Endocrinol Metab Clin North Am.* 1990;19:345–360.

Jialal I. A practical approach to the laboratory diagnosis of dyslipidemia. *Am J Clin Pathol.* 1996;106:128–138.

Jones PH. A clinical overview of dyslipidemias: Treatment strategies. *Am J Med.* 1992;93:187–198.

Krauss RM. Triglycerides and atherogenic lipoproteins: Rationale for lipid management. *Am J Med.* 1998; 105(1A):58S–62S.

LaRosa JC, et al. The cholesterol facts. A summary of evidence relating dietary fats, serum cholesterol, and coronary heart disease. A joint statement by the American Heart Association and the National Heart, Lung, and Blood Institute. *Circulation.* 1990;81:1721–1733.

Lavie CJ, et al. High density lipoprotein cholesterol: Recommendations for routine testing and treatment. *Postgrad Med.* 1990;87:36–51.

Levy RI, Troendle AJ, Fattu JM. A quarter century of drug treatment of dyslipoproteinemia, with a focus on the new HMG-CoA reductase inhibitor fluvastatin. *Circulation.* 1993;87:III-45–III-53.

Lipid Research Clinics Program. The Lipid Research Clinics coronary primary prevention trial results: I. Reduction in incidence of coronary heart disease. *JAMA.* 1984;251:351–364.

Lipid Research Clinics Program. The Lipid Research Clinics coronary primary prevention trial results: II. The relationship of reduction in incidence of coronary heart disease to cholesterol lowering. *JAMA.* 1984;251:365–374.

Lipsky H, Gloger M, Frishman WH. Dietary fiber for reducing blood cholesterol. *J Clin Pharmacol.* 1990;30:699–703.

Malenka DJ, Baron JA. Cholesterol and coronary heart disease: The attributable risk reduction of diet and drugs. *Arch Intern Med.* 1989;149:1981–1985.

Mancini M, et al. Acquired (secondary) forms of hypertriglyceridemia. *Am J Cardiol.* 1991;68:17A–21A.

McNamara DJ, Howell WH. Epidemiologic data linking diet to hyperlipidemia and arteriosclerosis. *Semin Liver Dis.* 1992;12:347–355.

Miller VT. Dyslipoproteinemia in women: Special considerations. *Endocrinol Metab Clin North Am.* 1990;19:381–398.

Montalto SJ. Lovastatin and cataracts: An update. *Clin Eye Vision Care.* 1989;1:212–217.

National Center for Health Statistics: National Heart, Lung, and Blood Institute Collaborative Lipid Group. Trends in serum cholesterol levels among U.S. adults aged 20 to 74 years. *JAMA.* 1987;257:937–942.

National Heart, Lung, and Blood Institute Consensus Development Panel. Treatment of hypertriglyceridemia. *JAMA.* 1984;281:1196–1200.

Nishimoto JH, et al. Corneal arcus as an indicator of hypercholesterolemia. *J Am Optom Assoc.* 1990;61:44–49.

Pearson TA. Therapeutic management of triglycerides: An international perspective. *Am J Cardiol.* 1992;70:26H–31H.

Phillips CI, Tsukahara S, Gore SM. Corneal arcus: Some morphology and applied pathophysiology. *Jpn J Ophthalmol.* 1990;34:442–449.

Rekhraj S, Hsia J. Evaluation and management of lipid disorders. *Curr Opin Cardiol.* 1999;14:298–302.

Schonfeld G. Inherited disorders of lipid transport. *Endocrinol Metab Clin North Am.* 1990;19:229–257.

Scott D, Kurenitz M. Using lipid lowering agents effectively: When diet is not enough. *Postgrad Med.* 1990;87:171–186.

Segal P et al. The Lipid Research Clinics Program Prevalence Study: The association of dyslipoproteinemia with corneal arcus and xanthelasma. *Circulation.* 1986;73(suppl I): 108–118.

Sempos C, et al. The prevalence of high blood cholesterol levels among adults in the United States. *JAMA.* 1989; 262:45–52.

Simmons LA. Choosing the most appropriate therapy for lipid disorders. *Aust Fam Physician.* 2000;29:199–203.

Stamler J, et al. Is the relationship between serum cholesterol and risk of premature death from coronary heart disease continuous and graded? *JAMA.* 1986;256:2823–2838.

Stein EA. Management of hypercholesterolemia: Approach to diet and drug therapy. *Am J Med.* 1989;87(suppl 4A): 20S–27S.

Stein EA, Steiner PM. Triglyceride measurement and its relationship to heart disease. *Clin Lab Med.* 1989;9:169–185.

Steiner G, Shafrir E. *Primary Hyperlipoproteinemias.* New York: McGraw-Hill; 1991.

Varnek L, Schnohr P, Jensen G. Presenile corneal arcus in healthy persons. A possible cardiovascular risk indicator in younger adults. *Acta Ophthalmol.* 1979;57:755–765.

Wilson PWF. The epidemiology of hypercholesterolemia: A global perspective. *Am J Med.* 1989;87(suppl 4A): 5S–13S.

Working Group on Management of Patients with Hypertension and High Blood Cholesterol. National Education Programs Working Group Report on the Management of Patients with Hypertension and High Blood Cholesterol. *Ann Int Med.* 1991;114:224–237.

Yeshurun D, Gotto AM. Hyperlipidemia: Perspectives in diagnosis and treatment. *South Med J.* 1995;88:379–391.

Chapter 59

ALBINISM

Jerome Sherman, Sherry J. Bass

Albinism is a congenital deficiency in pigment that has been recognized since ancient times. Early writings suggest that Noah of the Biblical period was an albino. In contrast to the generalized or universal form of albinism, albinism affecting only the eye was not recognized until the beginning of the 20th century.

When the enzyme tyrosinase is present and functioning properly, tyrosine is converted into melanin, resulting in normal skin and eye color. In all forms of albinism, melanocytes are present but are amelanotic due to absent, relatively deficient, or poorly functional tyrosinase (Carr & Siegel, 1981). When tyrosinase is absent, the term used is tyrosinase-negative. In this case, hair, skin, and ocular findings are more prominent than in the tyrosinase-positive form, in which at least some tyrosinase can be demonstrated. Other forms of albinism exist, such as cutaneous albinism, ocular albinism, and the rarer Hermansky–Pudlak (HP) and Prader–Willi (PW) syndromes.

EPIDEMIOLOGY

Cutaneous Albinism

No epidemiological data are available in the literature concerning cutaneous albinism.

Oculocutaneous Albinism

There are four subtypes of oculocutaneous albinism. All are inherited as autosomal recessive traits. Each subtype is relatively rare, and the incidence in the United States and Europe ranges from 1 in 10,000 to 1 in 40,000.

Ocular Albinism

Ocular albinism had been thought to be inherited as an X-linked trait. In the late 1970s, a new form of ocular albinism, inherited as an autosomal recessive trait, was reported (O'Donnell et al, 1976). The incidence of X-linked ocular albinism is 1 in 50,000, and although the incidence of autosomal recessive ocular albinism is not known with certainty, it is probably the more common form of ocular albinism (O'Donnell & Green, 1987).

Hermansky–Pudlak and Prader–Willi Syndromes

In Puerto Rico the prevalence of HP syndrome is 1 in 1800 people with albinism. The incidence of PW syndrome is estimated to be 1 in 25,000 people with albinism.

PATHOPHYSIOLOGY/DISEASE PROCESS

Cutaneous Albinism

Although not frequently encountered by the eyecare practitioner, these individuals typically have hypopigmentation of the skin but normally pigmented and functioning eyes. The most obvious finding is a white frontal hair lock with occasional hypopigmentation on the forehead. Visual function is normal.

Oculocutaneous Albinism

The hereditary pattern is mostly autosomal recessive, although the tyrosinase-negative and tyrosinase-positive forms represent different genotypes. Thus, it is possible for a tyrosinase-negative albino married to a tyrosinase-positive albino to have all "normal" children, although they will all be carriers of two different recessive genes. In Caucasians the skin is quite light and sometimes described as milk white (Figure 59–1). In African-American albinos, the skin color is lighter than unaffected family members but slightly darker than most Caucasians.

Most individuals with oculocutaneous albinism (especially the complete or tyrosinase-negative type) burn in the sun and never tan. Slow tanning does occur, however, in the mild forms of the tyrosinase-positive or incomplete albinism. Although the underlying condition changes little over time, continued exposure to ultraviolet rays may lead to precancerous keratosis, and squamous and basal cell carcinoma. Amelanotic malignant melanomas also have been reported. Those with the mild form of tyrosinase-positive albinism who tan slowly, appear to be at a lower risk of serious dermatologic consequences.

The hair of the tyrosinase-negative albino is usually described as straw or platinum in color. The hair of the tyrosinase-positive albino may be nearly as light in the early years of life, but generally darkens with age.

Ocular findings include reduced central vision, nystagmus, iris transillumination (Figure 59–2), decreased pigmentation of the fundus, poor foveal development, and ill-defined macular landmarks (Figure 59–3).

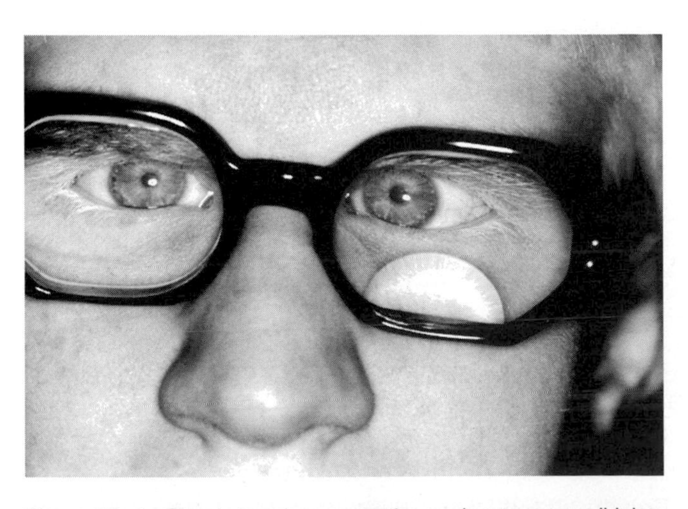

Figure 59–1. Classic tyrosinase-negative oculocutaneous albinism showing hair, skin, eyes. *(Courtesy of Bruce Rosenthal, OD.)*

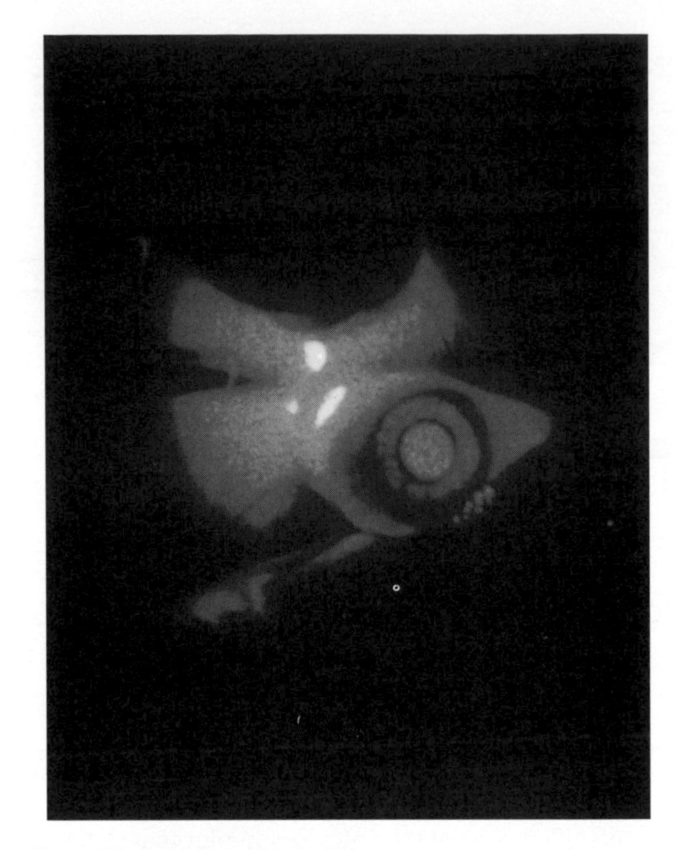

Figure 59–2. Iris transillumination.

Ocular Albinism

Although the skin and hair appear normal in ocular albinism, the same ocular manifestations seen in oculocutaneous albinism are clearly present. Some patients with ocular albinism have jet-black hair, dark skin, brown eyes that demonstrate iris transillumination, and macular hypoplasia with resultant nystagmus and reduced visual acuity.

Clinically, ocular albinism appears limited to the eyes, but skin biopsies reveal unusual macromelanosomes (abnormally formed melanin granules) in the dermis and epidermis. These diagnostic macromelanosomes appear only in X-linked ocular albinism and have not been found in autosomal recessive ocular albinism (Creel et al, 1974).

The impaired ocular function in autosomal recessive ocular albinism may be due to altered neuroectoderm (the retinal and iris pigment epithelium), whereas the skin, hair, and iris stroma are normal due to intact neural-crest derived melanocytes.

On rare occasion, nystagmus may decrease slowly in time, with subtle improvement in visual acuity. Clin-

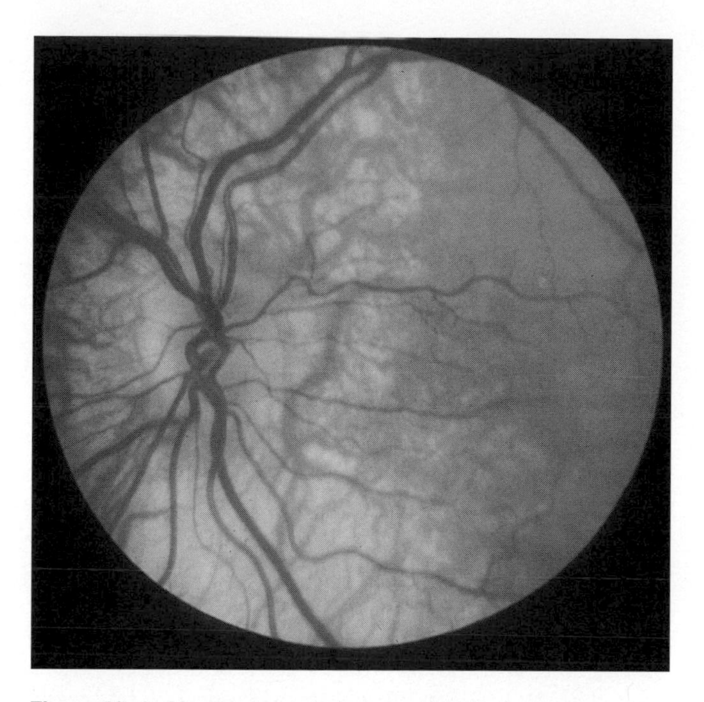

Figure 59–3. Macular hypoplasia in an albinotic fundus.

ically, overall visual function generally remains unchanged, in spite of electroretinogram (ERG) amplitudes that begin supernormal in the early years and slowly decrease to an abnormal range. This suggests slow destruction of the photoreceptors, most likely due to excessive light exposure.

HP and PW Syndromes

Several rare syndromes with life-threatening manifestations exist. HP syndrome is the association of oculocutaneous albinism with defective platelet function leading to an increased bleeding tendency. Easy bruisability and gum bleeding are common in HP syndrome.

HP in Puerto Rican albinos should be suspected because they appear to be at a higher risk. Aspirin use can be life threatening in HP patients, and death can be caused by fibrotic restrictive pulmonary disease. Ceroid (yellowish-brown lipid end-products of unsaturated fatty acid metabolism) may accumulate in tissues in HP, and an enteropathic disorder resembling Crohn disease has also been reported (Simon et al, 1982). It is unclear whether this disorder is actually caused by the ceroid.

PW syndrome is characterized by muscular hypotonia, hypogenitalism, obesity, mental retardation, short stature, and diminished sensitivity to pain. A single chromosomal abnormality has been demonstrated as a frequent cause of PW (Ledbetter et al, 1981). This subtle abnormality, an interstitial deletion on the proximal long arm of one of the number 15 chromosomes, can be easily missed unless specifically considered during chromosomal analysis. In 1982, a previously missed component of the PW syndrome was recognized, that of oculocutaneous albinoidism (Hittner et al, 1982). Nine patients were found with PW who also had decreased tyrosinase activity in isolated hair bulbs, light hair and skin, decreased pigmentation of the iris stroma, and variable amounts of iris translucency. However, none had reduced vision, nystagmus, photophobia, or foveal hypoplasia; hence the term "albinoidism."

> Any patient presenting with reduced visual acuity and nystagmus should have iris transillumination testing performed, regardless of skin and hair color, to rule out albinism.

DIAGNOSIS

When a patient presents with congenital nystagmus and reduced best corrected visual acuity, albinism is one of several conditions to consider in the differential diagnosis (Table 59–1). The tyrosinase-negative oculocutaneous albino, with platinum hair and diaphanous blue eyes, is easily diagnosed. However, albinism is best considered a syndrome with a variety of clinical expressions (Table 59–2). Some patients with albinism present with findings so subtle that the correct diagnosis is often overlooked. Occasionally the examination of family members becomes essential if the actual

TABLE 59–1. DIFFERENTIAL DIAGNOSIS OF ALBINISM—OTHER DISEASES CAUSING NYSTAGMUS OR IRIS TRANSILLUMINATION

Condition	Clinical Characteristics
Aniridia	Nystagmus, absence or maldevelopment of iris tissue, reduced VA
Congenital optic atrophy	Nystagmus, pale optic nerve heads, reduced VA
Leber congenital amaurosis	Nystagmus, flat electroretinogram (ERG), very poor VA
Achromatopsia	Nystagmus, poor color vision, reduced or flat photopic ERG, reduced VA
Pigmentary dispersion syndrome	Iris transillumination, concave iris, heavy pigmented trabeculum, normal VA

TABLE 59–2. SYSTEMIC MANIFESTATIONS OF ALBINISM

Cutaneous Albinism
- White frontal hair lock
- Hypopigmentation of skin—occasionally of forehead

Oculocutaneous Albinism
- **Tyrosinase negative**
  - Light skin (burns easily)
  - White hair
  - (−) tyrosinase activity in hair bulbs
  - No melanin
- **Tyrosinase positive**
  - Light skin (burns easily)
  - White to yellow hair
  - Normal to increased tyrosinase activity in hair bulbs
  - Trace melanin

Ocular Albinism
- **X-linked**
  - Light skin (may or may not tan)
  - Normal hair
  - Normal tyrosinase activity in hair bulbs
  - Abnormally formed melanin
- **Autosomal recessive**
  - Light skin (may or may not tan)
  - Normal hair
  - Normal tyrosinase activity in hair bulbs
  - Normal melanosomes in skin

HP Syndrome
- Light skin (freckles, burns easily)
- White to brown hair
- Normal tyrosinase activity in hair bulbs
- Incompletely melanized melanosomes in skin
- Other: easy bruisability, gum bleeding, platelet function defect (prolonged bleeding time), enteropathic disorder

PW Syndrome
- Light skin
- Light hair
- Decreased tyrosinase activity in hair bulbs
- Other: interstitial deletion on long arm of chromosome #15, muscular hypotonia, hypogenitalism, obesity, mental retardation, short stature, diminished sensitivity to pain

diagnosis is ever to be appreciated. If viewed as a syndrome, as few as two but often all of the components listed in Table 59–3 under "oculocutaneous form" will be identifiable.

The typical patient with albinism presents at a young age with photophobia and reduced vision. Nystagmus is usually of the horizontal pendular variety, but a rotary component may be observed. The nystagmus may lessen at near, and with a very reduced reading distance the child may be able to distinguish reading material. This may be due to the accommodative and vergence system coming into play as well as the change in head position. Color vision testing and visual fields are generally normal and are most useful in ruling out some other conditions causing nystagmus and reduced visual acuity, such as achromatopsia, optic nerve hypoplasia, retinal degeneration (Leber congenital amaurosis), and macular scar.

TABLE 59–3. CRITERIA FOR DIAGNOSIS OF ALBINISM

Oculocutaneous Form
- Light skin, hair, and fundus color
- Nystagmus
- Reduced visual acuity
- Iris transillumination
- Foveal hypoplasia

Ocular Form
- Nystagmus
- Reduced visual acuity
- Iris transillumination
- Foveal hypoplasia

Iris transillumination is a translucency of the iris due to defects in the iris pigment epithelium (Table 59–4). Variable amounts of iris transillumination should be present in every albino. Testing should occur in a completely black room after 30 seconds of dark adaptation, and a well-charged halogen transilluminator should be ideally placed directly on the globe near the equator. Grading the transillumination is useful, because the greater the transillumination, the more likely the diagnosis of albinism. None, trace, and 1+ through 4+ are the grades suggested.

Although a positive iris transillumination is most helpful in diagnosing the subtle forms of albinism, it

TABLE 59–4. OCULAR MANIFESTATIONS OF ALBINISM

Cutaneous Albinism
- Normal ocular structures and normal visual functioning

Oculocutaneous Albinism (OCA)
- Light blue irides
- Nystagmus—congenital, bilateral and usually pendular
- Reduced visual acuity (20/20− to 20/800−), almost always bilateral
- Photophobia
- Iris transillumination, occasionally very subtle
- Foveal hypoplasia
- Macular hypoplasia
- Small capillary free zone in posterior pole
- Hypopigmentation of choroid and retinal pigment epithelium
- Prominent observable choroidal vessels
- Bihemispheric VEP asymmetries

Ocular Albinism
- Normal irides *plus* any of the other manifestations listed under OCA

HP Syndrome
- Blue to brown irides *plus* any of the other manifestations listed under OCA

PW Syndrome
- Blue to brown irides
- Variable iris transillumination

is not pathognomonic. It may occur in pigmentary glaucoma, pigmentary dispersion syndrome, pseudoexfoliation, chronic open-angle glaucoma, and chronic recurrent uveitis (Krill, 1972). Lightly pigmented, nonalbinotic patients may exhibit trace to 1+ iris transillumination as well.

Visual acuity is quite variable in albinism and ranges from 20/20 to 20/800. Most albinos have visual acuity in the 20/100 to 20/400 range. The patient with only trace nystagmus, and visual acuity of 20/20, 3 to 4+ transillumination, poor foveal and macular landmarks, and siblings with albinism might be considered a forme fruste albino by some. Others may use the term "albinoidism" to describe this clinical presentation. Of particular interest are a few asymptomatic individuals with normal visual acuity but no identifiable fovea among family members with albinism.

Most patients with albinism have no clinically demonstrable fovea, poorly defined macular landmarks, and capillaries that appear to traverse the macula, sometimes encroaching on the spot where the foveal reflex should be present. Minimal retinal and choroidal pigment allows the large choroidal vessels to be easily observed.

Refractive error measurements in albinism are widely scattered and thus are not diagnostic. Fonda (1962) reported that well over one third of nearly 300 albino eyes had astigmatism greater than three diopters. In addition, over one third had moderate to high myopia and over one third had mild to moderate hyperopia. Strabismus was also present in over one third of the sample as well, with exotropia diagnosed in 83 patients and esotropia in 28.

In questionable cases, the diagnosis can be supported by a specific electrophysiological profile. The electroretinogram (ERG) shows large supernormal responses in essentially all young albinos. This is probably due to the light energy of the flash bouncing around the eye until much of it is eventually absorbed by the photoreceptors. In a normally pigmented eye, light absorbed by the retinal and choroidal pigment has no influence on the size of the ERG. As the albino ages, the ERG amplitude gradually drops to the normal range and then often to the subnormal range, possibly due to chronic overexposure to light and eventual retinal degeneration.

Clinically, ERGs are not particularly useful in the diagnosis of albinism, and reductions in amplitude over time do not appear to have a clinical correlate with age. Most albinos report that their vision either has remained the same or has actually gotten somewhat better as they get older. Visual acuity measurements generally appear unchanged with time. Occasionally, an albino may form pigment at the macula as he or she grows older, and demonstrate an improvement in visual acuity.

The electrooculogram (EOG) is the best clinical test of retinal pigment epithelial function. Available data suggest large amplitudes during light adaptation and larger than normal Arden ratios. Like the ERG, the EOG is not used for the clinical diagnosis of albinism.

The visual evoked potential (VEP), in contrast to ERGs and EOGs and when performed under appropriate conditions, is quite useful in the diagnosis of albinism (Table 59–5). Standard pattern VEPs using only one occipital electrode will reveal the typical VEP profile found in any macular abnormality. VEPs to fine checks or gratings will be flat because under these conditions, VEPs reflect the foveal and macular pathways. As the pattern size increases, generally the VEP amplitude increases. But albinos have a unique feature that can be elegantly demonstrated with VEPs using bihemispheric recordings. During the past three decades a wealth of scientific reports have shown that the human albino, like the albino rat, pig, and Siamese cat, have disorganized uncrossed retinogeniculate striate projections. In normal humans, about half of the optic nerve crosses at the chiasm, allowing all nasal fibers to decussate. However, in albinos not only do the nasal fibers cross, but many temporal fibers do as well. VEPs recorded from both occipital hemispheres in normal patients are quite symmetric, because half of the optic nerve fibers project to the right hemisphere while the other half project to the left hemisphere. Asymmetry of the VEPs using bihemispheric recordings appears to be a universal finding in all forms of albinism. Some clinical researchers claim they can diagnose all cases of albinism solely on the basis of bihemispheric VEP recordings (P. Apkarian, personal communication). Although brain tumors, cerebrovascular accidents, and aneurysms can also cause asymmetric VEPs, the diagnosis of albinism is generally made in the very young, who are not likely to be suffering from such neurological problems. In addition, these conditions can be diagnosed based on other signs and symptoms.

Mutations in several genes have been reported to be responsible for the various forms of oculocutaneous and ocular albinism. The tyrosinase gene (TYR), the

TABLE 59–5. DIAGNOSTIC TESTING FOR ALBINISM

Diagnosis is made primarily based upon clinical characteristics (eg, nystagmus and iris transillumination).

Visual evoked potential (VEP)

May reveal asymmetry between hemispheres due to abnormal decussation of some temporal fibers along with the nasal fibers in the chiasm.

OCA2 gene, the tyrosinase-related protein-1 gene (TYRP1), the HPS gene (Hermansky–Pudlak syndrome), the CHS gene (CHS1) in Chediak–Higashi syndrome, and the X-linked ocular albinism gene have all been identified. However, the functions of only the TYR and TYRP1 gene are known. These genes are enzymes in the melanin biosynthetic pathway.

The importance of viewing albinism as a continuum has been well demonstrated by a study of albinotic characteristics of 13 family members who were graded clinically, electrophysiologically, and biochemically. The authors (Simon et al, 1982) point out that the correlation between visual acuity and nystagmus was "particularly strong," and suggest that nystagmus imposes a visual deficit beyond that related to foveal hypoplasia alone. Thus the "variable expression of albinism," an expression used by Simon and associates (1982), should be recognized by clinicians, and in difficult cases examination of family members is clearly indicated. Even monocular albinism appears possible (Sherman, 1991).

HP and PW

HP syndrome should be considered in Puerto Rican albinos and in those albinos who bruise easily and report excessive bleeding. A hematologist should be consulted. The diagnosis is based upon prolonged bleeding time with a normal platelet count, normal prothrombin time (PT), normal partial thromboplastin time (PTT), and normal factor VIII determinations accompanied by a platelet function defect characterized by diminished platelet aggregation and serotonin uptake (Simon et al, 1982). The diagnosis of PW can be supported by chromosome analysis (Hittner et al, 1982).

TREATMENT AND MANAGEMENT

Table 59–6 summarizes the treatment and management of albinism.

TABLE 59–6. TREATMENT AND MANAGEMENT OF ALBINISM

Cutaneous Albinism
• **Systemic**
Protective sunwear
Sunblock lotion
• **Ocular**
None
Oculocutaneous Albinism
• **Systemic**
Protective sunwear
Sunblock lotion
• **Ocular**
Protective sunshades with side shields
Correction of refractive error
Low-vision devices
Auditory feedback to reduce nystagmus
Ocular Albinism
• **Systemic**
Protective sunwear
Sunblock lotion
• **Ocular**
Protective sunshades with side shields
Correction of refractive error
Low-vision devices
Auditory feedback to reduce nystagmus
HP Syndrome
• **Systemic**
Protective sunwear
Sunblock lotion
Hematology consult
Avoidance of antiplatelet drugs (eg, aspirin)
Avoidance of surgery unless essential
• **Ocular**
Protective sunshades with side shields
Correction of refractive error
Low-vision devices
Auditory feedback to reduce nystagmus
PW Syndrome
• **Systemic**
Protective sunwear
Sunblock lotion
• **Ocular**
Protective sunshades with side shields

Systemic

Due to unpredictable breaks in the ozone layer, essentially everyone should limit exposure to sunlight and artificial sources of ultraviolet rays. However, the albino is at an even greater risk of precancerous keratosis, squamous cell and basal cell carcinoma, and amelanotic malignant melanomas. The use of sunscreen products, umbrellas, hats, and other protective clothing should be emphasized.

If the diagnosis of HP syndrome is established, antiplatelet drugs such as aspirin must be avoided. Surgery should be avoided unless essential. There are no known treatment recommendations for PW syndrome. However, because of the chromosomal abnormality found in this disease, genetic counseling should be offered to affected patients.

Ocular

Various absorptive lenses in addition to frames with side shields should be considered or advised. Light tints are sometimes adequate to lessen photophobia and occasional glare. Many albinos have large refractive errors requiring correction with spectacles or contact lenses. The young albino generally needs only to move closer to printed material. Based upon the patient's age and visual acuity, adds from +2.00 to +10.00 should be attempted. Telescopes and microscopes are often helpful. Low-vision specialists (B. Rosenthal, personal communication) report that virtually all albinos can be helped visually with various tints and low-vision devices.

Auditory biofeedback for the amelioration of nystagmus has met with some success (S. Goldrich, personal communication).

CONCLUSION

Albinism is actually a spectrum of diseases with many different presentations. Although all forms of albinism have in common some problem with pigmentation in the skin and eye, these structures may be variably affected. Even within families, members may be affected differently.

The eyecare practitioner must consider albinism when presented with any patient with either reduced vision from birth and/or nystagmus. Albinos, especially the ocular types, are easy to miss. Because some forms of albinism are associated with other systemic problems, the proper diagnosis becomes extremely important.

REFERENCES

Butler MG. Prader–Willi syndrome. Current understanding of cause and diagnosis. *Am J Med Genet.* 1990;35:319–332.

Carr RE, Siegel IM. The retinal pigment epithelium in ocular albinism. In: Duane TD, ed. *Clinical Ophthalmology.* Philadelphia: Harper & Row; 1981;4:413–423.

Creel D, O'Donnell E Jr, Witkop C Jr. Visual system anomalies in human ocular albinos. *Science.* 1978;201:931–933.

Creel D, Witkop C Jr, King RA. Asymmetric visually evoked potentials in human albinos: Evidence for visual system anomalies. *Invest Ophthalmol.* 1974;13:430–440.

Donaldson DD. Transillumination of the iris. *Trans Am Ophthalmol Soc.* 1974;72:89–105.

Fonda G. Characteristics and low vision corrections in albinism. *Arch Ophthalmol.* 1962;68:754.

Hittner HM, King RA, Riccardi VM, et al. Oculocutaneous albinoidism as a manifestation of reduced neural crest derivatives in the Prader–Willi syndrome. *Am J Ophthalmol.* 1982;94:328–337.

Krill AE. Albinism. In: Krill AE, ed. *Krill's Hereditary Retinal and Choroidal Diseases.* Philadelphia: Harper & Row; 1972:645–663.

Ledbetter DH, Riccardi VM, Airhardt SD, et al. Deletions of chromosome 15 as a cause of the Prader–Willi syndrome. *N Engl J Med.* 1981;304:325.

O'Donnell FE, Green WR. The eye in albinism. In: Duane TD, ed. *Clinical Ophthalmology.* Philadelphia: Harper & Row; 1987;4:6.

O'Donnell FE, Hambrick GW Jr, Green WR, et al. X-linked ocular albinism. An oculotaneous macromelanosomal disorder. *Arch Ophthalmol.* 1976;94:1883–1892.

Oetting WS, King RA. Molecular basis of albinism: Mutations and polymorphisms of pigmentation genes associated with albinism. *Hum Mutat.* 1999;13:99–115.

Sherman J. Patient management: The case of the colorful patient. *Optom Management.* 1991;26:56–57.

Simon JW, Adams RJ, Calhoun JH, et al. Ophthalmic manifestations of the Hermansky–Pudlak syndrome (oculocutaneous albinism and hemorrhage diathesis). *Am J Ophthalmol.* 1982;93:71–77.

Witkop CJ, Pineiro B, Almadovar C, Nunez-Babcock M. Hermansky–Pudlak syndrome. An epidemiologic study. *Ophthal Pediatr Genet.* 1990;11:250–295.

Chapter 60

WILSON DISEASE

Kelly H. Thomann

Wilson disease, also called hepatolenticular degeneration, is an inherited autosomal recessive disorder of copper metabolism and excretion. The liver's ability to transport and store copper in the bile is impaired, resulting in toxic accumulations in the liver, central nervous system, cornea, kidney, and other organs.

The systemic manifestations and severity of Wilson disease are variable. These include liver, neurologic, psychiatric, blood, kidney, bone, and joint disturbances. Females present more often with liver disease and males with neurological features.

The Kayser–Fleischer ring, a deposition of copper in the cornea, is the classic feature of Wilson disease. Copper deposition is also seen in the lens and is known as a "sunflower cataract."

EPIDEMIOLOGY

Systemic

- Incidence ranges from 1 in 30,000 to 1 in 200,000 live births.
- Prevalence is approximately 15 to 30 million persons.
- Gene frequency varies between 0.3 and 0.7%, which corresponds to a heterozygous carrier rate of slightly greater than 1 in 100.
- There is no ethnic or geographic predisposition.
- The distribution is equal male to female.

Ocular

- The Kayser–Fleischer ring is present in 100% of cases with neurologic findings and 70 to 90% of cases with liver disease.
- The sunflower cataract is present in 15 to 20% of patients.

PATHOPHYSIOLOGY/DISEASE PROCESS

Systemic

- Patients with Wilson disease exhibit impaired biliary excretion of copper.
- The biochemical defect is present at birth, but most patients become symptomatic during adolescence or from their twenties to thirties.
- An abnormal gene, located on chromosome 13, is responsible for the sequence of events leading to the abnormal transport of copper in varying degrees at different cellular sites.
- The harmful effects of excess copper are mediated by the generation of free radicals, which disrupts a number of intracellular systems.
- The primary defect is located in the liver lysosome. It results in a reduction of copper incorporated into ceruloplasmin, the major copper transport protein. Excess copper leads to toxicity, manifested as acute or chronic liver disease.

- Excess copper is released into the blood and excreted through the kidneys, where it can become deposited in the brain, kidneys, and eyes.
- Most patients with Wilson disease first present with hepatic and/or neurologic dysfunction (Table 60–1).
- Hepatic manifestations follow three major patterns:

1. Cirrhosis
2. Chronic active hepatitis
3. Fulminant hepatic failure

- Neurologic and psychiatric complications occur later.
- Motor (neurologic) abnormalities include bradykinesia, rigidity, tremor, ataxia, drooling, and difficulty controlling speech and writing.
- Psychiatric abnormalities include behavioral and cognitive impairment, affective disorder, and psychosis.
- Clinical manifestations can be reversible if treated prior to permanent damage to the brain and liver.
- The disease can be fatal if treatment is delayed.

Detection of the Kayser–Fleischer ring through biomicroscopy is a simple screening tool to detect Wilson disease in symptomatic patients (it is present in 100% of patients with neurologic findings and up to 90% of patients with liver disease) and in asymptomatic patients with a positive family history.

Ocular

- The Kayser–Fleischer ring (Figure 60–1) appears as a golden brown, ruby-red, or green-brown band (Table 60–2).
- The rings are often visible grossly (without the use of a biomicroscope).
  - The size ranges from 1.0 to 3.0 mm.
  - It starts at the limbus, at the level of Descemet membrane.
  - The ring consists of nonuniform layers of unequal-size granules rich in copper and sulfur; they are separated by clear intervals of variable width.

TABLE 60–1. SYSTEMIC MANIFESTATIONS OF WILSON DISEASE

Organ or System	Systemic Manifestations
Liver	• Deposition of copper in the liver is always the first expression of the disease • Liver damage may present as: Asymptomatic Acute hepatitis (self-limited) Fulminant hepatitis (usually lethal) Chronic acute hepatitis (parenchymal liver disease) Cirrhosis (chronic, progressive liver disease)
Nervous system	• Extrapyramidal dysfunction and/or cerebellar dysfunction: May be the first clinical expression; possible symptoms: resting and intention tremor, spasticity, rigidity, choreic movements, slowness of movement, excess salivation, dysphagia, dysarthria, hoarseness • "Classic" neurologic syndrome noted after disease progression: dysphagia, drooling, rigidity, slowness of limb movements, fixed posture/facial muscles, dysarthria, wing beating tremor
Psychiatric	• May manifest as: Schizophrenia Mania Depression Psychosis Neuroses Bizarre behavioral disturbances
Other	• Blood disorders • Joint and bone disorders • Kidney disease • Primary or secondary amenorrhea • Spontaneous abortion

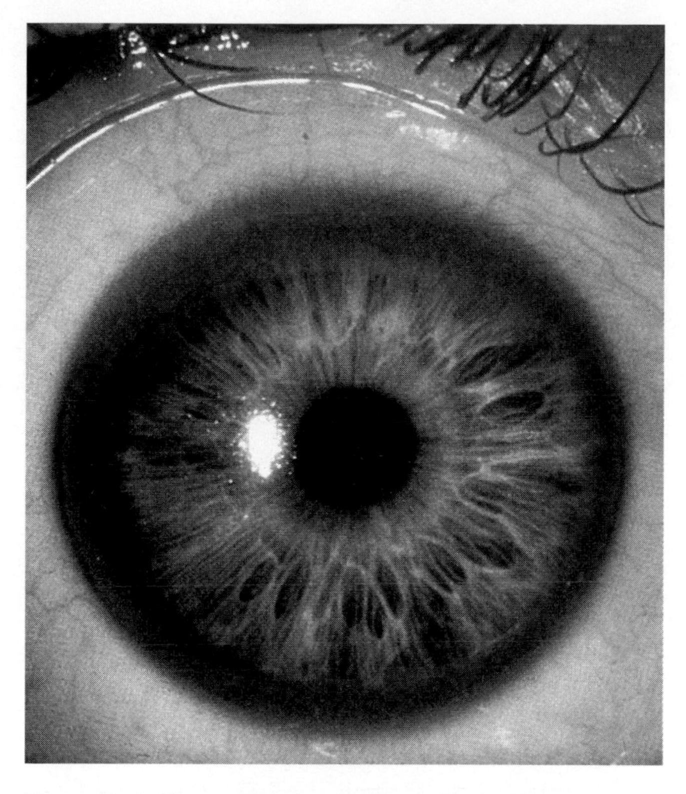

Figure 60–1. Kayser–Fleischer ring located in the Descemet membrane can be identified by external inspection. *(Reprinted with permission from Finley TF.* Wilson disease. J Am Optom Assoc. *1988; 59:1119.)*

- The ring begins in the superior periphery of the cornea from 10 to 2 o'clock and spreads slowly toward the horizontal plane while gradually broadening; later it begins inferiorly from 5 to 7 o'clock and in time the arcs meet. Therefore, it fades toward the center of the cornea and is more pronounced peripherally.
- The "sunflower" cataract is less common than the Kayser–Fleischer ring.
  - It appears as a centrally pigmented opacity of the lens with tapering extensions that resemble the petals of a sunflower.
  - It consists of copper granules located in the anterior subcapsular lens and occasionally the posterior lens capsule.
  - It does not impair vision.

TABLE 60–2. OCULAR MANIFESTATIONS OF WILSON DISEASE

- Kayser–Fleischer corneal pigment ring
- Sunflower cataract

DIAGNOSIS

Systemic

- Slit-lamp biomicroscopy is the simplest screening test for Wilson disease.
- The diagnosis is conclusive when the triad of liver disease, Kayser–Fleischer rings, and extrapyramidal motor disorders is present.
- The diagnosis is also conclusive if a similar syndrome exists in a sibling.
- Diagnosis is not always straightforward because systemic manifestations often vary; differential diagnoses must be ruled out (Table 60–3).
- The diagnosis is rarely established based upon a single test; clinical and laboratory data must be correlated.
- The diagnostic criteria vary according to clinical signs and symptoms (Table 60–4).
- Twenty percent of chronic liver disease between the ages of 4 and 16 is secondary to Wilson disease; therefore, it should be ruled out in any young person with liver disease.
- Wilson disease should be considered in any patient with liver, neurologic, or psychiatric disease who fails to respond to therapy.
- The most reliable diagnostic test is a liver biopsy that exhibits a high copper content. It is recommended in all patients with high clinical suspicion and negative laboratory test findings or children with chronic liver disease.
- Siblings of patients with Wilson disease should be tested with 24-hour urinary copper level, serum ceruloplasmin assay, and biomicroscopy; a liver biopsy is indicated if there is a high clinical suspicion and other tests are negative (Table 60–5).

Ocular

- The Kayser–Fleischer ring is seldom noted unless neurologic findings are evident.

TABLE 60–3. DIFFERENTIAL DIAGNOSES OF WILSON DISEASE

Organ(s) or System	Differential Diagnoses
Liver	• Viral hepatitis • Infectious mononucleosis
Psychiatric/nervous system	• Schizophrenia • Mania • Depression • Psychoses • Neuroses • Behavior disturbances

TABLE 60–4. DIAGNOSIS OF WILSON DISEASE

Clinical Signs and/or Symptoms	Indicated Test(s)	Follow-up Test(s)
Neurologic signs/symptoms present	Biomicroscopy to look for Kayser–Fleischer rings	Serum ceruloplasmin levels <20 mg/dL confirms diagnosis; if ceruloplasmin level *normal*, must do liver biopsy to quantify hepatic copper
Isolated liver disease, no neurologic signs/symptoms	Serum ceruloplasmin <20 mg/dL Urinary copper excretion >100 μg/24 hours	Liver biopsy: hepatic copper concentration >250 μg/g dry weight confirms diagnosis
Child with liver disease	Liver biopsy	—
Sibling of patient with Wilson disease	Biomicroscopy 24-hour urinary copper excretion Serum ceruloplasmin	Liver biopsy if clinical suspicion high and indicated tests negative

- Establishing the presence of a Kayser–Fleischer ring is a simple screening test that is a useful adjunctive measure when diagnosing Wilson disease.
- Slit-lamp biomicroscopy should be done to rule out the presence of a Kayser–Fleischer ring in patients with the new onset of liver disease of unknown etiology with or without neuropsychiatric manifestations.
- It is also useful to look for the presence of a Kayser–Fleischer ring in patients with a family history of Wilson disease.

TREATMENT AND MANAGEMENT

Systemic

- The goal of treatment (Table 60–6) is to reduce the body's accumulation of copper. This can be accomplished by decreasing the body's intestinal absorption of copper or by enhancing the urinary excretion of copper.
- Treatment is life-long.
- Neurologic signs improve with treatment, but clinical improvement may not be evident for weeks to months.
- D-Penicillamine (a copper chelating agent) is the most commonly used medication.
- Changes in diet and eating habits are recommended, including dietary reduction of liver, mushrooms, cocoa, chocolate, nuts, and shellfish, plus drinking and cooking with distilled water.
- Oral zinc supplements may be used as an adjunct therapy; zinc blocks copper absorption from the intestional mucosa, thus leading to a higher level of copper excreted through the fecal route.
- Genetic counseling is indicated; siblings of patients with Wilson disease should be examined.

Ocular

- There is no treatment necessary for Kayser–Fleischer rings or sunflower cataracts.

TABLE 60–5. DIAGNOSTIC TESTING OF WILSON DISEASE

Test	Diagnostic Criteria	Normal Values	Comments
Serum copper level	>150 μg/dL	15–55 μg/dL	Finding normal values effectively excludes the diagnosis of untreated disease
Serum ceruloplasmin	<20 mg/dL	20–40 mg/dL	Levels are low in newborns and gradually increase during the first 2 years of life (coincident with postnatal decline in hepatic copper concentration)
24-hour urinary copper excretion rate	>100 μg/24 hours	<40 μg/24 hours	Not a very valuable screening test, but may be more useful as a means of confirming the diagnosis and in the evaluation of compliance and response to chelation therapy

TABLE 60–6. TREATMENT AND MANAGEMENT OF WILSON DISEASE

Drug or Action	Dosage	Indications	Side Effects	Notes
D-Penicillamine	150 to 500 mg qid on an empty stomach	Initial treatment, maintenance treatment, presymptomatic patients, pregnancy	Systemic: initial neurological worsening, toxicity, fever, rash, kidney dysfunction, decrease in blood platelets, zinc deficiency, taste and smell disorders, connective tissue disease, polyarthritis, lupus-like and myasthenia-like syndromes, aplastic anemia	Gold standard of therapy in Wilson disease
Trientine	250 to 500 mg tid on an empty stomach	Initial treatment, maintenance treatment, presymptomatic patients, pregnancy	Iron deficiency anemia, anorexia, abdominal pain, skin rash, rhabdomyolysis (disintegration of muscle); more clinical research needed to indicate all side effects	
Zinc acetate	50 mg tid on an empty stomach	Maintenance treatment, presymptomatic patients, pregnancy	Dehydration, electrolyte imbalance, lethargy, dizziness, muscular incoordination, impairment of lymphocyte and neutrophil functions, increase in LDL cholesterol; limited clinical experience has not fully explored the usefulness of this treatment modality	
Dietary reduction of copper		Maintenance treatment adjunct with medical treatment	Further research needed to indicate its full usefulness as a treatment modality Foods very rich in copper: liver, chocolate, nuts, mushrooms, legumes, shellfish should be avoided Drinking distilled water is recommended; water from domestic softeners should be avoided	Complete restriction is impractical as copper is ubiquitous in most food
Liver transplant		Treatment of choice when end-stage liver cirrhosis and fulminant hepatic failure are present		Some currently advocate liver transplantation prior to liver damage but when intractable, neurologic manifestations are present

- The Kayser–Fleischer rings may regress with appropriate therapy; however, this has not been found to be a good predictor of clinical improvement in patients with neuropsychiatric manifestations.

REFERENCES

Affra RC. *Grayson's Diseases of the Cornea.* 3rd ed. St. Louis: Mosby–Year Book; 1991.

Anderson LA, Hakojarvi SL, Boudreaux SK. Zinc acetate treatment in Wilson's disease. *Ann Pharmacother.* 1998;32:78–87.

Brewer GJ, Yuzbasiyan-Gurkan V, Lee DY. Use of zinc-copper metabolic interactions in the treatment of Wilson's disease. *J Am College Nutr.* 1990;9:487–491.

Cairns JE, Walshe JM. The Kayser-Fleischer ring. *Trans Ophthalmol Cos UK.* 1970;90:187–190.

Cartwright GE. Current concepts: Diagnosis of treatable Wilson's disease. *N Eng J Med.* 1983;298:1347–1350.

Crumley FE. Case study, pitfalls of diagnosis in the early stages of Wilson's disease. *J Am Acad Child Adolesc Psychiatr.* 1990;29:470–471.

Danks DM. Copper and liver disease. *Eur J Pediatr.* 1991; 150:142–148.

Dobyns WM, Goldstein NP, Gordon H. Clinical spectrum of Wilson's disease (hepatolenticular degeneration). *Mayo Clin Proc.* 1979;54:35–42.

Emery AEH, Rimoin DL. *Principles and Practice of Medical Genetics.* New York: Churchill Livingstone; 1990:2.

Esmaeli B, et al. Regression of Kayser-Fleischer rings during oral zinc therapy: Correlation with systemic manifestations of Wilson's disease *Cornea.* 1996;15:582–588.

Gollan JL, Gollan TJ. Wilson disease in 1998: Genetic, diagnostic, and therapeutic aspects. Hepatol. 1998;28(suppl 1):28–36.

Schumacher G, et al. Liver transplantation: Treatment of choice for hepatic and neurological manifestations of Wilson's disease. *Clin Transplant.* 1997;1:217–224.

Smithgal JM. The copper-controlled diet: Current aspects of dietary copper restriction in management of copper metabolism disorders. *J Am Diet Assoc.* 1985;85:609–611.

Starosta-Runinstein S, Young AB, Kluin K, et al. Clinical assessment of 31 patients with Wilson's disease. *Arch Neurol.* 1987;44:365–379.

Sternlieb I. Perspectives on Wilson's disease. *Hepatology.* 1990;12:1234–1239.

Tankanow RM. Pathophysiology and treatment of Wilson's disease. *Clin Pharm.* 1991;10:839–849.

Walshe JM. The physiology of copper in man and its relation to Wilson's disease. *Brain.* 1967;90:149–176.

Wiebers DO, Hollenhorst RW, Goldstein NP. The ophthalmologic manifestations of Wilson's disease. *Mayo Clin Proc.* 1977;52:409–416.

Woods SE, Colon VF. Wilson's disease. *Am Fam Pract.* 1989; 40:171–178.

Chapter 61

GOUT

Esther S. Marks

The term "gout" represents a group of disorders generally characterized by hyperuricemia (elevated uric acid levels), leading to acute attacks of monosodium urate crystal-induced inflammatory arthritis. This may be followed by the development of chronic aggregated deposits of these crystals (tophi) in and around the joints of the extremities, the skin, and in some cases the kidneys. Permanent joint and kidney damage may result.

Recognized for hundreds of years, gout was even referred to by the Greek physician Hippocrates in the fifth century B.C. The term comes from the Latin word "gutta" meaning a drop. It was thought that drops of "humors" would flow into a joint, setting off an acute attack of inflammation (Jayson & St. J Dickson, 1974).

In the past, gout was associated with ocular inflammation termed gouty iritis. Under more recent scrutiny, this association has been seriously questioned. However, there clearly remain ocular manifestations of gout, in particular bilaterally chronic red eyes.

EPIDEMIOLOGY

Systemic

In the United States the prevalence of gout varies with the source. Wyngaarden (1988) lists it as 130 to 370 per 100,000, with a positive family history in 6 to 18% of cases. It appears to be much more common in middle-aged men (95%) than in women (5%), who are almost always postmenopausal (Wyngaarden, 1988). However, some sources now list the frequency of gout in women to be as high as 15 to 30% of newly diagnosed cases. Women usually have a milder course of the disease (Macfarlane & Dieppe, 1985).

Gout represents 5% of all arthritis (Wyngaarden, 1988), and is the most common form of inflammatory joint disease in males over 40 (Roubenoff, 1990). It is associated with many other conditions such as obesity, diabetes mellitus, hyperlipidemia (especially hypertriglyceridemia), hypertension, and atherosclerotic cardiovascular disease.

Ocular

There are few epidemiologic data available in the literature on the prevalence or incidence of ocular manifestations of gout. The most commonly noted finding is chronic bilateral injection of the conjunctiva and episclera (Ferry et al, 1985).

PATHOPHYSIOLOGY/DISEASE PROCESS

Systemic

In the human body, purine (a component of cell nuclei) metabolism results in uric acid as an end product. This is excreted almost exclusively by the kidneys. Hyperuricemia may be caused by either overproduction or underexcretion of uric acid. Overproduction may be due to a purine-rich diet, an inborn metabolic defect, or disorders characterized by increased cell turnover (e.g., psoriasis, polycythemia vera, myeloid metaplasia, multiple myeloma, and acute leukemia) (Boss & Seegmiller, 1979). Underexcretion of uric acid may be due to kidney abnormalities, drugs (eg, thiazide diuretics, aspirin, ethambutol, pyrazinamide, alcohol, levodopa–carbidopa, and nicotinic acid), and lead poisoning, as well as several other conditions such as uncontrolled diabetes, starvation, exercise, hypothyroidism, and hyperparathyroidism (Harris et al, 1999). Other conditions, such as hypertension, obesity, hyperlipidemia, atherosclerosis, sarcoidosis, and Down syndrome have been associated with gout (Pittman & Bross, 1999).

Patients may live with hyperuricemia for years without symptoms, until monosodium urate crystals spontaneously, or triggered by dietary or alcoholic overindulgence, trauma, illness, or surgery, precipitate in and around a joint. In an unsuccessful attempt to metabolize the indigestible crystals, engulfing leukocytes burst, releasing lysosomes and other enzymes into the joint and surrounding tissue. This results in a severe inflammatory reaction—acute gouty arthritis.

A single joint is affected in 75 to 90% of initial attacks, and more than 50% will involve the first metatarsophalangeal joint of the big toe—referred to as podagra (Wyngaarden, 1988). There are many theories as to why the big toe is so commonly affected. The most widely accepted theory is that crystal precipitation is favored in joints with lower temperatures and local degenerative changes. This is particularly true of the big toe, located distant from the heart and required to withstand strong forces (Jayson & St. J Dixon, 1974). The big toe is followed in frequency by the foot, ankle, knee, wrist, and fingers (Harris et al, 1999). Subsequent attacks may involve more than one joint and may affect the elbow and even larger joints, such as the hip. As many as 60% of patients will have a second attack within the first year (Cardenosa & Deluca, 1990).

The acute attack often occurs at night, beginning with a feeling of discomfort in the joint, followed by significant swelling, redness, and tenderness. The patient may be awakened with pain so excruciating that just the weight of a sheet on the joint is intolerable. Without treatment, the mild to moderate attack may last several hours to days, and the severe attack sometimes weeks, but both fully resolve. The patient then enters a symptom-free period of varying duration, referred to as intercritical gout. The self-limited nature of the acute attack of gout is somewhat of a mystery. One possible factor may be that the inflammation in the joint increases the local temperature, resulting in increased urate solubility (Kelley & Schumacher, 1993).

The patient may experience only one or two acute episodes, or develop multiple acute attacks of increasing duration and severity, until permanent joint damage occurs caused by clumps of monosodium urate crystals (tophi) forming within and around the joints and elsewhere (Figure 61–1). This is termed chronic tophaceous gouty arthritis (Table 61–1). At this point, polyarticular involvement is common.

About 20% of gout patients develop tophi, leading to a destructive arthritis (Scott, 1980). The skin over a tophaceous joint may become quite thinned to the point of ulceration, with discharge of the solid urates as a white chalky substance. Tophi may also occur in other tissues such as the skin of the elbows and hands, cartilage of the ears, Achilles tendon, and kidneys.

Kidney involvement is a common extra-articular manifestation of gout. It may take several forms. Gouty or urate nephropathy—the deposition of urate crystals in the interstitial tissue of the kidney—is not believed to contribute significantly to renal dysfunction in the majority of patients with gout. However, acute uric acid nephropathy—uric acid crystal obstruction of the collecting ducts and distal tubules—does lead to acute renal failure. This is especially common in patients

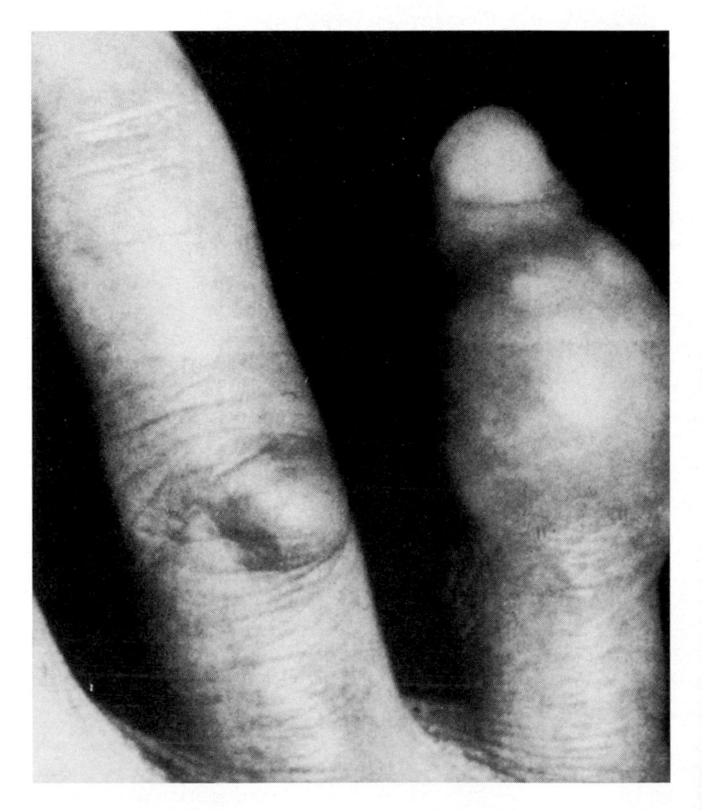

Figure 61–1. Tophus of fifth digit, with smaller tophus over fourth proximal interphalangeal joint. *(Reprinted with permission from Kelly WN, Schumacher HR.* Gout *In: Kelley WN, Harris ED, Ruddy S, Sledge CB (eds.)* Textbook of Rheumatology. *Philadelphia: Saunders; 1993:1295.)*

TABLE 61–1. SYSTEMIC MANIFESTATIONS OF GOUT

Acute Gouty Arthritis
- Hyperuricemia
- Sodium urate crystal deposition in joint
- Most commonly affects the big toe, followed by foot, ankle, knee, wrist, finger, elbow, hip
- Significant swelling, tenderness, redness of joint
- Excruciating pain

Intercritical Gout
- Hyperuricemia
- Asymptomatic

Chronic Tophaceous Gout
- Hyperuricemia
- Tophi deposition
  - In and around joints leading to bony erosions, calcification, and narrowing of joint space
  - In skin of elbows and hands, cartilage of the ears—may ulcerate and discharge contents
  - In kidney leading to urate nephropathy, acute uric acid nephropathy, nephrolithiasis, and renal failure

with high cell turnover (e.g., in leukemias). Nephrolithiasis—uric acid kidney stones —occurs in about 1% of established gouty arthritis patients per year (Kelley & Schumacher, 1993). Renal damage from crystal or stone formation may lead to a failure to clear waste products, secondary hypertension, heart disease, or cerebrovascular accidents.

Ocular

Chronic bilateral conjunctival injection is the most commonly associated ocular manifestation of gout (Table 61–2). Described as "dusky red," it has been reported that the bulbar and palpebral injection can be aggravated by manipulation of the tissue during ocular examination. Unfortunately, it does not appear to be an indicator of blood urate levels, and interestingly does not necessarily subside when urate levels are lowered medically (Ferry et al, 1985). Episcleritis and scleritis have also been associated with gout.

Asteroid hyalosis (Figure 61–2) is considered a possible ocular manifestation of gout. Safir and coworkers (1990) reported 7 of 76 (9.2%) patients with asteroid hyalosis had gout, far exceeding the prevalence of gout in the general population (0.13 to 0.37%).

TABLE 61–2. OCULAR MANIFESTATIONS OF GOUT

- Chronic bilateral conjunctival injection
- Episcleritis
- Scleritis
- Asteroid hyalosis
- Crystal deposition: cornea, sclera, lens, tarsal plates, extraocular muscles, tendons
- Uveitis (?)
- Elevated intraocular pressure (?)

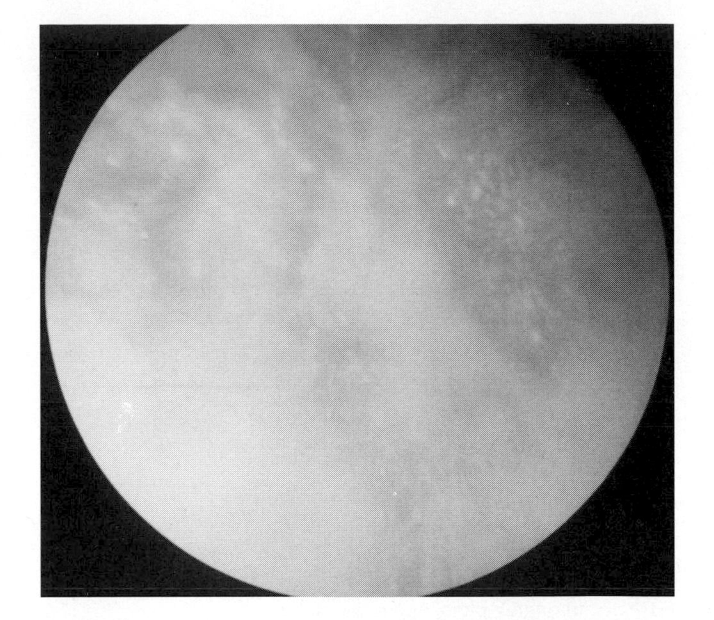

Figure 61–2. Asteroid hyalosis in a patient with gout.

Ferry and associates (1985) reported 3 out of 69 (4.3%) patients with gout had asteroid hyalosis. This also far exceeds the typically reported prevalence of asteroid hyalosis (0.042 to 0.50%) (Safir et al, 1990).

> Chronically injected conjunctiva, episcleritis, scleritis, or asteroid hyalosis can be ocular signs of gout.

Uveitis was once believed to be strongly associated with gout. However, in a study of 69 patients with severe gout, Ferry and associates (1985) found no patients with uveitis. Yet it continues to be reported in the literature despite no recent studies supporting the association (Berman, 1995). Elevated intraocular pressure has been reported, although again, no studies have been able to substantiate this association.

Crystal and tophi deposition in ocular tissues, although rare, has been reported. It is theorized that this deposition occurs in poorly vascularized or avascular tissues such as the cornea, sclera, lens, tarsal plates, and extraocular muscle tendons (Bloch & Henkind, 1992). Corneal crystal deposition has been variably described in the epithelial and subepithelial layers.

DIAGNOSIS

Systemic

The diagnosis of gout (Table 61–3) includes a thorough history and physical examination in order to rule out

TABLE 61–3. DIAGNOSTIC TESTS FOR GOUT

Systemic
- Complete blood count (CBC)
- Serum creatinine
- Blood urea nitrogen (BUN)
- Serum uric acid
- Urinalysis
- Synovial fluid evaluation for the presence of monosodium urate crystals[a]
- X-ray of involved joint
- MRI

Ocular
- CBC
- Serum uric acid level
- Fasting blood sugar
- Antinuclear antibodies
- Rheumatoid factor
- Erythrocyte sedimentation rate
- Rapid plasma reagin and fluorescent treponemal antibody absorption
- PPD with anergy panel and chest x-ray
- Serum antineutrophilic cytoplasmic antibody

[a]Gold standard for diagnosis.

other disorders such as pseudogout (a calcium crystal–induced arthropathy) (Table 61–4), as well as to establish any associated conditions. Tests for complete blood count, serum chemistry, and analysis of renal function are recommended.

The clinical presentation of hyperuricemia (serum urate concentration greater than 7 mg/dL) alone does not make the diagnosis, since some patients demonstrate normal serum uric acid levels. The presence of monosodium urate crystals in synovial fluid aspirated from affected joints is the gold standard. The presence of polymorphonuclear leukocytes in this fluid, as well as negative cultures for infectious micro-organisms, supports the diagnosis.

TABLE 61–4. DIFFERENTIAL DIAGNOSIS OF GOUT

Systemic
- Pseudogout
- Septic arthritis
- Rheumatoid arthritis
- Erosive osteoarthritis
- Spondyloarthropathies

Ocular (conjunctivitis, episcleritis, scleritis)
- Rosacea
- Collagen vascular disease
- Syphilis
- Tuberculosis
- Herpes simplex
- Herpes zoster
- Leukemia
- Metastases of systemic malignancies
- Lyme disease
- Wegener granulomatosis

> The gold standard for the diagnosis of gout is the presence of monosodium urate crystals in aspirated synovial fluid from an involved joint.

Radiography is usually not of much diagnostic help for early acute gouty arthritis, as it takes years of untreated or poorly treated gout for a patient to develop the punched-out bony erosions and chronic arthritis visible on film (Pittman & Bross, 1999). Round or oval in shape, these erosions usually occur on the long axes of bones. There may also be an increase in density in the areas of soft tissue swelling due to repeated attacks, and eventual uniform narrowing of the joint space (Cardenosa & Deluca, 1990). Although rare, tophi may appear to be infectious or neoplastic, prompting evaluation by magnetic resonance imaging (MRI) (Pittman & Bross, 1999).

Ocular

There are no ocular manifestations pathognomic for gout. However, gout should be considered in patients presenting with chronic bilateral conjunctival injection, recurrent episcleritis, or scleritis of unknown etiology. Asteroid hyalosis may also be a potential warning sign of gout.

TREATMENT AND MANAGEMENT

Systemic

The correct diagnosis of hyperuricemia and gout is critical, since the medications used to treat these disorders have potentially serious side effects. Some rheumatologists feel that gout is overdiagnosed or misdiagnosed by primary care physicians (Wolfe & Cathey, 1991). This may be partly due to equating hyperuricemia with gout and thus treating it as gout. Although treatment is clearly warranted in symptomatic hyperuricemic patients with evidence of renal damage, frequent acute attacks, and chronic joint changes or tophi, treatment of the asymptomatic idiopathic hyperuricemic patient is questionable. Serum uric acid levels of greater than 11 mg/dL warrant a 24-hour urine uric acid level and close renal monitoring but do not require immediate treatment (Kelley, 1993).

The treatment of gout (Table 61–5) must address both the acute and chronic aspects of this disorder. An acute attack of gout requires rest and medication to reduce inflammation as quickly as possible. The drugs of choice include nonsteroidal anti-inflammatory drugs (NSAIDs), colchicine, and corticosteroids. Colchicine, an antimitotic drug, was for years the drug of choice.

TABLE 61–5. TREATMENT AND MANAGEMENT OF GOUT

Systemic

Acute gouty arthritis

- Rest ***PLUS***
- NSAID (one of the following)
  - Indomethacin 25–100 mg qid until relieved, then taper
  - Naproxen 500 mg bid until relieved, then taper
  - Ibuprofen 800 mg qid until relieved, then taper
  - Sulindac 200 mg bid until relieved, then taper
  - Ketoprofen 75 mg qid until relieved, then taper ***OR***
- Colchicine 0.5–0.6 mg qh, D/C after maximum 6 mg ***OR***
- Corticosteroid
  - Intra-articular:
    - Small joints: 5–20 mg triamcinolone acetonide or methylprednisolone
    - Large joints: 10–40 mg triamcinolone hexacetonide
  - Oral: prednisone 0.5 mg/kg first day, then taper
  - Intramuscular: 60 mg triamcinolone acetonide

Intercritical and chronic tophaceous gout

- Diet moderation, e.g., avoid high-purine foods and alcohol ***PLUS***
- Weight reduction ***PLUS***
- Urate-lowering drugs:
  - Probenecid 250 mg bid increase to max 3 g/day ***OR***
  - Sulfinpyrazone 50 mg tid increase to 200–400 mg/day ***OR***
  - Allopurinol 50–100 mg qd increase to max 200–300 mg/day ***PLUS***
- Surgical removal of large tophi if necessary

Ocular

Chronic bilateral conjunctival injection

- Artificial tears prn ***OR***
- Topical vasoconstrictors—very limited use advised

Episcleritis

- Warm/cold compresses ***PLUS***
- Artificial tears qid ***OR***
- Mild topical steroids, e.g., prednisolone acetate 0.125% qid

Scleritis

- Topical steroids (prednisolone acetate 1% qid to q4h) ***PLUS***
- NSAIDs, e.g., indomethacin 75–100 mg PO daily
- If severe, ***ADD*** prednisone 60–80 mg daily, taper then D/C after 2 weeks
- If unresponsive, use immunosuppressives

Abbreviations: bid, twice a day; D/C, discontinue; PO, orally; prn, as required; qd, every day; q4h, every 4 hours; qh, every hour; qid, four times daily; tid, three times a day.

However, because of the overwhelming number of patients who experience gastrointestinal toxicity (nausea, diarrhea, vomiting) at therapeutic doses, NSAIDs have become the favored first-line drug (Harris et al, 1999). The majority of patients treated with an NSAID immediately after the onset of symptoms, or at the time of diagnosis, experience complete resolution of the acute attack. Unfortunately, the side effects of NSAID use (GI disturbances, nephropathy, liver dysfunction, central nervous system dysfunction, platelet dysfunction, exacerbation of congestive heart failure) limit its use.

Corticosteroids have been found to be useful in treating acute attacks of gout. Patients presenting with one or two accessible inflamed joints have been found to respond quite well to intra-articular injections. Diagnostic joint aspiration should precede the injections. Interestingly, aspiration alone has been reported to greatly alleviate joint pain from acute gout (Emmerson, 1996). Systemic corticosteroid therapy is utilized when NSAIDs and colchicine are contraindicated or have been ineffective. Colchicine and NSAIDs do not prevent future attacks or alter the amount of uric acid in the body, nor do they alter uric acid deposition. Therefore, once the acute attack is over, long-term or chronic treatment must be considered to prevent recurrent arthritis and tophaceous gout.

The medications for long-term treatment decrease serum uric acid either by increasing excretion from the kidney with uricosuric agents (e.g., probenecid or sulfinpyrazone) or by decreasing the formation of uric acid with xanthine oxidase inhibitors (e.g., allopurinol). Patients also should be instructed on proper diet. The strict exclusion of foods and alcohol is unnecessary, and usually results in poor patient compliance. Therefore, the key is moderation. Weight reduction is also recommended because it may help lower plasma urate levels. If necessary, surgical removal of large tophi may be performed once serum uric acid levels are controlled. Patients on medications that alter uric acid metabolism may need to be closely monitored, or have their medications changed. For example, thiazide diuretics, which cause the undersecretion of uric acid, may need to be replaced with beta-blockers or calcium channel blockers in patients with gout and hypertension.

Ocular

The available literature does not address treatment of the gout-related chronic bilateral conjunctival injection (see Table 61–3). Artificial tears may be used for symptomatic relief. Topical vasoconstrictors may be considered for cosmesis, but chronic use should be strongly discouraged to avoid rebound hyperemia.

Episcleritis should be treated with standard modalities: warm/cold compresses, artificial tears, or if moderate to severe, topical steroids. Scleritis should also be treated with standard regimens: topical steroids combined with NSAIDs, oral steroids, and immunosuppressive agents if unresponsive to treatment.

Chronic bilateral conjunctival injection, recurrent episcleritis, or scleritis of unknown etiology may warrant a test for serum uric acid level. The presence of asteroid hyalosis in patients with no other known associated disease (e.g., diabetes and hypercholesterolemia) also may warrant evaluation for gout.

Systemic treatment for gout may alleviate some of the ocular manifestations (Berman, 1995). However,

Liu and colleagues (1988) found that patients on long-term allopurinol therapy had anterior subcapsular lens changes, including opacities and thinning of the anterior clear zone.

CONCLUSION

Historically, gout was considered almost exclusively a "disease of kings," caused purely by overindulgence in food and alcohol. Now, recognized genetic and environmental factors, as well as changes in diet, have altered the face of gout worldwide. An eminently treatable disorder, gout should no longer be a cause of debilitating arthritis. Although relatively few ocular manifestations of gout exist, an alert eyecare provider may aid in the initial diagnosis.

REFERENCES

Becker MA. Rheumatology. *JAMA.* 1989;261:2287–2289.

Berman EL. Clues in the eye: Ocular signs of metabolic and nutritional disorders. *Geriatrics.* 1995;50:34–37.

Bloch RS, Henkind P. Ocular manifestations of endocrine and metabolic disease. In: Tasman W, Jaeger EA, eds. *Duane's Clinical Ophthalmology.* Vol. 5. Hagerstown, MD: Harper & Row; 1992:20–21.

Boss GR, Seegmiller JE. Hyperuricemia and gout: Classification, complications and management. *N Engl J Med.* 1979; 300:1459–1468.

Cardenosa G, Deluca SA. Radiographic features of gout. *Am Fam Physician.* 1990;41:539–542.

Emmerson, BT. The management of gout. *N Engl J Med.* 1996; 334:445–451.

Ferry AP, Safir A, Melikian HE. Ocular abnormalities in patients with gout. *Ann Ophthalmol.* 1985;17:632–635.

Fishman RS, Sunderman FW. Band keratopathy in gout. *Arch Ophthalmol.* 1966;75:367–369.

Harris MD, Siegel LB, Alloway JA. Gout and hyperuricemia. *Am Fam Physician.* 1999;59:925–934.

Jayson M, St. J Dixon A. Gout and pseudogout. In: *Understanding Arthritis and Rheumatism: A Complete Guide to the Problems and Treatment.* New York: Pantheon; 1974:105–117.

Kelley WN. Hyperuricemia. In: Kelley WN, Harris ED, et al, eds. *Textbook of Rheumatology.* Vol. 1. Philadelphia: WB Saunders; 1993:498–506.

Kelley WN, Schumacher HR. Gout. In: Kelley WN, Harris ED, et al, eds. *Textbook of Rheumatology.* Vol. 2. Philadelphia: WB Saunders; 1993:1291–1336.

Liu CSC, Brown NAP, et al. The prevalence and morphology of cataracts in patients on allopurinol treatment. *Eye.* 1988; 2:600–606.

Macfarlane DG, Dieppe PA. Diuretic induced gout in elderly women. *Br J Rheum.* 1985;24:155–157.

Pittman JR, Bross MH. Diagnosis and management of gout. *Am Fam Physician.* 1999;59:1799–1806.

Roubenoff R. Gout and hyperuricemia. *Rheum Dis Clin North Am* 1990;16:539–550.

Safir A, Dunn SN, et al. Is asteroid hyalosis ocular gout? *Ann Ophthalmol.* 1990;22:70–77.

Scott JT. Gout and other related forms of arthritis. In: Scott JT, ed. *Arthritis and Rheumatism.* Oxford: Oxford University Press; 1980:67–75.

Slansky HH, Kuwabara T. Intranuclear urate crystals in corneal epithelium. *Arch Ophthalmol.* 1968;80:338–344.

Wolfe F, Cathey MA. The misdiagnosis of gout and hyperuricemia. *J Rheumatol.* 1991;18:1232–1234.

Wyngaarden JB. Gout. In: Wyngaarden JB , Smith LH, eds. *Cecil Textbook of Medicine.* Philadelphia: WB Saunders; 1988:1161–1170.

Zell SC, Carmichael JM. Evaluation of allopurinol use in patients with gout. *Am J Hosp Pharm.* 1989;46:1813–1816.

Chapter 62

CYSTINOSIS

Thu-ha Dao Easter

Cystinosis is a rare inherited metabolic disorder characterized by accumulation of intracellular nonprotein cystine crystals in multiple organs including the eyes. Cystinosis can be categorized as nephropathic or nonnephropathic. All patients with cystinosis have ocular involvement; however, post–kidney transplant nephropathic patients are at risk for the more severe ocular complications.

EPIDEMIOLOGY

Cystinosis is a rare autosomal recessive disorder with an estimated incidence of 2.5 per 100,000. The disease affects approximately 2000 individuals worldwide and about 400 individuals in the United States. There is no sexual predilection. The prevalence of cystinosis in French Canada is the highest in the world probably because of the small French Canadian gene pool. The incidence and prevalence of all types of cystinosis are probably underreported because of lack of recognition and reporting of the disease.

PATHOPHYSIOLOGY/DISEASE PROCESS

Systemic

The etiology of cystinosis is a defect in the lysosomal membrane transport system of cystine. In this condition, nonprotein cystine cannot be transported from lysosomes into the cytoplasm, resulting in accumulation and crystallization of free cystine within the lysosomes. The plasma cystine level is usually well below saturation, indicating that the defect is at the cellular level. There are three phenotypes of cystinosis: infantile (nephropathic), adolescent, and adult (nonnephropathic/benign). Each form has different systemic manifestations (Table 62–1). Accumulation of cystine results in multiple organ damage with renal dysfunction being most pronounced in the first decade in infantile cystinosis. Of the three types, adult cystinosis is probably most underreported since patients are usually asymptomatic and ocular manifestations are incidental findings during routine eye examination.

Infantile and adolescent cystinosis have an autosomal recessive inheritance. The mode of inheritance in adult cystinosis is unknown. The cystinosis gene, CTNS, was isolated in 1998 and mapped to chromosome 17p13. The CTNS gene has 367 amino acids with seven transmembrane domains and is thought to transport cystine out of lysosomes. As of 1999, 32 mutations associated with infantile cystinosis, three with the adolescent type, and two with the adult type were described. Researchers have found that mutation and deletion of certain loci related to cystinosis are specific for different ethnic gene populations. Deletion and mutation can be heterozygous or homozygous. However, there is only a 50/50 probability that a patient

TABLE 62–1. SYSTEMIC MANIFESTATIONS OF CYSTINOSIS

Infantile:Pre-Renal Transplantation
- Fanconi syndrome—renal tubular dysfunction
  - Episodes of vomiting, weakness, unexplained fever
  - Anorexia, dehydration, constipation
  - Polydipsia, polyuria
  - Failure to thrive and grow
  - Rickets
- End-stage renal failure

Infantile:Post-Renal Transplantation
- Myopathy, especially oral-motor
- Diabetes
- Hypothyroidism
- Cerebral atrophy
- Liver enlargement
- Pancreatic endocrine insufficiency
- Epistaxis
- Hypohidrosis
- Late sexual maturation

Adolescent
- Renal glomerular dysfunction

Adult
- None

with cystinosis will have the specific deletion. Gene research is ongoing by the Cystinosis Collaborative Research Group.

Infantile cystinosis has an onset between 6 to 18 months of age and is associated with the most severe systemic complications. Systemic complications include renal Fanconi syndrome followed by glomerular failure, leading to end-stage renal failure by the end of the first decade. Fanconi renal failure is due to dysfunction of the proximal tubules. They are affected first because this is the site of amino acid reabsorption. Children with cystinosis appear normal at birth, but by 10 months of age they are shorter than their peers, urinate more frequently, have excessive thirst, and are picky eaters. At 12 months, they have difficulty bearing their weight and therefore are slower to walk. Since the intervention of dialysis and renal transplantation, patients with infantile cystinosis are now surviving into the second and third decade. There is no accumulation of cystine in the grafted kidney; however, cystine continues to accumulate in other organs and tissues, causing new long-term complications after renal transplantation. Hypothyroidism, diabetes mellitus, late sexual maturation, pancreatic endocrine insufficiency, liver enlargement with portal hypertension, epistaxis (nose bleed), central nervous system disorders, and severe myopathy (especially oral motor dysfunction) have all been reported in patients who survive into their second or third decade after renal transplantation.

Adolescent cystinosis is also nephropathic; however, this form of cystine nephropathy manifests itself first at age 10 to 12 with proteinuria due to glomerular damage rather than the tubular damage that occurs first in infantile cystinosis. Therefore, symptoms associated with Fanconi syndrome are not present. Life expectancy is related to renal dysfunction, which is managed by kidney dialysis or transplantation.

Cogan and co-workers first described adult cystinosis in 1957. These patients have normal renal function and life expectancy. Cystine crystal deposits are found predominantly in the cornea and/or conjunctiva. Cystine crystals are also found in white cells and bone marrow; however, no systemic manifestation has been reported.

Ocular

All three types of cystinosis display ocular involvement (Table 62–2). Crystal accumulation can occur in the cornea, conjunctiva, uvea, anterior lens surface, and retina.

Corneal deposits start in the peripheral anterior stroma and proceed more centrally and deeper into the tissue as the patient ages. Although not common, there have been reports of crystal deposits in the epithelium causing superficial punctate keratopathy and corneal erosion in certain patients with cystinosis. The crystals are fine, needle-like, refractile deposits homogeneously distributed in the stroma (Figure 62–1). Although visual acuity is usually unaffected by the corneal crystals, they can cause glare disability, decreased contrast sensitivity, and photophobia. Conjunctival deposits are

TABLE 62–2. OCULAR MANIFESTATIONS OF CYSTINOSIS

Cornea
- Superficial punctate keratitis
- Band keratopathy
- Recurrent corneal erosion

Uveal Tract
- Posterior synechiae
- Pupillary block glaucoma

Retina
- RPE retinopathy

Long-Term Complications
- Photophobia
- Blepharospasm
- Decreased visual acuity
- Decreased contrast sensitivity
- Decreased color vision
- Abnormal ERG

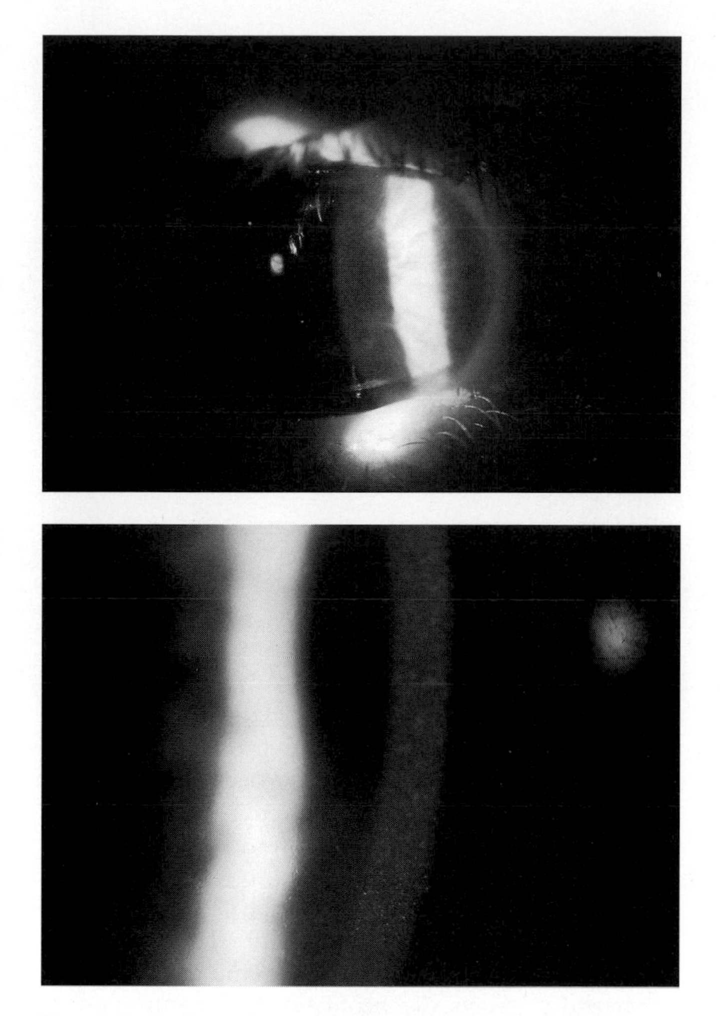

Figure 62–1. Corneal crystals in cystinosis.

more whitish with a ground-glass appearance. Band keratopathy in cystinosis is likely due to associated renal failure. Glistening polymorphous crystal deposits on the iris can cause the iris stroma to thicken, leading to posterior synechiae and pupillary block glaucoma. Retinal changes have only been reported in infantile cystinosis. These range from patchy depigmentation of the retinal pigment epithelium (RPE) to subtle mottling and pigment clumping. Retinal changes are usually peripheral, symmetrical, and bilateral; however, some patients also develop atrophic macular changes.

Cystine crystals do not accumulate in the new kidney after renal transplantation; however, they continue to accumulate in the eye and other tissues. Long-term ocular complications of cystinosis in patients who survive into their second and third decade after renal transplantation include massive accumulation of crystals in corneal stroma, iris, anterior lens surface, and surface of the retina. Continued deposition of cystine in the RPE has been suggested as the etiology of abnormal color vision and electroretinograms (ERGs). Debilitating photophobia and blepharospasm can significantly decrease quality of life. The degree of ocular involvement varies from patient to patient; however Kaiser-Kupfer and co-workers (1986) reported that there appeared to be some correlation between early onset of renal failure and the severity of long-term ocular complications.

DIAGNOSIS

Systemic

Diagnosis of cystinosis (Table 62–3) is made based on increased intracellular cystine levels in certain tissues. Measurement of lysosomal cystine content in acid-stabilized leukocytes is the routine method for diagnosing cystinosis and for evaluating efficacy of a treatment regimen for cystinosis. White blood cells are used because cystine levels are not elevated in the red blood cells or plasma of patients with cystinosis. Cystine levels may be elevated in urine; however, this is not diagnostic. The normal value for intracellular cystine is generally less than 0.2 nmol half cystine/mg white cell protein. In cystinosis patients, the value is generally greater than 2 nmol half cystine/mg white cell protein. When the cystine level in leukocytes is inconclusive for diagnosis, measurement of intracellular cystine in a cultured skin fibroblast can be used. This method is more costly and time-consuming; however, confirmation using fibroblasts is definitive for cystinosis. For diagnosis of cystinosis in the newborn, the placenta can be sampled and assayed for intracellular cystine.

Prenatal diagnosis of cystinosis can be made from chorionic villus or amniocyte cultures. The cystine values will be more than 10 times greater than normal.

Ocular

Corneal crystals are the most common ocular manifestation of cystinosis and are sufficiently unique and

TABLE 62–3. DIAGNOSTIC CRITERIA FOR CYSTINOSIS

Systemic

- White blood cells: cystine level greater than 2 nmol half cystine/mg protein
- Cultured fibroblast with increased cystine levels
- Placental assay in newborn for increased intracellular cystine
- Chorionic villus or amniocyte cultures in fetus: cystine level more than 10 times normal

Ocular

- Fine, needle-like, refractile corneal crystals
- Conjunctival crystals and biopsy

TABLE 62–4. DIFFERENTIAL DIAGNOSIS OF CYSTINOSIS

Systemic
- Hereditary progressive nephritis
- Cystic diseases of the kidney
- Diffuse mesangial sclerosis of the kidney

Ocular
- Multiple myeloma
- Schnyders crystalline dystrophy
- Bietti crystalline dystrophy
- Gout

characteristic to form the basis for diagnosis of the disease. These fine, needle-like, refractile deposits in the stroma will be noted on slit-lamp biomicroscopy. The next most common ocular finding is white ground-glass–like conjunctival crystals. Conjunctival biopsy for cystine can also be done to determine the exact mechanism for the accumulation of crystals. Other ocular findings include cystine crystal deposits on the iris, lens, and retinal pigment epithelium; however, these tissues are not generally biopsied for diagnosis. Other conditions with corneal crystals, such as multiple myeloma, Schnyders crystalline dystrophy, Bietti crystalline dystrophy, and gout, must be ruled out (Table 62–4).

TREATMENT AND MANAGEMENT

Systemic

Patients with cystinosis are treated symptomatically (Table 62–5). Medical therapy is aimed at reducing or depleting accumulation of cystine crystals in tissues, especially in the kidney to delay kidney dysfunction.

Renal tubular dysfunction causes increased loss of electrolytes and fluid due to excessive urination. To prevent dehydration and maintain the normal electrolyte balance, patients require a high intake of fluids and oral electrolyte supplements in the form of sodium bicarbonate, sodium citrate, and potassium citrate. Depletion of phosphate, which can lead to rickets, is treated with a combination of sodium or potassium phosphate and vitamin D. Hypothyroidism is treated with thyroxin. Carnitine may help to replace muscular carnitine deficiency. Aminothiol therapy, which depletes lysosomal cystine, is used to prolong glomerular function and improve growth. Cystagon (cysteamine bitartrate) is an aminothiol which was approved by the FDA in August 1994 for use in the United States. This agent is capable of depleting cystine from body tissues and can be used systemically to ameliorate the course of the disease. It delays renal failure and improves growth, but it does not reverse existing renal tubular or glomerular damage. There is evidence that indomethacin increases appetite, decreases urine volume, and also improves growth in pretransplantation patients with cystinosis. Renal dialysis or transplantation is required for end-stage renal failure. After kidney transplantation, cystine crystals continue to accumulate in tissues other than the kidney. Given the effectiveness of cysteamine therapy and the harmful effects of chronic cystine accumulation, oral cysteamine should be considered for use in post-kidney transplant patients.

TABLE 62–5. TREATMENT AND MANAGEMENT OF CYSTINOSIS

Systemic
- Increased fluid intake
- Electrolyte supplements
- Potassium phosphate and vitamin D
- Carnitine
- Oral cysteamine
- Indomethacin
- Renal dialysis
- Renal transplant

Post–Renal Transplantation
- Oral and topical cysteamine
- Carnitine

Ocular
- Artificial tears
- Bandage contact lens
- Penetrating keratoplasty
- Topical cysteamine

Ocular

Artificial tears, bandage contact lens, and penetrating keratoplasty (PK) can be used to treat corneal complications of cystinosis, depending on the severity of involvement or degree of photophobia. Recurrence of cystinosis in the grafted cornea is inconclusive. Topical cysteamine has been reported to reverse corneal crystal deposits with stromal clearing through hourly use in young patients. However, compliance with this treatment regimen is difficult since cysteamine is a malodorous, foul-tasting substance with a prolonged aftertaste. Oral cysteamine may prevent further crystal deposits in ocular structures; however, there is no evidence that it reverses any damage or deposition that has already occurred. In post–renal transplantation patients, oral cysteamine should be considered in addition to topical therapy since it may decrease long-term accumulation of crystals, leading to decreased photophobia and blepharospasm and improved visual function.

CONCLUSION

Cystinosis is a disease caused by a defect in the cellular membrane cystine transport system. It is characterized by cystine crystal deposits in multiple organs, initially manifesting as kidney dysfunction. There is a wide range of systemic manifestations in cystinosis depending upon the phenotype. The most common ocular findings in all types are corneal and conjunctival crystals. Management involves treating conditions associated with kidney failure through renal transplantation when end-stage renal failure occurs. Treatment of ocular manifestations centers on the corneal involvement, which includes cysteamine therapy, bandage contact lens, and PK. With the advent of renal transplantation, nephropathic cystinosis patients are surviving longer and are faced with long-term ocular complications that must be managed in order to improve their quality of life.

REFERENCES

Cogan G, Kowabara T, Kimoshita J, et al. Cystinosis in an adult. *JAMA.* 1957;164:394.

Kaiser-Kupfer M, Caruso R, Minkler D, Gahl W. Long-term ocular manifestations in nephropathic cystinosis. *Arch Ophthalmol.* 1986;104:706–711.

Kaiser-Kupfer M, Fujikawa L, Kurvabara T, et al. Removal of corneal crystals by topical cysteamine in nephropathic cystinosis. *N Engl J Med.* 1987;316:775–779.

Kaiser-Kupfer M, Gazzo M, Datiles M, et al. A randomized placebo-controlled trial of cysteamine eye drops in nephropathic cystinosis. *Arch Ophthalmol.* 1990;108:689–693.

Katz B, Melles R, Schneider A. Contrast sensitivity function in nephropathic cystinosis. *Arch Ophthalmol.* 1987;105: 1667–1669.

Katz B, Melles R, Schneider A. Glare disability in nephropathic cystinosis. *Arch Ophthalmol.* 1987;105:1670–1671.

Markello TC, Bernardidni IM, Gahl WA. Improved renal function in children with cystinosis treated with cysteamine. *N Engl J Med.* 1993;16:1157–1162.

Richler M, Milot J, Quigley M, O'Regan S. Ocular manifestation of nephropathic cystinosis. *Arch Ophthalmol.* 1991; 109:359–362.

Wan W, Minckler D, Rao N. Pupillary block glaucoma associated with childhood cystinosis. *Am J Ophthalmol.* 1986; 101:700–705.

Wong V, Schulman J, Seegmiller J. Conjunctival biopsy for the biochemical diagnosis of cystinosis. *Am J. Ophthalmol.* 1970;70:278–280.

http://medicine.ucsd.edu/cystinosis

http://cystinosis.org

http://mcrcr2.med.nyu.edu/murphp01/lysosome/dischart.html

Section XIV

CHROMOSOMAL DISORDERS

Chapter 63

DOWN SYNDROME

Lyndon C. Wong

Down syndrome (DS), the manifestation of a common chromosomal abnormality in the human population, is the result of extra chromosomal material located on chromosome 21. Ocular abnormalities exist in almost all individuals with DS; however, the majority can be managed with minimal adverse sequelae. In the past, the majority of patients with DS remained in institutions most of their lives. However, over the past 20 years, a greater number of individuals with DS have been mainstreamed into schools, jobs, and the home. This has resulted in more parental involvement in the care of DS individuals, and a greater need for healthcare practitioners to understand and recognize their medical needs.

EPIDEMIOLOGY

Systemic

The prevalence of DS is approximately 1 per 600 live births (Frynes, 1987). The only risk factor is increased maternal age. Gaynon and Schimek's (1977) study reported the incidence of DS in teenage mothers to be 1 per 1850 live births. In contrast, DS is observed in 1 per 368 live births of women over 35 years of age (Palomaki, 1996). The incidence increases to 1 per 50 live births in females giving birth in their late forties (Gaynon & Schimek, 1977). In addition, the number of males exceeds the number of females among live born infants with DS. Race or ethnicity does not appear to be a risk factor for DS (Bishop et al, 1997). In the absence of any life-threatening congenital abnormalities, over 90% of individuals with DS live into adulthood (Rudolph & Hoffmann, 1987). Approximately 50% of DS individuals will have some type of hearing loss (Rudolph & Hoffmann, 1987). In addition, about 50% of DS infants are born with a simian palmar crease (Walker, 1958). Congenital heart defects are present in approximately 30 to 50% of DS infants (Goldhaber et al, 1986). The incidence of leukemia in DS children is 10 to 20 times greater than the general population (Van Dyke et al, 1990). With advancements in prenatal diagnosis and the opportunity to abort DS fetuses, a substantial reduction in the number of live DS births has been observed.

Ocular

The most outstanding ocular clinical feature of DS is the oblique and short palpebral fissures (Lowe, 1949). Shapiro and France (1985) found that 89% of DS patients have palpebral slants of 6 degrees or more. Prominent epicanthal folds are present in 60% of the DS population and tend to decrease with age (Davis, 1996). Blepharitis has been reported to be present in DS individuals with varying frequency, ranging from 2% (Cullen & Butler, 1963) to 67% (Skeller & Oster, 1951). In one study, the presence of lacrimal duct obstruction was observed in 30% of the DS population (Da Cunha

& De Castro Moreira, 1996). Keratoconus has been reported in 5 to 15% of patients with DS (Frantz et al, 1990). Brushfield spots are observed in approximately 85% of the irides of DS patients and in 24% of the "normal" population (Donaldson, 1961). Strabismus has been reported to occur in about 23 to 43% of DS individuals. Of these, 90% are esotropes compared to exotropes (4%) or hypertropes (6%). The most common type of esotropia in this patient population is accommodative (Davis, 1996). Jaeger (1980) reported only 12.5% of his patients with an ocular misalignment were amblyopic. Nystagmus is present in about 5 to 30% of the DS population. "Coronary cerulean" or isolated punctate lenticular opacities have been noted in 25 to 85% of the patients with DS (Eissler & Longenecker, 1962). The most common retinal abnormality in DS individuals is a high number of retinal vessels crossing the margin of the optic nerve head, along with an unusual spoke-like appearance of the vasculature in nearly 75% of DS patients (Down, 1866). The incidence of glaucoma is less than 5% (Davis, 1996).

TABLE 63–1. SYSTEMIC MANIFESTATIONS OF DOWN SYNDROME

- Mental retardation
- Congenital heart defects
- Musculoskeletal disturbances
- Gastrointestinal abnormalities
- Greater incidence of leukemia

Characteristic features:

- Small brachycephalic skull
- Flat nasal bridge
- Low-set ears
- Dental hypoplasia
- Thick, protruding tongue
- Redundant skin around the neck
- Short, broad hands
- Simian palmar crease
- Abdominal protuberance

PATHOPHYSIOLOGY/DISEASE PROCESS

Systemic

The etiology of DS is attributed to the presence of extra genetic material, which can be transmitted in three ways. The first, and most common anomaly, affecting 90 to 95% of DS individuals, is called trisomy 21. These individuals demonstrate an extra complete chromosome 21 (Catalano, 1990). Second and less common is a translocation of genetic material. Translocation occurs when part of chromosome 21 breaks off during cell division and attaches itself to another chromosome (Polani et al, 1960). Third, mosaic DS is a rare disorder resulting from a nondisjunction in cell division after fertilization. This causes a mixture of two types of cells, some with 46 chromosomes and others with 47 chromosomes. Hence, the "mosaic" pattern of cells. The mosaic DS child demonstrates less intellectual impairment as compared with children in the first two categories (Clarke et al, 1961).

Systemic characteristics (Table 63–1) include abnormalities in the development of the cranium, face, teeth, neck, heart, and dermatoglyphics (markings of the surface markings of the skin), as well as in the musculoskeletal and gastrointestinal systems. Neurologically, DS individuals usually have some form of developmental delays. IQ is variable but averages about 50. Social skills are typically closer to normal and once learned, these skills are never extinguished (Catalano, 1990). The typical DS individual has a small brachycephalic skull with frontal and perinasal sinus hypoplasia, a flat occiput, and delayed closure of the fontanelles (Martin, 1970). Characteristically, by 6 months of age, the DS infant will have an open mouth with a thick, rugged, and protruding tongue. Other craniofacial manifestations include dental hypoplasia, a flattened nasal bridge, and redundant skin around neck, and ears that are often small and low set. Dental problems include malocclusion, a protrusion of the mandible in relation to the upper jaw. Interestingly, DS individuals have fewer dental caries than the general population; however, the presence of gingivitis is more common (Van Dyke et al, 1990).

Since heart defects are quite common in DS persons, in adulthood there is an increased occurrence of mitral valve prolapse and aortic regurgitation (Goldhaber et al, 1986). Additionally, duodenal atresia and obstruction occurs in 8% of DS infants. Imperforate anus has also been reported (Behrman et al, 1987). Dermatoglyphics refers to a skin pattern of whorls, loops, and arches that are found on the palms, soles, and fingers. The most notable is a simian palmar crease (Figure 63–1).

Musculoskeletal abnormalities in DS infants include hypotonia and hyperextensibility of the joints. Hands are usually short, broad, and stubby, with incurving and dysplasia of the middle phalanx of the fifth finger. Typically, the feet have poorly developed arches and wide spaces between the first and second toes (Holmes et al, 1972). Hypotonic muscles often result in abdominal protuberance.

Ocular

Ocular manifestations are numerous in DS; however, they are rarely sight-threatening (Table 63–2). Slanting of the palpebral fissures is characteristic of DS. Shapiro and France (1985) found that DS individuals have palpebral slants of 6 degrees or more. In contrast, the

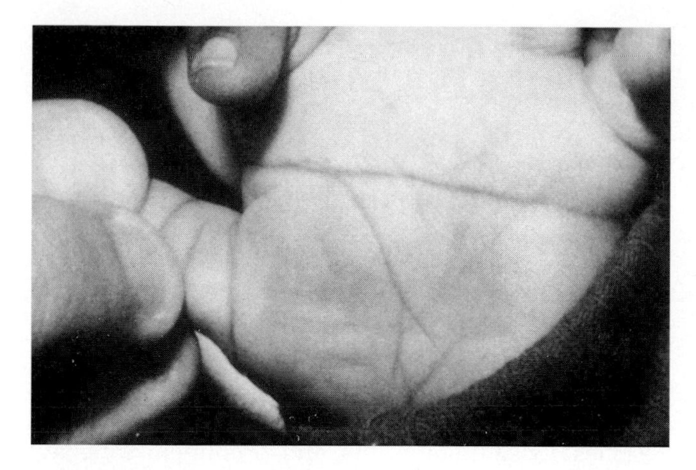

Figure 63–1. Simian palmar crease.

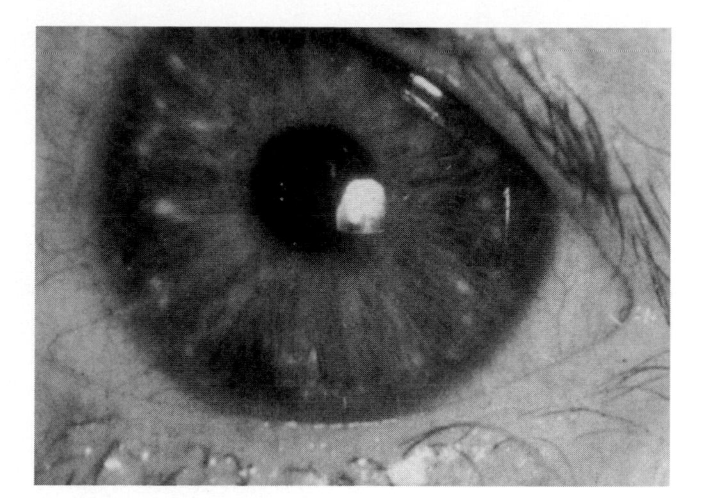

Figure 63–2. Brushfield spots.

slant observed in "normals" is less than 5 degrees. Woodhouse and associates (1997) compared the refractive status of 96 DS infants and children with a corresponding group of age-matched normals. A similar distribution of refractive errors was observed between the two groups. However, there was a wider distribution of refractive errors in children with DS, especially astigmatism.

Spotting of the iris is a frequent ocular manifestation observed in DS patients. These lesions appear as white elevated speckles. Histologic studies characterize the lesions to be densely packed stromal fibers. The speckle patterns were first described by Brushfield. Thus, the lesions have been termed Brushfield spots (Figure 63–2). These lesions are more numerous and distinct at the pupillary margin in DS individuals. In contrast, these spots are typically located in the periphery and appear less distinct in the "normal" population (Donaldson, 1961).

The high incidence of blepharitis in DS patients is likely due to their susceptibility to infections (Berk et al, 1996). The great variability in frequency of diagnosing blepharitis may be attributed to the different criteria being used. Accommodative esotropia is the most common type of strabismus found in DS individuals. Despite the prevalence of strabismus, amblyopia is very uncommon. Usually DS patients with nystagmus do not have any ocular pathology. The nystagmus, in general, is horizontal, fine, rapid, and pendular in nature (Davis, 1996). Congenital cataracts that are isolated punctate lenticular opacities are very common in DS patients. The most common retinal abnormality is a high number of retinal vessels crossing the margin of the optic nerve head with an unusual spoke-like appearance. The next most common retinal findings are high myopic degenerative changes. Keratoconus and glaucoma have also been found to a lesser extent in DS patients.

TABLE 63–2. OCULAR MANIFESTATIONS OF DOWN SYNDROME

- Slanting of palpebral fissures
- Prominent epicanthal folds
- Blepharitis
- Lacrimal duct obstruction
- Keratoconus
- Refractive errors
- Brushfield spots
- Strabismus
- Nystagmus
- Amblyopia
- Cataracts
- Retinal abnormalities
- Glaucoma

DIAGNOSIS

Systemic

Prenatal tests for DS involve either screening or diagnostic tests (Table 63–3). Typically, prenatal screening for DS is recommended when maternal age is more than 34 years, because of the increased risk. DS pregnancies

TABLE 63–3. DIAGNOSIS OF THE DOWN SYNDROME FETUS

Test	Normal Reference Range
Prenatal Screening	
Alpha-fetoprotein	0–15 ng/mL
Human chorionic gonadotropin	<5 mU/mL
Unconjugated estriol	50–125 pg/mL
Diagnostic Tests	
• Amniocentesis	
• Chorion villus biopsy	

can be screened by the use of biochemical markers. The best predictors are human chorionic gonadotropin (hCG), followed by unconjugated estriol (uE3), and then, alpha-fetoprotein (AFP) (Takashima, 1997). These screening tests measure the levels of various substances in the maternal blood. The concentration of hCG in maternal blood rises exponentially until 9 to 10 weeks of gestation. Thereafter, it decreases to approximately 20% of the maximum level in normal pregnancies. Therefore, high concentrations of hCG in the maternal blood found during the second trimester indicate an increased risk for DS. Low levels of AFP in maternal blood during the second trimester suggests a DS fetus (Loncar et al, 1995). This is because the DS fetus tends to be smaller and thus has a smaller placenta secreting less AFP. If AFP is tested alone, 20% of DS fetuses will be detected. AFP and hCG together will determine 50 to 60% of DS fetuses and AFP and hCG with uE3 will detect about 60 to 70% of DS fetuses.

> Pregnant women over 34 years of age are recommended to have prenatal screening for DS.

Definitive diagnosis requires either amniocentesis or chorion villus sampling (CVS). Amniocentesis is usually performed at 14 to 16 weeks of gestation and involves a sampling of amniotic fluid. CVS is usually done at 10 to 11 weeks of gestation and involves the collection of trophoblastic tissue from the placenta. Both procedures involve the culturing and karyotyping of chromosomes. Amniocentesis and CVS carry a small risk for miscarriage; however, diagnosis of DS is 98 to 99% accurate (Catalano, 1990).

Fetal ultrasound has also been used in the early detection of DS. Amniocentesis is suggested when thickening of the nuchal skin fold is present. A nuchal (nape of the neck) skin fold of 6 mm or greater is found in 8.5% of normal chromosome fetuses and 38% of those with DS (Grandjean et al, 1995). Lockwood and colleagues (1987) suggested that the biparietal diameter to femur length ratio is increased in DS fetuses. However, this type of screening test for DS is less than ideal because the measurements are subjective and subject to variances in imaging techniques among technicians.

The incidence of births of children with DS increases with the age of the mother; however, DS infants are more commonly born to mothers less than 35 years of age. This is because pregnant women who are over the age of 34 are highly recommended to have a prenatal screening for DS. Bishop and associates (1997) found an approximate 20% reduction of live births with DS as the result of elective abortion of diagnosed fetuses for all maternal ages. In mothers aged over 35 years, Bishop's group found a reduction of approximately 49% live births with DS as the result of elective abortion.

Differential diagnosis (Table 63–4) of DS includes fragile X syndrome, cerebral palsy, and Eagle–Barrett syndrome. Fragile X syndrome is an inherited genetic condition associated with mental retardation. The etiology is a break in the long arm of the X chromosome. This is a "sex-linked" abnormality in which the mother is a carrier and the sons are at risk of being affected. Physical features include a long narrow face, enlarged testicles, loose finger joints, and prominent ears, jaw, and forehead (Hagerman & Silverman, 1991).

Cerebral palsy (CP) is a motor impairment resulting from brain damage in the young child. The damage occurs because of a congenital malformation of the brain and not during the birthing process. Physical findings include abnormal muscle tone, abnormal movements, abnormal reflexes, and persistent infantile reflexes. CP is usually suspected when a child does not reach normal developmental milestones such as sitting (6 months) and walking (12 months). Typically, a diagnosis of CP can not be made until the child is 18 months of age (Bass, 1999).

Eagle–Barrett syndrome, commonly known as the prune-belly syndrome, consists of a triad of features: (1) anterior abdominal wall musculature that is deficient or absent, (2) urinary tract abnormalities, and (3) bilateral cryptorchidism (testes not descended into the scrotum). The incidence is 1 in 40,000 live births and 95% of cases occur in males. The cause is believed to be a multisystem disease complex that arises from a defect in the mesodermal development (Sutherland et al, 1995).

> Most strabismic DS individuals are esotropes, typically accommodative.

Ocular

Ocular manifestations are common in DS individuals. Examination should include a detailed case history with an emphasis on squinting, eye turn, epiphora, and

TABLE 63–4. DIFFERENTIAL DIAGNOSIS OF DOWN SYNDROME

- Fragile X syndrome
- Cerebral palsy
- Eagle–Barrett syndrome

eye rubbing. Visual acuity can be assessed with the use of Teller cards, forced preferential looking, Lighthouse cards, broken wheel, and/or tumbling E. Refractive errors are very common and can be assesed with retinoscopy and keratometry. The use of a corneal topographer may be necessary in aiding the diagnosis of keratoconus. If cover testing is difficult to perform, one can try Hirshberg or Bruckner tests to assess ocular misalignment. Since most esotropes in DS individuals are accommodative, the addition of plus lenses for near can be used to determine if a reduction in ocular misalignment is possible.

> Astigmatism is common in DS individuals.

A slit-lamp examination should be performed with an emphasis on nasolacrimal duct obstruction or any signs of congenital glaucoma (megalocornea). The use of atropine for dilated fundus examination is contraindicated in these patients because of an increased incidence of vagolytic action as well as a more rapid and sustained pupillary dilation (Catalano, 1990).

TREATMENT AND MANAGEMENT

Treatment and management of DS patients is outlined in Table 63–5.

Systemic

DS individuals may present with many systemic manifestations. The key to management is the cooperation between professionals across various disciplines. Congenital heart disease is found in 40 to 50% of patients with DS. Once the diagnosis is made, it is managed with digoxin, diuretics, and/or surgery. Dental problems are treated with proper oral hygiene, teeth cleaning, dental rinses, diet, and regular dental visits. Treatment of musculoskeletal abnormalities includes the use of foot orthoses to improve gait and balance. Gross motor and fine skills can be treated by a physical therapist (Van Dyke et al, 1990). Children with DS who are reared at home seem to have higher IQs and improved social skills compared to their counterparts in institutions. In addition, early intervention has been found to accelerate the process of obtaining developmental skills (Pueschel, 1980).

TABLE 63–5. TREATMENT AND MANAGEMENT OF DOWN SYNDROME

Systemic
- Congenital heart disease: digoxin, diuretics, surgery (if necessary)
- Dental manifestations: proper oral hygiene, regular dental visits/cleaning
- Musculoskeletal abnormalities: orthoses, physical therapy

Ocular
- Blepharitis: lid hygiene
- Epiphora: dilation and irrigation of puncta, lacrimal intubation, or dacryocystorhinostomy (if necessary)
- Refractive error: correction with polycarbonate lenses
- Strabismus: spectacle correction, vision therapy, surgery
- Nystagmus: prism therapy (if severe)

Ocular

Investigating a patient with special needs requires the examiner to concentrate on the individual rather than the disability. Woodhouse (1998) recommends the following guidelines: (1) be aware of correct terminology, (2) avoid the word "normal" when making comparisons of an individual's performance, (3) communicate with other professionals and parents, (4) always emphasize the positives, and (5) try to be flexible in the testing approach.

Blepharitis is treated with lid hygiene and antibiotics when indicated. The presence of epiphora may indicate lacrimal duct obstruction requiring dilation and irrigation. In some cases, lacrimal intubation or dacryocystorhinostomy may be necessary.

Refractive errors should be corrected with polycarbonate lenses. The management of strabismus may involve the use of spectacles, vision therapy, amblyopia therapy, and/or strabismus surgery. Treatment of nystagmus may involve the use of prisms to direct the eyes toward a null point.

Brushfield spots and vessel changes at the optic nerve head have no pathological significance. The presence of a cataract may require surgery if it reduces vision. Often an intraocular lens implant is used since contact lenses are not readily tolerated by DS individuals. DS patients with keratoconus usually develop hydrops that requires penetrating keratoplasty to prevent loss of vision. Initially, glaucoma can be managed medically. However, in most cases, surgical intervention is ultimately required.

CONCLUSION

Down syndrome is the manifestation of a common chromosomal abnormality. Persons with DS carry a wide range of manifestations, both systemic and ocular. With increased mainstreaming of DS individuals, they may be encountered more frequently by the eyecare provider. A thorough understanding of DS and its systemic and ocular manifestations can allow for the proper management of these patients.

REFERENCES

Bass N. Cerebral palsy and neurodegenerative disease. *Curr Opin Pediatr.* 1999;6:504–507.

Behrman RE, Vaughan VC III, Nelson WE. *Textbook of Pediatrics.* Philadelphia: WB Saunders; 1987:254–256.

Berk AT, Saatci AO, Ercal MD, et al. Ocular findings in 55 patients with Down's syndrome. *Ophthalmic Genet.* 1996; 17:15–19.

Bishop J, Huether CA, Torfs C, et al. Epidemiologic study of Down syndrome in a racially diverse California population, 1989–1991. *Am J Epidemiol.* 1997;145:134–147.

Catalano RA. Down syndrome. *Surv Ophthalmol.* 1990;34: 385–398.

Clarke CM, Edwards JH, Smallpeice V. 21 trisomy/normal mosaicism in an intelligent child mongoloid. *Lancet.* 1961; 1:1028–1030.

Cullen JF, Butler HG. Mongolism and keratoconus. *Br J Ophthalmol.* 1963;47:321.

Da Cunha RP, De Castro Moreira JB. Ocular findings in Down's syndrome. *Am J Ophthalmol.* 1996;122:236–244.

Davis JS. Ocular manifestations in Down syndrome. *Pennsylvania Med.* 1996;(suppl):67–70.

Donaldson DD. The significance of spotting of the iris in mongoloids. *Arch Ophthalmol.* 1961;4:26–31.

Down JLH. Observations on an ethnic classification of idiots. *Lond Hosp Rep.* 1866;3:259–262.

Eissler R, Longenecker LP. The common eye findings in mongolism. *Am J Ophthalmol.* 1962;54(suppl 3):398–406.

Frantz JM, Insler MS, Hagenah M, et al. Penetrating keratoplasty for keratoconus in Down's syndrome. *Am J Ophthalmol.* 1990;109:143–147.

Frynes JP. Chromosomal anomalies and autosomal syndromes. *Birth Defects.* 1987;23:7–32.

Gaynon MW, Schimek RA. Down's syndrome: A ten-year group study. *Ann Ophthalmol.* 1977;9:1493–1497.

Goldhaber SJ, Rubin IL, Brown W, et al. Valvular heart disease among institutionalized with Down's syndrome. *Am J Cardiol.* 1986;57:278–281.

Grandjean H, Sarramon M, AFDPHE Study Group. Sonographic measurement of skinfold thickness for detection of Down syndrome in the second-trimester fetus: A multicenter prospective study. *Obstet Gynecol.* 1995;85:103–106.

Hagerman RJ, Silverman AC, eds. *Fragile X Syndrome: Diagnosis, Treatment and Research.* Baltimore: John Hopkins University Press; 1991.

Hershey DW. Maternal serum α-fetoprotein screening and Down's syndrome. *Am J Obstet Gynecol.* 1988;158:215–217.

Holmes LB, Mosher HW, Halldorsson S, et al. *Mental Retardation: An Atlas of Diseases with Associated Physical Abnormalities.* New York: Macmillan; 1972.

Jaeger EA. Ocular findings in Down's syndrome. *Trans Am Ophthalmol Soc.* 1980;158:808–845.

Lockwood C, Benacerraf B, Krinsky A, et al. A sonographic screening method for Down's syndrome. *Am J Obstet Gynecol.* 1987;157:803–808.

Loncar J, Barnabei VM, Larsen JW. Advent of maternal serum markers for Down syndrome screening. *Obstet Gynecol Surv.* 1995;50:316–320.

Lowe RF. The eyes in mongolism. *Br J Ophthalmol.* 1949;33: 131–174.

Martin HP. Microcephaly and mental retardation. *Am J Dis Child.* 1970;119:128–131.

Palomaki GE. Down's syndrome epidemiology and risk estimation. *Early Hum Dev.* 1996;47(suppl):S19–S26.

Polani PE, Briggs JH, Ford CE. A mongol girl with 46 chromosomes. *Lancet.* 1960;1:721–724.

Pueschel SM. *Down's Syndrome, Growing and Learning.* Kansas City: Andrews & McMeel; 1980:1–25.

Rudolph AM, Hoffmann JIE. *Pediatrics.* Norwalk, CT. Appleton & Lange; 1987:234–235.

Shapiro MB, France TD. The ocular features of Down's syndrome. *Am J Ophthalmol.* 1985;99:659–663.

Skeller E, Oster J. Eye symptoms in mongolism. *Acta Ophthalmol.* 1951;29:149.

Sutherland RS, Mevorach RA, Kogan BA. The prune-belly syndrome: Current insights. *Pediatr Nephrol.* 1995;6: 770–778.

Takashima S. Down syndrome. *Curr Opin Neurol.* 1997;10: 148–152.

Van Dyke DC, Lang DJ, Heide F, et al, eds. *Clinical Perspective in the Management of Down Syndrome.* New York: Springer-Verlag; 1990:3–54.

Walker NF. The use of dermal configurations in the diagnosis of mongolism. *Pediatr Clin North Am.* 1958;5:531–543.

Woodhouse JM. Investigating and managing the child with special needs. *Ophthalmic Physiol Opt.* 1998;18:147–152.

Woodhouse JM, Pakeman VH, Cregg M, et al. Refractive errors in young children with Down syndrome. *Optom Vis Sci.* 1997;74:844–851.

Section XV

NUTRITIONAL DEFICIENCIES

Chapter 64

VITAMIN DEFICIENCIES

Dawn N. Tomasini, Tanya L. Carter

Nutritional deficiencies can result in clinically evident ocular manifestations. They are more common in developing nations than in North America. Although the relationship between socioeconomic status and diet is the primary factor in nutritional deprivation, other secondary causes of deprivation must be considered, such as inadequate absorption, storage, and transport. Despite primary and secondary causes of vitamin deficiency, the general level of nutrition is high in much of the technologically developed world. In other areas of the world, vitamin deficiencies resulting from famine or poor nutrition can have devastating or even fatal results.

The recommended daily allowance (RDA) is the minimum amount below which nutritional problems may occur. Many nutritionists are now recommending a suggested optimal intake (SOI) that is usually well above the RDA. The therapeutic dose of a nutrient is usually 10 to 50 times the RDA. Therapeutic doses are gradually decreased upon resolution of signs and symptoms.

The six basic classes of substances that are considered essential nutrients are proteins, carbohydrates, fats, fiber, minerals, and vitamins. The next two chapters will focus on the more common vitamin and mineral deficiencies.

Vitamins are organic compounds that are necessary for normal growth, development, and sustenance of health. They serve as components of enzymes that metabolize energy from food, as antioxidants to neutralize damaging free radicals, and as structural components of bones, teeth, and skin. They play an important role in red blood cell (RBC) formation, hormone function, the production of genetic material, and the proper function of the immune, gastrointestinal, respiratory, nervous, and muscular systems.

There are two categories of vitamins: fat-soluble (vitamins A, D, E, and K) and water-soluble (B-complex vitamins, vitamin C, carotenes, folic acid, and bioflavonoids). Fat-soluble vitamins are stored in the body and therefore are more prone to reach toxic levels. The water-soluble vitamins are easily lost in cooking, and must be replenished daily because excesses are excreted in the urine. They are usually nontoxic except in extremely high quantities.

Free-radical pathology is an important concept in understanding the role of many vitamins and minerals in maintaining good health. A free radical is an atom or molecule that has an unpaired electron. Although essential for biological systems, they may be destructive. Free radicals are used to kill invading bacteria, release energy, and detoxify chemicals. Yet they can act to destroy cell membranes, genetic material, and enzymes, as well as to promote cross-linkage of collagen molecules. Vitamins A, C, and E and zinc serve as free-radical scavengers. Our bodies are burdened with an overabundance of free radicals due to pollution, radiation exposure, and unknowingly eating rancid foods. Thus it is possible that under conditions of stress, even a mild nutrient deficiency may affect the body's ability to perform this function.

Preventive nutrition has become a primary objective for many health-conscious consumers. Changing dietary practices and including dietary supplements for the purpose of reducing the risk of disease and improving health outcomes have become a standard in healthcare today. Public health policies have adapted preventive nutritional strategies such as the inclusion of iodine in salt for the prevention of iodine deficiency disease. As healthcare providers, it is essential that we understand how vitamin deficiencies manifest systemically as well ocularly.

VITAMIN A (RETINOL)

Vitamin A is a naturally occurring fat-soluble substance. It plays an important role in maintaining the integrity of epithelial membranes in many tissues, including the mucous membranes of the eyes, skin, and respiratory, gastrointestinal, reproductive, and genitourinary systems. Beta-carotene, the provitamin A, is an antioxidant. Retinol is necessary for normal cell growth, bone development, resistance to infection, and maintenance of ocular health.

Epidemiology

Systemic

The exact prevalence and incidence of vitamin A deficiency in developed countries is not known. In the United States, many nutritionists feel that the amount of vitamin A for optimal health is not obtained. Vitamin A deficiency is a common problem in underdeveloped countries like Asia, the Caribbean, India, Central and South America, and Africa. Children are more commonly affected and suffer from a high incidence of associated morbidity and mortality.

Ocular

Sommer (1982) reported vitamin A deficiency to be the leading cause of childhood blindness in many underdeveloped countries. Xerophthalmia, a condition in which the cornea and conjunctiva become keratinized from excessive dryness, is estimated to occur in 10 million children yearly with a quarter million suffering from blindness. The mortality in untreated cases of xerophthalmia ranges between 50 and 90%. Even children with mild xerophthalmia are reported to die at a rate of three to nine times the norm.

According to Sommer (1989), there is evidence that a "subclinical" vitamin A deficiency involving conjunctival epithelium is more pervasive than clinical xerophthalmia.

Pathophysiology/Disease Process

Systemic

The onset of vitamin A deficiency is insidious. As the disease becomes more advanced, it will progress more rapidly, resulting in irreversible damage (Table 64–1). An early clinical sign of deficiency in children is the absence of the "spring growth spurt." Sommer (1989) proposed that vitamin A influences mortality, at least in part, by altering resistance to infections like measles, respiratory disease, and diarrhea. The mechanism for altered resistance is possibly related to the disrupted epithelial linings of the respiratory, gastrointestinal, and genitourinary tracts that occur early in deficiency. Borderline deficiencies may manifest if compounded by illness like measles or diarrhea, in which the body's nutritional demand increases. Measles can cause a sudden and severe depletion in the circulating levels of serum retinol. It has been linked to 50 to 80% of childhood blindness in some underdeveloped countries. In the United States, marked deficiency is more often seen in association with fad diets; diseases causing malabsorption (gastroenteritis, cystic fibrosis, celiac disease); problems with storage (liver disease); and deficiency in retinol-binding protein (RBP), which affects transport. Systemic manifestations include diseases producing hard, dry, flaky skin and hyperkeratosis, as in psoriasis, and problems with respiratory, gastrointestinal, and genitourinary function. The mucous membrane atrophy of these organs results in decreased resistance to infections. In particular, there may be increased susceptibility to respiratory infections like pneumonia or tonsillitis. Severe chronic deficiency can result in death when cellular growth is inhibited, the lysosome membranes are disrupted, or there is an altered resistance to infection.

Ocular

Since vitamin A plays a vital role in the function of many organs, systemic signs of vitamin A deficiency are nonspecific. However, the ocular signs of nyctalopia and xerophthalmia are unequivocal indications of vitamin A deficiency. Nyctalopia, or night blindness, is a well-known consequence of vitamin A deficiency (Table 64–2). It is an early symptom that may be experienced even in mild cases of deprivation. Retinol, a form of vitamin A, is a component of the rod and cone visual pigments (rhodopsin and iodopsin, respec-

TABLE 64–1. SYSTEMIC MANIFESTATIONS OF VITAMIN DEFICIENCIES

Vitamin A
- Psoriasis
- Keratosis follicularis
- Ichthyosis
- Arrested growth
- Respiratory dysfunction
- Gastrointestinal dysfunction
- Genitourinary dysfunction
- Lowered resistance to infection

Thiamine/B_1
- Beriberi
- Wernicke encephalopathy
- Korsakoff syndrome
- Learning disability
- Indigestion, anorexia, constipation
- Fatigue, weakness, neurosensory and motor deficits
- Cardiac dysfunction
- Depression
- Decreased mental alertness

Riboflavin/B_2
- Tissue hypoxia
- Glossitis
- Angular stomatitis
- Seborrheic dermatitis

Niacin/B_3
- Glossitis
- Pellagra
- Diarrhea
- Dementia, memory loss, disorientation, psychosis, decreased mental alertness
- Chronic fatigue and weakness
- Headache
- Insomnia
- Anorexia

Pyridoxine/B_6
- Seborrheic dermatitis
- Glossitis
- Angular stomatitis
- Peripheral neuropathy
- Lymphocytopenia

Vitamin B_{12}
- Macrocytic (dietary) anemia
- Pernicious (absorption defect) anemia
- Leukopenia
- Thrombocytopenia

Vitamin C
- Tendency to bruise easily
- Petechial and broad-based hemorrhages into the skin
- Low resistance to infection
- Scurvy

Vitamin D and Calcium
- Muscular cramping and twitching
- Rickets
- Osteomalacia
- Hyperparathyroidism
- Inefficient blood coagulation
- Insomnia
- Sensitivity to pain
- Poor bone healing

Vitamin E
- Skin wrinkling
- Poor wound healing
- Respiratory failure
- Myocardial infarction, stroke
- Neurological deficit
  Hyporeflexia, gait disturbance, ataxia, vertigo

tively). The onset of night blindness is insidious, with rod function affected earlier and to a greater extent than cone function. Initially, one may have trouble seeing in the dark or at dusk, which is a result of a lengthened dark adaptation time. In chronic cases the cones will be affected, leading to impairment of central acuity and defects in color vision. Also, bright lights in the dark may be momentarily blinding. Night blindness is usually reversible with oral supplements.

When hypovitaminosis is not corrected in its early stage, xerophthalmia may occur. Xerophthalmia is an excessive dryness of the conjunctiva and cornea in which they lose their luster and become keratinized. This results from a lack of vitamin A that subsequently affects the mucin-secreting goblet cells present in the conjunctival epithelium. Without mucin to coat the hydrophobic surface of the cornea, tear break-up time is greatly diminished, leading to the formation of keratinized plaques. As a result, corneal xerosis and keratomalacia can occur. Bilateral corneal ulcers have been reported in patients with a secondary vitamin A deficiency. Bitot spots are another common ocular entity that is associated with vitamin A deficiency. These are seen as small greyish-white deposits that first appear on the temporal bulbar conjunctiva adjacent to the cornea. In young children, Bitot spots are considered pathogonomic for present or past vitamin A deficiency. Other associated findings include cataracts, glaucoma, and retinal pigment epitheliopathy. Early stages of vitamin A deficiency are often referred to as subclinical, because marked xerophthalmia is not present yet structural damage has occurred as evidenced by conjunctival cell cytology. As the disease progresses, severe ocular drying (xerosis) occurs.

A patient may first present with typical dry eye symptoms along with conjunctival inflammation. As the disease becomes more severe and chronic, the classic signs of xerosis manifest as conjunctival looseness,

TABLE 64–2. OCULAR MANIFESTATIONS OF VITAMIN DEFICIENCIES

Vitamin A
- Dermatitis (eyelid)
- Dry eyes
- Xerophthalmia
- Night blindness
- Bitot spot
- Diffuse conjunctival infection
- Cataract
- Peripheral pigment epitheliopathy
- Macular degeneration
- Glaucoma[a]

Vitamin B_1
- Restricted EOM motility, ophthalmoplegia
- Anterior or retrobulbar optic neuropathy
- Nystagmus

Vitamin B_2
- Angular or seborrheic blepharoconjunctivitis
- Dermatitis (eyelid)
- Dry eyes
- Diffuse conjuctival injection
- Limbal injection
- Phlyctenular keratoconjuctivitis
- Corneal vascularization
- Keratitis/infiltrates
- Cataract
- Photophobia

Vitamin B_3
- Dermatitis (eyelid)
- Hyperpigmentation, hyperkeratosis (eyelid)
- Madarosis
- Diffuse conjunctival injection
- Corneal epithelial erosions
- Photophobia
- Pigment maculopathy
- Optic neuropathy

Vitamin B_6
- Blepharitis (angular or sebhorreic)
- Dermatitis (eyelid)
- Dry eyes

Vitamin B_{12}
- Subconjunctival hemorrhages
- Retinal hemorrhages
- Cotton-wool spots
- Retinal venous tortuosity
- Optic neuropathy

Vitamin C
- Conjunctival petechial hemorrhages
- Recurrent subconjunctival hemorrhages
- Retinal hemorrhages
- Orbital hemorrhages
- Hyphema
- Glaucoma[b]

Vitamin D and Calcium
- Band keratopathy
- Cataract
- EOM dysfunction

Vitamin E
- Cataract
- Pigmentary retinopathy
- Macular degeneration
- EOM dysfunction
- Nystagmus
- Night blindness

[a]The exact role is still under investigation.
[b]Due to its role in maintaining or enhancing the use of vitamin A.

folds, pigmentation, decreased luster, dry granular patches, and poor wetting (Figure 64–1). The loss of goblets cells leads to squamous cell metaplasia and epithelial keratinization. This forms a diffuse skin-like appearance that is not always reversible with therapy.

The Bitot spot is described as a sequela of conjunctival xerosis. It appears as an oval or triangular, shiny, gray spot and is usually found bilaterally near the temporal limbus. A foamy substance may be scraped from the surface, leaving a chalky conjunctival bed (Figure 64–2). The exact role that vitamin A plays in the development of the Bitot spot is not entirely clear. Bitot spots have been found in individuals who were not deficient in vitamin A. Also, in some individuals there is no response to vitamin A therapy. However, this may be due to chronic vitamin A deficiency that has resulted in irreversible squamous cell metaplasia.

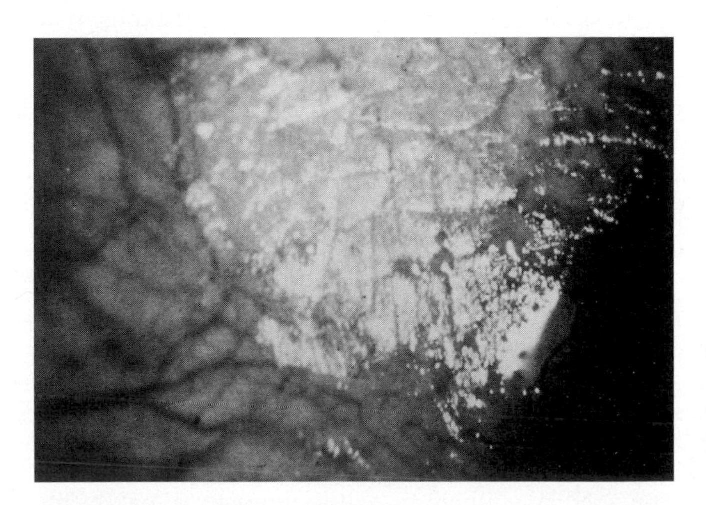

Figure 64–1. In vitamin A deficiency, a dry lusterless conjunctiva with a crocodile pattern and failure to wet the tears. *(Reprinted with permission from Fells P, Bors F. Ocular complications of self-induced vitamin A deficiency.* Trans Ophthamol Soc UK. *1969;89:222.)*

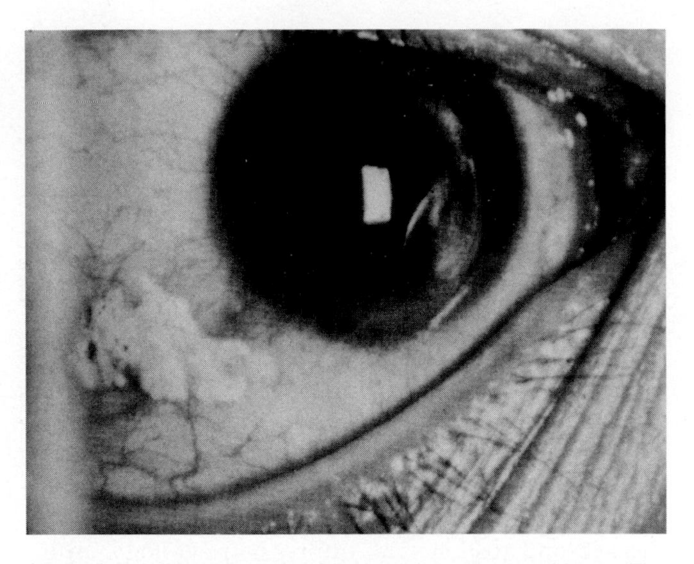

Figure 64–2. Nonresponsive Bitot spot in a 20-year-old man. The superior margin has a foamy appearance, the remainder has a cheesy appearance. *(Reprinted with permission from Sommer A, Emran N, Tjakrasudjatma S. Clinical characteristics of vitamin A responsive and nonresponsive Bitot's spots.* Am J Ophthamol. *1980;90:163.)*

Corneal xerosis may develop as the xerophthalmia progresses. A dry granular appearance with loss of luster and superficial punctate staining will occur early. This is often described as "orange peel" or "pebble like" and can progress to marked keratinization. Corneal ulcers can range in size and location. They tend to start small and peripherally, extending only partly into the cornea, but can become large, central, and full thickness. Some peripheral full-thickness ulcers may be plugged up by the iris, thereby maintaining an intact anterior chamber. Scattered gray or yellow areas of opacification can form, which may coalesce, leading to "liquefactive" stromal necrosis and ulceration, termed "keratomalacia." The changes that occur in keratomalacia are irreversible. Phthisis bulbi may be the final stage of this process.

The antioxidant property of beta-carotene is a factor in protecting the lens proteins from oxidation. It is well documented that nutritional factors play a role in the development of cataracts. Studies have found that the formation of insoluble lens proteins occurs earlier and faster in undernourished subjects.

Normally, the retinal pigment epithelium (RPE) stores vitamin A for utilization by the photoreceptors. According to Fells and Bors (1969), retinal pigment epitheliopathy can occur in chronic vitamin A deficiency. The exact mechanism for the pigmentary disturbance is not well established. It appears as small, white intraretinal opacities and pigment mottling in the periphery (Figure 64–3). They tend to appear in the equatorial regions of both eyes, staying outside the vascular arcades. The opacities eventually fade with treatment but can recur.

Vitamin A may play a role in primary open angle glaucoma. Krishna and Pramod (1982) found serum levels significantly lower in patients with glaucoma compared with normals. It is speculated that lowered vitamin A levels increased the resistance to aqueous outflow because of decreased enzyme activity in the trabecular meshwork. Further research is needed to substantiate the role of vitamin A in glaucoma. People with a predisposition to glaucoma may need more vitamin A.

Diagnosis

Systemic

The key to diagnosis of vitamin A deficiency is observation of the clinical signs and associated symptoms. These include dry, irritated skin, indigestion, problems with breathing, or frequent colds. The best diagnostic laboratory test (Table 64–3) is the serum vitamin A assay. Levels less than 20 μg/100 mL are considered deficient. However, vitamin A status is not solely determined by serum levels of retinol and therefore may not be the most accurate way to diagnose vitamin A deficiency. Liver vitamin A concentration is a more direct

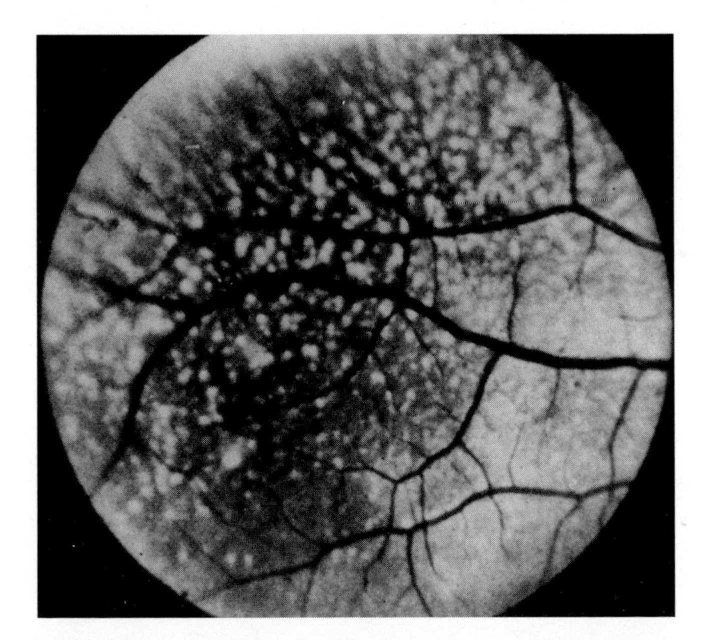

Figure 64–3. Photograph of superotemporal area of right fundus showing discrete white dots apparently deep to the vessels, secondary to vitamin A deficiency. *(Reprinted with permission from Fells P, Bors F. Ocular complications of self-induced vitamin A deficiency.* Trans Ophthamol Soc UK. *1969;89:225.)*

TABLE 64–3. DIAGNOSTIC TESTING FOR VITAMIN DEFICIENCY

Deficient Vitamin	Systemic Test	Ocular Test
A	Serum vitamin A assay	ERG
	Liver vitamin A concentration	Dark adaptometry
	Serum RBP levels	Schirmer test
		Fluorescein staining
		Rose bengal staining
		Impression cytology
B_1	Erythrocyte transketolase activity	Same as systemic
B_2	Serum erythrocyte fluorometric assay	Fluorescein staining
	Urine analysis	Rose bengal staining
B_3	Serum microbial assay	Same as systemic
	Urine analysis	
B_6	Urine fluorometric assay of 4-pyridoxic acid	Same as systemic
	Serum assay of alanine (SGPT) transaminase	
	Serum assay of aspartic (SGOT) transaminase	
	Serum microbial assay utilizing *T. thermophilia*	
B_{12}	Blood serum levels	Same as systemic
	Urinary methylmalonic acid	
	Schilling test	
C	Serum ascorbic acid concentration	Same as systemic
	Leukocyte ascorbic acid concentration	
	Urinary excretion test	
D	Serum calcium levels	Same as systemic
	Serum phosphorous levels	
	Serum alkaline phosphatase activity	
E	Serum vitamin E levels	Dark adaptometry
	Erythrocyte tocopherol levels	ERG

measure of vitamin A status. Since 90% of vitamin A is stored in the liver, biopsy specimens provide the most accurate estimate of liver stores of vitamin A. Although accurate, liver biopsy is not a practical test for vitamin A deficiency because it is so invasive. Assessing the level of serum retinol-binding protein (RBP) is used to rule out transport of vitamin A as a source of deficiency.

Ocular

Symptoms of night blindness or difficulty driving during dusk can be supported by electroretinography (ERG) and dark adaptometry (Table 64–3). The ERG response will show early loss of the a-wave followed by disappearance of the remaining waves. Genest and co-workers (1967) reported that both a-waves and b-waves are equally affected by low serum vitamin A. Dark adaptation time is lengthened. Patients may also complain of being blind after exposure to a bright light, such as the headlights of a car or a light turned on in a dark room. Dark adaptometry can also be used to diagnose subclinical vitamin A deficiency. ERG values return to normal if vitamin A therapy is implemented early on.

The clinical signs of conjunctival xerosis, corneal xerosis, keratomalacia, Bitot spot, and retinal pigment epitheliopathy may be seen along with dry eye symptoms of burning, irritation, and lacrimation in vitamin A deficiency. An early dry eye condition can be diagnosed with the Schirmer test or staining using fluorescein and rose bengal. Impression cytology, an important tool in diagnosis, can determine if goblet cells are absent. Visual acuity and color vision deficits along with photophobia may also be evident.

Treatment and Management

Systemic

The recommended mode of therapy for vitamin A deficiency is retinyl palmitate given orally (Table 64–4). If there is a problem with absorption, an intramuscular injection is suggested. Additionally, vitamin B-complex and systemic antibiotics are also recommended because of the role of vitamins B_2, B_3, and B_6 in maintaining mucous membranes and promoting tissue repair. Also, the disrupted epithelial linings of the respiratory, gastrointestinal, and genitourinary tracts can increase the incidence of infections.

Ocular

Retinyl palmitate is given orally to reverse night blindness and conjunctival xerosis. The effective oral dose of vitamin A to treat corneal xerosis is the dose that causes a rapid increase in blood plasma levels (Table 64–4). Conjunctival and corneal xerosis responds to systemic therapy in 1 to 4 days. Topical vitamin A therapy is still under investigation. Weeks of therapy are needed when topical treatments are used. Topical retinoic acid has been shown to speed healing, but is reserved for opacities on the visual axis because of its potential for scarring. Rengstorff and associates (1988) reported that Vit-A-Drops, which contain 5000 IU of retinol and polysorbate 80, are effective in the treatment of various dry eye disorders. Topical antibiotics may be indicated in cases of epithelial erosion. Keratomalacia is treated in the same manner as corneal xerosis; however, it may not respond to therapy. Bitot

TABLE 64–4. TREATMENT AND MANAGEMENT OF VITAMIN DEFICIENCIES

Vitamin A
- Oral: 200,000 IU retinyl palmitate × 2 days
- IM: 100,000 IU
- RDA: 1400–3300 IU: Infancy–10 years
  4000 IU: Female adult
  5000 IU: Male adult
  6000 IU: Pregnancy/lactation
- Vitamin A toxicity can occur with greater than 30,000 IU/d

Beta-Carotene
- RDA: 2400 μg
- Night blindness
  Oral: 30,000 IU/d × 2–3 weeks
- Conjunctival xerosis
  Oral: 30,000 IU/day × 2–3 weeks
  Topical: 0.01% retinoic ointment 1–3 × /d
  Vit-A-Drops 3–4 × /d
- Bitot spot
  Oral: 200,000 IU
- Corneal xerosis
  Oral: Dose that causes rapid increase in serum levels
  Topical: See conjunctival xerosis
- Keratomalacia
  See corneal xerosis

Thiamine/B_1
- Oral: 500 mg/d
- RDA: 0.5 mg: Infants
  1.2 mg: Children
  1.5 mg: Adults
  1.6 mg: Pregnancy/lactation

Riboflavin/B_2
- Oral: 6 mg/d
- IM: 1 single 25-mg dose
- RDA: 0.6 mg: Infants
  1.2 mg: Children
  1.7 mg: Adults
  2.0 mg: Pregnancy
  2.2 mg: During lactation
- Cataract
  50–100 mg daily

Niacin/B_3
- Oral: 50–250 μg nicotinamide/d
- RDA: 8 mg: Infants
  9 mg: Children
  20 mg: Adults

Pyridoxine/B_6
- Oral: 100–150 mg/d
- RDA: 1.2 mg: Children
  2.0 mg: Adults
  2.5 mg: Pregnancy/lactation

Vitamin B_{12}
- RDA: 10 μg: Adolescents and adults
  15 μg: Pregnancy/lactation
- Not obtained from fruits or vegetables but mainly from meats and meat products
- Pernicious anemia
  1–30 μg parenteral injections/d followed by 100 μg IM monthly for life

Vitamin C
- RDA: 35 mg: Infants
  40 mg: Children
  60 mg: Adults
- SOI: 150 mg/d
- During stress or sickness: 1000 mg/d
- Cataracts
  1000 mg/d in time-release capsules
- Corneal ulcers
  1500 mg/d

Vitamin D
- RDA: 400 IU
- Exposure to sunlight
- Rickets
  2200 IU daily
- Osteomalacia
  1600 IU × 1 month

Calcium
- RDA: 400–600 mg: Infants
  800 mg: Children 1–10 years
  1300 mg: Adults and children 10–18 years
  1300 mg: Pregnancy/lactation
- The elderly may need higher amounts

Vitamin E
- Oral: 400–1800 IU/d
- RDA: 5 IU: Infants
  10 IU: Children
  30 IU: Adults
- SOI: 30–400 IU/day

Reprinted with permission from Food and Nutrition Board Commission on Life Sciences National Research Council. Recommended Daily Allowances. *Washington, DC: National Academy Press; 1989.*

spots may be treated as well. Semba and colleagues (1990) reported cases of Bitot spots that showed a response as soon as 2 weeks.

Beta-carotene can be obtained from fruits and vegetables, and good sources of vitamin A include animal liver, eggs, fish liver oils, and milk. Megadoses of vitamin A can be toxic because it is fat-soluble. Up to approximately 30,000 IU daily is usually safe. The RDA as put forth by the Food and Nutrition Board is outlined in Table 64–4.

VITAMIN B_1

Vitamin B_1 (thiamine) is important to the normal functioning of the heart, muscles, digestive system, and nervous system. It serves as a co-enzyme for converting carbohydrates into glucose and therefore plays a role in the Krebs cycle. It is also necessary for the synthesis of acetylcholine, which is critical in some nerve functions. The more common systemic manifestations of thiamine deficiency include beriberi, Wernicke encephalopathy, and Korsakoff syndrome. The ocular manifestations of deficiency include extraocular muscle palsies, optic neuropathy, and nystagmus.

Epidemiology

Thiamine deficiency is endemic in the Orient and Pacific Islands. It generally occurs in populations relying heavily on polished rice or unenriched white flour that has lost thiamine in the milling process. In North America, it is estimated that 5% of adults over 60 years of age are deficient because of poor dietary intake. The prevalence is even higher among the poor, the institutionalized, alcoholics, and patients with chronic GI syndromes. Fever, exercise, hyperthyroidism, pregnancy, and lactation increase the thiamine requirement.

Pathophysiology/Disease Process

Systemic

Thiamine deprivation may develop in a short period of time because depletion of body stores can occur in just 12 to 14 days. As caloric consumption is increased, more thiamine is necessary. Deficiency can manifest itself in three different forms: anorexia, cardiac involvement, and neurologic involvement. Signs of early deficiency may include impaired digestion of carbohydrates and constipation (Table 64–1). Chronic deficiency can lead to beriberi syndrome. The classic symptoms of beriberi are anorexia, cardiac enlargement that can lead to tachycardia, muscular weakness that can lead to ataxia, paresthesia (abnormal sensation), and dyspnea on exertion. Cardiac and cerebral abnormalities become evident in severe, chronic deficiency. Wernicke encephalopathy can result from severe, acute deficiency; however, it is more commonly found in association with chronic alcoholism or chronic malnutrition. This syndrome is characterized by dementia, ataxia, ophthalmoplegia with nystagmus, and neurologic dysfunction ranging from mild confusion to coma. Resolution of signs and symptoms may begin 24 hours after intiating therapy. Damage to the cerebral cortex can lead to Korsakoff psychosis, and untreated cases can lead to death.

Ocular

Chronic thiamine deficiency can cause restricted extraocular muscle motility, anterior or retrobulbar optic neuropathy, and nystagmus (Table 64–2). The optic neuropathy is due to an alteration in myelin sheath that results in axoplasmic flow stasis. There is a slow, progressive, bilateral, yet often asymmetric involvement of the optic nerves. Toxic optic neuropathy may arise as a result of increased vulnerability to toxicity from exogenous substances such as tobacco and alcohol. The administration of thiamine can improve the condition even if the alcohol and tobacco abuse continues. The ophthalmoplegia associated with Wernicke encephalopathy includes lateral rectus muscle weakness, impaired conjugate gaze, partial third nerve palsies, ptosis, and nystagmus.

Diagnosis

Systemic

Along with the signs already outlined, a patient with thiamine deficiency may complain of fatigue, weakness, muscle tenderness, paresthesia, loss of appetite, indigestion, palpitation, sleep disturbances, poor memory, irritability, and other personality changes. The best laboratory test for assessing thiamine status is the evaluation of the erythrocyte transketolase activity (a thiamine-dependent enzyme) after stimulation by thiamine pyrophosphate (Table 64–3). A significant increase in enzyme activity reflects a thiamine deficiency. Direct serum thiamine assay is not a useful diagnostic tool because only small quantities of thiamine are found in the blood. Urinary microbial or chemical assays are not valuable for assessing thiamine status mainly because of problems obtaining a satisfactory sample size.

Ocular

Ocular diagnosis of thiamine deficiency is based on clinical observation of the signs and correlated symptoms. The most common complaint is a gradual decline in vision ("nutritional amblyopia"). The visual acuity loss is usually bilateral and rarely falls below 20/200. Pain behind the eye, diplopia, and color vision defects also arise in deficiency states. Bilateral centrocecal scotomas are the classic visual field defects associated with nutritional optic neuropathy; however, central scotomas have been reported. The scotomas may be more easily detected with colored targets, especially red.

Treatment and Management

The recommended therapy for thiamine deficiency is oral daily dosing until resolution of signs and symptoms, followed by a daily maintenance dose that meets the RDA as outlined in Table 64–4. Most foods contain low concentrations of thiamine, but good dietary sources of thiamine include whole grain cereals, plant and animal tissue, beans, nuts, peas, oranges, and brewer's yeast.

VITAMIN B_2 (RIBOFLAVIN)

Vitamin B_2 (riboflavin) is essential in the metabolism of carbohydrates, fatty acids, and amino acids. It is necessary for transporting hydrogen and assisting in the transfer of oxygen from plasma to tissues. Riboflavin is important in tissue repair, formation of antibodies, maintaining mucous membranes, and enhancing the efficacy of vitamin D. It also plays a role in light adaptation and promoting ocular lens clarity. Deficiency can result in restricted cellular growth and tissue hypoxia, leading to dermatitis, glossitis, angular stomatitis, circumcorneal injection, superficial keratitis, corneal vascularization, and keratoconjunctivitis sicca.

Epidemiology

Riboflavin deficiency is more commonly found in underdeveloped countries. However, in the United States reports indicate that one third of women over age 65 and men over age 75 have diets deficient in vitamin B_2. As with thiamine deficiency, riboflavin deprivation is associated with low socioeconomic status, the elderly recluse, and chronic alcoholism because of inadequate dietary consumption. Other depleting factors that have been indicated are the use of oral contraceptives, diuretics, and hemodialysis along with cooking styles, processed foods, exposure to UV light, and stress.

Pathophysiology/Disease Process

Systemic

Signs of riboflavin deficiency can manifest after 3 to 4 months of deprivation. Systemic signs include a purplish-red, inflamed, or shiny tongue (glossitis), cracking in the corners of the lips (angular stomatitis), greasy skin, and seborrheic dermatitis (Table 64–1). Initially the corners of the mouth will be pale followed by hyperkeratosis, inflammation, and local ulceration, which progresses to cracks or fissures. The dermatitis commonly involves the nasolabial folds and forms a butterfly distribution involving the cheeks and skin around the ears. Some individuals have proposed the concept of a deficiency syndrome that is characterized by angular stomatitis, glossitis, seborrheic dermatitis, and corneal vascularization.

Ocular

The early signs of riboflavin deficiency are usually ocular. Conjunctival injection with subsequent proliferation and anastomosis of the limbal vessels followed by corneal vascularization is one of the earliest signs of riboflavin deprivation (Table 64–2). Prolonged deficiency can lead to keratitis sicca, interstitial infiltration, and even ulceration. The underlying causes of these ocular changes are tissue hypoxia and mucous membrane dysfunction. The corneal changes will respond to oral riboflavin therapy.

Phlyctenular keratoconjunctivitis, rosacea keratitis, and seborrheic and angular blepharoconjunctivitis also occur in association with riboflavin deficiency. Riboflavin and niacin are present with vitamin A in retinal tissue and are thought to work synergistically to produce efficient visual function. These B vitamins are implicated as necessary components for light adaptation; however, their exact role is not clear.

Riboflavin deficiency also has a controversial role in cataract formation. Riboflavin serves as the coenzyme for glutathione reductase, which catalyses the reduction of oxidized glutathione in the lens. Researchers postulate that because oxidized glutathione is a free radical, its reduction may serve to protect the lens proteins against free-radical damage. Additionally, studies have shown that glutathione reductase activity is decreased in cataractous lenses. Bhat (1987) supported this association with a study in which riboflavin deficiency was found in 81% of cataract patients and only 12.5% of control subjects.

Diagnosis

Systemic

Diagnosis is based on the clinical signs and associated symptoms, which include dry irritated skin and sore tongue. There are two different laboratory tests that clinically measure the presence and degree of riboflavin deprivation (Table 64–3). One test is the serum erythrocyte fluorometric assay to measure the level of reduced glutathione. The other test is the serum microbial assay that utilizes an organism (*Tetrahymena thermophilia*) that requires riboflavin for growth. Urine analysis will show deficiency if values fall below 27 μg/g creatinine for an adult. For children between the ages of 1 and 15, values are considered deficient if they fall below 70 to 150 μg/g creatinine.

Ocular

Riboflavin deficiency should be considered when faced with the common ocular signs and corresponding symptoms. The patient will complain of irritation, lacrimation, and burning. Keratitis may lead to decreased visual acuity and photophobia. Corneal and conjunctival fluorescein and rose bengal staining may be present.

Treatment and Management

The recommended therapeutic approach is a single intramuscular dose or daily oral doses until resolution of the signs and symptoms, after which the RDA should be maintained as outlined in Table 64–4. To manage or prevent cataract formation, some suggest much higher daily doses.

Good dietary sources of riboflavin include milk products, whole grain cereals, dairy products, liver, beef, and eggs.

VITAMIN B_3

Vitamin B_3 (niacin) is also known as nicotinic acid or nicotinamide. As a component of two important coenzymes, it plays an essential role in electron transfer for cellular respiration, and is a necessary component for the metabolism of carbohydrates, fats, proteins, and amino acids. However, niacin is most known for its role in the neurologic and dermatologic systems. Pellagra is a well-known consequence of niacin deficiency. It is characterized by cutaneous, gastrointestinal, mucosal, neurologic, and mental disturbances. This classic deficiency syndrome is described as the three Ds: dermatitis, diarrhea, and dementia. The associated dermatitis can involve the eyelids. Central nervous system involvement may manifest ocularly as external ophthalmoplegia and optic neuropathy.

Epidemiology

Niacin deficiency is still endemic in areas of the world that rely heavily on corn as their principal food source, because corn is deficient in nicotinic acid. In the United States, niacin deficiency is associated with the poor dietary intake of alcoholics, the elderly recluse, and the impoverished. Tryptophan and leucine are two amino acids that affect the supplies of niacin. A deficiency of tryptophan, the amino acid precursor to niacin, will result in a deficiency of niacin. Although the etiology is unclear, excessive leucine may antagonize the synthesis and utilization of niacin, resulting in pellagra.

There are also two hereditary diseases that involve impaired niacin function: schizophrenia and Hartnup disease. Patients with schizophrenia oxidize nicotinamide and excrete it more readily than healthy individuals, resulting in niacin deficiency. Hartnup disease involves a malabsorption of tryptophan.

Pathophysiology/Disease Process

Systemic

One of the earliest signs of niacin deficiency is glossitis (Table 64–1). This begins as a burning sensation of the tongue followed by erythema and edema. As the disease progresses, the classic syndrome, pellagra, may develop, manifesting as dermatitis, diarrhea, and dementia. The most pronounced sign of pellagra involves the skin lesions. The skin will be erythematous followed by vesicle formation, crusting, scaling, and desquamation. The dermatitis tends to be most severe in sun-exposed areas. The diarrhea is caused by intestinal mucous membrane atrophy. Central nervous system involvement will manifest as anxiety, depression, and fatigue in the early stages, and as apathy, dizziness, irritability, and tremors in the more advanced stages.

Ocular

Advanced stages of deficiency may result in eyelid dermatitis, hyperpigmentation, hyperkeratosis, inflammation, and madarosis (Table 64–2). Additionally, conjunctival hyperemia, epithelial erosions, small lymphocytic and leukocytic infiltrates, optic neuropathy, and pigment maculopathy are signs associated with deficiency states. The optic neuropathy may be anterior or retrobulbar and typically is bilateral. Further neuronal involvement may manifest as external ophthalmoplegia.

Diagnosis

Systemic

Diagnosis is based on the signs and their corresponding symptoms, which include chronic fatigue and weakness, hallucinations, and distortions of perception. The more common laboratory tests (Table 64–3) employed are the serum microbial assay that utilizes the *T. thermophilia* organism (which requires nicotinic acid for growth) and urine analysis that measures the level of N-methylnicotinamide (a metabolite of niacin). The normal daily excretion is at least 0.5 mg/g creatinine.

Ocular

Niacin deficiency should be suspected when classic dermatological signs are found along with conjunctival, corneal, and retinal signs as previously outlined. Possible niacin deficiency should be considered in the presence of unexplained gradual loss of visual acuity ("nutritional amblyopia"). The acuity loss is usually bilateral and rarely progresses below 20/200. The patient may also complain of photophobia and aching behind the eyeball that worsens with strong light. Color vision testing may reveal dyschromotopsia, and central or centrocecal scotomas may be evident on visual field testing.

Treatment and Management

Niacin deficiency will respond to a daily oral therapeutic regimen of nicotinamide. Once resolution of signs and symptoms is achieved, at least the RDA, as outlined in Table 64–4, should be maintained. Parenteral therapy is necessary in the presence of malabsorption. Good dietary sources of niacin include brewer's yeast, meats, bran, liver, and legumes.

VITAMIN B_6

Vitamin B_6 (pyridoxine) is a water-soluble co-enzyme that is primarily involved in metabolism, particularly in the metabolism of amino acids, and is required for the release of glucose from glycogen. Pyridoxine is important in the production of neurotransmitters such as serotonin, epinephrine, and GABA, and therefore is essential in maintaining the health of neuronal tissue. It also plays a role in antibody production, and dermatological functions. Deficiency can cause problems similar to vitamin B_2 and B_3 deprivation. Low vitamin B_6 intake is implicated in the onset of cancer, coronary heart disease, eyelid dermatitis, and angular blepharitis.

Epidemiology

The exact incidence and prevalence of pyridoxine deficiency is not known; however, it is observed in association with chronic alcoholism. Pyroxidine has also been shown to have interactions with medications, such as oral contraceptives, antihypertensives, postmenopausal estrogen, isonicotinic acid hydrazide (INH) used to treat tuberculosis, and L-dopa used to treat Parkinson's disease. Vitamin B_6 deprivation can occur in congenital disorders such as homocysteinuria and GABA deficiency. Recent studies show a high prevalence of pyridoxine deficiency in the elderly.

Pathophysiology/Disease Process

Systemic

Small amounts of vitamin B_6 are stored in the body and any excess is excreted in the urine; therefore, adequate dietary intake is essential. Exposure to heat, sunlight, or air causes rapid inactivation. Signs of pyridoxine deficiency are usually dermatological or neurological, including seborrhea-like lesions around the eyes, nasolabial folds, mouth, and forehead, and behind the ears. Glossitis, angular stomatitis, peripheral neuropathy, and lymphocytopenia may also be present (Table 64–1). Symptoms of pyridoxine deficiency are similar to riboflavin and niacin deficiency.

Ocular

Most ocular manifestations of vitamin B_6 deprivation are dermatological, including eyelid dermatitis and angular blepharoconjunctivitis (Table 64–2). The fissuring and cracking at the outer canthi are frequently associated with similar changes at the angles of the mouth. Periocular seborrheic dermatitis that does not respond to riboflavin or niacin therapy may respond to pyridoxine.

Diagnosis

Systemic

Nausea, vomiting, weakness, sleeplessness, irritability, and nervous disorders are signs and symptoms of vitamin B_6 deficiency. The most common laboratory tests (Table 64–3) are the urine fluorometric assay of 4-pyridoxic acid (principal excreted metabolite of vitamin B_6), serum assay of alanine (SGPT) and aspartic (SGOT) transaminases, and the serum microbial assay utilizing *T. thermophilia.* To determine short- versus long-term dietary intake, urine analysis is a better test; however, its reliability as an indicator of vitamin B_6 status is questionable. Vitamin B_6 deficiency causes decreased plasma SGPT and SGOT. The radioenzymatic serum assay will result in a mean B_6 level of 3.6 to 18.0 μg/L of whole blood.

Ocular

A vitamin B_6–deficient patient may complain of ocular burning, irritation, and foreign-body sensation. Eyelid dermatitis and angular blepharoconjunctivitis may be evident on clinical examination along with fissuring and cracking of the outer canthi.

Treatment and Management

Vitamin B_6 deficiency is treated with an oral daily regimen until resolution of signs and symptoms, followed by the RDA as outlined in Table 64–4. If angular blepharoconjunctivitis is present, the differential diagnosis must include the more common cause, *Staphylococcus aureus.*

Good dietary sources of vitamin B_6 include meats, whole grains, nuts, vegetables such as cabbage and peas, and fruits such as bananas and pears.

VITAMIN B_{12}

Vitamin B_{12} (cobalamin) is active in all cells. It is essential in cellular replication and therefore has a great effect on cells that rapidly reproduce, such as those in the bone marrow and GI tract. It is a co-enzyme in the initial stages of DNA synthesis and plays a major role in myelin sheath formation and the metabolism of folates. Vitamin B_{12} is mainly synthesized by bacteria found in water, soil, and the intestines of animals. Therefore, good sources of vitamin B_{12} are foods that are bacterially fermented or animal tissue, such as liver, which accumulates vitamin B_{12}. It is not found in fruits and vegetables except in the legume nodules of root vegetables. Pernicious anemia is the major consequence of deficiency states. The most common ocular manifestation of vitamin B_{12} deficiency is optic neuropathy. Subconjunctival and retinal hemorrhages, cotton-wool spots, and congested vessels may be present in association with anemia.

Epidemiology

Vitamin B_{12} deficiency is predominantly a disease of the elderly, strict vegetarians, and chronic alcoholism, because of poor dietary intake. However, Combs (1992) reported that inadequate dietary intake is rarely a cause of deficiency except in cases of strict vegetarianism. He stated that deficiency occured mostly from inadequate absorption of vitamin B_{12} caused most commonly by inadequate production and secretion of intrinsic factor by the gastric mucosa. Pernicious anemia, an inherited disorder most commonly affecting northern Europeans 40 to 80 years of age, is caused by a lack of intrinsic factor. Other causes of malabsorption are pancreatic insufficiency, intestinal parasitism, and competition for receptor sites from drugs like birth control pills and alcohol. Other depleting factors include inherited disorders of intracellular metabolism, as well as pregnancy and hyperthyroidism, which increase vitamin B_{12} requirements.

Pathophysiology/Disease Process

Systemic

Vitamin B_{12} deficiency takes at least a few years to develop because the depletion of liver stores occurs gradually. Deficiency delays or prevents normal cell division, particularly in the bone marrow and intestinal mucosa. Systemic manifestations of deficiency include anemia, leukopenia, and thrombocytopenia (Table 64–1). With the rate of mitosis reduced, abnormally large cells are formed, giving rise to megaloblastic anemia. Vitamin B_{12} anemias are characterized by large, irregularly shaped red blood cells that have a short life span. The characteristic symptoms of vitamin B_{12} deprivation include fatigue, weakness, dypsnea, and vertigo. The GI tract is also affected, resulting in epithelial changes along the entire digestive tract, including glossitis, diarrhea, and constipation. Neurological abnormalities usually occur later in the course of deprivation because of effective storage and conservation. Nerve demyelination occurs, giving rise to a progressive neuropathy that starts peripherally and causes muscle weakness and paresthesia, ultimately leading to mental confusion, memory loss, hallucinations, and dementia. The symptoms of vitamin B_{12} deficiency are very similar to folate deficiency but can be differentiated by urinary excretion of specific metabolites. A distinction should be made between these similar deficiencies if they are to be properly managed.

Ocular

Optic nerve involvement occurs from damage to its myelin sheath. Early stages may manifest as bilateral retrobulbar neuropathy, which progresses to temporal pallor and eventually anterior optic atrophy. Optic neuropathy may precede, coincide with, or follow the signs and symptoms of megaloblastic anemia (Table 64–2). The primary eyecare provider may play a crucial role in diagnosing vitamin B_{12} deficiency because optic neuropathy can precede anemia and neural involvement in one out of three cases. Prognosis for recovery of visual loss and visual field defects is enhanced if therapy is initiated early in the course of optic nerve involvement; however, recovery is usually slow. Cases have been reported of recovery occurring after 10 months of therapy.

Vitamin B_{12} deficiency is commonly associated with "toxic optic neuropathy" caused by tobacco abuse in which the optic nerve becomes vulnerable to toxicity from the cyanide. Alcohol abuse may also lead to vitamin B_{12} deficiency, because of associated malnutrition and interference by alcohol with B_{12} absorption. In this case the associated optic nerve involvement is known as nutritional optic neuropathy. See Chapter 66 for further discussion of this topic.

Retinal hemorrhages, cotton-wool spots, and congested/tortuous vessels may also appear in the presence of severe chronic anemia.

Diagnosis

Systemic

Diagnosis of vitamin B_{12} deficiency is based on the clinical signs and symptoms, along with blood serum levels (Table 64–3). If deficiency is suspected, a serum microbial assay should be obtained. The normal values range between 200 and 900 pg/mL. Serum levels may be normal because the presence of a biologic inactive analogue of vitamin B_{12} will interfere with the assay. Urinary methylmalonic acid (MMA) levels may also be used for differential diagnosis of vitamin B_{12} deficiency and folate deficiency. MMA levels are elevated in vitamin B_{12} deprivation, but not in folate deprivation. Vitamin B_{12} anemia is diagnosed by obtaining a complete blood count (CBC). This will show reduced quantities of erythrocytes, white blood cells (WBCs), and platelets. The hemoglobin and hematocrit levels will be decreased, whereas the mean corpuscular volume and mean corpuscular hemoglobin will be increased. A serum smear will reveal large oval RBCs and hypersegmented neutrophils. The Schilling test for gastrointestinal absorption should be obtained to specifically rule out pernicious anemia. In the first stage of this test, vitamin B_{12} labeled with radioactive cobalt is given orally. Measurements are based on how much is recovered in the urine in 24 hours. Normal measurements usually range between 7 and 38%. In the second stage, intrinsic factor is added to the vitamin B_{12} doses. A lower amount recovered in stage one versus stage two implies that the malabsorption is a result of a deficiency in the intrinsic factor. A bone marrow smear may show megaloblastic changes and erythroid hyperplasia secondary to an increase in the number of immature erythroid cells.

Ocular

Ocular diagnosis is based on direct observation of the retinal signs as previously outlined. The main complaint with optic nerve involvement will be a gradual decrease in visual acuity. Photophobia and pain behind the eyeball that is made worse by strong light has also been reported. This is believed to be caused by abnormal conduction within the nerve fibers due to myelin sheath dysfunction. The neural response becomes disseminated, resulting in increased sensitivity. Color vision defects will occur, and perimetry or Amsler grid testing may reveal a central or centrocecal scotoma. True "toxic amblyopia" from tobacco abuse may manifest with larger areas of the visual field affected.

The ocular manifestations of vitamin B_{12} anemia include retinal hemorrhages, cotton-wool spots, venous dilation, and tortuosity. Peripheral capillary microaneurysms have also been reported.

Treatment and Management

Dietary vitamin B_{12} deficiency is treated by enhancing the diet with naturally occurring vitamin B_{12} as well as with supplements (Table 64–4). Vitamin B_{12} is not found in plants except for in the roots of certain legumes that contain microorganisms that synthesize the B_{12}. It can be obtained from meats and meat products including red meat, fish, poultry, milk, and eggs. Only 10 to 20% of dietary vitamin B_{12} is absorbed. The intake of iron and folic acid should be increased, because they too are involved in the production of red blood cells. Pernicious anemia is treated with parenteral injections of vitamin B_{12}. It is recommended that approximately 1 to 30 μg be given daily until levels increase followed by monthly injections for life. When managing nutritional optic neuropathy, the recommended therapy is to supplement the entire B complex rather than B_{12} alone.

VITAMIN C

Vitamin C (ascorbic acid) is a water-soluble compound found in plasma, WBCs, and platelets. Ascorbic acid is not produced by the body and therefore must be ingested. It is necessary in the formation of connective tissue and to protect the basement membrane of capillaries. Along with the bioflavinoids, it functions to reduce the permeability of capillaries, thereby strengthening them and minimizing the occurrence of hemorrhages. The presence of vitamin C enhances iron absorption and the ability to fight infection. It also promotes wound healing and healthy gums, teeth, and bones; converts food to energy; recycles vitamin E; and is one of the primary antioxidants. Scurvy is a well-documented consequence of vitamin C deprivation. It is characterized by hemorrhages and abnormal formation of bones and teeth. In the eye, vitamin C deficiency has been associated with hemorrhages, cataracts, and possibly glaucoma.

Epidemiology

Although the classic vitamin C deficiency syndrome, scurvy, is rarely found today, various levels of deprivation often occur in the United States. Studies suggest that the prevalence of vitamin C deficiency is higher in the institutionalized elderly. Ascorbic acid is so easily destroyed that food storage and cooking styles found in institutions may contribute to this deprivation.

Pathophysiology/Disease Process

Systemic

Under normal circumstances, body stores can sustain periods of vitamin C deprivation for up to 3 to 4 months. During periods of increased stress, surgery, burns, smoking, and infection, the demand for vitamin C increases dramatically. Certain drugs like aspirin, antibiotics, cortisone, and oral contraceptives deplete body stores or increase the demand for this nutrient. Cooking, processing, and storage affect the vitamin content of many foods. Vitamin C is particularly vulnerable, showing losses of up to 80%.

A subclinical vitamin C deficiency can exist prior to developing the classic signs and symptoms. This usually develops 2 to 3 months after the onset of dietary deficiency. Ascorbic acid deficiency manifests as hemorrhages from capillary damage and weakening of collagenous structures. The earliest clinical signs of vitamin C deficiency may include a tendency to bruise easily with petechial or ecchymotic hemorrhages into the skin, weakened hair or nails, and a low resistance to infection. Vitamin C is responsible for stimulating the production of interferons, proteins which protect cells against viral attacks and promote the production of IgG and IgM antibodies. Therefore, the body becomes more susceptible to infections during deficiency.

In more advanced stages the classic deficiency syndrome known as scurvy may develop, resulting in defects in collagen formation that manifest as intermittent reductions in growth; impaired wound healing; edema; arthritis; bleeding into the joints and muscles; swollen, bleeding gums with tooth loss; impaired digestion; brittle bones; and psychological changes such as hysteria and depression. If left untreated, death may occur. Prasad and Rama (1985) presented one of many reports suggesting that the antioxidant properties of vitamins A, C, and E and selenium may be necessary for preventing cancer because they reduce the formation and effectiveness of cancer-causing agents (Table 64–1).

Ocular

There is an abundance of vitamin C in the eye. The normal aqueous humor level is 25 times that of plasma. The more common ocular manifestations of vitamin C deficiency are conjunctival petechial hemorrhages and recurrent subconjunctival hemorrhages (Table 64–2). Prolonged deficiency may lead to retinal and orbital hemorrhages and hyphemas. Because vitamin C reduces capillary permeability and fragility, it is recommended in the management of diabetic retinopathy, macular degeneration, and central serous maculopathy. Some researchers have found that adequate levels seemed to decrease the risk of subcapsular cataracts via the role of vitamin C as an antioxidant. This association is supported by the fact that the normally high concentration of vitamin C in the lens decreases with cataract formation. The lack of vitamin C may slow healing of corneal ulcers and other wounds due to its role in collagen formation. The role of vitamin C in glaucoma is still under investigation. It has been reported that megadoses of vitamin C (100 to 150 mg/kg three to five times daily) decreased intraocular pressure (IOP) in patients with glaucoma. Lane (1980) observed that the average IOP was significantly lower in subjects with a mean daily intake of 1200 mg versus 75 mg. The most obvious problem is that megadoses often are not tolerated, and the duration and magnitude of the IOP decrease is limited.

Diagnosis

Systemic

The symptoms of vitamin C deficiency may include weakness, headaches, shortness of breath, impaired digestion, and swollen or painful joints. Measuring the serum and leukocyte ascorbic acid concentrations directly assesses vitamin C status. Serum levels of less than 0.2 mg/dL are considered deficient. The urinary excretion test involves giving an oral dose of ascorbic acid and then measuring the amount released in the urine in 6 hours. Those with deficiency will excrete less of a given dose than those with adequate intake. Measuring urinary ascorbate levels is more effective at detecting excesses of vitamin C than it is at detecting deficiencies.

Ocular

Observation of the clinical signs as previously outlined is the key to diagnosing ocular vitamin C deficiency. Retinal hemorrhages that involve the macula, hyphemas, or cataracts may lead to decreased vision.

Treatment and Management

Some nutritionists suggest that the optimal intake should be greater than the RDA (Table 64–4). This should be increased further when ill or during stress. Body stores are increased through ingestion of 500 mg daily. Since vitamin C is a water-soluble nutrient, toxicity does not occur. However, by taking megadoses, the increased activity can result in allergic reactions, diarrhea, or kidney stones. It is suggested that if supplements are taken, a buffered form should be used.

Todd (1987) reported successfully reversing cataracts with large daily doses in time-release capsules. Other studies report that megadoses will speed the healing of corneal ulcers.

Citrus fruits, papaya, cantaloupes, strawberries, broccoli, green leafy vegetables, spinach, tomatoes, potatoes, and peppers are good dietary sources of vitamin C.

VITAMIN D AND CALCIUM

Vitamin D is a fat-soluble micronutrient that is essential in the absorption and utilization of calcium and phosphorous. It primarily serves to elevate plasma levels of calcium and phosphorous by activating intestinal absorption, enhancing renal absorption, and mobilizing these minerals from the bone. Exposure to ultraviolet radiation stimulates the synthesis of vitamin D in the skin from endogenous or dietary cholesterol. In adults, the body's requirement is usually met by its own synthesis via exposure to sunlight. The liver and the kidney are essential in the activation of vitamin D; therefore, hypocalcemia can occur in patients with chronic renal failure.

Calcium is a macromineral that constitutes about 85% of the mineral matter in bones as calcium phosphate. Calcium plays many roles in the body, such as promoting bone growth, metabolism, and healthy teeth, controlling muscle contraction and neuromuscular excitability, and maintaining membrane permeability. It is also essential for maintaining plasma pH balance, activating enzymes, and blood coagulation. It is a factor in efficient brain function, energy storage in muscles, and healthy digestive, circulatory, and immune systems. Vitamin D and the parathyroid hormone are the primary factors controlling calcium homeostasis.

Hypocalcemia and vitamin D deficiency are associated with rickets in children, osteomalacia in adults, hyperparathyroidism, zonular cortical cataracts, band keratopathy, conjunctival calcification, and impaired oculomotor function.

Epidemiology

Traditionally, vitamin D is naturally found in low amounts in many foods. As a result, countries have made a practice of enriching common and frequently consumed foods with vitamin D. However, vitamin D deficiency may still be found because of decreased sun exposure, GI disorders, lead poisoning, or hereditary disorders of vitamin D metabolism. Even certain drugs, namely anticonvulsants, have been found to reduce the circulating levels of vitamin D.

Before such fortification of foods, rickets, a childhood disease caused by vitamin D deficiency, was found in approximately 75% of children of working-class parents in industrialized countries. Today rickets exists in children living at impoverished levels. Milder cases of calcium deficiency occur in association with hypoparathyroidism, nursing mothers, and poor dietary intake. Calcium absorption is more efficient in males than in females, and the elderly may require a higher intake because inactivity, which often occurs with aging, causes skeletal demineralization.

Pathophysiology/Disease Process

Systemic

A small drop in the concentration of serum calcium can lead to muscular cramping and uncontrolled muscle contractions known as tetany. When the serum levels of calcium become low, compensatory mechanisms attempt to increase calcium levels. Secondary hyperparathyroidism may result from an increase in the secretion of parathyroid hormone, which enhances mobilization of calcium from bone stores (Table 64–1). Excessive parathyroid hormone causes phosphaturia, which interferes with bone calcification, resulting in rickets or osteomalacia. Rickets is a childhood disease caused by inadequate deposition of calcium in developing cartilage and newly formed bone. It is characterized by imperfect skeletal formation, bone pain, muscle tenderness, unhealthy teeth, an enlarged odd-shaped head secondary to late closure of the fontanelle, and enlargement of liver and spleen. Convulsions, hemorrhaging, and tetany mark severe cases. The prognosis is favorable, with deformity disappearing in 90% of treated cases. However, some bone deformations may require surgery.

Osteomalacia is the adult form of rickets, but its signs and symptoms are more generalized. Because the longitudinal growth has stopped, only the shafts of the long and flat bones are affected. The bone mass is still of normal volume, but there is loss of bone density. Its symptoms include muscular weakness and bone tenderness, especially in the spine, shoulder, ribs, and pelvis. Osteomalacia is associated with an increased risk for fractures. It is most often related to diseases causing calcium malabsorption, such as chronic pancreatitis, Crohn disease, chronic ulcerative colitis, and gastric and small bowel resections. Other signs of vitamin D and calcium deficiency include insomnia, pale skin, pain sensitivity, and poor healing of bone injuries.

Ocular

Zonular cortical cataracts may appear months to years after the onset of hypocalcemia (Table 64–2). Typically they develop gradually, forming small, punctate, discrete refractile opacities that are separated from the capsule by a clear zone. These are usually bilateral and seldom interfere with vision. Extraocular muscle deficits are also associated with later stages of deficiency.

Secondary hyperparathyroidism is associated with band keratopathy and conjunctival calcification because calcium is mobilized from the body reserve, resulting in calcium deposition into various body tissues.

Diagnosis

Adults that are deficient in vitamin D or calcium will complain of rheumatic pain in the limbs, spine, thorax, and pelvis; progressive weakness; nervous system hyperirritability; depression; headaches; and insomnia. A child with rickets may exhibit restlessness, slight fever at night, diffuse soreness and tenderness throughout the body, and headaches. Radiographs will show characterisitc body deformities or decrease in bone density. The status of vitamin D is indirectly measured by serum calcium, phosphorous, and alkaline phosphatase activity. Analysis will show normal or low plasma calcium (norms: 8.5 to 10.5 mg/dL), low phosphorous levels (below 2.5 mg/dL), and increased plasma alkaline phosphatase activity. A direct measure of vitamin D status is now available that assesses the plasma level of the vitamin D metabolite, hydroxyvitamin D.

Normal serum calcium levels range from 8.9 to 10.1 mg/dL. Serum calcium is not a useful indicator of dietary calcium intake. Urinary calcium reflects intake to some extent, but further research is needed regarding the nature of this relationship. Hair analysis is a useful method for obtaining the average level of the body's mineral content over a period of several months. Trace elements are accumulated in hair at a rate 10 times higher than in blood serum or urine. The areas where it is most useful is in showing inefficient absorption and toxic levels of minerals such as calcium, magnesium, zinc, manganese, and chromium. This mode of diagnostic testing is often criticized because comparisons of data from different laboratories often show large variations. Also, hair and serum values do not always correlate well, because serum levels give an instantaneous picture of mineral status. Hair analysis indicates the average level over the last 2 to 3 months, yet it can be a useful addition to serum and urine analysis as a diagnostic tool.

Treatment and Management

Exposure to sunlight along with oral vitamin D is the suggested therapy for rickets. Osteomalacia is treated with vitamin D for approximately 1 month followed by the normal daily requirement of vitamin D, calcium, and phosphorous, as outlined in Table 64–4.

Normally, 800 to 1300 mg of calcium daily is sufficient to prevent deficiency. Only about 30 to 60% of the normal dietary calcium is absorbed. In cases of malabsorption, dietary fat should be restricted to 30 g daily.

Good dietary sources of vitamin D include beans, cheese, egg yolk, milk, shellfish, tuna, salmon, cod liver oil, and watercress. Calcium can be obtained from nuts, beets, rhubarb, bran, green vegetables, cauliflower, carrots, milk, cheese, yogurts, lemons, and oranges.

VITAMIN E

There are seven naturally occurring forms of vitamin E. The most active form is tocopherol. Vitamin E is essential for the maintenance of membrane integrity of nearly all cells in the body. As an antioxidant, it serves to protect vitamin A from oxidation. It also serves an important role in maintaining vascular health by protecting red blood cells from lysis, stabilizing blood vessel cell walls, and reducing thrombin formation. It also plays roles in the reproductive, neurological, and muscular systems. Vitamin E is especially important in people who exercise because it provides the body with extra energy for muscle contraction.

The National Institutes of Health reported in 1983 that vitamin E was an essential nutrient in retinal function because it prevents the oxidation of vitamin A and the peroxidation of photoreceptor lipoproteins. Its role in retinopathy of prematurity is well documented. Vitamin E deficiency is also implicated in cataract formation, eye movement abnormalities, pigmentary retinopathy, and central serous retinopathy.

Epidemiology

Clinical vitamin E deficiency has only been reported in premature and low-birth-weight infants, and in association with conditions causing fat malabsorption, such as cystic fibrosis or diseases of the pancreas. Yet many more Americans may be deficient, because lifestyles that produce an abundance of free radicals will increase the need for vitamin E. The National Institutes of Health reported that the average American diet only contains approximately 10 IU daily. In addition, cooking over high heat and food processing lead to oxidation and loss of vitamin E.

Pathophysiology/Disease Process

Systemic

Free-radical damage can affect many systems (Table 64–1). However, vitamin E deficiency targets the neuromuscular, vascular, and reproductive systems. Its manifestations arise secondary to cell membrane dysfunction. The vascular system may respond with strokes, hemorrhages, and poor wound healing. There may be respiratory difficulties or an increased susceptibility to myocardial infarction. The occurrence of a progressive neurological syndrome is believed to occur if vitamin E is deficient during the development of the nervous system. This syndrome is characterized by hyporeflexia, gait disturbance, truncal ataxia, vertigo, transient loss of vision, decreased adduction, nystagmus on adduction, and limited superior gaze.

Ocular

Vitamin E deficiency can result in night blindness and visual dysfunction because one of its roles is to maintain the integrity of vitamin A (Table 64–2). Because vitamin E is highly concentrated in the photoreceptor outer segments, it is thought to protect its photoreceptor membranes from oxidative damage. Therefore, when vitamin E is deficient, it may initiate the process of lipofuscin formation within the retinal pigment epithelial cell with subsequent damage to the RPE cell membrane. This may lead to inefficient metabolism of the rod and cone outer segments and cell death. The cell's contents are then deposited extracellularly in the form of drusen. Drusen that forms in the macular region and other risk factors (genetic traits, UV exposure, presence of cardiovascular disease, and cigarette smoking) may result in macular degeneration.

Berger and colleagues (1991) reported a generalized retinal pigment epithelium dropout and pigment clumping in chronic vitamin E deficiency in the presence of normal vitamin A levels (Figure 64–4). The mechanism for the occurrence of this pigmentary retinopathy is thought to be same mechanism that causes macular degeneration.

In the presence of increased oxygen, vitamin E deficiency can enhance oxidative injury to retinal capillaries forming in the developing eye. This results in retinopathy of prematurity.

Jacques and co-workers (1988) and others have reported a statistically significant relationship between vitamin E deficiency and lens opacification. Because the oxidative process causes unfolding and cross-linkages with other proteins, they postulate that vitamin E serves to stabilize lens protein oxidation.

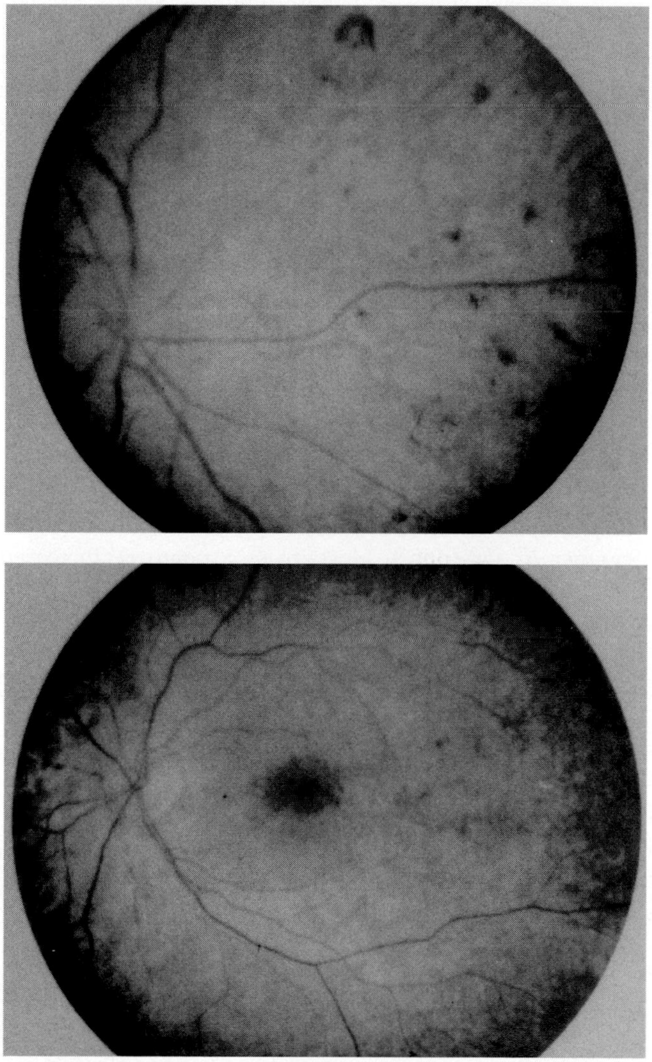

Figure 64–4. Widespread depigmentation, pigment clumping **A**, narrowing of retinal arterioles, and scalloped foci of pigment dropout within the vascular arcades, and loss of the foveal reflex **B**, secondary to vitamin E deficiency. *(Reprinted with permission from Berger AS, Tychsen E, Rosenblum JL. Retinopathy in human vitamin E deficiency.* Am J Ophthalmol. *1991;3:774.)*

The ocular manifestations of progressive neurologic dysfunction related to vitamin E deficiency include decreased adduction, nystagmus on adduction, and limited superior gaze.

Diagnosis

Systemic

Systemic manifestations include hyperreflexia, gait disturbance, and vertigo. The available diagnostic tests (Table 64–3) are serum vitamin E levels and erythrocyte tocopherol levels.

Ocular

Ocular diagnosis of vitamin E deficiency is suspected when a patient complains of night vision problems, decreased visual acuity that is not correctable with a refractive prescription, transient loss of vision, and limited ability to adduct or elevate the eyes. Examination may reveal constricted and depressed visual fields, reduced color vision, increased dark adaptation threshold, or attenuated electroretinogram signals.

Treatment and Management

Daily doses of vitamin E are recommended until resolution of the signs and symptoms, followed by RDA requirements (Table 64–4). However, nutritionists recommend a larger daily intake. Good dietary sources are green leafy vegetables, whole grains, vegetable and seed oils, sweet potatoes, seeds, and peanuts.

REFERENCES

Bendrich A, Deckelbaum R. *Preventive Nutrition: The Comprehensive Guide for Health Professionals.* Totowa, NJ: Humana Press; 1997.

Berger AS, Tychsen E, Rosenblum JL. Retinopathy in human vitamin E deficiency. *Am J Ophthalmol.* 1991;3:774–775.

Bhat R, Raja T, Barrad A, Evens M. Disposition of vitamin E in the eye. *Pediatr Res.* 1987;22:16–20.

Combs G. *The Vitamins: Fundamental Aspects in Nutrition and Health.* San Diego: Academic Press; 1992.

Day PL, Langston WC, O'Brien CS. Cataract and other ocular changes in vitamin G deficiency: An experimental study on albino rats. *Am J Ophthalmol.* 1931;14:1005–1009.

Fells P, Bors F. Ocular complications of self-induced vitamin A deficiency. *Trans Ophthalmol Soc UK.* 1969;89:221–228.

Frei B, England L, Ames BN. Ascorbate is an outstanding antioxidant in human blood plasma. *Proc Natl Acad Sci USA.* 1989;86:6377–6381.

Genest AA, Sarwono D, Gyorgy P. Vitamin A blood serum levels and electroretinogram in five to fourteen year old age groups in Indonesia and Thailand: A preliminary report. *Am J Clin Nutrition.* 1967;20:1275–1279.

Goodhart RS, Shils ME. *Modern Nutrition in Health and Disease.* 6th ed. Philadelphia: Lea & Febiger; 1980.

Hamilton HE, Ellis PP, Sheets RF. Visual impairment due to optic neuropathy in pernicious anemia: Report of a case and review of the literature. *Blood.* 1959;14:378–385.

Hittner HM, Rudolph AJ, Kretzer FL. Suppression of severe retinopathy of prematurity with vitamin E therapy: Ultrastructural mechanism of clinical efficacy. *Ophthalmology.* 1984;91:1512.

Jacques PF, Hartz SC, Chylack LT, et al. Nutritional status in persons with and without senile cataract: Blood vitamin and mineral levels. *Am J Clin Nutr.* 1988;48:152–158.

Johnson L, Quinn GE, Abbasi S, et al. Effect of sustained pharmacologic vitamin E levels on incidence and severity of retinopathy of prematurity: A controlled clinical trial. *J Pediatr.* 1989;114:827.

Ibrahim K, Kara RY, Zuberi SJ. Hypercarotenemia: A case report. *JPMA.* 1976;224–225.

Krishna SM, Pramod KS. Vitamin A and primary glaucoma. *Glaucoma.* 1982;4:226–227.

Kutsky R. *Handbook of Vitamins and Hormones.* New York: Van Nostrand Reinhold; 1973.

Lamand M, Favier A, Pineau A. Determination of trace elements in the hair: Significance and limitations. *Ann Biologie Clinique.* 1990;48:433–442.

Lane BC. Evaluation of intraocular pressure with daily, sustained closework stimulus to accommodation to lowered tissue chromium and dietary deficiency of ascorbic acid. PhD dissertation, 1980, New York University.

Lane BC. Nutrition and vision. In: Bland J, ed. *1984–85 Yearbook of Nutritional Medicine.* New Canaan, CT: Keats; 1985:273.

Lascari AD. Carotenemia. *Clin Pediatr.* 1981;20:25.

Maugh TH. Hair: A diagnostic tool to complement blood serum and urine. *Science.* 1978;202:1271.

Mueller JF, Vilter RW. Pyridoxine deficiency in human beings induced with desoxypyridoxine. *J Clin Invest.* 1950; 29:193.

Murray MT. Iron: Deficiencies and supplements. *Health Counselor.* Nov/Dec 1991:31–33.

Paton D, Mclaren DS. Bitot spots. *Am J Ophthalmol.* 1960; 50:568.

Pihl RO, Parks M. Hair element content in learning-disabled children. *Science.* 1977;198:204–206.

Prasad K, Rama B. Nutrition and cancer. In: Bland J, ed. *1984–85 Yearbook of Nutritional Medicine.* New Canaan, CT: Keats; 1985, 179–211.

Rapp J. Nutrition in the vision of children. *J Am Opt Assoc.* 1979;50:1107–1111.

Rengstorff RH, Krall CC, Westerhout DI. Topical antioxidant treatment for dry-eye disorders and contact lens-related complications. *Afro-Asian J Ophthalmol.* 1988;7:81–83.

Rodger F. The ocular effects of vitamin A deficiency in man in the tropics. *Exp Eye Res.* 1964;3:367–372.

Rosenblum JD, Keating JP, Prensky AL, Nelson JS. A progressive neurologic syndrome in children with chronic liver disease. *N Engl J Med.* 1991;304:503.

Russel RM, Smith VC, Multack R, et al. Dark adaptation testing for diagnosis of subclinical vitamin A deficiency. *Lancet.* 1973;2:1161–1163.

Semba R, Sopandi W, Natadisastra M, Sommer A. Response of Bitot's spot in preschool children to vitamin A treatment. *Am J Ophthalmol.* 1990;110:416–420.

Senile cataract and vitamin nutrition. *Nutr. Rev.* 1989;47: 326–328.

Sommer A. New imperatives for an old vitamin (A). *J Nutrition.* 1989;119:96–100.

Sommer A. *Nutritional Blindness.* New York: Oxford; 1982: 51–52.

Sommer A. Treatment of corneal xerophthalmia with topical retinoic acid. *Am J Ophthalmol.* 1983;95:349–352.

Sommer A. Xerophthalmia and vitamin A status. *Prog Retinal Eye Res.* 1998;17:9–31.

Sommer A, Emran N, Tjakrasudjatma S. Clinical characteristics of vitamin A responsive and nonresponsive Bitot's spots. *Am J Ophthalmol.* 1980;90:160.

Sommer A, Quesada J, Doty M, Faich G. Xerophthalmia and anterior segment blindness among preschool children in El Salvador. *Am J Ophthalmol.* 1975;80:1066.

Sommer A, Sugana T, Djunaedi E, Green R. Vitamin A responsive panocular xerophthalmia in healthy adult. *Arch Ophthalmol.* 1978;96:1630–1634.

Sommer A, Tarwotjo I, Hussaini G, Susanto D. Increased mortality in mild vitamin A deficiency. *Lancet.* 1983;2: 585–588.

Stern JJ. Nutrition in ophthalmology. In: Goodhart R, Shils M, eds. *Modern Nutrition in Health and Disease.* 5th ed. Philadelphia: Lea & Febiger; 1973:1009.

Todd GP. *Nutrition in Health and Disease.* Norfolk, VA: Donning; 1987.

Tomasi LG. Reversibility of human myopathy caused by vitamin E deficiency. *Neurology.* 1979;29:1182–1186.

Wohbach S, Howe P. Tissue changes following deprivation of fat soluble vitamin A. *J Exp Med.* 1925;42:753–777.

Chapter 65

MINERAL DEFICIENCIES

Sharon L. Feldman, Tanya L. Carter

Minerals are important components of hormones and enzymes. They are vital for cellular function and also serve as building blocks for bones, teeth, muscles, plasma cells, and neuronal tissue. As electrolytes, they serve to control neuromuscular contractions and help maintain osmotic pressure as well as the acid–base balance of internal fluids. Minerals also play a role in the digestive and reproductive systems. Calcium (see Chapter 64), chloride, magnesium, potassium, phosphorus, sodium, and sulfur are classified as macrominerals; while copper, cobalt, chromium, fluorine, iodine, iron, manganese, selenium, and zinc are the trace minerals. The Senate Select Committee on Nutrition reported that 99% of the American population is deficient in at least one mineral.

IODINE

Iodine is important in the development and function of the thyroid gland and in manufacturing the hormone thyroxine, which controls the rate at which cells utilize energy from food. It also is essential in the proper functioning of the heart and immune systems as well as protein synthesis. Additionally, iodine deficiency is the most common cause of endemic goiter. Associated hypothyroidism may lead to photophobia, cataracts, eyelid edema, and optic neuropathy.

Epidemiology

Iodine deficiency is more prevalent in areas near freshwater lakes as opposed to those near the seacoast. In many highland areas of America, like states bordering Canada and areas between the Rocky and Appalachian Mountains, the soil is not rich in iodine and many people suffer from dietary deprivation. The process of putting iodine in salt has significantly decreased the incidence of deficiency. Yet it is estimated that approximately 200 million people throughout the world suffer from goiter caused by iodine deficiency.

Pathophysiology/Disease Process

Systemic

Almost 80% of dietary iodine is absorbed by the thyroid gland and is bound with the amino acid tyrosine to form triiodothyronine (T3) and thyroxine (T4). The main function of these thyroid hormones is to control the basal metabolic rate. Iodine deficiency is one cause of goiter, characterized by thyroid enlargement and hypothyroidism (Table 65–1). Physical, sexual, and mental development may be inhibited, and there is lowered resistance to infection and lowered basal metabolism. Signs include obesity, dry skin, dry hair, poor complexion, unhealthy nails, low blood pressure, slow pulse, sluggishness of all functions, and nervous irritability.

TABLE 65–1. SYSTEMIC AND OCULAR MANIFESTATIONS OF IODINE DEFICIENCIES

Systemic
Goiter/hypothyroidism
- Enlarged thyroid gland, obesity, dry skin and hair, poor complexion, unhealthy nails, sluggishness of all functions, nervous irritability, lowered resistance to infection, hypotension, slow pulse, inhibitions of physical, sexual, and mental development

Ocular
- Edema (periorbital or eyelid)
- Photophobia
- Cataract
- Optic neuropathy

Ocular
The ocular manifestations of hypothyroidism include photophobia, cataracts, periorbital or eyelid edema, and optic neuropathy (Table 65–1).

Diagnosis
Iodine deficiency is diagnosed by assessing urinary iodine. Levels that are less than 25 μg/g creatine are considered deficient. In primary hypothyroidism, laboratory evaluation will show high levels of serum thyroid-stimulating hormone (TSH) and decreased levels of T3 and T4 hormones. It is important to remember that changes in the serum-binding protein levels will affect measured T3 and T4. T3 uptake reflects the level of unsaturated thyroid hormone binding sites. The ability of the thyroid gland to take up radioactive iodine is also used as a diagnostic tool.

Treatment and Management
Table 65–2 describes the RDA for the treatment and management of iodine deficiency. Good dietary sources of iodine include fresh seafish, seaweed, garlic, leafy greens, celery, tomatoes, radishes, carrots, onions, and iodized salt. Oral potassium iodide given at a dose of 30 mg monthly or 8 mg twice weekly has been proven to prevent iodine deficiency in areas where iodine deficiency is endemic. Oral supplementation for prophylaxis has been recommended in addition to the universal iodization of salt. If iodine deficiency is suspected, a referral to an endocrinologist or internist is recommended.

TABLE 65–2. TREATMENT AND MANAGEMENT OF IODINE DEFICIENCY

- RDA: Infants: 40 μg
  Children: 50–120 μg
  Adults: 150 μg
  Pregnant: 200 μg

Reprinted with permission from Food and Nutrition Board Commission of Life Sciences National Research Council. Recommended Daily Allowances. *Washington, DC: National Academy Press; 1989.*

IRON

Iron is needed for the production of erythrocytes. It also binds oxygen to hemoglobin for transport to body tissues. The body has a high demand for iron, and this often is not satisfied by the average American diet. There are two different types of iron, nonheme (mainly from vegetables) and heme (from meat and fish), which is absorbed more efficiently. Microcytic anemia is produced in deficiency states. Iron deficiency is also associated with alterations in cellular function, growth, motor development, behavior, and cognitive function. The gastrointestinal and other organ systems are affected. Ocular manifestations may include subconjunctival or flame-shape retinal hemorrhages, retinal ischemia, and distended/tortuous veins.

Epidemiology
Iron deficiency is considered the most common chronic disease of humankind and the most common cause of anemia throughout the world. It is more prevalent in countries where there are meat shortages; however, it is estimated that at least 18 million people in the United States are iron deficient. The primary cause of iron deficiency is inadequate dietary intake, malabsorption, and chronic blood loss. In food, iron is bound to proteins and amino acids and must be reduced for absorption. Vitamin C and other gastric acids serve to reduce the complex, thereby enhancing absorption. The absorption of heme iron is not affected by gastric acid; however, nonheme iron demonstrates reduced absorption in the presence of low acidity. Many components in foods, such as phytates (a carbohydrate in whole grains), fiber, egg yolks, and tea, may bind iron, thereby making it unavailable for absorption. This is true for many other minerals. Females are very susceptible to iron deficiency because of blood loss during menstruation and the high iron demand during pregnancy.

Pathophysiology/Disease Process

Systemic
Early stages of iron deficiency result in malfunctioning of the iron-dependent enzymes involved in energy production and metabolism. Marginal deficiency can affect immune function, which can lead to an increased incidence and chronicity of infections such as *Candida albicans* and colds. The long-term and final stage of iron

deficiency is anemia (Table 65–3), which usually develops very gradually. Chronic iron deficiency can also lead to menorrhagia (excessive menstrual flow). Signs of anemia include chronic fatigue, dyspnea, palpitation, tachycardia, pale skin, opaque or brittle nails, increased rate of infections, and lymphatic tissue shrinkage. Iron deficiency has also been implicated in learning disabilities because of the effect on brain function. It is associated with decreased attentiveness, narrower attention span, and decreased voluntary activity.

Ocular

Severe anemia can lead to subconjunctival and flame-shape retinal hemorrhages, cotton-wool spots, retinal pallor, and distended, tortuous veins (Table 65–3).

Diagnosis

Systemic

Iron deficiency is diagnosed through observation of the clinical signs and symptoms, which include chronic fatigue, shortness of breath, and headache. If deficiency is suspected, appropriate laboratory testing should be obtained. The more commonly used procedures include serum iron assay, serum ferritin assay, total iron-binding capacity (TIBC), percent serum transferrin saturation, and complete blood count (normal values are summarized in Table 65–4). The serum iron assay measures the amount of iron bound to transferrin (plasma iron-transport protein) The direct measurement of serum iron can be unreliable, because levels vary considerably over a short period of time. Serum ferritin is the chief iron-storage protein in the body and correlates with total body iron stores. Detecting low ferritin levels is specific for iron deficiency, because only two other conditions will cause a decrease in ferritin: hypothyroidism and ascorbate deficiency. Unfortunately, this test is not always available. The total iron binding capacity (TIBC) test is also used diagnostically. This is thought to be the most sensitive diagnostic test. The normal TIBC value ranges from 150 to 300 μg/dL. In deficiency states the TIBC value will increase from 350 to 500 μg/dL. TIBC is also used to determine the percentage of transferrin saturation (serum iron value divided by the TIBC). Normally, transferrin is about 30% saturated.

A complete blood count (CBC) includes an assessment of the number of red blood cells, hematocrit (Hct), and hemoglobin (Hgb), along with various morphologic indices that are used to differentiate the type of anemia. These indices include mean corpuscular volume (MCV), mean corpuscular hemoglobin (MCH), and mean corpuscular hemoglobin concentration (MCHC). A fall in the RBC count below 2.5 million/mm^3 is diagnostic for anemia. The MCV reflects the size of the red blood cells; those produced during iron deficiency are usually smaller (microcytic). An MCV of less than 80 μm^3 is diagnostic for microcytic cells. The Hct count is a measure of the number of cells in a given volume of blood. The Hct may drop by as much as 30% before signs or symptoms manifest. The Hgb status is reflected in the overall Hgb concentration and the MCH. The normal Hgb concentration is 12 to 16 g/dL of blood for females and 14 to 18 g/dL

TABLE 65–3. SYSTEMIC AND OCULAR MANIFESTATIONS OF IRON DEFICIENCY

Systemic
- Microcytic anemia
  - Chronic fatigue
  - Dyspnea
  - Palpitations, tachycardia
  - Pale skin, opaque or brittle nails
  - Increased rate of infections
  - Lymphatic tissue shrinkage
- Menorrhagia
- Learning disabilities

Ocular
- Subconjunctival hemorrhages
- Retinal hemorrhages
- Cotton wool spots
- Retinal venous tortuosity
- Retinal pallor

TABLE 65–4. DIAGNOSTIC TESTS UTILIZED IN THE DIAGNOSIS OF MINERAL DEFICIENCIES

Mineral	Test	Normal Values[a]
Iodine	Free urinary iodine	100–460 μg/24 hours
Iron	Serum iron assay	Males: 75–175 μg/dL Females: 65–165 μg/dL
	Serum ferritin assay	Males: 20–300 μg/L Females: 20–120 μg/L
	Total iron-binding capacity (TIBC)	240–450 μg/dL
	CBC	
	RBC	>2.5 million/mm^3
	Hct	Males: 42–52% Females: 37–47%
	Hgb concentration	Males: 14–18 g/dL Females: 12–16 g/dL
	MCV	Males: 80–94 μm^3 Females: 81–99 μm^3
	MCH	27–31 pg
	MCHC	32–36%
Potassium	Serum analysis	3.5–5.1 mEq/L
	Urine analysis	25–125 mmol/24 hours
Zinc	Serum analysis	0.75–1.4 μg/mL

[a]Values vary with the laboratory used.

in males. MCH is a measure of the hemoglobin content of each RBC, which determines the color. MCH level below 26 pg is diagnostic and is termed hypochromic. MCHC is also a measure of chronicity. Normal MCHC levels range from 32 to 36%. The white blood cell count and function may also be altered in deficiency states.

Urinary iron tests are not useful because iron is not normally excreted in the urine. Hair analysis may be useful as a compliment to serum analysis; however, its validity is still questionable. Studies by Lamand and associates (1990) indicate that caution must be taken when using data from hair analysis because the environmental minerals will be absorbed by the hair and the different steps in the hair analysis process may modify the mineral composition.

Treatment and Management

Most cases of iron deficiency are managed with oral ferrous sulfate or ferrous gluconate along with a balanced diet (Table 65–5). In cases of poor absorption, nonheme iron is more effective than the ferrous sulfate salts. In severe deficiency, iron injections or transfusions may be necessary. Iron supplements are highly recommended and the demand usually is not met with the average diet, because only 10% of dietary iron is absorbed. In addition to initiating iron supplements, the exact cause of the iron deficiency should be determined to rule out a slow-bleeding cancer or ulcer. A referral to a hematologist or internist is recommended to best manage the anemia.

When treating iron deficiency, it is important to realize that after menopause, women build up their iron stores. Therefore, women who are taking supplements may develop an abundance of iron. Excess iron acts as a catalyst in certain reactions that produce free radicals, and it competes with chromium for blood protein-binding sites. A shortage of chromium may lead to various metabolic disorders such as an inability to maintain appropriate blood glucose levels. Excess iron has been linked to cirrhosis, diabetes, heart failure, and hepatic carcinoma.

TABLE 65–5. TREATMENT AND MANAGEMENT OF IRON DEFICIENCY

- RDA: Adult males: 10 μg
  Adult females: 18 μg
  Pregnant: 30–60 μg
- With malabsorption, the nonheme iron is more effective than ferrous sulfate salts.

Reprinted with permission from Food and Nutrition Board Commission of Life Sciences National Research Council. Recommended Daily Allowances. *Washington, DC: National Academy Press; 1989.*

Dietary sources of iron include egg yolks, leafy green vegetables, dried beans, peaches, apricots, dates, prunes, raisins, cherries, figs, and blackstrap molasses.

POTASSIUM

Potassium is an electrolyte that regulates osmotic pressure and helps maintain the alkaline pH of internal body fluids. The proper balance of potassium, calcium, and magnesium is necessary for the conduction of nerve impulses and for neuromuscular contractions. It is also necessary for the normal health of the adrenal glands and the generalized electrophysiology of cells. Low potassium intake has been associated with renal dysfunction, hypertension, possibly strokes, weakness of extraocular muscles, dry eyes, and deposits on contact lenses.

Epidemiology

There are no available data on the incidence and prevelance of potassium deprivation. However, adequate levels of dietary potassium are most often easily maintained. Yet potassium deprivation does occur due to various disorders that produce excess urinary or gastrointestinal loss and dietary deficiency of meat and vegetables. The more common depleting factors include alcohol abuse, stress, laxatives, diarrhea, enemas, excess salt, diabetic acidosis, renal disease, and the widespread use of steroids and diuretics.

Pathophysiology/Disease Process

Systemic

Potassium deficiency leads to functional and structural changes in the kidneys. Renal disease may develop after short periods of deprivation and severe, prolonged deficiency can lead to irreversible damage. Clinical signs include an inability to concentrate and acidify urine, nocturia, muscle weakness or paralysis, unhealthy-looking skin, slow-healing injuries, and edema (Table 65–6). These signs can occur rapidly and are easily reversible with oral potassium chloride. When the gastrointestinal system is the site for potassium loss, clinical signs and symptoms may not develop for many years.

Ocular

Potassium deficiency is associated with fatigue and weakness of the extraocular muscles (Table 65–6). Lane (1985) reported that potassium deficiency plays a role in contact lens coating, dry-eye syndrome, and oculomotor as well as accommodative dysfunction.

TABLE 65–6. SYSTEMIC AND OCULAR MANIFESTATIONS OF POTASSIUM DEFICIENCY

Systemic
- Renal disease
- Hypertension
- Possible strokes
- Unhealthy skin
- **Signs and symptoms**
  Nocturia, muscle weakness, edema, slow-healing injuries, irregular heartbeat, poor reflexes, nervousness, lethargy; constipation, insomnia

Ocular
- Dry eyes
- Oculomotor and accomodative dysfunction

Diagnosis

Systemic

Patients may complain of muscle weakness, irregular heartbeat, impaired neuromuscular function, poor reflexes, nervousness, dizziness, lethargy, insomnia, and constipation. The more commonly utilized diagnostic laboratory tests are serum and urinary analysis. A basic blood chemistry analysis, which includes a fasting potassium assay, should be performed. Urinary analysis of electrolytes is usually of limited value because the wide range of water and electrolyte intake from the diet leads to a wide range of normal values. Hair analysis may be obtained as a complement to the serum and urinary analysis.

Ocular

The symptoms associated with potassium deficiency include burning, tearing, inability to successfully wear contact lenses, and diplopia.

Treatment and Management

The RDA for potassium is summarized in Table 65–7. Good dietary sources include oranges, bananas, cantaloupes, avocados, dates, prunes, dried apricots, raisins, watermelon, whole grains, seeds, nuts, peas, beans, milk, fresh fish, beef, and poultry.

TABLE 65–7. TREATMENT AND MANAGEMENT OF POTASSIUM DEFICIENCY

- RDA:
  Adults: 2000 mg
  Children 7–10 years: 1600 mg
  Infants: 500–700 mg
  Pregnant and lactating women: 2000 mg

ZINC

Zinc is an important component of several enzyme systems that are involved in the metabolism of nucleic acids, proteins, carbohydrates, and alcohol. It is a coenzyme that is required in DNA/RNA synthesis and vitamin A use. It serves as an antioxidant in protecting cell membranes against peroxidative damage. The ocular manifestations of zinc deficiency can include macular degeneration, optic neuropathy, night blindness, low intraocular pressure, and possibly cataracts.

Epidemiology

Zinc deficiency in humans was first reported in 1961 in the Middle East in people whose diet was high in breads and low in animal protein. The Senate Select Committee on Nutrition reported that 85% of the population is deficient in zinc. Factors that can lead to deficiency include poor dietary intake; stress; deficient soils used to grow food; excessive levels of copper and cadmium that compete with zinc for cellular sites; the use of EDTA in foods for chelation of certain metals; the use of drugs and foods that contain phytic acid or fiber that will chelate zinc; excessive loss of body fluids as in perspiration and increased urination (often associated with alcohol abuse and diuretics); and diseases that affect zinc metabolism like alcoholic cirrhosis and acrodermatitis enteropathica (a disease of the skin of the extremities that is caused by a genetically determined malabsorption of zinc). Zinc deficiency is also a common finding in Crohn disease.

Pathophysiology/Disease Process

Systemic

Zinc deficiency can manifest as atherosclerosis, failure to grow, anorexia, testicular atrophy, skin lesions, skin stretch marks, acne, psoriasis, opaque fingernails, brittle hair, and lowered levels of plasma vitamin A (Table 65–8). Zinc's role in protein synthesis has lead to the controversial association between zinc deficiency and learning disabilities.

Ocular

The high concentration in ocular tissues has lead to much research regarding ocular findings (Table 65–8). The literature varies on the importance of zinc in cataract formation. Animal studies found cataract development correlated with zinc-deficient diets. Todd (1987) found that 20 mg of zinc daily would reverse cataract in humans. Todd claimed a 67% success rate using zinc along with other vitamins. Other mineral

TABLE 65–8. SYSTEMIC AND OCULAR MANIFESTATIONS OF ZINC DEFICIENCY

Systemic
- Growth failure
- Testicular atrophy
- Skin disease: acne, psoriasis, opaque fingernails, brittle hair, skin stretch marks
- Learning disability
- Atherosclerosis
- Lack of taste and smell

Ocular
- Dry eyes
- Cataracts
- Macular degeneration
- Optic neuropathy
- Night blindness
- Dyschromotopsia
- Low IOP

deficiencies that have been associated with cataracts are calcium, chromium, magnesium, and selenium. These minerals are components of antioxidative enzymes and therefore have an antioxidative role.

Recent research suggests that macular degeneration may be associated with a lack of zinc-dependent enzyme. This enzyme is responsible for the metabolism of retinal byproducts by the RPE cells. Newsome and associates (1988) reported less visual loss in a group of patients with macular degeneration given 100 mg bid zinc sulfate supplements, and also noted that those who developed macular degeneration had a tendency toward zinc deficiency.

Because of the high concentration of zinc in the retina and optic nerve, there is speculation that zinc's role in axoplasmic transport may lead to optic neuropathy in deficiency states. Certain toxic optic neuropathies may be associated with zinc deficiency, because many of the associated drugs are zinc chelators. These toxic neuropathies begin with red/green dyschromatopsia and retrobulbar neuropathy in their early states.

Zinc's role in vitamin A metabolism may cause signs and symptoms that are common to vitamin A deficiency. Zinc helps maintain normal serum levels of vitamin A by mobilizing it from the liver. Zinc also plays a role in transforming retinol to retinaldehyde for utilization by the rods, thus playing a role in night blindness even in the presence of adequate vitamin A.

Low levels of zinc have been associated with low intraocular pressure. As a coenzyme of carbonic anhydrase, zinc is involved in aqueous production. Decreased zinc levels may lead to reduced carbonic anhydrase activity, thus lowering the IOP.

Diagnosis

Systemic

Symptoms of zinc deficiency include lack of taste or smell, dry irritated skin, poor appetite, and fatigue. Normal serum zinc values range from 0.75 to 1.4 μg/mL. Dietary zinc deficiency may not result in lowered plasma levels because blood zinc is sensitive to a wide range of nondietary factors. The use of hair analysis as a diagnostic tool is becoming more widespread. Kobayashi and associates (1991) reported that marginal zinc deficiencies can be assessed through hair analysis.

Ocular

The corresponding symptoms associated with zinc deprivation are decreased visual acuity, dyschromatopsia, and night blindness.

Treatment and Management

Systemic

Therapeutic daily doses of zinc are suggested in deficiency states (Table 65–9). This type of therapy should be closely monitored by a trained nutritionist, because zinc toxicity may occur with doses greater than 45 mg/d. Excessive zinc interferes with the metabolism of other minerals like iron and copper, and can distort the ratio of HDL/LDL cholesterol levels. Therefore it is recommended that iron and copper be given in conjunction with zinc therapy. Good dietary sources include milk, eggs, poultry, seafood, red meat, onions, peas, soybeans, mushrooms, whole grains, nuts, and seeds. Soils are often deficient in zinc, making supplements an important source.

Ocular

Specific treatment regimens relative to zinc have been outlined for the management of cataracts and macular

TABLE 65–9. TREATMENT AND MANAGEMENT OF ZINC DEFICIENCY

- Oral:15–45 mg/d
- RDA: Infants: 3 mg
  Children: 10 mg
  Adults: 20 mg
  Pregnant/lactating: 30 mg
- Cataracts: 20 mg/d
- Macular degeneration: 30 mg/d as preventative therapy
  100 mg/d therapeutic dose
- Must monitor closely because toxicity may occur with doses greater than 45 mg/d.
- Todd (1987) suggests 25,000 IU vitamin A, 400 IU vitamin E and vitamin C, 1000 μg Biotin, 50 mg L-glutathione, 1 tbsp lecithin granules, and reducing dietary fat.

degeneration (Table 65–9). The recommended dosage of zinc for the treatment of macular degeneration varies among investigators. Todd (1987) suggests managing macular degeneration with a daily vitamin and mineral regimen (Table 65–9), as well as reducing fat consumption as much as possible in order to reduce free-radical damage.

CONCLUSION

Good nutritional status is required for adequate biological function, and the ocular structures are no exception. Nutritional deficiencies are more common in the elderly, chronic illness, endocrine imbalances, inability to chew, physical handicaps, and fad diets, and in those impoverished and institutionalized. It is important to realize that it is prudent to maintain an overall good nutritional balance, because nutrients function interdependently and sometimes synergistically. Therefore, eyecare practitioners should be aware of the ocular manifestations of nutritional deficiency, and should consider obtaining a good nutritional history in addition to a medical history when indicated. If a deficiency is suspected, a referral for laboratory analysis and nutritional counseling should be considered. Before nutritional therapy is initiated, an evaluation from a family physician or internist should be obtained to rule out any contraindications or conflict with existing medical management.

REFERENCES

Bhat KS. Distribution of HMW proteins and crystallins in cataractous lenses from undernourished and well-nourished subjects. *Exp Eye Res.* 1983;37:267–271.

Bhat KS. Nutritional status of thiamine, riboflavin and pyridoxine in cataract patients. *Nutr Rep Int.* 1987;36:685–692.

Brown NA, Bron AJ, Harding JJ, Dewar HM. Nutrition supplements and the eye. *Eye.* 1998;12:127–133.

Frei B, England L, Ames BN. Ascorbate is an outstanding antioxidant in human blood plasma. *Proc Natl Acad Sci USA.* 1989;86:6377–6381.

Goodhart RS, Shils ME. *Modern Nutrition in Health and Disease.* 6th ed. Philadelphia: Lea & Febiger; 1980.

Hamilton HE, Ellis PP, Sheets RF. Visual impairment due to optic neuropathy in pernicious anemia: Report of a case and review of the literature. *Blood.* 1959;14:378–385.

Ibrahim K, Kara RY, Zuberi SJ. Hypercarotenemia: A case report. *JPMA.* 1976;224–225.

Jacques PF, Hartz SC, Chylack LT, et al. Nutritional status in persons with and without senile cataract: Blood vitamin and mineral levels. *Am J Clin Nutr.* 1988;48:152–158.

Kobayashi S, et al. Determination of zinc in very small body hair samples by one-drop flame atomic absorption spectrophotometry. *Jpn J Hygiene.* 1991;46:762–768.

Kutsky R. *Handbook of Vitamins and Hormones.* New York: Van Nostrand Reinhold; 1973.

Lamand M, Favier A, Pineau A. Determination of trace elements in the hair: Significance and limitations. *Ann Biologie Clinique.* 1990;48:433–442.

Lane BC. Evaluation of intraocular pressure with daily, sustained closework stimulus to accommodation to lowered tissue chromium and dietary deficiency of ascorbic acid. PhD dissertation, 1980, New York University.

Lane BC. Nutrition and vision. In: Bland J, ed. 1984–85 *Yearbook of Nutritional Medicine.* New Canaan, CT: Keats; 1985:273.

Lascari AD. Carotenemia. *Clin Pediatr.* 1981;20:25.

Leopold IH. Zinc deficiency and visual impairment. *Am J Ophthalmol.* 1978;85:871–874.

Maugh TH. Hair: A diagnostic tool to complement blood serum and urine. *Science.* 1978;202:1271.

Mueller JF, Vilter RW. Pyridoxin deficiency in human beings induced with desoxypyridoxine. *J Clin Invest.* 1950;29:193.

Murray MT. Iron: Deficiencies and supplements. *Health Counselor.* Nov/Dec 1991:31–33.

Myung SJ, Yang SK, Jung HY, et al. Zinc deficiency manifested by dermatitis and visual dysfunction in a patient with Crohn's disease. *J Gastroenterol.* 1998;33:876–879.

Newsome DA, Swartz M, Leone NC, et al. Oral zinc in macular degeneration. *Arch Ophthalmol.* 1988;106:192–198.

Paton D, Mclaren DS. Bitot spots. *Am J Ophthalmol.* 1960; 50:568.

Pihl RO, Parks M. Hair element content in learning-disabled children. *Science.* 1977;198:204–206.

Prasad AS. *Essential and Toxic Trace Elements in Human Health and Disease: An Update.* New York: Wiley–Liss; 1993.

Prasad K, Rama B. Nutrition and cancer. In: Bland J, ed. *1984–85 Yearbook of Nutritional Medicine.* New Canaan, CT: Keats; 1985.

Rapp J. Nutrition in the vision of children. *J Am Opt Assoc.* 1979;50:1107–1111.

Rengstorff RH, Krall CC, Westerhout DI. Topical antioxidant treatment for dry-eye disorders and contact lens-related complications. *Afro-Asian J Ophthalmol.* 1988;7:81–83.

Rosenblum JD, Keating JP, Prensky AL, Nelson JS. A progressive neurologic syndrome in children with chronic liver disease. *N Engl J Med.* 1991;304:503.

Sommer A. *Nutritional Blindness.* New York: Oxford; 1982: 51–52.

Sommer A. Treatment of corneal xerophthalmia with topical retinoic acid. *Am J Ophthalmol.* 1983;95:349–352.

Sommer A, Quesada J, Doty M, Faich G. Xerophthalmia and anterior segment blindness among preschool children in El Salvador. *Am J Ophthalmol.* 1975;80:1066.

Stern JJ. Nutrition in ophthalmology. In: Goodhart R, Shils M, eds. *Modern Nutrition in Health and Disease.* 5th ed. Philadelphia: Lea & Febiger; 1973:1009.

Todd GP. *Nutrition in Health and Disease.* Norfolk, VA: Donning; 1987.

Van Gossum A, Neve J. Trace element deficiency and toxicity. *Curr Opin Clin Nutr Metab Care.* 1998;1:499–507.

Yolton DP. Nutritional effects of zinc on ocular and systemic physiology. *J Am Optom Assoc.* 1981;52:409–414.

Section XVI

DRUG AND ALCOHOL ABUSE

Chapter 66

DRUG AND ALCOHOL ABUSE

Jean Y. Jung

Drug abuse is defined as the inappropriate and usually excessive self-administration of a drug or substance for nonmedical purposes. Drug abuse in the United States poses many concerns relating to social, economic, and medical factors. The medical considerations may involve stroke, cerebral hemorrhages, and cardiovascular and pulmonary problems. Likewise, the visual system is not immune to these drugs. Ocular manifestations of drugs, both legal and illegal, have been well documented. Some of these manifestations are from the drugs themselves and their toxicity. Others are due to embolic processes (talc retinopathy) and/or infection (endophthalmitis) secondary to the invasive methods of administration. Other ocular manifestations may be the result of trauma or other activities that the patient undertakes while under the influence.

ALCOHOL

Ethanol or ethyl alcohol is an organic, volatile, and flammable substance that is obtained, in its pure form, by fermentation and distillation of grain. It is present in fermented or distilled liquor and is used in preparing essences, tinctures, and extracts, as well as in manufacturing ether, ethylene, rubbing compounds, antiseptics, and other industrial products. It is also given intravenously to stop premature labor. Alcohol acts as a depressant to the central nervous system and causes potent psychoactive effects when taken in excessive amounts. Psychological and physiological dependence can occur. The physiological dependence, or physical dependence as it is often called, will result in withdrawal signs and symptoms.

Methanol is an organic, poisonous, volatile, and flammable liquid that is obtained from distillation of wood. It is also known as carbinol, methyl alcohol, or wood alcohol, and is more commonly found in bootleg whiskey. Unlike ethanol, it is not intended for human consumption. It is used as a solvent, as an additive for denaturing ethyl alcohol, as an antifreeze agent, in fuel, and in the preparation of formaldehyde.

Epidemiology

Ethanol is the most widely abused drug in the world and the most frequently abused drug in the United States. According to the 1997 National Household Survey on Drug Abuse from the Substance Abuse and Mental Health Services Administration (SAMHSA) (1998), approximately 111 million Americans 12 years and older have used alcohol. This is 51% of the population. Of these Americans, 11.2 million admit to being heavy drinkers, which is defined as five or more drinks on the same occasion at least five different days in the month.

Pathophysiology/Disease Process

Systemic

Alcoholism is a chronic, progressive, and potentially fatal disease. It is characterized by physiological dependence resulting in physical, emotional, and social changes that progressively worsen as the abuse continues. Tolerance is common, whereby higher and higher concentrations are needed for an effect. The exact mechanism for the onset of alcoholism is not fully understood. It is felt that psychological, physiological, sociological, and genetic factors play an important role. The role of genetics in alcoholism is uncertain, but alcoholism does run in families, regardless of whether the child is raised by alcoholic parents or nonalcoholic surrogate parents.

Alcohol is a central nervous system (CNS) depressant that is absorbed throughout the gastrointestinal tract and metabolized in the liver. In small concentrations, it may have the effect of a stimulant, causing talkativeness, aggressiveness, and decreased social inhibition. The main consequence of acute ethanol poisoning is irregularly descending CNS depression that causes peripheral vasodilation with flushing of the skin, rapid pulse, hypotension, tachycardia, hypothermia, polyneuritis, coma, and death from respiratory or circulatory failure (Table 66–1). The probable lethal dose for acute ethanol poisoning varies among individuals from 1 pint to more than 1 quart when ingested at one time. The subsequent "hangover" is also very common.

TABLE 66–1. SYSTEMIC MANIFESTATIONS OF ALCOHOL ABUSE

- Alcoholism
- Respiratory failure
- Circulatory failure
- Mental disturbances
- Liver cirrhosis
- Gastritis
- Pancreatitis
- Neurological disorders
- Wernicke–Korsakoff syndrome
- Skin flushing
- Tachycardia
- Muscular incoordination
- Drowsiness
- Stupor, delirium
- Tremulousness
- Seizures
- Hallucinations
- Emotional instability
- Slurred speech
- Poor comprehension, memory
- Irritability
- Cerebral and cerebellar atrophy
- Bad judgement
- Hypotension
- Cardiomyopathy
- Anemia
- Cerebral and cerebellar atrophy

Chronic alcohol abuse affects many organs, particularly the liver, brain, peripheral nervous system, and gastrointestinal tract. Direct tissue toxicity may cause permanent tissue and organ damage. Cirrhosis of the liver, cardiomyopathy, gastritis, pancreatitis, peripheral neuropathy, anemia, and cerebral and cerebellar atrophy are consistent with chronic alcohol abuse. Neurological disorders such as tremulousness, hallucinosis, seizures, and delirium can occur with alcohol abuse. Wernicke–Korsakoff syndrome is a neurological and psychological dysfunction associated with chronic alcoholism secondary to thiamine deficiency. It is characterized by encephalopathy, loss of memory, disorientation, psychosis, polyneuritis, ataxia, delirium, insomnia, illusions, and hallucinations. Chronic alcoholism interferes with the absorption and metabolism of certain essential nutrients such as zinc, folate, vitamin A, and the B complex vitamins including B_1 (thiamine), B_3 (niacin), B_6 (pyridoxine), and B_{12}. Gastrointestinal and pancreatic problems further affect nutritional absorption. Additionally, hepatitis and cirrhosis alter the nutritional storage capacity of the liver. Other consequences of nutritional deficiency are outlined in Chapters 64 and 65.

The manifestations of methanol abuse are more severe than those of ethanol abuse. The major consequence of methanol poisoning is a severe metabolic acidosis with progressive cerebral dysfunction, circulatory collapse, and respiratory failure. The signs and symptoms include exhilaration accompanied by headache, muscular weakness, weak and rapid pulse, rapid and shallow breathing, nausea, vomiting, and abdominal pain. Direct toxicity to the nervous system may lead to convulsions and coma. Respiratory failure can result in cyanosis (bluish, grayish, or dark purple discoloration to the skin) and death from a lack of oxygen and an excess of carbon dioxide in the blood. The lethal dose for methanol poisoning is approximately 500 to 5000 mg per kilogram of body weight for adults.

Ocular

Acute alcohol intoxication can affect the eye via its effects on the CNS (Table 66–2). Both smooth pursuits and saccades are affected and manifest as slow, jerky, and inefficient eye movements when blood alcohol levels reach 60 to 100 mg/dL. Patients may report diplopia, and extraocular muscle (EOM) palsies may

TABLE 66–2. OCULAR MANIFESTATIONS OF ALCOHOL ABUSE

Ethanol
- Nystagmus
- Altered motilities, EOM palsies
- Accommodative insufficiency
- Color vision defects
- Decreased rate of recovery from bright lights
- Ptosis
- Decreased intraocular pressure
- Nutritional optic neuropathy
    - Retrobulbar or anterior optic nerve/disc pallor
    - Centrocecal or central scotoma
    - Decreased vision

Methanol
- Decreased vision
- Mydriasis
- Retinal edema
- Toxic optic neuropathy
    - Anterior disc edema
    - Disc hyperemia
    - Optic atrophy
    - Centrocecal or central scotoma

occur. Esophoria, intermittent esotropia, and altered stereopsis have been reported with acute alcohol intoxication. Intoxication can also cause decreased accommodation, nystagmus, transient changes in color vision, and decreased rate of recovery from bright light exposure. Ethanol has been associated with decreased intraocular pressure (IOP). The effect is greater in open-angle glaucoma patients than in normal eyes.

> Alcohol most often affects the oculomotor system. Jerky inefficient eye movements are classic signs.

Chronic alcohol abuse can affect the oculomotor, abducens, and vestibular nuclei, giving rise to ophthalmoplegia, ptosis, lateral rectus muscle palsies, diplopia, and nystagmus. This may be observed in Wernicke–Korsakoff syndrome. Alcohol amblyopia is a well-known consequence of chronic alcoholism. It usually is associated with drinking excessively and steadily for many years. It is now known that the associated nutritional deficiency, primarily in the vitamin B complex—thiamine (B_1), niacin (B_3), B_{12}, and folate—is the major underlying factor. Other nutrients that are involved are iodine, zinc, and vitamin A.

Nutritional optic neuropathy may manifest initially as a bilateral, yet often asymmetric, retrobulbar neuropathy that progresses slowly to anterior optic atrophy. Visual acuity loss ranges from a mild decrease in acuity to amaurosis. The classic visual field defect is a centrocecal scotoma, yet central scotomas and occasional peripheral constrictions have also been reported. Prognosis for recovery of vision loss and visual field defects is a function of the severity of the loss and is enhanced if therapy is initiated early in the course of optic nerve involvement. Vitamin B complex therapy was found to improve the optic neuropathy in many instances despite continuation of the alcohol abuse. Nutritional deficiencies that are associated with alcohol abuse may also lead to cataracts, macular degeneration, and ophthalmoplegia. More details on the ocular manifestations of nutritional deficiencies can be found in Chapters 64 and 65.

True toxicity to the optic nerve also occurs in chronic alcohol abuse and is found mainly in association with methanol poisoning. Sharpe (1982) showed that the pathophysiology is related to myelin damage with axonal preservation in the retrolaminar portion of the optic nerve. The mechanism for this disturbance is thought to be caused by anoxia. Toxic optic neuropathy will manifest in the same manner as nutritional optic neuropathy. However, methanol intoxication may present initially with disc edema, which can lead to optic atrophy. The initial amaurosis may occur suddenly and improve, and then increase again but with permanent vision loss. The central scotoma is large, dense, and irregular, and is not reversible. Methanol intoxication can also cause pupillary dilatation and sluggishness, optic nerve hyperemia, and retinal edema. These signs may manifest within 2 months of the visual acuity decline. Prognosis for visual recovery is poor when vision is severely affected. Temporary blindness attributed to ethanol is usually rare.

Diagnosis

Systemic

The diagnosis of alcohol as well as other drug abuse is often based upon suspicion and guesswork. The abusers usually do not volunteer this information; however, a careful history is often revealing. Questioning patients about alcohol and other drug abuse should be approached gingerly. It may be best to first ask about prescription drugs, cigarettes, alcohol, and then illicit drugs. Suspicions should be raised in the presence of certain characteristic signs and symptoms such as changes in mood and emotional instability, impaired motor coordination, slurred speech, ataxia, sweating, nausea, vomiting, drowsiness, and stupor. Other diagnostic signs of alcohol abuse include a patient who has a history of difficulty maintaining employment or appears manipulative as well as evasive. Suspicions should be confirmed with urine and blood analysis. Urine testing will detect drug use within the preceding 7 days, whereas blood analysis can determine an approximate quantity of alcohol intake. Table 66–3 lists objective tests to diagnose recent substance use. Breath alcohol analyzers are used by law enforcement officials to determine alcohol intoxication. However, one cannot diagnose alcohol intoxication on the basis of odor of alcohol on the breath alone because certain conditions such as diabetic ketoacidosis will present with the same odor. Certain questionnaires such as the CAGE questionnaire or Brief Michigan Alcoholism Screening Test can be used as an indirect means of detecting alcohol use. The content of these questionnaires is outlined in Speicher (1989).

Ocular

In acute intoxication, the patient may have decreased vision and accommodation, poor extraocular motilities, and nystagmus. It may be best to postpone testing until the patient is sober.

In chronic alcoholism, the patient may present with decreased acuity that ranges from mild blurring to total blindness. Occasionally, chronic alcoholics experience an acute amaurosis lasting 24 hours with no sound pathologic basis. Although methanol poisoning is associated more frequently with blindness, the patient usually does not survive to complain about it. Visual field changes caused by direct toxicity may show larger areas of defects than nutritional optic neuropathy. Also, the visual field defect is smaller, more central, and steeper than in tobacco amblyopia. According to Harrington (1962), centrocecal defects will have the area of greatest density near fixation. Red-colored targets may more easily detect incipient scotomas. Other ocular symptoms include pain behind the eye, diplopia, red-green dyschromatopsia, impaired depth perception, and near point blur. Knave et al (1974) and others have shown that disturbances exist in the electroretinogram (ERG). The diagnosis of alcohol-induced nutritional optic neuropathy should be one of exclusion. Orbital and cerebral CT scans or MRIs are warranted to rule out compressive lesions, and laboratory tests should be done to rule out optic neuritis.

The presence of severe end-gaze nystagmus, the onset of nystagmus prior to 45-degree lateral gaze, and jerky pursuits are signs used by the National Highway Traffic Safety Administration to help detect drivers who are intoxicated (Halperin & Yolton, 1986).

TABLE 66–3. TESTING FOR SUBSTANCE ABUSE

Substance	Test
Alcohol	Blood and urine analysis Severe end-stage nystagmus and nystagmus prior to 45-degree lateral gaze with jerky pursuits Breath alcohol analyzer
Marijuana	Blood and urine toxicology
Tobacco	Increased levels of thiocyanate in urine
Stimulants	Blood and urine analysis Nasal swabs
Depressants	Blood and urine analysis EEG may show nonspecific depression
Opiates	Blood and urine analysis (0.1–0.4 mg naloxone will reverse respiratory depression in opiate overdose)
Hallucinogens	LSD Observation (panic reaction) and history Phencyclidine Blood and urine analysis Irregular, bidirectional nystagmus
Inhalants	Urine analysis or Breathalyzer

Treatment and Management

Table 66–4 summarizes the treatment and management of substance overdose and abuse for all substances in this chapter.

Systemic

For all cases of overdose, the ABCs of emergency care (airway, breathing, circulation) are the first step. In cases of acute ethanol intoxication, the airway is opened, and artificial respiration and circulatory support are provided as needed. This should be followed by intravenous saline for circulatory collapse and dehydration.

Chronic alcoholism is best treated through rehabilitation programs. Detoxification may require medical supervision as tremors, seizures, hyperthermia, hallucinations, and autonomic hyperactivity are common with alcohol withdrawal. Nutritional supplements (vitamin A, vitamin B complex, and zinc) may be required. To decrease the desire to drink, aversion therapy is sometimes used. This involves taking prescribed drugs, such as disulfiram, which causes headaches, nausea, vomiting, respiratory difficulties, and chest pain among other symptoms when alcohol is ingested. The purpose is to associate alcohol ingestion with such undesirable consequences that the patient no longer wishes to drink. Currently, anticraving drugs are also being developed.

Treatment for methanol poisoning is counteraction of the acidosis. The standard treatment is to pro-

TABLE 66–4. SYSTEMIC TREATMENT AND MANAGEMENT OF SUBSTANCE OVERDOSE AND ABUSE

For all overdoses:
- Airway must be opened and secured
- Breathing must be monitored and artificial respiration must be used if needed
- Circulation must be stabilized
- Send blood for studies
- Use IV glucose or dextrose to rule out hypoglycemia

Ethanol
- IV saline or hypertonic glucose
- Hemodialysis

Methanol
- Oral or IV ethanol or fomepizole
- Sodium bicarbonate to counter acidosis
- Hemodialysis

Tobacco, Marijuana
- Supportive care

Stimulants
- Ice bath for hyperthermia
- Benzodiazepines (diazepam) or barbiturates for CNS symptoms, seizures, and sedation
- Haldol for hallucinations
- Supportive care—prevent patients from harming themselves

Depressants
- Activated charcoal; if ingested depressants within 6 hours
- Gastric lavage
- CNS stimulants

Opiates
- Keep patient awake
- Antagonist treatment (naloxone or nalmefene)

Hallucinogens
- IV hydration
- Ice packs for hyperthermia
- Benzodiazepines to sedate and for seizures
- Reorient to reality and reassure in quiet, dim room

Inhalants
- Supportive care—talk patients down in quiet room and prevent them from hurting themselves
- Treatment for all chronic substance abuse is discontinuation, detoxification, and rehabilitation

tect the airway, monitor breathing with artificial respiration if necessary, and give IV or oral ethanol or fomepizole (4-methylpyrazole, an alcohol dehydrogenase inhibitor), followed by hemodialysis. Since ethanol has a higher affinity for alcohol dehydrogenase than methanol, it will bind with the enzyme, preventing the methanol from oxidizing into toxic formic acid and allowing it to be excreted unchanged. Similarly, fomepizole inhibits alcohol dehydrogenase, thus preventing the methanol from oxidizing and allowing it to be excreted. Sodium bicarbonate may be necessary to counter the acidosis. Activated charcoal to decrease absorption is generally not effective since most alcohols are 80 to 90% absorbed within 30 to 60 minutes.

Ocular

The first step in reversing the ocular manifestations of alcohol abuse is to remove the alcohol. This should be followed by vitamin therapy including vitamin B complex, vitamin A, and zinc. It is recommended that a hematologist, internist, or nutritionist manage the nutritional deficiency.

TOBACCO

Tobacco is the dried leaves of the nicotiana plant and is often used for smoking or chewing. Most of the 4000 active substances in tobacco smoke, including nicotine, cyanide, and carbon monoxide, are hazardous to human health. Tobacco lowers plasma antioxidant levels, causing increased oxidative stress and arteriosclerosis.

Epidemiology

Tobacco is the second most abused substance in the United States after alcohol. The 1997 National Household Survey on Drug Abuse estimated that 64 million Americans over the age of 12 years are current smokers. This represents 30% of the household population. Current smokers were more likely to be drinkers or illicit drug users.

Pathophysiology/Disease Process

Systemic

Tobacco smoking is considered a major risk factor for 6 of the 15 leading causes of death including cardiovascular disease, cancer, and respiratory disorders. A smoker has twice the risk of premature death as a nonsmoker and the heavier the tobacco use, the higher the risk. Table 66–5 lists many of the systemic effects of tobacco.

Nicotine is the most active constituent of tobacco and is highly addictive. It causes transient stimulation followed by subsequent CNS depression. Nicotine

TABLE 66–5. SYSTEMIC MANIFESTATIONS OF TOBACCO ABUSE

- Cancer (mouth, throat, lung)
- Cardiovascular disease
- Bronchopulmonary disease (emphysema)
- Allergies
- Lack of appetite, digestive disturbance
- Insomnia
- Constipation
- Decreased sexual desire
- Fatigue
- Depression

decreases appetite and lowers estrogen levels in female smokers, making them more at risk for osteoporosis.

Although nicotine is physically and psychologically addicting, smokers have a compulsion to smoke even when their nicotine levels are maintained. Withdrawal symptoms such as anxiety, confusion, blurred vision, headache, restlessness, irritability and gastrointestinal upset can occur within a few hours of the last cigarette, peak within 24 to 48 hours, and then dissipate over 2 weeks. After a month, symptoms are gone, but cigarette cravings and increased appetite continue.

Ocular

Tobacco smoking is a major risk factor in ocular ischemic disorders and age-related macular degeneration (ARMD) (Table 66–6). It has also been linked with increased risk of cataract development. Tobacco amblyopia has been reported but usually as tobacco–alcohol amblyopia without differentiating the two, so it is unknown if it is the tobacco or the combination of the two that causes the optic atrophy.

Studies have shown increased choroidal vascular resistance in rats exposed to cigarette smoke inhalation, thereby decreasing blood supply to the choroid. Anterior ischemic optic neuropathy (AION) is usually due to a disruption in the posterior ciliary circulation. Smoking has been strongly associated with vasoconstriction of these arteries and has been identified as a risk factor for nonarteritic AION. Smoking-induced ischemia can affect ocular muscles and may result in ophthalmoplegia.

> Tobacco smoking is a major risk factor for ARMD, cataract, AION, ocular ischemic syndrome, and Graves ophthalmopathy.

Tobacco amblyopia has been reported in the literature. It may be a result of AION in each eye, or it may be due to a nutritional deficiency. Most investigators agree that it is not the tobacco alone that causes the amblyopia. Actually, many cases of tobacco amblyopia have been later diagnosed as Leber optic neuropathy, which causes some to doubt its existence. Rare cases of it still are reported. Table 66–7 lists differential diagnoses of tobacco amblyopia.

TABLE 66–6. OCULAR CONDITIONS FOR WHICH TOBACCO ABUSE IS A RISK FACTOR

Age-related macular degeneration
Anterior ischemic optic neuropathy
Ocular ischemic syndrome
Cataract
Tobacco amblyopia (nutritional versus toxic)
Graves disease

TABLE 66–7. TOBACCO AMBLYOPIA AND DIFFERENTIAL DIAGNOSIS

Tobacco Amblyopia
- Tends to occur in males 40–60 years old
- Pale nerves
- VA 20/30–5/200
- Decreased color vision
- Visual field defects—bilateral centrocecal scotomas

Differential Diagnosis
- Leber optic neuropathy
- Nutritional amblyopia
- Toxic amblyopia
- Anterior ischemic optic neuropathy
- Bilateral optic neuritis

Tobacco amblyopia tends to occur in males between the ages of 40 and 60. Visual acuity may range between 20/30 and 5/200. Centrocecal scotomas may be noted on visual fields, as well as color vision defects, indicating optic nerve involvement (Table 66–7). The optic neuropathy is usually retrobulbar, but may progress to optic atrophy. Vision usually improves, especially with discontinuation of smoking and improved nutrition.

Because tobacco smoking causes ischemia to the choroid and increases oxidative stress, it makes the macula more susceptible to damage and has been identified as a major risk factor for age-related macular degeneration. The Pola Study found smokers had an increased risk of late ARMD, which was defined as neovascular ARMD or geographic atrophy 175 microns or larger within 3000 microns of the fovea. The increased risk among smokers does not decline until 20 years after quitting. There was no significant correlation of smoking habits with early ARMD.

Several studies have linked the development of cataracts, particularly nuclear sclerotic opacities, with smoking. It has been suggested that the cataracts are a result of the oxidative stress from the cigarette smoke in addition to the toxic effect of some of the heavy metals contained in tobacco.

Graves disease is thought to be an autoimmune disease, but it is influenced by certain genetic and environmental factors. Smoking seems to be one of them and is more associated with the ophthalmologic findings of Graves disease. Smokers with Graves disease are more likely than nonsmokers to have Graves ophthalmopathy and more severe eye disease. Pfeilschifter and Zeigler (1996) found current tobacco use a risk factor for proptosis and diplopia in patients with Graves disease.

Diagnosis

Systemic

Smokers usually have the characteristic smell of smoke on their breath. Heavy long-term smokers often have yellow club fingers. However, in order to clinically diagnose tobacco intoxication, urinary levels of thiocyanate must be measured (Table 66–3). These levels are elevated in smokers. Systemic symptoms may also include a lack of appetite, digestive disturbance, insomnia, constipation, diminution of sexual desire, and feelings of fatigue and depression.

Ocular

It would be difficult to state that cataracts, age-related macular degeneration, anterior ischemic optic neuropathy, and Graves disease were solely due to tobacco use. It is best to educate patients that smoking is a risk factor for these entities and recommend quitting.

Tobacco amblyopia is usually diagnosed by the characteristic bilateral centrocecal scotoma with sloping edges and an area of increased density within the scotoma between the blindspot and fixation, as described by Harrington (1962).

Treatment and Management

The best treatment for tobacco use and abuse is to discontinue its use. When nutritional deficiencies are present, a balanced diet with emphasis on vitamin B complex and folic acid, 300 mg thiamine per week for 10 weeks, and 1000 μg IV of vitamin B_{12} per week for 10 weeks should be recommended. Smoking cessation programs are available, as are nicotine patches to help curtail the addiction.

MARIJUANA

Marijuana and its related products are derived from the cannabis (hemp) plant. The primary constituent in cannabis is delta-9-tetrahydrocannabinol (THC). Although all portions of the cannabis plant contain THC, the flowering tops have the highest concentrations. Marijuana, made from the dried tops of the plant, and hashish, the dried flowers, leaves, and stalks of the plant, are the most common forms of marijuana in the United States. Hashish is five to eight times more potent than marijuana. Hashish is most often smoked but can be eaten, as well as crushed and boiled to make hashish oil.

Marijuana affects the cardiovascular system by increasing heart rate. A sense of euphoria, followed by sedation, occurs after smoking a "joint," a marijuana cigarette. Each joint contains 2.5 to 5.0 mg of THC. Smoking THC has a quicker onset but shorter duration of action than taking the drug orally. Pharmacological effects may be noticed within minutes after smoking and last up to 4 hours, whereas oral administration may delay effects for 30 minutes and last up to 5 hours. Hallucinations may occur in high doses.

Cannabis has been used medicinally in several countries and therapeutic use of THC has been reported for several conditions including migraines, glaucoma, hypertension, and multiple sclerosis. However, it is only approved in the United States for the treatment of nausea caused by chemotherapy for cancer. THC is being considered for treatment of AIDS wasting syndrome since it does increase appetite and may induce weight gain.

Epidemiology

Marijuana is the most widely abused illicit drug in the United States. The 1997 National Household Survey on Drug Abuse reported that 32.9% of Americans over the age of 12 have used marijuana and 11.1 million were current users of marijuana/hashish. This represents 5.1% of the population. Nearly 10% of youth aged 12 to 17 years were current users of marijuana in 1997. The number of first-time users of marijuana has increased steadily since 1991, and the increased incidence seems to be due to the initiation of marijuana use among the youth.

Pathophysiology/Disease Process

Systemic

The systemic manifestations of marijuana use (Table 66–8) are dose dependent. The effects occur rapidly and may peak within 10 to 30 minutes after inhalation. Acute intoxication causes a period of euphoria, excitement, and restlessness followed by calm and sedation. Motor skills and judgment are impaired, making it dangerous to drive. Perception of time, comprehension, and short-term memory are also affected. Muscle tremors and weakness may be noted. Higher doses may cause hallucinations. The euphoria that occurs at lower doses may become anxiety and paranoia at higher doses. Changes in mood or transient episodes of confusion and toxic delirium may occur. Eventually, sleep is induced. Users wake up with a clear memory and often have dry mouth.

Although marijuana does not depress the respiratory system, chronic abuse can lead to bronchitis, chronic cough, and emphysema-like lung changes.

TABLE 66–8. SYSTEMIC MANIFESTATIONS OF MARIJUANA ABUSE

Initial
- Excitement, euphoria
- Restlessness
- Talkativeness
- Hyperactivity

Late
- Calm, sedation
- Altered perception
- Psychomotor incoordination
- Impaired learning, memory, thinking, and comprehension
- Anxiety
- Auditory hallucinations
- Heightened sexual arousal
- Enhanced sense of taste, touch, smell, and hearing

Chronic
- CNS damage (seizures and dementia)
- Psychological effects (paranoia)
- Respiratory disease
- Reproductive dysfunction (altered menstrual cycle and temporary infertility)

This may be due to the nature of the administration (smoke containing hydrocarbons) or to the concomitant use of tobacco that is common in users. Hypotension and increased heart rate, sometimes even tachycardia, can occur with marijuana use. Chronic, heavy use may cause behavioral disorders and CNS damage, causing epileptic seizures or dementia. Altered menstrual cycles have been reported as well. No deaths have been reported due to marijuana use. Marijuana is both physically and psychologically addicting. Tolerance develops slowly, with less perceptual and motor impairment in experienced users. Users do not require higher doses since the subjective effects are not reduced with increased use.

Ocular

Marijuana smoking causes conjunctival hyperemia and decreased lacrimation. Bloodshot eyes are the most prominent ocular sign of marijuana use. Chronic users may develop congestion of the lids. Diplopia, decreased accommodation, photophobia, nystagmus, and blepharospasm have been noted as side effects. Visual hallucinations can occur. These are often brightly colored flashes of light, shapes, or scenes. Dyschromatopsia, yellow vision, and heightened color perception are associated with chronic use. Table 66–9 lists common ocular manifestations of marijuana use.

Smoking 2% marijuana cigarettes has the beneficial side effect of decreasing intraocular pressure (IOP) 25 to 30% in 60 to 65% of patients. Duration of the IOP reduction is 3 to 4 hours. Maximum absorption occurs with smoking. To maintain the IOP at this lower level, a patient would need to smoke 8 to 10 marijuana cigarettes per day. The short duration and systemic toxic effects of smoking marijuana make this a poor choice for glaucoma treatment. However, oral and topical cannabinoids show promise as possible glaucoma treatment. These forms of delivery can provide reduced IOP without the psychoactive effects of the drug.

> The most common sign of marijuana use is bloodshot eyes. Users often wear sunglasses secondary to photophobia and red eyes.

Diagnosis

Systemic

Bloodshot eyes and the scent of marijuana on the patient may raise suspicion of marijuana intoxication. Blood toxicology can denote marijuana use within the past 60 days and urine screens can denote use within the past 3 to 30 days depending on the level of usage and the user's amount of body fat. Because THC is stored in fat cells, the more fat a user has, the longer it stays in the body and can be detected (Table 66–3).

Ocular

The visual hallucinations associated with marijuana use are described as brightly colored light flashes or amorphous forms that develop into shapes, faces, or scenes. Patients may report symptoms of diplopia or photophobia with acute intoxication. CNS involvement can cause accommodative insufficiency, leading to the complaint of near vision blur.

TABLE 66–9. OCULAR MANIFESTATIONS OF MARIJUANA ABUSE

- Conjunctival hyperemia
- Lid congestion
- Increase or decrease in tear production
- Diplopia
- Nystagmus
- Blepharospasm
- Decreased accommodation
- Photophobia
- Dyschromatopsia, yellow vision
- Decreased intraocular pressure
- Visual hallucinations

Treatment and Management

Since marijuana does not affect the respiratory or circulatory system severely, no treatment is necessary to combat acute intoxication. Drug rehabilitation programs can help chronic users stop using the drug.

STIMULANTS

Stimulants are a category of drugs that augment the action of the neurotransmitter norepinephrine, thereby stimulating the sympathetic nervous system. They may also stimulate the release of dopamine in the brain. Stimulants are easily found in our society. Almost everyone has used stimulants in the form of caffeine present in coffee, tea, and cola beverages, or in the form of nicotine in tobacco products. Stimulants are often used by athletes, students, and truck drivers because they increase short-term physical and mental performance. The more commonly abused stimulants include tobacco, amphetamines, methamphetamine, methylphenidate (Ritalin), and cocaine. Because of the high potential for abuse, medical use of these drugs has declined considerably. However, newer drugs that are being used in place of amphetamines (especially appetite suppressants) have potential for abuse.

Amphetamines are synthetic stimulants used to elevate mood and to treat narcolepsy (inability to stay awake), as well as certain types of mental depression. Because they also act as an appetite suppressant, they are sometimes used to treat obesity. Amphetamines are also used to manage hyperkinesis or "attention deficit disorder," in children, and athletes use them to enhance performance. Large doses are toxic, and chronic use has led to drug dependence. The more commonly used amphetamines include methamphetamine hydrochloride (Desoxyn) and dextroamphetamine sulfate (Dexedrine). Amphetamine abuse usually begins after becoming habituated to a medical prescription, but the substance is often purposely sought after for its euphoric effect.

Methamphetamines are a class of drugs that are chemically related to amphetamines. The more commonly used methamphetamine is methadrine, also known as "speed." Amphetamines and methamphetamines are usually taken orally or injected intravenously.

Methylphenidate (Ritalin) is a mild CNS stimulant. It is more often used, instead of amphetamines, to treat hyperkinesis in children because the adverse effects are milder. This drug is often abused by intravenous injection. Like other injected drugs, there is a risk for embolic retinopathy and respiratory as well as cerebral complications.

Cocaine is derived from the leaves of the coca plant and is the most potent of the nonsynthetic stimulants. Cocaine was first used medically in the 1800s as a topical anesthetic. It blocks nerve conduction by inhibiting the reuptake of norepinephrine. Its use as an anesthetic has subsided because it is not metabolized as fast as other synthetic stimulants.

Illicit cocaine is usually sniffed or snorted but can be injected. Cocaine vaporizes at too low a temperature to be smoked, but crack, a "free base" form, can be smoked. It is made by mixing cocaine hydrochloride with water and baking soda and then heating the mixture to evaporate the water. A white powder is left that can be smoked. Because it makes a crackling sound when it is smoked, it became known as "crack." Crack is a cheaper yet more potent form of cocaine. IV administration of cocaine and smoking of crack produce a rapid intense state of euphoria. This is short lasting (about a half hour). Intranasal administration has a longer duration but causes a less intense euphoria. Illicit cocaine is usually "cut" or adulterated with other substances like sugar, talc, cornstarch, procaine, quinine, and amphetamines, which decreases its strength.

Ecstasy (3,4-methylene dioxymethamphetamine) belongs to a family of drugs that fall between amphetamines and hallucinogens. Originally used as an appetite suppressant, it was banned in 1985. Onset of action is 20 to 60 minutes. It produces the effects of a stimulant, but users also get the calm euphoria that is an effect similar to that obtained from the hallucinogens.

Epidemiology

The 1997 National Household Survey on Drug Abuse estimates that 4.5% of the population over the age of 12 has used stimulants other than cocaine and another 10.5% has used cocaine. In 1997, 1.5 million Americans admitted to being current cocaine users. Although this is a decline from its peak in 1985, it represents 0.7% of the population over age 12. The highest incidence of cocaine users is among 18 to 25-year-olds. Men are more often current users than women.

It is estimated that 0.3% of the population are current crack users. This relatively inexpensive form of cocaine makes it a popular street drug.

Over 5 million Americans have tried methamphetamine. This is an increase from 1994 although the number of active users has declined.

Pathophysiology/Disease Process

Systemic

All stimulants affect the nervous system and accelerate most of the body's functions. Table 66–10 lists systemic manifestations of stimulant abuse. Body tem-

TABLE 66–10. SYSTEMIC MANIFESTATIONS OF STIMULANT ABUSE

Cardiovascular
- Tachycardia
- Arrhythmia
- Increased blood pressure
- Circulatory collapse
- Cerebral hemorrhage
- Vasospasm

CNS
- Sympathomimetic
- Convulsions
- Coma
- Hallucinations
- Headaches
- Needle track marks, inflammation of nasal mucosa
- Hyperthermia

Manifestations in Pregnant Women
- Increased rate of spontaneous abortion
- Congenital malformation
- Perinatal mortality
- Neurobehavioral problems in children

Psychological
- Excitement, euphoria
- Increased energy
- Talkativeness
- Restlessness
- Aggressiveness
- Anxiety/suspicion/paranoia
- Delirium
- Wakefulness
- Increased concentration/confusion in higher doses

perature increases and tremors are often present. Stimulants cause a sense of euphoria, increased energy, alertness, feelings of sexuality, and decreased appetite. Sense of time and mental processing is faster so 5 minutes may seem like 15 to a person under the influence.

Patients under the influence of amphetamines tend to be restless and talkative, yet their ability to concentrate is improved. These effects usually last up to 4 hours. Higher doses may have a more intense, less desirable effect. The euphoria may turn into aggressiveness, and the increased alertness may become suspicion. The increased concentration seen at lower doses may become compulsive behavior at higher doses, with patients focusing all their attention on one task for hours at a time. Periods of paranoia progressing to toxic paranoid psychosis can occur with higher doses and chronic abuse. This can be difficult to differentiate from acute paranoid schizophrenia, but stimulants found in the urine and disappearance of the psychosis within approximately 7 days help to assist in the diagnosis. Hallucinations, delusions of persecution or grandeur, and combative behavior often occur.

Tolerance, requiring larger and more frequent doses, is common and psychological dependence develops quickly. Often users will go on "speed runs" or binges. Because of tolerance, they will use increased amounts of stimulants for days without sleeping to obtain their high. They may get acute psychosis until they eventually burn out and fall asleep. The rebound effect occurs when the drug level drops and the patient becomes lethargic, irritable, hungry, and depressed.

Since stimulants cause hyperfunction, high doses can lead to tachycardia, arrhythmias, delirium, convulsions, coma, cerebral hemorrhages, and death. The lethal dose is approximately 5 to 50 mg per kilogram of body weight and varies among individuals.

Delusions may persist after the drug abuse is discontinued. Withdrawal produces convulsions, delirium, depression, fatigue, hypotonia, and sleep disturbance.

Cocaine causes CNS stimulation by blocking the re-uptake of norepinephrine. The sense of euphoria is often more intense albeit more fleeting than amphetamine or methamphetamine. To maintain the "high," cocaine would have to be injected every half hour. Smoking crack has a similar onset and duration as injecting cocaine, whereas snorting cocaine has a longer onset of action. Overall, the stimulating effects of cocaine last around 2 hours. The other symptoms of cocaine are the same as for other stimulants, and the rebound effect of depression is similar. Chronic abuse can also lead to paranoia and toxic pychosis. Psychological dependence can occur and is often faster with the crack version.

Cocaine has an acute effect on the vascular system, causing vasospasm and thrombosis. In the cardiovascular system, tachycardia, increased blood pressure, myocarditis, and myocardial infarctions can occur with cocaine abuse. Vascular events and changes such as cerebral vascular accidents, pulmonary hemorrhage, and atherosclerosis/arteriosclerosis of coronary, thoracic, abdominal, and renal vessels have been implicated with cocaine abuse. Autopsy reports have shown increased coronary artery disease and arteriosclerosis in cocaine abusers versus nonabusers of the same age. Crack abuse usually causes more frequent pulmonary and cerebrovascular complications, including pulmonary edema and bronchiolitis. The lethal dosage may vary from 30 mg to 1.2 g.

Because of the popularity of the intranasal mode of administration of cocaine, irritation of the mucosal lining of the upper respiratory tract, chronic osteolytic sinusitis, and nasoseptal perforation are common. Cocaine has a deleterious effect on pregnancy. Women using cocaine have a higher rate of spontaneous abortion

> The lethal dose of stimulants varies from 5 to 50 mg per kilogram of body weight. The lethal dose of crack varies from 30 mg to 1.2 g.

than nonusers. Infants exposed to cocaine have higher rates of congenital malformations, perinatal mortality, and neurobehavioral problems. Sexual dysfunction has been reported with chronic cocaine abuse.

Ocular

The classic ocular sign of stimulant use is mydriasis with a decreased pupillary response to light. Stimulants can also cause lid retraction, decreased accommodation, convergence insufficiency, eyelid tremors when the eyes are closed, and color vision defects. Table 66–11 lists common ocular signs of stimulants. Retinal vasoconstriction, microaneurysms, central retinal artery occlusions, retinal hemorrhages, and secondary optic neuropathy have all been reported with amphetamine and cocaine abuse. Chronic nasal cocaine abuse can cause erosion of the bones of the maxillary sinus and orbit. This has been reported to lead to preseptal and orbital cellulitis.

Corneal epithelial defects have been reported after crack use including corneal abrasions, ulcers, and superficial punctate keratitis, giving rise to the term "crack eye." Rofsky and associates (1995) reported sparkling white dust particles in the superficial retinal layers of the posterior pole in free-basing cocaine users that they have termed "microtalc retinopathy." They suggest that the adulterants in the crack are inhaled as a vapor. They enter the pulmonary circulation and vascularized mucous membranes of the lungs, eventually lodging in the retinal microcirculation. "Rake" nerve fiber defects similar to those seen in glaucoma are often noted in these crack users.

TABLE 66–11. OCULAR MANIFESTATIONS OF STIMULANT ABUSE

- Lid retraction
- Eyelid tremors
- Mydriasis and decreased pupillary response
- Accommodative insufficiency
- Convergence insufficiency
- Retinal vasoconstriction and microaneurysms
- Corneal epithelial defects
- Microtalc retinopathy
- Color vision defects
- Preseptal and orbital cellulitis

Diagnosis

Systemic

Urine or blood testing will reveal stimulant use within the past 2 to 4 days (Table 66–3). Diagnosis can be based on observation. Nasal swabs can detect intranasal usage of stimulants. All stimulants can produce tremor of the hands and feet, restlessness, and hyperactivity.

> Tremors of hands and feet in young healthy patients may indicate stimulant use.

They can also cause dizziness, headaches, palpitations, fever, nausea, diarrhea, hallucinations, and dehydration. The hallucinations may be visual, auditory, or olfactory. Needle marks or "pop" scars on the skin may indicate intravenous or subcutaneous use of stimulants. Constant sniffling caused by inflammation of the nasal mucosa may indicate intranasal administration of these drugs. Often, users keep pinky fingernails long to use as spoons to sniff cocaine.

> Constant sniffling in hyperactive patients with no allergies or viral infection may indicate cocaine use.

> Single long pinky fingernails may be used as spoons to sniff cocaine.

Ocular

Ocular involvement is diagnosed by observation and through systemic signs. In addition, the dilated pupil with a poor response to light is a classic ocular sign of stimulant abuse. Patients may complain of photophobia and wear sunglasses even in dim light. Patients may also complain about near blur and near point asthenopia.

> Dilated pupils with poor response to light are a classic sign of stimulant use.

Treatment and Management

The standard ABCs (airway, breathing, and circulation) are the first order of treatment (Table 66–4). Depending on the patient's condition, ice baths are used for hyperthermia and benzodiazepines for seizures, CNS symptoms, and sedation. Antipsychotic agents such as haloperidol can decrease the hallucinations but do not affect the paranoia.

Chronic abuse is best treated by rehabilitation programs. However, the prognosis for patients psychologically addicted to stimulants is poor because the rebound depression can last for months and recurrence is very common. Stimulant abstinence syndrome is a three-phase pattern that needs to occur for the patient to recover. The three phases are crash (intense depression, agitation, and anxiety), withdrawal (decreased energy and disinterest in environment), and extinction (decreased craving for the drug). Medical treatment is not necessary for stimulant abuse; however, psychotherapy to break the psychological dependence on the drugs can help.

Minimal treatment is necessary for the ocular manifestations of stimulant use. Infectious keratitis and corneal epithelial defects should be treated, if warranted. No treatment, other than monitoring, is necessary for microtalc retinopathy.

DEPRESSANTS

CNS depressants are generally prescribed to relieve anxiety, produce sleep, and treat epilepsy. They are among the most commonly prescribed drugs in the United States. For healthy individuals, their use is short term, but for patients with mental illness, use may be life-long. CNS depressants include barbiturates, benzodiazepines, and azapirones. Benzodiazepines are prescribed for muscle spasms and to decrease rigidity in cerebral palsy since they relax muscles. Nearly all CNS depressants suppress seizures. Clonazepam (Klonopin) and diazepam (Valium) are most common in the treatment of epilepsy and seizure disorders.

Benzodiazepines have replaced barbiturates as the antianxiety drugs of choice since they are less likely to cause a fatal overdose. Barbiturates continue to be used to treat sleep disorders and for surgical anesthesia. On the street, they are generally called "downers," but they are also given more specific names correlating to the color of their dosage forms, such as "yellow jackets" for pentobarbital and "purple hearts" for phenobarbital.

CNS depressants are taken orally. Onset of action and duration vary with the drug, but onset usually is about 30 minutes with duration lasting several hours. Tolerance develops slowly. Chronic use of barbiturate-like substances requires larger doses to achieve the desired subjective effects. Cross-tolerance with alcohol and other antianxiety agents occurs as well.

The more common barbiturates include pentobarbital (Nembutal), phenobarbital (Luminal), and secobarbital (Seconal). The more common nonbarbiturate sedatives are zolpidem (Ambien), temazepam (Restoril), and flurazepam (Dalmane).

Epidemiology

The National Household Survey on Drug Abuse 1997 estimates over 4 million Americans over the age of 12 years have used sedatives and another 6.9 million have taken tranquilizers in their lifetime. They estimate that 0.1% of the population is currently using sedatives and 0.4% are taking tranquilizers for nonmedical purposes.

Pathophysiology/Disease Process

Systemic

Systemic manifestations of depressants are listed in Table 66–12. At low therapeutic levels, CNS depressants produce a calming, relaxed feeling. At higher doses, intoxication similar to alcohol is produced. Poor motor coordination, slurred and slow speech, drowsiness, and difficulty with comprehension and attention are also exhibited. Physiologically, there is decreased

TABLE 66–12. SYSTEMIC MANIFESTATIONS OF DEPRESSANT ABUSE

Systemic
- Calmness, relaxation
- Motor incoordination
- Slurred speech
- Drowsiness
- Difficulty with comprehension and attention
- Respiratory depression
- Hypotension
- Decreased body temperature
- Decreased heart rate
- CNS depression
- Decreased REM sleep
- Death

Withdrawal Symptoms
- Anxiety
- Weakness
- Decreased appetite
- Tremors
- Tachycardia
- Hyperthermia
- Convulsions
- Delirium
- Hallucinations
- Cardiovascular collapse

respiration, blood pressure, body temperature, and heart rate. The depressants will depress the CNS, but they have no analgesic properties. Although they are used to treat sleep disturbances, they depress REM (rapid eye movement) sleep. The lethal dose for barbiturates is 50 to 500 mg per kilogram of body weight when taken as a single dose. Death is due to cardiovascular collapse and respiratory depression. Benzodiazepines require a larger difference between doses that cause sleep and doses that cause death, making them safer than barbiturates. Overdoses are common but fatalities rare with benzodiazepines.

> Withdrawal symptoms from depressants begin 12 to 24 hours after the last dose.

Withdrawal symptoms from depressants may begin within 12 to 24 hours after the last dose in chronic users. Symptoms include anxiety, weakness, decreased appetite, and tremors. Withdrawal symptoms reach peak intensity within 24 to 48 hours. Physiologically at this time, the user will experience increased blood pressure, tachycardia, and increased body temperature (fever). Users may also have tonic–clonic convulsions. Delirium may develop between 4 and 7 days after last dose. At this time, users may experience hallucinations; cardiovascular collapse can occur secondary to hyperthermia and tachycardia. With longer-acting depressants, the withdrawal symptoms may be delayed but they will occur unless another dose of the drug is administered. Withdrawal symptoms are reversible with another dose unless delirium has already developed, in which case the symptoms are relatively irreversible.

The severity of the withdrawal symptoms is related to the dose and duration of use. The minimum dose of barbiturates to produce a clinically significant degree of physical dependence is 400 mg/day for 2 to 3 months.

> The most common ocular side affects of CNS depressants are extraocular motility dysfunction, decreased convergence, and nystagmus.

Ocular

The most common ocular side effects of CNS depressants are EOM dysfunction, decreased convergence, and nystagmus (Table 66–13). Chronic users may have ptosis and blepharoclonus. Normally, a tapping on the glabella area of the forehead (glabella tap test) produces a few blinks, but in users, it causes a fluttering of the eyelids. Other ocular side effects include diplopia, visual field defects and constrictions, color vision defects, visual hallucinations, decreased accommodation, dry eye, and decreased intraocular pressure. Pupil size may vary, but pupils are miotic in barbiturate coma. They may react poorly to light. Transient or permanent loss of vision can occur in patients in barbiturate coma. These agents decrease sympathetic inhibition, which is believed to cause poor perfusion of the optic nerve leading to optic neuropathy and subsequent optic atrophy. Allergic conjunctivitis and dermatitis have been reported with barbiturate use.

TABLE 66–13. OCULAR MANIFESTATIONS OF DEPRESSANT ABUSE

- Extraocular motility dysfunction
- Ptosis
- Convergence insufficiency
- Nystagmus
- Blepharoclonus
- Diplopia
- Visual field defects and constrictions
- Color vision defects
- Visual hallucinations
- Decreased accommodation
- Dry eye
- Decreased intraocular pressure
- Allergic conjunctivitis/lid dermatitis
- Optic neuropathy/atrophy (in patients recovering from barbiturate coma)

Diagnosis

Systemic

Blood and urine testing for CNS depressants will detect intoxication (Table 66–3). An EEG may show nonspecific depression. Dependence on these agents can be diagnosed with the administration of two 200-mg doses of pentobarbital 6 hours apart. This will not cause CNS depression in addicts because of their high level of tolerance but will cause CNS depression in nonusers. Patients exhibiting drowsiness, slurred speech, and impaired motor coordination should raise the suspicion of CNS depressant or alcohol use. However, during the euphoric stage, patients may present with an elevated mood or rapid mood swings. Early signs of withdrawal such as anxiety and tremors should also raise suspicion.

Ocular

In the early stages of depressant abuse, the subtle oculomotor pursuit deficits may only be observable with electronystagmography. While tracking an optokinetic nystagmus (OKN) stimulus, the smooth pursuits will be replaced with jerky, saccadic movements. As blood levels increase, cogwheel-type movements may be more easily observed with the naked eye. The glabellar tap test can also be used in the diagnosis of barbiturate abuse. For those who recover from coma, decreased visual acuity may be present. This visual disturbance will usually improve; however, permanent optic atrophy has been reported in some cases. Complaints of diplopia, dyschromatopsia, yellow or green tinge to vision, and visual hallucinations may occur.

Treatment and Management

Treatment of acute barbiturate intoxication (Table 66–4) involves stabilizing respiration with mechanical ventilation (airway, breathing, and circulation). Activated charcoal may be given to decrease drug absorption if the depressants were ingested within 6 hours. Gastric lavage may be performed once the airway is secured. CNS stimulants may be given in cases of nonbarbiturate sedative intoxication.

Withdrawal from CNS depressants is best done in a hospital because of the severe and possibly life-threatening complications. Pentobarbital or phenobarbital is administered until the patient exhibits mild barbiturate intoxication. This initial dose is maintained until the patient stabilizes, and then it is reduced until the patient is drug-free. If the withdrawal symptoms occur, the dose is increased to mild intoxication again and then decreased slowly. Psychological and social rehabilitation should begin during detoxification and continue after the patient is drug-free to prevent relapse.

OPIATES

The opiates are narcotic analgesics, which include any drug that is derived from or contains opium. Raw opium is a naturally occurring substance that is derived by air-drying the juice from the poppy plant. There are twenty different alkaloids that contain up to 25% opium. The more commonly known alkaloids include morphine, codeine, heroin, and papaverine. Opiate receptors on cell surfaces interact with opiate drugs, resulting in sedation and anesthesia. The analgesic property of opiates is due to their action in the part of the brain that interprets the nerve message rather than by blocking transmission of the pain impulse. Thus, the subjective perception of pain is relieved, yet the ability to feel and have sensation is not altered. They are often used to treat chronic malignant pain as well as severe acute pain. Opiates possess a significant potential for abuse because they also relieve anxiety and promote a feeling of well-being. Long-term use results in both a psychological and physiological dependence, thereby producing withdrawal signs and symptoms. Unfortunately, the physical dependence occurs with therapeutic dosages.

Morphine is a naturally occurring opiate that contains approximately 10% raw opium by weight, and is considered one of medicine's strongest analgesics. It is administered subcutaneously, intramuscularly, or intravenously. Morphine was used extensively in medicine until 1850, when its use declined due to the significant potential for opiate addiction and illicit use. Currently it is reserved for moderate to severe pain relief only when other nonnarcotic analgesics are ineffective.

Codeine is a naturally occurring opiate that is less potent than morphine. It contains approximately 0.7 to 2.5% raw opium. It is commonly used in tablet or liquid form to relieve mild to moderate pain and as an antitussive (cough suppressant) agent. Physical dependence usually does not result with typical therapeutic use.

Heroin is a semisynthetic derivative of morphine. It is produced by chemically mixing morphine with acetic acid. The name developed because it was thought to be the "heroic" cure for morphine addiction. However, heroin is three times as potent as morphine, and the potential for addiction is greater than with any other drug. Heroin can be administered orally, nasally ("snorting"), subcutaneously ("skin-popping"), or intravenously ("mainlining"), which is the preferred route. Most illicit heroin is cut with fillers.

> Heroin has the highest potential for addiction than any other drug.

There is a class of synthetic narcotic analgesics known as opioids. This term signifies any drug whose pharmacologic actions resemble those of morphine. Opioids in common use include meperidine (Demerol), methadone (Dolophine), fentanyl (Sublimaze), butorphenol (Stadol), and nalbuphine (Nubain). These drugs are used medically as pain relievers and in relieving the symptoms of morphine and heroin withdrawal. Recently, some of these drugs have also become widely abused.

Epidemiology

The opium poppy plant is native to ancient civilizations in Asia. The East Indians typically confined its use to medical and ritual purposes, whereas the Chinese often smoked opium for social reasons. Abuse was first recorded in the seventeenth century, making it the second oldest abused drug after alcohol. Morphine was more commonly used in the West because raw opium is not legally permitted in the United States.

Lifetime heroin prevalence was estimated to be 2 million in 1997 with about 71% sniffing, smoking, or snorting the drug and 55% injecting it. Abusers may use several different modes of administration, which is why the total percentage is larger than 100 percent.

Pathophysiology/Disease Process

Systemic

Narcotic analgesics such as the opiates depress the CNS, causing a dreamy euphoric state with a decrease in pain sensation (Table 66–14). However, new users of opiates often experience nausea, vomiting, and dysphoria such that less than half of the people who have tried heroin continue using it.

After IV administration, the user initially gets a "rush," which is reported to be intense pleasure similar to sexual orgasm. There is a warm flushing of the skin and sensation in the lower abdomen. The user then gets a sense of relaxation, contentment, and tranquility known as the "nod." Physiologically, during this phase, the user experiences drowsiness, lethargy, hypoventilation, hypotension, decreased body temperature, and heart rate. The patient may appear asleep even when standing up. Onset of action is very rapid when the drug is administered by IV and can be as short as 20 minutes when taken orally. The overall duration of action also depends on the mode of administration, but usually ranges from 3 to 6 hours.

Although opiates can cause euphoria in some patients, they usually produce sedation in most patients. These sedative effects are additive when opiates are used with alcohol or barbiturates. Constipation occurs with opiate use since they inhibit intestinal tract motility. Because opiates suppress brainstem respiratory centers, respiratory depression and failure can occur with 100 to 200 mg. The medical dose for analgesia for heroin in England is 3 mg subcutaneously, whereas the typical addict uses up to 100 mg daily. Decreased libido and altered REM (rapid eye movement) sleep and menstrual cycles have been reported in users.

Users quickly develop tolerance towards opiates and require increased amounts to obtain the subjective effects. Opiates also cause physiological and psychological dependence. The minimum amount of heroin needed to produce dependence is considered to be 24 mg daily.

TABLE 66–14. SYSTEMIC MANIFESTATIONS OF OPIATE AND OPIOID ABUSE

- **"Rush"**
  - Euphoria
  - Skin flushing
  - Warm sensation in lower abdomen
  - Nausea, vomiting in new users
- **"Nod"**
  - Relaxation
  - Contentment
  - Tranquility
  - Apathy
  - Floating feeling
  - Drowsiness
  - Lethargy
  - Hypotension
  - Hypothermia
  - Decreased heart rate
- CNS depression
- Decreased pain sensation
- Constipation
- Respiratory failure
- Circulatory failure
- Decreased libido
- Altered REM sleep pattern
- Altered menstrual cycles
- **Withdrawal Symptoms**
  - Anxiety
  - Craving
  - Perspiration
  - Chills
  - Gastrointestinal disturbances
  - Hyperthermia
  - Cramps/diarrhea
  - Hypertension
  - Tachycardia
  - Irritability
  - Depression
  - Sleep disturbances

Within 4 to 6 hours after the last dose of morphine or heroin, the addict may get withdrawal symptoms of anxiety, craving, perspiration, chills, rhinitis, gastrointestinal disturbances, hyperthermia, cramps, and diarrhea. These symptoms reach peak intensity within 48 hours of the last dose if another dose of narcotic is not received. Withdrawal symptoms may be so severe that users will try to keep a maintenance dose in order to avoid the rebound effect. Hypertension, tachycardia, irritability, depression, sleep disturbances, and paresthesia can occur in severe withdrawal.

> Withdrawal symptoms begin 4 to 6 hours after the last dose of morphine or heroin and peak within 48 hours.

Pure heroin is generally "cut" or mixed with many adulterants, including sugar, talc, and quinine, before being sold on the street. These adulterants can cause ocular and systemic manifestations.

Ocular

The classic ocular manifestation of opiate use is extreme miosis (often less than 3 mm in the dark), known as "pinpoint" pupils (Table 66–15). Initially after use there is a 20-second mydriasis followed by pinpoint pupils that may not react to light. However, "speed balls," heroin and cocaine combinations, will give variable pupil findings. During withdrawal after prolonged use, anisocoria, mydriasis, or irregular pupils are sometimes noted. Bilateral ptosis is common with opiate use. Horner syndrome has been reported in chronic addicts. Studies have found lower intraocular pressure in opium users than in nonusers, and the longer the duration of opium addiction, the lower the mean intraocular pressure.

> The classic ocular manifestation of opiate use is "pinpoint pupils" (<3mm in the dark).

> Bilateral ptosis is common in heroin abusers.

TABLE 66–15. OCULAR MANIFESTATIONS OF OPIATE ABUSE

- Pinpoint pupils
- Ptosis
- Decreased intraocular pressure
- Accommodative excess
- Horner syndrome in chronic addicts

Withdrawal Symptoms

- Excessive tearing
- Accommodative insufficiency
- Diplopia

In addition to the pupillary effects, opiate withdrawal can also cause ocular manifestations. Excessive tearing, decreased or paresis of accommodation, and diplopia have been reported.

Diagnosis

Systemic

Blood and urine toxicology is used to diagnose opiate use (Table 66–3). However, over 90% of the dose of most opiates is excreted in the urine within 24 hours. Administration of Narcan (naloxone), a narcotic antagonist, is a reliable albeit possibly risky means of determining physical opiate overdose. It is usually given to unconscious patients with respiratory depression. If a patient starts breathing with 0.1 to 0.4 mg naloxone, the diagnosis of opiate overdose is made, but some opiate-dependent patients may get withdrawal signs such as mydriasis, nausea, vomiting, and profuse sweating within 15 minutes. Opiate overdose in nonopiate-dependent patients may require up to 10 mg naloxone to resume breathing, and nonopiate overdoses (benzodiazepines, phencyclidine) will not respond to naloxone. Tachycardia, increased blood pressure, and seizures may occur with naloxone in users. Nonnarcotic users and users who are not physically dependent will have no withdrawal signs.

The presence of needle tracks and signs of thrombophlebitis and toxic dermatitis over injection sites often indicate IV drug use. Opiate abusers may also appear to be asleep when they actually are not.

Ocular

Pinpoint pupils or poorly reactive pupils in an otherwise healthy patient may raise suspicion of opiate use. Ptosis, decreased accommodation, and convergence may support the suspicion. The presence of talc retinopathy, discussed later in the chapter, would be indicative of chronic IV drug abuse.

Treatment and Management

Acute overdose that is causing severe respiratory depression can be treated with naloxone (Table 66–4). This drug, which is used in diagnosing opiate overdose, will also help reverse the sedation, CNS, and respiratory effects of the opiate. Monitoring with mechanical ventilation and patient stimulation is necessary until respiration stabilizes.

Like all substance abuse conditions, discontinuing the drug use is the treatment. However, opiates actually cause a physical addiction such that the withdrawal symptoms must also be treated. Withdrawal therapy and maintenance therapy are two methods to treat the opiate addiction. The optimal withdrawal strategy is in a hospital, attempting to get the patient drug-free quickly. It involves giving enough oral methadone to suppress most of the withdrawal symptoms. Once the patient stabilizes, the dose is halved every other day until it is stopped within 6 to 10 days. With a methadone maintenance program, a "maintenance" dose of oral methadone is given to prevent withdrawal symptoms. This allows the patient to work or go to an outpatient drug program. The maintenance program usually lasts for a minimum of 3 months and may continue for life. Drug rehabilitation programs that include behavioral therapy help patients deal with their addiction. Still, there is a high incidence of relapse with opiate abusers.

HALLUCINOGENS

Hallucinogens are a class of drugs that distort one's perception. There are three major classes of hallucinogens—indolealkylamines (eg, LSD), phenethylamines (eg, mescaline), and phencyclidine (eg, angel dust). These substances are found naturally in certain mushrooms, cacti, and hemp plants, but synthetic substances such as LSD (acid) and ecstasy (3,4-methylene dioxymethamphetamine) are more common. The mechanism of action of the indolealkylamines and phenethylamines is not certain. These two classes produce CNS stimulation and distortion of sensory perception. These substances have no accepted medical use. Phencyclidines were initially used as anesthetic agents but because of the high incidence of patients emerging from anesthesia with disorientation, hallucinations, and delirium, their use has been discontinued. Phencyclidines are still available on the street for recreational use. In powder form, it is known as angel dust and is snorted or mixed with marijuana or other leaves and smoked. Tablets and capsules are ingested. The liquid form can either be injected intravenously or put on leaves and smoked.

Epidemiology

Natural hallucinogens have been used since antiquity but abuse was first reported in the mid-1900s and became widespread during the 1960s, mainly with LSD. According to the 1997 National Household Survey on Drug Abuse, 9.6% of the population over the age of 12 years have used hallucinogens in their lifetime, but only 0.8% are current users. LSD is the most common hallucinogen. Hallucinogens are more often used by white males 18 to 25 years of age. Use is more prevalent in the western United States.

Pathophysiology/Disease Process

Systemic

Table 66–16 lists systemic manifestations of hallucinogens. Hallucinations are false perceptions and hallucinogens distort sensory perception, especially visual perception, giving rise to kaleidoscope-like hallucinations. Perceptions of size, distance, time, and body images are distorted. With low doses of LSD-like drugs, users may get feelings of euphoria and relaxation and heightened awareness of sensory input. This is known as a "trip." "Bad" or "bum trips" tend to occur with higher doses. Anxiety occurs and the user experiences severe disorientation. There have been reports of self-inflicted injury while under the influence of the hallucinogens. This is most likely due to toxic psychosis. Physiologically, an increase in blood pressure, tachycardia, hyperthermia, increased respiratory rate, and nausea occur. After 2 to 4 days of daily dosing, tolerance may develop. Overdoses can cause seizures, convulsions, delirium, and circulatory collapse. Onset of action ranges from minutes to hours after ingestion. Duration is about 8 to 10 hours. Physical dependence

TABLE 66–16. SYSTEMIC MANIFESTATIONS OF HALLUCINOGEN ABUSE

- **Indolealkylamines and Phenethylamines**
  - **Psychological**
    - Hallucinations
    - Altered judgement, concentration, sense of time, size, and space
    - Euphoria
    - Relaxation
    - Heightened sensory input
    - Anxiety, paranoia, aberrant behavior on "bad trips"
    - Delirium
    - Toxic psychosis
  - **Physiological**
    - Hypertension
    - Tachycardia
    - Circulatory collapse
    - Hyperthermia
    - Increased respiration rate
    - Sweating
    - Nausea
    - Seizures, convulsions
- **Phencyclidine (angel dust)**
  - **Psychological**
    - Mood swings
    - Combativeness
    - Confusion
    - Schizophrenia
    - Paranoia
    - Delirium
  - **Physiological**
    - Hypertension
    - Tachycardia
    - Decreased sense of pain
    - Myoclonic jerks
    - Muscle rigidity
    - Seizures, convulsions
    - Ataxia
    - Coma
    - Respiratory depression
    - Cardiac arrest
    - Death

does not occur so there are no withdrawal symptoms after discontinuing the drugs. Psychological dependence is usually weak, and tolerance is lost quickly after discontinuing the drug.

Phencyclidine (PCP or "dust") also causes feelings of euphoria and detachment from the environment. At low doses (2 to 10 mg), the user's mood may swing from euphoria to depression. Visual hallucinations can occur, and the user may get a sense of invulnerability. Larger doses and/or chronic use cause more dramatic mood swings, confusion, combativeness, schizophrenic episodes, and paranoia. Physiologically, PCP causes increased blood pressure, tachycardia, salivation, sweating, CNS depression or stimulation, decreased sense of pain and touch, and myoclonic jerks. Increased muscle rigidity also occurs with increased PCP use and may present as facial grimacing or a blank stare. With PCP overdose, seizures, convulsions, delirium, ataxia, coma, respiratory depression, and cardiac arrest leading to death have been reported. Onset of action is 2 to 5 minutes if smoked and 15 to 30 minutes if ingested. Duration of action is about 4 to 6 hours with moderate doses.

Ocular

Much emphasis is placed on the occurrence of spectacular hallucinations with the use of indolealkylamines like LSD. However, according to Krill and associates (1960) and Cohen and Ditman (1963), one will usually experience abnormal visual perceptions rather than true hallucinations (Table 66–17). The altered perceptions include changes in color vision; positive or negative afterimages; illusions of movement (objects may move in a wave-like fashion or melt); halos around objects; shimmering of images; micropsia or macropsia; metamorphopsia; teleopsia (perceptual disturbance involving an apparent increase in distances between objects); motion–perception defects like the "strobe light effect," in which a moving object is seen in serial momentary stationary positions; and palinopsia (visual perseveration), whereby there is "streaking" of moving objects that is termed the trailing effect. One may also experience visual hallucinations in the form of intense colored geometric patterns that appear to move kaleidoscopically with an iridescent quality. The hallucination or altered visual perception episodes are not dose-related, and flashbacks may last up to a few years after discontinuation of drug use.

In addition to these images, hallucinogens may cause decreased accommodation, blurred vision, and color vision defects. Pupils may be mydriatic with decreased reaction to light caused by the drug's effect on the autonomic nervous system. It has been reported that better "trips" can be experienced by staring at bright lights or the sun while using LSD-like hallucinogens. Because of this, many cases of solar retinopathy have been associated with LSD use. The mydriatic effect of the drug makes the user more susceptible to the thermal burn that can occur within 30 to 60 seconds of staring at the sun. Patients usually complain of decreased vision, metamorphopsia, and a central scotoma the day after the sun-gazing. Depending on the time between the sun-gazing and the examination, the ophthalmoscopic appearance may vary from extensive macula edema to a hole-like lesion with RPE mottling. Vision usually improves with time or may remain mildly reduced.

TABLE 66–17. OCULAR MANIFESTATIONS OF HALLUCINOGEN ABUSE

- **Indolealkylamines and Phenethylamines**
  - Hallucinations (abnormal visual perceptions rather than true hallucinations)
    - Intense colored geometric patterns
    - Altered color perception
    - Positive or negative afterimages
    - Prolongation of afterimages
    - Illusions of movement
    - Halos around objects
    - Shimmering images
    - Micropsia
    - Macropsia
    - Metamorphopsia
  - Blurred vision
  - Decreased accommodation
  - Solar retinopathy secondary to sun-gazing
  - Mydriasis
- **Phencyclidine**
  - Hallucinations associated with delirium
  - Ptosis
  - Miosis
  - Decreased convergence
  - Abnormal extraocular motilities—jerky pursuits
  - Irregular nystagmus in horizontal and vertical gazes
  - Papilledema and retinal hemorrhages associated with hypertensive encephalopathy

> Many cases of solar retinopathy associated with LSD use are caused by the reports of better "trips" when users stare at the sun or bright lights.

Phencyclidine also causes visual hallucinations often related to delirium. However, ocular side effects of PCP are actually secondary to the CNS depression caused by the drug. Horizontal, vertical, and rotary nystagmus are nearly always noted, even in low doses. Primary gaze is normal, but bursts of irregular jerk nystagmus occur. Ptosis, decreased convergence, difficulty with extraocular motility resulting in jerky pursuits, and diplopia are common. Miosis is common, but pupils may still respond well to light. Because phencyclidine is an acute vasopressor, hypertensive encephalopathy can occur, resulting in papilledema and retinal hemorrhages.

> Nystagmus is the most common finding with phencyclidine use.

Diagnosis

Systemic

Diagnosis usually is made by observation and history because blood and urine toxicology are not widely available. The test to detect phencyclidines in the urine must be requested specifically because it is not part of the drug toxicology screen (Table 66–3). Patients will only test positive when the drug is still in their system. Patients experiencing flashbacks will test negative. Users of LSD-like hallucinogens may have panic reactions with visual hallucinations or they may report a feeling of oneness with the universe. Users of phencyclidine may be very combative or confused and because of the anesthetic effect of the drug may continue fighting after they have already broken bones. They may present with rigidity, motor restlessness, and gross ataxia. In an acute overdose of phencyclidine, users may go into a coma with possible motor seizures.

Ocular

Users of hallucinogens may complain of blurred vision, and difficulty reading or driving. Jerky pursuits and irregular nystagmus may raise suspicion of phencyclidine use, but the diagnosis of these signs and symptoms as due to drug abuse must be one of exclusion. A careful history and full neurological workup including visual field, CT, or MRI is needed unless blood, urine, or history prove hallucinogens to be the cause.

Solar maculopathy varies in appearance depending on the number of days after exposure. Macula edema is usually noted shortly after the burn and will resolve within 14 days. A central yellow spot with a gray halo around it is seen within the first 4 days. Later, the appearance of a small macula hole may be evident. This is not a true hole but a psuedolamellar hole with all retinal layers intact. RPE mottling with a ring of hyperpigmentation giving rise to a honeycomb appearance may also be noted (Figures 66–1 and 66–2). In these cases, the patient should be asked about sungazing. He or she may admit to watching an eclipse or a welding light, and a tactful question concerning drug history may be informative.

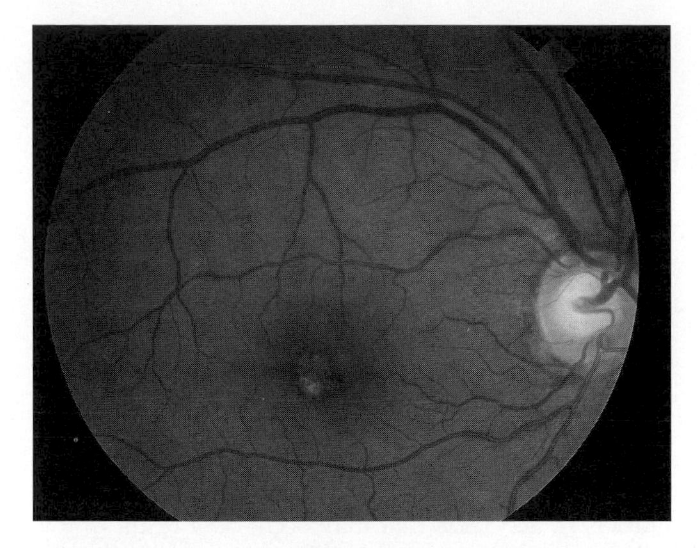

Figure 66–1. Solar retinopathy, right eye.

A patient with solar maculopathy might notice a decrease in vision a day after sun-gazing, and visual acuity is usually at the 20/40 level. Solar maculopathy is bilateral in about 47% of cases although studies have indicated a range from 0 to 97%. If unilateral, the lesion is always in the dominant eye. Metamorphopsia and central or paracentral scotoma may also be present. Fluorescein angiography may reveal late-stage choroidal fluorescence. Vision may improve over time with most of the improvement occurring within 1 month. Subjective visual disturbances often remain

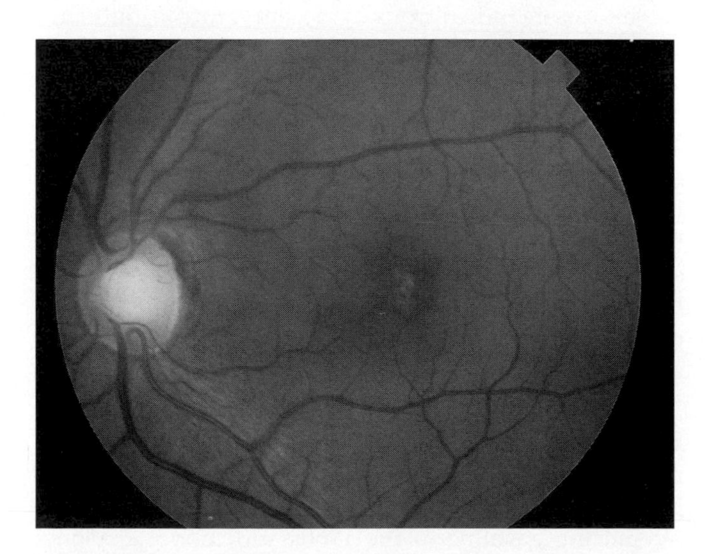

Figure 66–2. Solar retinopathy, left eye.

and can be quantified as metamorphopsia or scotoma on the Amsler grid. Solar maculopathy rarely decreases visual acuity more than 3 Snellen lines, but the associated central or paracentral scotomas can be noticeable to patients.

Treatment and Management

In acute overdose, vital signs need to be monitored and mechanical ventilation may be required (Table 66–4). Gastric lavage and activated charcoal will help decrease absorption if the drugs were ingested. IV hydration and ice packs may be administered to decrease hyperthermia. Benzodiazepines (usually diazepam), are often used for sedation and seizures. The patient needs to be monitored to prevent attempts at suicide, self-inflicted injuries, or accidents that may occur as a result of the hallucinations and delirium. Phenothiazines may be used to treat psychosis and hallucinations, but this is not recommended because of adverse effects such as hypotension and reduction in seizure threshold. The patient should be managed in a psychiatric ward and reoriented in a quiet, dimly lit room to keep sensory stimulation to a minimum until he or she is calmed.

INHALANTS

Inhalants are substances such as organic solvents, degreasers, and aerosol propellants that produce psychological and physiological effects when inhaled. These substances act as stimulants or depressants, and are easily obtained from common household products such as aerosols (whipped cream, pan coating sprays), nail polish, glue, paint thinner, transmission fluid, and room deodorizers. The desired chemicals within these substances include nitrous oxide, amyl nitrite, butyl nitrite, esters, acetone, aromatic hydrocarbons, alcohols, and many others. Nitrous oxide, which is commonly referred to as laughing gas, is a well-known inhalant. These substances are abused for their euphoric and excitatory effects. They are usually ingested by inhaling into a cloth that has been soaked or sprayed or by inhaling from a bag or balloon that has the chemical sprayed into it. A secondary danger from abusing inhalants is that they often contain compounds that are even more toxic than the chemical that produces the desired effect.

Epidemiology

Abuse of nitrous oxide as "laughing gas" was first reported as early as the 19th century. This was followed by sniffing gasoline in the 1950s and model airplane glue in the 1960s. In 1960, amyl nitrite abuse rose when it became available over the counter in ampules that were crushed and inhaled. Approximately 10 years later it was reclassified as prescription only, but was replaced with butyl nitrite. Butyl nitrite was packaged as a room odorizer or liquid incense and was easily available at drug paraphernalia stores. Around this time inhaling a variety of aerosol sprays containing alcohol also became popular. Inhalants are most commonly abused by adolescents probably because of their easy accessibility. The 1997 National Household Survey on Drug Abuse estimated that 5.7% of the population over the age of 12 have used inhalants. There has been an increase in the number of inhalant users among 12- to 25-year-olds in the past few years with an increased rate of incidence in younger users. Most inhalant use occurs before the 9th grade. It is more frequently used in middle school and less in high school. It has been suggested that inhalants are "gateway drugs," like alcohol and tobacco, to harder drugs like cocaine and marijuana as the adolescents age.

> Inhalants are most commonly used by the 12- to 25-year-old population and usually while they are in middle school.

Pathophysiology/Disease Process

Systemic

The onset and duration of action of inhalants are rapid because of the large surface area of the lungs. The chemicals are transported across the pulmonary capillary membrane. The systemic manifestations vary according to the chemical that is inhaled (Table 66–18). The effects most often reported (Wilford, 1981) involve an initial cortical disinhibition followed by generalized CNS depression resulting in transient ataxia, slurred speech, vomiting, slow and shallow respiration, and local irritation to the mucous membranes that may present as a watery discharge from the nose. Manifestations of acute intoxication with low doses may also include laryngospasm or airway freezing due to rapid vaporization as well as obstruction of the passage of oxygen across the capillary membrane. Unpleasant breath odor may also be apparent. Inhaling certain substances like hydrocarbons or fluoroalkene gases may cause respiratory depression, arrhythmias, loss of consciousness, and sudden death. Other physiological changes that occur from certain substances involve myocardial infarction, hepatic or renal toxicity, bone marrow suppression, and encephalopathy. The psy-

TABLE 66–18. SYSTEMIC MANIFESTATIONS OF INHALANT ABUSE

Generalized CNS depression
Airway freezing
Respiratory depression
Arrhythmias
Tachycardia
Hypotension
Irritation of mucous membranes
Euphoria
Drunkenness (slurred speech, transient ataxia)
Impulsiveness
Hyperactivity
Confusion, cognitive and perceptual impairments
Numbness
Death due to asphyxiation
- Chronic
  - Polyneuropathy
  - Encephalopathy
  - Damage to liver, kidneys, bone marrow, respiratory system

chological effects may resemble the early stages of alcohol intoxication or they may take on the characteristics of anesthesia. There may be signs of impulsiveness, excitement, hyperactivity, and exhilaration or feelings of numbness or weightlessness. Cerebral involvement can progress to mental confusion, clumsiness, cognitive and perceptual impairments, delirium, and sometimes irreversible brain damage. Altered behavior may result in recklessness that causes self-inflicted injury or danger. Death may also occur from asphyxiation due to an intense inhalation from a bag or ingestion of other toxic ingredients.

Ocular

Inhalants are irritating to the conjunctiva and cornea, resulting in conjunctival hyperemia, lacrimation, and decreased vision (Table 66–19). Direct contact can lead to corneal epithelial erosion and edema. The effects are of short duration and are reversible. The organic solvents have been reported to cause optic atrophy and nystagmus. The optic atrophy is secondary to optic neuritis and toxicity; it is not reversible.

TABLE 66–19. OCULAR MANIFESTATIONS OF INHALANT ABUSE

- Conjunctival hyperemia and irritation
- Corneal epithelial erosion due to direct contact
- Blurry vision
- Diplopia
- Lacrimation
- Nystagmus
- Optic neuritis/atrophy

Diagnosis

Systemic

Diagnosis of inhalant abuse is based upon clinical signs and symptoms. A user may experience symptoms of drunkenness with inability to concentrate, unsteady gait, sleepiness, confusion, and impaired judgements. Other consequences include headaches, dizziness, insomnia, delusions of unusual strength and ability to fly, auditory hallucinogens, and feelings of giddiness. Chemicals that are typically found in inhalants may be evident in the urine or with a Breathalyzer test (Table 66–3).

Ocular

Symptoms of ocular involvement include blurry vision, diplopia, lacrimation, visual hallucinations, and distortions of visual perceptions.

Treatment and Management

Treatment involves mechanical ventilation, if necessary; otherwise, it is strictly supportive (Table 66–4). Breathing should be monitored until stable and efforts made to prevent self-inflicted injuries. Since most of these patients are young, parental counseling is necessary.

INTRAVENOUS DRUG ABUSE AND ADVERSE SEQUELAE

There are a variety of systemic and ocular manifestations of intravenous drug abuse (Tables 66–20 and 66–21). This mode of administration carries high risk for infection from sharing of needles, nonsterile conditions, and contamination. In addition, the drugs are often adulterated with fillers that can embolize and cause vascular occlusion.

TABLE 66–20. COMPLICATIONS OF INTRAVENOUS DRUG ABUSE

- HIV
- Pulmonary—emboli, pneumonia, lung abscess, edema
- Cerebrovascular emboli
- Granulomas in lungs, liver, kidneys, lymph nodes
- Fungal infection
  - Disseminated, endocarditis, arthritis, mucocutaneous vasculitis, glomerulonephritis
- Bacterial infection
  - Disseminated, endocarditis, circulating immune complexes
- Hepatitis
- Tetanus
- Talc retinopathy

TABLE 66–21. OCULAR MANIFESTATIONS OF INTRAVENOUS DRUG ABUSE

- **AIDS (see Chapter 45)**
- **Talc Retinopathy**
- **Fungal Infection**
  - Endophthalmitis
  - Focal chorioretinitis
  - Uveitis
  - Papillitis
  - Vitreitis
- **Bacterial Infection**
  - Endophthalmitis
  - Retinitis
  - Vasculitis
  - Uveitis
  - Papillitis
  - Vitreitis

Acquired Immune Deficiency Syndrome

AIDS is the most serious consequence of intravenous drug abuse. Needle sharing is common with IV drug abuse and is a risk factor for transmitting the human immunodeficiency virus (HIV). In addition, users tend to participate in risky behavior while under the influence and in order to obtain funds to pay for the drugs. The systemic and ocular manifestation of AIDS are described in Chapter 45.

Talc Retinopathy

Talc retinopathy occurs as a result of embolization of talc, cornstarch, or other particles to the retina as a result of IV drug abuse. Drugs such as cocaine and heroin are often adulterated with talc or cornstarch and sold on the street. Tablets meant for oral consumption such as Ritalin and methamphetamine also contain talc and are commonly injected for recreation. These drugs or tablets are crushed, dissolved in boiling water, filtered through cotton or other homemade filters, and injected intravenously. Often, the filtrate still contains talc and other insoluble particles that can embolize to the lung. Most of the particles are larger than 5 microns, which is large enough to cause capillary occlusion. As the embolization continues, pulmonary hypertension develops and collateral vessels form. The collateral vessels allow the emboli to bypass the lungs and go directly to the heart, where they can get pumped to various organs including the eye. Particles smaller than 5 microns may pass through the pulmonary circulation on their own and lodge in the smaller capillaries of the eye and the brain. Talc retinopathy is only found in chronic abusers. Tse and Ober (1980) did not note any retinopathy in patients who injected less than 3500 tablets or used IV drugs less than 1 year. Most of these patients have injected about 20 to 35 tablets daily for 1 to 10 years. The severity of the talc retinopathy correlates with the duration of drug abuse and cumulative injections.

Epidemiology

The incidence of talc retinopathy has been reported to be 28 to 48%. Tse and Ober (1980) reported the incidence to be as high as 82%. Talc retinopathy is more prevalent in users who inject tablets meant for oral consumption, such as Ritalin (methylphenidate hydrochloride), methamphetamines, or methadone rather than in users who inject heroin sold on the street. When the drugs are injected on a more frequent or chronic basis and the filtration process prior to injection is not meticulous, talc retinopathy is more likely to occur.

Pathophysiology/Disease Process

Systemic. Pulmonary emboli can occlude the capillaries and small vessels of the lungs. Endothelial proliferation and granulomas occur with secondary occlusion of the capillaries, arterioles, and arteries. Initially, there is obstruction to the blood flow to the distal lung with subsequent constriction of the air spaces and airways. Pulmonary hypertension develops and collateral vessels form to bypass the lung. Acute and chronic impairment of pulmonary function is common, but complete pulmonary infarction rarely occurs.

Emboli that pass through the collateral vessels of the lung or emboli small enough to pass through the pulmonary capillaries and reach the systemic circulation can lodge in the vessels of various organs. Occlusion of the cerebral vasculature can lead to transient ischemic attacks, strokes, and cerebral hemorrhages. Talc granulomas have been found in the lungs, liver, kidneys, and lymph nodes of IV drug abusers. These granulomas are more often associated with IV administration of oral medications rather than with street heroin.

Ocular. When the talc particles reach the eye, they can embolize to the small capillaries of the retina and to the choriocapillaris. They appear as tiny yellow or white glistening, crystalline deposits in the small arterioles of the posterior pole, usually along the perifoveal arcade (Figure 66–3). They lodge primarily at this location as a result of the dense capillary net of the posterior pole. In the acute stage, retinal hemorrhages and cotton-wool spots may be present. Microaneurysms and venous tortuosity may form. Retinal and macula ischemia can occur as the emboli disrupt blood flow and cause capillary nonperfusion.

The emboli can also lodge in the peripheral vessels of the retina, causing areas of nonperfusion. The result-

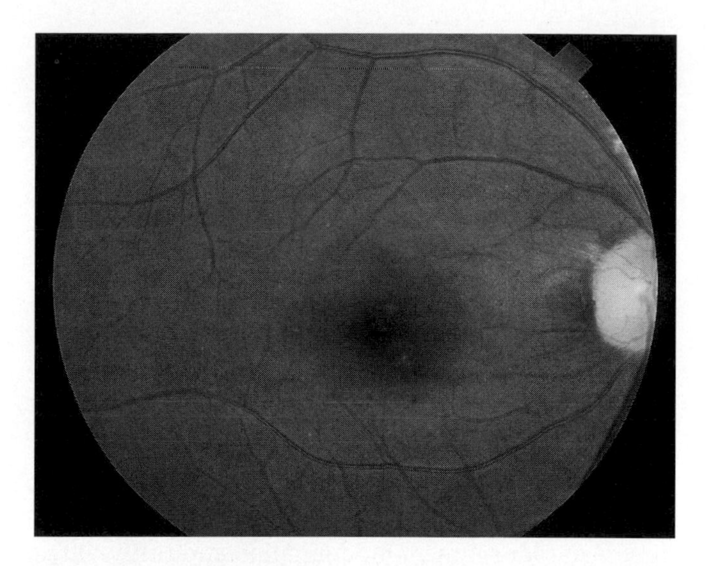

Figure 66–3. Talc retinopathy.

ing ischemia can cause vasoproliferation. Neovascularization in the form of seafans can occur between the areas of perfusion and nonperfusion, resembling sickle-cell retinopathy. Vitreal hemorrhages and retinal detachments may occur as a result of the neovascularization. Neovascularization of the optic disc in patients with talc retinopathy has been reported in rare incidences.

Diagnosis

Systemic. Patients with pulmonary emboli may complain of difficulty breathing. Chest x-ray (which may reveal parenchymal infiltrate), pulmonary function tests, and pulmonary angiography can confirm the diagnosis. Biopsy of granulomas will confirm if talc or cornstarch is present. Pare and Fraser (1979) reported 60% of IV drug abusers had talc retinopathy. Fundus evaluation had a higher diagnostic yield than chest x-ray or pulmonary function testing. Cerebral involvement is diagnosed by observing the typical signs and symptoms. Cerebral angiography will show scattered areas of nonperfusion as well as narrowing and fragmentation of arterioles and capillaries.

Ocular. Most patients with talc retinopathy are asymptomatic with VA 20/30 or better. Some individuals will present with complaints of decreased vision secondary to microvascular occlusion of retinal arterioles and capillary nonperfusion. Central scotomas corresponding to the ischemic areas may be found on Amsler grid testing or perimetry. The talc emboli in the retinal arterioles are easily seen on fundus evaluation (Figure 66–3). The classic appearance is glistening yellow particles in the superficial layers of the retina in the perifoveal area. Differential diagnosis of talc retinopathy (Table 66–22) include drusen, cholesterol emboli, exudates, tamoxifen, and fundus flavimaculatus. They can be differentiated from drusen, exudates, and cholesterol emboli by their superficial location in the smaller retinal vessels of the posterior pole. In addition to this, exudates are often accompanied with hemorrhages, and it is rare to have several cholesterol emboli such that they would resemble talc. The good vision will differentiate it from fundus flavimaculatus. Tamoxifen, a chemotherapy agent for the treatment of breast cancer, also deposits in the paramacular area but is easily ruled out by history. A red-free filter may highlight the emboli on fundus photography. Fluorescein angiography will show precapillary arteriolar occlusions, capillary nonperfusion, and vascular leakage. It will also help differentiate emboli from drusen and fundus albipunctatus. Focal electroretinography will show a reduced amplitude of the foveal signal. Hematologic testing will rule out sickle-cell retinopathy as the cause for the peripheral neovascularization.

Treatment and Management

Systemic and Ocular. Talc retinopathy is a static condition. The emboli are insoluble and cannot be metabolized. Martidis and co-workers (1997) suggest that the emboli may be subjected to endothelialization, limiting their mobility in the retinal capillaries. Therefore, treatment is limited to discontinuing the IV drug abuse and making the proper referrals. The presence of talc retinopathy indicates significant damage to the lungs; therefore, a pulmonary workup is indicated. A neurological workup may also be warranted to rule out and manage cerebral complications. If neovascularization is noted, fluorescein angiography should be done and a retinal consultation obtained for photocoagulation.

TABLE 66–22. TALC RETINOPATHY AND DIFFERENTIAL DIAGNOSIS

Talc Retinopathy
Tiny white-yellow crystals in the perimacular capillaries
Microaneurysms
Hemorrhages
Venous tortuosity
Retinal ischemia
VA usually 20/30 or better
Differential Diagnosis
Drusen
Exudates
Cholesterol emboli
Stargardt disease
Tamoxifen retinopathy

Fungal Infection

Fungal infections occur more often when sharing dirty, unsterilized needles and when the proper aseptic precaution of cleaning the skin prior to intravenous injection is not followed. *Candida* and *Aspergillus* are ubiquitous in the environment and are the most common fungal infections in IV drug abusers. *Candida* occurs in the eye, skeleton, heart, and CNS. Endocarditis is a frequent complication of parenteral drug addiction, with the endocardium of the aortic and mitral valves most often affected. Disseminated fungal infection may also occur. Endophthalmitis associated with intravenous drug abuse develops as a result of invasion of the organism into the eye from the bloodstream, metastasis from other tissues, or septic emboli from infected heart valves that lodge intraocularly.

Epidemiology

Fungal infection accounts for 5 to 50% of serious infections in IV drug users. Approximately 10 to 15% of the cases of endocarditis associated with IV drug abuse are due to *Candida*, but infection with multiple organisms is common.

> *Candida* and *Aspergillus* are the most common fungal infections in IV drug abusers.

Pathophysiology/Disease Process

Systemic. Infectious endocarditis associated with IV drug abuse develops acutely. This disease is characterized by vegetations growing on valves or other parts of the endocardium. Often the organism is localized on sterile vegetations of platelets and fibrin that are already present. These vegetations may occlude the valve orifices or stimulate an immune reaction, with subsequent scar formation resulting in conduction abnormalities. Pieces of the vegetation may break off, forming emboli to the brain, kidney, spleen, liver, extremities, and lung with subsequent infarction. Myocarditis may develop from coronary artery emboli, extension of the infection to the myocardium with abscess formation, or immune complex vasculitis. Circulating immune complexes may also result in glomerulonephritis, arthritis, and mucocutaneous vasculitis. There is a high rate of mortality associated with endocarditis if left untreated. However, fewer cases of mortality are reported with intravenous drug abuse than with cases associated with immunodeficiency.

Ocular. Ocular manifestations may occur days to weeks after the use of intravenous drugs. Ocular involvement may range from a localized lesion (abcess of granulomatous inflammatory material) to endophthalmitis. Both *Candida* and *Aspergillus* will give similar signs that are characterized by a choroidal or chorioretinal white cotton-like circumscribed exudate (Figure 66–4). Lesions are approximately 1 mm in diameter and most often located in the posterior pole. An overlying vitreal haze is usually present when the predisposing factor is IV drug abuse. The lesion typically originates in the choroid. It can progress to the RPE and eventually into the overlying retina. Retinal detachment may occur because of the retinal and subretinal exudates. Hemorrhages, Roth spots (white-centered hemorrhages), and retinal edema may be noted first. Anterior segment inflammation and fluffy vitreal infitrates containing the organism known as "string of pearls" may follow. These two signs are more common among drug abusers who may lack typical retinal lesions and other systemic signs of disseminated candidiasis. Papillitis may also occur. Visual prognosis is poor once the vitreous is involved, but vision may improve if treatment is initiated early. Phthisis bulbi may result in intractable cases.

> Fungal infection appears as a choroidal or chorioretinal white cotton-like circumscribed exudate with accompanying uveitis or vitreitis.

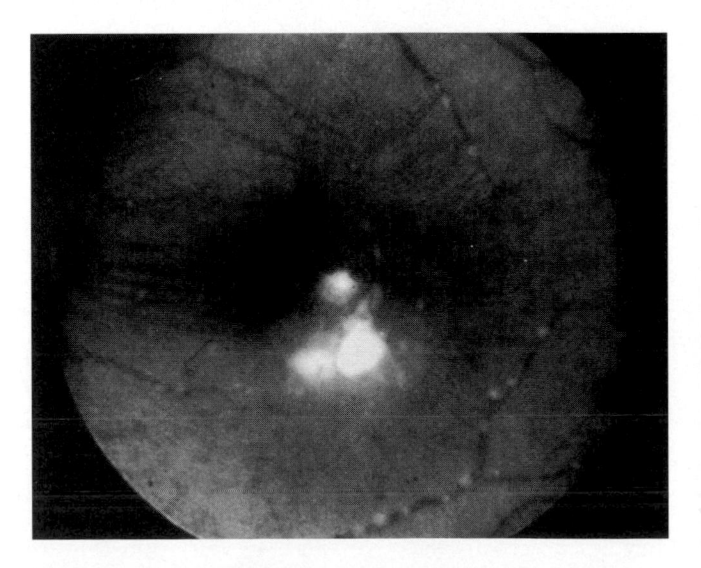

Figure 66–4. *Candida* retinitis. *(Courtesy of Dr. Scott Richter.)*

Fungal endophthalmitis occurs and progresses at a much slower rate than bacterial endophthalmitis. Embolization from the heart valves in infectious endocarditis may result in retinal and conjunctival hemorrhages and central or branch retina artery occlusions.

Diagnosis

Systemic. Endocarditis and endophthalmitis in an otherwise healthy person should raise the suspicion of possible drug abuse. Blood and urine toxicology testing should be obtained to detect the presence of abused substances, antibody titers, circulating immune complexes, and fungal organisms. Blood cultures for fungal organisms may be negative because multiple samples are often needed to enhance fungal growth.

An echocardiogram is needed to visualize the internal cardiac structures. Needle tracks and thrombophlebitis, as well as dermatitis overlying the injection site, are supportive signs. Diagnostic symptoms of endocarditis will generally start 2 weeks after the acute infection and include fever, malaise, and on occasion, joint pain. Unlike other causes of endocarditis, heart murmurs are usually absent in cases associated with IV drug abuse.

Ocular. Any white retinal infiltrate extending into the vitreous in an immunocompromised patient or a patient with a history of IV drug abuse should raise the suspicion of fungal retinitis or endophthalmitis. This is especially true if there is an accompanying uveitis. The patient may complain of blurry vision, photophobia, and generalized ocular pain. A systemic workup may be negative because disseminated fungal infection may not show up concurrently with endophthalmitis. Vitreous biopsies and new techniques to detect anti-*Candida* antibody titers in anterior chamber fluid may help diagnose fungal endophthalmitis.

Treatment and Management

Systemic. Disseminated systemic *Candida* infections are treated with amphotericin B with or without oral flucytosine. Ketoconazole is still used, but fluconazole is able to penetrate into the cerebral spinal fluid and may soon become the drug of choice for *Candida* infections. Acute endocarditis is managed with bed rest, antifungal agents, and prophylactic antibiotics.

Ocular. There are many variations as to how to manage fungal endophthalmitis. However, it is generally agreed that treatment should commence even before the diagnosis is confirmed. For those who do treat with antifungal agents, intravitreal injection is required, because systemic administration does not result in sufficient penetration into the vitreous. Pars plana vitrectomy may also be performed with or without intraocular or systemic antifungal agents. The safety and efficacy of this regimen is still questionable. The use of topical or systemic corticosteroids is controversial.

Bacterial Infections

Bacterial infections associated with IV drug abuse usually arise from microorganisms on the skin. Disseminated infection and endocarditis are life-threatening consequences. The heart, gastrointestinal tract, and genitourinary tract are the most common sources for infection. Endophthalmitis associated with IV drug abuse develops from spread from an endogenous site of infection.

Epidemiology

Fifty percent of endocarditis cases associated with IV drug abuse are caused by *Staphylococcus,* while *Streptococcus* makes up about 15% of the cases. However, infection with multiple organisms is common. Ocular manifestations of bacterial infection are less common than fungal infections in IV drug users.

> Fifty percent of bacterial infections associated with IV drug abuse are due to *Staphylococcus.*

Pathophysiology/Disease Process

Systemic. *Staphylococcus aureus* usually causes acute endocarditis. This characteristically develops on a normal heart valve, is rapidly destructive, produces metastatic foci, and can cause fatality in 6 weeks if left untreated. *Streptococcus* is more commonly associated with subacute endocarditis. It characteristically occurs on a damaged heart valve, does not produce metastases, and has a longer onset of fatality if left untreated (sometimes up to a year). The clinical features are similar to fungal endocarditis in that vegetations can lead to occlusion of valve orifices, development of immune reactions, scar formation with valvular stenosis, and myocardial involvement from coronary artery emboli, myocardial abscesses, or immune complex vasculitis. Emboli to the pulmonary, cerebral, renal, liver, and peripheral vasculature may occur with resultant infarction. Other manifestations include glomerulonephritis, arthritis, mucocutaneous vasculitis, skin petechiae, nodules on the finger or toes, small hemorrhages on the palms and soles of the feet, and clubbing of the fingers in chronic cases. Prognosis for recovery is good in treated cases; however, fatality may occur from heart failure, rupture of mycotic aneurysm, or renal failure. See Chapter 4 for a more detailed discussion.

Ocular. Endophthalmitis may present acutely with rapid progression. Signs are usually evident in the first 24 to 48 hours. The posterior chamber is the site most involved, with retinitis the most common ocular manifestation. The retinal lesions may be found centrally or peripherally and are characterized by a white cotton-like infiltrate with fluffy borders extending into the vitreous. Roth spots may occur in 5% of cases. A "candle-wax" vasculitis similar to that found in sarcoidosis may also be evident. Advanced cases will manifest with lid swelling, conjuctival edema, injection, petechiae, corneal edema, uveitis (often with hypopyon), papillitis, and vitritis. Banks and co-workers (1973) reported three cases of unilateral, purulent panophthalmitis in 28 heroin addicts. Prognosis is enhanced if treatment occurs early and prior to vitreal involvement.

> In endophthalmitis, retinal cotton-like infiltrates may extend into the vitreous and progress rapidly.

Embolization from the heart valves in endocarditis can result in retinal and conjunctival hemorrhages and central or branch retinal artery occlusion, resulting in retinal edema and ischemia.

Diagnosis

Systemic. The diagnosis of bacterial infection is based on blood assays of antibody titers to the organism, serum titers to teichoic acid (a cell-wall antigen in *S. aureus*), circulating immune complexes, and the presence of microorganisms. Bacteremia (widespread dissemination by way of the bloodstream) may be evident. An echocardiogram may not always detect the vegetations. Diagnostic symptoms include fever, malaise, and possibly joint pain.

Ocular. Retinitis will mainly cause decreased visual acuity. Severe endophthalmitis involving the uvea will cause blurry vision, photophobia, and pain. Bacterial endophthalmitis should be suspected whenever rapidly progressive chorioretinal infiltrates are noted. A vitrectomy with culture should be performed for confirmation, because many of the therapeutic medications are toxic.

Treatment and Management

Systemic. Intravenous antibiotics, especially directed at *S. aureus,* are used to treat bacterial endocarditis and bacteremia associated with IV drug abuse. Therapy is initiated prior to knowing the results of culture and altered as needed once results are available. Good results are seen with parenteral penicillin, gentamicin, cephalosporin, and vancomycin given for long durations.

Ocular. The management of bacterial endophthalmitis, although controversial, usually involves administering intravitreal, subconjunctival, topical, and systemic broad-spectrum antibiotics simultaneously. Vitrectomy and corticosteroids may also be necessary.

CONCLUSION

The systemic and ocular manifestations of drug and alcohol abuse are many. Those eyecare practitioners working in drug rehabilitation clinics should be well aware of the effects of illicit drugs on the visual system. Since most patients outside of rehabilitation clinics will not volunteer information on drug use, eyecare practitioners should be familiar with the ocular manifestations of such use because they may resemble other disease processes. A review of ocular signs of drug intoxication can be found in Table 66–23.

TABLE 66–23. OCULAR SIGNS OF DRUG INTOXICATION

	VA Decrease	EOM Dysfunction	Decreased Accommodation	Decreased Convergence	Color Defects	Pupil	Nystagmus
Alcohol	Yes	Yes	Yes	Yes	Yes	Dilated	Yes
Cannabis			Yes	Yes	Yes	Dilated	Yes
Stimulants			Yes	Yes	Yes	Dilated	Maybe
Depressants		Yes	Yes	Yes	Yes	Variable	Yes
Hallucinogens	Yes		Yes	No	Yes	Dilated	No
Phencyclidine	Yes	Yes		Yes		Miotic	Yes
Opiates			Yes	Yes		Miotic	No
Inhalants	Yes			Yes		Normal	Yes

REFERENCES

Adams AJ, Brown B. Marijuana, alcohol, and combined drug effects on the time course of glare recovery. *Psychopharmacology.* 1978;56:81–86.

Apter JT, Pfeiffer CC. Effect of hallucinogenic drugs on the ERG. *Am J Ophthalmol.* 1956;42:206–210.

Banks T, Fletcher R, et al. Infective endocarditis in heroin addicts. *Am J Med.* 1973;55:444–451.

Brown E, Prager J, et al. CNS complications of cocaine abuse: Prevalence, pathophysiology and neuroradiology. *Am J Radiol.* 1992;159:137–147.

Brown GC, Brown RH, et al. Peripheral proliferative retinopathies. *Int Ophthalmol.* 1987;11:41–50.

Burns MJ, Graudins A, et al. Treatment of methanol poisoning with intravenous 4-methylpyrazole. *Ann Emerg Med.* 1997;30:829–832.

Chasnoff ID, Burns WJ, et al. Cocaine use in pregnancy. *N Engl J Med.* 1985;313:666–669.

Chiang WK. Amphetamines. In: Goldfrank LR, Flomenbaum NE, eds. *Goldfrank's Toxicologic Emergencies.* 6th ed. Stamford, CT: Appleton & Lange; 1998:1091–1103.

Cohen S, Ditman KS. Prolonged adverse reactions to lysergic acid diethylamide. *Arch Gen Psychiatry.* 1963;8:475–480.

Colasanti BK, Martin B. Contemporary drug abuse. In: Craig CR, Stitzel RE, eds. *Modern Pharmacology.* 4th ed. Boston: Little, Brown & Company; 1990:459–474.

Cregler LL. Cocaine: The newest risk factor for cardiovascular disease. *Clin Cardiol.* 1991;14:449–456.

Cregler LL, Mark H. Medical complications of cocaine abuse. *N Engl J Med.* 1986:315;1495–1500.

Delcourt C, Diaz JL, et al. Smoking and age-related macular degeneration: The Pola Study. *Arch Ophthalmol.* 1998; 116:1031–1035.

Diaz-Calderon E, Del Brutoo OH, et al. Bilateral internuclear ophthalmoplegia after smoking "crack" cocaine. *J Clin Neuroophthalmol.* 1991;11:297–299.

Fogo A, Superdock KR, et al. Severe arteriosclerosis in the kidney of a cocaine addict. *Am J Kidney Dis.* 1992;20: 513–515.

Foulds WS, Pettigrew AR. The biochemical basis of the toxic amblyopias. In: Perkins ED, Hill DW, eds. *Scientific Foundations of Ophthalmology.* London: Heinemann; 1977:50–54.

Fraunfelder FT. *Drug-Induced Ocular Side Effects and Drug Interactions.* Philadelphia: Lea & Febiger; 1989.

Friberg TR, Gragoudas ES, et al. Talc emboli and macular ischemia in intravenous drug abuse. *Arch Ophthalmol.* 1979; 97:1089–1091.

Girault C, Tamion F, et al. Fomepizole (4-methylpyrazole) in fatal methanol poisoning with early CT scan cerebral lesions. *J Toxicol Clin Toxicol.* 1999;37:777–780.

Glaser JS. Topical diagnosis: Prechiasmal visual pathways. In: Tasman W, Jaeger EA, eds. *Duane's Clinical Ophthlamology.* Philadelphia: Lippincott; 1991;2:69–74.

Goldfrank LR, Flomenbaum NE. Phencyclidine. In: Goldfrank LR, Flomenbaum NE, eds. *Goldfrank's Toxicologic Emergencies.* 6th ed. Stamford, CT: Appleton & Lange; 1998:1105–1110.

Goldfrank LR, Flomenbaum NE. Toxic alcohols. In: Goldfrank LR, Flomenbaum NE, eds. *Goldfrank's Toxicologic Emergencies.* 6th ed. Stamford, CT: Appleton & Lange; 1998:1049–1060.

Goodwin DW. Alcoholism and genetics: The sins of the fathers. *Arch Gen Psychiatry.* 1985;42:171–174.

Halperin E, Yolton RL. Is the driver drunk? Oculomotor sobriety testing. *J Am Optom Assoc.* 1986;57:654–657.

Hanson WB, Rose LA. Recreational use of inhalant drugs by adolescents: A challenge for family physicians. *Fam Med.* 1995;27:383–387.

Harrington DO. Amblyopia due to tobacco, alcohol and nutritional deficiency. Differential diagnosis with special reference to the character of the visual field defect. *Am J Ophthalmol.* 1962;53:967–972.

Hepler RS, Frank IR. Marihuana smoking and intraocular pressure. *JAMA.* 1971;217:1392.

Herskowitz J, Oppenheimer EY. More about poisoning by phencyclidine (PCP, angel dust). *N Eng J Med.* 1977; 297:1405.

Hill AD, Toner ME, et al. Talc lung in a drug abuser. *Ir J Med Sci.* 1990;159:147–148.

Hoffman A, Barth A, et al. Vascular risk factors in patients with ophthalmoplegia. *J Med Klin.* 1990;85:459–462.

Hogan RE, Linfield PB. The effects of moderate doses of ethanol on heterophoria and other aspects of binocular vision. *Ophthalmic Physiol Opt.* 1983;3:21–31.

Holdeman NR, Bartlett JD. Analgesics for treatment of acute ocular pain. In: Bartlett JD, Jaanus SD, eds. *Ocular Pharmacology.* 3rd ed. Boston: Butterworth Heinemann 1995: 131–150.

Hollander JE, Hoffman RS. Cocaine. In: Goldfrank LR, Flomenbaum NE, eds. *Goldfrank's Toxicologic Emergencies.* 6th ed. Stamford, CT: Appleton & Lange; 1998:1071–1089.

Holzman PS, Levy DL, et al. Smooth pursuit eye movements, and diazepam, CPZ, and secobarbital. *Psychopharmacologia.* 1975;44:111–115.

Howells DE. Nystagmus as a physical sign in alcoholic intoxication. *Br Med J.* 1956;1:1405–1406.

Hunt WA. Ethanol and other aliphatic alcohols. In: Craig CR, Stitzel RE, eds. *Modern Pharmacology.* 4th ed. Boston: Little, Brown & Company 1990:451–457.

Kaye D. Infective endocarditis. In: Wilson JD, Braunwald E, Isselbacher KJ, et al, eds. *Harrison's Principles of Internal Medicine,* 12th ed. New York: McGraw-Hill; 1991:508–512.

Klee A, Willinger R. Disturbances of visual perception in migraine. *Acta Neurol Scand.* 1966;42:400–414.

Knave B, Persson HE, et al. A comparative study on the effects of barbiturates and ethyl alcohol on retinal functions. *Acta Ophthalmol.* 1974;52:254–259.

Kosnoski EM, Yolton RL, et al. The drug evaluation classification program: Using ocular and other signs to detect drug intoxication. *J Am Optom Assoc.* 1998;69:211–227.

Krill AE, Wieland AM, et al. The effect of two hallucinogenic agents on human retinal function. *Arch Ophthalmol.* 1960;64:724–733.

Levi L, Miller NR. Visual illusions associated with previous drug abuse. *J Clin Neuroophthalmol.* 1990;10:103–110.

Martidis A, Yung C, et al. Talc embolism: A static retinopathy. *Am J Opthalmol.* 1997;124:841–843.

McLane NJ, Carroll DM. Ocular manifestations of drug abuse. *Surv Ophthalmol.* 1986;30:298–313.

McLaren D. *Nutritional Ophthalmology: Malnutrition & the Eye.* New York: Academic Press; 1980.

Michelson JB, Freedman SD, et al. *Aspergillus* endophthalmitis in a drug abuser. *Ann Ophthalmol.* 1982;14:1051–1054.

Michelson JB, Friedlaender MH. Endophthalmitis of drug abuse. *Int Ophthalmol Clin.* 1987;27:120–126.

Michelson JB, Robin HS, Nozik RA. Nonocular manifestations of parenteral drug abuse. *Surv Ophthalmol.* 1986;30:314–320.

Miller TA. Crack and gastroduodenal perforation. *Gastroenterology.* 1992;102:1431–1432.

Morse RM, Flavin DK. The definition of alcoholism. *JAMA.* 1992;268:1012–1014.

Moser KM. Pulmonary thromboembolism. In: Wilson JD, Barunwald E, Isselbacher KJ, et al, eds. *Harrison's Principles of Internal Medicine.* 12th ed. New York: McGraw-Hill; 1991:1090–1096.

National Consensus Development Panel on Effective Medical Treatment of Opiate Addiction. Effective medical treatment of opiate addiction. *JAMA.* 1998;280:1936–1943.

Nicotine. In: Gosselin RE, Smith RP, Hodge HC, eds. *Clinical Toxicology of Commercial Products.* 5th ed. Baltimore: Williams & Wilkins; 1984:311–313.

Otten EJ. Marijuana. In: Goldfrank LR, Flomenbaum NE, eds. *Goldfrank's Toxicologic Emergencies.* 6th ed. Stamford, CT: Appleton & Lange, 1998;1121–1125.

Pare JA, Fraser RG. Pulmonary 'mainline' granulomatosis: Talcosis of intravenous methadone abuse. *Medicine.* 1979; 58:229–239.

Parsian A, Todd RD, et al. Alcoholism and alleles of the human D2 dopamine receptor locus: Studies of association and linkage. *Arch Gen Psychiatry.* 1991;48:655–663.

Parsons JH. Action of nicotine upon nerve cells. *J Physiol (Lond).* 1901;26:38–39.

Pettigrew AR, Fell GS. The simplified colorimetric determination of thiocyanate in biological fluids, and its application to investigation of the toxic amblyopias. *Clin Chem.* 1972;18:996–998.

Pezcon JD, Grant M. Glaucoma, alcohol and intraocular pressure. *Arch Opthalmol.* 1965;73:495–501.

Pfeilschifter J, Zeigler R. Smoking and endocrine opthalmoplegia: Impact of smoking severity and current vs lifetime cigarette consumption. *Clin Endocrinol (Oxf).* 1996; 45:477–481.

Rizzo JF, Lessell S. Tobacco amblyopia. *Am J Ophthalmol.* 1993;116:84–87.

Rofsky JE, Townsend JC, et al. Retinal nerve fiber layer defects and microtalc retinopathy secondary to free-basing "crack" cocaine. *J Am Optom Assoc.* 1995;66:712–720.

Russell RM, Carney EA, et al. Acute ethanol administration causes transient impairment of blue-yellow color vision. *Alcohol Clin Exp Res.* 1980;4:396–399.

Sachs R, Zagelbaum BM, et al. Corneal complications associated with the use of crack cocaine. *Ophthalmology.* 1993; 100:187–191.

Schatz H, Mendelblatt F. Solar retinopathy from sun-gazing under the influence of LSD. *Brit J Ophthalmol.* 1973;57: 270–274.

Sharpe JA. Methanol optic neuropathy: A histopathological study. *Neurology.* 1982;32:1093–1100.

Shimozono M, Townsend JC, et al. Acute vision loss resulting from ethanol. *J Am Optom Assoc.* 1998;69:293–303.

Silvette H, Haag HB, et al. Tobacco amblyopia: The evolution and natural history of a "tobaccogenic" disease. *Am J Ophthalmol.* 1960;50:71–100.

Smith W, Mitchell P, et al. Smoking and age-related maculopathy. The Blue Mountains Eye Study. *Arch Ophthalmol.* 1996;114:1518–1523.

Solberg Y, Rosner M, et al. The association between cigarette smoking and ocular diseases. *Surv Ophthalmol.* 1998;42: 535–547.

Speicher CE. Screening. In: Dyson J, ed. *The Right Test: A Physician's Guide to Laboratory Medicine.* Philadelphia: WB Saunders; 1989:29–37.

Srinivasan BD. Bacterial endophthalmitis. In: Srinivasan BD, ed. *Ocular Therapeutics.* Kinderhook, NY: Masson; 1980: 59–63.

Stokkermans TJ, Dunbar MT. Solar retinopathy in a hospital-based primary care clinic. *J Am Optom Assoc.* 1998; 69:625–636.

Substance Abuse and Mental Health Services Administration. *Preliminary Results from the 1997 National Household Survey on Drug Abuse.* Rockville, MD: Department of Health and Human Services; 1998.

Summerskill WHJ, Molnar GD. Eye signs in hepatic cirrhosis. *N Engl J Med.* 1962;226:1244–1248.

Traquair HM. Tobacco amblyopia. *Lancet.* 1928;2:1173–1177.

Traquair HM. Toxic amblyopia. *Trans Ophthalmol Soc UK.* 1931;50:372–385.

Tse DT, Ober RR. Talc retinopathy. *Am J Ophthalmol.* 1980; 90:624–640.

Tucker JR, Fern RP. Lysergic acid diethylamide and other hallucinogens. In: Goldfrank LR, Flomenbaum NE, eds. *Goldfrank's Toxicologic Emergencies.* 6th ed. Stamford, CT: Appleton & Lange, 1998;1111–1119.

Underdahl JP, Chiou AG. Preseptal cellulitis and orbital wall destruction secondary to nasal cocaine abuse. *Am J Ophthalmol.* 1998;125:266–268.

Urey JC. Some ocular manifestations of systemic drug abuse. *J Am Optom Assoc.* 1991;62:832–842.

Wallace RT, Brown GC, et al. Sudden retinal manifestations of intranasal cocaine and methamphetamine abuse. *Am J Ophthalmol.* 1992;114:158–160.

Walsh FB. *Clinical Neuro-ophthalmology.* 2nd ed. Baltimore: Williams & Wilkins;1957:1180–1230.

Wilford BB. *Drug Abuse. A Guide for the Primary Physician.* Chicago: American Medical Association, 1981.

Wilkinson IMS, Kime R, Purnell M. Alcohol and human eye movement. *Brain.* 1974;97:785–792.

Witherspoon CD, Feist FW, et al. Ocular self-mutilation. *Ann Ophthalmol.* 1989;21:255–259.

Appendix

OCULAR MANIFESTATIONS OF SYSTEMIC DISEASE

	Lids, Lashes, Adnexa	Conjunctiva, Sclera	Cornea	Iris, Uvea, Ciliary Body, Anterior Chamber	Lens	Vitreous
Acquired immunodeficiency syndrome	Molluscum contagiosum, herpes zoster ophthalmicus, Kaposi sarcoma	Nonspecific conjunctivitis, Kaposi sarcoma, microvasculopathy	Ocular surface disease; HSV, HZV, and microsporidial keratitis, fungal and bacterial ulcers	Primary HIV uveitis		
Addison disease, *see* Adrenal gland dysfunction						
Adrenal gland dysfunction	Pigmentation (Addison disease)	Pigment of conjunctiva (Addison disease)		Increased IOP (Cushing syndrome)		
Albinism	White lashes, poliosis			Light blue to brown irides, iris transillumination		
Alzheimer disease						
Anemia		Conjunctival pallor/hemorrhage, subconjunctival hemorrhage		Hyphema (aplastic)		Blood in vitreous from retinal internal limiting membrane breaks
Ankylosing spondylitis				Iridocyclitis		
Aplastic anemia, *see* Anemia						
Arnold Chiari malformations, *see* Chiari malformations						
Arteriosclerosis						

Optic Nerve	Macula	Retina, Choroid	Extraocular Muscles, Eye Movements	Higher Cortical Function	Other
Neuritis, neuropathy, papilledema		Noninfectious retinopathy, CMV retinitis, syphilitic retinitis	3,4,6 CN palsy, abnormal saccades, abnormal pursuits, and eye movements	Visual field defects	Pupil abnormalities, lymphoma
Chiasmal compression (Cushing syndrome, adrenal insufficiency), papilledema (neuroblastoma)		Hypertensive retinopathy (Cushing syndrome, primary aldosteronism, pheochromocytoma)			Exophthalmos (Cushing syndrome), Horner syndrome (neuroblastoma), proptosis with ecchymosis (neuroblastoma)
	Hypoplasia	Small capillary free zone in posterior pole, prominent choroidal vessels	Nystagmus	Bihemispheric VEP asymmetries	Reduced VA
Degeneration			Impaired ocular motility	Visuospatial disorientation, agnosia, apraxia, hallucinations, optic ataxia	Dyschromatopsia, decreased contrast sensitivity
Pallor (aplastic, pernicious), swelling (aplastic), neuropathy (pernicious)		Dilated/tortuous veins, hemorrhages (retinal/preretinal), exudates, cotton-wool spots, pallor of fundus, retinal edema, CRVO	CN palsies (iron deficient)		
		Hyalinization of arterioles, broadening of arterial light reflex, copper to silver wire appearance, CRVO/BRVO, hypoperfusion retinopathy			

	Lids, Lashes, Adnexa	Conjunctiva, Sclera	Cornea	Iris, Uvea, Ciliary Body, Anterior Chamber	Lens	Vitreous
Atopic dermatitis	Prominent lower eyelid fold, pruritis, foreign-body sensation, blepharitis, thickened lid margins	Keratoconjunctivitis, symblepharon	Superficial punctate keratitis, increased susceptibility to herpes simplex, keratoconus	Uveitis, ocular hypertension	Cataracts	
Behçet syndrome	Ulcerative eyelid lesions	Conjunctivitis, episcleritis, scleritis	Keratitis	Bilateral granulomatous anterior uveitis, hypopyon, iris neovascular-ization, posterior synechiae, secondary glaucoma	Cataracts	Cells, hemorrhage
Cancer, *see* specific type						
Cardiac disorders, *see* specific valvular disease						
Cerebrovascular disease				Anterior segment ischemia (carotid disease)		
Chiari malformations			Exposure keratitis			
Chlamydia	Edematous lids, lid deformities (late complication), pseudoptosis	Follicular/papillary conjunctivitis, dry eye	Ulceration and scarring secondary to trichiasis (trachoma), superior keratitis, vascularization, limbal swelling, micropannus (inclusion conjunctivitis)	Mild anterior uveitis		
Chronic progressive ophthalmoplegia	Ptosis					
Cicatricial pemphigoid	Severe dry eye, entropion, trichiasis	Chronic conjunctivitis, symblepharon, ankyloblepharon, shrinkage	Vascularization			
Crohn disease, *see* Inflammatory bowel disease						

Optic Nerve	Macula	Retina, Choroid	Extraocular Muscles, Eye Movements	Higher Cortical Function	Other
		BRVO, RD, central serous choroidopathy			
Papillitis, papilledema, atrophy	Edema, hemorrhage	Focal retinal lesions, RD, RPE hypertrophy, retinal atrophy, CRVO/BRVO, peripheral vasculitis, choroidal vasculitis, sheathing	CN 3,4,6 palsies		
		Plaques, emboli, cotton-wool spots, asymmetric retinopathy, hypoperfusion retinopathy (carotid disease)	Motility abnormalities (vertebrobasilar disease)	Bilateral hemianopsia (vertebrobasilar disease), transient visual obscuration (carotid disease)	Horner syndrome (vertebrobasilar disease)
Papilledema			CN 6 palsy, INO, nystagmus		
		Pigmentary retinopathy	Ophthalmoplegia		Orbicularis oculi weakness, reduced saccadic velocity

	Lids, Lashes, Adnexa	Conjunctiva, Sclera	Cornea	Iris, Uvea, Ciliary Body, Anterior Chamber	Lens	Vitreous
Cushing syndrome, *see* Adrenal dysfunction						
Cystinosis		Conjunctival crystals	Stromal crystals, band keratopathy	Iris crystals		
Diabetes	Decreased tear production, periorbital edema		Decreased sensitivity, abrasions, erosions, slow and defective re-epithelialization	Rubeosis iridis, ectropion uveae, neovascular glaucoma, increased incidence of COAG	Premature or diabetic cataract	
Diffuse large-cell lymphoma			Keratic precipitates	Posterior or anterior uveitis, hypopyon, neovascular glaucoma		Vitreitis
Down syndrome	Slanting of palpebral fissures, prominent epicanthal folds, blepharitis, lacrimal duct obstruction		Keratoconus	Brushfield spots	Congenital cataracts	
Drug and alcohol abuse, *see* Tables 66–2, 66–11, 66–17, 66–6, 66–13, 66–19, 66–9, 66–15, 66–23						
Dysproteinemias, *see* Waldenstroms macroglobulinemia, multiple myeloma						
Ehlers–Danlos syndrome	Prominent epicanthal folds	Blue sclera	Microcornea, keratoconus or globus, haze at Bowman membrane, rupture with minimal trauma		Ectopia lentis	
Erythema multiforme	Lid edema, focal ulcerations, dry eye	Conjunctival pseudo or true membranes, scarring		Iritis, iridocyclitis		
Erythema nodosum				Uveitis (if associated with systemic inflammatory disease)		
Fabry disease, *see* Sphingolipidoses						
Gaucher disease, *see* Sphingolipidoses						
Giant-cell arteritis				Rubeosis irides with secondary glaucoma		
Gout	Crystal deposition in tarsal plates	Chronic bilateral conjunctival injection, episcleritis, scleritis, crystal deposition in sclera	Crystal deposition		Crystal deposition	Increased incidence of asteroid hyalosis

Optic Nerve	Macula	Retina, Choroid	Extraocular Muscles, Eye Movements	Higher Cortical Function	Other
	Edema	Diabetic retinopathy (nonproliferative/ proliferative)	3,4,6 CN palsy		Decreased accommodation, fluctuating vision or refraction, tritan color defect
Optic nerve sheathing		Exudative RD, subretinal infiltrates	CN palsies (with CNS involvement)		Blurred vision
		Myopic degeneration			Strabismus, nystagmus, amblyopia
		RD, angioid streaks, vitreoretinal degeneration	Strabismus		Myopia
AION		CRAO	CN 3,6 palsy	Cortical blindness (occipital infarction)	Ocular pain
			Crystal deposition in EOM tendons		

	Lids, Lashes, Adnexa	Conjunctiva, Sclera	Cornea	Iris, Uvea, Ciliary Body, Anterior Chamber	Lens	Vitreous
Guillain–Barré syndrome	Ectropion, ptosis, lagophthalmos		Keratoconjunctivitis sicca, exposure keratitis, neurotrophic ulceration			
Hansen disease	Brow/lash loss, thickened lids, ptosis, ectropion, lagophthalmos, dacryoadenitis, dacryocystitis	Palpebral and limbal lepromas, episcleritis, scleritis, staphyloma or scleromalacia	Hypesthesia, beaded and thickened corneal nerves, neurotrophic keratitis, secondary infection, pannus or avascular interstitial keratitis	Iris pearls, iris atrophy with miotic pupil, acute or chronic anterior uveitis, secondary glaucoma	Secondary cataract	
Herpes simplex	Blepharitis	Conjunctivitis	Epithelial or stromal keratitis, trophic ulcer	Uveitis, secondary glaucoma		
Herpes zoster	Skin lesions, ptosis, secondary *Staphylococcus aureus* infection, complications secondary to scarring, dacryoadenitis, canaliculitis	Conjunctivitis, mucous membrane lesions, conjunctival vesicles, petechial hemorrhages, episcleritis, scleritis	Punctate epithelial keratitis, pseudodendrite, anterior stromal infiltrates, mucous adherent plaques, keratouveitis, disciform keratitis, neurotrophic keratitis, exposure keratitis, scarring	Iritis, pupil distortion, iris atrophy, cyst formation, hypopyon, heterochromia irides, anterior chamber hemorrhage, hypotony, acute or chronic glaucoma	Cataract	
Histoplasmosis						
HIV, *see* AIDS						
Homocystinuria				Blue irides, iridodonesis, secondary glaucoma	Ectopia lentis, phakodonesis, congenital cataracts	
Hyperlipidemia	Xanthelasma		Arcus			
Hypertension						
Hyperthyroidism, *see* Thyroid dysfunction						

Optic Nerve	Macula	Retina, Choroid	Extraocular Muscles, Eye Movements	Higher Cortical Function	Other
Papilledema			External ophthalmoplegia		
			Retinitis		
			CN 3,4,6 palsy		Ophthalmic division of CN 5 involved: frontal, lacrimal, nasociliary; Horner syndrome; light-near dissociation; proptosis
	Exudative maculopathy	Circumpapillary choroiditis, peripheral atrophic choroidal scars, linear streak lesions			
Atrophy, staphyloma		CRAO, RD, peripheral retinal degeneration	Strabismus		Progressive myopia
		Lipemia retinalis			
Bilateral disc edema		Retina: vasoconstriction, sclerosis, exudation; choroid: Elschnig spots, Siegrist spots, BRVO/CRVO, BRAO/CRAO, macroaneurysm			

	Lids, Lashes, Adnexa	Conjunctiva, Sclera	Cornea	Iris, Uvea, Ciliary Body, Anterior Chamber	Lens	Vitreous
Hypothyroidism, *see* Thyroid dysfunction						
Inflammatory bowel disease		Episcleritis (Crohn disease), scleritis		Uveitis (Crohn disease)		
Intracranial tumors						
Iron deficient anemia, *see* Anemia						
Juvenile rheumatoid arthritis			Band keratopathy	Uveitis, secondary glaucoma	Cataract	
Kawasaki disease		Bilateral conjunctival hyperemia, subconjunctival hemorrhage	Superficial punctate keratitis	Bilateral iridocyclitis		Opacities
Kearns–Sayre syndrome	Ptosis		Clouding of endothelium			
Leprosy, *see* Hansen disease						
Leukemia	Lacrimal gland infiltration, dacryocystitis, infiltration of lid, exophthalmos	Infiltrates, swelling, subconjunctival hemorrhage, necrosis secondary to ischemia, episcleritis	Sterile peripheral corneal ulcers	Infiltration, iris color change, pseudo hypopyon		Infiltrates
Lyme disease	Periorbital edema	Conjunctivitis, episcleritis	Keratitis	Granulomatous iritis		Vitreitis
Marfan syndrome	Down-slanting palpebral fissures	Blue sclera		Iridodonesis, Reiger anomaly, deep anterior chamber angle, heterochromic irides, hypoplastic iris dilator, transillumination defects, secondary glaucoma	Ectopia lentis	

Optic Nerve	Macula	Retina, Choroid	Extraocular Muscles, Eye Movements	Higher Cortical Function	Other
Papilledema			CN 3,4,6, palsy	Visual field defects	Pupil abnormality, color vision defect
Bilateral disc edema		Chorioretinal inflammation			
		Salt-and-pepper retinopathy, peripapillary changes, visible choroid vessels	Progressive ophthalmoplegia with ptosis		
Infiltrates, papilledema		Infiltrates, serous sensory RD, RPE changes, cystoid retinal edema, drusen, dilated tortuous veins, yellowing of the vascular reflex, hemorrhages, cotton-wool spots, microaneurysm, peripheral retinal neovascularization	Extraocular muscle infiltrates		
Optic neuropathy, optic neuritis, bilateral disc edema, pseudotumor cerebri		Retinitis	CN 3,4,6 palsies		Photophobia, facial nerve palsy
		RD, peripheral retinal degenerations	Strabismus		Amblyopia, anisometropia, enophthalmos, colobomas

	Lids, Lashes, Adnexa	Conjunctiva, Sclera	Cornea	Iris, Uvea, Ciliary Body, Anterior Chamber	Lens	Vitreous
Metastases of systemic malignancies	Ptosis	Conjunctival erythema				Floaters
Multiple myeloma	Orbital bone involvement	Sludging of blood, iridescent crystalline deposits	Iridescent crystalline deposits	Ciliary body cysts		
Multiple sclerosis				Granulomatous uveitis		
Myasthenia gravis	Ptosis, lid twitch, incomplete lid closure		Decreased corneal sensitivity			
Myopathies, *see* Oculopharyngeal muscular dystrophy, Kearns–Sayre syndrome, Chronic progressive ophthalmoplegia						
Myotonic dystrophy	Ptosis				Opacity	
Neuroblastoma, *see* Adrenal dysfunction						
Neurofibromatosis	Neurofibromas of lids, café au lait spots on lids	Neurofibromas, schwannomas	Neurofibromas, schwannomas, corneal nerve thickening, decreased sensitivity, exposure keratitis	Iris: Lisch nodules, hamartoma of anterior chamber, congenital glaucoma, neovascular glaucoma	Cataracts	
Niemann–Pick disease, *see* Sphingolipidoses						
Nutritional deficiency, *see* Tables 64–1, 65–1, 65–3, 65–6, 65–8						

Optic Nerve	Macula	Retina, Choroid	Extraocular Muscles, Eye Movements	Higher Cortical Function	Other
			Diplopia	Visual field defects	Decreased vision, headaches/head pain, proptosis
Compression		Retinopathy		CN 3,4,6 palsy secondary to compression	
Optic neuritis			INO/BINO, impaired smooth pursuits or saccades, nystagmus		Uhtoff sign
			Ophthalmoplegia, diplopia, nystagmus, pseudo internuclear ophthalmoplegia, convergence difficulties, saccadic quiver		Blurred vision, orbicularis weakness, decreased accommodation
	Pigment changes	Peripheral pigment changes, epiretinal membrane	Motility disturbances, exotropia/ exophoria, convergence insufficiency		Hypotony, orbicularis oculi weakness, poor Bell phenomenon
Nerve or chiasmal gliomas					Orbital meningiomas, neurofibromas, schwannomas, CN 5,7 palsy

	Lids, Lashes, Adnexa	Conjunctiva, Sclera	Cornea	Iris, Uvea, Ciliary Body, Anterior Chamber	Lens	Vitreous
Oculopharyngeal muscular dystrophy	Ptosis					
Osteogenesis imperfecta		Blue sclera	Corneal collagen irregularities	Congenital glaucoma	Dislocation, zonular cataract	Subhyaloid hemorrhage
Paget disease	Epiphora secondary to lacrimal duct obstruction			Glaucoma		
Parathyroid disease (Pth dx)		Conjunctival calcification (hyper Pth dx)	Band keratopathy (hyper Pth dx), pannus (hyper Pth dx), keratoconjunctivitis (hypo Pth dx)		Polychromatic cataract (hypo Pth dx)	
Parkinson disease	Blepharospasm, blepharoplegia, Myerson sign, Wilson sign					
Pernicious anemia, *see* Anemia						
Pheochromocytoma, *see* Adrenal dysfunction						
Pituitary dysfunction						
Polyarteritis nodosa		Conjunctival hyperemia, inflammation, scleritis		Iridocyclitis		
Polycythemia		Dilated/tortuous conjunctival vessels				
Polymyalgia rheumatica						
Pseudotumor cerebri						

Optic Nerve	Macula	Retina, Choroid	Extraocular Muscles, Eye Movements	Higher Cortical Function	Other
			Ophthalmoplegia		
Compression		Choroidal sclerosis			Partial color blindness
Neuropathy		Angioid streaks	EOM palsy		Exophthalmos
Papilledema (hypo Pth dx)					
			Abnormal saccades and/or pursuits, convergence insufficiency		Decreased contrast sensitivity, abnormal VEP
Compression of optic nerve, chiasm, or tract, optic atrophy			Compression of CN 3,4,6		Compression of first or second division of trigeminal nerve
Bilateral disc edema, ischemic optic neuropathy		Ischemic retinopathy, choroidal vasculitis	EOM palsy		Photophobia, intraocular pain, decreased visual acuity, exophthalmos
Florid color, edema		Deep purple hue of fundus, small, scattered superficial and deep hemorrhages; retinal edema; darkened, dilated, tortuous veins; bilateral CRVO		Cerebrovascular insufficiency with secondary amaurosis fugax, visual field loss	
AION (when associated with giant-cell arteritis)					Diplopia and/or transient visual obscuration (when associated with giant-cell arteritis)
Papilledema			CN 6 palsy		

	Lids, Lashes, Adnexa	Conjunctiva, Sclera	Cornea	Iris, Uvea, Ciliary Body, Anterior Chamber	Lens	Vitreous
Pseudoxanthoma elasticum			Nonspecific opacities, keratoconus, wrinkles in Descemet membrane		Subluxation, cataract	
Psoriatic arthritis		Mucopurulent conjunctivitis, episcleritis		Anterior uveitis		
Reiter syndrome		Conjunctivitis		Uveitis, secondary glaucoma	Cataract secondary to chronic uveitis	Vitreitis secondary to chronic uveitis
Rheumatoid arthritis		Episcleritis, scleritis (non or necrotizing)	Keratitis sicca, filamentary keratitis, secondary bacterial keratitis, furrowing of peripheral cornea			
Rosacea	Blepharitis, meibomianitis, disrupted tear film, hordeola, chalazia	Conjunctival hyperemia	Punctate keratitis, epithelial erosions, vascularization, thinning, ulceration, perforation	Anterior uveitis		
Rubella (congenital)			Clouding, microcornea	Miotic/irregular pupil, iridocyclitis, transillumination defects, glaucoma	Cataract	
Sarcoidosis	Granulomatous lid lesions, lacrimal gland enlargement	Conjunctival granulomas	Keratoconjunctivitis sicca	Anterior uveitis, secondary glaucoma	Secondary cataract	Vitreal opacities
Scleroderma	Lagophthalmos, tightening of lids, ptosis, decreased tear production	Conjunctival microvascular abnormalities	Keratoconjunctivitis sicca	Anterior uveitis	Early cataracts	
Sickle hemoglobinopathies		Conjunctival sickling		Focal iris atrophy, microhyphema, rubeosis irides		Hemorrhage
Sjögren syndrome			Keratitis sicca, filamentary sicca, bacterial keratitis			

Optic Nerve	Macula	Retina, Choroid	Extraocular Muscles, Eye Movements	Higher Cortical Function	Other
Drusen, optic atrophy secondary to optic nerve drusen		Angioid streaks, drusen, peripheral punched-out lesions	EOM paralysis		Exophthalmos
	Edema secondary to chronic uveitis				
Pallor		Retinal pigment changes and folds, subretinal neovascularization	Nystagmus		Microphthalmia
Neovascularization of disc, direct optic nerve infiltration, papilledema secondary to intracranial lesions, optic atrophy		Periphlebitis or posterior uveitis with perivenous sheathing and exudates, retinal vein occlusion (rare), neovascularization of retina, choroidal granulomas	CN palsy		
Bilateral disc edema, neuropathy		Hypertensive retinopathy, choroidopathy			
Optic disc sign		Retinopathy (nonproliferative to proliferative), choroidal vascular occlusion, retinal arteriolar occlusion, arteriolo-venous anastomoses, retinal detachment			

	Lids, Lashes, Adnexa	Conjunctiva, Sclera	Cornea	Iris, Uvea, Ciliary Body, Anterior Chamber	Lens	Vitreous
Spasmus nutans						
Sphingolipidoses		Conjunctival angiokeratoma (Fabry disease), pigmented pingueculae (Gaucher disease)	Verticellata (Fabry disease), corneal opacification (Niemann–Pick disease)		Posterior cataracts (Fabry disease), lenticular opacities (Niemann–Pick disease)	
Sturge–Weber syndrome	Nevus flammeus of eyelid	Anomalous vessels of episclera and conjunctiva	Buphthalmos (with glaucoma at less than 3 years of age)	Iris heterochromia, glaucoma		
Syphilis	Gumma of lids and orbit, blepharo-ptosis	Conjunctivitis, episcleritis, scleritis, gumma of conjunctiva and sclera	Interstitial keratitis, gumma of cornea	Iris capillary abnormalities, anterior uveitis, gumma of iris and ciliary body, secondary glaucoma	Cataracts, dislocation	Vitreitis
Systemic lupus erythematosus		Nonspecific conjunctivitis, scleritis	Keratoconjunctivitis sicca, stromal/marginal infiltrates, ulceration, vascularization, superficial punctate keratitis, pannus	Nongranulomatous uveitis		Hemorrhage
Tay–Sach disease, *see* Sphingolipidoses						

Optic Nerve	Macula	Retina, Choroid	Extraocular Muscles, Eye Movements	Higher Cortical Function	Other
			Strabismus, pendular nystagmus		Amblyopia
	Cherry red spot (Tay–Sachs disease, Niemann–Pick type A and B)	Retinal angiokeratoma (Fabry disease), retinal white spots (Gaucher disease)	Ocular motor apraxia (Gaucher disease), eye movement paralysis (Gaucher disease), supranuclear gaze paresis (Niemann–Pick disease)		
Papilledema secondary to intracranial malformation		Choroidal hemangioma, serous/ exudative retinal detachment, retinal pigmentary atrophy/retinitis pigmentosa, choroidal coloboma, atrophic chorioretinitis, retinoblastoma		Homonymous hemianopsia secondary to intracranial malformation	
Neuritis, papillitis, perineuritis, neuroretinitis, optic atrophy, papilledema	Edema, stellate maculopathy, disciform detachment	Retinitis, chorioretinitis, retinal pigment epitheliitis, vasculitis, choroiditis, serous/exudative RD, subretinal neovasculariza- tion, retinal necrosis, CRAO, CRVO	CN 3,4,6 palsy	Arteritis with stroke- like effects to any part of the visual pathways	Pupil abnormalities: Argyll Robertson, tonic pupil
Neuritis, neuropathy, atrophy		Vasculitis, arterial occlusions, neovasculariza- tion, RD	EOM palsies, INO, nystagmus	Visual field loss, cortical blindness	Pupil abnormality

	Lids, Lashes, Adnexa	Conjunctiva, Sclera	Cornea	Iris, Uvea, Ciliary Body, Anterior Chamber	Lens	Vitreous
Thyroid dysfunction	Lid retraction, lid lag, lagophthalmos, proptosis, wide-eye stare (hyperfunction); madarosis, periorbital myxedema (hypofunction)	Edema (hyperfunction)	Exposure, photophobia (hyperfunction)	Increased IOP (hyperfunction)		
Toxocariasis						Vitreitis, white mass/granuloma, vitreous bands
Toxoplasmosis	Ptosis (congenital)			Anterior uveitis		Vitreitis
Tuberculosis	Granulomas of lid	Granulomas of conjunctiva and sclera, conjunctivitis, scleritis	Granulomas of cornea, phlyctenular keratoconjunctivitis, interstitial keratitis	Granulomas of uvea, uveitis with or without retinal vasculitis		
Tuberous sclerosis	Adenoma sebaceum of eyelids, poliosis			Iris hypopigmentation		
Ulcerative colitis, *see* Inflammatory bowel disease						
Valvular heart disease		Conjunctival petechiae (bacterial endocarditis)				
Varicella	Eyelid vesicular lesions	Conjunctivitis, limbal/conjunctival vesicles	Superficial punctate keratopathy, stromal disciform keratitis			
Vogt–Koyanagi–Harada disease	Poliosis, lacrimation	Perilimbal vitiligo	Keratic precipitates	Bilateral uveitis, posterior synechiae, iris nodules, iris neovascularization, secondary glaucoma	PSC cataracts	Cells

Optic Nerve	Macula	Retina, Choroid	Extraocular Muscles, Eye Movements	Higher Cortical Function	Other
Blurred margins (hyperfunction)			Restriction, diplopia (hyperfunction)		
Distorted optic nerve	Hypertrophic macula, macular granuloma	Retinitis, choroiditis, retinal traction, retinal folds, tortuous/dilated vessels			Endophthalmitis
Neuritis/papillitis		Retinochoroiditis, retinal tears, retinal detachment, chorioretinal scars	Nystagmus, strabismus (congenital)		Microphthalmia, enophthalmos
Granuloma, optic neuropathy					Granulomas of orbit
Astrocytic hamartoma, papilledema		Astrocytic hamartoma, pigment epithelial defects			Atypical coloboma
Neuritis (bacterial endocarditis)		Embolic CRAO, BRAO, Roth spots (bacterial endocarditis)	CN 3,4,6 palsy (bacterial endocarditis)		
Papilledema	Edema, scarring	Vessel sheathing, bilateral serous non-rhegamatogenous retinal detachment, chorioretinal scarring, diffuse RPE depigmentation, subretinal neovascularization			Blurred vision, photophobia, ocular pain

	Lids, Lashes, Adnexa	Conjunctiva, Sclera	Cornea	Iris, Uvea, Ciliary Body, Anterior Chamber	Lens	Vitreous
Von Hippel–Lindau disease						
Waldenström macroglobulinemia		Sludging of blood				
Wegener granulomatosis	Dacryocystitis or adenitis, nasolacrimal duct obstruction, eyelid erythema and edema	Episcleritis, scleritis	Subepithelial infiltrates, marginal infiltrates, circumlimbal ulceration/furrowing, exposure keratitis	Uveitis		
Wilm tumor			Pannus	Aniridia	Cataracts	
Wilson disease			Kayser–Fleischer pigment ring		Sunflower cataract	
Wyburn–Mason syndrome	Ptosis	Dilated conjunctival vessels secondary to orbital AVM				Hemorrhage secondary to retinal AVM

Optic Nerve	Macula	Retina, Choroid	Extraocular Muscles, Eye Movements	Higher Cortical Function	Other
Optic nerve or peripapillary angioma, papilledema secondary to CNS angioma		Angiomatosis retinae	CN palsy or nystagmus secondary to CNS angioma		
Compression		CRVO		EOM palsy secondary to compression of nerve	
Compression		Diffuse vasculitis, venous congestion, disseminated ischemic retinitis, retinal and choroidal detachments	Eye movement restrictions		Proptosis, orbital granulomatosis and vasculitis
Glaucoma, hypoplasia	Hypoplasia		Nystagmus, EOM palsy, esotropia		Anisocoria
Arteriovenous malformation, papilledema secondary to CNS AVM	Hemorrhage secondary to retinal AVM	Retinal arteriovenous malformation, BRVO/CRVO secondary to retinal AVM, ischemia secondary to retinal AVM	CN palsies secondary to orbital AVM		Proptosis secondary to orbital AVM

Index

ISBN 0-8385-8176-5
90000
9 780838 581766